FEATURES (continued)

Genes in Focus

Integrated Coverage of Diversity

Integrated Coverage of Student Research

www.wadsworth.com

wadsworth.com is the World Wide Web site for Wadsworth and is your direct source to dozens of online resources.

At *wadsworth.com* you can find out about supplements, demonstration software, and student resources. You can also send email to many of our authors and preview new publications and exciting new technologies.

wadsworth.com
Changing the way the world learns®

AN INVITATION TO HEALTH

Tenth Edition

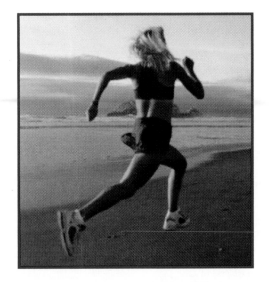

Dianne Hales

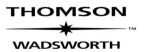

THOMSON

WADSWORTH

Australia · Canada · Mexico · Singapore · Spain · United Kingdom · United States

THOMSON

™

WADSWORTH

Publisher: Peter Marshall
Associate Editor: April Lemons
Assistant Editor: John Boyd
Editorial Assistant: Andrea Kesterke
Executive Technology Project Manager: Donna M. Kelley
Marketing Manager: Jennifer Somerville
Marketing Assistant: Mona Weltmer
Advertising Project Manager: Shemika Britt
Project Manager, Editorial Production: Sandra Craig
Print/Media Buyer: Barbara Britton

Permissions Editor: Joohee Lee
Production: The Book Company
Text and Cover Design: Hespenheide Design
Photo Researcher: Myrna Engler
Copy Editor: Pat Brewer
Illustrator: Hespenheide Design
Cover Image: © 2002 Joe Patronite/Getty Images/The Image Bank
Cover Printer: Phoenix Color
Compositor: Parkwood Composition
Printer: Quebecor World/Dubuque

For more information about our products, contact us at:
Thomson Learning Academic Resource Center
1-800-423-0563
For permission to use material from this text, contact us by:
Phone: 1-800-730-2214   **Fax:** 1-800-730-2215
Web: http://www.thomsonrights.com

Wadsworth/Thomson Learning
10 Davis Drive
Belmont, CA 94002-3098
USA

Asia
Thomson Learning
60 Albert Street, #15-01
Albert Complex
Singapore 189969

Australia
Nelson Thomson Learning
102 Dodds Street
South Melbourne, Victoria 3205
Australia

Canada
Nelson Thomson Learning
1120 Birchmount Road
Toronto, Ontario M1K 5G4
Canada

Europe/Middle East/Africa
Thomson Learning
Berkshire House
168-173 High Holborn
London WC1 V7AA
United Kingdom

Latin America
Thomson Learning
Seneca, 53
Colonia Polanco
11560 Mexico D.F.
Mexico

Spain
Paraninfo Thomson Learning
Calle/Magallanes, 25
28015 Madrid, Spain

*To my husband, Bob, and my
daughter, Julia, who make every
day an invitation to joy.*

Brief Contents

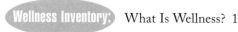

Contents

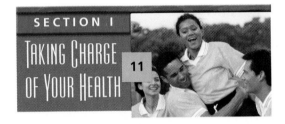

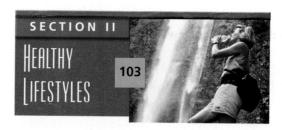

SECTION II
HEALTHY
LIFESTYLES
103

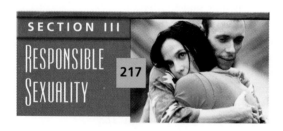

SECTION III
RESPONSIBLE SEXUALITY
217

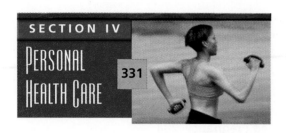

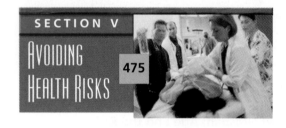

SECTION V
AVOIDING HEALTH RISKS
475

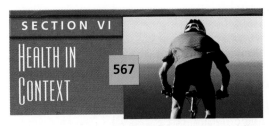

SECTION VI
HEALTH IN CONTEXT
567

Preface

To the Student

This textbook is an invitation to you—an invitation to a healthier, happier, fuller life. Every day you make choices that can affect both how long and how well you live. The knowledge you acquire in this course will help you make better choices, ones that will have a direct impact on how you look, feel, and function—now and for decades to come.

Perhaps you are in good health and think that you know all that you need to know about how to take care of yourself. If so, take a minute and ask yourself some questions:

- How well do you understand yourself? Are you able to cope with emotional upsets and crises? Do you often feel stressed out?
- How nutritiously do you eat? Are you always going on—and off—diets? Do you exercise regularly?
- How solid and supportive are your relationships with others? Are you conscientious about birth control and safe-sex practices?
- Do you get drunk or high occasionally? Do you smoke?
- Are you a savvy health-care consumer? Do you know how to evaluate medical products and health professionals?
- How much do you know about complementary and alternative medicine?
- If you needed health care, do you know where you'd turn or how you'd pay? What do you know about your risk for infectious diseases, heart problems, cancer, or other serious illnesses?
- Have you taken steps to ensure your personal safety at home, on campus, or on the streets?
- What are you doing today to prevent physical, psychological, social, and environmental problems in the future?

As you consider these questions, chances are there are some aspects of health you haven't considered before—and others you feel you don't have to worry about for years. Yet the choices you make and the actions you take now will have a dramatic impact on your future.

Your health is your personal responsibility. Over time, your priorities and needs will inevitably change, but the connections between various dimensions of your well-being will remain the same: The state of your mind will affect the state of your body, and vice versa. The values that guide you through today can keep you mentally, physically, and spiritually healthy throughout your lifetime. Your ability to cope with stress will influence your decisions about alcohol and drug use. Your commitment to honest, respectful relationships will affect the nature of your sexual involvements. Your eating and exercise habits will determine whether you develop a host of medical problems.

An Invitation to Health, Tenth Edition, is packed with information, advice, recommendations, and research, and provides the first step in taking full charge of your own well-being. An important theme of this book is prevention. Ultimately, the power of prevention belongs to you—and it's a lot easier than you might think. You could simply add a walk or workout to your daily routine. You could snack on fruit instead of high-fat foods. You could cut back on alcohol. You could buckle your seat belt whenever you get in a car. These things may not seem like a big deal now, yet they could make a crucial difference in determining how active and fulfilling the rest of your life will be.

Yet knowledge alone can't assure you of a lifetime of well-being. The rest depends on you. The skills you acquire, the habits you form, the choices you make, the ways you live day by day will all shape your health and your future. You cannot simply read this book and study health the way you study French or chemistry. You must decide to make it part of your daily life.

This is our invitation to you.

Dianne Hales

To the Instructor

This is the tenth edition of *An Invitation to Health*, a textbook that some of you know well from the past and that others may be looking at for the first time. A great deal has changed over the lifetime of this book—in medical research, in the field of health, on college and university campuses, in the nation and the world. What has not changed is the commitment we share to prepare students to make informed, thoughtful choices that will help them live longer, healthier, happier, fuller lives.

For the last twenty years, it's been my privilege to work closely with health educators around the country toward this goal. *An Invitation to Health* contains the insights, perspectives, and wisdom of many people. Each edition has been enriched by what we've learned before. In this landmark tenth edition, much has changed—but the essentials remain the same.

As I point out to students, health—unlike physics or history—is not a subject that they must memorize and master, but one to be both learned and lived. Often for the first time in their lives, students in a university health class become aware of the importance of personal responsibility for their health and acquire the skills they need to protect their well-being and prevent serious health problems.

By its very nature, health is an interactive course. Every topic of every lecture prompts questions. Every week brings health news that students are eager to discuss and debate. This edition of *An Invitation to Health* offers even more features designed to intrigue and involve your students. Every chapter begins with a campus-based vignette illustrating the relevance of the material to a stu-

dent's life. Every chapter incorporates research on college students or college-age individuals; these findings are highlighted by a new icon. In addition, "Student Snapshot" uses tables and graphs to report recent data on the health, habits, and concerns of today's college students.

As always, this edition defines health in the broadest sense of the word—not as an entity in itself but as a process of discovering, using, and protecting all possible resources within the individual, family, community, and environment. It presents the most recent, state-of-the-science information on medical research, along with the fundamental background students need to understand and apply these findings. Some chapters, such as Chapter 12 "Keeping Your Heart Healthy," have been rewritten to present the latest information and insight into what students should know and can do to protect their health. I've

also updated and expanded the coverage of diversity in health, which is integrated throughout every chapter and highlighted by another icon. The "Across the Lifespan" fea-

ture in every chapter also has been expanded to present more material related to age and aging.

As I tell students, *An Invitation to Health* can serve as an owner's manual to their bodies and minds. By using this book and taking your course, they can acquire a special type of power—the power to make good decisions, to assume responsibility, and to create and follow a healthy lifestyle. This textbook is our invitation to them to live what they learn and make the most of their health and of their lives.

This textbook also is an invitation to you as an instructor. I invite you to share your passion for education and to enter into a partnership with the editorial team at Wadsworth. We welcome your feedback and suggestions. Please let us hear from you at http://health.wadsworth.com. I personally look forward to working with you toward our shared goal of preparing a new generation for a healthful future.

Overview of the Tenth Edition

On September 11, 2001, I was immersed in working on this edition. Like millions around the world, I stopped and watched the unimaginable happen. In the following months, I had the opportunity to interview specialists involved in the emotional and physical aftermath of the terrorist attacks. "Forget a return to normalcy," they told me. "Life will never be the same again." They were right. We all have had to adjust to a new reality in which the only certainty is uncertainty.

The students in your health courses are different because of the events of September 11. This edition of *An Invitation to Health* also is different. In relevant sections throughout the book, I cover topics that I never even thought of including in the past, including the use of infectious agents as weapons of bioterrorism and living in a dangerous world. Chapter 18, "When Life Ends," begins with a reflection on the painful lessons in grief and mortality that we all learned on a September day. Other references to issues related to health and terrorism appear throughout the book.

The tenth edition carries *An Invitation to Health* into the twenty-first century with a wealth of new research, references, and features. Yet the basic themes remain the same: personal responsibility, a commitment to prevention, practical applications of knowledge, and a focus on behavioral change.

The nineteen chapters in this edition are organized into six sections. One new chapter, Chapter 3 "Psychological Health," combines material on emotional and spiritual well-being, mental health, and mental disorders, with an emphasis on those most common among college students. Several chapters—such as Chapter 4 "The Joy of Fitness," Chapter 9 "Reproductive Choices," and Chapter 12 "Keeping Your Heart Healthy"—have been rewritten because so much has changed in these fields.

The new features in the tenth edition include "Savvy Consumer," which offers specific advice on getting the best possible health care and services, whether the student is interested in spotting nutrition misinformation or evaluating the risks of contraceptives. Every section also includes "Genes in Focus," a feature that reports on cutting-edge research in genetics, including genetic disorders and cancer genes. In addition, we've retained, updated, and enhanced other popular features, including the chapter "FAQs," "Across the Lifespan," "Self-Surveys," "Strategies for Change" / "Strategies for Prevention," "The X & Y Files," "Pulse Points," "Student Snapshot," and "Making This Chapter Work for You."

Because the health sciences advance so rapidly, all of the chapters have been updated with the most current research, including hundreds of citations published in 2000 and 2001 and incorporating the latest available statistics. The majority come from primary sources, including professional books, medical, health, and mental health journals, health education periodicals, scientific meetings, federal agencies and consensus panels, publications from research laboratories and universities, and personal interviews with specialists in a number of fields. In addition, "Sites & Bytes" presents reliable Internet addresses where students can turn for additional information and Suggested Readings from InfoTrac® College Edition, an online library of literally hundreds of academic journals and popular periodicals.

Following is a chapter-by-chapter listing of some of the key topics that have been added, expanded, or revised for the tenth edition:

Chapter 1: An Invitation to Health for the Twenty-first Century

- Expanded discussion of spiritual health
- Updated discussion of "Healthy People 2010"
- New data on average life expectancy
- New section on health in the United States compared to the rest of the world
- Expanded discussion of the health of college students
- New section discussing the future of medicine
- New research on genetic risks

Chapter 2: Personal Stress Management

- Expanded discussion on the effects of stress on physical health
- Updated discussion on minorities and stress
- New research on coping with stress
- New section on desk rage

Chapter 3: Psychological Health

- New section and strategies for leading a fulfilling life
- New discussion on diversity and mental health among college students
- Expanded discussion on why so many people are depressed
- Expanded section on suicide
- New section on alternative mind-mood products

Chapter 4: The Joy of Fitness

- Expanded discussion on who exercises and who doesn't
- Updated section on why exercise is important
- New Physical Activity Pyramid
- New research on how much exercise is enough
- New section on motivation and psyching yourself to work out
- Expanded aerobic options including walking and cycling
- New aerobic fitness program
- New discussion on performance-enhancing drugs such as creatine and steroids
- New research on stretching versus warming up
- New section on the role of sleep and how much is enough
- Updated discussion on sports safety

Chapter 5: Personal Nutrition

- Updated discussion on how to follow the Food Guide Pyramid
- New section on functional foods
- New discussion on food safety including foodborne illnesses and mad-cow disease
- New research on gender differences in relation to nutritional needs
- New discussion on evaluating nutrition information

Chapter 6: Eating Patterns and Problems

- New discussion on body composition and age
- Updated discussion on the eating patterns and problems of college students
- New research on the genetics of obesity
- New research on gender differences in relation to weight

Chapter 7: Communication and Relationships

- New research on gender differences in communication
- Expanded discussion of friendship and dating
- New section on seniors looking for love
- New discussion on types of marriages
- New discussion on two-career couples
- Updated statistics on the current divorce rate
- New discussion on the do's and don'ts of online dating
- New discussion on men, women, and marital preferences

Chapter 8: Personal Sexuality

- New section on premenstrual dysphoric disorder (PMDD)
- New statistics regarding sexual activity among college students
- New discussion on sexuality and aging
- Expanded discussion of homosexuality
- Expanded discussion of abstinence
- New discussion of cybersex on campus

Chapter 9: Reproductive Choices

- Updated discussion of prescription and nonprescription contraceptives

Chapter 10: Consumerism, Complementary/Alternative Medicine, and the Health-Care System

- Expanded discussion of oral health
- Updated section on elective treatments including laser vision and cosmetic surgery
- Expanded discussion on the use and benefits of complementary and alternative medicine

Chapter 11: Protecting Yourself from Infectious Diseases

- Updated section on the common cold
- Updated section on meningitis
- Revised discussion on hepatitis
- Revised discussion on Lyme disease
- New section on biological terrorism
- New research on STDs among adolescents and young adults

- New research on the progress being made in treating HIV/AIDS

Chapter 12: Keeping Your Heart Healthy

- Expanded discussion on how to prevent heart problems
- Updated discussion on risk factors you can control
- New research on novel risk factors including homocysteine, C-reactive protein, and lipoprotein a
- Expanded discussion on stroke including risk factors and treatments

Chapter 13: Lowering Your Risk of Cancer and Other Major Diseases

- New research involving cancer genes and genetic screening
- New section on cancer and minorities
- Expanded discussion on skin and breast cancer
- Expanded discussion on diabetes mellitus and who is at risk
- New discussion on asthma among college students

Chapter 14: Drug Use, Misuse, and Abuse

- New discussion on the abuse of prescription painkillers
- New research on drug use on college campuses
- New section on club drugs including ecstasy and ketamine
- Expanded discussion on cocaine risks and withdrawal
- New discussion of gender differences in drug use

Chapter 15: Alcohol Use, Misuse, and Abuse

- New discussion of underage drinking
- Expanded discussion on binge drinking on campus
- New section on the genetics of alcoholism
- New section on drinking and race
- New section on alcohol and the elderly
- New research on gender differences in drinking

Chapter 16: Tobacco Use, Misuse, and Abuse

- Expanded discussion on smoking among women and minorities

• Expanded discussion on the families of smokers
• Revised section on the politics of tobacco

Chapter 17: Staying Safe: Preventing Injury, Violence, and Victimization

• Updated discussion on road safety
• Expanded section on repetitive motion injury
• Updated statistics on teen violence and crime on campus
• Updated statistics on hate crimes
• Expanded discussion of sexual harassment on campus and sexual victimization of students

Chapter 18: When Life Ends

• Expanded discussion of the dying process
• New research on why men die sooner than women
• Expanded discussion of funeral cost

Chapter 19: Working Toward a Healthy Environment

• Expanded discussion of global warming
• Expanded discussion of acid rain
• Revised section on protecting your hearing and the effects of noise
• New research on cellular phone safety

Features and Pedagogy

Chapter Opening Vignettes—new to this edition, are found at the beginning of every chapter and engage students with stories and experiences to further stimulate their interest in the chapter content. These practical vignettes mirror the information, advice, and recommendations of the text.

Genes in Focus—new to this edition, are found in each section of the text and report on cutting-edge research on how our genes may influence personal health. Topics include the genetics of obesity (Ch 6), childbirth and genetic disorders (Ch 9), and genetic screening for cancer (Ch 13).

FAQ—Frequently Asked Questions appear at the beginning of each chapter, immediately engaging students with questions such as "Should I use butter or margarine?" (Ch 5) "How much exercise is enough?" (Ch 4) and "Who's at highest risk of infectious diseases?" (Ch 11). Page references are included after each question, and each

corresponding heading is marked with an icon, signaling that the answer can be found there.

Student Snapshot—a popular feature formerly Campus Focus that appears in every chapter, uses graphs and charts to illustrate eye-catching data on college populations. Topics include student stress levels, mental disorders on campus, condoms on campus, and the social life of college students. Campus data have been completely revised for this edition

X & Y Files—are found throughout the text and present scientific findings on health-related differences between men and women. Much of this truly groundbreaking research has shattered stereotypes about sex and gender and challenged the traditional assumption that women are essentially smaller, shorter, rounder versions of men. Among the topics covered: differences in nutritional needs; differences in vulnerabilities to tobacco and alcohol; differences in physical fitness and eating patterns; and differences in risk for heart attacks, cancer, and infectious diseases.

Pulse Points—is a popular feature that appears in every chapter, offering a list of relevant and practical motivators to help students achieve their personal health goals. Examples include "Top Ten Ways to Take Care of Your Mind" (Ch 3), "Ten Ways to Eat Smart" (Ch 5), "Ten Ways to Prevent STDs" (Ch 11), and "Ten Ways to Protect the Planet."

Self Surveys—appear in every chapter and allow students to assess themselves on various aspects of health. Examples: "Stress Scale" (Ch 2) "Is Something Wrong?" (Ch 3) "Are You a Savvy Medical Consumer?" (Ch 10) "Are You at Risk for Cancer?" (Ch 13).

Strategies for Change—appear throughout the text and provide practical, checklist-format behavioral change strategies for achieving better health.

Strategies for Prevention—appear throughout the text and provide effective, checklist-format strategies for preventing health problems and reducing health risks.

Savvy Consumer—focuses on consumer-related health topics and provides guidelines for critical thinking about health care and services. Topics include "Do Stress Relief Products Work for you?" (Ch 2) "Do's and Don'ts of On-line Dating" (Ch 7), and "Getting the Most Out of Medications" (Ch 14).

Across the Lifespan—integrated throughout each chapter, this text focuses on health issues as they relate to childhood or aging, as well as how health changes now can result in benefits later in life. Examples include "The Aging Brain" (Ch 3), "Seniors Looking for Love" (Ch 7), "Seniors at the Wheel" (Ch 17).

Sites & Bytes—presents more engaging and reliable Internet resources than you will find in any other college textbook on the market. Every chapter includes three websites relevant to chapter topics (along with descriptions of each) and a suggested reading from the InfoTrac online library—a terrific way to have students research topics on the Internet from *trusted and credible* sources. Moreover, students can go to **http://health.wadsworth.com** to find link updates, over 500 additional health-related links (researched by a health professor), and additional suggested readings on InfoTrac, complete with review/discussion questions.

The Wellness Inventory—is a self-inventory that precedes Chapter 1. It allows students to assess and rate their lifestyles in various areas of wellness, providing a useful springboard for deciding which areas they would like to pay special attention to and improve.

Hales Health Almanac—appears at the end of the text and includes resources related to finding health information on the Internet; a comprehensive, completely updated health directory of contact information for various health organizations; what to do in an emergency; a consumer's guide to medical tests; and tables for counting calories and fat in specific foods.

In addition:

- *Learning Objectives* open each chapter and outline the most essential information for students.
- *Key Terms* are boldfaced when they first appear in the chapter and are listed at the end of each chapter with page references. They are also defined in the Glossary at the end of the book.
- *Integrated Coverage of Diversity* related to race and ethnicity is highlighted with an icon throughout each chapter.
- *Integrated Coverage of Student Research* is highlighted with an icon throughout each chapter.
- *Critical Thinking* questions are included at the end of each chapter and ask the students to consider some applications of the chapter's coverage, or weigh in on a health-related controversy.
- *CNN Video Discussion Question,* included at the end of each chapter, is designed to work in conjunction with the video of CNN health clips that has been developed with this edition. The CNN health video is complimentary with adoption of this textbook.
- *Making This Chapter Work for You.* This completely revamped end-of-chapter section both summarizes key content and tests students' understanding and knowledge with multiple-choice questions.

Ancillary Package

Instructor's Manual The Instructor's Manual provides chapter outlines, learning objectives, classroom handouts, discussion questions, a video list, keyword transparency masters, a resource integration guide, a free supplement on alternative medicine, and more. A section for Canadian instructors is also included.

Test Bank The test bank for the new edition contains a variety of questions to test students' understanding and comprehension of the text. It contains at least 75 questions per chapter, with 50 multiple-choice questions, 20 fill-in-the-blank questions, and no fewer than 5 essay questions.

ExamView® Computerized Testing Create, deliver, and customize the thorough Test Bank in minutes with this easy-to-use assessment and tutorial system. *ExamView* offers both a *Quick Test Wizard* and an *Online Test Wizard* that guide you step-by-step through the process of creating tests, while it allows you to see the test you are creating on the screen exactly as it will print or display online. You can build tests of up to 250 questions using up to 12 question types. Using *ExamView's* complete word-processing capabilities, you can enter an unlimited number of new questions or edit existing questions.

Multimedia Manager for Health, Fitness, and Wellness: A Microsoft® PowerPoint® Link Tool This comprehensive CD-ROM contains more than 100 PowerPoint slides, featuring text art and art from numerous Wadsworth health, fitness, and wellness titles.

Transparency Acetates More than 100 transparency acetates of art taken from the text enhance lectures and provide visual support in the classroom.

WebTutor™ Advantage and WebTutor™ Advantage Plus *WebTutor Advantage's* text-specific content allows instructors to create and manage a personal website! *WebTutor Advantage's* course management tool gives you the ability to provide virtual office hours, post syllabi, set up threaded discussions, track student progress with the quizzing material, and much more. For students, *WebTutor Advantage* offers real-time access to a full array of study tools, including chapter outlines, summaries, learning objectives, glossary flashcards (with audio), practice quizzes, web links, *InfoTrac® College Edition* exercises, animations, and videos. *WebTutor Advantage Plus* offers all these great features, as well as the entire text in electronic format.

Study Guide The Study Guide is an excellent aid to the student's understanding of the text. It contains learning objectives, key terms, chapter review questions, and a detailed practice test for each chapter.

InfoTrac College Edition Student Guide for Health This 24-page booklet offers detailed guidance for students on how to use the *InfoTrac® College Edition* database. Includes log-in help, a complete search tips "cheat sheet," and a topic list of key word search terms for health, fitness, and wellness. Available FREE when packaged with the text. The text also features InfoTrac Activities for each chapter that challenge the student to critically read articles and studies relating to key topics in the chapters. These activities help guide students through the vast database and answer questions relating to specific articles.

Telecourse Study Guide For use with the Dallas County Community College Telecourse, the telecourse guide contains a brief summary of each lesson, followed by learning objectives, study assignments for the text and video, key terms, a list of the experts interviewed with their affiliations, video focus points, individual health plan assignments, enrichment opportunities, and practice tests with page-referenced answers.

Health, Fitness, and Wellness Internet Explorer A handy full-color trifold brochure contains dozens of useful health, fitness, and wellness Internet links.

Personal Daily Log The Personal Daily Log contains an exercise pyramid, study and exercise tips, a goal setting worksheet, cardiorespiratory exercise record form, strength training record form, a daily nutrition diary, helpful Internet links, and more.

Wellness Worksheets These detachable self-assessments and wellness worksheets are handy, easy to use, and make a terrific bundle item.

Integrative Medicine: The Mind-Body Prescription This interesting supplement, written by Dr. John Janowiak from Appalachian State University, explains the relationship between Western medical practice and more traditional therapies. The supplement explains the evolution of integrative medicine, provides a detailed list of Internet resources, a comprehensive list of herbs and their interactions, and more.

Profile Plus 2003 The most comprehensive software pack available with any health textbook, *Profile Plus* allows students to generate personalized fitness and wellness profiles, conduct self-assessments, analyze their diets, tailor exercise prescriptions to their individual needs, keep an exercise log, and much more.

Diet Analysis 6.0 This unique assessment tool provides students with experience in the estimation and analysis of dietary patterns and practices. It allows students to track their food intake for up to seven days and to create a personal dietary profile based on height, weight, age, gender, and activity level. *Diet Analysis Plus* calculates Dietary Reference Intakes, goal percentages, and actual percentages of essential nutrients, vitamins, and minerals. Comprehensive dietary data is displayed in attractive, easy-to-read reports that enhance learning. Students can view data as a bar graph or spreadsheet, in Food Pyramid form, or as a Nutrition Fact Panel Report. They can then identify dietary habits, correct nutritional deficiencies, and truly appreciate the impact of nutrient dense foods.

http://health.wadsworth.com When you adopt *An Invitation to Health*, Tenth Edition, you and your students will have access to a rich array of teaching and learning resources that you won't find anywhere else. This outstanding site features both student resources for the text, including quizzes, web links, suggested online readings, and discussion forums, and instructor resources, including downloadable supplementary resources and multimedia presentation slides. You will also find an online catalog of Wadsworth's health, fitness, wellness, and physical education books and supplements.

CNN Today: Health and Wellness Video, Volumes I, II and III. A Wadsworth exclusive—updated yearly!

An exclusive agreement between Wadsworth Group and Turner Learning! Launch your lectures with riveting footage from CNN, the world's leading 24-hour global news television network. The *CNN Today: Health and Wellness* videos allow you to integrate the newsgathering and programming power of CNN into the classroom to show students the relevance of course topics to their everyday lives. The videos include news clips correlated directly with the Hales text and cover such topics as the role of vegetables in cancer prevention, abuse of Ritalin on college campuses, gambling addiction, and stress and the immune system.

Relaxation: A Guide to Personal Stress Management This 30-minute video shows students how to manage their stress and what is a healthy stress level in their life. Experts explain relaxation techniques and guide the student through progressive relaxation, guided imagery, breathing, and physical activity.

Trigger Video Series: Fitness This 60-minute video focuses on changing concepts of fitness, contains five 8–10 minute clips followed by questions for answer or discussion, and material appropriate to the fitness chapters in the text.

Trigger Video Series: Stress This 60-minute video focuses on stress, contains five 8–10 minute clips followed by questions for answer or discussion, and material appropriate to the text chapters concerning stress and its positive and negative effects on health.

Spiritual Health: The Faith Factor, Developing a Personal Plan This unique ancillary covers a variety of important issues and useful topics dealing with spirituality's relationship to overall health. As Dianne Hales writes, "Health involves more than physical well-being." It covers such topics as an introduction to spiritual health, religion's positive and negative roles in health, and setting up a personal spiritual plan. The book includes more than a dozen exercises, a detailed set of Internet resources, a complete text reference guide, and religious perspectives from seven major religions.

Acknowledgments

Ten editions of a textbook mean hundreds of contributors to thank. I remain deeply indebted to all the instructors, students, reviewers, editors, artists, and others who have made this project so successful and so satisfying for so long. I have learned a great deal from all of you, and I am grateful.

For the tenth edition, I was fortunate to work with a terrific team at Wadsworth, with Peter Marshall at its helm. April Lemons, the health editor, brought new energy, great expertise, and endless enthusiasm to the project. It was a special pleasure for me to work again with developmental editor Deborah Gale, whose wit, creativity, and professionalism have enriched several editions of *An Invitation to Health*. Once again, I applaud and admire the production team, headed by Sandra Craig of Wadsworth and Dusty Friedman of The Book Company. Time and again they outdo themselves in their ability to produce stunning books on nearly impossible schedules.

I also am grateful to Hespenheide Design, who have given this edition and the evocative cover the look and feel of a new century; and to Myrna Engler, for her work on photos and permissions. My thanks go to Pat Brewer, who skillfully edited the final manuscript. I also am appreciative of Shemika Britt's work in preparing promotional materials and of Jennifer Somerville's marketing efforts on behalf of the book. Thanks also to editorial assistant Andrea Kesterke.

Finally, I would like to thank the reviewers whose input has been so valuable through these many editions. For the tenth edition, I thank the following for their comments and helpful assistance:

Jeremy Barnes, Southeast Missouri State University
Carol Biddington, California University of Pennsylvania
Richard Capriccioso, University of Phoenix
Lori Dewald, Shippensburg University of Pennsylvania
Harold Horne, University of Illinois at Springfield
Jessica Middlebrooks, University of Georgia
Kris Moline, Lourdes College
Richard Morris, Rollins College
Rosanne Poole, Tallahassee Community College
Sadie Sanders, University of Florida
Debra Secord, Coastline College
Teresa Snow, Georgia Institute of Technology

For their help as reviewers or focus group participants from previous editions, I want to thank the following:

Ghulam Aasef, Kaskaskia College
Andrea Abercrombie, Clemson University
Judy Baker, East Carolina University
Marcia Ball, James Madison University
Rick Barnes, East Carolina University
Lois Beach, SUNY-Plattsburg
Betsy Bergen, Kansas State University
Nancy Bessette, Saddleback College
David Black, Purdue University
Jill M. Black, Cleveland State University
Cynthia Pike Blocksom, Cincinnati Health Department
James Brik, Willamette University
Mitchell Brodsky, York College
Jodi Broodkins-Fisher, University of Utah
James G. Bryant, Jr., Western Carolina University
Marsha Campos, Modesto Junior College
James Lester Carter, Montana State University
Patti Cost, Weber State University
Maxine Davis, Eastern Washington University

Lori Dewald, Shippensburg University of Pennsylvania
Julie Dietz, Eastern Illinois University
Robert Dollinger, Florida International University
Gary English, Ithaca College
Michael Felts, East Carolina University
Kathie C. Garbe, Kennesaw State College
Gail Gates, Oklahoma State University
Dawn Graff-Haight, Portland State University
Carolyn Gray, New Mexico State University
Mary Gress, Lorain County Community College
Janet Grochowski, University of St. Thomas
Stephen Haynie, College of William and Mary
Ron Heinrichs, Central Missouri State University
Michael Hoadley, University of South Dakota
Linda L. Howard, Idaho State University
Kim Hyatt, Weber State University
Dee Jacobsen, Southeastern Louisiana University
John Janowiak, Appalachian State University
Peggy Jarnigan, Rollins College
Jim Johnson, Northwest Missouri State University
Chester S. Jones, University of Arkansas
Herb Jones, Ball State University
Jane Jones, University of Wisconsin, Stevens Point
Lorraine J. Jones, Muncie, Indiana
Becky Kennedy-Koch, Ohio State University
Mark J. Kittleson, Southern Illinois University
Darlene Kluka, University of Central Oklahoma
Debra A. Krummel, West Virginia University
Roland Lamarine, California State University, Chico
David Langford, University of Maryland, Baltimore County
Beth Lanning, Baylor University
Norbert Lindskog, Harold Washington College
Loretta Liptak, Youngstown State University
S. Jack Loughton, Weber State University
Rick Madson, Palm Beach Community College
Ashok Malik, College of San Mateo
Michele P. Mannion, Temple University
Esther Moe, Oregon Health Sciences University
Anne O'Donnell, Santa Rosa Junior College
Randy M. Page, University of Idaho
Carolyn P. Parks, University of North Carolina
Anthony V. Parrillo, East Carolina University
Miguel Perez, University of North Texas
Pamela Pinahs-Schultz, Carroll College
Janet Reis, University of Illinois at Urbana-Champaign
Steven Sansone, Chemeketa Community College
Andrew Shim, Southwestern College
Steve Singleton, Wayne State University
Larry Smith, Scottsdale Community College
Carl A. Stockton, Radford University
Linda Stonecipher, Western Oregon State College
Emogene Johnson Vaughn, Norfolk State University
David M. White, East Carolina University

Sabina White, University of California—Santa Barbara
Robert Wilson, University of Minnesota
Roy Wohl, Washburn University
Martin L. Wood, Ball State University

About the Author

Dianne Hales, one of the most widely published and honored health journalists in the country, is a contributing editor for *Parade, Ladies Home Journal,* and *Working Mother* and has written more than 1,000 articles for national publications. Her trade books include *Just Like a Woman: How Gender Science Is Redefining What Makes Us Female* and the award-winning compendium of mental health information, *Caring for the Mind: The Comprehensive Guide to Mental Health.* Dianne Hales is one of the few journalists to be honored with national awards for excellence in magazine writing by both the American Psychiatric Association and the American Psychological Association. She also has won the "EMMA" (Exceptional Media Merit Award) for health reporting from the National Women's Political Caucus and Radcliffe College, and numerous writing awards from various organizations, including the Arthritis Foundation, California Psychiatric Society, CHAAD, Council for the Advancement of Scientific Education, National Easter Seal Society, and the New York City Public Library.

What is Wellness?*

by John W. Travis, M.D.

Most of us think in terms of illness, and assume that the absence of illness indicates wellness. There are actually many degrees of wellness, just as there are many degrees of illness. The Wellness Inventory is designed to stir up your thinking about many areas of wellness.

While people often lack physical symptoms, they may still be bored, depressed, tense, anxious, or generally unhappy with their lives. Such emotional states often set the stage for physical and mental disease. Even cancer may be brought on through the lowering of the body's resistance from excessive stress. These same emotional states can also lead to abuse of the body through smoking, overdrinking, and overeating. Such behaviors are usually substitutes for other, more basic human needs such as recognition from others, a more stimulating environment, caring and affection from friends, and greater self-acceptance.

Wellness is not a static state. High-level wellness involves giving good care to your physical self, using your mind constructively, expressing your emotions effectively, being creatively involved with those around you, and being concerned about your physical, psychological and spiritual environments.

Instructions

Set aside a half hour for yourself in a quiet place where you will not be disturbed while taking the Inventory. Record your responses to each statement in the columns to the right where:

2 = Yes, usually
1 = Sometimes, maybe
0 = No, rarely

Select the answer that best indicates how true the statement is for you presently.

After you have responded to all the appropriate statements in each section, compute your average score for that section and transfer it to the corresponding box provided around the Wellness Inventory Wheel on page 3. Your completed Wheel will give you a clear presentation of the balance you have given to the many dimensions of your life.

You will find some of the statements are really two in one. We do this to show an important relationship between the two parts—usually an awareness of an issue, combined with an action based on that awareness. Mentally average your score for the two parts of the question.

Each statement describes what we believe to be a wellness attribute. Because much wellness information is subjective and "unprovable" by current scientific methods, you (and possibly other authorities as well), may not agree with our conclusions. Many of the statements have further explanation in a footnote (noted with an asterisk). We ask only that you keep an open mind until you have studied available information, then decide.

This questionnaire was designed to educate more than to test. All statements are worded so that you can easily tell what we

*Abridged from the Wellness Index in *The Wellness Workbook*, Travis & Ryan, Ten Speed Press, 1988. Used with the permission of John Travis.

think are wellness attributes (which also makes it easy to "cheat" on your score). This means there can be no trick questions to test your honesty or consistency—the higher your score, the greater you believe your wellness to be. Full responsibility is placed on you to answer each statement as honestly as possible. It's not your score but what you learn about yourself that is most important.

If you decide that a statement does not apply to you, or you don't want to answer it, you can skip it and not be penalized in your score.

Transfer your average score from each section to the corresponding box around the Wheel. Then graph your score by drawing a curved line between the "spokes" that define each segment. (Use the scale provided—beginning at the center with 0.0 and reaching 2.0 at the circumference.) Last, fill in the corresponding amount of each wedge-shaped segment, using different colors if possible.

Conclusions

When you have completed the Wellness Inventory, study your wheel's shape and balance. How smoothly would it roll? What does it tell you? Are there any surprises in it? How does it feel to you? What don't you like about it? What do you like about it?

We recommend that you use colored pens to go back over the questions, noting the ones on which your scores were low and choosing some areas on which you are interested in working. It is easy to overwhelm yourself by taking on too many areas at once. Ignore, for now, those of lower priority to you. Remember, if you don't enjoy at least some aspects of the changes you are making, they probably won't last.

Sample Questions

	Yes, usually	Sometimes, maybe	No, rarely
	2	**1**	**0**
1. I am an adventurous thinker.	✔		
2. I have no expectations, yet look to the future optimistically.		✔	
3. I am a nonsmoker.	✔		
4. I love long, hot baths.			✔

Total points for this section = 5 | 4 + 1 + 0

Divided by __4__ (number of statements answered) = __1.3__ Average score for this section.

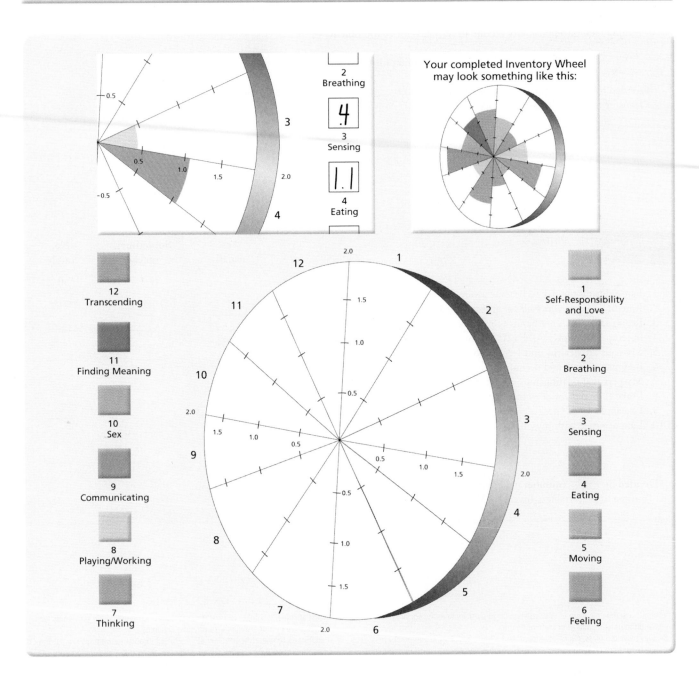

Your completed Inventory Wheel may look something like this:

12 Transcending
11 Finding Meaning
10 Sex
9 Communicating
8 Playing/Working
7 Thinking

1 Self-Responsibility and Love
2 Breathing
3 Sensing
4 Eating
5 Moving
6 Feeling

Section 1 Wellness, Self-Responsibility and Love	Yes, usually	Sometimes, maybe	No, rarely
	2	1	0
1. I believe how I live my life is an important factor in determining my state of health, and I live it in a manner consistent with that belief.			
2. I vote regularly.[1]	_____	_____	_____
3. I feel financially secure.	_____	_____	_____
4. I conserve materials/energy at home and at work.[2]	_____	_____	_____
5. I protect my living area from fire and safety hazards.	_____	_____	_____
6. I use dental floss and a soft toothbrush daily.	_____	_____	_____
7. I am a nonsmoker.	_____	_____	_____
8. I am always sober when driving or operating dangerous machinery.	_____	_____	_____
9. I wear a safety belt when I ride in a vehicle.	_____	_____	_____
10. I understand the difference between blaming myself for a problem and simply taking responsibility (ability to respond) for that problem.	_____	_____	_____

Total points for this section = ☐ _____ + _____ + _____

Divided by ____ (number of statements answered) = ____ Average score for this section.
(Transfer to the Wellness Inventory Wheel on **p. 3**)

Section 2 Wellness and Breathing	Yes, usually	Sometimes, maybe	No, rarely
	2	1	0
1. I stop during the day to become aware of the way I am breathing.	_____	_____	_____
2. I meditate or relax myself for at least 15 to 20 minutes each day.	_____	_____	_____
3. I can easily touch my hands to my toes when standing with knees straight.[3]	_____	_____	_____
4. In temperatures over 70° F (21° C), my fingers feel warm when I touch my lips.[4]	_____	_____	_____
5. My nails are healthy and I do not bite or pick at them.	_____	_____	_____
6. I enjoy my work and do not find it overly stressful.	_____	_____	_____
7. My personal relationships are satisfying.	_____	_____	_____
8. I take time out for deep breathing several times a day.	_____	_____	_____
9. I have plenty of energy.	_____	_____	_____
10. I am at peace with myself.	_____	_____	_____

Total points for this section = ☐ _____ + _____ + _____

Divided by _____ (number of statements answered) = ____ Average score for this section.
(Transfer to the Wellness Inventory Wheel on **p. 3**)

---

[1] Voting is a simple measure of your willingness to participate in the social system, which ultimately impacts your state of health.

[2] Besides recycling glass, paper, aluminum, and other recyclables, if you purchase products that are reusable rather than disposable, and are packaged with a minimum of material, you will reduce the drain of resources and the toxic load on the environment caused by the disposal of wastes.

[3] A lack of spinal flexibility is usually a symptom of chronic muscle tension as well as indicative of a poor balance of physical activities.

[4] If your hand temperature is below 85° F (30° C) in a warm room, you're cutting off circulation to your hands via an overactive sympathetic nervous system. You can learn to warm your hands with biofeedback and to thereby better relax.

Section 3	Wellness and Sensing	Yes, usually	Sometimes, maybe	No, rarely
		2	1	0
1.	My place of work has mostly natural lighting or full-spectrum fluorescent lighting.[5]	_____	_____	_____
2.	I avoid extremely noisy areas or wear protective ear covers.[6]	_____	_____	_____
3.	I take long walks, hikes, or other outings to actively explore my surroundings.	_____	_____	_____
4.	I give myself presents, treats, or nurture myself in other ways.	_____	_____	_____
5.	I enjoy getting, and can acknowledge, compliments and recognition from others.	_____	_____	_____
6.	It is easy for me to give sincere compliments and recognition to other people.	_____	_____	_____
7.	At times I like to be alone.	_____	_____	_____
8.	I enjoy touching or hugging other people.[7]	_____	_____	_____
9.	I enjoy being touched or hugged by others.[8]	_____	_____	_____
10.	I get and enjoy backrubs or massages.	_____	_____	_____

Total points for this section = ☐   _____ + _____ + _____

Divided by _____ **(number of statements answered)** = _____ **Average score for this section.**
(Transfer to the Wellness Inventory Wheel on **p. 3**)

Section 4	Wellness and Eating	Yes, usually	Sometimes, maybe	No, rarely
		2	1	0
1.	I am aware of the difference between refined carbohydrates and complex carbohydrates and eat a majority of the latter.[9]	_____	_____	_____
2.	I think my diet is well balanced and wholesome.	_____	_____	_____
3.	I drink fewer than five alcoholic drinks per week.	_____	_____	_____
4.	I drink fewer than two cups of coffee or black (nonherbal) tea per day.[10]	_____	_____	_____
5.	I drink fewer than five soft drinks per week.[11]	_____	_____	_____
6.	I add little or no salt to my food.[12]	_____	_____	_____
7.	I read the labels for the ingredients of all processed foods I buy and I inquire as to the level of toxic chemicals used in production of fresh foods—choosing the purest available to me.	_____	_____	_____
8.	I eat at least two raw fruits or vegetables each day.	_____	_____	_____
9.	I have a good appetite and am within 15% of my ideal weight.	_____	_____	_____
10.	I can tell the difference between "stomach hunger" and "mouth hunger," and I don't stuff myself when I am experiencing only "mouth hunger."[13]	_____	_____	_____

Total points for this section = ☐   _____ + _____ + _____

Divided by _____ **(number of statements answered)** = _____ **Average score for this section.**
(Transfer to the Wellness Inventory Wheel on **p. 3**)

---

[5] Full-spectrum light, like sunlight, contains many different wavelengths. Most eyeglasses, and the glass windows in your home or car, block the "near" ultra-violet light needed by your body. Special bulbs and lenses are available.

[6] Loud noises that leave your ears ringing cause irreversible and cumulative nerve damage over time. Ear plugs/muffs, obtained in sporting goods stores, should be worn around power saws, heavy equipment, and rock concerts!

[7,8] Long recognized by hospitals as therapeutic, touch can be a powerful preventative as well.

[9] Refined carbohydrates (white flour, sugar, white rice, alcohol, and others) are burned up by the body very quickly and contain no minerals or vitamins. Complex carbohydrates (fruits and vegetables) burn evenly and provide the bulk of dietary nutrients.

[10] Coffee and nonherbal teas contain stimulants that, when overused, abuse your body's adrenal glands.

[11] Besides caffeine, the empty calories in these chemical brews may cause a sugar "crash" shortly after drinking. Artificially sweetened ones may be worse. Consider the other nutrients you won't be getting, and the prices!

[12] In addition to having a presumed connection with high blood pressure, the salt-ing of foods during cooking draws out minerals, which are lost when the water is poured off.

[13] Stomach hunger is a signal that your body needs food. Mouth hunger is a signal that it needs something else (attention/acknowledgement), which you are not getting, so it asks for food, a readily available "substitute."

Section 5	Wellness and Moving	Yes, usually	Sometimes, maybe	No, rarely
		2	**1**	**0**
1.	I climb stairs rather than ride elevators.[14]	⎯⎯	⎯⎯	⎯⎯
2.	My daily activities include moderate physical effort.[15]	⎯⎯	⎯⎯	⎯⎯
3.	My daily activities include vigorous physical effort.[16]	⎯⎯	⎯⎯	⎯⎯
4.	I run at least 1 mile three times a week (or equivalent aerobic exercise).[17]	⎯⎯	⎯⎯	⎯⎯
5.	I run at least 3 miles three times a week (or equivalent aerobic exercise).	⎯⎯	⎯⎯	⎯⎯
6.	I do some form of stretching/limbering exercise for 10 to 20 minutes at least three times per week.[18]	⎯⎯	⎯⎯	⎯⎯
7.	I do some form of stretching/limbering exercise for 10 to 20 minutes at least six times per week.	⎯⎯	⎯⎯	⎯⎯
8.	I enjoy exploring new and effective ways of caring for myself through the movement of my body.	⎯⎯	⎯⎯	⎯⎯
9.	I enjoy stretching, moving, and exerting my body.	⎯⎯	⎯⎯	⎯⎯
10.	I am aware of and respond to messages from my body about its needs for movement.	⎯⎯	⎯⎯	⎯⎯

Total points for this section = ☐ ⎯⎯ + ⎯⎯ + ⎯⎯

Divided by ⎯⎯ **(number of statements answered)** = ⎯⎯ **Average score for this section.**
(Transfer to the Wellness Inventory Wheel on **p. 3**)

Section 6	Wellness and Feeling	Yes, usually	Sometimes, maybe	No, rarely
		2	**1**	**0**
1.	I am able to feel and express my anger in ways that solve problems, rather than swallow anger or store it up.[19]	⎯⎯	⎯⎯	⎯⎯
2.	I allow myself to experience a full range of emotions and find constructive ways to express them.	⎯⎯	⎯⎯	⎯⎯
3.	I am able to say "no" to people without feeling guilty.	⎯⎯	⎯⎯	⎯⎯
4.	I laugh often and easily.	⎯⎯	⎯⎯	⎯⎯
5.	I feel OK about crying and allow myself to do so when appropriate.[20]	⎯⎯	⎯⎯	⎯⎯
6.	I listen to and consider others' criticisms of me rather than react defensively.	⎯⎯	⎯⎯	⎯⎯
7.	I have at least five close friends.	⎯⎯	⎯⎯	⎯⎯
8.	I like myself and look forward to the rest of my life.	⎯⎯	⎯⎯	⎯⎯
9.	I easily express concern, love and warmth to those I care about.	⎯⎯	⎯⎯	⎯⎯
10.	I can ask for help when needed.	⎯⎯	⎯⎯	⎯⎯

Total points for this section = ☐ ⎯⎯ + ⎯⎯ + ⎯⎯

Divided by ⎯⎯ **(number of statements answered)** = ⎯⎯ **Average score for this section.**
(Transfer to the Wellness Inventory Wheel on **p. 3**)

---

[14] If a long elevator ride is necessary, try getting off five flights below your destination. Urge building managers to keep stair doors unlocked.

[15] Moderate = rearing young children, gardening, scrubbing floors, brisk walking, and so on.

[16] Vigorous = heavy construction work, farming, moving heavy objects by hand, and so on.

[17] An aerobic exercise (like running) should keep your heart rate at about 60% of its maximum (120–150 bpm) for 12–20 minutes. Brisk walking for 20 minutes every day can produce effects similar to aerobic exercise.

[18] The stretching of muscles is important for maintaining maximum flexibility of joints and ligaments. It feels good, too.

[19] Learning to take charge of your emotions and using them to solve problems can prevent disease, improve communications, and increase your self-awareness. Suppressing emotions or using them to manipulate others is destructive to all.

[20] Crying over a loss relieves the body of pent-up feelings. In our culture males often have a difficult time allowing themselves to cry, while females may have learned to cry when angry, using tears as a means of manipulation.

Section 7	Wellness and Thinking	Yes, usually	Sometimes, maybe	No, rarely
		2	1	0
1.	I am in charge of the subject matter and the emotional content of my thoughts, and am satisfied with what I choose to think about.[21]	_____	_____	_____
2.	I am aware that I make judgments wherein I think I am "right" and others are "wrong."[22]	_____	_____	_____
3.	It is easy for me to concentrate.	_____	_____	_____
4.	I am conscious of changes (such as breathing pattern, muscle tension, skin moisture, and so on) in my body in response to certain thoughts.[23]	_____	_____	_____
5.	I notice my perceptions of the world are colored by my thoughts at the time.[24]	_____	_____	_____
6.	I am aware that my thoughts are influenced by my environment.	_____	_____	_____
7.	I use my thoughts and attitudes to make my reality more life-affirming.[25]	_____	_____	_____
8.	Rather than worry about a problem when I can do nothing about it, I temporarily shelve it and get on with the matters at hand.	_____	_____	_____
9.	I approach life with the attitude that no problem is too big to confront, and some mysteries aren't meant to be solved.	_____	_____	_____
10.	I use my creative powers in many aspects of my life.	_____	_____	_____

Total points for this section = ☐   _____ + _____ + _____

Divided by _____ **(number of statements answered)** = _____ **Average score for this section.**
(Transfer to the Wellness Inventory Wheel on **p. 3**)

Section 8	Wellness and Playing/Working	Yes, usually	Sometimes, maybe	No, rarely
		2	1	0
1.	I enjoy expressing myself through art, dance, music, drama, sports, or other activities, and make time to do so.	_____	_____	_____
2.	I regularly exercise my creativity "muscles."	_____	_____	_____
3.	I enjoy spending time without planned or structured activities and make the effort to do so.	_____	_____	_____
4.	I can make much of my work into play.	_____	_____	_____
5.	At times I allow myself to do nothing.[26]	_____	_____	_____
6.	At times I can sleep late without feeling guilty.	_____	_____	_____
7.	The work I do is rewarding to me.	_____	_____	_____
8.	I am proud of my accomplishments.	_____	_____	_____
9.	I am playful and the people around me support my playfulness.	_____	_____	_____
10.	I have at least one activity, hobby, or sport that I enjoy regularly but do not feel compelled to do.	_____	_____	_____

Total points for this section = ☐   _____ + _____ + _____

Divided by _____ **(number of statements answered)** = _____ **Average score for this section.**
(Transfer to the Wellness Inventory Wheel on **p. 3**)

---

[21] When you are unconscious of the content of your thoughts, they are more likely to control you. Observing them objectively develops self-awareness and strengthens your ability to take charge.

[22] Rather than trying to completely stop yourself from judging, you can observe your judgments as efforts by your ego to avoid getting on with life and hiding behind "right/wrong" game playing.

[23] Both biofeedback and the field of psycho-neuro-immunology have shown the connections between the mind, nervous system and body. The more you become consciously aware of that connection, the greater responsibility you can take for your health.

[24] Being aware of your internal distortion of perceptions can allow you to step back and reassess a situation more objectively.

[25] Honesty, tempered with care and concern, clears out many negative thoughts that can clutter up your mind, thus making your reality more fun. "Positive thinking" without honesty and truthfulness can backfire by suppressing valid concerns that must be addressed.

[26] Doing "nothing" can give us access to the more creative and nonverbal aspects of our being, so from another perspective, doing nothing becomes doing much more.

Section 9	Wellness and Communicating	Yes, usually	Sometimes, maybe	No, rarely
		2	1	0
1.	In conversation I can introduce a difficult topic and stay with it until I've gotten a satisfactory response from the other person.	___	___	___
2.	I enjoy silence.	___	___	___
3.	I am truthful and caring in my communications with others.	___	___	___
4.	I assert myself (in a nonattacking manner) in an effort to be heard, rather than be passively resentful of others with whom I don't agree.[27]	___	___	___
5.	I readily acknowledge my mistakes, apologizing for them if appropriate.	___	___	___
6.	I am aware of my negative judgments of others and accept them as simply judgments—not necessarily truth.[28]	___	___	___
7.	I am a good listener.	___	___	___
8.	I am able to listen to people without interrupting them or finishing their sentences for them.	___	___	___
9.	I can let go of my mental "labels" (for example, this is good, that is wrong) and judgmental attitudes about events in my life and see them in light of what they offer me.	___	___	___
10.	I am aware when I play psychological "games" with those around me and work to be truthful and direct in my communications.[29]	___	___	___

Total points for this section = [ ] ___ + ___ + ___

Divided by _____ (number of statements answered) = ____ Average score for this section.
(Transfer to the Wellness Inventory Wheel on **p. 3**)

Section 10	Wellness and Sex	Yes, usually	Sometimes, maybe	No, rarely
		2	1	0
1.	I feel comfortable touching and exploring my body.	___	___	___
2.	I think it's OK to masturbate if one chooses to do so.	___	___	___
3.	My sexual education is adequate.	___	___	___
4.	I feel good about the degree of closeness I have with men.	___	___	___
5.	I feel good about the degree of closeness I have with women.	___	___	___
6.	I am content with my level of sexual activity.[30]	___	___	___
7.	I fully experience the many stages of lovemaking rather than focus only on orgasm.[31]	___	___	___
8.	I desire to grow closer to some other people.	___	___	___
9.	I am aware of the difference between needing someone and loving someone.	___	___	___
10.	I am able to love others without dominating or being dominated by them.	___	___	___

Total points for this section = [ ] ___ + ___ + ___

Divided by _____ (number of statements answered) = ____ Average score for this section.
(Transfer to the Wellness Inventory Wheel on **p. 3**)

---

[27] Attacking others rarely accomplishes your goals in the long run. Persisting in your convictions without using force is more effective and usually solves the problem without creating new ones.

[28] It is important to recognize that our internal judgments of others are based on personal biases that often have little objective basis.

[29] Psychological games, defined by Eric Berne in Games People Play, are complex unconscious manipulations that result in the players getting negative attention and feeling bad about themselves.

[30] Including the choice to have no sexual activity.

[31] A common problem for many people is an overemphasis on performance and orgasm, rather than on enjoying a close sensual feeling with their partner whether or not they experience orgasm.

Section 11	Wellness and Finding Meaning	Yes, usually	Sometimes, maybe	No, rarely
		2	1	0
1.	I believe my life has direction and meaning.	_____	_____	_____
2.	My life is exciting and challenging.	_____	_____	_____
3.	I have goals in my life.	_____	_____	_____
4.	I am achieving my goals.	_____	_____	_____
5.	I look forward to the future as an opportunity for further growth.	_____	_____	_____
6.	I am able to talk about the death of someone close to me.	_____	_____	_____
7.	I am able to talk about my own death with family and friends.	_____	_____	_____
8.	I am prepared for my death.	_____	_____	_____
9.	I see my death as a step in my evolution.[32]	_____	_____	_____
10.	My daily life is a source of pleasure to me.	_____	_____	_____

Total points for this section = ☐ _____ + _____ + _____

Divided by _____ **(number of statements answered)** = _____   Average score for this section.
(Transfer to the Wellness Inventory Wheel on **p. 3**)

This portion of the Inventory goes beyond the scope of most generally accepted "scientific" principles and expresses the values and beliefs of the authors. It is intended to stimulate interest in these areas. If you have strong beliefs to the contrary, you can skip the questions or make up your own.

Section 11	Wellness and Transcending	Yes, usually	Sometimes, maybe	No, rarely
		2	1	0
1.	I perceive problems as opportunities for growth.	_____	_____	_____
2.	I experience synchronistic events in my life (frequent "coincidences" seeming to have no cause-effect relationship).[33]	_____	_____	_____
3.	I believe there are dimensions of reality beyond verbal description or human comprehension.	_____	_____	_____
4.	At times I experience confusion and paradox in my search for understanding of the dimensions referred to above.	_____	_____	_____
5.	The concept of god has personal definition and meaning to me.	_____	_____	_____
6.	I experience a sense of wonder when I contemplate the universe.	_____	_____	_____
7.	I have abundant expectancy rather than specific expectations.	_____	_____	_____
8.	I allow others their beliefs without pressuring them to accept mine.	_____	_____	_____
9.	I use the messages interpreted from my dreams.	_____	_____	_____
10.	I enjoy practicing a spiritual discipline or allowing time to sense the presence of a greater force in guiding my passage through life.	_____	_____	_____

Total points for this section = ☐ _____ + _____ + _____

Divided by _____ **(number of statements answered)** = _____   Average score for this section.
(Transfer to the Wellness Inventory Wheel on **p. 3**)

[32] Seeing your death as a stage of growth and preparing yourself consciously is an important part of finding meaning in your life.

[33] Modern physics reveals that the idea of cause and effect may be as limited as Newton's theory of a mechanical universe. It suggests that we must expand our view to see that everything in the universe is connected to everything else. (Synchronicity describes that experience.)

TAKING CHARGE OF YOUR HEALTH

Health may be a science; living is an art. The principles that can help you understand the science and practice the art are simple and timeless and form the basic premise of this book: You have more control over your life and well-being than does anything or anyone else. Through the decisions you make and the habits you develop, you can influence how well—and perhaps how long—you will live. This section defines health and wellness and provides the information you need to take charge of your well-being now and in the years to come.

1

An Invitation to Health for the Twenty-First Century

"How are you?" You may hear that question dozens of times each day. "Fine," you answer, without thinking. But how often do you ask yourself how you *really* are? How do you feel about yourself and your life? Are you under pressure to get good grades? Are you eating well and exercising regularly? Do you have close friends with whom to share your triumphs and traumas? If you choose to be sexually active, what do you do to prevent unwanted pregnancy or sexually transmitted illnesses? Do you smoke or use drugs? How much do you drink? Are you taking steps to prevent major illnesses? Do you get regular health checkups? Are you aware of safety and environmental threats to your health? How are you going to make the most of your life? What do you hope to accomplish before you die?

This book asks these questions and many more. It is a book about you: your mind and your body, your spirit and your social ties, your needs and your wants, your past and your potential. It will help you explore options, discover possibilities, and find new ways to make your life worthwhile.

This book is also about living in a human body, thinking with a human mind, responding to a world of ideas and experiences with a human spirit. You are designed to move, to think, to act—to stretch yourself in every way. If you don't make the most of what you are, you risk never discovering what you might become.

Health involves more than physical well-being. It is a state of body, mind, and spirit that must be viewed within the context of community, society, and environment. By providing the information and understanding you need to take care of your own health, *An Invitation to Health* can help you live more fully, more happily, and more healthfully. It also goes beyond the basics of health maintenance. Its primary themes—prevention of health problems, protection from health threats, and promotion of the health of others—can establish the basis for good health now and in the future.

The invitation to health that we extend to every reader is one offer you literally cannot afford to refuse: The quality of your life depends on it.

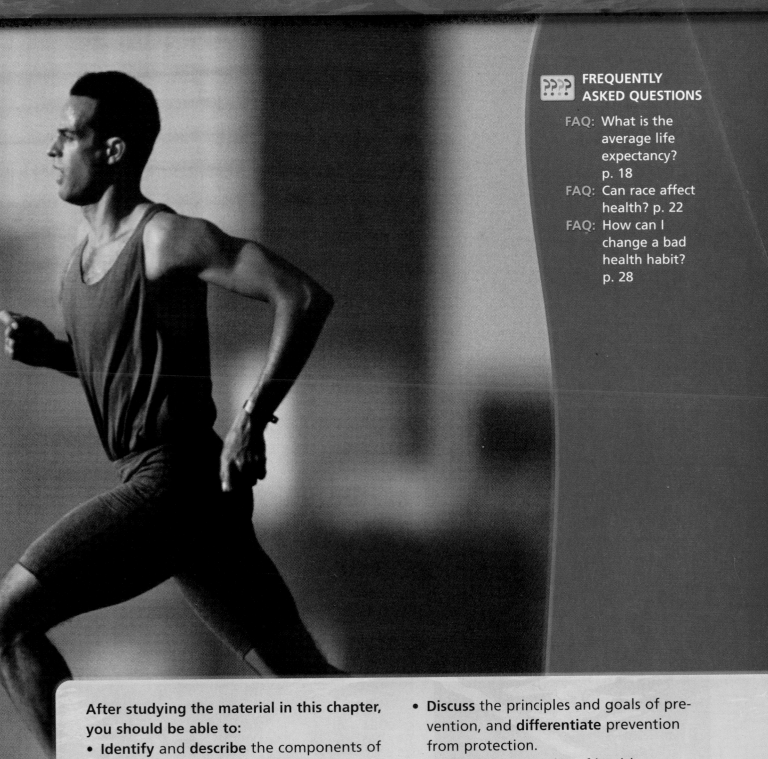

FAQ: What is the average life expectancy? p. 18

FAQ: Can race affect health? p. 22

FAQ: How can I change a bad health habit? p. 28

After studying the material in this chapter, you should be able to:

- **Identify** and **describe** the components of health and how they relate to total wellness.
- **Describe** how gender, race, and ethnicity can influence health and access to health care.
- **List** the factors that influence the development of health behaviors.
- **Discuss** the principles and goals of prevention, and **differentiate** prevention from protection.
- **Explain** the principles of health promotion.
- **Create** a complete plan to change or develop a health behavior.
- **Discuss** the factors and actions influencing an individual's longevity.

Health and Wellness

By simplest definition, **health** means being sound in body, mind, and spirit. The World Health Organization defines health as "not merely the absence of disease or infirmity," but "a state of complete physical, mental, and social well-being."[1] Health is the process of discovering, using, and protecting all the resources within our bodies, minds, spirits, families, communities, and environment.

Health has many components: physical, psychological, spiritual, social, intellectual, and environmental. This book takes a *holistic* approach, one that looks at health and the individual as a whole, rather than part by part. Your own definition of health may include different elements, but chances are that you and your classmates would agree that it includes at least some of the following:

▶ A positive, optimistic outlook.
▶ A sense of control over stress and worries; time to relax.
▶ Energy and vitality; freedom from pain or serious illness.
▶ Supportive friends and family, and a nurturing intimate relationship with someone you love.
▶ A personally satisfying job.
▶ A clean environment.

Wellness can be defined as purposeful, enjoyable living or, more specifically, a deliberate lifestyle choice characterized by personal responsibility and optimal enhancement of physical, mental, and spiritual health. Wellness means more than not being sick; it means taking steps to prevent illness and to lead a richer, more balanced, and more satisfying life.

Although physical well-being is essential to health, the term *wellness,* as used by health professionals, has a broader meaning. To understand how the concepts of wellness and health fit together, think of an automobile transmission: Having a disease (illness) is like being in reverse; absence of disease (health) puts you in neutral; but positive health changes (wellness) push you into drive—forward motion. When your entire lifestyle is based on health-enhancing behaviors, you're in high gear and going at top speed—and you've achieved total wellness.

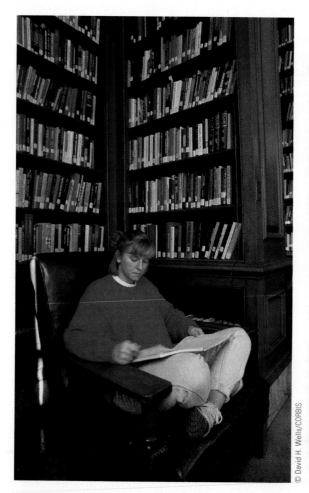
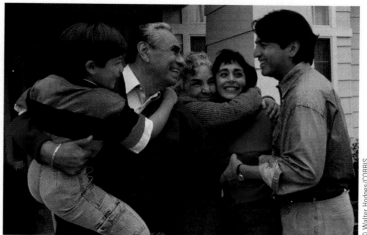
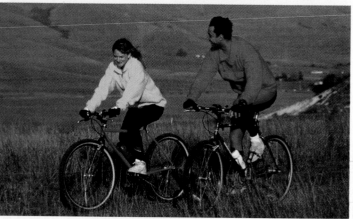

▲ Health is the process of discovering, using, and protecting all the resources within our bodies, minds, spirits, families, communities, and environment.

John Travis, M.D., creator of the Wellness Inventory (see p. 1), compares the various dimensions of wellness to an iceberg (see Figure 1-1). Only about one-tenth of the mass of an iceberg is visible; the rest is submerged. Your current state of health is like the tip of the iceberg—the part that shows.

"To understand all that creates and supports your current state of health," says Travis, "you have to look 'underwater.'" The first hidden level—the "lifestyle/behavioral" level—consists of what you eat, how active you are, how you manage stress, and how you protect yourself from hazards. Below this dimension is the "cultural/psychological/motivational" level, the often-invisible influences that lead us to choose a certain lifestyle. The foundation of the iceberg is the "spiritual/being/meaning" realm, which encompasses issues such as your reason for being, the meaning of your life, and your place in the universe. "Ultimately," says Travis, "this realm determines whether the tip of the iceberg, representing your state of health, is one of disease or wellness."

In wellness, health, and sickness, there is considerable overlap in the functions of the mind, body, and spirit. As scientists have shown again and again in recent decades, psychological factors play a major role in enhancing physical well-being and preventing illness, but they can also trigger, worsen, or prolong physical symptoms.

"The mind clearly can have a profound effect on every aspect of physiologic functioning," says James Gordon, M.D., Director of the Center for Mind-Body Studies in Washington, DC. "Individuals who are chronically pessimistic, angry, anxious or depressed are clearly more susceptible to stress and illness, including heart disease and cancer."[2] Similarly, almost every medical illness affects people psychologically as well as physically.

Physical Health

The various states of good and ill physical health can be viewed as points on a continuum (see Figure 1-2). At one end is early and needless death; at the other is optimal wellness, in which you feel and perform at your very best. In the middle, individuals are neither sick enough to need medical attention nor well enough to live each day with zest and vigor. For the sake of optimal physical health, we must take positive steps away from illness and toward well-being. We must feed our bodies nutritiously, exercise them regularly, avoid harmful behaviors and substances, watch out for early signs of sickness, and protect ourselves from accidents.

Psychological Health

Like physical well-being, psychological health is more than the absence of problems or illness. Psychological health refers to both our emotional and mental states—that is, to our feelings and our thoughts. It involves awareness and acceptance of a wide range of feelings in oneself and others, the ability to express emotions, to function independently, and to cope with the challenges of daily stressors. (Chapter 3 provides more information on psychological health.)

Spiritual Health

Spiritually healthy individuals identify their own basic purpose in life; learn how to experience love, joy, peace, and fulfillment; and help themselves and others achieve their full potential. As they devote themselves to others' needs more than their own, their spiritual development produces a sense of greater meaning in their lives.

Americans tend to be both spiritual and religious. According to the most recent in a series of national Gallup polls conducted over the last 60-plus years, 95 percent of Americans believe in God—an all-time high. Most Americans also say that prayer is an important part of their lives, that they believe that miracles are performed by a divine power, and that they are sometimes conscious of the presence of God.[3] Faced with physical or psychological difficulties, most Americans turn to prayer, reading the Bible, or meditation as a way of coping.[4]

Prayer is the most commonly used form of complementary/alternative medicine (discussed in Chapter 10). Being prayed for also may have some benefits. In a

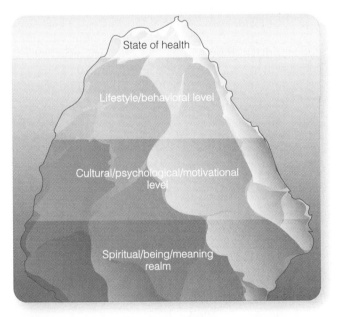

▲ **Figure 1-1** The iceberg model of wellness.
Like an iceberg, only a small part of your total wellness is visible: your current state of health. Just as important are hidden dimensions, including lifestyle habits, cultural and psychological factors, and the realm of spiritual meaning and being. Used with permission of John Travis.

Source: Adapted from Travis and Ryan, *The Wellness Workbook,* 2nd ed. Berkeley, CA, Ten Speed Press, 1988. Used with permission of John Travis.

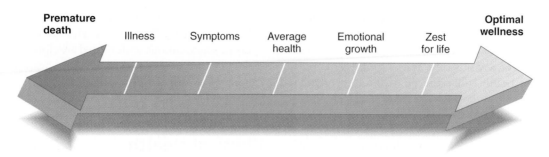

Premature death | Illness | Symptoms | Average health | Emotional growth | Zest for life | Optimal wellness

▲ **Figure 1-2** The wellness-illness continuum.

controlled study of 40 adults with moderately severe rheumatoid arthritis, those who were the recipients of intense praying aloud and "laying on of hands," followed by educational sessions on spirituality and healing, showed improvements in joint swelling and other symptoms. However, blood tests showed no changes in inflammatory markers, a finding suggesting that prayer changed perceptions of illness rather than the illness itself.[5]

The data on the health effects of spirituality and health have mounted steadily in recent years. Using data from some 126,000 people, scientists at the National Institute for Healthcare Research found that those with some religious involvement, such as attending worship services, were almost 30 percent more likely to live longer than less involved men and women.[6] Open-heart surgery patients who reported drawing strength and comfort from religion had only a third the risk of dying within six months of the surgery as those who didn't. Believers also have recovered from depression earlier,[7] and believers became pregnant sooner than other patients at a fertility clinic.[8] Frequent churchgoers also have lower blood pressures and more rigorous immune systems and report fewer physical symptoms.[9]

Are religious people simply healthier to begin with? At the very least, they're well enough to get to church. By avoiding sin, they may stay away from harmful habits, such as excessive drinking, taking drugs, smoking, or risky sexual practices.[10] In addition, belonging to a religious congregation may broaden and cement social bonds that buffer the harmful effects of stress, anxiety, and depression. Prayer itself may have a therapeutic effect, inducing the relaxation responses by producing a tranquil state of mind. Faith also may help people understand and interpret negative life situations so they can cope better with unexpected upsets.[11]

In one survey of family practitioners 99 percent said they believe that religious beliefs can heal; 75 percent believe that others' prayers can promote healing. However, more than half felt uncertain about how to ask about a patient's spirituality.[12] About half of America's medical schools now offer courses on spirituality and healing. And a growing number of doctors, while not endorsing or pre-

scribing any one approach to religion, are encouraging patients to cultivate a spiritual commitment—for the sake of their mortal bodies as well as their immortal souls.[13]

Some health professionals have long recognized the power and potential of spirituality. For 30 years, Herbert Benson, M.D., head of the Mind/Body Medical Institute at Harvard Medical School, has conducted rigorous experiments to document the influence of the spirit on health. His conclusion: The combination of relaxation and behavioral methods, such as prayer and meditation, with standard surgical and medical treatments can help relieve a host of medical problems, including chronic pain, arthritis, insomnia, and premenstrual symptoms. Improving spiritual health may not cure an illness, but it may help patients feel better, prevent certain illnesses, and cope with disease or death.[14]

"Religion is very, very good for you," says psychiatrist David B. Larson, M.D., president of the National Institute for Healthcare Research.[15] In an extensive review of the medical literature, he found not only that faith, belief, and religious commitment are positive influences on physical

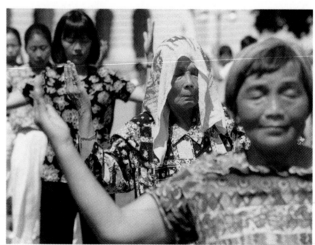

▲ In every culture, religious rituals play an important role in the lives and health of individuals.

and mental health, but also that a lack of religious practice constitutes a clear and consistent health risk factor.

"Deeply religious people of all faiths appear to benefit in five major areas," reports Dale Matthews of Georgetown School of Medicine, who reviewed more than 300 studies on healing and religion.[16] These are: less substance abuse; lower rates of depression and anxiety, especially among women; enhanced quality of life; quicker recovery from injury or illness; and longer life expectancy.

Skeptics point out that none of the research has pinpointed religion rather than another alternative as the direct cause of health benefits. As they note, meditation, exercise, healthful habits, and a strong social network may provide similar benefits.

Social Health

Social health refers to the ability to interact effectively with other people and the social environment, to develop satisfying interpersonal relationships, and to fulfill social roles. It involves participating in and contributing to your community, living in harmony with fellow human beings, developing positive interdependent relationships with others (discussed in Chapter 7), and practicing healthy sexual behaviors.

For Americans, the terrorist attacks of September 11, 2001 dramatically demonstrated the importance of social connections. As the routines of everyday life stopped, people checked on the safety of loved ones and gathered

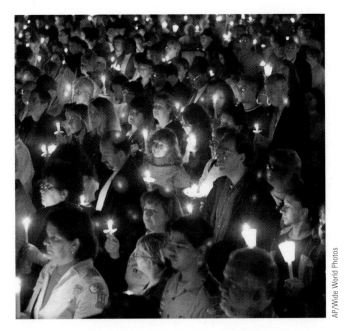

AP/Wide World Photos

▲ In the aftermath of the terrorist attacks of September 11, 2001, hundreds of thousands of people throughout the world came together for both social and spiritual comfort.

together in churches, synagogues, university centers, living rooms, parks, or plazas. In times of crisis, social connections provide comfort and support. "Ultimately, community helps us heal from trauma," says psychiatrist Robert Ursano, M.D., author of *The Psychiatric Aspects of Terrorism.*[17]

Even in tranquil times, social isolation increases the risk of sickness and mortality. In a landmark study of 4,725 men and women in Alameda County, California, death rates were twice as high for "loners" as for those with strong social ties. In other studies, social isolation greatly increased the risk of dying of a heart attack. Heart attack patients have a better chance of long-term survival if they believe they have adequate help in performing daily tasks from family and friends. People with spouses, friends, and a rich social network may outlive isolated loners by as much as 30 years.[18]

Health educators are placing greater emphasis on social health in its broadest sense as they expand the traditional individualistic concept of health to include the complex interrelationships between one person's health and the health of the community and environment. This change in perspective has given rise to a new emphasis on **health promotion,** which enhances health by building knowledge and skills among individuals and modifying their environment to foster healthier lifestyles.

Intellectual Health

Your brain is the only one of your organs capable of self-awareness. Every day you use your mind to gather, process, and act on information; to think through your values; to make decisions, set goals, and figure out how to handle a problem or challenge. Intellectual health refers to your ability to think and learn from life experience, your openness to new ideas, and your capacity to question and evaluate information. Throughout your life, you'll use your critical thinking skills, including your ability to evaluate health information to safeguard your well-being.

Another important component of intellectual well-being is "emotional intelligence," which is discussed in Chapter 3.

Environmental Health

You live in a physical and social setting that can affect every aspect of your health. Environmental health refers to the impact that your world has on your well-being. It means protecting yourself from dangers in the air, water, and soil, and in products you use—and also working to preserve the environment itself. (Chapter 19 offers a thorough discussion of environmental health.)

???? What Is the Average Life Expectancy?

A hundred years ago, the average white American could expect to live for only 48 years; nonwhites to age 38.[19] Infectious diseases, such as smallpox and tuberculosis, claimed tens of thousands of lives, particularly among the young and the poor. A high percentage of women died during childbirth or shortly afterward. By 1900, the average American woman could expect to live to an age of 50.9 years, compared with 47.9 years for a man.

At the beginning of the twenty-first century, life expectancy reached a record high of 76.9 years. Both gender and race affect how long we live. (See Figure 1-3.) As discussed in The X & Y Files: "Do Sex and Gender Matter?" there is a gap of 5.4 years between male and female life expectancy. A white girl born in the year 2000 can expect to live to 79.5 years; a black girl, to 75 years. A white baby boy's life expectancy is 74.8 years; a black baby boy's, 68.3 years.[20]

At the turn of the last century, 30.4 percent of all deaths were among children younger than age 5, and pneumonia, tuberculosis, and diarrhea were leading causes of death. However, scientists note that gains in life expectancy are slowing, primarily because adding decades, or even years, to the lives of people who have already lived for 70 years is much more difficult than adding decades to the lives of children who might otherwise die of infectious diseases. According to current predictions, the practical upper limit for life expectancy is 88 years for women and 82 for men. The French may reach this limit in the year 2033; the Japanese, in 2035; Americans, not until 2182.[21]

Chronic diseases, such as heart disease, cancer, and diabetes, currently account for 75 percent of deaths in the United States.[22] However, fewer people are dying of heart disease and cancer, according to the Centers for Disease Control and Prevention (CDC). Death rates from murder, suicide, accidents, stroke, diabetes, chronic respiratory disease, chronic liver disease, and AIDS also have fallen.[23]

Homicide and suicide have declined as causes of death for the total population, but among young persons 15 to 24 years of age, they remain, respectively, the second and third leading causes of death. Accidents are the number-one cause of death in this age group.

Is U.S. Health the Best in the World?

You may assume that it is. However, this isn't the case. In a comparison of 13 countries, the United States ranks an average of twelfth, second from the bottom. The nations that rank higher are Japan, Sweden, Canada, France, Australia, Spain, Finland, the Netherlands, the United

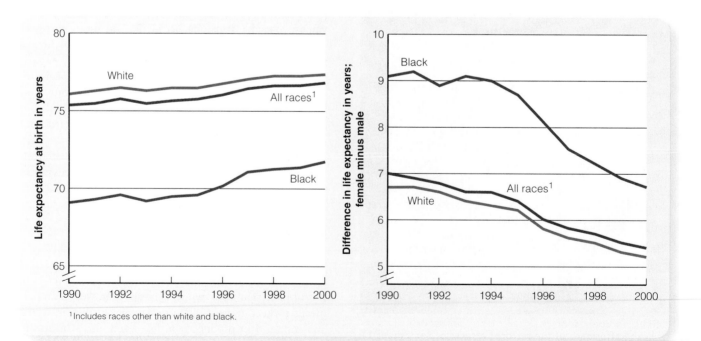

▲ **Figure 1-3** Increases in life expectancy in the United States: 1990–2000.

Source: National Vital Statistics Report, Vol. 49, No. 12, October 9, 2001.

Kingdom, Denmark, and Belgium. Here is the U.S. ranking on some indicators:

▶ 13th (last) for percentage of low-birthweight babies.

▶ 13th for mortality at birth and during infancy (although infant mortality has fallen to its lowest ever in the United States: 6.9 deaths per 1,000 live births).[24]

▶ 13th for years of potential life lost (excluding intentional and nonintentional injury).

▶ 11th for life expectancy for females at age one; 12th for males.

▶ 10th for life expectancy at age 40 for females; 9th for males.

▶ 7th for life expectancy at age 65 for females and males.

▶ 10th for age-adjusted mortality.[25]

The X&Y Files — Do Sex and Gender Matter?

"Sex does matter. It matters in ways that we did not expect. Undoubtedly, it also matters in ways that we have not begun to imagine." This was the conclusion of the Institute of Medicine Committee on Understanding the Biology of Sex and Gender Differences in the first significant review of the status of sex and gender differences in biomedical research.

"Sex," the committee stated, is "a classification, generally as male or female, according to the reproductive organs and functions that derive from the chromosomal complement." Gender refers to "a person's self-representation as male or female, or how that person is responded to by social institutions on the basis of the individual's gender presentation." Rooted in biology, gender is shaped by environment and experience.

In animals other than humans, sex alone influences the prevalence and severity of a broad range of diseases, disorders, and conditions. In human beings, gender also matters. The experience of being male or female in a particular culture and society can and does have an effect on physical and psychological well-being. In fact, sex and gender may have a greater impact than any other variable on how our bodies function, how long we live, and the symptoms, course, and treatment of the diseases that strike us.

This realization is both new and revolutionary. For centuries, scientists based biological theories solely on a male model and viewed women as shorter, smaller, and rounder versions of men. Even modern medicine is based on the assumption that, except for their reproductive organs, both sexes are biologically interchangeable. We now know that this simply isn't so. Sex begins in the womb, but sex and gender differences affect behavior, perception, and health throughout life.

As "The X & Y Files" features throughout the book show, virtually every part and organ system of the body differs in men and women (see Figure 1-4). A man's core body temperature runs lower than a woman's; his heart beats at a slower rate. A woman takes 9 breaths a minute; a man averages 12. Her blood carries higher levels of protective immunoglobulin; his has more oxygen-rich hemoglobin. Her ears are more sensitive to sound; his eyes are more sensitive to light. Male brains are 10 percent larger, but certain areas in female brains contain more neurons.

Gender differences persist in sickness as well as in health. Before age 50, men are more prone to lethal diseases, including heart attacks, cancer, and liver failure. Women show greater vulnerability to chronic but non–life-threatening problems such as arthritis and autoimmune disorders. Women are twice as likely to suffer depression; men have a fivefold greater rate of alcoholism. Women outlive men by more than six years, yet they're more prone to age-related problems, such as osteoporosis and Alzheimer's disease. Health behaviors—patterns of drinking, smoking, or using seat belts—also are different in men and women.

More than half of men between ages 18 and 29 do not have a regular physician, compared with a third of women. Seven in ten of those who have not visited a doctor in more than five years are men. Men get fewer dental as well as medical checkups. They're less likely to seek psychiatric services, to have their cholesterol levels and blood pressure checked regularly, and to undergo some form of screening for colon cancer. More women than men are overweight, and fewer women are physically active. Although college men are among those at highest risk of testicular cancer, three out of four do not know how to perform a self-examination. Male undergraduates are much less likely to examine their testicles than female students are to examine their breasts. College-age men also are significantly more likely to engage in risky and physically dangerous behaviors—and to suffer more injuries, including fatal ones, as a result.

Recognition of these gender differences is transforming medical research and practice. A new science called gender-specific medicine is replacing "good-enough," one-size-fits-all health care with new definitions of what is normal in both men and women, more complex concepts of disease, more precise diagnostic tests, and more effective treatments.

Sources: Committee on Understanding the Biology of Sex and Gender Differences. *Exploring the Biological Contributions to Human Health: Does Sex Matter?* Washington, DC: Institute of Medicine—National Academy of Sciences, 2001. Courtenay, Will. "Behavior Factors Associated with Disease, Injury and Death Among Men: Evidence and Implications for Prevention," *Journal of Men's Studies,* Vol. 9, No. 1, Fall 2000. Hales, Dianne. *Just Like a Woman.* New York: Bantam, 2000.

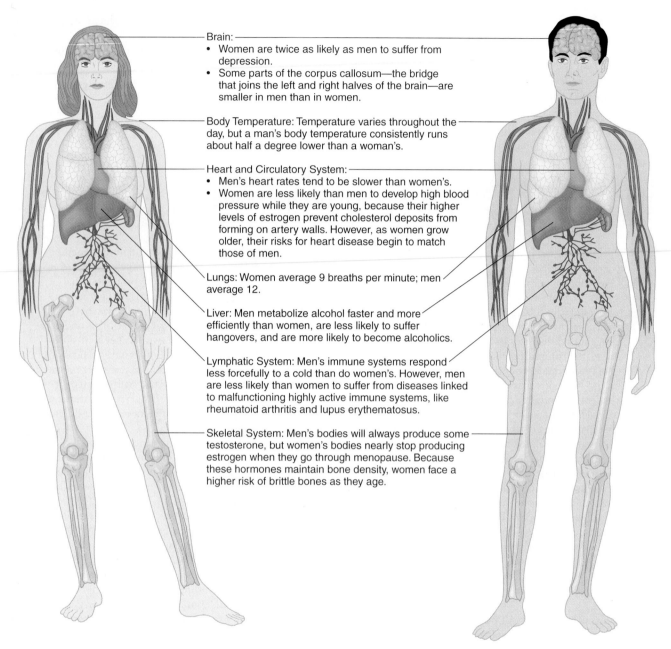

Brain:
• Women are twice as likely as men to suffer from depression.
• Some parts of the corpus callosum—the bridge that joins the left and right halves of the brain—are smaller in men than in women.

Body Temperature: Temperature varies throughout the day, but a man's body temperature consistently runs about half a degree lower than a woman's.

Heart and Circulatory System:
• Men's heart rates tend to be slower than women's.
• Women are less likely than men to develop high blood pressure while they are young, because their higher levels of estrogen prevent cholesterol deposits from forming on artery walls. However, as women grow older, their risks for heart disease begin to match those of men.

Lungs: Women average 9 breaths per minute; men average 12.

Liver: Men metabolize alcohol faster and more efficiently than women, are less likely to suffer hangovers, and are more likely to become alcoholics.

Lymphatic System: Men's immune systems respond less forcefully to a cold than do women's. However, men are less likely than women to suffer from diseases linked to malfunctioning highly active immune systems, like rheumatoid arthritis and lupus erythematosus.

Skeletal System: Men's bodies will always produce some testosterone, but women's bodies nearly stop producing estrogen when they go through menopause. Because these hormones maintain bone density, women face a higher risk of brittle bones as they age.

▲ **Figure 1-4** Sex differences in health.

Why does American health get such poor marks? Some point to the fact that more than 40 million people have no health insurance. Others observe that among those who can afford health care, 20 to 30 percent receive treatments that may be more harmful than beneficial.[26]

Are health behaviors to blame? Not necessarily. The proportion of men and women who smoke is higher in many other nations. The United States ranks fifth lowest in alcohol consumption. Americans also have relatively low consumption of animal fats. However, our nation has the dubious distinction of outranking all others in deaths due to motor vehicle accidents and violence.

Americans are living healthier lifestyles than they did 25 years ago. Fewer smoke. More have lowered their blood pressure and cholesterol levels. But Americans in small towns and rural areas lag behind others. They tend to smoke more, lose more teeth as they age, exercise less, and die sooner than residents of suburbs and big cities.[27]

Healthy People 2010

Americans entered the twenty-first century in fairly good shape but with a way to go to attain optimal wellness and fitness. *Healthy People 2000*, a federal initiative for health promotion and disease prevention, announced that Americans had achieved or "nearly met" about 60 percent of its health goals. On 18 percent of the objectives, however, the nation did worse rather than better. For example, the number of overweight persons increased in the last decade, and physical activity levels decreased.

Healthy People 2010 has more than 450 health objectives organized into 28 areas and two overarching goals: to increase years of healthy life and to eliminate racial and ethnic health disparities.[28] To track the nation's progress, the government has set up key health indicators that it will follow closely in the coming decade (see Table 1-1).

Among the specific goals related to wellness and fitness in *Healthy People 2010* are the following:

▶ Increase the number of adolescents engaging in vigorous physical activity three or more days per week for 20 or more minutes per occasion.

▶ Encourage adults to engage in moderate physical activity for at least 30 minutes on a regular basis, if not daily.

▶ Reduce the proportion of obese adults from 23 percent of the population to 15 percent. (See Chapter 6 for a definition of obesity based on body mass index.)

▶ Reduce the proportion of obese children and adolescents from 11 percent to 5 percent.

▶ Reduce the number of adolescents and adults using illegal substances.

▶ Reduce the proportion of adults engaging in binge drinking.

▶ Reduce the percentage of teens and adults who report having smoked cigarettes in the past month.[29]

Diversity and Health

We live in the most diverse nation on Earth, and in one that is becoming increasingly diverse. During the 1990s, the Hispanic and Asian populations of the United States surged, growing by 35 and 40 percent, respectively. The number of African Americans grew by almost 13 percent.

For society, this variety can be both enriching and divisive. Tolerance and acceptance of others have always been part of the American creed. By working together, Americans have created a country that remains a symbol of opportunity around the world. Yet members of different ethnic groups still have to struggle against discrimination. Today, in this country's third century, all Americans still aren't equal in their access to health care. Poverty remains a major barrier to good health care for minorities in the United States. Without adequate insurance or ability to pay, many cannot afford the tests and treatments that could prevent illness or overcome it at the earliest possible stages. Some groups, particularly African Americans, also rate the health services in their communities as lower than those available to white Americans and have more negative opinions of the health care they receive.

The growing influence of diverse racial and ethnic groups on our culture will affect national health priorities for many decades. As medical scientists are learning, there are clear differences with regard to disease and disability among different peoples. However, as public health experts explore the links between race, culture, and health, they are moving beyond any narrow definition of "minority" to the broader concept of "undeserved," a group made up of many cultures that also includes the homeless, rural Americans, and women. Special problems also exist for illegal Americans, who often live in extreme poverty; perform difficult, hazardous jobs; and have little or no access to health services. Even when they desperately need medical care, they may be so fearful of deportation that they do not seek help.[30]

Diversity poses special challenges in health care. Racial and ethnic minority communities have a disproportionately high burden of disability from inadequately treated mental health problems and illnesses.[31] In some cultures, physicians are seen as less effective than other healers, who are believed to cure illness caused by bad karma or evil spirits. American physicians, trained to believe that high-tech medicine is best, may not understand or appreciate traditional healing practices. In many

---

▼ **Table 1-1   Healthy People 2010: Lifestyle Indicators**

To monitor the progress the nation makes in meeting new health objectives, *Healthy People 2010* has identified the following ten key health indicators that will serve as indicators of how Americans are doing in terms of improving health and enhancing wellness:

Lifestyle Indicators	Health system indicators
• Physical activity	• Immunication rates for children and adults
• Obesity and nutrition	• Access to health care
• Tobacco use	• Injury and violence prevention
• Substance abuse	• Environmental health
• Responsible sexual behavior	• Mental health

Source: www.health.gov.healthypeople

communities, innovative programs have begun to educate patients from other cultures about the American health-care system, as well as to educate American health-care providers about the beliefs and health practices of their diverse patients.

???? Can Race Affect Health?

Different racial and ethnic groups often face different health risks. Consider the following statistics:

▶ The infant mortality rate for African-American babies remains higher than that for white babies.[32]

▶ Life expectancy for African Americans, though increasing, is seven years lower than that for whites.[33]

▶ African Americans have higher rates of high blood pressure (hypertension), develop this problem earlier in life, suffer more severe hypertension, and have higher rates of strokes and hypertension-related deaths than whites. Cardiovascular risk is higher in minority than white youth.

▶ African Americans have higher rates of glaucoma, systemic lupus erythematosus, liver disease, and kidney failure than whites.

▶ The death rate for heart disease among middle-aged black women is 150 percent higher than among white women the same age; among those with diabetes, their death rate is 134 percent higher than white female diabetics.

▶ Cardiologists are 60 percent less likely to refer a black woman for cardiac catheterization (a test of the heart's blood vessels) than a white woman of the same age.

▶ Among young African-American women, breast cancer is a special threat. Of all black women diagnosed with breast cancer, 37 percent are younger than 50—compared with 22 percent of white women. Older black and Latino women have fewer mammograms than their white counterparts.

▶ Native Americans have the highest rates of diabetes in the world. Among the Pima Indians, half of all adults have diabetes.

▶ Southeast Asian men have a higher incidence of lung and liver cancer than the population as a whole.

▶ Native Hawaiian women have a higher rate of breast cancer than women from other racial and ethnic groups.

▶ Native Americans, including those indigenous to Alaska, are more likely to die young, primarily as the result of accidental injuries, cirrhosis of the liver, homicide, pneumonia, and the complications of diabetes than the population as a whole.[34]

▶ The suicide rate among American Indians/Alaska Natives is 50 percent higher than the national rate. The rates of co-occurring mental illness and substance abuse (especially alcohol) are also higher among Native American youth and adults.[35]

▶ Disproportionate numbers of African Americans are among the groups most vulnerable to mental illness: the homeless, incarcerated, those in the child welfare system, and victims of trauma.

Are these increased susceptibilities the result of racial or ethnic background, the stress of living with discrimination, an unhealthy lifestyle, lack of access to health services, or poverty? It is hard to say precisely. Certainly, poverty presents a major barrier to seeking preventive care and getting timely and effective treatment.

Genetic and environmental factors also may play a role. Take, for example, the high rates of diabetes among the Pima Indians. Until 50 years ago, these Native Americans were not notably obese or prone to diabetes. However, after World War II, the tribe started trading handmade baskets for lard and flour. Their lifestyle became more sedentary, and their diet, higher in fats. In addition, researchers have discovered that many Pima Indians have an inherited resistance to insulin that increases their susceptibility to diabetes. The combination of a hereditary predisposition and environmental factors may explain why the Pimas now have epidemic levels of diabetes.

Other groups have other vulnerabilities. Caucasians, for instance, are prone to osteoporosis (progressive weakening of bone tissue); cystic fibrosis; skin cancer; and phenylketonuria (PKU), a metabolic disorder that can lead to mental retardation. Women with Chinese or Latino backgrounds face a significantly greater risk of developing diabetes during pregnancy than African Americans or whites. Asians and Asian Americans metabolize some medications faster than whites and thus require much smaller doses. Latinos have higher rates of death from diabetes and infectious and parasitic diseases than African Americans or whites. (See Table 1-2.)

Health-care providers often fail to recognize such factors, in part because the discussion of ethnicity in health is politically controversial. Some fear that it could lead to misconceptions about genetic superiority or inferiority. Yet recognition of different health needs and risks is the first step toward overcoming the health problems of many Americans.

Closing the Minority Health Gap

In the words of a National Institutes of Health (NIH) report, minorities have carried "an unequal burden with respect to disease and disability, resulting in a lower life expectancy." Each year minorities in the United States—African Americans, Latinos, Asian Americans, Pacific Islanders, Native Americans, and other groups—experience as many as 75,000 more deaths than they would if they lived under the same health conditions as the white population.

But race itself isn't the primary reason for the health problems faced by minorities in the United States. Poverty

▼ Table 1-2	Diversity and Genetic Disorders	
Ethnic Group	**Genetic Disorder**	**Typical Features**
Africans (blacks)	African-type adult lactase deficiency	Milk intolerance
Afrikaners (white South Africans)	Porphyria variegata	Neurological problems
Amish or Mennonites	Ellis-Van Creveld syndrome	Dwarfism and extra digits
Armenians	Familial Mediterranean fever	Inflammation and fever
Ashkenazi Jews	Tay-Sachs disease	Brain degeneration
Chinese	Thalassemia (alpha)	Anemia
Finns	Dystrophic retinae dysacusis syndrome	Blindness
French Canadians	Familial hypercholesterolemia	Coronary heart disease
Irish	Neural-tube defects	Spina bifida
Italians	Fucosidosis	Mental retardation
Japanese and Koreans	Oguchi disease	Night blindness
Maori (Polynesians)	Clubfoot	Foot deformity
Mediterraneans	Glycogen-storage disease (type III)	Liver disease
Norwegians	Cholestasis-lymphedema	Liver problems

Source: Milansky, Aubrey. *Your Genetic Destiny.* New York: Perseus Publishing, 2001.

is. One in three Hispanics under age 65 has no health insurance.[36] According to public health experts, low income may account for one-third of the racial differences in death rates for middle-aged African-American adults. High blood pressure, high cholesterol, obesity, diabetes, and smoking are responsible for another third. The final third has been blamed on "unexplained factors," which may well include poor access to health care and the stress of living in a society in which skin color remains a major barrier to equality. Language, too, can create communication barriers.

NIH has established an Office of Research on Minority Health (ORMH) with the goal of "closing the gap that cur-

rently exists between the health of minorities and the majority population." It has provided funds for research and prevention efforts aimed at improving minority health. Some focus on prenatal care to improve survival rates. Others are educating minority youths about HIV infection and AIDS.

The Health of College Students

As one of the nation's 12 million full- or part-time college students, you belong to one of the most diverse groups in America. A quarter of all 18- to 24-year-olds in the United States—some 7.1 million in all—are enrolled at one of the nation's 3,600 colleges and universities. Some of you are reentry students, back on campus for the second time; half of all college dropouts return to school within 15 years.

As shown in the "Student Snapshot" features throughout this book, college students often engage in behaviors that put them at risk for serious health problems. Student health behaviors also show gender differences. (See Student Snapshot: "The American Freshman.")

College-age men are more likely than women to engage in risk-taking behaviors—to use drugs and alcohol, to engage in risky sexual behaviors, such as having multiple partners and having sex while under the influence of alcohol, and to drive dangerously than college women. Men also are more likely to be hospitalized for injuries and to commit suicide. Three-fourths of the deaths in the 15- to 24-year age range are men.[37] However, college students of both sexes can and often do make permanent, life-enhancing changes.[38]

College itself can seem hazardous to health. Dormitories have proven to be breeding grounds for serious infectious diseases, such as meningitis (discussed in Chapter 11). Secondhand smoke can present a long-term threat to smokers' roommates. Binge drinking imperils not only the drinkers but those in their immediate environment, including anyone on the road if an intoxicated student gets behind the wheel of a car.[39]

Undergraduates also face risks to their psychological health. In a Canadian survey, college students reported more distress than the general Canadian population and than same-age peers not enrolled in college.[40] Nearly a third of more than 7,500 undergraduates surveyed had significantly elevated psychological distress—women more than men, younger students more than upperclassmen.

As discussed in Chapter 2, the sources of stress on campus are many: academic pressures, financial worries, adjustment to new people and expectations, anxieties about the future. One often-overlooked stressor is unpleasant interaction with others. In a recent study of students, hostile or upsetting exchanges with friends, ex-friends, loved ones, and even strangers—in person, by phone, or

Student Snapshot The American Freshman

What is our racial background?[1]

White/Caucasian	76.1%
African American/Black	10.4%
Hispanic	7.0%
Asian American/Asian	7.1%
Native American	1.9%

[1] Some respondents checked more than one category.

How many hours per week do we spend on homework?

None	2.3%
Less than one	11.8%
1 to 2	21.1%
3 to 5	28.7%
6 to 10	20.0%
11 to 15	8.8%
16 to 20	4.2%
More than 20	3.0%

On what issues do more than half of us strongly agree or somewhat agree?

The federal government should do more to control handguns.	82.0%
Employers should be able to require drug tests.	76.5%
Our society shows too much concern for criminals.	66.5%
Colleges should prohibit racist/sexist speech.	61.8%
Abortion should be legal.	53.9%
The wealthy should pay more taxes than they do now.	52.2%

Source: Adapted from Sax, Linda, et al. *The American Freshman: National Norms for Fall 2000.* Los Angeles: Higher Education Research Institute, UCLA, 2000.

online—strongly correlated with both emotional and physical well-being.[41] Students who endure harassment or abuse of any sort are more likely to report health-related symptoms. Those most at risk include minority students as well as gay, lesbian, and bisexual undergraduates.[42]

Colleges and universities can take varied steps to protect students' well-being. These range from offering vaccination against meningitis to banning alcohol at athletic and social events.[43] Reliable health-related information also can make a difference. Although the majority of college students report receiving some health information, only 6 percent in one recent survey had gotten information on a comprehensive range of health topics. Full-time, single students between ages 18 and 25 are most likely to receive health information. Students who are black, Hispanic, or belong to another racial or ethnic group are more likely than white students to have gotten information from campus sources.[44]

Yet, despite potential health risks, the great majority of students not only survive college but, simply by acquiring more years of schooling, increase their chances of a long and healthful life. Many risk factors for disease—including high blood pressure, elevated cholesterol, and cigarette smoking—decline steadily as education increases, regardless of how much money people make. Education may be good for the body as well as the mind by influencing lifestyle behaviors, problem-solving abilities, and values. People who earn college degrees gain positive attitudes about the benefits of healthy living, learn how to gain access to preventive health services, join peer groups that promote healthy behavior, and develop higher self-esteem and greater control over their lives.

Do healthy behaviors have an effect on academic performance? In a study of 200 students living in on-campus residence halls at a large private university, researchers weighed the impact of various health-related variables on first-year students' grade point averages (GPAs). Those associated with higher grades include female gender, age, studying spiritually oriented material, eating breakfast, and using a planner to organize time. Students with lower GPAs were more likely to stay up and wake up later on weekdays and weekends, sleep more on weekend nights, and work longer hours.[45]

Becoming All You Can Be

Your choices and behaviors affect how long and how well you live. (See Pulse Points: "Ten Simple Changes to Improve Your Health.") Nearly half of all deaths in the United States are linked to behaviors such as tobacco use, improper diet, abuse of alcohol and other drugs, use of firearms, motor vehicle accidents, risky sexual practices, and lack of exercise. Yet doctors rarely counsel patients about behavior changes.[46] Among young Americans ages 10 to 24, three causes are responsible for 73 percent of deaths: motor vehicle accidents, homicides, and suicides.[47]

What aspects of your life could use some attention and improvement? As Savvy Consumer: "Too Good to Be True?" points out, there are no easy answers or quick solutions. Use this course as an opportunity to zero in on at least one less-than-healthful behavior and improve it. The following sections discuss some of the processes you'll have to go through in order to make a successful change for the better.

Understanding Health Behavior

Behaviors that affect your health include exercising regularly, eating a balanced, nutritious diet, seeking care for

PULSE POINTS

Ten Simple Changes to Improve Your Health

1. **Use seat belts.** In the last decade seat belts have saved more than 40,000 lives and prevented millions of injuries.

2. **Eat an extra fruit or vegetable every day.** Adding more fruit and vegetables to your diet can improve your digestion and lower your risk of several cancers.

3. **Get enough sleep.** A good night's rest provides the energy you need to make it through the following day.

4. **Take regular stress breaks.** A few quiet minutes spent stretch-
ing, looking out the window, or simply letting yourself unwind are good for body and soul.

5. **Lose a pound.** If you're overweight, you may not think a pound will make a difference, but it's a step in the right direction.

6. **If you're a woman, examine your breasts regularly.** Get in the habit of performing a breast self-examination every month after your period (when breasts are least swollen or tender).

7. **If you're a man, examine your testicles regularly.** These simple self-exams can spot the
early signs of cancer when they're most likely to be cured.

8. **Get physical.** Just a little exercise will do some good. A regular workout schedule will be good for your heart, lungs, muscles, bones—even your mood.

9. **Drink more water.** Eight glasses a day are what you need to replenish lost fluids, prevent constipation, and keep your digestive system working efficiently.

10. **Do a good deed.** Caring for others is a wonderful way to care for your own soul and connect with others.

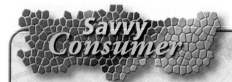

Too Good To Be True?

Almost every week you're likely to come across a commercial or an ad for a new health product that promises better sleep, more energy, clearer skin, firmer muscles, lower weight, brighter moods, longer life—or all of these combined. As the "Savvy Consumer" features throughout this book point out, you can't believe every promise you read or hear. Keep these general guidelines in mind the next time you come across a health claim:

- If it sounds too good to be true, it probably is. If a magic pill could really trim off excess pounds or banish wrinkles, the world would be filled with thin people with unlined skin. Look around, and you'll realize that's not the case.

- Look for objective evaluations. If you're watching an infomercial for a treatment or technique, you can be sure that the enthusiastic endorsements have been skillfully scripted and rehearsed. Even ads that claim to

be presenting the science behind a new "breakthrough" are really sales pitches in disguise.

- Consider the sources. Research findings from carefully controlled scientific studies are reviewed by leading experts in the field and published in scholarly journals. The fact that someone has conducted a study doesn't mean it was a valid scientific investigation.

- Check credentials. Anyone can claim to be a "scientist" or a "health expert." Find out if advocates of any type of therapy have legitimate degrees from recognized institutions and are fully licensed in their fields.

- Do your own research. Check with your doctor or with the student health center. Go to the library or do some online research to gather as much information as you can. (See Chapter 10 for more on evaluating health information and the Health Almanac on finding information on the Internet.)

symptoms, and taking necessary steps to overcome illness and restore well-being. If there is one health behavior that you would like to improve, you have to realize that change isn't easy. Between 40 and 80 percent of those people who try to kick bad health habits lapse back into their unhealthy ways within six weeks. To make lasting beneficial changes, you have to understand the three types of influences that shape behavior: predisposing, enabling, and reinforcing factors (Figure 1-5).

Predisposing Factors

Predisposing factors include knowledge, attitudes, beliefs, values, and perceptions. Unfortunately, knowledge isn't enough to cause most people to change their behavior; for example, people fully aware of the grim consequences of smoking often continue to puff away. Nor is attitude—one's likes and dislikes—sufficient; an individual may dislike the smell and taste of cigarettes but continue to smoke regardless.

Beliefs are more powerful than knowledge and attitudes, and researchers report that people are most likely to change health behavior if they hold three beliefs:

▶ **Susceptibility.** They acknowledge that they are at risk for the negative consequences of their behavior.
▶ **Severity.** They believe that they may pay a very high price if they don't make a change.
▶ **Benefits.** They believe that the proposed change will be advantageous to their health.

There can be a gap between stated and actual beliefs, however. Young adults may say they recognize the very real dangers of casual, careless sex in this day and age. Yet, rather than act in accordance with these statements, they may impulsively engage in unprotected sex with individuals whose health status and histories they do not know.

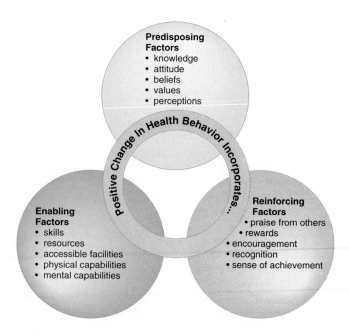

▲ **Figure 1-5** Factors that shape positive behavior.

The reason: Like young people everywhere and in every time, they feel they are invulnerable, that nothing bad can or will happen to them, that if there were a real danger, they would somehow know it. Often it's not until something happens—a former lover may admit to having a sexually transmitted disease (STD)—that their behaviors become consistent with their stated beliefs.

Young people, especially young men, are the greatest risk takers, a fact reflected in their high rates of auto accidents, binge drinking, drug use, and pathological gambling.[48] The death rates for injuries related to swimming, boating, driving, cycling, and even crossing the street are higher in college-age men than women.[49]

The value or importance we give to health also plays a major role in changing behavior. Many people aren't concerned about their health just for the sake of being healthy. Usually they want to look or feel better, be more productive or competitive, or behave more independently. They're more likely to change, and to stick with a change, if they can see that the health benefits also enhance other important aspects of their lives.

Perceptions are the way we see things from our unique perspective; they vary greatly with age. As a student, you may not think that living a few hours longer is a significant gain; as you grow older, however, you may prize every additional second.

Enabling Factors

Enabling factors include skills, resources, accessible facilities, and physical and mental capacities. Before you initiate a change, assess the means available to reach your goal. No matter how motivated you are, you'll become frustrated if you keep encountering obstacles. That's why breaking a task or goal down into step-by-step strategies is so important in behavioral change.

Reinforcing Factors

Reinforcing factors may be praise from family and friends, rewards from teachers or parents, or encouragement and recognition for meeting a goal. Although these help a great deal in the short run, lasting change depends not on external rewards, but on an internal commitment and sense of achievement. To make a difference, reinforcement must come from within.

A decision to change a health behavior should stem from a permanent, personal goal, not from a desire to please or impress someone else. If you lose weight for the homecoming dance, you're almost sure to regain pounds afterward. But if you shed extra pounds because you want to feel better about yourself or get into shape, you're far more likely to keep the weight off.

Making Decisions

Every day you make decisions that have immediate and long-term effects on your health. You decide what to eat, whether to drink or smoke, when to exercise, and how to cope with a sudden crisis. Beyond these daily matters, you decide when to see a doctor, what kind of doctor, and with what sense of urgency. You decide what to tell your doctor and whether to follow the advice given, whether to keep up your immunizations, whether to have a prescription filled and comply with the medication instructions, and whether to seek further help or a second opinion. The entire process of maintaining or restoring health depends on your decisions; it cannot start or continue without them.

The small decisions of everyday life—what to eat, where to go, when to study—are straightforward choices. Larger decisions—which major to choose, what to do about a dead-end relationship, how to handle an awkward work situation—are more challenging. However, if you think of decision making as a process, you can break down even the most difficult choices into manageable steps:

▶ **Set priorities.** Rather than getting bogged down in details, step back and look at the big picture. What matters most to you? What would you like to accomplish in

STRATEGIES FOR PREVENTION

Setting Realistic Goals

Here's a framework for setting goals and objectives, the crucial preliminary step for prevention:

✔ Determine your goal or objective. Define it in words and on paper. Then test your definition against your own value system. Can you attain your goal and still be the person you want to be?

✔ Think in terms of evolution, not revolution. Revolutionary changes only inspire counterrevolutions. If you want to change the way you eat, start by changing just one meal a week.

✔ Identify your resources. Do you have the knowledge, skills, finances, time—whatever it takes? Find out from others who know. Be sure you're ready for the next step.

✔ Systematically analyze barriers. How can missing resources be acquired? Identify and select alternative plans. List solutions for any obstacles you foresee.

✔ Choose a plan. Think it through, step by step, trying to anticipate what might go wrong and why.

the next week, month, year? Look at the decision you're about to make in the context of your values and goals.

▶ **Inform yourself.** The more you know—about a person, a position, a place, a project—the better you'll be able to evaluate it. Gathering information may involve formal research, such as an online or library search for relevant data, or informal conversations with teachers, counselors, family members, or friends.

▶ **Consider all your options.** Most complex decisions don't involve simple either-or alternatives. List as many options as you can think of, along with the advantages and disadvantages of each.

▶ **Tune in to your gut feelings.** After you've gotten the facts and analyzed them, listen to your intuition. While it's not infallible, your "sixth sense" can provide valuable feedback. If something just doesn't feel right, try to figure out why. Are there any fears you haven't dealt with? Do you have doubts about taking a certain path?

▶ **Consider a worst-case scenario.** When you've pretty much come to a final decision, imagine what will happen if everything goes wrong—the workload becomes overwhelming, your partner betrays your trust, your expectations turn out to be unrealistic. If you can live with the worst consequences of a decision, you're probably making the right choice.

How Can I Change a Bad Health Habit?

Change is never easy—even if it's done for the best possible reasons. When you decide to change a behavior, you have to give up something familiar and easy for something new and challenging. Change always involves risk—and the prospect of rewards.

Researchers have identified various approaches that people use in making beneficial changes. In the moral model, you take responsibility for a problem (such as smoking) and its solution; success depends on adequate motivation, while failure is seen as a sign of character weakness. In the enlightenment model, you submit to strict discipline in order to correct a problem; this is the approach used in Alcoholics Anonymous. The behavioral model involves rewarding yourself when you make positive changes. The medical model sees the behavior as caused by forces beyond your control (a genetic predisposition to being overweight, for example) and employs an expert to provide advice or treatment. For many people, the most effective approach is the compensatory model, which doesn't assign blame but puts responsibility on individuals to acquire whatever skills or power they need to overcome their problems.

Before they reach the stage where they can and do take action to change, most people go through a process comparable to religious conversion. First, they reach a level of accumulated unhappiness that makes them ready for change.

Then they have a moment of truth that makes them want to change. One pregnant woman, for instance, felt her unborn baby quiver when she drank a beer and swore never to drink again. As people change their behavior, they change their lifestyles and identities as well. Ex-smokers, for instance, may start an aggressive exercise program, make new friends at the track or gym, and participate in new types of activities, like racquetball games or fun runs.

Social and cultural **norms**—behaviors that are expected, accepted, or supported by a group—can make change much harder if they're constantly working against a person's best intentions. You may resolve to eat less, for instance, yet your mother may keep offering you homemade fudge and brownies because your family's norm is to show love by making and offering delicious treats. Or you might decide to drink less, yet your friends' norm may be to equate drinking with having a good time.

If you're aware of the norms that influence your behavior, you can devise strategies either to change them (by encouraging your friends to dance more and drink less at parties, for example) or adapt to them (having just a bite of your mother's sweets). Another option is to develop relationships with people who share your goals and whose norms can reinforce your behavior.

Successful Change

Awareness of a negative behavior is always the first step toward changing it. Once you identify what you'd like to change, keep a diary for one or two weeks, noting what you do, when, where, and what you're feeling at the time. If you'd like, enlist the help of friends or family to call attention to your behavior. Sometimes self-observation in itself proves therapeutic: Just the act of keeping a diary can be enough to help you lose weight or kick the smoking habit.

Once you've identified the situations, moods, thoughts, or people that act as cues for a behavior, identify the most powerful ones and develop a plan to avoid them. For instance, if you snack continuously when studying in your room, try working in the library, where food is forbidden.

Planning ahead is a crucial part of successful change. If you can't avoid certain situations, anticipate how you can cope with the temptation to return to your old behavior. Develop alternatives. Visualize yourself walking past the desserts in the cafeteria or chewing gum instead of lighting a cigarette.

Some people find it helpful to sign a "contract," a written agreement in which they make a commitment to change, with their partner, parent, or health educator. Spelling out what they intend to do, and why, underscores the seriousness of what they're trying to accomplish (see Figure 1-6).

Above all else, change depends on the belief that you can and will succeed. In his research on **self-efficacy,** psychologist Albert Bandura of Stanford University found

STRATEGIES FOR CHANGE

How to Make a Change

✔ Get support from friends, but don't expect them to supply all the reinforcement you need. You may join a group of overweight individuals and rely on their encouragement to stick to your diet. That's a great way to get going; but in the long run, your own commitment to losing weight has got to be strong enough to help you keep eating right and light.

✔ Focus on the immediate rewards of your new behavior. You may stop smoking so that you'll live longer, but take note of every other benefit it brings you—more stamina, less coughing, more spending money, no more stale tobacco taste in your mouth.

✔ To boost your self-confidence, remind yourself of past successes you've had in making changes. Give yourself pep talks, commending yourself on how well you've done so far and how well you'll continue to do.

✔ Reward yourself regularly. Plan a pleasant reward as an incentive for every week you stick to your new behavior—sleeping in on a Saturday morning, going out with some friends, or spending a sunny afternoon outdoors. Small, regular rewards are more effective in keeping up motivation than one big reward that won't come for many months.

✔ Expect and accept some relapses. The greatest rate of relapse occurs in the first few weeks after making a behavior change. During this critical time, get as much support as you can. In addition, work hard on self-motivation, reminding yourself daily of what you have to gain by sticking with your new health habit.

My Contract For Change

Date: _____

Personal Goal: _____

_____

Motivating Factors: _____

Change(s) I Promise to Make to Reach This Goal: ___

Plan for Making This Change: _____

_____

Start Date: _____

Assessment Plan: _____

If I Need Help: _____

_____

Target Date for Reaching Goal: _____

Reward for Achieving Goal: _____

Penalty for Failing to Achieve Goal: _____

Signed: _____

Witnessed By: _____

▲ **Figure 1-6** A sample health-change contract.

that the individuals most likely to reach a goal are those who believe they can. The more strongly they feel that they can and will change their behavior, the more energy and persistence they put into making the change. Other researchers have linked positive health change with optimism. Individuals who see themselves as optimists may underestimate their susceptibility to problems, such as hypertension, because they always expect things to turn out well. Individuals who perceive themselves as suscepti-ble—that is, who anticipate potentially negative conse-quences—may be more cautious.

Another crucial factor is **locus of control.** If you believe that your actions will make a difference in your health, your locus of control is internal. If you believe that external forces or factors play a greater role, your locus of control is external. Individuals with an external locus of control for health are less likely to seek preventive health care, are less optimistic about early treatment, rate their own health as poorer, and spend more time in bed because of illness than those with an internal locus of control.

Reinforcements—either positive (a reward) or negative (a punishment)—also can play a role. If you decide to set up a regular exercise program, for instance, you might reward yourself with a new sweat suit if you stick to it for three months or you might punish yourself for skipping a day by doing an extra ten minutes of exercises the following day.

Your **self-talk**—the messages you send yourself—also can play a role. In recent decades, mental health professionals have recognized the conscious use of positive self-talk as a powerful force for changing the way individuals think, feel, and behave. "We have a choice about how we think," explains psychologist Martin Seligman, Ph.D., author of *Learned Optimism.* As he notes, by learning to challenge automatic negative thoughts that enter our brains and asserting our own statements of self-worth, we can transform ourselves into optimists who see what's right rather than pessimists forever focusing on what's wrong. "Optimism is a learned set of skills," Seligman contends. "Once learned, these skills persist because they feel so good to use. And reality is usually on our side."

A New Era in Health Education

In the past, health education focused on individual change. Today many educators are using a new framework in which behavior change occurs within the context of the entire environment of a person's life. Its primary themes—prevention of health problems and protection from health threats—can establish the basis for good health now and in the future.

The Power of Prevention

No medical treatment, however successful or sophisticated, can compare with the power of **prevention.** Two out of every three deaths and one in three hospitalizations in the United States could be prevented by changes in six main risk factors: tobacco use, alcohol abuse, accidents, high blood pressure, obesity, and gaps in screening and primary health care. Preventive efforts have already proved helpful in increasing physical activity, quitting smoking, reducing dietary fat, preventing STDs and unwanted pregnancy, reducing intolerance and violence, and avoiding alcohol and drug abuse.

Prevention can take many forms. Primary or "before-the-fact" prevention efforts might seek to reduce stressors and increase support in order to prevent problems in healthy people. Consumer education, for instance, provides guidance about how to change our lifestyle—the way we care for the basic needs of body and mind—to prevent problems and enhance well-being. Other preventive programs identify people at risk and empower them with information and support so they can avoid potential problems. Prevention efforts may target an entire community and try to educate all of its members about the dangers of alcohol abuse, for instance, or environmental hazards, or they may zero in on a particular group (for instance, seminars on safer sex practice offered to teens) or an individual (one-on-one counseling about substance abuse).

In the past, physicians did not routinely incorporate prevention into their professional practices. Instead, consumers played the role of Humpty-Dumpty: As long as they sat quietly on the wall, they were ignored. When they fell, the medical equivalents of all the king's horses and all the king's men came running to put them back together again. Often, however, even the best these professionals could provide was still too little, too late.

But times have changed. Medical schools are providing more training in preventive care. A growing number of studies have demonstrated that prevention saves not only money but also productivity, health, and lives. As many as 50 to 80 percent of the deaths caused by cardiovascular disease, strokes, and cancer could be avoided or delayed by preventive measures. Eliminating smoking could prevent more than 300,000 deaths each year, for instance, while changes in diet could prevent 35 percent of unnecessary deaths from heart disease.

The Potential of Protection

There is a great deal of overlap between prevention and **protection.** Some people might think of immunizations (discussed in Chapter 11) as a way of preventing illness; others see them as a form of protection against dangerous diseases. In many ways, protection picks up where prevention leaves off. You can prevent STDs or unwanted pregnancy by abstaining from sex. But if you decide to engage in potentially risky sexual activities, you can protect yourself by means of condoms and spermicides (discussed in Chapter 9). Similarly, you can prevent many automobile accidents by not driving when road conditions are hazardous. But if you do have to drive, you can protect yourself by wearing a seat belt and using defensive driving techniques (discussed in Chapter 17).

The very concept of protection implies some degree of risk—immediate and direct (for instance, the risk of intentional injury from an assailant or unintentional harm from a fire) or long-term and indirect (such as the risk of heart disease and cancer as a result of smoking). To know how best to protect yourself, you have to be able to assess risks realistically.

Assessing Risks

Today's young people face a host of risks, from the danger of being the victim of violence to the hazards of self-destructive behaviors like drinking and drugs. The CDC's Youth Risk Behavior Surveys show a decline in some risky behaviors, such as carrying a weapon and not wearing a bicycle helmet, but an increase in others, including cigarette smoking and marijuana use.

At any age, the greatest health threats stem from high-risk behaviors—smoking, excessive drinking, not getting enough exercise, eating too many high-fat foods, and not getting regular medical checkups, to name just a few. That's why changing unhealthy habits is the best way to reduce risks and prevent health problems.

Environmental health risks are the stuff newspaper headlines are made of (see Chapter 19). Every year brings calls of alarm about a new hazard to health: electromagnetic radiation, fluoride in drinking water, hair dyes, silicone implants, radon, lead. Often the public response is panic. Consumers picket and protest. Individuals arrange for elaborate testing. Yet how do we know whether or not alleged health risks are acceptable? Some key factors to consider:

▶ **Possible benefits.** Advantages or payoffs—such as the high salary paid for working with toxic chemicals or radioactive materials—may make some risks seem worthwhile.

▶ **Whether the risk is voluntary.** All of us tend to accept risks that we freely choose to take, such as playing a sport that could lead to injuries, as opposed to risks imposed on us, such as threats of terrorism.

▶ **Is it fair?** The risk of skin cancer, which is increasing because of ozone depletion (see Chapter 19), affects us all. We may worry about it and take action to protect ourselves and our planet, but we don't resent it the way we resent living with the risk of violent crime because the only housing we can afford is in a high-crime area.

▶ **Are there alternatives?** As consumers, we may become upset about cancer-causing pesticides or food additives when we learn about safer chemicals or methods of preservation.

▶ **"Framing."** Our thinking about risks often depends on how they're presented or framed—for instance, if we're told that a new drug may kill 1 out of every 100 people, instead of that it may save the lives of 99 percent of those who use it.

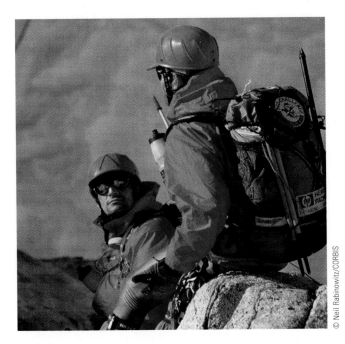

▲ Wearing a helmet is a health choice that diminishes your risk of serious injury.

The Promise of Promotion

If the best defense is a good offense, health promotion represents the ultimate form of prevention and protection. The World Health Organization defines health promotion as the process of enabling people to improve and increase control over their health. Other health specialists define it as "a science and an art devoted to helping people achieve a state of optimal health."

Health promotion programs emphasize health-enhancing behaviors, such as exercising regularly; eating nutritious foods; managing stress well; avoiding tobacco, excess alcohol, and drugs; forming fulfilling relationships with friends; living in a community with clean air; and having purpose in life. They may focus on risk avoidance, such as staying out of the sun at midday, and risk reduction, such as using sunscreen.

One of the best examples of how effective health promotion can be is the dramatic reduction in smoking among young African Americans. In the past, black male teenagers started smoking earlier and in much greater numbers than white adolescents. But the African-American community began to send messages to its youth. Some people whitewashed billboards advertising cigarettes. Black musicians, athletes, and celebrities stopped using cigarettes in a public, glamorized way. Most powerful of all were the messages sent from teen to teen: that smoking was a bad, uncool habit that exploited the African-American community. As discussed in Chapter 16, African-American adolescents now smoke much less than white teens.

Peer counseling—support offered by one student to another—has proven effective in many areas, from awareness of the dangers of casual, unprotected sex to education about what constitutes sexual harassment and coercion. However, often it's not enough to provide information and focus on an individual's responsibility to practice safer sex, eat less fat, exercise regularly, or stop a dangerous behavior. The reality is that all health decisions are made within the complex context of culture and community.

Increasingly, health educators are realizing that overemphasizing individual responsibility sets people up to fail and, with repeated failures, to blame themselves, even in circumstances beyond their control. A college student, for instance, may decide to eat more nutritiously. However, if the only available choices are high-fat foods in vending machines and campus cafeterias, all the good intentions and willpower in the world won't lead to success.

Many health promotion efforts look beyond the campus to make the same opportunities for nutritious food, leisure, exercise, and support open to others. To develop social responsibility in students, they encourage volunteering at community centers, homeless shelters, nursing homes, environmental agencies, and advocacy groups. Their goal is to help students define health, not only in terms of their own behaviors and well-being, but also in terms of what they can

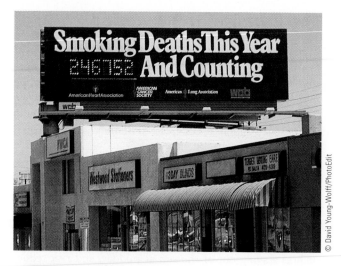

Smoking Deaths This Year And Counting

▲ Education about health choices is a major aspect of health promotion.

do to reach out and help others in the broader community make healthier choices and changes.

The Future of Medicine

Medical science is moving ahead at astounding speed. Every week seems to bring a new discovery or breakthrough. In their quest for new cures for deadly or disabling disease, scientists have ventured into uncharted and highly controversial territory. The ethics of cloning, whether of animals or of human embryos, and the use of embryonic stem cells (which have the potential to grow into any type of cell, such as muscle, bone, or skin) have stirred passionate debate among legislators, scientists, religious leaders, and patient advocacy groups. Gene therapy, which replaces defective genes with normal ones, also has come under attack after the death of a volunteer in an experimental program. The federal government has restricted funding for certain types of research and has set up a panel of doctors, lawyers, and ethicists to advise the president on stem cells, cloning, and other challenging research issues.

Genetic Research

One of the most exciting scientific frontiers has been genetic research. The "Genes in Focus" features in this book provide insight into some recent findings. The completion of the mapping of the human genome sequence in 2001 was a milestone in biological science. Two teams of scientists identified 26,588 human genes for sure, with another 12,731 possible others. The total—probably somewhere

between 30,000 and 40,000 genes—is far less than the estimated 100,000 genes that scientists had predicted.[50]

In addition to tens of thousands of genes, the human genome contains hundreds of thousands of proteins used

GENES IN FOCUS

Would You Want to Know Your Genetic Risks?

In the future, millions of Americans may be able to undergo tests to find out if they have genes that increase their risk of cancer, heart disease, alcoholism, and other common problems. But how many will want to know their possible fate? "That may depend on the type of problem," says geneticist Helga Toriello, M.D., of the American Society of Human Genetics. "Knowledge can be frightening when little, if anything, can be done to alter the course of a disease. But in most cases, forewarned is forearmed."[51]

Yet genetic testing may never be able to tell individuals all they want to know. A test can tell only whether you have a gene or a predisposition for a disorder, not when you might develop the disease, how it might affect you, whether your symptoms will be mild or severe, or what the course of the illness will be. Consumers aren't the only ones eager to find out about inherited risks. Insurance companies and employers also want to know who may be vulnerable. In this way, testing could lead to genetic discrimination.

Testing also may provide false reassurance. "If you discover that you don't have the gene that's been linked to alcoholism, does that give you permission to drink as much as you want?" asks Toriello, pointing out that among 70 people in a recent study, 28 percent of those without the gene became alcohol-dependent and 23 percent of those with the gene did not.

Given the complexities and varied implications of learning about genetic risks, how much would you want to know? The answer is always profoundly personal. Knowledge can give you the power to prevent some problems or to seek early treatment for others. Yet it also can be a burden. As one woman at risk for a potentially fatal genetic disorder puts it, "You have to decide which is worse: the awful uncertainty of not knowing or the possibility of finding out that your worst fears will come true."

to transmit messages by our seemingly versatile genes.[52] "The human genome has been called the Book of Life," observed an editorial in *Science*. "Rather it is a library, in which . . . we can find many of the books that will help define us and our place in the great tapestry of life."[53]

When all human genes are identified, scientists will have the tools to study the details of human development and disease.[54] In addition to the classic genetic disorders, genes contribute to common and deadly disorders, such as heart disease and cancer.

Each individual carries about 20 abnormal genes, including 7 or 8 deadly ones. Most are hidden, but in combination with other genes or in certain environmental conditions, they can become dangerous. (See Genes in Focus: "Would You Want to Know Your Genetic Risks?") According to the American Society of Human Genetics, about 5 percent of adults under age 25 have a genetically linked disease; among adults over 25, 60 percent develop a genetically influenced disorder. In addition to rare genetic syndromes, hereditary diseases include common problems such as certain types of cataracts, glaucoma, gallbladder disease, hypertension, nearsightedness, ulcers, and dyslexia.

Most adult-onset illnesses, such as cancer, heart disease, and alcoholism, are caused by the interaction of multiple genes and environmental factors. Other disorders can be traced to a single gene. If the gene is stronger, or dominant (as is the case for Huntington's chorea, a progressive, incurable brain disorder), each child of a carrier faces a 50 percent risk of inheriting the disease. If the gene is weaker, or recessive (as in cystic fibrosis, a disorder of the mucous and sweat glands), each child faces a 25 percent chance of having the disease and a 50 percent chance of becoming a carrier. If the X gene contributed by the mother—which joins with a Y gene from the father to create a boy or an X gene from the father to create a girl—has the harmful trait (as in hemophilia), each son has a 50 percent risk of inheriting the disorder; each daughter has a 50 percent risk of being a carrier.

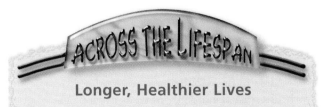

Longer, Healthier Lives

The number of Americans living long enough to blow out 100 birthday candles has increased 35 percent from a decade ago. Among senior citizens, the most rapid growth in the last decade has been in the oldest age groups.[55] (See Figure 1-7.)

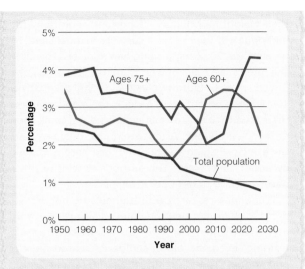

▲ **Figure 1-7** Average annual percent growth of total population and older population in America.

Source: National Institute on Aging.

Americans are not only living longer, but staying healthy and independent longer. More than eight in ten elderly Americans are able to take care of themselves on their own. For the first time, the rate of disability among Americans older than age 85 has dropped below 20 percent. Among the factors contributing to a longer "healthspan" are improved medical care, diet, exercise, and public health advances.[56]

Genes, as studies of identical twins have revealed, influence only about 30 percent of the rate and ways in which we age. "The rest is up to us," says Michael Roizen, M.D., of the University of Chicago, author of *RealAge,* who notes that it's possible to become healthier, fitter, and biologically younger with time. "With relatively simple changes, someone whose chronological age is 69 can have a physiological age of 45. And the most amazing thing is that it's never too late to live younger—until one foot is 6 feet under."[57]

Staying Strong

In 1966 researchers tested the aerobic fitness of five healthy 20-year-old men before and after three weeks of bed rest. This relatively brief period without any activity had the effect of aging the men by three decades—or so the researchers thought.[58] Then the researchers studied the same men again after 30 years had passed.

The men had not kept up their youthful fitness levels. On average, over the course of three decades, their weight had climbed 25 percent; their body fat had doubled; their aerobic capacity had declined 11 percent. Yet 30 years of aging had done less to lower the men's aerobic power than the three weeks they'd spent in bed as 20-year-olds. Starting with a 15-minute workout twice a week, the men increased their activity to approximately one hour a week four or five days a week. After six months, they reversed the effects of aging and boosted their aerobic power by about 15 percent. The author's conclusion: "It's never too late to get back in shape."[59]

Landmark research with frail nursing home residents in their eighties and nineties also proved this point. After just eight to ten weeks of strength training, even the oldest seniors increased muscle and bone, speeded up their metabolic rate, improved sleep and mobility, boosted their spirits, and gained in self-confidence.

We start losing a third to a half pound of muscle in our mid-thirties. Regular resistance training—lifting handheld weights or working on weight machines for at least ten minutes three times a week—can maintain muscle mass, prevent bone loss, and help control weight.

Thinking Young

The healthiest seniors are "engaged" in life, resilient, optimistic, productive, and socially involved, observe John Rowe, M.D., and Robert Kahn, Ph.D., of the MacArthur Foundation Research Network on Successful Aging, authors of *Successful Aging*.[60] While they are not immune to life's slings and arrows, successful agers bounce back after a setback and have a "can-do" attitude about the challenges they face. They also tend to be lifelong learners who may take up entirely new hobbies late in life—pursuits that stimulate production of more connections between neurons and may slow aging within the brain.

Just as with muscles, the best advice for keeping your brain healthy as you age is "use it or lose it." Some memory losses among healthy older people are normal, but these are reversible with training in simple methods, such as word associations, that improve recall. The National Institute on Aging has launched a study of Vitamin E and an experimental medication, Aricept (donepezil), as potential treatments for age-related mild cognitive impairment.

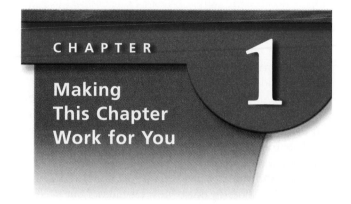

CHAPTER

1

Making This Chapter Work for You

1. The components of health include all of the following except
   a. supportive friends and family.
   b. a well-paying job.
   c. energy and vitality.
   d. a clean environment.

2. Wellness is defined as
   a. purposeful, enjoyable living, characterized by personal responsibility and enhancement of physical, mental, and spiritual health.
   b. a state of complete physical, mental, and social well-being.
   c. attitudes and beliefs that contribute to a healthy state of mind.
   d. the absence of physical or mental illness.

3. Which of the following statements about the dimensions of health are true?
   a. Spirituality provides solace and comfort for those who are severely ill, but it has no health benefits.
   b. The people who reflect the highest levels of social health are usually among the most popular individuals in a group and are often thought of as the "life of the party."
   c. Intellectual health refers to one's academic abilities.
   d. Optimal physical health requires a nutritious diet, regular exercise, avoidance of harmful behaviors and substances, and self-protection from accidents.

4. The goals of the *Healthy People 2010* initiative include all of the following except
   a. reduce the proportion of obese adults and children in the population.
   b. decrease the number of teens using illegal substances.
   c. increase the number of adults engaging in daily vigorous physical activity for 30 minutes per occasion.

d. reduce the percentage of teens and adults who report smoking cigarettes in the past month.

5. Health risks faced by different ethnic and racial groups include all of the following except:
   a. Whites have higher rates of hypertension, lupus, liver disease, and kidney failure than African Americans.
   b. Native Hawaiian women have a higher rate of breast cancer than women from other racial and ethnic groups.
   c. Southeast Asian men have a higher rate of lung and liver cancers than the population as a whole.
   d. Chinese and Latino women are at greater risk of developing diabetes during pregnancy than African-American and white women.

6. Which of the following health hazards faced by college students can be avoided?
   a. binge drinking
   b. unprotected sex
   c. smoking
   d. all of the above

7. The development of health behaviors is influenced by all of the following except
   a. reinforcing factors, which involve external recognition for achieving a goal.
   b. preexisting health factors, which take into account the individual's current position on the wellness continuum.
   c. predisposing factors, which include knowledge, attitudes, and beliefs.
   d. enabling factors, which are related to an individual's skills and capabilities to make behavior changes.

8. If you want to change unhealthy behavior, which of the following strategies is least likely to promote success?

a. Believe that you can make the change.
b. Reward yourself regularly.
c. During self-talks, remind yourself about all your faults.
d. Accept that you are in control of your health.

9. Which of the following statements is incorrect?
   a. The main objective of health promotion programs is to evaluate whether certain health behaviors are risky and then to provide medical attention to those individuals practicing these behaviors.
   b. Protection involves specific actions that an individual can take when participating in risky behavior to prevent health threats.
   c. You can prevent health problems by educating yourself about them and then avoiding the risky behavior that may cause them.
   d. An example of a preventive measure is to avoid driving in icy, snowy conditions, and an example of a protective measure is to put chains on your tires.

10. Behaviors that can help you live a longer and healthier life includes all of the following except
    a. a diet rich in fruits and vegetables.
    b. involvement in your community.
    c. daily flossing.
    d. genetic testing.

Answers to these questions can be found on page 640.

 Why is taking the stairs a healthier alternative over elevators?

Critical Thinking

1. What is the definition of health according to the text? Does your personal definition differ from this, and if so, in what ways? How would you have defined health before reading this chapter?

2. Talk to classmates from different racial or ethnic backgrounds than yours about their culture's health attitudes. Ask them what is considered healthy behavior in their culture? For example, is having a good appetite a sign of health? What kinds of self-care practices did their parents and grandparents use to treat colds, fevers, rashes, and other health problems? What are their attitudes about the health-care system?

3. Where are you on the wellness-illness continuum? What variables might affect your place on the scale? What do you consider your optimum state of health to be?

4. In what ways would you like to change your present lifestyle? What steps could you take to make those changes?

SITES & BYTES

LiveWell Health Risk Appraisal
http://wellness.uwsp.edu/Health_Service/services/livewell
This colorful and comprehensive site was created by the National Wellness Institute and features a series of questions to help you identify what specific lifestyle factors can impair your health and longevity. This self-assessment asks 10 questions in a variety of wellness dimensions, including physical fitness, nutrition, self-care, drugs and driving, emotional health, as well as social, intellectual, occupational, and spiritual wellness.

Health Calculators by Dr. Koop
http://www.drkoop.com/tools/calculator
Take at least 10 of the 21 quick health risk assessments to learn how to best manage your health and decrease risk factors. Some of the areas covered by these personal health calculators include diabetes, pregnancy due date, fitness (BMI, target heart rate, calorie-burned by activity), diet and nutrition (various nutrients), smoking, sleep, stress, HIV risk, and heart disease risk.

The Transtheoretical Model
http://www2.msstate.edu/~bhunt/Stages_of_Change_Theory/transtheoretical.html
This excellent site features self-assessment tools to help you personally determine what stage of change you are in based on the transtheoretical model for the following behaviors: smoking, exercise, eating and diet, alcohol and drug behaviors, and condoms and HIV prevention.

Please note that links are subject to change. If you find a broken link, use a search engine such as **http://www.yahoo.com** *and search for the website by typing in key words.*

InfoTrac Activity   You can find additional readings related to health and wellness with InfoTrac College Edition, an online library of more than 900 journals and publications. Follow the instructions for accessing InfoTrac that were packaged with your textbook; then search for articles using a key word search.

Suggested Article: Cynthia G. Wagner. "Minority Health." *The Futurist*, Vol. 35, No. 3, May 2001, p. 12.

(1) What are five diseases that are more prevalent in minorities?

(2) According to the article, why do minorities have a higher incidence of chronic diseases?

For additional links, resources, and suggested readings on InfoTrac, visit our Health & Wellness Resource Center at **http://health.wadsworth.com**.

Key Terms

The terms listed here are used within the chapter on the page indicated. Definitions of terms are in the Glossary at the end of the book.

health 14	**prevention** 30	**self-talk** 29
health promotion 17	**protection** 30	**wellness** 14
locus of control 29	**reinforcements** 29	
norms 28	**self-efficacy** 28	

References

1. "Constitution of the World Health Organization." *Chronicle of the World Health Organization*. Geneva, Switzerland: WHO, 1947.

2. Gordon, James. Personal interview.

3. Amandarajah, Gowri, and Ellen Hight. "Spirituality and Medical

Practice." *American Family Physician,* Vol. 63, No. 1, January 1, 2001.

4. Ferraro, Kenneth, et al. "Religious Consolation Among Men and Women: Do Health Problems Spur Seeking?" *Journal for the Scientific Study of Religion,* Vol. 39, No. 2, June 2000, p. 220.

5. "Can Your Prayer Heal Others?" *Spirituality & Health,* Fall 2001, p. 15.

6. "Spiritual Matters, Earthly Benefits." *Tufts University Health & Nutrition Letter,* Vol. 19, No. 6, August 2001, p. 1.

7. Schnittker, Jason. "When Is Faith Enough?" *Journal for the Scientific Study of Religion,* Vol. 40, No. 3, September 2001, p. 393.

8. Nagourney, Eric. "A Study Links Prayer and Pregnancy." *New York Times,* October 2, 2001.

9. Garfield, A. M., et al. "Religion/Spirituality, Education and Physical Health in Mid-Life Adults." *Gerontologist,* October 15, 2001, p. 160.

10. Strawbridge, William, et al. "Frequent Religious Attendance May Encourage Better Health Behaviors." *Annals of Behavioral Medicine,* February 2001.

11. "Spiritual Matters, Earthly Benefits."

12. Larrimore, Walter. "Providing Basic Spiritual Care for Patients: Should It Be the Exclusive Domain of Pastoral Professionals?" *American Family Physician,* Vol. 63, No. 1, January 1, 2001.

13. Sloan, Richard, and Emilia Bagiella. "Spirituality and Medical Practice: A Look at the Evidence." *American Family Physician,* Vol. 63, No. 1, January 1, 2001.

14. "Spirituality and Health." *American Family Physician,* Vol. 63, No. 1, January 1, 2001.

15. Larson, David. Personal interview.

16. Matthews, Dale. Personal interview.

17. Ursano, Robert. Personal interview.

18. Roizen, Michael. *RealAge: Are You as Young as You Can Be?* New York: HarperCollins, 2000.

19. "America Then and Now: It's All in the Numbers." *New York Times,* December 31, 2000.

20. Minino, Arialdi, et al. "Deaths: Preliminary Data for 2000." *National Vital Statistics Reports,* Vol. 49, No. 12, October 9, 2001.

21. Olshanky, S. Jay, et al. "Life Expectancy." *Science,* Vol. 291, No. 5508, February 23, 2001.

22. Gorin, Stephen. "Inequality and Health: Implications for Social Work." *Health and Social Work,* Vol. 25, No. 4, November 2000.

23. Minino, et al., "Deaths: Preliminary Data for 2000."

24. Ibid.

25. Starfield, Barbara. "Is U.S. Health Really the Best in the World?" *Journal of the American Medical Association,* Vol. 284, No. 4, July 26, 2000.

26. *Crossing the Quality Chasm: A New Health System for the 21st Century.* Washington, DC: Institute of Medicine, 2001.

27. http://www.cdc.gov/nchs.

28. Healthy People 2010 Fact Sheet: "Healthy People in Healthy Communities." Healthy People 2010 is available on the Internet at www.health.gov.healthypeople.

29. Ibid.

30. Swanbrow, Diane. "Black-White Health Gap Is as Large as It Was in 1950." University of Michigan News Service, February 24, 2000.

31. *Mental Health: Culture, Race, and Ethnicity.* Washington, DC: Office of the Surgeon General, August 2001. www.surgeongeneral.gov/library/mentalhealth/cre/

32. Scanlan, James. "Race and Mortality." *Society,* Vol. 37, No. 2, January 2000.

33. Guyer, Bernard, et al. "Annual Summary of Vital Statistics: Trends in the Health of Americans During the 20th Century." *Pediatrics,* Vol. 106, No. 6, December 2000.

34. Department of Health and Human Services.

35. *Mental Health: Culture, Race, and Ethnicity.*

36. Vitucci, Jeff. "The State of Hispanic Health." *Hispanic Business,*

Vol. 21, No. 6, June 1999.

37. Davies, Jon, et al. "Identifying Male College Students' Perceived Health Needs, Barriers to Seeking Help, and Recommendations to Help Men Adopt Healthier Lifestyles." *Journal of American College Health,* Vol. 48, No. 5, May 2000.

38. Keeling, Richard. "Resiliency and Prevention in College Health." *Journal of American College Health,* Vol. 49, No. 1, July 2000.

39. Keeling, Richard. "Is College Dangerous?" *Journal of American College Health,* Vol. 50, No. 2, September 2001, p. 53.

40. Adlaf, Edward, et al. "The Prevalence of Elevated Psychological Distress Among Canadian Undergraduates: Findings from the 1998 Canadian Campus Survey." *Journal of American College Health,* Vol. 50, No. 2, September 2001, p. 67.

41. Edwards, Kevi, et al. "Stress, Negative Social Exchange, and Health Symptoms in University Students." *Journal of American College Health,* Vol. 50, No. 2, September 2001, p. 75.

42. Bowen, Anne, and Martin Bourgeois. "Attitudes Toward Lesbian, Gay, and Bisexual College Students." *Journal of American College Health,* Vol. 50, No. 2, September 2001, p. 91.

43. Bormann, Carol, and Michael Stone. "The Effects of Eliminating Alcohol in a College Stadium: The Folsom Field Beer Ban." *Journal of American College Health,* Vol. 50, No. 2, September 2001, p. 81.

44. Brener, Nancy, and Vani Gowda. "U.S. College Students' Reports of Receiving Health Information on College Campuses." *Journal of American College Health,* Vol. 49, No. 5, March 2001, p. 223.

45. Trockel, Mickey, et al. "Health-Related Variables and Academic Performance Among First-Year College Students: Implications for Sleep and Other Behaviors." *Journal of American College Health,* Vol. 49, No. 3, November 2000.

46. Gruman, Jessie. "Integration of Health Behavior Counseling in Routine Medical Care." Washington, DC: Center for the Advancement of Health, 2001. This report is also available at www.cfah.org.

47. "Social and Emotional Competence: Healthy Behaviors for Youth." *Facts of Life: Issue Briefing for Health Reporters,* May 2001, Vol. 6, No. 4, p. 1.

48. Zuckerman, Marvin. "Are You a Risk Taker?" *Psychology Today,* November/December 2000.

49. Courtenay, Will. "Behavioral Factors Associated with Disease, Injury and Death Among Men: Evidence and Implications for Prevention." *Journal of Men's Studies,* Vol. 9, No. 1, Fall 2000.

50. Venter, J. Craig, et al. "The Sequence of the Human Genome." *Science,* Vol. 291, No. 5507, February 15, 2001.

51. Toriello, Helga. Personal interview.

52. Knowles, James. "Genetics," *Textbook of Psychiatry.* Washington, DC: American Psychiatric Association, 2002.

53. Jasny, Barbara, and Donald Kennedy. "The Human Genome." *Science,* Vol. 291, No. 5507, February 16, 2001.

54. Peltonen, Leena, and Victor A. McKusick. "Genomics and Medicine: Dissecting Human Disease in the Postgenomic Era." *Science,* Vol. 291, No. 5507, February 16, 2001.

55. U.S. Census Bureau.

56. Manton, Kenneth, and XiLing Gu. "Changes in the Prevalence of Chronic Disability in the United States Black and Nonblack Population Above Age 85 from 1982 to 1999." *Proceedings of the National Academy of Sciences of the United States,* Vol. 98, No. 11, May 22, 2001, p. 6354.

57. Roizen, *Real Age.*

58. McGuire, Darren, et al. "A 30-Year Follow-Up of the Dallas Bed Rest and Training Study II. Effect of Age on Cardiovascular Adaptation to Exercise Training." *Circulation,* Vol. 104, September 17, 2001, p. 1356.

59. Ibid., p. 1337.

60. Rowe, John. Personal interview.

2

Personal Stress Management

Two months into her freshman year, Maria feels as if a tornado has torn through her life. She is living thousands of miles from her family and the friends who share her culture and ethnic background. Her dormmates range from different to downright difficult. Her professors expect her to read and learn more in a week than in an entire month of high school. After blowing her budget decorating her room, she took on a part-time job—only to end up so exhausted that she dozes off in lectures. Stress? Maria considers it a way of life.

Like Maria, you live with stress every day, whether you're studying for exams, meeting people, facing new experiences, or figuring out how to live on a budget. You're not alone. Everyone, regardless of age, gender, race, or income, has to deal with stress—as an individual and as a member of society.

As researchers have demonstrated time and again, stress has profound effects, both immediate and long-term, on our bodies and minds. While stress alone doesn't cause disease, it triggers molecular changes throughout the body that make us more susceptible to many illnesses. Its impact on the mind is no less significant. The burden of chronic stress can undermine ability to cope with day-to-day hassles and can exacerbate psychological problems like depression and anxiety disorders.

Yet stress in itself isn't necessarily bad. What matters most is not the stressful situation itself, but an individual's response to it. By learning to anticipate stressful events, to manage day-to-day hassles, and to prevent stress overload, you can find alternatives to running endlessly on a treadmill of alarm, panic, and exhaustion. As you organize your schedule, find ways to release tension, and build up coping skills, you will begin to experience the sense of control and confidence that makes stress a challenge rather than an ordeal.

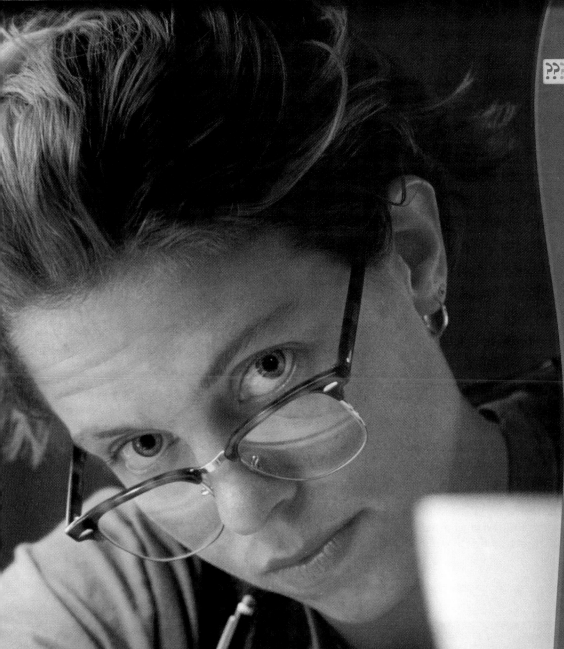

After studying the material in this chapter, you should be able to:

- **Define** stress and stressors and **describe** how the body responds to stress according to the general adaptation syndrome theory.
- **List** the physical changes associated with frequent or severe stress and **discuss** how stress can affect the cardiovascular, immune, and digestive systems.
- **Describe** some personal causes of stress, especially those experienced by students, and **discuss** how their effects can be prevented or minimized.
- **Discuss** the major social issues that can cause stress.
- **Identify** ways of managing time more efficiently.
- **Describe** some techniques to help manage both short-term and long-term stress.
- **Explain** how stressful events can affect psychological health and **describe** the factors contributing to posttraumatic growth.

What Is Stress?

People use the word *stress* in different ways: as an external force that causes a person to become tense or upset, as the internal state of arousal, and as the physical response of the body to various demands. Dr. Hans Selye, a pioneer in studying physiological responses to challenge, defined **stress** as "the nonspecific response of the body to any demand made upon it." In other words, the body reacts to **stressors**—the things that upset or excite us—in the same way, regardless of whether they are positive or negative.

Stress can be acute, episodic, or chronic, depending on the nature of the stressors or external events that cause the stress response. Acute or short-term stressors, which can range from a pop quiz to a bomb threat in a crowded stadium, trigger a brief but intense response to a specific incident. Episodic stressors like monthly bills or quarterly exams cause regular but intermittent elevations in stress levels. Chronic stressors include everything from rush-hour traffic to a learning disability to living with an alcoholic parent or spouse.

Not all stressors are negative. Some of life's happiest moments—births, reunions, weddings—are enormously stressful. We weep with the stress of frustration or loss; we weep, too, with the stress of love and joy. Selye coined the term **eustress** for positive stress in our lives (*eu* is a Greek prefix meaning "good"). Eustress challenges us to grow, adapt, and find creative solutions in our lives. **Distress** refers to the negative effects of stress that can deplete or even destroy life energy. Ideally, the level of stress in our lives should be just high enough to motivate us to satisfy our needs and not so high that it interferes with our ability to reach our fullest potential.

What Causes Stress?

Of the many biological theories of stress, the best known may be the **general adaptation syndrome (GAS),** developed by Hans Selye. He postulated that our bodies constantly strive to maintain a stable and consistent physiological state, called **homeostasis.** Stressors, whether in the form of physical illness or a demanding job, disturb this state and trigger a nonspecific physiological response. The body attempts to restore homeostasis by means of an **adaptive response. Allostasis** describes the body's ability to adapt to constantly changing environments.

Selye's general adaptation syndrome, which describes the body's response to a stressor—whether threatening or exhilarating—consists of three distinct stages:

1. *Alarm.* When a stressor first occurs, the body responds with changes that temporarily lower resistance. Levels of certain hormones may rise; blood pressure may increase (see Figure 2-1). The body quickly makes internal adjustments to cope with the stressor and return to normal activity.
2. *Resistance.* If the stressor continues, the body mobilizes its internal resources to try to sustain homeostasis. For example, if a loved one is seriously hurt in an accident, we initially respond intensely and feel great anxiety. During the subsequent stressful period of recuperation, we struggle to carry on as normally as possible, but this requires considerable effort.
3. *Exhaustion.* If the stress continues long enough, we cannot keep up our normal functioning. Even a small amount of additional stress at this point can cause a breakdown.

© CORBIS

▲ An automobile accident is an example of an acute stressor. Getting married is an example of a positive stressor.

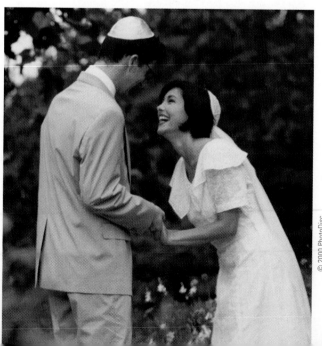

© 2000 PhotoDisc

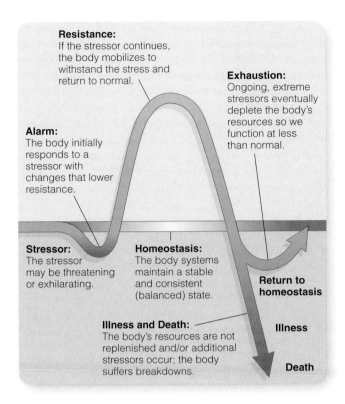

Resistance:
If the stressor continues, the body mobilizes to withstand the stress and return to normal.

Exhaustion:
Ongoing, extreme stressors eventually deplete the body's resources so we function at less than normal.

Alarm:
The body initially responds to a stressor with changes that lower resistance.

Stressor:
The stressor may be threatening or exhilarating.

Homeostasis:
The body systems maintain a stable and consistent (balanced) state.

Return to homeostasis

Illness and Death:
The body's resources are not replenished and/or additional stressors occur; the body suffers breakdowns.

Illness

Death

▲ **Figure 2-1** The three stages of Selye's General Adaptation Syndrome (GAS): alarm, resistance, exhaustion.

Among the nonbiological theories is the cognitive-transactional model of stress, developed by Richard Lazarus, which looks at the relation between stress and health. As he sees it, stress can have a powerful impact on health. Conversely, health can affect a person's resistance or coping ability. Stress, according to Lazarus, is "neither an environmental stimulus, a characteristic of the person, nor a response, but a relationship between demands and the power to deal with them without unreasonable or destructive costs."[1] Thus, an event may be stressful for one person but not for another, or it may seem stressful on one occasion but not on another. For instance, one student may think of speaking in front of the class as extremely stressful, while another relishes the chance to do so—except on days when he's not well-prepared.

At any age, some of us are more vulnerable to life changes and crises than are others. The stress of growing up in families troubled by alcoholism, drug dependence, or physical, sexual, or psychological abuse may have a lifelong impact—particularly if these problems are not recognized and dealt with. Other early experiences, positive and negative, also can affect our attitude toward stress—and our resilience to it. Our general outlook on life, whether we're optimistic or pessimistic, can determine whether we expect the worst and feel stressed or anticipate a challenge and

feel confident. The when, where, what, how, and why of stressors also affect our reactions. The number and frequency of changes in our lives, along with the time and setting in which they occur, have a great impact on how we'll respond.

Our level of ongoing stress affects our ability to respond to a new day's stressors. Each of us has a breaking point for dealing with stress. A series of too-intense pressures or too-rapid changes can push us closer and closer to that point. That's why it's important to anticipate potential stressors and plan how to deal with them.

Stress experts Thomas Holmes, M.D., and Richard Rahe, M.D., devised a scale to evaluate individual levels of stress and potential for coping, based on *life-change units* that estimate each change's impact. The death of a partner or parent ranks high on the list, but even changing apartments is considered a stressor. People who accumulate more than 300 life-change units in a year are more likely to suffer serious health problems. Scores on the scale, however, represent "potential stress"; the actual impact of the life change depends on the individual's response. (See Self-Survey: "Student Stress Scale," on page 47.)

Holmes has evaluated variations in life events among many groups, including college students, medical students, football players, pregnant women, alcoholics, and heroin addicts. Heroin addicts and alcoholics have the highest totals of life-change units, followed by college students. In general, younger people experience more life changes than do older people; factors such as gender, education, and social class also have a strong impact.[2] Marriage seems to promote greater stability and fewer changes.

If you score high on the Student Stress Scale, think about the reasons your life has been in such turmoil. Are there any steps you could take to make your life more stable? Of course, some changes, such as your parents' divorce or a friend's accident, are beyond your control. Even then, you can respond in ways that may protect you from disease.

Is Stress Hazardous to Physical Health?

These days we've grown accustomed to warning labels advising us of the health risks of substances like alcohol and cigarettes. Medical researchers speculate that another component of twenty-first-century living also warrants a warning: stress.[3] In recent years, an every-growing number of studies has implicated stress as a culprit in a range of medical problems. While stress itself may not kill, it clearly undermines our ability to stay well.[4]

Stress triggers complex changes in the body's endocrine, or hormone-secreting, system. The scientific field of **psychoneuroimmunology** has been exploring these intricate interconnections. When you confront a stressor, the adrenal glands, two triangle-shaped glands that sit atop the kidneys, respond by producing stress hormones, including catecholamines, cortisol (hydrocortisone), and epinephrine (adrenaline), that speed up heart rate and blood pressure and prepare the body to deal with the threat. This "fight-or-flight" response prepares you for quick action: Your heart works harder to pump more blood to your legs and arms. Your muscles tense, your breathing quickens, and your brain becomes extra alert. And because they're nonessential in a crisis, your digestive and immune systems practically shut down.

Unlike many other molecules in the body (such as the neurotransmitters that transmit messages in the brain), most stress hormones are water-insoluble, which means that they remain in the bloodstream longer. The effects of neurotransmitters disappear within seconds or milliseconds; stress hormones persist in the blood for hours. Cortisol remains elevated for the longest period and has the most important long-term effects on our health.

One effect of cortisol and the other stress hormones, for example, is to speed the conversion of proteins and fats into carbohydrates, the body's basic fuel, so we have the energy to fight or flee from a threat. Another effect is to increase appetite and food-seeking behavior. Cortisol can cause excessive central or abdominal fat, which heightens the risk of diseases such as diabetes, high blood pressure, and stroke.[5] Even slender, premenopausal women faced with increased stress and lacking good coping skills are more likely to accumulate excess weight around their waists, thereby increasing their risk of heart disease and other health problems.[6]

In the brain, stress hormones linked to powerful emotions may help create long-lasting memories of events such as the Colombine shootings. But very prolonged or severe stress can damage the brain's ability to remember and can actually cause brain cells, or neurons, to atrophy and die.

As Figure 2-2 illustrates, persistent or repeated increases in the stress hormones can be hazardous throughout the body. Catecholamines cause a rise in blood

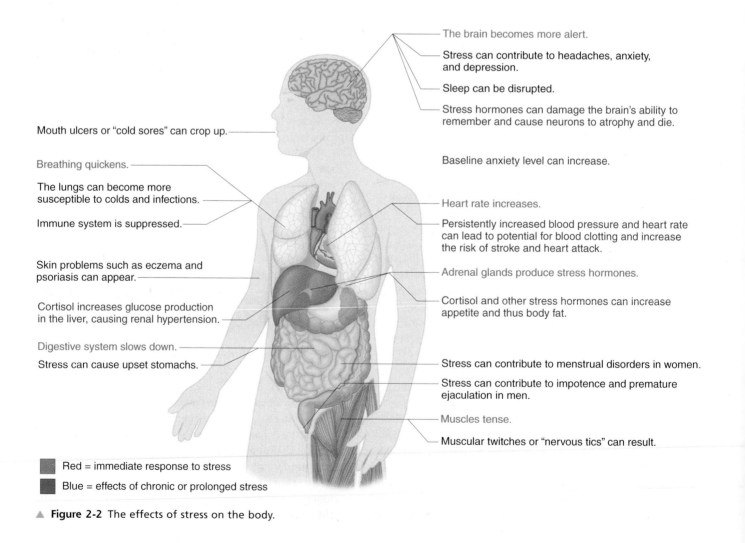

The brain becomes more alert.

Stress can contribute to headaches, anxiety, and depression.

Sleep can be disrupted.

Stress hormones can damage the brain's ability to remember and cause neurons to atrophy and die.

Baseline anxiety level can increase.

Heart rate increases.

Persistently increased blood pressure and heart rate can lead to potential for blood clotting and increase the risk of stroke and heart attack.

Adrenal glands produce stress hormones.

Cortisol and other stress hormones can increase appetite and thus body fat.

Stress can contribute to menstrual disorders in women.

Stress can contribute to impotence and premature ejaculation in men.

Muscles tense.

Muscular twitches or "nervous tics" can result.

Mouth ulcers or "cold sores" can crop up.

Breathing quickens.

The lungs can become more susceptible to colds and infections.

Immune system is suppressed.

Skin problems such as eczema and psoriasis can appear.

Cortisol increases glucose production in the liver, causing renal hypertension.

Digestive system slows down.

Stress can cause upset stomachs.

Red = immediate response to stress

Blue = effects of chronic or prolonged stress

▲ **Figure 2-2** The effects of stress on the body.

pressure and heart rate, make breathing short and shallow, and increase the potential for blood clotting, upping the risk for stroke and heart attack. Cortisol increases glucose production in the liver, causes renal hypertension (which also raises blood pressure), and suppresses the immune system. Chronically elevated stress hormones raise the baseline anxiety level, making it harder to cope with daily annoyances.

Hundreds of studies over the last 20 years have shown that stress contributes to approximately 80 percent of all major illnesses: cardiovascular disease, cancer, endocrine and metabolic disease, skin rashes, ulcers, ulcerative colitis, emotional disorders, musculoskeletal disease, infectious ailments, premenstrual syndrome (PMS), uterine fibroid cysts, and breast cysts. As many as 75 to 90 percent of visits to physicians are related to stress.

The first signs of stress include muscle tightness, tension headaches, backaches, upset stomach, and sleep disruptions (caused by stress-altered brain-wave activity). Some people feel fatigued, their hearts may race or beat faster than usual at rest, and they may feel tense all the time, easily frustrated and often irritable. Others feel sad; lose their energy, appetite, or sex drive; and develop psychological problems, including depression, anxiety, and panic attacks (discussed in Chapter 3). Stress can lead to self-destructive behaviors, such as drinking, drug use, and reckless driving. Some people see such acts as offering an escape from the pressure they feel. Unfortunately, they end up adding to their stress load.

Stress and the Heart

In the 1970s, cardiologists Meyer Friedman, M.D., and Ray Rosenman, M.D., suggested that excess stress could be the most important factor in the development of heart disease. They compared their patients to individuals of the same age with healthy hearts and developed two general categories: Type A and Type B.

Hardworking, aggressive, and competitive, Type A's never have time for all they want to accomplish, even though they usually try to do several tasks at once. Type B's are more relaxed, though not necessarily less ambitious or successful. Type-A behavior has been found to be the major contributing factor in the early development of heart disease.

The degree of danger associated with Type-A behavior remains controversial. According to a 22-year follow-up study of 3,000 middle-aged men by researchers at the University of California, Berkeley, both smoking and high blood pressure proved to be much greater threats than Type-A behavior with respect to heart attack risk. Of all the personality traits linked with Type-A behavior, the one that has emerged as most sinister is chronic hostility or cynicism. People who are always mistrustful, angry, and

suspicious are twice as likely to suffer blockages of their coronary arteries.

Depression, a mental disorder often linked with stress, clearly affects the prognosis of individuals who suffer heart attacks. (See Chapter 12.) The National Heart, Lung, and Blood Institute currently is studying 2,000 cardiac patients to determine if treating their depression may improve the quality of their lives and their survival odds.

Stress and the Immune System

The powerful chemicals triggered by stress dampen or suppress the immune system—the network of organs, tissues, and white blood cells that defend against disease. Impaired immunity makes the body more susceptible to many diseases, including infections (from the common cold to tuberculosis) and disorders of the immune system itself.

As psychoneuroimmunology research has shown, traumatic stress, such as losing a loved one through death or divorce, can impair immunity for as long as a year. Even minor hassles take a toll. Under exam stress, students experience a dip in immune function and a higher rate of infections. Ohio State University researchers found a significant drop in the immune cells that normally ward off infection and cancer in medical students during exam periods.[7]

Scientists have identified what may be an important biological link between stress and the common cold: interleukin-6 (IL-6), a chemical pathway used by the immune system. In a 1999 study, researchers at the Children's Hospital of Pittsburgh measured the levels of 55 volunteers before infecting them with an influenza virus. While all developed flu symptoms, the concentration of IL-6, as measured from nasal secretions, was higher in those reporting greater psychological stress before being infected.[8]

The immune response induced by vaccination against pneumococcal pneumonia is lower in people under stress, such as caregivers to relatives with dementia.[9] Studies of university students and staff in the United States and in Spain have implicated stress and a generally negative outlook as increasing susceptibility to the common cold, even in individuals taking vitamin C and zinc to ward off infection.[10]

Stress also interferes with the body's ability to heal itself. By inflicting small cuts in volunteers who are then subjected to controlled stressful situations, researchers have shown a significant delay in healing among those under stress.[11]

Stress hormones also may play a role in the progression of breast cancer. In research on women with metastatic breast cancer, psychiatrist David Spiegel of Stanford University, correlated variations in cortisol secretion with survival rates. The average survival time of women with normal cortisol patterns (high levels in the early morning and progressively lower concentrations during the day) was significantly longer than that of the women whose cortisol remained high all day (a stress indicator).[12]

Aging seems to compound the negative impact of stress on health. Older adults show even greater immunological impairments associated with stress or depression than younger adults and face a greater risk of illness and death.[13]

Certain uplifts, including humor and altruism, may buffer the harmful effects of stress. In studies of college students, watching videotapes of comedians bolstered immune function. Students who provided services to others show a temporary boost in immunity.

Writing about stressful events also can improve the health of people suffering from immune disorders such as chronic asthma or rheumatoid arthritis. In one study, volunteers who wrote about "the most stressful event they had ever undergone" for 20 minutes on three consecutive days showed significant improvements compared with those who spent the same amount of time writing about neutral topics. It is not known why writing about traumatic experiences can relieve immune system disorders, but the researchers theorize that it may help patients make sense of what had happened to them and come to terms with its impact.[14]

Stress and the Digestive System

Do you ever get butterflies in your stomach before giving a speech in class or before a big game? The digestive system is, as one psychologist quips, "an important stop on the tension trail." To avoid problems, pay attention to how you eat: Eating on the run, gulping food, or overeating results in poorly chewed foods, an overworked stomach, and increased abdominal pressure. The combination of poor eating habits and stress can add up to real pain in the stomach.

As noted in Chapter 13, scientists, after identifying the bacterium *H. pylori* as a cause of most peptic ulcers, had downplayed the role of stress. However, more recent studies suggest that stress may indeed be a factor. About 80 percent of people carrying the *H. pylori* bacteria do not get ulcers; about 30 percent of patients who do have ulcers test negative for the bacteria. Researchers now contend that stress does contribute to the development of ulcers, hamper their healing, and increase the likelihood of their recurrence.[15]

Good nutrition can help soothe a stressed-out stomach. Complex carbohydrates are an ideal antistress food because they boost the brain's level of the mood-enhancing chemical serotonin. Good sources include broccoli, leafy greens, potatoes, corn, cabbage, spinach, whole-grain breads and pastas, muffins, crackers, and cereals. Leafy vegetables, whole grains, nuts, and seeds also are rich in other important nutrients, including magnesium and vitamin C.

Some simple strategies can help you avoid stress-related stomachaches. Many people experience dry mouth or sweat more under stress. By drinking plenty of water, you replenish lost fluids and prevent dehydration. Fiber-rich foods counteract common stress-related problems, such as cramps and constipation. Do not skip meals. If you do, you're more likely to feel fatigued and irritable.

Be wary of overeating under stress. Some people eat more because they scarf down meals too quickly. Others reach for snacks to calm their nerves or comfort themselves. Watch out for caffeine. Coffee, tea, and cola drinks can make your strained nerves jangle even more. Also avoid sugary snacks. They'll send your blood sugar levels on a roller coaster ride—up one minute, down the next.

Other Stress Symptoms

Stress can affect any organ system in the body, causing painful symptoms or a flare-up of chronic conditions such as asthma. By interfering with our alertness and ability to concentrate, stress also increases the risk of accidents at home, at work, and on the road.

Headaches are one of the most common stress-related conditions. The most common type, tension headache, is caused by involuntary contractions of the scalp, head, and neck muscles. **Migraine headache** is the result of constriction (narrowing), then dilation (widening) of blood vessels within the brain; chemicals leak through the vessel walls, inflame nearby tissues, and send pain signals to the brain. Surveys of college women show that Type-A behavior can trigger both types of headache.

Stress also is closely linked to skin conditions. If you break out the week before an exam, you know firsthand that skin can be extremely sensitive to stress. Skin conditions worsened by stress include acne, psoriasis, herpes, hives, and eczema. With acne, increased touching of the face, perhaps while cramming for a test, may be partly responsible. Other factors, such as temperature, humidity, and cosmetics and toiletries, may also play a role.

Stress and the Student

You've probably heard that these are the best years of your life, but being a student—full-time or part-time, in your late teens, early twenties, or later in life—can be extremely stressful. You may feel pressure to perform well to qualify for a good job or graduate school. To meet steep tuition payments, you may have to juggle part-time work and coursework. You may feel stressed about choosing a major, getting along with a difficult roommate, passing a particularly hard course, or living up to your parents' and teachers' expectations. If you're an older student, you may have children, housework, and homework to balance. Your days may seem so busy and your life so full that you worry about coming apart at the seams. One thing is for certain: You're not alone. (See Student Snapshot: "Freshman Stress.")

Stress levels among college students have been rising steadily, especially among women. (See the X & Y Files: "Men, Women, and Stress.") According to surveys of students at colleges and universities around the country and the world, stress levels are consistently high and stressors are remarkably similar.[16] Among the most common are:

- Test pressures.
- Financial problems.
- Frustrations, such as delays in reaching goals.
- Problems in friendships and dating relationships.
- Daily hassles.
- Academic failure.

- Pressures as a result of competition, deadlines, and the like.
- Changes, which may be unpleasant, disruptive, or too frequent.
- Losses, whether caused by the breakup of a relationship or the death of a loved one.

Many students bring complex psychological problems with them to campus, including learning disabilities and mood disorders like depression and anxiety. "Students arrive with the underpinnings of problems that are brought out by the stress of campus life," says one counselor. Some have grown up in broken homes and bear the scars of family troubles. Others fall into the same patterns of alcohol abuse that they observed for years in their families or suffer lingering emotional scars from childhood physical or sexual abuse.

The X & Y Files — Men, Women, and Stress

Women, who make up 56 percent of today's college students, also shoulder the majority of the stress load. In a nationwide survey of students in the class of 2004, freshmen women were twice as likely to be anxious as men. More women (36.4 percent) described themselves as "overwhelmed by all I have to do," compared with just 17.9 percent of men. More women than men reported feeling depressed, insecure about their physical and mental health, and worried about paying for college. More men—60.2 percent, compared with 48.6 percent of women—considered themselves above average or in the top 10 percent of people their age in terms of emotional health.

Gender differences in lifestyle may help explain why women feel so stressed. College men, the survey revealed, spend significantly more time doing things that are fun and relaxing: exercising, partying, watching TV, and playing video games. Women, on the other hand, tend to study more, do more volunteer work, and handle more household and child-care chores.

The stress gender gap, which appeared in the mid-1980s, is "one of the ironies of the women's movement," says Alexander Astin of UCLA, founder of the annual American Freshman Survey, which has tracked shifting student attitudes for 35 years. "It's an inevitable consequence of women adding more commitments and responsibilities on top of all the other things they have to cope with." He believes that college women are experiencing an early version of the stress that "supermoms" feel later in life when they pursue a career, care for children, and maintain a household.

Where can stressed-out college women turn for support? The best source, according to University of California research, is other women. In general, the social support women offer their friends and relatives seems more effective in reducing the blood pressure response to stress than that provided by men.

At all ages, women and men tend to respond to stress differently. While males (human and those of other species) react with the classic "fight-or-flight" response, females under attack try to protect their children and seek help from other females—a strategy dubbed "tend-and-befriend." When exposed to experimental stress (such as a loud, harsh noise), women show more affection for friends and relatives; men show less. When working mothers studied by psychologists had a bad day, they coped by concentrating on their children when they got home. Stressed-out fathers were more likely to withdraw.

The gender difference in stress responses may be the result of hormones and evolution. While both men and women release stress hormones, men also secrete testosterone, which tends to increase hostility and aggression. For prehistoric women, who were usually pregnant, nursing, or caring for small children, neither fight nor flight was a wise strategy. Smaller and weaker than males, women may long ago have reached out to other women to form a social support system that helped ensure their safety and that of their children.

Sources: Sax, Linda, et al. *The American Freshman: National Norms for Fall 2000.* Los Angeles: Higher Education Research Institute, UCLA, 2000. Glynn, Laura, et al. "Women's Social Support More Beneficial than Men's." *Psychosomatic Medicine,* Vol. 61, April 1999. "How Women Handle Stress: Is There a Difference?" *Harvard Mental Health Letter,* Vol. 17, No. 10, April 2001.

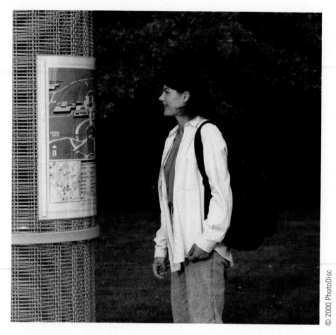

© 2000 PhotoDisc

▲ The first year of college can be overwhelming as you learn your way around the campus, become acquainted with new people, and strive to succeed.

For many students, the first year at college is the most stressful. Many have to deal with issues like sexism, racism, and financial difficulties for the first time in their lives. They may experience social discrimination in cafeterias and dorms. Older students may feel out of place taking the same classes as 18-year-olds and worry about going into debt to pay for tuition after years of earning their own money. Students of all ages feel intense pressure to succeed and may worry about not being able to manage their time, get good grades, or decide on a major and a career.

While the self-esteem of college freshmen typically falls, students recover their self-confidence in their second year. They become more positive, introspective, and independent and have a stronger sense of their own intellectual ability. It may well be that as students acclimate to college, they experience less stress and therefore view themselves more positively.

Students say they react to stress in various ways: physiologically (by sweating, stuttering, trembling, or developing physical symptoms); emotionally (by becoming anxious, fearful, angry, guilty, or depressed); behaviorally (by crying, eating, smoking, being irritable or abusive); or

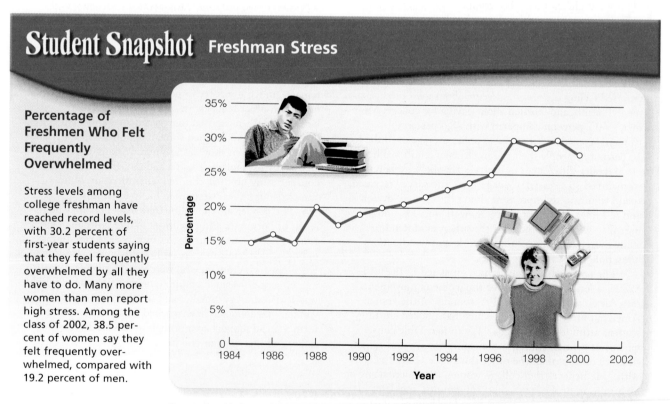

Student Snapshot Freshman Stress

Percentage of Freshmen Who Felt Frequently Overwhelmed

Stress levels among college freshman have reached record levels, with 30.2 percent of first-year students saying that they feel frequently overwhelmed by all they have to do. Many more women than men report high stress. Among the class of 2002, 38.5 percent of women say they felt frequently overwhelmed, compared with 19.2 percent of men.

Source: Sax, Linda, et al. *The American Freshman: National Norms for Fall 2000.* Los Angeles: Higher Education Research Institute, UCLA, 2000.

SELF SURVEY

Student Stress Scale

The Student Stress Scale, an adaptation of Holmes and Rahe's Life Events Scale for college-age adults, provides a rough indication of stress levels and possible health consequences.

In the Student Stress Scale, each event, such as beginning or ending school, is given a score that represents the

1.	Death of a close family member	100
2.	Death of a close friend	73
3.	Divorce of parents	65
4.	Jail term	63
5.	Major personal injury or illness	63
6.	Marriage	58
7.	Getting fired from a job	50
8.	Failing an important course	47
9.	Change in the health of a family member	45
10.	Pregnancy	45
11.	Sex problems	44
12.	Serious argument with a close friend	40
13.	Change in financial status	39
14.	Change of academic major	39
15.	Trouble with parents	39
16.	New girlfriend or boyfriend	37
17.	Increase in workload at school	37
18.	Outstanding personal achievement	36
19.	First quarter/semester in college	36
20.	Change in living conditions	31
21.	Serious argument with an instructor	30
22.	Getting lower grades than expected	29
23.	Change in sleeping habits	29
24.	Change in social activities	29
25.	Change in eating habits	28
26.	Chronic car trouble	26
27.	Change in number of family get-togethers	26
28.	Too many missed classes	25
29.	Changing colleges	24
30.	Dropping more than one class	23
31.	Minor traffic violations	20

Total Stress Score _____

amount of readjustment a person has to make as a result of the change. In some studies, using similar scales, people with serious illnesses have been found to have high scores.

To determine your stress score, add up the number of points corresponding to the events you have experienced in the past 12 months.

Here's how to interpret your score: If your score is 300 or higher, you're at high risk for developing a health problem. If your score is between 150 and 300, you have a 50–50 chance of experiencing a serious health change within two years. If your score is below 150, you have a 1-in-3 chance of a serious health change.

Making Changes

Coping with Life Changes

If you're going through a lot of change, you can take steps to minimize harmful effects. Here are some suggestions:

▶ Review the Student Stress Scale often so you're familiar with different life events and the amount of stress they can cause.

▶ When change occurs, think about its meaning and your feelings about it.

▶ Try to come up with different ways of adjusting to the change.

▶ Don't rush into action; take time to make a careful decision.

▶ Pace yourself. Even if you have a lot to do, stick to a reasonable schedule that allows you some time off to relax.

▶ Look at each change as a part of life's natural flow, rather than as a disruption in the way things should be.

Source: Mullen, Kathleen, and Gerald Costello. *Health Awareness Through Discovery.*

cognitively (by thinking about and analyzing stressful situations and strategies that might be useful in dealing with them).

 Social support makes a difference. Students with a truly supportive network of friends and family available to them report greater satisfaction and less psychological distress. Effective time management, discussed later in this chapter, helps buffer academic stress.[17] Higher levels of positive

experiences, such as forming close friendships, also reduce stress and compensate for the depressive effects of negative experiences, such as failing a test.[18]

Campuses are providing more "frontline services" than they have in the past, including career-guidance workshops, telephone hot lines, and special social programs for lonely, homesick freshmen. At a growing number of schools, peer mentors provide companionship and psychological support. These programs may be particularly beneficial for minorities and women, who most often feel excluded in the academic world.[19]

Test Stress

For many students, midterms and final exams are the most stressful times of the year. Studies at various colleges and universities found that the incidence of colds and flu soared during finals. Some students feel the impact of test stress in other ways—headaches, upset stomachs, skin flare-ups, or insomnia.

Test stress affects people in different ways. Sometimes students become so preoccupied with the possibility of failing that they can't concentrate on studying. Others, including many of the best and brightest students, freeze up during tests and can't comprehend multiple-choice questions or write essay answers, even if they know the material.

The students most susceptible to exam stress are those who believe they'll do poorly and who see tests as extremely threatening. Unfortunately, such negative thoughts often become a self-fulfilling prophecy. As they study, these students keep wondering, "What good will studying do? I never do well on tests." As their fear increases, they try harder, pulling all-nighters. Fueled by caffeine, munching on sugary snacks, they become edgy and find it harder and harder to concentrate. By the time

of the test, they're nervous wrecks, scarcely able to sit still and focus on the exam.

Can you do anything to reduce test stress and feel more in control? Absolutely. One way is to defuse stress through relaxation. In a study by researchers Janice Kiecolt-Glaser and Ron Glaser of Ohio State University, one group of students was taught relaxation techniques—such as controlled breathing, meditation, progressive relaxation, and guided imagery (visualization)—a month before finals. The more the students used these "stress busters," the higher were their levels of immune cells during the exam period. The extra payoff was that they felt calmer and in better control during their tests.[20] (See Pulse Points: "Top Ten Stress Busters.")

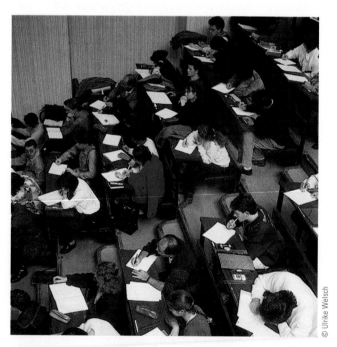

▲ Test stress can affect your immune system, cause digestive problems, and even cause you to freeze during the exam. But you can take control of your stress responses by practicing relaxation techniques, avoiding cramming, and being positive about your performance on the test.

STRATEGIES FOR PREVENTION

Defusing Test Stress

✔ *Plan ahead.* A month before finals, map out a study schedule for each course. Set aside a small amount of time every day or every other day to review the course materials.

✔ *Be positive.* Picture yourself taking your final exam. Imagine yourself walking into the exam room feeling confident, opening up the test booklet, and seeing questions for which you know the answers.

✔ *Take regular breaks.* Get up from your desk, breathe deeply, stretch, and visualize a pleasant scene. You'll feel more refreshed than you would if you chugged another cup of coffee.

✔ *Practice.* Some teachers are willing to give practice finals to prepare students for test situations, or you and your friends can test each other.

✔ *Talk to other students.* Chances are that many of them share your fears about test taking and may have discovered some helpful techniques of their own. Sometimes talking to your adviser or a counselor can also help.

✔ *Be satisfied with doing your best.* You can't expect to ace every test; all you can and should expect is your best effort. Once you've completed the exam, allow yourself the sweet pleasure of relief that it's over.

PULSE POINTS

Top Ten Stress Busters

1. **Strive for balance.** Review your commitments and plans, and if necessary, scale down.

2. **Get the facts.** When faced with a change or challenge, seek accurate information, which can bring vague fears down to earth.

3. **Talk with someone you trust.** A friend or a health professional can offer valuable perspective as well as psychological support.

4. **Exercise.** Even when your schedule gets jammed, carve out 20 or 30 minutes several times a week to walk, swim, bicycle, jog, or work out at the gym.

5. **Express yourself in writing.** Keeping a journal is one of the best ways to put your problems into perspective.

6. **Take care of yourself.** Get enough sleep. Eat a balanced diet. Limit your use of sugar, salt, and caffeine, which can compound stress by leading to fatigue and irritability. Watch your alcohol intake. Drinking can cut down on your ability to cope.

7. **Set priorities.** Making a list of things you need to do and rank-ing their importance help direct your energies so you're more efficient and less stressed.

8. **Help others.** One of the most effective ways of dealing with stress is to find people in a worse situation and do something positive for them.

9. **Cultivate hobbies.** Pursuing a personal pleasure can distract you from the stressors in your life and help you relax.

10. **Master a form of relaxation.** Whether you choose meditation, yoga, mindfulness, or another technique, practice it regularly.

Minorities and Stress

Regardless of your race or ethnic background, college may bring culture shock. You may never have encountered such a degree of diversity in one setting. You probably will meet students with different values, unfamiliar customs, entirely new ways of looking at the world—experiences you may find both stimulating and stressful.

Mental health professionals have long assumed that minority students may feel a double burden of stress. Many undergraduates experience emotional difficulties (see Chapter 3), and researchers have theorized that students from a racial or ethnic minority would be especially likely to develop psychological symptoms, such as anger, anxiety, and depression, as a result of increased stress.

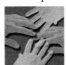 Racism has indeed been shown to be a source of stress that can affect health and well-being.[21] In the past, some African-American students have described predominately white campuses as hostile, alienating, and socially isolating and have reported greater estrangement from the campus community and heightened estrangement in interactions with faculty and peers.[22] However, the generalization that all minority students are more stressed may not be valid.

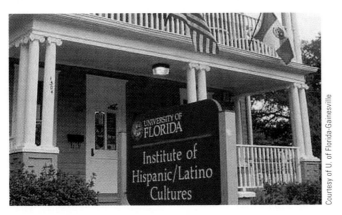
Courtesy of U. of Florida-Gainesville

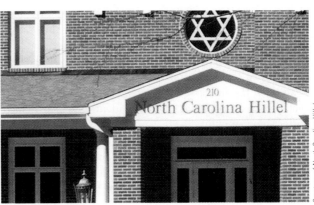
Courtesy of North Carolina Hillel

▲ Although minority students may perceive interpersonal tensions between themselves and nonminority students, they can often find culturally sensitive support services on campus.

A review of the eleven objective studies of ethnic differences among college students conducted in the last decade and a half has found that the number of minority students included was too small to warrant conclusions about their mental health and that the results were not consistent.[23] A more recent study conducted at a racially diverse university in a large metropolitan area in the Northeast evaluated 595 freshmen, including students of both genders and various racial and ethnic backgrounds, including Asians, African Americans, and Latino/Hispanics.[24] Less than 15 percent of these students—whether Asian, African American, Latino/Hispanic, white, or another ethnic minority—reported clinically significant levels of anger, anxiety, and depression, and there was no correlation between these stress-linked symptoms and ethnicity or race.

"Diversity, in and of itself, is unlikely to be related to higher levels of reported psychological symptoms on campus," the researchers concluded, theorizing that minority students "may have developed strengths while growing up within their particular cultures, subcommunities, and families that have often gone unrecognized or unnoted." They called for more research into "the psychosocial dynamics of stress, psychological symptoms, and resilience among racial and ethnic minority," as well as greater emphasis on developing culturally sensitive ways of providing support to those minority students who may need them.[25]

All minority students do share some common stressors. In one study of minority freshmen entering a large, competitive university, Asian, Latino, Filipino, African-American, and Native-American students all felt more sensitive and vulnerable to the college social climate, to interpersonal tensions between themselves and nonminority students and faculty, to experiences of actual or perceived racism, and to racist attitudes and discrimination (discussed later in this chapter, under Societal Stressors). Despite scoring above the national average on the SAT, the minority students in this study did not feel accepted as legitimate students and sensed that others viewed them as unworthy beneficiaries of affirmative action initiatives. While most said that overt racism was rare and relatively easy to deal with, they reported subtle pressures that undermined their academic confidence and their ability to bond with the university. Balancing these stressors, however, was a strong sense of ethnic identity, which helped buffer some stressful effects.

Latino students have identified three major types of stressors in their college experiences: academic (related to exam preparation and faculty interaction), social (related to ethnicity and interpersonal competence), and financial (related to their economic situation). Some Asian students who recently immigrated to the United States report feeling ostracized by students of similar ancestry who are second- or third-generation Americans. While they take pride in being truly bicultural and bilingual, the newcomers feel ambivalent about mainstream American culture. "My parents stress the importance of traditions; my friends tell me to get with it and act like an American," says one Asian-born student who has spent five years in the United States. "I feel trapped between cultures."

Other Personal Stressors

At every stage of life, you will encounter challenges and stressors. Among the most common are those related to anger, conflict, work, and overwork.

❓❓❓ Why Is Everyone So Angry?

According to the AAA Foundation for Traffic Safety, violent aggressive driving—which some dub "mad driver disease"—has been rising by 7 percent per year.[26] Sideline rage at amateur and professional sporting events has become so widespread that a Pennsylvania midget football game ended in a brawl involving more than 100 coaches, players, parents, and fans.

No one seems immune. Women fly off the handle just as often as men, although they're less likely to get physical. The young and the infamous, including several rappers and musicians sentenced to anger management classes for violent outbursts, may seem more volatile, but ordinary senior citizens have erupted into "line rage" and pushed ahead of others simply because they feel they've "waited long enough" in their lives.

"Everyone everywhere seems to be hotter under the collar these days," observes Sybil Evans, a conflict resolution expert who singles out three primary culprits: time, technology, and tension. "Americans are working longer hours than anyone else in the world. The cell phones and pagers that were supposed to make our lives easier have put us on call 24-7-365. Since we're always running, we're tense and low on patience, and the less patience we have, the less we monitor what we say to people and how we treat them."[27]

The sheer somplexity of our lives also has shortened our collective fuse. We rely on computers that crash, drive on roads that gridlock, place calls to machines that put us on endless hold. "It's not any one thing but lots of little things that make people feel they don't have control of their lives," comments consultant Jane Middleton-Moz, author of *Boiling Point: The High Cost of Unhealthy Anger to Individuals and Society*. "A sense of helplessness is what triggers rage. It's why people end up kicking ATM machines."[28]

Getting a Grip

For years therapists encouraged people to "vent" their anger. However, recent research shows that letting anger out only makes it worse. "Catharsis is worse than useless," says psychology professor Brad Bushman of Iowa State University, whose research has shown that letting anger out makes people more aggressive, not less. "Many people think of anger as the psychological equivalent of the steam in a pressure cooker that has to be released or it will explode. That's not true. People who react by hitting, kicking, screaming, and swearing aren't dealing with the underlying cause of their anger. They just feel more angry."[29]

Over time, temper tantrums sabotage physical health as well as psychological equanimity. By churning out stress hormones, chronic anger revs the body into a state of combat readiness, multiplying the risk for stroke and heart attack—even in healthy individuals. In one study by Duke University researchers, young women with "Jerry-Springer type anger," who tended to slam doors, curse, and throw things in fury, had higher cholesterol levels than those who reacted more calmly.

The first step to dealing with anger is figuring out what's really making you mad. Usually the jammed soda machine is the final straw that unleaches bottled-up fury over a more difficult issue, such as a recent breakup or a domineering parent. Also monitor yourself for early signs of exhaustion and overload. While stress alone doesn't cause a blowup, it makes you more vulnerable to overreacting.

"People blame anyone and everything for their anger, but there's never any justification for an outburst," says therapist Doris Helmering of St. Louis, author of *Sense Ability: Expanding Your Sense of Awareness for a Twenty-First Century Life.* "It's not easy, but you can learn to control your anger rather than letting it control you. Like any other feeling, anger lasts only about three seconds. What keeps it going is your own negative thinking." As long as you focus on who or what irritated you—like the oaf who rammed his grocery cart into your heels—you'll stay angry. "Once you come to understand that you're driving your own anger with your thoughts," says Helmering, "you can stop it."[30]

Conflict Resolution

Disagreements are inevitable; disagreeable ways of dealing with them are not. One of the most important skills in any setting—from dormitory floor to staff meeting to corporate boardroom—is resolving conflicts. The key is to focus on the problem, not the individual. Try to put aside unconscious biases, such as assuming a person is difficult to deal with, or preconceived notions about what others really want. Rather than planning what you might say, focus your attention on what others are saying.

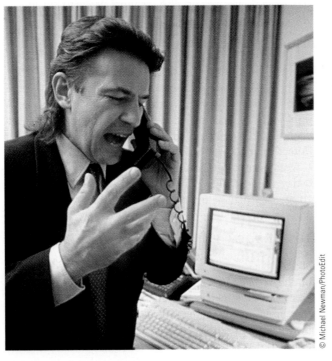

© Michael Newman/PhotoEdit

▲ How you manage your anger has consequences for your health and personal and professional relationships.

STRATEGIES FOR CHANGE

How to Deal with an Angry Person

✔ Become an impartial observer. Act as if you were watching someone else's two-year-old have a temper tantrum at the supermarket.

✔ Stay calm. Letting your emotions loose only adds fuel to fury. Talk quietly and slowly; let the person know you understand that he or she is angry.

✔ Refuse to engage. Step back to avoid invading his or her space. Retreat further if need be until the person is back in control.

✔ Find something to agree with. Look for common ground, if only to acknowledge that you're both in a difficult situation.

Professionals recommend the following steps:

▶ **Listen.** To work through a conflict, you need to understand the other person's point of view. This demands careful listening in a quiet, private setting, away from activity and background noise. If conflict erupts in a public place, move the discussion elsewhere.

▶ **Assimilate.** Rather than taking a position and focusing only on defending it, try not to shut yourself off to other possibilities. Keep open the possibility that no one party is completely right or completely wrong. To get a fresh perspective, consider the situation from the "third person." If you were seeing the conflict from the outside, what would you think about the information? Once you've taken in all available information, ask yourself: What do I know now about the overall situation? Has my opinion changed?

▶ **Respond.** Especially if another person is responding in anger, give a calm, well-reasoned response. It will help defuse a highly emotional situation. Try to find a common goal that will benefit you both. Restate the other person's position when both of you are finished speaking so you both know you've been heard and understood.

Job Stress

More so than ever, many people find that they are working more and enjoying it less. Many people, including working parents, spend 55 to 60 hours a week on the job. More people are caught up in an exhausting cycle of overwork, which causes stress, which makes work harder, which leads to more stress. Even the workplace itself can contribute to stress. A noisy, open-office environment can increase levels of stress without workers realizing it.[31]

Yet work in itself is not hazardous to health. Attitudes about work and habits related to how we work are the true threats. In fact, a job—stressful or not, enjoyable or not—can be therapeutic.

Workaholism and Burnout

People who become obsessed by their work and careers can turn into *workaholics,* so caught up in racing toward the top that they forget what they're racing toward and why. In some cases they throw themselves into their work to mask or avoid painful feelings or difficulties in their own lives. One consequence is **burnout,** a state of physical, emotional, and mental exhaustion brought on by constant or repeated emotional pressure. Particularly in the helping professions, such as social work or nursing, men and women who've dedicated themselves to others may realize they have nothing left in themselves to give.

Early signs of burnout include exhaustion, sleep problems or nightmares, increased anxiety or nervousness, muscular tension (headaches, backaches, and the like), increased use of alcohol or medication, digestive problems, such as nausea, vomiting, or diarrhea, loss of interest in sex, frequent body aches or pain, quarrels with family or friends, negative feelings about everything, problems concentrating, job mistakes and accidents, and feelings of depression, hopelessness, and helplessness.

Who Experiences Burnout?

Age is the one variable most consistently associated with burnout: Younger employees between ages 30 and 40 report the highest rates. Both men and women are susceptible to burnout. Unmarried individuals, particularly men, seem more prone to burnout than married workers. Single employees who've never been married have higher burnout rates than those who are divorced.

North American workers are more likely to experience burnout than employees in Western Europe. High burnout also has been reported in Japan, Taiwan, and other Asian countries. Certain occupations, particularly the helping professions, such as social work and nursing, have been linked with a greater risk of burnout. However, burnout also is common in teaching, law enforcement, and medicine.

People who have an external locus of control—that is, who attribute events to chance or forces beyond themselves—have higher burnout rates than those with an internal locus of control, who attribute achievements to their own ability and effort. Workers who have little participation in decision-making and who receive little feedback from their superiors also are more prone to burnout.[32]

Preventing Burnout

Personal satisfaction with your work helps avoid burnout. In a recent study of physicians, researchers found that hard work and fatigue can be countered by job satisfaction. A high sense of accomplishment was associated with an increase in the number of T cells, the white blood cells that protect the body against disease.[33] However, the best way to avoid burnout is learning to cope well with smaller, day-to-day stresses. Then, tiny frustrations won't smolder into a blaze that may be impossible to put out.

Desk Rage

Job stress has intensified into a more intense and dangerous condition that has been dubbed "desk rage." According to a survey of 1,305 men and women, 42 percent of employees have witnessed yelling or verbal abuse; 29 percent yelled at coworkers themselves; 23 percent cried over work-related issues; 10 percent reported physical violence.[34]

Why are workers so upset? Experts blame corporate downsizing, intense competition, longer hours, economic insecurity, and nonstop electronic communication. "Many employees today have a sense of voiceless overload," says Ken Jacobsen, an expert in workplace distress at the University of Northern Iowa, "Each is doing the job of two or two-and-a-half people, and the demands on them may be completely unrealistic. In the past, there was a belief that if you worked harder or longer, you'd be rewarded. That's no longer the case, and it flies in the face of an employee's sense of fairness."[35]

While rage can smolder in any workplace, it is most likely to reach a boiling point when job responsibilities are ambiguous or unpredictable or when many people think they can hold a worker accountable. Frustration and anger also intensify when employees think they can't or shouldn't express negative feelings. The perpetrators of desk rage typically feel they're not listened to, heard or respected. They're often afraid to speak up for fear of being labeled as a squeaky wheel and missing out on a promotion or a raise.

However, those who try to ignore their negative emotions suffer on the job and off. Employees may procrastinate or indulge in "toxic" gossip with other disgruntled colleagues. Many develop physical symptoms, such as insomnia or indigestion, or take up self-destructive habits, like eating or drinking too much. As resentment turns to hostility, workers may fantasize about what they might do to get even with those who've wronged them. Withdrawing from their coworkers, they direct their anger outward—pounding their desks, firing off irate e-mails, flinging a coffee mug (or, in some cases, an entire computer) across the room, getting into shouting matches or name-calling. Verbal aggression can escalate into physical violence. Coworkers or former employees account for aboug 15 percent of violent incidents in the workplace.

Illness and Disability

Just as the mind can have profound effects on the body, the body can have an enormous impact on our emotions. Whenever we come down with the flu or pull a muscle, we feel under par. When the problem is more serious or persistent—a chronic disease like diabetes, for instance, or a lifelong hearing impairment—the emotional stress of constantly coping with it is even greater.

A common source of stress for college students is a learning disability, which may affect one of every ten Americans. Most learning-disabled have average or above-average intelligence, but they rarely live up to their ability in school. Some have only one area of difficulty, such as reading or math. Others have problems with attention, writing, communicating, reasoning, coordination, social

---

STRATEGIES FOR PREVENTION

Defusing Desk Rage

Desk rage builds in little steps, so you can take it away in little steps. Here are suggestions on how to do so:

✔ Take better care of yourself. Get enough sleep. Schedule a softball game or work out at the end of the day to release physical tension. Avoid excess caffeine and alcohol.

✔ If you sense a problem, monitor the situation for a week. Write down when you're feeling hungry, tired, overloaded. Try to identify the triggers that might cause you to do something you'll later regret.

✔ Get feedback from friends. An objective person who knows you well can provide a fresh take on a troubling situation.

✔ If your irritation stems from a coworker, approach him or her in a nonthreatening way. You might say, "Could you hear me out for a few minutes?" To lower the hostility level, start by stating something you have in common, such as "We both want this project to work."

✔ If you fly off the handle, learn from the experience. Do immediate damage control by apologizing to coworkers and explaining that you've been under stress. Plan what you might do differently the next time someone sets you off.

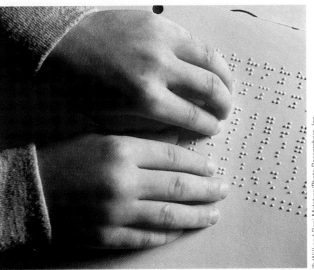

▲ The blind college student has unique challenges and stressors that sighted students do not.

competence, and emotional maturity—all of which may make it difficult, if not impossible, for them to find and keep jobs. Special training and a better understanding of what's wrong can make an enormous difference.

Learning disorders can be hard to recognize in adults, who often become adept at covering up or compensating for their difficulties. However, someone with a learning disability may be

- Unable to engage in a focused activity such as reading.
- Extremely distractible, forgetful, or absentminded.
- Easily frustrated by waiting, delays, or traffic.
- Disorganized, unable to manage time efficiently and complete tasks on time.
- Hot-tempered, explosive, constantly irritated.
- Impulsive, making decisions with little reflection or information.
- Easily overwhelmed by ordinary hassles.
- Clumsy, with a poor body image and poor sense of direction.
- Emotionally immature.
- Physically restless.

Individuals with several of these characteristics should undergo diagnostic tests to evaluate their skills and abilities and to determine whether remedial training, available through state offices of vocational rehabilitation, can help.

Societal Stressors

Not all stressors are personal. Centuries ago the poet John Donne observed that no man is an island. Today, on an

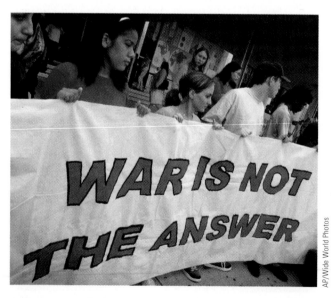

AP/Wide World Photos

▲ Protest marches are one way in which college students have often responded to national and international crises, including acts of terrorism.

increasingly crowded and troubled planet, these words seem truer than ever. Problems such as discrimination and terrorism can no longer be viewed only as economic or political issues. Directly or indirectly, they affect the well-being of all who inhabit the Earth—now and in the future. Even more mundane stressors, such as traffic, can lead to outbursts of anger that have come to be known as "road rage."[36] (This common stress-related response is discussed in Chapter 17.)

Discrimination

Discrimination can take many forms—some as subtle as not being included in a conversation or joke, some as blatant as threats scrawled on a wall, some as violent as brutal beatings and other hate crimes. Because it can be hard to deal with individually, discrimination is a particularly sinister form of stress. By banding together, however, those who experience discrimination can take action to protect themselves, challenge the ignorance and hateful assumptions that fuel bigotry, and promote a healthier environment for all.

In the last decade, there have been reports of increased intolerance among young people and greater tolerance of expressions and acts of hate on college campuses. To counteract this trend, many schools have set up programs and classes to educate students about each other's backgrounds and to acknowledge and celebrate the richness diversity brings to campus life. Educators have called on universities to make campuses less alienating and more culturally and emotionally accessible, with programs and policies targeted not only at minority students but also at the university as a whole.

Violence and Terrorism

The deliberate use of physical force to abuse or injure is a leading killer of young people in the United States—and a potential source of stress in all our lives. Chances are that you or someone you know has been the victim of a violent crime, and awareness of our own vulnerability adds to the stress of daily living. After the terrorist attacks on New York and Washington DC, on September 11, 2001, 44 percent of Americans in a national survey conducted several days later reported one or more substantial symptoms of stress. They coped with their increased sense of vulnerability by talking with others, turning to religion, participating in group activities, and making donations.[37]

Stress Survival

Although stress is a very real threat to emotional and physical well-being, its impact depends not just on what happens to you, but on how you handle it. If you tried to predict who would become ill based simply on life-change units or other stressors, you'd be correct only about 15 percent of the time.

The key to coping with stress is realizing that your *perception* and *response* to a stressor are crucial. Changing the way you interpret events or situations—a skill called *reframing*—makes all the difference. An event, such as a move to a new city, is not stressful in itself. A move becomes stressful if you see it as a traumatic upheaval rather than an exciting beginning of a new chapter in your life.

To get a sense of your own stress level, ask yourself the following questions about the preceding week of your life:

- How often have you felt out of control?
- How often have you felt confident that you'd be able to handle personal problems?
- How often have you felt things were generally going your way?
- How often have you felt that things were piling up so high you'd never be able to catch up?

Think through your answers. If the experiences of being out of control or overwhelmed outnumbered those of confidence and control, it's time to develop a stress-management plan and put it into action.

To achieve greater control over the stress in your life, start with some self-analysis: If you're feeling overwhelmed, ask yourself: Are you taking an extra course that's draining your last ounce of energy? Are you staying up late studying every night and missing morning classes? Are you living on black coffee and jelly doughnuts? While you may think that you don't have time to reduce the stress in your life, some simple changes can often ease the pressure you're under and help you achieve your long-term goals.

Relieving Short-Term Stress

Acute stress strikes every day: You forget your wallet. You show up late for work—again. You blow a big test. The computer crashes just as you're about to print out a term paper. Frustrated and anxious, you'd love to start the day all over again. Unfortunately, no one can undo the past. However, you can control how you react in the present. Simple exercises, like the following examples, can stop the stress buildup inside your body and help you regain a sense of calm and control:

- **Breathing.** Deep breathing relaxes the body and quiets the mind. Draw air deeply into your lungs, allowing your chest to fill with air and your belly to rise and fall. You will feel the muscle tension and stress begin to melt away. When you're feeling extremely stressed, try this calming breath: Sit or lie with your back straight and place the tip of your tongue on the roof of your mouth behind your teeth. Exhale completely through the mouth, then inhale through the nose for 4 seconds. Hold the breath for 7 seconds, then exhale audibly through the mouth for 8 seconds. Repeat four times.

- **Refocusing.** Thinking about a situation you can't change or control only increases the stress you feel. Force your mind to focus on other subjects. If you're stuck in a long line, distract yourself. Check out what other people are buying or imagine what they do for a living. In the car, turn on the radio to a music station you like. Imagine that you're in a hot shower and a wave of relaxation is washing your stress down the drain.

- **Serenity breaks.** Build moments of tranquility into your day. For instance, while waiting for your computer to warm up or a file to download, look at a photograph of someone you love or a poster of a tropical island. If none is available, close your eyes and visualize a soothing scene, such as walking in a meadow or along a beach.

- **Stress signals.** Learn to recognize the first signs that your stress load is getting out of hand: Is your back bothering you? Do you have a headache? Do you find yourself speeding or misplacing things? Whenever you spot these early warnings, force yourself to stop and say, "I'm under stress. I need to do something about it."

- **Reality checks.** To put things into proper perspective, ask yourself: Will I remember what's made me so upset a month from now? If you had to rank this problem on a scale of 1 to 10, with worldwide catastrophe as 10, where would it rate?

- **Stress inoculation.** Rehearse everyday situations that you find stressful, such as speaking in class. Think of how you might make the situation less tense, for instance, by breathing deeply before you talk or jotting down notes beforehand. Think of these small "doses" of stress as the psychological equivalent of allergy shots: They immunize you so you feel less stressed when bigger challenges come along.[38]

- **Rx: Laughter.** Humor counters stress by focusing on comic aspects of difficult situations and may, as various studies have shown, lessen harmful effects on the immune system and overall health. However, humor may have different effects on stress in men and women. In a study of 131 undergraduates, humor buffered stress-related physical symptoms in men and women. However, it reduced stress-linked anxiety only in men. The researchers theorized that men may prefer humor as a more appropriate way of expressing emotions such as anxiety, whereas women are more likely to use self-disclosure, that is, to confide in friends.[39]

- **Spiritual coping.** Saying a prayer under stress is one of the oldest and most effective ways of calming yourself. Other forms of spiritual coping, such as putting trust in

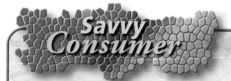

Savvy Consumer

Can Stress-Relief Products Help?

You're stressed out, and you see an ad for a product—an oil, candle, cream, herbal tea, pill, or potion—that promises to make all your cares disappear. Should you soak in an aromatic bath, have a massage, try kava, squeeze foam balls? In most cases, you're probably not doing yourself much harm, but you aren't necessarily doing yourself much good either. Keep these considerations in mind:

• Be wary of instant cures. Regardless of the promises on the label, it's unrealistic to expect any magic ingredient or product to make all your problems disappear.

• Focus on stress-reducing behavior, rather than a product. An aromatic candle may not bring instant serenity, but if you light a candle and meditate, you may indeed feel more at peace. A scented pillow may not be a cure

for a stress, but if it helps you get a good night's sleep, you'll cope better the next day.

• Experiment with physical ways to work out stress. Exercise is one of the best ways to lower your stress levels. Try walking, running, swimming, cycling, kickboxing—anything physical that helps you release tension.

• Don't make matters worse by smoking (the chemicals in cigarettes increase heart rate, blood pressure, and stress hormone), consuming too much caffeine (it speeds up your system for hours), eating snacks high in sugar (it produces a quick high followed by a sudden slump), or turning to drugs or alcohol (they can only add to your stress when their effects wear off.)

• Remember that stress is a matter of attitude. Remind yourself of some basic words of wisdom: Don't sweat the small stuff—and it's all small stuff.

God and doing for others (for instance, by volunteering at a shelter for battered women) also can provide a different perspective on daily hassles and stresses.

▶ **Sublimation.** This term refers to the redirection of any drives considered unacceptable into socially acceptable channels. Outdoor activity is one of the best ways to reduce stress through sublimation. For instance, if you're furious with a friend who betrayed your trust or frustrated because your boss rejects all of your proposals, you might go for a long run or hike to sublimate your anger.

Dealing with Long-Term Stress

If you're going through a transition or you're coming to terms with a setback or loss, you need time to regain a sense of perspective. Any major change, positive or negative, triggers a mixed array of feelings, and you have to sort these out by thinking through what happened, why, and where it might lead.

Journaling

One of the simplest, yet most effective, ways to work through stress is by putting your feelings into words that only you will read. The more honest and open you are as you write, the better. According to the research of psychologist James Pennebaker of the University of Texas, Austin, college students who wrote in their journals about trau-

matic events felt much better afterward than those who wrote about superficial topics. Recording your experiences and feelings on paper or audiotape may help decrease stress and enhance well-being.[40]

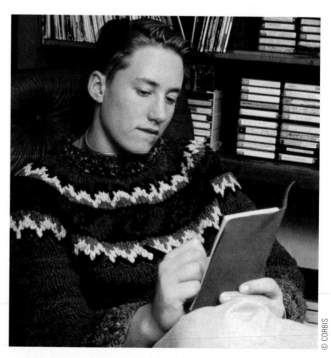

▲ Writing in your journal about feelings and difficulties is a simple and very effective way to help control your stress.

© CORBIS

As noted earlier in this chapter, recent research has shown that writing about stressful events can actually ease the symptoms of chronic illnesses like asthma and arthritis. As psychiatrist David Spiegel, M.D., of Stanford University notes, stress affects both mind and body, and illness may trigger associations to past stressful events that were beyond individual control. Writing about traumatic experience may alter the way people think about the event, giving it order and structure and enhancing their own feelings of control.[41]

A "stress journal" can serve a similar purpose. Focus on intense emotional experiences and "autopsy" them to try to understand why they affected you the way they did. Rereading and thinking about your notes may reveal the underlying reasons for your response.

???? What Can Help Me Relax?

Relaxation is the physical and mental state opposite that of stress. Rather than gearing up for fight or flight, our bodies and minds grow calmer and work more smoothly. We're less likely to become frazzled and more capable of staying in control. The most effective relaxation techniques include progressive relaxation, visualization, meditation, mindfulness, and biofeedback.

Progressive relaxation works by intentionally increasing and then decreasing tension in the muscles. While sitting or lying down in a quiet, comfortable setting, you tense and release various muscles, beginning with those of the hand, for instance, and then proceeding to the arms, shoulders, neck, face, scalp, chest, stomach, buttocks, genitals, and so on, down each leg to the toes. Relaxing the muscles can quiet the mind and restore internal balance.

Visualization, or **guided imagery,** involves creating mental pictures that calm you down and focus your mind. Some people use this technique to promote healing when they are ill (see Chapter 10). Visualization skills require practice and, in some cases, instruction by qualified health professionals.

Meditation has been practiced in many forms over the ages, from the yogic techniques of the Far East to the Quaker silence of more modern times.

Brain scans have shown that meditation activates the sections of the brain in charge of the autonomic nervous system, which governs bodily functions, such as digestion and blood pressure, that we cannot consciously control.[42] Although many studies have documented the benefits of meditation for overall health, it may be particularly helpful for people dealing with stress-related medical conditions such as high blood pressure.

 In a study of African Americans with atherosclerosis, or hardening of the arteries, those who meditated showed a marked decrease in the thickness of their artery walls, while the nonmeditators showed an increase. This benefit is particularly important because African Americans are twice as likely to die from cardiovascular disease as are whites.[43]

Meditation helps a person reach a state of relaxation, but with the goal of achieving inner peace and harmony. There is no one right way to meditate, and many people have discovered how to meditate on their own, without even knowing what it is they are doing. Among college students, meditation has proven especially effective in increasing relaxation. Most forms of meditation have common elements: sitting quietly for 15 to 20 minutes once or twice a day, concentrating on a word or image, and breathing slowly and rhythmically. If you wish to try meditation, it often helps to have someone guide you through your first sessions. Or try tape recording your own voice (with or without favorite music in the background) and playing it back to yourself, freeing yourself to concentrate on the goal of turning the attention within.

Mindfulness is a modern form of an ancient Asian technique that involves maintaining awareness in the present moment. You tune in to each part of your body, scanning from head to toe, noting the slightest sensation. You allow whatever you experience—an itch, an ache, a feeling of warmth—to enter your awareness. Then you open yourself to focus on all the thoughts, sensations, sounds, and feelings that enter your awareness. Mindfulness keeps you in the here-and-now, thinking about what *is* rather than about *what if* or *if only.*

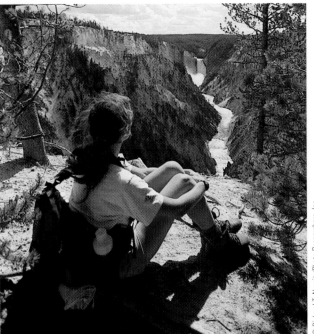

▲ Spending time outdoors is a great way to leave behind daily tensions.

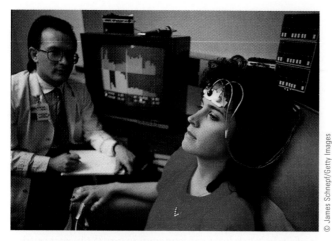

▲ Biofeedback training uses electronic monitoring devices to teach conscious control over heart rate, body temperature, and muscle tension. Once the technique is learned, the electronic devices are unnecessary.

© James Schnepf/Getty Images

Biofeedback, discussed in Chapter 10, is a method of obtaining feedback, or information, about some physiological activity occurring in the body. An electronic monitoring device attached to the body detects a change in an internal function and communicates it back to the person through a tone, light, or meter. By paying attention to this feedback, most people can gain some control over functions previously thought to be beyond conscious control, such as body temperature, heart rate, muscle tension, and brain waves. Biofeedback training consists of three stages:

1. Developing increased awareness of a body state or function.
2. Gaining control over it.
3. Transferring this control to everyday living without use of the electronic instrument.

The goal of biofeedback for stress reduction is a state of tranquility, usually associated with the brain's production of alpha waves (which are slower and more regular than normal waking waves). After several training sessions, most people can produce alpha waves more or less at will.

Time Management

We live in what some sociologists call hyperculture, a society that moves at warp speed. Information bombards us constantly. The rate of change seems to accelerate every year. Our "time-saving" devices—pagers, cell phones, modems, faxes, palm-sized organizers, laptop computers—have simply extended the boundaries of where and how we work.

As a result, more and more people are suffering from "timesickness," a nerve-racking feeling that life has become little more than an endless to-do list. The best antidote is time management, and hundreds of books, seminars, and experts offer training in making the most of the hours in the day. Yet these well-intentioned methods often fail, and sooner or later most of us find ourselves caught in a time trap.

Poor Time Management

Every day you make dozens of decisions, and the choices you make about how to use your time directly affect your stress level. If you have a big test on Monday and a term paper due Tuesday, you may plan to study all weekend. Then, when you're invited to a party Saturday night, you go. Although you set the alarm for 7:00 A.M. on Sunday, you don't pull yourself out of bed until noon. By the time you start studying, it's 4:00 P.M., and anxiety is building inside you.

How can you tell if you've lost control of your time? The following are telltale symptoms of poor time management:

▶ Rushing.
▶ Chronic inability to make choices or decisions.
▶ Fatigue or listlessness.
▶ Constantly missed deadlines.
▶ Not enough time for rest or personal relationships.
▶ A sense of being overwhelmed by demands and details and having to do what you don't want to do most of the time.

One of the hard lessons of being on your own is that your choices and your actions have consequences. Stress is just one of them. But by thinking ahead, being realistic about your workload, and sticking to your plans, you can gain better control over your time and your stress levels.

⁇⁇ How Can I Better Manage My Time?

Time management involves skills that anyone can learn, but they require commitment and practice to make a difference in your life. It may help to know the techniques that other students have found most useful:

▶ **Schedule your time.** Use a calendar or planner. Beginning the first week of class, mark down deadlines for each assignment, paper, project, and test scheduled that semester. Develop a daily schedule, listing very specifically what you will do the next day, along with the times. Block out times for working out, eating dinner, calling home, and talking with friends as well as for studying.

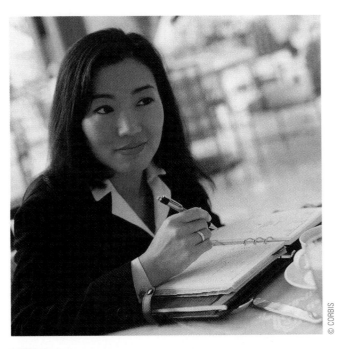

▲ A calendar or planner is an important tool in time management. You can use it to keep track of assignment due dates, class meetings, and other "to do's."

margins, which will help you retain more information. Even if you're racing to start a paper, take a few extra minutes to prepare a workable outline. It will be easier to structure your paper when you start writing.

▷ **Focus on the task at hand.** Rather than worrying about how you did on yesterday's test or how you'll ever finish next week's project, focus intently on whatever you're doing at any given moment. If your mind starts to wander, use any distraction—the sound of the phone ringing or a noise from the hall—as a reminder to stay in the moment.

▷ **Turn elephants into hors d'oeuvres.** Cut a huge task into smaller chunks so it seems less enormous. For instance, break down your term paper into a series of steps, such as selecting a topic, identifying sources of research information, taking notes, developing an outline, and so on.

▷ **Keep your workspace in order.** Even if the rest of your room is a shambles, try to keep your desk clear. Piles of papers are distracting, and you can end up wasting lots of time looking for notes you misplaced or an article you have to read by morning. Try to spend the last ten minutes of the day getting your desk in order so you get a fresh start on the new day.

▷ **Develop a game plan.** Allow at least two nights to study for any major exam. Set aside more time for researching and writing papers. Make sure to allow time to type and print out a paper—and to deal with emergencies like a computer breakdown. Set daily and weekly goals for every class. When working on a big project, don't neglect your other courses. Whenever possible, try to work ahead in all your classes.

▷ **Identify time robbers.** For several days keep a log of what you do and how much time you spend doing it. You may discover that disorganization is eating away at your time or that you have a problem getting started. (See the following section on Overcoming Procrastination.)

▷ **Make the most of classes.** Read the assignments before class rather than waiting until just before you have a test. By reading ahead of time, you'll make it easier to understand the lectures. Go to class yourself. Your own notes will be more helpful than a friend's or those from a note-taking service. Read your lecture notes at the end of each day or at least at the end of each week.

▷ **Develop an efficient study style.** Some experts recommend studying for 50 minutes, then breaking for 10 minutes. Small incentives, such as allowing yourself to call or visit a friend during these 10 minutes, can provide the motivation to keep you at the books longer. When you're reading, don't just highlight passages. Instead, write notes or questions to yourself in the

Overcoming Procrastination

 Putting off until tomorrow what should be done today is a habit that creates a great deal of stress for many students. It also takes a surprising toll. In studies with students taking a health psychology course, researchers found that although procrastinating provided short-term benefits, including periods of low stress, the tendency to dawdle had long-term costs, including poorer health and lower grades. Early in the semester, the procrastinators reported less stress and fewer health problems than students who scored low on procrastination. However, by the end of the semester, procrastinators reported more health-related symptoms, more stress, and more visits to health-care professionals than nonprocrastinators. They also received significantly lower grades on term papers and exams.[44]

The three most common types of procrastination are: putting off unpleasant things, putting off difficult tasks, and putting off tough decisions. Procrastinators are most likely to delay by wishing they didn't have to do what they must or by telling themselves they "just can't get started," which means they never do.

To get out of the procrastination trap, keep track of the tasks you're most likely to put off, and try to figure out why you don't want to tackle them. Think of alternative ways to get tasks done. If you put off library readings, for instance, is the problem getting to the library or the reading itself? If it's the trip to the library, arrange to walk over with a friend whose company you enjoy.

Develop daily time-management techniques, such as a to-do list. Rank items according to priorities: A, B, C, and schedule your days to make sure the A's get accomplished. Try not to fixate on half-completed projects. Divide large tasks, such as a term paper, into smaller ones, and reward yourself when you complete a part.

Do what you like least first. Once you have it out of the way, you can concentrate on the tasks you do enjoy. You also should build time into your schedule for interruptions, unforeseen problems, unexpected events, and so on, so you aren't constantly racing around. Establish ground rules for meeting your own needs (including getting enough sleep and making time for friends) before saying yes to any activity. Learn to live according to a three-word motto: Just do it!

PPPP Is Stress Hazardous to Psychological Health?

The lifetime prevalence of major stressful events is high. In one study of 1,000 adults in four cities in the southeastern United States, 21 percent of the sample reported a traumatic event (such as a robbery, assault, or traumatic death of a loved one) during the previous year, and 69 percent reported at least one such event in their lifetime.[45] Such stressors always take a toll on an individual, and it's normal to feel sad, tense, overwhelmed, angry, or incapable of coping with the ordinary demands of daily living. Usually such feelings and behaviors subside with time. The stressful event fades into the past, and those whose lives it has touched adapt to its lasting impact. But sometimes individuals remain extremely distressed and unable to function as they once did. While the majority of individuals who survive a trauma recover, at least a quarter of such individuals later develop serious psychological symptoms.[46]

Posttraumatic Stress Disorder

In the past, **posttraumatic stress disorder (PTSD)** was viewed as a psychological response to out-of-the-ordinary stressors, such as captivity or combat. However, other experiences can also forever change the way people view themselves and their world. Thousands of individuals experience or witness traumatic events, such as fires or floods. Children, in particular, are likely to develop PTSD symptoms when they live through a traumatic event or witness a loved one or friend being assaulted. Sometimes an entire community, such as the residents of a town hit by a devastating hurricane, develops symptoms.

STRATEGIES FOR PREVENTION

Recognize the Warning Signals of Stress Overload

✔ Experiencing physical symptoms, including chronic fatigue, headaches, indigestion, diarrhea, and sleep problems.

✔ Having frequent illness or worrying about illness.

✔ Self-medicating, including nonprescription drugs.

✔ Having problems concentrating on studies or work.

✔ Feeling irritable, anxious, or apathetic.

✔ Working or studying longer and harder than usual.

✔ Exaggerating, to yourself and others, the importance of what you do.

✔ Becoming accident-prone.

✔ Breaking rules, whether it's a curfew at home or a speed limit on the highway.

✔ Going to extremes, such as drinking too much, overspending, or gambling.

According to recent research, almost half of car accident victims may develop PTSD. Individuals who were seriously injured are especially vulnerable.[47] The main symptoms are re-experiencing the traumatic event, avoiding the site of the accident, refraining from driving in weather and road conditions similar to those on the day of the accident, and feeling a general increase in distress.

A history of childhood sexual abuse can greatly increase the likelihood of developing PTSD.[48] An episode that repeats the abuse, such as a sexual assault or rape, can trigger an intense reaction as individuals "re-experience" the initial trauma. Childhood abuse—physical, sexual, or emotional—can affect student dropout rates. In one study that followed 210 freshmen (aged 17–21 years) for four years, those suffering PTSD symptoms in the second week of their freshman year were less likely to remain enrolled through their senior years. Half of those who'd been sexually abused and 65 percent of those who'd experienced multiple forms of abuse dropped out.[49]

In PTSD, individuals re-experience their terror and helplessness again and again in their dreams or intrusive thoughts. To avoid this psychic pain, they may try to avoid anything associated with the trauma. Some enter a state of emotional numbness and no longer can respond to people and experiences the way they once did, especially when it comes to showing tenderness or affection. Those who've been mugged or raped may be afraid to venture out by themselves.

The sooner trauma survivors receive psychological help, the better they are likely to fare. Often talking about what happened with an empathic person or someone who's shared the experience as soon as possible—preferably before going to sleep on the day of the event—can help an individual begin to deal with what has occurred. Group sessions, ideally beginning soon after the trauma, allow individuals to share views and experiences. Behavioral, cognitive, and psychodynamic therapy (described in Chapter 3) can help individuals suffering PTSD.

Resilience: Bouncing Back from Adversity

Adversity—whether in the form of a traumatic event or chronic stress—has different effects on individuals. Some people never recover and continue on a downward slide that may ultimately prove fatal. Others return, though at different rates, to their prior level of functioning. In recent years researchers have focused their attention on a particularly intriguing group: those people who not only survive stressful experiences but also thrive, that is, who actually surpass their previous level of functioning.

Resilience can take many forms.[50] A father whose child is kidnapped and killed may become a nationwide advocate for victims' rights. A student whose roommate dies in a car crash after a party may campaign for tougher

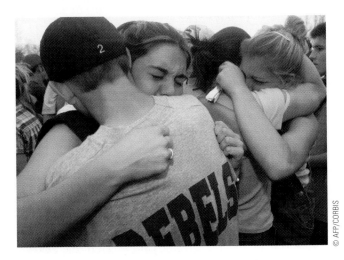

▲ Trauma survivors can often find support and comfort from those who have shared the experience.

laws against drunk driving. A couple whose premature baby spends weeks in a neonatal intensive care unit may find that their marriage has grown closer and stronger. Even though their experiences were painful, the individuals often look back at them as bringing positive changes into their lives.

Researchers have studied various factors that enable individuals to thrive in the face of adversity. These include:

▶ **An optimistic attitude.** Rather than reacting to a stressor simply as a threat, these men and women view stress as a challenge—one they believe they can and will overcome. Researchers have documented that individuals facing various stressors, including serious illness and bereavement, are more likely to report experiencing growth if they have high levels of hope and optimism.
▶ **Self-efficacy.** A sense of being in control of one's life can boost health, even in times of great stress.
▶ **Stress inoculation.** People who deal well with adversity often have had previous experiences with stress that toughened them in various ways, such as teaching them skills that enhanced their ability to cope and boosting their confidence in their ability to weather a rough patch.
▶ **Secure personal relationships.** Individuals who know they can count on the support of their loved ones are more likely to be resilient.
▶ **Spirituality or religiousness.** Religious coping may be particularly related to growth and resilience. In particular, two types seem most beneficial: spiritually based religious coping (receiving emotional reassurance and guidance from God) and good-deeds coping (living a better, more spiritual life that includes altruistic acts).

Resilience sometimes means developing new skills simply because, in order to get through the stressful experience, people had to learn something they hadn't known how to do before—for instance, wrangling with insurance companies or other bureaucracies. By mastering such skills, they become more fit to deal with an unpredictable world and develop new flexibility in facing the unknown.

Along with new abilities comes the psychological sense of mastery. "I survived this," an individual may say. "I'll be able to deal with other hard things in the future." Such confidence keeps people actively engaged in the effort to cope and is itself a predictor of eventual success. Stress also can make individuals more aware of the fulfilling aspects of life, and they may become more interested in spiritual pursuits. Certain kinds of stressful experiences also have social consequences. If a person experiencing a traumatic event finds that the significant others in his or her life can be counted on, the result can be a strengthening of their relationship.

Researchers are trying to determine ways in which more people can derive positive benefits from stressful experiences. One important step, they believe, is to encourage people to view a traumatic situation as an opportunity for personal growth, rather than a test of whether or not they "have what it takes" to survive.

In a study of the life narratives of midlife adults (aged 35–65 years) and college students (aged 18–24), both groups reported greater psychological well-being when the stories of low points and turning points in their lives contained images of redemption and they were able to find benefits and lessons in their experiences of adversity.[51]

Focusing on finding meaning in their experience—what some call "cognitive coping"—can help individuals move beyond initial emotional responses such as anxiety, distress, and confusion. Over time, some people may develop what may be the ultimate "gift" of a stressful experience: wisdom.

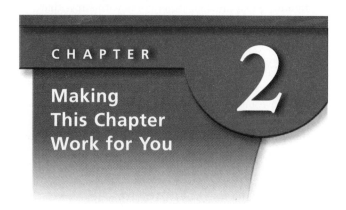

CHAPTER

Making This Chapter Work for You

2

1. Stress can be defined as
   a. a negative emotional state related to fatigue and similar to depression.
   b. the physiological and psychological response to any event or situation that either upsets or excites us.
   c. the end result of the general adaptation syndrome.
   d. a motivational strategy for making life changes.

2. According to the general adaptation syndrome theory, how does the body typically respond to an acute stressor?
   a. The heart rate slows, blood pressure declines, and eye movement increases.
   b. The body enters a physical state called eustress and then moves into the physical state referred to as distress.
   c. If the stressor is viewed as a positive event, there are no physical changes.
   d. The body demonstrates three stages of change: alarm, resistance, and exhaustion.

3. Over time, increased levels of stress hormones have been shown to increase a person's risk for which of the following conditions?

   a. diabetes, high blood pressure, memory loss, and skin disorders
   b. stress fractures, male pattern baldness, and hypothyroidism
   c. hemophilia, AIDS, and hay fever
   d. none of the above

4. Stress levels in college students
   a. may be high due to stressors such as academic pressures, financial concerns, learning disabilities, and relationship problems.
   b. are usually low because students feel empowered, living independently of their parents.
   c. are typically highest in seniors because their self-esteem diminishes during the college years.
   d. are lower in minority students because they are used to stressors such as a hostile social climate and actual or perceived discrimination.

5. Which of the following statements about anger is true?
   a. The healthiest way to deal with anger is to express the rage.
   b. When confronted by an angry person, you can usually defuse the situation quickly by explaining that he or she is acting immaturely and inappropriately.
   c. Venting anger can adversely affect one's physical health over time.
   d. Statistics show that anger-related public behaviors such as aggressive driving and workplace outbursts have been on the decrease.

6. One consequence of job stress is burnout, which can be defined as
   a. injuries caused by computer overuse.
   b. company initiatives to enhance employee's work-life balance.
   c. lack of career advancement.
   d. physical and psychological exhaustion resulting from work pressures.

7. Which of the following situations is representative of a societal stressor?
   a. Peter has been told that his transfer application has been denied because his transcripts were not sent in by the dealine.
   b. Nia and Kwame find an unsigned note pinned to the door of their new home, ordering them to move out or face the consequences.
   c. Kelli's boyfriend drives her car after he had been drinking and has an accident.
   d. Joshua, who is the leading basketball player on his college varsity team, has just been diagnosed with diabetes.

8. If you are stuck in a traffic jam, which of the following actions will help reduce your stress level?
   a. deep slow breathing
   b. honking your horn

c. berating yourself for not taking a different route

d. getting on your cell phone to reschedule appointments

9. A relaxed peaceful state of being can be achieved with which of the following activities?

a. an aerobic exercise class

b. playing a computer game

c. meditating for 15 minutes

d. attending a rap concert

10. A person suffering from posttraumatic stress disorder may experience which of the following symptoms?

a. procrastination

b. constant thirst

c. drowsiness

d. terror-filled dreams

Answers to these questions can be found on page 640.

 What is the difference between short term and long term stress? How does stress affect your health?

Critical Thinking

1. Stress levels among college students have reached record highs. What reasons can you think of to account for this? Consider possible social, cultural, and economic factors that may play a role.

2. Identify three stressful situations in your life and determine whether they are examples of eustress or distress. Describe both the positive and negative aspects of each situation.

3. Can you think of any ways in which your behavior or attitudes might create stress for others? What changes could you make to avoid doing so?

4. What advice might you give an incoming freshman at your school about managing stress in college? What techniques have been most helpful for you in dealing with stress? Suppose that this student is from a different ethnic group than you? What additional suggestions would you have for this student?

SITES & BYTES

Stress Assess

http://wellness.uwsp.edu/Health_Service/services/stress

This three-part outline educational tool was developed by the National Wellness Institute at the University of Wisconsin—Steven's Point. Designed to increase your knowledge about stress, this questionnaire features separate evaluations for stress sources, distress symptoms, and stress-balancing strategies.

Stress4Teens

http://health4teens.org/stress/index.html

This site describes signs of stress as well as strategies to cope with stress, written for adolescents.

How to Survive Unbearable Stress

http://www.teachhealth.com

This comprehensive website is written specifically for college students by Steven Burns, M.D. It features the following topics: signs of how to recognize stress, two stress surveys for adults and college students, information on the pathophysiology of stress, the genetics of stress and stress tolerance, and information on how to best manage and even treat stress.

Please note that links are subject to change. If you find a broken link, use a search engine such as http://www.yahoo.com and search for the website by typing in key words.

InfoTrac Activity "How Women Handle Stress: Is There a Difference?" *Harvard Mental Health Letter*, April 2001, Vol. 17, No. 10.

(1) Name two reasons for the observed differences in how men cope with stress when compared to women's coping mechanisms.

(2) When exposed to stress, how do men and women deal with family conflict?

(3) How can different hormones result in the observed gender differences in coping with stress?

For additional links, resources, and suggested readings on InfoTrac, visit our Health & Wellness Resource Center at http://health.wadsworth.com.

Key Terms

The terms listed here are used within the chapter on the page indicated. Definitions of the terms are in the Glossary at the end of the book.

adaptive response 40
allostasis 40
biofeedback 58
burnout 52
distress 40
eustress 40
general adaptation syndrome
    (GAS) 40

guided imagery 57
homeostasis 40
meditation 57
migraine headache 44
mindfulness 57
posttraumatic stress disorder
    (PTSD) 60
progressive relaxation 57

psychoneuroimmunology 41
stress 40
stressor 40
visualization 57

References

1. Lazarus, R., and R. Launier. "Stress-Related Transactions Between Person and Environment" in *Perspectives in Interactional Psychology*. New York: Plenum, 1978.
2. Gadzella, Bernadette. "Student-Life Stress Inventory: Identification of and Reactions to Stressors." *Psychological Reports,* Vol. 74, No. 2, April 1994.
3. Senior, Kathryn. "Should Stress Carry a Health Warning?" *Lancet,* Vol. 357, No. 9250, January 13, 2001, p. 126.
4. Booth, Roger, et al. "The State of the Science: The Best Evidence for the Involvement of Thoughts and Feelings in Physical Health." *Advances in Mind-Body Medicine,* Vol. 17, No. 1, Winter 2001, p. 2.
5. Davis, Mary, et al. "Body Fat Distribution and Hemodynamic Stress Responses in Premenopausal Obese Women: A Preliminary Study." *Health Psychology* Vol. 18, No. 6, November 1999, p. 625.
6. Epel, Elissa. "Can Stress Shape Your Body? Stress and Cortisol Reactivity Among Women with Central Body Fat Distribution." *Yale University, U.S. Dissertation Abstracts International: Section B: The Sciences & Engineering,* Vol. 60, No. 5-B, December 1999, p. 2403.
7. Glaser, Ronald, and Janice Kiecolt-Glaser. *Handbook of Human Stress and Immunity.* San Diego: Academic Press, 1994.
8. Cohen, Sheldon, et al. "Susceptibility to the Common Cold." *Psychosomatic Medicine,* March 1999.
9. Glaser, Ronald, et al. "Chronic Stress Modulates the Immune Response to a Pneumococcal Pneumonia Vaccine." *Psychosomatic Medicine,* Vol. 62, No. 6, November–December 2000, p. 804.
10. Takkouche, Bahi, et al. "Stress and Susceptibility to the Common Cold." *Epdiemiology,* Vol. 11, April 2001, p. 345.
11. Rubin, Aaron, and Karageanes, Steven. "Stress, Cytokine Changes, and Wound Healing." *Physician and Sportsmedicine,* Vol. 28, No. 5, May 2000, p. 21.
12. Turner-Cobb, Julie, et al. "Social Support and Salivary Cortisol in Women with Metastatic Breast Cancer." *Psychosomatic Medicine,* Vol. 62, No. 3, May–June 2000, p. 337.
13. Kiecolt-Glaser, Janice, and Ronald Glaser. "Stress and Immunity: Age Enhances the Risks." *Current Directions in Psychological Science,* Vol. 10, No. 1, February 2001, p. 18.
14. Smyth, Joshua, et al. "Effects of Writing About Stressful Experiences on Symptom Reduction in Patients with Asthma or Rheumatoid Arthritis: A Randomized Trial." *Journal of the American Medical Association,* Vol. 281, No. 14, April 14, 1999.
15. Senior, "Should Stress Carry a Health Warning?"
16. "Stressed Out on Campus." *Techniques,* Vol. 75, No. 3, March 2000.
17. Misra, Ranjita, and Michelle McKean. "College Students, Academic Stress and Its Relation to Their Anxiety, Time Management and Leisure Satisfaction." *American Journal of Health Studies,* Vol. 16, No. 1, Winter 2000.
18. Dixon, Wayne, and Reid, Jon. "Positive Life Events as a Moderator of Stress-Related Depressive Symptoms." *Journal of Counseling and Development,* Vol. 78, No. 3, Summer, 2000.
19. Murray, Bridget. "Peer Mentoring Gives Rookies 'Inside Advice.'" *American Psychological Monitor,* Vol. 29, No. 12, December 1998.
20. Glaser and Kiecolt-Glaser, *Handbook of Human Stress and Immunity.* Hornig-Rohan, Mary. "Stress, Immune-Mediators, and Immune-Mediated Disease." *Advances: The Journal of Mind-Body Health,* Vol. 11, No. 2, Spring 1995.
21. Harrell, Shelly. "A Multidimensional Conceptualization of Racism-Related Stress: Implications for the Well-Being of People of Color." *American Journal of Orthopsychiatry,* Vol. 70, No. 1, January 2000.
22. Launier, Raymond. "Stress Balance and Emotional Life Complexes in Students in a Historically African American College." *Journal of Psychology,* Vol. 131, No. 2, March 1997.
23. Rosenthal, Beth Spenciner, and Schreiner, Arleen Cedeno. "Prevalence of Psychological Symptoms Among Undergraduate Students in an Ethnically Diverse Urban Public College." *Journal of American College Health,* Vol. 49, No. 1, July 2000.
24. Ibid.
25. Ibid.
26. AAA Foundation for Traffic Safety website. http://www.aaafts.org
27. Evans, Sybil. Personal interview.
28. Middleton-Moz, Jane. Personal interview.
29. Bushman, Brad. Personal interview.
30. Helmering, Doris. Personal interview.
31. Evans, Gary, and Dana Johnson. "Stress and Open-Office Noise." *Journal of Applied Psychology,* Vol. 85, No. 5, October 2000.
32. Maslach, Christina, et al. "Job Burnout." *Annual Review of Psychology,* 2001, p. 397.
33. Bargellinia, Annalisa, et al. "Relation Between Immune Variables and Burnout in a Sample of Physicians." *Occupational and Environmental Medicine,* Vol. 57, July 2000.
34. Maslach, "Job Burnout."
35. Jacobsen, Ken. Personal interview.
36. "Driving-Induced Stress in Urban College Students." *Perceptual and Motor Skills,* Vol. 90, No. 2, April 2000.
37. Schuster, Mark et al. "A National Survey of Stress Reactions after the September 11, 2001, Terrorist Attacks," New England Journal of Medicine, Vol. 345, No. 20, November 15, 2001, p. 1507.
38. Saunders, Teri, et al. "The Effect of Stress Inoculation Training on Anxiety and Performance." *Journal of Occupational Health Psychology,* Vol. 1, No. 2, pp. 170–186.

39. Abel, Millicent. "Interaction of Humor and Gender in Moderating Relationships Between Stress and Outcomes." *Journal of Psychology,* Vol. 132, No. 3, May 1998.

40. Pennebaker, James. "Putting Stress into Words: Health, Linguistic and Therapeutic Implications." *Behavioral Research,* Vol. 31, No. 6, 1993.

41. Spiegel, David. "Healing Words: Emotional Expression and Disease Outcome." *Journal of the American Medical Association,* Vol. 281, No. 14, April 14, 1999.

42. Barbar, Cary. "The Science of Meditation." *Psychology Today,* May–June 2001, p. 54.

43. "Is Meditation Good Medicine?" *Harvard Women's Health Watch,* Vol. 8, No. 5, January 2001, p. 1.

44. "Procrastinators Always Finish Last, Even in Health," *American Psychological Monitor,* Vol. 20, No. 1, January 1998.

45. Calhoun, Lawrence, and Richard Tedeschi. "Beyond Recovery from Trauma: Implications for Clinical Practice and Research." *Journal of Social Issues,* Vol. 54, No. 2, Summer 1998.

46. Spiegel, David, and Jose Maldonado. "Dissociative Disorders" in *American Psychiatric Press Textbook of Psychiatry,* 3rd ed., Robert Hales et al. (eds.). Washington, DC: American Psychiatric Press, 1999.

47. Schnyder, Ulrich, et al. "Incidence and Prediction of Posttraumatic Stress Disorder Symptoms in Severely Injured Accident Victims." *American Journal of Psychiatry,* Vol. 158, No. 4, April 2001, p. 594.

48. Wijma, Klaas, et al. "Prevelance of Post-traumatic Stress Disorder Among Gynecological Patients with a History of Sexual and Physical Abuse." *Journal of Interpersonal Violence,* Vol. 15, No. 9, September 2000, p. 944.

49. Duncan, Renae. "Childhood Maltreatment and College Drop-out Rates: Implications for Child Abuse Researchers." *Journal of Interpersonal Violence,* Vol. 15, No. 9, September 2000, p. 987.

50. Lindstroem, Bengt. "The Meaning of Resilience." *International Journal of Adolescent Medicine & Health,* Vol. 13, No. 1, January–March 2001, p. 7.

51. McAdams, Dan, et al. "When Bad Things Turn Good and Good Things Turn Bad: Sequences of Redemption and Contamination in Life Narrative and Their Relation to Psychosocial Adaptation in Midlife Adults and in Students." *Personality & Social Psychology Bulletin,* Vol. 27, No. 4, April 2001, p. 474.

3

Psychological Health

For years, Travis put on his "happy face" around his friends and family. Popular and athletic in high school, he never let anyone know how desperately unhappy he actually felt. "Whatever I was doing during the day, nothing was on my mind more than wanting to die," he recalls. On a perfectly ordinary day in his senior year, Travis tried to kill himself with an overdose of pills. Rushed to a hospital, Travis recovered, resumed his studies, and entered college. By the middle of his freshman year, he was struggling once more with feelings of hopelessness. This time he realized what was happening and sought help from a therapist. "I thought college was supposed to be the happiest time of your life," he said. "What went wrong?"

This is a question many young people might ask. Although youth can seem a golden time, when body and mind glow with potential, the process of becoming an adult is a challenging one in every culture and country. Psychological health can make the difference between facing this challenge with optimism and confidence or feeling overwhelmed by expectations and responsibilities.

Unlike physical health, psychological well-being cannot be measured, tested, X-rayed, or dissected. Yet psychologically healthy men and women generally share certain characteristics: They value themselves and strive toward happiness and fulfillment. They establish and maintain close relationships with others. They accept the limitations as well as the possibilities that life has to offer. And they feel a sense of meaning and purpose that makes the gestures of living worth the effort required.

Feeling good does not depend on money, success, recognition, or status. At any age, at any level of education and achievement, regardless of disability or disease, it is possible to find happiness and fulfillment in life. Achieving the highest possible level of psychological well-being, like achieving peak physical well-being, depends primarily on assuming responsibility for yourself.

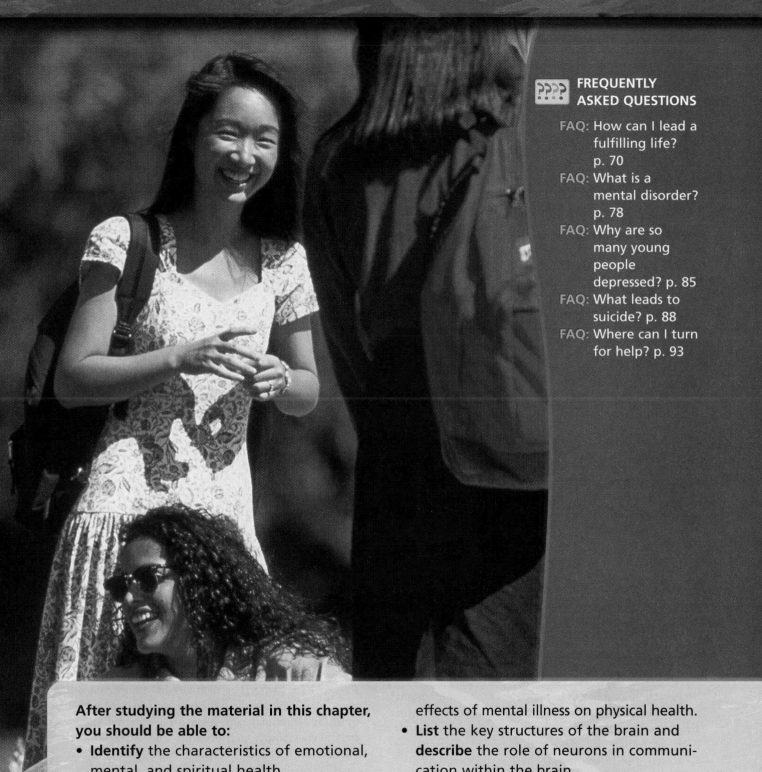

After studying the material in this chapter, you should be able to:

- **Identify** the characteristics of emotional, mental, and spiritual health.
- **Discuss** the concepts of emotional and spiritual intelligence.
- **Describe** the relationship of needs, values, self-esteem, optimism, a sense of control, and relationships to psychological health.
- **Identify** effective coping strategies that promote positive attitudes and actions.
- **Explain** the differences between mental health and mental illness and **list** some effects of mental illness on physical health.
- **List** the key structures of the brain and **describe** the role of neurons in communication within the brain.
- **Describe** the major mental illnesses—anxiety disorders, depressive disorders, attention disorders, and schizophrenia—and the characteristic symptoms of each type.
- **Discuss** some of the factors that may lead to suicide as well as strategies for prevention.
- **Describe** the treatment options available for those with psychological problems.

This isn't always easy. At some point in life, one of every three people develops an emotional disorder. Young adulthood—the years from the late teens to the mid-twenties—is a time when many serious disorders, including bipolar illness (manic depression) and schizophrenia, often develop. The saddest fact is not that so many feel so bad, but that so few realize they can feel better. Only one of every five men and women who could use treatment ever seeks help. Yet 80 to 90 percent of those treated for psychological problems recover, most within a few months.[1]

By learning about psychological disorders, you may be able to recognize early warning signals in yourself or your loved ones so you can deal with potential difficulties or seek professional help for more serious problems.

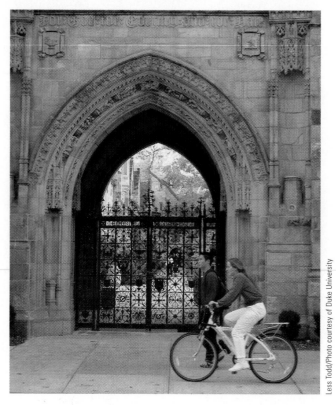

Less Todd/Photo courtesy of Duke University

▲ Psychologically healthy people can adapt to a variety of circumstances, have the ability to form relationships, and strive to achieve their full potential.

What Is Psychological Health?

"A sound mind in a sound body is a short but full description of a happy state in this world," the philosopher John Locke wrote in 1693. More than 300 years later his statement still rings true. Both physical and psychological well-being are essential to total wellness. However, modern theorists have gone beyond these general requirements to analyze other components of well-being, including coping styles, goals, and adaptation to stress and change.[2]

Psychological health encompasses both our emotional and mental states—that is, our feelings and our thoughts. **Emotional health** generally refers to feelings and moods, both of which are discussed later in this chapter. Characteristics of emotionally healthy persons, identified in an analysis of major studies of emotional wellness, include the following:

▶ Determination and effort to be healthy.
▶ Flexibility and adaptability to a variety of circumstances.
▶ Development of a sense of meaning and affirmation of life.
▶ An understanding that the self is not the center of the universe.

▶ Compassion for others.
▶ The ability to be unselfish in serving or relating to others.
▶ Increased depth and satisfaction in intimate relationships.
▶ A sense of control over the mind and body that enables the person to make health-enhancing choices and decisions.[3]

Mental health describes our ability to perceive reality as it is, to respond to its challenges, and to develop rational strategies for living. The mentally healthy person doesn't try to avoid conflicts and distress but can cope with life's transitions, traumas, and losses in a way that allows for emotional stability and growth. The characteristics of mental health include:

▶ The ability to function and carry out responsibilities.
▶ The ability to form relationships.
▶ Realistic perceptions of the motivations of others.
▶ Rational, logical thought processes.
▶ The ability to adapt to change and to cope with adversity.[4]

There is considerable overlap between psychological and **spiritual health,** which involves our ability to identify our basic purpose in life and to experience the fulfillment of achieving our full potential. However, many people consider the two separate. "We like to think that emotional problems have to do with the family, childhood, and trauma—with personal life but not with spirituality," observes Thomas Moore, author of *Care of the Soul,* "Yet it is obvious that the soul, seat of the deepest emotions, can benefit greatly from the gifts of a vivid spiritual life and can suffer when it is deprived of them."[5]

In addition, **culture** helps to define psychological health. While, in one culture, men and women may express feelings with great intensity, shouting in joy or wailing in grief, in another culture such behavior might be considered abnormal or unhealthy. In our diverse society, many cultural influences affect Americans' sense of who they are, where they came from, and what they believe. Cultural rituals help bring people together, strengthen their bonds, reinforce the values and beliefs they share, and provide a sense of belonging, meaning, and purpose.

Emotional Intelligence

Once a person's "IQ"—or intelligence quotient—was considered the leading determinant of achievement. However, psychologists have determined that another "way of knowing," dubbed **emotional intelligence,** may make an even greater difference in a person's personal and professional success. In his international best-seller on what some call "EQ" (for emotional quotient), psychologist Daniel Goleman identified five components of emotional intelligence: self-awareness, altruism, personal motivation, empathy, and the ability to love and be loved by friends, partners, and family members. People who possess high emotional intelligence are the people who truly succeed in work as well as play, building flourishing careers and lasting, meaningful relationships.[6]

Men and women, who vary more in the intensity of their emotional experiences than in the nature of their emotions, are equally capable of cultivating greater emotional intelligence. Emotional intelligence isn't fixed at birth, nor is it the same as intuition. Among the emotional competencies that most benefit students are focusing on clear, manageable goals and identifying and understanding emotions rather than relying on "gut" feelings.[7]

Spiritual Intelligence

Spiritual approaches to knowledge and well-being have recently become the focus of scholarly interest and research. As noted in Chapter 1, a growing number of research studies are assessing the impact of spirituality on health, and nearly 30 medical schools include courses on religion, spirituality, and health in their curricula.[8]

Mental health professionals also are recognizing the power of **spiritual intelligence,** which some define as "the capacity to sense, understand, and tap into the highest parts of ourselves, others, and the world around us." What distinguishes spiritual intelligence from spirituality is that it does not center on the worship of a God above, but on the discovery of a wisdom within. All of us are born with the potential to develop spiritual intelligence, but relatively few do. Yet its dividends are many. As one minister put it, this way of knowing provides solutions—often surprising and unexpected—to problems that had seemed insolvable.[9]

Here are some guidelines for tapping into your own spiritual intelligence:

▷ Build silence and solitude into your daily life. Even a few stolen moments in the early morning or evening hours can help quiet the hum of constant distractions. "There is an inner wisdom," says cardiologist

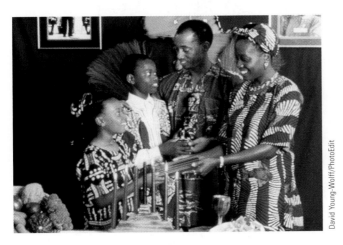
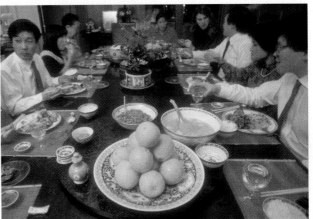

▲ Special holidays, such as Kwanzaa and Chinese New Year, bring people together in cultural celebration.

Dean Ornish, "but it speaks very, very softly." He suggests ending each session with a question like "What am I not paying attention to that's important?"[10]

▶ Spend time in nature. A walk on the beach, a stroll through a park, or simply looking up at the night sky has value—perhaps because nature helps put our mostly man-made problems into perspective.

▶ Keep company with the wise—either in person or through their words. Inspirational people or their writings provide both factual knowledge and insight that enable us to examine serious issues.

▶ Reflect on the nature of life and death. You don't need a doctorate in philosophy for this task, because the basic principles are simple: Life is precious. Life is short. Death is certain. While life involves difficulties, these can be transcended rather than avoided.

▶ Practice spiritual values. Spiritual intelligence is not a spectator sport. Rather than just contemplating kindness and honesty, we have to live them as best we can. One of the best places to learn and practice forgiveness is on the highway.

???? How Can I Lead a Fulfilling Life?

"What's it all about?" We all ask this question sooner or later. Whether dreams come true or fade away, whether we achieve our goals or not, we find ourselves confronting profound questions about the purpose of our time on Earth. There is no recipe that can guarantee a life worth living. Each of us must create life satisfaction on our own.

Psychology, a field that traditionally concentrated on what goes wrong in our lives and in our minds, has shifted its focus to the study of what goes right. "Positive psychology" emphasizes building personal strengths rather than treating weaknesses. One of its key beliefs is that young people who learn to be optimistic and resilient are less likely to suffer from mental disorders and more likely to lead happy, productive lives.

Positive attitudes may even prolong life In a study that has followed 678 Catholic nuns into old age, those who expressed more positive emotions, such as joy, love, hope, and happiness in autobiographies written in their twenties, lived as much as ten years longer than those expressing fewer positive emotions.[11]

Knowing Your Needs

Newborns are unable to survive on their own. They depend on others for the satisfaction of their physical needs for food, shelter, warmth, and protection, as well as their less tangible emotional needs. In growing to maturity, children take on more responsibility and become more independent. No one, however, becomes totally self-sufficient. As adults, we easily recognize our basic physical needs, but we often fail to acknowledge our emotional needs. Yet they, too, must be met if we are to be as fulfilled as possible.

The humanist theorist Abraham Maslow believed that human needs are the motivating factors in personality development. First, we must satisfy basic physiological needs, such as those for food, shelter, and sleep. Only then can we pursue fulfillment of our higher needs—for safety and security, love and affection, and self-esteem. Few individuals reach the state of **self-actualization,** in which one functions at the highest possible level and derives the greatest possible satisfaction from life. (See Figure 3-1.)

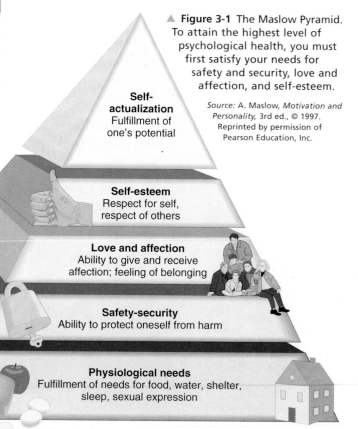

▲ **Figure 3-1** The Maslow Pyramid. To attain the highest level of psychological health, you must first satisfy your needs for safety and security, love and affection, and self-esteem.

Source: A. Maslow, *Motivation and Personality,* 3rd ed., © 1997. Reprinted by permission of Pearson Education, Inc.

Self-actualization
Fulfillment of one's potential

Self-esteem
Respect for self, respect of others

Love and affection
Ability to give and receive affection; feeling of belonging

Safety-security
Ability to protect oneself from harm

Physiological needs
Fulfillment of needs for food, water, shelter, sleep, sexual expression

Clarifying Your Values

Your **values** are the criteria by which you evaluate things, people, events, and yourself; they represent what's most important to you. In a world of almost dizzying complexity, values can provide guidelines for making decisions that are right for you. If understood and applied, they help give life meaning and structure.

Social psychologist Milton Rokeach distinguished between two types of values. *Instrumental* values represent ways of thinking and acting that we hold important, such as being loving or loyal. *Terminal* values represent goals, achievements, or ideal states that we strive toward, such as happiness. Instrumental and terminal values form the basis for your attitudes and your behavior.

There can be a large discrepancy between what people say they value and what their actions indicate about their values. That's why it's important to clarify your own values, making sure you understand what you believe so that you can live in accordance with your beliefs. To do so, follow these steps:

1. Carefully consider the consequences of each choice.
2. Choose freely from among all the options.
3. Publicly affirm your values by sharing them with others.
4. Act out your values.

Values clarification is not a once-in-a-lifetime task, but an ongoing process of sorting out what matters most to you. If you believe in protecting the environment, do you shut off lights, or walk rather than drive, in order to conserve energy? Do you vote for political candidates who support environmental protection? Do you recycle newspapers, bottles, and cans? Values are more than ideals we'd like to attain; they should be reflected in the way we live day by day.

Boosting Self-Esteem

Each of us wants and needs to feel significant as a human being with unique talents, abilities, and roles in life. A sense of **self-esteem,** of belief or pride in ourselves, gives us confidence to dare to attempt to achieve at school or work and to reach out to others to form friendships and close relationships. Self-esteem is the little voice that whispers, "You're worth it. You can do it. You're okay."

Self-esteem is based, not on external factors like wealth or beauty, but on what you believe about yourself. It's not something you're born with; self-esteem develops over time. It's also not something anyone else can give to you, although those around you can either help boost or diminish your self-esteem.

The seeds of self-esteem are planted in childhood when parents provide the assurance and appreciation youngsters need to push themselves toward new accomplishments: crawling, walking, forming words and sentences, learning control over their bladder and bowels.

Adults, too, must consider themselves worthy of love, friendship, and success if they are to be loved, to make friends, and to achieve their goals. Low self-esteem is more common in people who have been abused as children and in those with psychiatric disorders, including depression, anxiety, alcoholism, and drug dependence. Feeling one did not receive love and encouragement as a child can also lead to poor self-esteem. Adults with poor self-esteem may

STRATEGIES FOR CHANGE

Being True to Yourself

✔ Take the tombstone test: What would you like to have written on your tombstone? In other words, how would you like to be remembered? Your honest answer should tell you, very succinctly, what you value most.

✔ Describe yourself, as you are today, in a brief sentence. Ask friends or family members for their descriptions of you. How would you have to change to become the person you want to be remembered as?

✔ Try the adjective test: Choose three adjectives that you'd like to see associated with your reputation. Then list what you've done or can do to earn such descriptions.

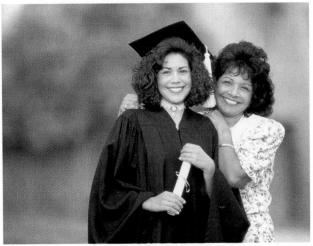

© 2000 Bob Torrez/Stone

▲ Self-esteem is based on what you believe about yourself, and it tends to increase when you experience success.

unconsciously enter relationships that reinforce their self-perceptions and may prefer and even seek out people who think poorly of them.

One of the most useful techniques for bolstering self-esteem and achieving your goals is developing the habit of positive thinking and talking. While negative observations, such as constant criticisms or reminders of the most minor of faults, can undermine self-image, positive affirmations—compliments, kudos, encouragements—have proven effective in enhancing self-esteem and psychological well-being. Individuals who fight off negative thoughts fare better psychologically than those who collapse when a setback occurs or who rely on others to make them feel better.

 True self-esteem requires an honest sense of your own worth. In a study of college students, psychology professors followed "self-enhancers" who began their freshman year with an inflated sense of their own academic ability. These students expected to get much higher college grades than might be expected based on their high school grades and test scores. While they felt confident and happy for a while, they did no better academically and were no more likely to graduate than their realistic or self-deprecating peers. In fact, the short-term benefits of their self-illusions took a toll over the long term: Their self-esteem and interest in school declined with each passing year.[12]

Managing Your Moods

Feelings come and go within minutes. A **mood** is a more sustained emotional state that colors our view of the world for hours or days. According to surveys by psychologist Randy Larsen, of the University of Michigan, bad moods descend upon us an average of three out of every ten days. "A few people—about 2 percent—are happy just about every day," he says. "About 5 percent report bad moods four out of every five days."[13]

There are gender differences in mood management: Men typically try to distract themselves (a partially successful strategy) or use alcohol or drugs (an ineffective tactic). Women are more likely to talk to someone (which can help) or to ruminate on why they feel bad (which doesn't help).[14] Learning effective mood-boosting, mood-regulating strategies can help both men and women pull themselves up and out of an emotional slump. (See "Pulse Points: Ten Ways to Pull Yourself out of a Bad Mood.")

The most effective way to banish a sad or bad mood is by changing what caused it in the first place—if you can figure out what made you upset and why. "Most bad moods are caused by loss or failure in work or intimate relationships," says Larsen. "The questions to ask are: What can I do to fix the failure? What can I do to remedy the loss? Is there anything under my control that I can change? If there is, take action and solve it." Rewrite the report. Ask to take a make-up exam. Apologize to the friend whose feelings you hurt. Tell your parents you feel bad about the argument you had.

If there's nothing you can do, accept what happened and focus on doing things differently next time. "In our studies, resolving to try harder actually was as effective in improving mood as taking action in the present," says Larsen. You also can try to think about what happened in a different way and put a positive spin on it. This technique, known as *cognitive reappraisal,* or "reframing," helps you look at a setback in a new light: What lessons did it teach you? What would you have done differently? Could there be a silver lining or hidden benefit?

If you can't identify or resolve the problem responsible for your emotional funk, the next-best solution is to concentrate on altering your negative feelings. For example, try setting a quick, achievable goal that can boost your spirits with a small success. Clean out a closet; sort through

STRATEGIES FOR CHANGE

How to Talk to Yourself

✔ To make sure you're sending yourself the right messages, tune into the unspoken commentary playing in your head.

✔ If you spot a self-put-down (e.g., "What a klutz!" or "I screwed up again!"), scream (silently) "STOP!" or "DELETE!" Then give yourself a compliment to replace the criticism.

✔ If you hear your mind replaying the same negative observations again and again, try to trace them back to their source. Did they come from your parents, teachers, siblings? Say, "That's what they think, but it's not necessarily true."

✔ Make a list of the qualities you like best about yourself. Replay the list in your mind when you're feeling down about yourself.

✔ Spend more time doing those activities you know you do best. For example, if you are a good cook, prepare a meal for someone; if you are good at writing, write a letter to someone.

✔ Separate what you do, especially any mistakes you make, from who you are. Instead of saying, "I'm so stupid," tell yourself, "That wasn't the smartest move I ever made, but I'll learn from it."

PULSE POINTS

Ten Ways to Pull Yourself Out of a Bad Mood

1. **Accentuate the positive.** Think of the parts of your life that are going well rather than mulling over what's not.

2. **Review past successes.** Remind yourself of what you've accomplished before to motivate yourself to accomplish more in the future.

3. **Pray.** In a Gallup poll of 1007 Americans, religious practices rated as the most effective way of relieving depression.

4. **Listen to music.** While many forms of distraction help, at least temporarily, this is one of the most popular and effective mood boosters.

5. **Treat yourself.** Indulgences—big or small, expensive or not—can bring you up when you're feeling down. The reason: They make you feel special.

6. **Volunteer.** A third of Americans—some 89 million people—give of themselves through volunteer work. By doing the same, you may feel better too.

7. **Exercise.** In various studies around the world, physical exertion ranks as one of the best ways to change a bad mood, raise energy, and reduce tension.

8. **Act happy.** Putting on a happy face doesn't make problems disappear, but it does improve mood.

9. **Focus on the future.** Although you can't rewrite the past, you can learn from it. Resolve to try harder and do better the next time around.

10. **Set a limit on self-pity.** Tell yourself, "I'm going to feel sorry for myself this morning, but this afternoon, I've got to get on with my life."

---

the piles of paper on your desk; write the letter to your aunt you've been putting off for weeks.

Another good option is to get moving. In studies of mood regulation, exercise consistently ranks as the single most effective strategy for banishing bad feelings. Numerous studies have confirmed that aerobic workouts, such as walking or jogging, significantly improve mood. Even nonaerobic exercise, such as weight lifting, can boost spirits; improve sleep and appetite; reduce anxiety, irritability, and anger; and produce feelings of mastery and accomplishment.

Although it's tempting to pull away from others when you're in a slump, it's better not to withdraw. "It's never a good idea to sulk by yourself when you're feeling down," says Larsen. "Pretend to be extroverted if you have to, but do spend time with other people." As he notes, friends often can help improve your mood by giving you good feedback. But be wary of seeking out companions solely for a gripe-and-groan session. You might end up feeling worse rather than better.

Taking your mind off your troubles, rather than mulling over what's wrong, is one of the most often used mood boosters, but it's only partly successful. Simple distractions—watching television, for instance, or reading—work only temporarily. Activities that engage the imagination, on the other hand, seem to have more lasting effects. Listening to music, for instance, is one of the most popular and effective ways of distracting people from their troubles and changing their bad moods.

Finding Happiness

Psychologist David Myers, author of *The Pursuit of Happiness: Who Is Happy—and Why*, defines happiness as "a sense of well-being, a feeling that life as a whole is going well."[15] This state depends not on big achievements, but on little pleasures. Happiness tends to be highest when people combine frequent good experiences—the daily joys of having a caring partner, a productive job, or enjoyable hobbies—with occasional very intense pleasures, such as a special vacation or a promotion.

An individual's happiness level may be largely genetic. In a study of sets of twins raised separately and together, psychologists concluded that, in the same way that humans may have a weight set point (discussed in Chapter 6), we also have a happiness set point. Although it fluctuates somewhat, it rarely changes radically.

Psychologists distinguish between two kinds of happiness: *feel-good* and *value-based*. Feel-good happiness is pleasure based on sensations, such as eating well or joking around with friends, and rarely lasts more than a few hours. Value-based happiness stems from our deeper purpose and values and represents a spiritual source of satisfaction that gives our lives lasting meaning.[16]

 Value-based happiness has a surprisingly small relationship to age, gender, or ethnicity. However, countries differ appreciably in the happiness of their people. In general, happiness is greater in more prosperous countries, but even in the more affluent nations there seems little relationship between wealth and happiness for people who have the basic necessities of life. In poor countries, the rich are significantly happier than the poor. Throughout the world, married people are happier than unmarried individuals, and religious people are happier than those who aren't religious.[17]

 Having an unhappy childhood does not doom anyone to a lifetime of misery, but it does increase the likelihood of unhappiness in adulthood. In a study of community college students, the vast majority reported a happy or very happy childhood. Only 9 percent of these students were unhappy as adults. About two-thirds of those reporting unhappy or very unhappy childhoods reported that they were unhappy or very unhappy adults. The risk of having an unhappy adulthood was two and a half times greater for those who'd been unhappy as children.[18]

The best predictors of happiness are the characteristics of good psychological health: high self-esteem, optimism, extroversion, and a sense of being in control. In addition to these four key traits, happy people are more likely to have healthy and fit bodies; realistic goals and expectations; supportive friendships; an intimate, sexually warm marriage; and a faith that provides support, purpose, and acceptance.

Although research indicates no clear relationship between wealth and happiness in developed countries, many people still equate more money with more happiness. Yet individuals who seek nonmaterial sources of fulfillment are far more likely to find joy, says psychologist Mihaly Csikszentmihalyi. By studying the lives of thousands of people, he discovered that the happiest regularly experienced what he calls "flow," a state of deep focus that occurs when individuals engage in challenging tasks that demand intense concentration and commitment. By this definition, a challenging game of chess can bring more happiness than a spin in a new sports car.[19]

Not even disability and illness are bars to happiness. One study of individuals who suffered accidents resulting in quadriplegia and paraplegia found that within six months the two groups reported nearly identical levels of happiness, despite the differences in the severity of their injuries.[20]

Happiness is not just a state of mind but quite literally a state of brain. By means of sophisticated imaging techniques, neuroscientists have discovered differences in brain chemistry and activity when people are experiencing happiness, sadness, and other moods. In both women and men, happiness activates a specific region in the area of the brain called the frontal cortex.[21]

 Happiness affects brain functions as well as the brain itself. Studies have found differences in basic information processing when individuals had to recognize or name certain words, depending on their perceived happiness.[22] It also matters whether people link their feelings of happiness to positive or negative life events. In a study of 89 college students, the "linkers" were most likely to see their happiness as contingent on attaining important goals in life.[23]

Becoming Optimistic

The dictionary defines **optimism** as "an inclination to anticipate the best possible outcome." For various reasons—because they believe in themselves, because they trust in a higher power, because they feel lucky—optimists expect positive experiences from life. When bad things happen, they tend to see setbacks or losses as specific, temporary incidents. In their eyes, a disappointment is "one of those things" that happens every once in a while, rather than the latest in a long string of disasters. And rather than blaming themselves ("I always mess things up," pessimists might say), optimists look at all the different factors that may have caused the problem.

Individuals aren't born optimistic or pessimistic; in fact, researchers have documented changes over time in the ways that individuals view the world and what they expect to experience in the future. The key is disputing the automatic negative thoughts that flood our brains and choosing to believe in our own possibilities.

Looking on the Light Side

Humor, which enables us to express fears and negative feelings without causing distress to ourselves or others, is one of the healthiest ways of coping with life's ups and downs. Laughter stimulates the heart, alters brain wave patterns and breathing rhythms, reduces perceptions of

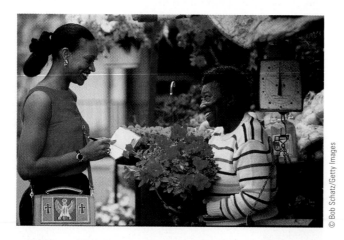

▲ Happiness and optimism go hand in hand. Small rewards can keep your spirits high and remind you that you are special.

© Bob Schatz/Getty Images

STRATEGIES FOR CHANGE

How to Be Happy

✔ Make time for yourself. It's impossible to meet the needs of others without recognizing and fulfilling your own.

✔ Invest yourself in closeness. Give your loved ones the gift of your time and caring.

✔ Work hard at what you like. Search for challenges that satisfy your need to do something meaningful.

✔ Be upbeat. If you always look for what's wrong about yourself or your life, you'll find it—and feel even worse.

✔ Organize but stay loose. Be ready to seize an unexpected opportunity to try something different.

✔ Despite inevitable highs and lows, strive for a sense of balance.

pain, decreases stress-related hormones, and strengthens the immune system. In psychotherapy, humor helps channel negative emotions toward a positive effect. Even in cases of critical or fatal illnesses, humor can relieve pain and help people live with greater joy until they die.[24]

Joking and laughing are ways of expressing honest emotions, of overcoming dread and doubt, and of connecting with others. They also can defuse rage. After all, it's almost impossible to stay angry when you're laughing. To tickle your funny bone, try keeping a file of favorite cartoons or jokes. Go to a comedy club instead of a movie. And when you see or hear something that makes you laugh out loud, don't keep it to yourself—multiply the mirth by sharing it with a friend.

Loving and Being Loved

"One can live magnificently in this world if one knows how to work and how to love, to work for the person one loves and to love one's work," Leo Tolstoy wrote. You may not think of love as a basic need like food and rest, but it is essential for both physical and psychological well-being.

Mounting evidence suggests that people who lack love and commitment are at high risk for a host of illnesses, including infections, heart disease, and cancer. "Love and intimacy are at the root of what makes us sick and what

makes us well," says cardiologist Dean Ornish, author of *Love & Survival: The Scientific Basis for the Healing Power of Intimacy.* "No other factor in medicine—not diet, not smoking, not exercise—has a greater impact."[25]

Doing Good

Altruism—helping or giving to others—enhances self-esteem, relieves physical and mental stress, and protects psychological well-being. Hans Selye, the father of stress research, described cooperation with others for the self's sake as altruistic egotism, whereby we satisfy our own needs while helping others satisfy theirs. This concept is essentially an updated version of the golden rule: Do unto others as you would have them do unto you. The important difference is that you earn your neighbor's love and help by offering them love and help.

Giving helps those who give as well as those who receive. People involved in community organizations, for instance, consistently report a surge of well-being called *helper's high,* which they describe as a unique sense of calmness, warmth, and enhanced self-worth. College students who provided community service as part of a semester-long course reported changes in attitude (including a decreased tendency to blame people for their misfortunes), self-esteem (primarily a belief that they can make a difference), and behavior (a greater commitment to do more volunteer work).

The options for giving of yourself are limitless: Volunteer to serve a meal at a homeless shelter. Collect donations for a charity auction. Teach in an illiteracy program. Perform the simplest act of charity: Pray for others.

Feeling in Control

Although no one has absolute control over destiny, we can do a great deal to control how we think, feel, and behave. By assessing our life situations realistically, we can make plans and preparations that allow us to make the most of our circumstances. By doing so, we gain a sense of mastery. In nationwide surveys, Americans who feel in control of their lives report greater psychological well-being than those who do not, as well as "extraordinarily positive feelings of happiness."[26]

Developing Autonomy

One goal that many people strive for is **autonomy**, or independence. Both family and society influence our ability to grow toward independence. Autonomous individuals are true to themselves. As they weigh the pros and cons of

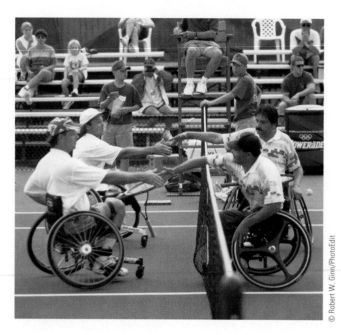

© Robert W. Ginn/PhotoEdit

▲ You may not have complete control over your destiny, but you can control how you respond to challenges. Even under the most difficult of circumstances, it is usually not impossible to gain a sense of mastery.

STRATEGIES FOR CHANGE

Asserting Yourself

✔ Use "I" statements to explain your feelings. This allows you to take ownership of your opinions and feelings without putting down others for how they feel and think.

✔ Listen to and acknowledge what the other person says. After you speak, find out if the other person understands your position. Ask how he or she feels about what you've said.

✔ Be direct and specific. Describe the problem as you see it, using neutral language rather than assigning blame. Also suggest a specific solution, but make clear that you'd like the lines of communication and negotiation to remain open.

✔ Don't think you have to be obnoxious in order to be assertive. It's most effective to state your needs and preferences without any sarcasm or hostility.

any decision, whether it's using or refusing drugs or choosing a major or career, they base their judgment on their own values, not those of others. Their ability to draw on internal resources and cope with challenges has a positive impact on both their psychological well-being and their physical health, including recovery from illness. Those who've achieved autonomy may seek the opinions of others, but they do not allow their decisions to be dictated by external influences. For autonomous individuals, their **locus of control**—that is, where they view control as originating—is *internal* (from within themselves) rather than *external* (from others).

Asserting Yourself

Being **assertive** means recognizing your feelings and making your needs and desires clear to others. Unlike aggression, a far less healthy means of expression, assertiveness usually works. You can change a situation you don't like by communicating your feelings and thoughts in nonprovocative words, by focusing on specifics, and by making sure you're talking with the person who is directly responsible.

Becoming assertive isn't always easy. Many people have learned to cope by being passive and not communicating their feelings or opinions. Sooner or later they become so irritated, frustrated, or overwhelmed that they explode in an outburst—which they think of as being

assertive. However, such behavior is so distasteful to them that they'd rather be passive. But assertiveness doesn't mean screaming or telling someone off. You can communicate your wishes calmly and clearly. Assertiveness is a behavior that respects your rights and the rights of other people even when you disagree.

Even at its mildest, assertiveness can make you feel better about yourself and your life. The reason: When you speak up or take action, you're in the pilot seat. And that's always much less stressful than taking a back seat and trying to hang on for dear life.

Connecting with Others

At every age, people who feel connected to others tend to be healthier physically and psychologically.[27] College students are no exception: Those who have a supportive, readily available network of relationships are less psychologically distressed and more satisfied with life. (See Chapter 7 for a comprehensive discussion of communication, friendship, and intimacy.)

The opposite of *connectedness* is **social isolation,** a major risk factor for illness and early death. Individuals with few social contacts face two to four times the mortality rate of others. The reason may be that their social isolation weakens the body's ability to ward off disease. Medical students with higher-than-average scores on a loneliness scale had lower levels of protective immune cells.[28] The end of a long-term relationship—through separation, divorce, or death—also dampens immunity.

It is part of our nature as mammals and as human beings to crave relationships. But invariably we end up alone at times. Solitude is not without its own quiet joys—time for introspection, self-assessment, learning from the past, and looking toward the future. Each of us can cultivate the joy of our company, of being alone without crossing the line and becoming lonely.

Overcoming Loneliness

More so than many other countries, we are a nation of loners. Recent trends—longer work hours, busy family schedules, frequent moves, high divorce rates—have created even more lonely people. Only 23 percent of Americans say they're never lonely. Loneliest of all are those who are divorced, separated, or widowed and those who live alone or solely with children. Among single adults who have never been married, 42 percent feel lonely at least sometimes. However, loneliness is most likely to cause emotional distress when it is a chronic rather than an episodic condition.[29]

To combat loneliness, people may join groups, fling themselves into projects and activities, or surround themselves with superficial acquaintances. Others avoid the effort of trying to connect, sometimes limiting most of their personal interactions to chat groups on the Internet.

The Internet may actually make people feel lonelier. In the first study of the social and psychological effects of Internet use at home, researchers at Carnegie Mellon University found that people who spend even a few hours a week online have higher levels of depression and loneliness than those who use the Internet less frequently. "Virtual" communication, it seems, does not provide the same benefits as old-fashioned, face-to-face relationships.[30]

The true keys to overcoming loneliness are developing resources to fulfill our own potential and learning to reach out to others. In this way, loneliness can become a means to personal growth and discovery.

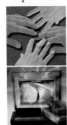 Race and gender also affect the experience of loneliness. In a study of 100 African-American undergraduates, having a best friend was the most important factor in low levels of emotional loneliness in men and high levels of feeling in control in women.[31] Some studies have found that men are lonelier than women. Others find no gender differences in loneliness, but researchers note that men, particularly those who score high on measures of mas-

culinity, are more hesitant than women to admit that they're lonely.[32]

 In cross-cultural studies, married people of all ages generally report less loneliness than single individuals and than unmarried individuals living together. In most nations, having children has little or no effect on how lonely people feel.[33] Even in middle and old age, the childless are not more vulnerable to loneliness or depression. Widowed and divorced men and women report higher levels of loneliness and depression than married people, regardless of whether they have children.[34]

 Loneliness also affects positive health practices among college students. Those who do not have a network of supportive relationships report feeling a sense of utter aloneness, of living in a barren environment, of feeling empty and hollow, and of frequently experiencing boredom and aimlessness. These students also feel least motivated to take the best possible care of their minds and bodies.

Facing Social Anxieties

Many people are uncomfortable meeting strangers or speaking or performing in public. In some surveys, as many as 40 percent of people describe themselves as shy, or socially anxious. Some shy people—an estimated 10 to 15 percent of children—are born with a predisposition to shyness. Others become shy because they don't learn proper social responses or because they experience rejection or shame. As a result, normal apprehension intensifies in situations in which they might be watched or criticized by others. They feel extremely self-conscious, embarrassed, and nervous. When attention is on them alone, they may tremble, breathe very rapidly (hyperventilate), sweat, or develop a dry mouth or nausea.

Social anxieties often become a problem in late adolescence. Students may develop symptoms when they go to a party or are called on in class. Some experience symptoms when they try to perform any sort of action in the presence of others, even such everyday activities as eating in public, using a public restroom, or writing a check. About 7 percent of the population could be diagnosed with a severe form of social anxiety, called **social phobia,** in which individuals typically fear and avoid various social situations.[35] Adolescents and young adults with severe social anxiety are at increased risk of major depression.[36] Phobias are discussed later in this chapter. The key difference between these problems and normal shyness and self-consciousness is the degree of distress and impairment that individuals experience.

If you're shy, you can overcome much of your social apprehensiveness on your own, in much the same way as you might set out to stop smoking or lose weight. For example, you can improve your social skills by pushing

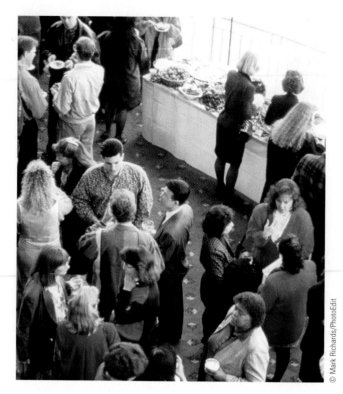

▲ Social situations can be extremely uncomfortable if you suffer from social anxieties. But over time you can overcome shyness by forcing yourself to interact with others.

yourself to introduce yourself to a stranger at a party or to chat about the weather or the food selections with the person next to you in a cafeteria line. Gradually you'll acquire a sense of social timing and a verbal ease that will take the worry out of close encounters with others.

Those with more disabling social anxiety may do best with professional guidance, which has proven highly effective. One common technique used by experts is role playing, in which individuals act out situations that normally produce butterflies in the stomach, such as returning a defective product to a store or calling for a date. With practice and time, most individuals are able to emerge from the walls that shyness has built around them and take pleasure in interacting with others.

Understanding Mental Health

Mentally healthy individuals value themselves, perceive reality as it is, accept their limitations and possibilities, carry out their responsibilities, establish and maintain close relationships, pursue work that suits their talent and training, and feel a sense of fulfillment that makes the efforts of daily living worthwhile (see Figure 3-2).

According to research conducted by the World Health Organization (WHO), mental disorders affect 400 million people around the world, and these numbers will surge even higher in the coming decades.[37] In its first-ever official report on mental health, the Office of the U.S. Surgeon General called for increased efforts to recognize, treat, and prevent mental disorders "We now realize that, just as things can go wrong with the heart, the lungs, the kidneys, and the liver, things can also go wrong with the human brain," observes Surgeon General David Satcher, M.D. "A person cannot be truly healthy overall without mental health."[38]

???? What Is a Mental Disorder?

While lay people may speak of "nervous breakdowns" or "insanity," these are not scientific terms. The U.S. government's official definition states that a serious mental illness is "a diagnosable mental, behavioral, or emotional disorder that interferes with one or more major activities in life, like dressing, eating, or working." According to the U.S. Surgeon General, one in five Americans experiences a mental disorder in the course of a year.[39]

The mental health profession's standard for diagnosing a mental disorder is the pattern of symptoms, or diagnostic criteria, spelled out for the almost 300 disorders in the American Psychiatric Association's *Diagnostic and Statistical Manual,* 4th edition (DSM-IV). It defines a **mental disorder** as "a clinically significant behavioral or psychological syndrome or pattern that occurs in an individual and that

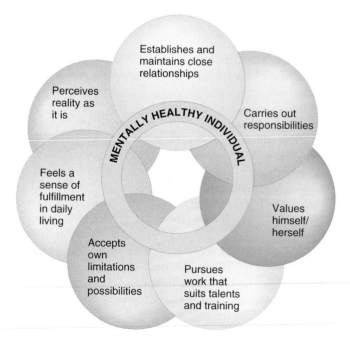

▲ **Figure 3-2** The mentally healthy individual. Mental well-being is a combination of many factors.

is associated with present distress (a painful symptom) or disability (impairment in one or more important areas of functioning) or with a significantly increased risk of suffering death, pain, disability, or an important loss of freedom."[40] (See Self-Survey: "Is Something Wrong?")

Does Mental Health Affect Physical Health?

Mental disorders affect not just the mind but also the body. **Anxiety** can lead to intensified asthmatic reactions, skin conditions, and digestive disorders. Stress can play a role in hypertension, heart attacks, sudden cardiac death, and immune disorders.

Depression has increasingly been recognized as a serious risk factor for physical illness. According to several studies by the Cardiovascular Health Study Research Group, individuals older than 65 with frequent symptoms of depression are as much as 40 percent more likely to develop heart disease and 60 percent more likely to die from any cause. The elderly aren't the only ones at risk. A study at Johns Hopkins University found that depressed male physicians were more than two times as likely to

---

SELF SURVEY

Is Something Wrong?

Which of the following apply to you? Think about how you've been feeling over the past month, and check all that apply. Be honest with yourself.

- Feel depressed or sad for several weeks ❏
- Lack energy or feel tired all the time ❏
- Take no joy or pleasure in normally enjoyable activities ❏
- Think or talk about suicide ❏
- Experience extreme mood swings ❏
- Feel helpless or hopeless ❏
- Feel excessively anxious ❏
- Abuse alcohol or drugs ❏
- Show a marked change in personality ❏
- Feel unable to cope with problems and daily activities ❏
- Show marked changes in eating or sleeping patterns ❏
- Feel extremely angry, hostile, or violent ❏
- Express bizarre or grandiose ideas ❏
- Am unable to control or stop destructive behavior, like gambling or drinking ❏
- Have troubling physical symptoms with no known medical cause ❏
- See things, experience sensations, or hear voices that don't exist ❏

The more boxes that describe what you (or someone close to you) have been experiencing in recent weeks, the more reason you have to be concerned that something may be wrong. This chapter provides information on common mental disorders, as well as guidance on finding and evaluating a therapist and advice on coping with everyday problems.

Psychological symptoms don't mean that you have a mental disorder, but they do indicate you need help in sorting out your life. Just as your body sometimes breaks down under the normal strain of day-to-day living, your mind also is vulnerable to dysfunction. Seeking help is the first step to feeling better and finding solutions to your problems. If you are struggling with a problem, you may want to schedule an appointment with a mental health professional at your school's counseling or student health-services facility.

Making Changes

Deciding If You Need Help

If you are still unsure about whether to seek help, the following questions may help in making the decision:

- Are emotional problems getting in the way of your work, relationships, or other aspects of your personal life?
- Have you been feeling less happy, less confident, and less in control than usual for a period of several weeks or longer?
- Have you reached the point of being so unhappy that you want to do something about it?
- Have trusted friends or family members commented on changes in your behavior and personality?
- Have your own efforts to deal with a problem failed to resolve the situation?
- Is dealing with everyday problems more of a struggle than it used to be?
- Do you feel emotionally "stuck" and helpless to change your own behavior or the circumstances you are in?

The key question to ask yourself is not, "Am I mentally ill?" or "Do I have serious problems?" but "Could I use some help right now?" If the answer is yes, do it. Therapy may turn out to be a catalyst and tool for change or a source of support when you need it most. At the very least, the psychological equivalent of a checkup can make sure that a problem isn't more serious than you may have realized.

develop heart disease as their colleagues. Together, depression and heart disease worsen a patient's prognosis more than either condition does alone. Depressed patients are two to five times more likely to die in the first six to twelve months following a heart attack.[41]

Depression increases other health risks as well. In a British study, cuts were slower to heal in depressed patients than in individuals who were not depressed.[42] Depression has been shown to hasten the changes in bone mass that lead to osteoporosis and to accelerate the progression of HIV infection in women, resulting in more complications and lower survival rates.[43] Since depression can and often does recur, physicians now view it as a chronic illness with lifelong implications for mental and physical health.[44]

By some estimates, as many as 60 percent of those who seek help from physicians suffer primarily from a psychological problem. Treating mental health problems leads not only to improved health but also to lower health-care costs. According to various studies, mental health care has reduced annual medical costs by 9.5 to 21 percent. Psychiatric treatment reduces hospitalizations, cuts medical expenses, and reduces work disability.

Diversity and Mental Health on Campus

College students have traditionally been viewed as psychologically troubled. Studies in the 1970s and 1980s concluded that half to three-quarters of students might have "significant emotional difficulties," while a smaller number—estimated from 10 to 40 percent—suffered more serious "psychological impairment." Many predicted that as campuses became more diverse in ethnicity and gender, rates of mental disorders would rise.

More recent studies of ethnic and gender differences challenged this assumption. The few that have looked into ethnic variations yielded conflicting or inconclusive results: Some found no differences; others suggested higher rates of depression among Korean and South Asian students. Studies comparing male and female students have also been inconclusive. Some reported higher rates of depression and anxiety in women; others showed no difference.

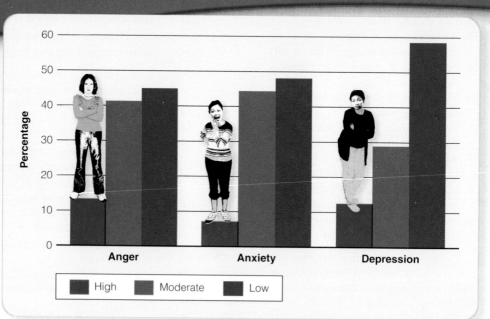

Student Snapshot Mental Disorders on Campus

Freshmen Reporting Psychological Symptoms

In a study of 595 ethnically diverse freshmen, the majority of participants reported experiencing moderate to low levels of anger, anxiety, and depression. Fewer than 15 percent indicated high levels of these symptoms.

Source: Rosenthal, Beth, et al. "Prevalence of Psychological Symptoms Among Undergraduate Students in an Ethnically Diverse Urban Public College." *Journal of American College Health*, Vol. 49, No. 1, July 2000.

A recent study of 595 freshmen at an ethnically diverse urban public college found that less than 15 percent reported high levels of anger, anxiety, and depression. (See Student Snapshot: "Mental Disorders on Campus.") There were no statistically significant differences among Asian, African-American, Latino/Hispanic, and white students on any of the three psychological symptoms. Although women reported higher levels of anger, anxiety, and depression, the differences compared with men were small.[45]

The Brain: The Last Frontier

The brain has intrigued scientists for centuries, but only recently have its explorers made dramatic progress in unraveling its mysteries. Leaders in **neuropsychiatry**—the field that brings together the study of the brain and the mind—remind us that 95 percent of what is known about brain anatomy, chemistry, and physiology has been learned in the last decade. These discoveries have reshaped our understanding of the organ that is central to our identity and well-being and have fostered great hope for more effective therapies for the more than 1,000 disorders—psychiatric and neurologic—that affect the brain and nervous system.

Inside the Brain

Each human brain contains hundreds of billions of nerve cells, or **neurons,** and support cells called **glia.** Most are present at birth, when the brain weighs less than a pound. In the first six years of life—the period when we acquire more knowledge more rapidly than ever again—the brain reaches its full weight of about 3 pounds (see Figure 3-3). From birth, male and female brains differ in a variety of ways. (See The X & Y Files: "Are Men's and Women's Brains Different?")

The neurons are the basic working units of the brain. Like snowflakes, no two are exactly the same. Each consists of a cell body containing the **nucleus;** a long fiber, called the **axon,** which can range from less than an inch to several feet in length; an **axon terminal,** or ending; and multiple branching fibers called **dendrites** (Figure 3-4 on page 83). The glia serve as the scaffolding for the brain, separate the brain from the bloodstream, assist in the growth of neurons, speed up the transmission of nerve impulses, and engulf and digest damaged neurons.

As the master control center for the body, the brain is constantly receiving information from the senses and relaying messages to various parts of the body. Some of these messages travel through the spinal cord, which extends from the neck about two-thirds of the way down

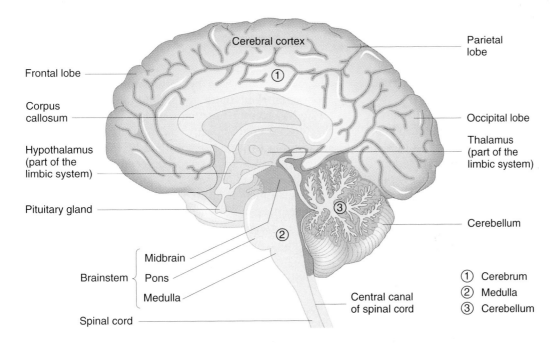

▲ **Figure 3-3** The brain.
The three major parts of the brain are the cerebrum, cerebellum, and brainstem. The cerebrum is divided into two hemispheres—the left, which regulates the right side of the body, and the right, which regulates the left side of the body. The cerebellum plays the major role in coordinating movement, balance and posture. The brainstem contains centers that control breathing, blood pressure, heart rate, and other physiological functions.

The X & Y Files

Are Men's and Women's Brains Different?

"The brain is not an organ of sex," the pioneering feminist and economist Charlotte Perkins Gilman declared in 1898. "[We might] as well speak of the female liver." These days, gender scientists do indeed speak of the female liver, describing it as one of the most gender-distinctive organs. What then of the brain? Consider these recent findings:

- **Men's brains are bigger; women use more neurons.** Overall, a woman's brain, like her body, is 10 to 15 percent smaller than a man's, yet the regions dedicated to higher cognitive functions such as language are more densely packed with neurons—and women use more of them. When a male puts his mind to work, neurons turn on in highly specific areas. When females set their minds on similar tasks, cells light up all over the brain.
- **Male and female brains perceive light and sound differently.** A man's eyes are more sensitive to bright light and retain their ability to see well at long distances longer in life. A woman hears a much broader range of sounds, and her hearing remains sharper longer.
- **The female brain responds more intensely to emotion.** According to neuroimaging studies, the genders respond differently to emotions, especially sadness, which activates, or turns on, neurons in an area eight times larger in women than men.
- **Male and female brains age in different ways.** The male brain loses tissue at almost three times the rate of the female brain. Because of this gender difference, the all-important frontal lobes, which are larger in men in youth and early adulthood, reach approximately the same size in men and women by the time they reach their forties. Other parts of men's brains—including the corpus callosum and the left hemisphere—also atrophy more rapidly.
- **Neither gender's brain is "better."** Intelligence per se appears equal in both. The greatest gender differences appear both at the top and bottom of the intelligence scales. Men outnumber women both as geniuses and as morons. Nevertheless, more than half the time, regardless of the type of test, most women and men perform more or less equally— even though they may well take different routes to arrive at the same answers. Cognitive skills show greater variability both among women and among men than between the genders. The best evaluation of all may have come from the essayist Samuel Johnson. When asked whether women or men are more intelligent, he responded, "Which man? Which woman?"

the backbone. Other signals are carried by nerves that connect the brain directly with certain parts of the body.

Historically, scientists have focused on the anatomy or structures of the brain in their attempts to understand how it functions and why it sometimes malfunctions. Modern neuropsychiatrists have shifted much of their attention to biochemical processes within the brain, particularly those involved in communication between neurons.

Communication Within the Brain

Neurons "talk" with each other by means of electrical and chemical processes (see Figure 3-4). An electric charge, or impulse, travels along an axon to the terminal, where packets of chemicals called **neurotransmitters** are stored. When released, these messengers flow out of the axon terminal and cross a **synapse,** a specialized site at which the axon terminal of one neuron comes extremely close to a dendrite from another neuron. On the surface of the dendrite are **receptors,** protein molecules designed to bind with neurotransmitters. It takes only about a ten-thousandth of a second for a neurotransmitter and a receptor to come together. Neurotransmitters that do not connect with receptors may remain in the synapse until they are reabsorbed by the cell that produced them—a process called **reuptake**—or broken down by enzymes.

A malfunction in the release of a neurotransmitter, in its reuptake or elimination, or in the receptors or secondary messengers may result in abnormalities in thinking, feeling, or behavior. Some of the most promising and exciting research in neuropsychiatry is focusing on correcting such malfunctions. The neurotransmitter serotonin and its receptors have been shown to affect mood, sleep, behavior, appetite, memory, learning, sexuality, and aggression and to play a role in several mental disorders. The discovery of a possible link between low levels of serotonin and some cases of major depression has led to the development of more precisely targeted **antidepressant** medications that boost serotonin to normal levels.

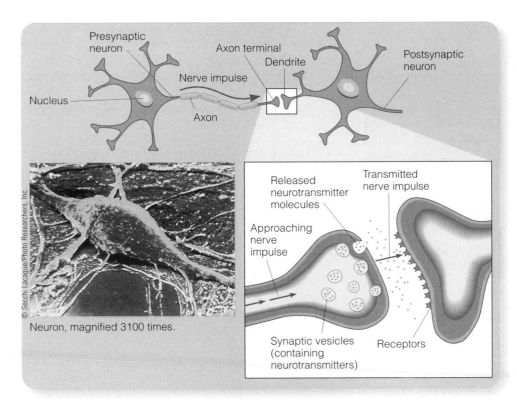

Nucleus
Presynaptic neuron
Nerve impulse
Axon terminal
Dendrite
Axon
Postsynaptic neuron

© Secchi Lacague/Photo Researchers, Inc.

Neuron, magnified 3100 times.

Released neurotransmitter molecules
Transmitted nerve impulse
Approaching nerve impulse
Synaptic vesicles (containing neurotransmitters)
Receptors

▲ **Figure 3-4** The neuron, the basic working unit of the brain. Neurotransmitters released across the synapse transmit the chemical nerve impulse from one neuron to another.

Anxiety Disorders

Anxiety disorders may involve inordinate fears of certain objects or situations **(phobias),** episodes of sudden, inexplicable terror **(panic attacks),** chronic distress **(generalized anxiety disorder, or GAD),** or persistent, disturbing thoughts and behaviors **(obsessive-compulsive disorder).** Over a lifetime, according to the National Comorbidity Survey, as many as one in four Americans may experience an anxiety disorder. Only one of every four of these individuals is ever correctly diagnosed and treated. Yet most who do get treatment, even for severe and disabling problems, improve dramatically.

Phobias

Phobias—the most prevalent type of anxiety disorder—are out-of-the-ordinary, irrational, intense, persistent fears of certain objects or situations. About two million Americans develop such acute terror that they go to extremes to avoid whatever it is that they fear, even though they realize that these feelings are excessive or unreasonable.[46] The most common phobias involve animals, particularly dogs, snakes,

insects, and mice; the sight of blood; closed spaces *(claustrophobia);* heights *(acrophobia);* air travel and being in places or situations from which they perceive it would be difficult or embarrassing to escape *(agoraphobia).*

Although various medications have been tried, none is effective by itself in relieving phobias. The best approach is behavior therapy, which consists of gradual, systematic exposure to the feared object (a process called *systematic desensitization*). Numerous studies have proven that exposure—especially in-vivo exposure, in which individuals are exposed to the actual source of their fear rather than simply imagining it—is highly effective. Medical hypnosis—the use of induction of an altered state of consciousness—also can help.

The characteristic symptoms of a phobia include:

▶ Excessive or unreasonable fear of a specific object or situation.
▶ Immediate, invariable anxiety when exposed to the object or situation.
▶ Recognition that the fear is excessive or unreasonable.
▶ Avoidance of the feared object or situation or enduring it only with intense anxiety or distress.
▶ Inability to function as usual at school or work or in social relationships because of the phobia.

Panic Attacks and Panic Disorder

Individuals who have had panic attacks describe them as the most frightening experiences of their lives. Without reason or warning, their hearts race wildly. They may become light-headed or dizzy. Because they can't catch their breath, they may start breathing rapidly and hyperventilate. Parts of their bodies, such as their fingers or toes, may tingle or feel numb. Worst of all is the terrible sense that something horrible is about to happen: that they will die, lose their minds, or have a heart attack. Most attacks reach peak intensity within ten minutes. Afterward, individuals live in dread of another one. **Panic disorder** develops when attacks recur or apprehension about them

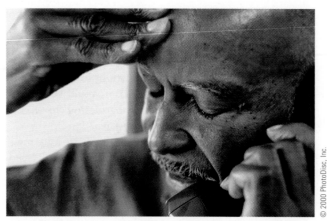

© 2000 PhotoDisc, Inc.

▲ Worry is a normal part of daily life, but individuals with generalized anxiety disorder worry constantly about everything and anything that might go wrong.

becomes so intense that individuals cannot function normally.

About one-third of all young adults experience at least one panic attack between the ages of 15 and 35. Full-blown panic disorder occurs in about 1.6 percent of all adults in the course of a lifetime and usually develops before age 30. Women are more than twice as likely as men to experience panic attacks, although no one knows why. Parents, siblings, and children of individuals with panic disorders also are more likely to develop them than are others.[47]

The two primary treatments for panic disorder are cognitive-behavioral therapy, which teaches specific strategies for coping with symptoms like rapid breathing, and medication. Treatment helps as many as 90 percent of those with panic disorder either improve significantly or recover completely, usually within six to eight weeks. Individuals who receive cognitive-behavioral therapy as well as medication are less likely to suffer relapses than those taking medication alone.

Generalized Anxiety Disorder

About 10 million adults in the United States suffer from a generalized anxiety disorder (GAD), excessive or unrealistic apprehension that causes physical symptoms and lasts for six months or longer. It usually starts when people are in their twenties.[48] Unlike fear, which helps us recognize and avoid real danger, GAD is an irrational or unwarranted response to harmless objects or situations of exaggerated danger. The most common symptoms are faster heart rate, sweating, increased blood pressure, muscle aches, intestinal pains, irritability, sleep problems, and difficulty concentrating.

Chronically anxious individuals worry—not just some of the time, and not just about the stresses and strains of ordinary life—but constantly, about almost everything: their health, families, finances, marriages, potential dangers. Treatment for GAD may consist of a combination of psychotherapy, behavioral therapy, and antianxiety drugs.

Obsessive-Compulsive Disorder

As many as 1 in 40 Americans has a type of anxiety called obsessive-compulsive disorder (OCD). Some of these individuals suffer only from an *obsession*, a recurring idea, thought, or image that they realize, at least initially, is senseless. The most common obsessions are repetitive thoughts of violence (e.g., killing a child), contamination (becoming infected by shaking hands), and doubt (wondering whether one has performed some act, such as having hurt someone in a traffic accident). Most people with OCD also suffer from a compulsion, repetitive behavior performed according to certain rules or in a stereotyped fashion. The most common compulsions involve hand-washing, cleaning, hoarding useless items, counting, or checking (for example, making sure dozens of times that a door is locked).[49]

Individuals with OCD realize that their thoughts or behaviors are bizarre, but they cannot resist or control them. Eventually, the obsessions or compulsions consume a great deal of time and significantly interfere with normal routine, job functioning, or usual social activities or relationships with others. A young woman who must follow a very rigid dressing routine may always be late for class, for example; a student who must count each letter of the alphabet as he types may not be able to complete a term paper.

OCD is believed to have biological roots. It may be a result of gene abnormalities, head injury, or even an autoimmune reaction after childhood infection with strep bacteria. Treatment may consist of cognitive therapy to correct irrational assumptions, behavioral techniques such as progressively limiting the amount of time someone obsessed with cleanliness can spend washing and scrubbing, and medication. About 70 to 80 percent of those with OCD improve with treatment.

Depressive Disorders

Depression, the world's most common mental ailment, affects the brain, the mind, and the body in complex ways. According to a survey of 2,000 adults, more than 20 percent of Americans feel unhappy or depressed. About 12 percent suffer from "clinical" depression and require psychiatric treatment.[50] Stress-related events may trigger half

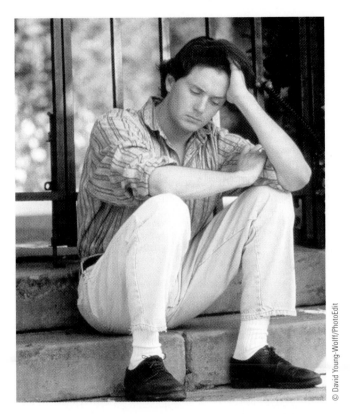

▲ A number of factors can contribute to the development of depression during your college years, including stressful events, poor academic performance, loneliness, and relationship problems.

of all depressive episodes; great trauma in childhood can increase vulnerability to depression later in life.[51] An estimated 15 to 40 percent of college-age men and women (18- to 24-year-olds) may develop depression.[52]

Comparing everyday "blues" to a **depressive disorder** is like comparing a cold to pneumonia. Major depression can destroy a person's joy for living. Food, friends, sex, or any form of pleasure no longer appeals. It is impossible to concentrate on work and responsibilities. Unable to escape a sense of utter hopelessness, depressed individuals may fight back tears throughout the day and toss and turn through long, empty nights. Thoughts of death or suicide may push into their minds.

But there is good news: Depression is a treatable disease. Psychotherapy is remarkably effective for mild depression. In more serious cases, antidepressant medication can lead to dramatic improvement in 40 to 80 percent of depressed patients.

Exercise also is a good way to both prevent and treat psychological problems. Several studies have shown that exercise effectively lifts mild to moderate depression; for some patients, it may be more effective than drug treatment for major depression.[53] In a study of 150 individuals diag-

nosed with major depression, one group was assigned to four months of walking, jogging, or cycling; another took antidepressant medication; and a third both exercised and took medication. At the end of four months, all had improved significantly. Six months later, the exercisers were in better shape physically and mentally—and much less likely to have suffered a relapse. At ten months, the chance of a patient still being depressed was reduced by 50 percent for every 50 minutes of current weekly exercise.[54] In older adults, low-intensity exercise that included weight training improved overall mood more than just aerobic exercise.[55]

Why Are So Many Young People Depressed?

Once young people were considered immune to sadness. Now mental health professionals know better. An estimated 5 to 10 percent of American teenagers suffer from a serious depressive disorder; girls are twice as susceptible as boys. Prior to puberty, girls and boys are equally likely to develop depression. Even preschoolers can develop symptoms of depression, such as irritability, sadness, and withdrawal.[56]

The risks of depression in the young are high. Four in ten of depressed adolescents think about killing themselves; two in ten actually try to do so. Every year an estimated 11 to 13 in every 100,000 teens take their own lives, twice as many as the number who die from all natural causes combined.

"Depression is the most common emotional problem in adolescence and the single greatest risk factor for teen suicide," says child psychiatrist Peter Jensen, M.D., director for the Center for the Advancement of Children's Mental Health at Columbia University, who notes that depression rates have been rising over the last half century. "Teens born in the 1980s are more likely to develop depression than those who were born in the 1970s, whose rate of depression is higher than for those born in the 1960s."[57]

No one knows the reason for this steady surge in sadness, but experts point to the breakdown of families, the pressures of the information age, and increased isolation. "Social environment doesn't cause depression," explains psychiatrist John March, M.D., of Duke University, who is heading a nationwide study of therapies for teen depression. "But environmental stress can bring out depression in people who are susceptible. Depression is more than teenage angst. It is an illness of the central nervous system that is common, impairing, and lethal."[58]

A family history of depression greatly increases a young person's vulnerability. In one recent study of high school students diagnosed with depression, family members of depressed adolescents had much higher rates of major depression.[59] However, the strongest predictor of depression is cigarette smoking. Depressed teens may smoke because they think smoking will make them feel better, but nicotine alters brain chemistry and actually worsens symptoms of depression.[60]

Depression can be hard to recognize in the young. Many depressed teens don't look or act sad. Rather than crying, they may snap grouchily at parents or burst into angry tirades. Some turn to alcohol or drugs in hopes of feeling better; others become depressed after they start abusing these substances. As they drop out of activities and pull away from friends, depressed teens spend more time alone. Their schoolwork suffers, and many are labeled as underachievers. Those whose anger explodes in public are branded as troublemakers

Only in the last decade have researchers in mental heath specifically studied treatments for teen depression. They now know that 60 to 75 percent of teenagers—the same percentage as adults—respond to treatment with the medications called SSRIs (a group of antidepressants that includes Prozac and Paxil). The use of these antidepressants in children and teenagers has increased three- to five-fold in recent years.[61] Older antidepressants called tricyclics, once the mainstay of treatment for adults, are not effective in adolescents. Some therapies are as effective as the SSRIs—particularly an approach called cognitive behavioral therapy (CBT), which focuses on teaching new ways to deal with stress and sadness, such as changing unrealistic or highly negative ways of thinking.

The National Institute of Mental Health has launched the Treating Adolescents with Depression Study (TADS) to compare the effectiveness of Prozac, cognitive-behavioral therapy, and a combination of both approaches. Other studies are focusing on prevention, particularly in youngsters who have some symptoms of depression but continue to function normally.

Major Depression

The simplest definition of **major depression** is sadness that does not end. The incidence of major depression has soared over the last two decades, especially among young adults. The National Comorbidity Survey found that major depression affects 10.3 percent of Americans in any given year.

The characteristic symptoms of major depression include:

- Feeling depressed, sad, empty, discouraged, tearful.
- Loss of interest or pleasure in once-enjoyable activities.
- Eating more or less than usual and either gaining or losing weight.
- Having trouble sleeping or sleeping much more than usual.
- Feeling slowed down or restless and unable to sit still.
- Lack of energy.
- Feeling helpless, hopeless, worthless, inadequate.
- Difficulty concentrating, forgetfulness.
- Difficulty thinking clearly or making decisions.
- Persistent thoughts of death or suicide.
- Withdrawal from others, lack of interest in sex.
- Physical symptoms (headaches, digestive problems, aches and pains).

Most cases of major depression can be treated successfully, usually with psychotherapy, medication, or both. Psychotherapy alone works in more than half of mild-to-moderate episodes of major depression. Psychotherapy helps individuals pinpoint the life problems that contribute to their depression, identify negative or distorted thinking patterns, explore behaviors that contribute to depression, and regain a sense of control and pleasure in life. Two specific psychotherapies—cognitive-behavioral therapy and interpersonal therapy (described later in this chapter)—have proved as helpful as antidepressant drugs in treating

---

STRATEGIES FOR PREVENTION

Recognizing the Signs of Teen Depression

✔ Mood changes, including feeling sad, irritable, or cranky; being easily angered; or having difficulty getting along with family members

✔ Loss of interest in hobbies, sports or social activities

✔ Lack of enjoyment even when involved in an activity they used to enjoy

✔ Changes in sleep patterns, such as difficulty falling asleep or staying asleep

✔ Changes in appetite; gaining or losing a lot of weight

✔ Changes in energy levels, such as feeling tired a lot of the time, moving more slowly, or being physical restless or agitated

✔ School difficulties, including problems concentrating or a decline in grades

✔ Personal criticism, such as saying they can't do anything right or blaming themselves for things that are not really their fault

✔ Self-harm, including thoughts or conversations about hurting themselves

mild cases of depression, although they take longer than medication to achieve results.

Antidepressant medications work for more than half of those with moderate-to-severe depression and may be useful in treating mild depression in individuals who do not improve with psychotherapy alone (see the section on psychiatric drug therapy, later in this chapter). These prescription drugs generally take three or four weeks to produce significant benefits and may not have their full impact for up to eight weeks.

Newer antidepressants that boost levels of the neurotransmitter serotonin have proven equally effective as older medications, but their side effects are different—patients report higher rates of diarrhea, nausea, insomnia, and headache.[62] The older drugs are more likely to adversely affect the heart and blood pressure and to cause dry mouth, constipation, dizziness, blurred vision, and tremors.

Modest exercise—30 minutes on a treadmill or stationary bicycle three times a week—also has proven effective.[63]

Eighty percent of people who have one episode of depression are likely to have another. Because of this high risk of recurrence, many psychiatrists now view depression as a chronic disease and advise ongoing treatment with antidepressants. However, little is known about the long-term effects of these medications.[64]

In individuals who cannot take antidepressant medications because of medical problems, or who do not improve with psychotherapy or drugs, *electroconvulsive therapy* (ECT)—the administration of a controlled electrical current through electrodes attached to the scalp—remains the safest and most effective treatment. About 50 percent of depressed individuals who do not get better with antidepressant medication and psychotherapy improve after ECT.

Bipolar Disorder (Manic Depression)

Bipolar disorder, or manic depression, consists of mood swings that may take individuals from *manic* states of feeling euphoric and energetic to depressive states of utter despair. In episodes of full mania, they may become so impulsive and out of touch with reality that they endanger their careers, relationships, health, or even survival. One percent of the population—about 2 million American adults—suffer from this serious but treatable disorder, which affects both genders and all races equally.

The characteristic symptoms of bipolar disorder include mood swings (from happy to miserable, optimistic to despairing, and so on); changes in thinking (thoughts speeding through one's mind; unrealistic self-confidence; difficulty concentrating; delusions; hallucinations); changes in behavior (sudden immersion in plans and projects; talk-ing very rapidly and much more than usual; excessive spending; impaired judgment; impulsive sexual involvement); and changes in physical condition (less need for sleep; increased energy; fewer health complaints than usual). During "manic" periods, individuals may make grandiose plans or take dangerous risks. But they often plunge from this highest of highs to a horrible low depressive episode, in which they may feel sad, hopeless, and helpless, and develop other symptoms of major depression. The risk of suicide is very real.

Professional therapy is essential in treating bipolar disorders. Mood-stabilizing medications are the keystone of treatment, although psychotherapy plays a critical role in helping individuals understand their illness and rebuild their lives. Most individuals continue taking medication indefinitely after remission of their symptoms because the risk of recurrence is high.

Suicide

Suicide is not in itself a psychiatric disorder, but it can be the tragic consequence of emotional and psychological problems. Every year 30,000 Americans—among them many young people who seem to have "everything to live for"—commit suicide. An estimated 752,000 attempt to take their own lives; there may be 4.5 million suicide "survivors" in the U.S.[65]

After rising steadily for decades, suicide rates among young people have remained stable since 1994. Despite what many people believe, young people between the ages of 15 and 24 have the lowest suicide rate in the nation (13.3 per 100,000), while white men in their eighties have the highest (63.1 per 100,000).[66]

Depressed teens are more likely to attempt suicide—and to die. "In psychological interviews after a teen suicide, we see that the warning signs were there," child psychiatrist Madelyn Gould, M.D., of Columbia University, notes, "but no one realized the underlying problem was depression."[67] Stresses that may contribute to the soaring suicide rates among the young are psychological problems, mental disorders, drug abuse, school pressures, social difficulties, concern and confusion about sexual orientation, and family problems.

At all ages, men commit suicide three times more frequently than women, but women attempt suicide much more often than men.[68] Elderly men are ten times more likely to take their own lives than older women. Native Americans have a suicide rate five times higher than that of the general population.

Suicide is the third leading cause of death among children and adolescents 10 to 19 years old in the United States. The age-adjusted death rate for suicide has decreased

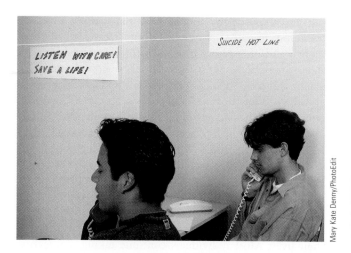

▲ About 20 percent of teenagers seriously consider suicide; a much smaller number actually attempt to take their own lives. Talking to a counselor at a suicide hot line may help a young person deal with his or her feelings of despondency.

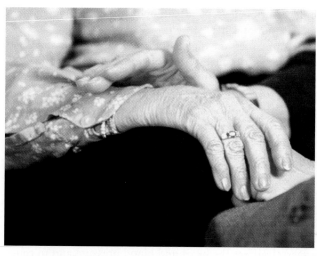

▲ Depression and suicidal thoughts are closely linked. If you know someone who is severely depressed, be willing to offer help and comfort during difficult times.

in recent years, but the death rate for suicide among children 10 to 14 years old has doubled. Although black youths have historically had lower suicide rates than whites, the gap between suicide rates for black and white youths has narrowed.[69] Among all young people under age 25, firearms-related deaths account for 67 percent of suicides.

Among the factors that increase the likelihood of teen suicide are a previous suicide attempt, violence (either as victim or perpetrator), and use of alcohol or marijuana. For girls, medical symptoms, having a friend attempt or complete suicide, illicit drug use, and a history of mental health problems also increase the risk. Among boys, risk factors include carrying a weapon at school, same-sex romantic attraction, a family history of suicide or suicide attemps, easy household access to guns, skipping school, and being held back or skipping a grade.

Researchers also have identified factors that protect young people from suicide. Number one for both boys and girls was feeling connected to their parents and family. For girls, emotional well-being was also protective; grade point average was an additional protective factor for boys. High parental expectations for their child's school achievement, more people living in the household, and religiosity were protective for some of the boys, but not for the girls. Availability of counseling services at school and parental presence at key times during the day were protective for some of the girls, but not for the boys.

Suicide is also the third leading cause of death among college-aged Americans.[70] Males in this age group have a suicide rate six times greater than that of females.[71]

Suicide is not inevitable. Appropriate treatment can help as many as 70 to 80 percent of those at risk for suicide. Among young people, early recognition and treatment for depressive disorders and alcohol and drug use could save thousands of lives each year.

???? What Leads to Suicide?

Researchers have looked for explanations for suicide by studying everything from phases of the moon to seasons (suicides peak in the spring and early summer) to birth order in the family.[72] They have found no conclusive answers. A constellation of influences—mental disorders, personality traits, biologic and genetic vulnerability, medical illness, and psychosocial stressors—may combine in ways that lower an individual's threshold of vulnerability. The risk of suicide is higher in people who live in cities, are single, have a low income, or are unemployed.[73] No one factor in itself may ever explain fully why a person chooses death.[74]

Mental Disorders

More than 95 percent of those who commit suicide have a mental disorder. Two in particular—depression and alcoholism—account for two-thirds of all suicides. Suicide also is a risk for those with other disorders, including schizophrenia and personality disorders.

Psychiatrists have revised the estimated risk of suicide among patients, which had been set on the basis of theoretical calculations at 15 percent—nearly 1 out of 6, or 30 times the lifetime rate in the general population. Suicide risk calculated from data on actual fatalities is lower: The average fatality rates were 2 percent for depressed patients outside of hospitals, 4 percent for depressed patients in hospitals, and 6 percent for hospitalized patients diagnosed as suicide. These figures are five or six (rather than 30) times the rate in the general population.[75]

Substance Abuse

Many of those who commit suicide drink beforehand, and their use of alcohol may lower their inhibitions. Since alcohol itself is a depressant, it can intensify the despondency suicidal individuals are already feeling. Alcoholics who attempt suicide often have other risk factors, including major depression, poor social support, serious medical illness, and unemployment. Drugs of abuse also can alter thinking and lower inhibitions against suicide.

Hopelessness

The sense of utter hopelessness and helplessness may be the most common contributing factors in suicide. When hope dies, individuals view every experience in negative terms and come to expect the worst possible outcomes for their problems. Given this way of thinking, suicide often seems a reasonable response to a life seen as not worth living.

Family History

One of every four people who attempt suicide has a family member who also tried to commit suicide. While a family history of suicide is not in itself considered a predictor of suicide, two mental disorders that can lead to suicide—depression and bipolar disorder (manic depression)—do run in families.

Physical Illness

People who commit suicide are likely to be ill or to believe that they are. About 5 percent actually have a serious physical disorder, such as AIDS or cancer. While suicide may seem to be a decision rationally arrived at in persons with serious or fatal illness, this may not be the case. Depression, not uncommon in such instances, can warp judgment. When the depression is treated, the person may no longer have suicidal intentions.

More than 80 percent of those who commit suicide have seen a physician about a medical complaint within the six months preceding suicide. To help general physicians identify people at risk of suicide, researchers at Johns Hopkins University developed a set of four crucial questions:

- Have you ever had a period of two weeks or more when you had trouble falling asleep, staying asleep, waking up too early, or sleeping too much?
- Have you ever had two weeks or more during which you felt sad, blue, depressed or when you lost interest and pleasure in things you usually cared about or enjoyed?
- Has there been a period of two weeks or more when you felt worthless, sinful, or guilty?
- Has there ever been a period of time when you felt that life was hopeless?

Anyone who answers yes to these questions should be referred immediately to a mental health professional.

STRATEGIES FOR PREVENTION

If You Start Thinking About Suicide

At some point, the thought of ending it all—the disappointments, problems, bad feelings—may cross your mind. This experience isn't unusual. But if the idea of taking your life persists or intensifies, you should respond as you would to other warnings of potential threats to your health—by getting the help you need:

✔ Talk to a mental health professional. If you have a therapist, call immediately. If not, call a suicide hot line.

✔ Find someone you can trust and talk with honestly about what you're feeling. If you suffer from depression or another mental disorder, educate trusted friends or relatives about your condition so they are prepared if called upon to help.

✔ Write down your more uplifting thoughts. Even if you are despondent, you can help yourself by taking the time to retrieve some more positive thoughts or memories. A simple record of your hopes for the future and the people you value in your life can remind you of why your own life is worth continuing.

✔ Avoid drugs and alcohol. Most suicides are the results of sudden, uncontrolled impulses, and drugs and alcohol can make it harder to resist these destructive urges.

✔ Go to the hospital. Hospitalization can sometimes be the best way to protect your health and safety.

Brain Chemistry

Investigators have found abnormalities in the brain chemistry of individuals who complete suicide, especially low levels of a metabolite of the neurotransmitter serotonin. There are indications that individuals with a deficiency in this substance may have as much as a ten times greater risk of committing suicide than those with higher levels.

Access to Guns

For individuals already facing a combination of predisposing factors, access to a means of committing suicide, particularly to guns, can add to the risk. Unlike other methods of suicide, guns almost always work. States with stricter gun-control laws have much lower rates of suicides than states with more lenient laws. Health professionals are urging parents whose children undergo psychological treatment or assessment to remove all weapons from their homes and to make sure their youngsters do not have access to potentially lethal medications and to alcohol.

Other Factors

Individuals who kill themselves often have gone through more major life crises—job changes, births, financial reversals, divorce, retirement—in the previous six months, compared with others. Long-standing, intense conflict with family members or other important people may add to the danger. In some cases, suicide may be an act of revenge that offers the person a sense of control—however temporary or illusory. For example, a husband whose wife has had an affair may rationalize that he can get back at her, and have the final word, by killing himself. Others may feel that, by rejecting life, they are rejecting a partner or parent who abandoned or betrayed them.

Suicide Prevention

If someone you know has talked about suicide, behaved unpredictably, or suddenly emerged from a severe depression into a calm, settled state of mind, don't rule out the possibility that he or she may attempt suicide.

▶ Encourage your friend to talk. Ask concerned questions. Listen attentively. Show that you take the person's feelings seriously and truly care.

▶ Don't offer trite reassurances. List reasons to go on living, try to analyze the person's motives, or try to shock or challenge him or her.

▶ Suggest solutions or alternatives to problems. Make plans. Encourage positive action, such as getting

away for a while to gain a better perspective on a problem.

▶ Don't be afraid to ask whether your friend has considered suicide. The opportunity to talk about thoughts of suicide may be an enormous relief, and—contrary to a long-standing myth—will not fix the idea of suicide more firmly in a person's mind.

▶ Don't think that people who talk about killing themselves never carry out their threat. Most individuals who commit suicide give definite indications of their intent to die.

Attention Disorders

Approximately 10 percent of boys and 2 percent of girls in the United States have **attention deficit/hyperactivity disorder (ADHD),** the most common psychiatric diagnosis of childhood.[76] Its causes are complex and include genetic and biological factors, including differences within the brain. Research has shown that children with ADHD often have smaller overall brain volumes than others, particularly in the right frontal region, an area of the brain associated with the processes of paying attention and focusing concentration.[77]

The diagnosis of ADHD in childhood remains controversial. Some critics charge that children with a variety of temperaments, neurological delays, and behavioral difficulties are being lumped together and labeled as being hyperactive or attention-disordered. Others feel that attention disorders are still under-diagnosed, especially in girls, who tend to develop a type of ADHD primarily characterized by inability to concentrate.

One-half to two-thirds of youngsters with ADHD do not outgrow their restless, reckless ways at puberty. In all, 1 to 2 percent of adult men and women—at least 5 million Americans—have problems sustaining attention or controlling their movements and impulses.

Adults with ADHD have one or more of three primary symptoms: hyperactivity, impulsivity, and distractibility. Rather than scooting around a room, they may tap their fingers or jiggle their feet. Some appear calm and organized but cannot concentrate long enough to finish reading a paragraph or follow a list of directions. Others, on a whim, go on buying sprees or take wild dares.

 An estimated 1 percent of college students have an attention disorder that can have a significant impact on their academic performance. At one midwestern university, for instance, the counseling service estimates that students with attention disorders have an average GPA of 2.4, compared to a university average mean of 3.1.

No specific test can detect attention disorders, and diagnosis, based on the patient's history and a therapist's interview, can be difficult. Adults with ADHD may take the same medications that children do—stimulant drugs that, paradoxically, can aid concentration and reduce restlessness. Some antidepressants are effective in treating adult ADHD and may be an alternative to stimulants. Medication often makes it possible for adults with ADHD to benefit from other treatments, such as psychotherapy, general counseling, vocational rehabilitation, and academic tutoring.

GENES IN FOCUS

The Genetics of ADHD

Attention deficit/hyperactivity disorder (ADHD), a problem that plagues many students, runs in families. The parents, brothers, and sisters of children with the disorder have a rate of ADHD three to five times the average. Which is the greater influence: the genes family members share or their environment? In research on adopted children with ADHD, their biological parents have had a much higher rate of the disorder than their adoptive parents, indicating that nature has a stronger influence than nurture. In a study comparing identical and fraternal twins, investigators found that the heritability of ADHD—the proportion of individual differences in susceptibility linked to genetic differences—was 80 percent.

Two genes related to the production of the neurotransmitter dopamine have been implicated by genetic research on families with ADHD. These genes are the dopamine transporter gene (or DAT gene) and the dopamine receptor gene (or DRD4 gene). They provide instructions for the synthesis, release, and reabsorption of dopamine. Genetically engineered mice that lack the DAT gene show symptoms of hyperactivity. The DRD4 gene has been found in novelty seekers—individuals drawn to new experiences and sensations—as are many people with ADHD.

Scientists are conducting more extensive studies to better understand the genetics of ADHD and to determine why different forms of the disorder appear in different families. Eventually this research may lead to specialized treatments and possibly even prevention of ADHD in children at risk.

Schizophrenia

Schizophrenia, one of the most debilitating mental disorders, profoundly impairs an individual's sense of reality. As the National Institute of Mental Health (NIMH) puts it, schizophrenia, which is characterized by abnormalities in brain structure and chemistry, destroys "the inner unity of the mind" and weakens "the will and drive that constitute our essential character." It affects every aspect of psychological functioning, including the ways in which people think, feel, view themselves, and relate to others.

The symptoms of schizophrenia include:

- Hallucinations.
- Delusions.
- Inability to think in a logical manner.
- Talking in rambling or incoherent ways.
- Making odd or purposeless movements or not moving at all.
- Repeating others' words or mimicking their gestures.
- Showing few, if any, feelings; responding with inappropriate emotions.
- Lacking will or motivation to complete a task or accomplish something.
- Functioning at a much lower level than in the past at work, in interpersonal relations, or in taking care of themselves.

Individuals with schizophrenia may hear, see, or feel things that do not exist—a voice telling them to jump from a bridge, a statue crying tears of blood, a spaceship beaming a light upon them. Frightened and vulnerable, they may devote all their energy to warding off the demons within. Unable to take care of themselves, they may look messy and disheveled. They often move in unusual ways, such as rocking or pacing, or repeat certain gestures again and again. They may believe that someone or something, such as the devil, is putting thoughts into their heads or controlling their actions. Some think they are reincarnations of Christ or Napoleon. About a third attempt to take their own lives, often in response to a command they hear inside their heads. Researchers have identified early markers of schizophrenia, including impaired social skills, intellectual ability, and capacity for organization.[78]

Schizophrenia is most likely to occur between the ages of 17 and 30 in men and between 20 and 40 in women.[79] Although symptoms do not occur until then, they are almost certainly the result of a failure in brain development that occurs very early in life. The underlying defect is probably present before birth. Schizophrenia has a strong genetic basis and is not the result of upbringing, social conditions, or traumatic experiences.[80]

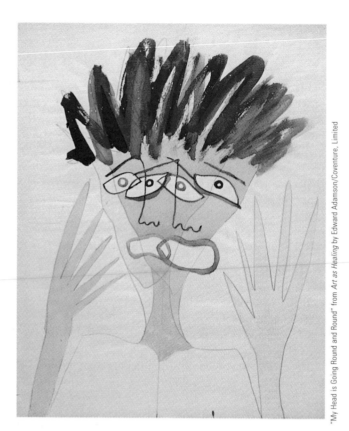

"My Head is Going Round and Round" from *Art as Healing* by Edward Adamson/Coventure, Limited

▲ *"My Head is Going Round and Round."* This drawing by a patient suffering from schizophrenia expresses the anxiety and agitation that may occur with this brain abnormality.

One-half to 1 percent of the population—about 1 in every 150 people—suffers from this disorder. Danish researchers have found that children born during late winter or in urban areas appear to be at greater risk of schizophrenia, possibly because their mothers were more likely to contract a viral infection during pregnancy that could have affected the developing fetal brain. Retroviruses (discussed in Chapter 11) also may play a role.[81] About half have a history of substance abuse or dependence, including alcoholism.[82] According to NIMH's epidemiological data, the total lifetime prevalence for schizophrenia in the United States ranges from 1 to 1.9 percent. This means that between 2.5 million and 4.75 million Americans may have schizophrenia at any one time.

Schizophrenia typically consists of several stages. During the *prodromal phase,* a period ranging from months to years, individuals withdraw from social interactions, pay less attention to keeping clean or dressing appropriately, or act in peculiar ways. In the acute, or *active phase,* individuals develop "positive symptoms." They may experience delusions and become convinced that space aliens have taken control of their bodies or hallucinate and hear voices mocking them. Some talk nonstop, rambling on without making any clear point; others repeatedly shake their heads, tap their feet, or assume odd postures or positions. After positive symptoms subside, individuals enter the *residual phase,* which is characterized by "negative symptoms," such as general apathy, flattened emotions, or inappropriate emotional reactions (for example, laughing when someone is hurt).

For centuries, the quest for a cure for this frightening and often tragic disease led to desperate methods, including spraying a strong stream of water at a patient's spine, injecting the patient with horse serum, and administering huge doses of vitamins. Today, for the vast majority of individuals with schizophrenia, antipsychotic drugs are the foundation of treatment. They make most people with schizophrenia feel more comfortable and in control of themselves, help organize chaotic thinking, and reduce or eliminate delusions or hallucinations, allowing fuller participation in normal activities. Those who do not improve significantly on medication almost invariably do even worse without it.

Most of the antipsychotic drugs have a similar mode of action. While some may act more quickly than others, almost all are equally effective. But they can have problematic side effects, including uncontrollable facial tics, tongue tremors, and jaw movements known as tardive dyskinesia. Lowering the dose may help. Nearly one-third of individuals given conventional antipsychotics continue to have residual symptoms, such as apathy. In the past, little, if anything, could be done to relieve these negative symptoms. However, new "atypical" antipsychotics, such as Clozaril (clozapine) and Zyprexa (olanzapine), can relieve such symptoms and help individuals who do not improve with standard medications or who develop intolerable side effects. They are less likely to cause abnormal body movements, such as muscle spasms and restless pacing.[83]

Some individuals with schizophrenia recover completely. However, many thousands—perhaps as many as 200,000—live on the street or in homeless shelters.

Overcoming Problems of the Mind

Mental illness costs our society an estimated $150 billion a year in lost work time and productivity, employee turnover, disability payments, and death. Yet many Americans do not have access to mental health services, nor do they have insurance for such services. Despite the fact that treatments for mental disorders have a higher success rate than those for many other diseases, employers often restrict mental health benefits. HMOs and health insurance plans are much more likely to limit psychotherapy visits and psychiatric hospitalizations than treatments for medical illnesses.

Even when cost is not a barrier, many people do not seek treatment because they see psychological problems as a sign of weakness rather than illness. They also may not realize that scientifically proven therapies can bring relief, often in a matter of weeks or months.

Because an individual's perception of a problem is "culture-specific"—that is, influenced by his or her cultural, social, and religious beliefs—immigrants to the United States may treat symptoms of psychological distress in different ways. For instance, Asian-American college students tend to seek medical care for physical symptoms, such as aches, pains, or sleep problems, but forgo counseling for a mental disorder, because it is more appropriate in their native cultures to do so.

???? Where Can I Turn for Help?

As a student, your best contact for identifying local services may be your health education instructor or department. The health instructors can tell you about general and mental health counseling available on campus, school-based support groups, community-based programs, and special emergency services. On campus, you can also turn to the student health services or the office of the dean of student services or student affairs.

Within the community, you may be able to get help through the city or county health department and neighborhood health centers. Local hospitals often have special clinics and services; and there are usually local branches of national service organizations, such as United Way or Alcoholics Anonymous, other 12-step programs, and various support groups. You can call the psychiatric or psychological association in your city or state for the names of licensed professionals. (Check the telephone directory for listings.) Your primary physician may also be able to help.

The telephone book is another good resource. Special programs are often listed either by the nature of the service, by the name of the neighborhood or city, or by the name of the sponsoring group. In some places, the city's name may precede a listing: the New York City Suicide Hot Line, for instance. In addition to suicide-prevention programs, other listings usually include crisis intervention, violence prevention, and child-abuse prevention programs; drug-treatment information; shelters for battered women; senior citizen centers; and self-help and counseling services. Many services have special hot lines for coping with emergencies. Others provide information as well as counseling over the phone.

Types of Therapists

Many people refer to anyone in the mental health field as a "psychotherapist," but this is not an official designation, and anyone can advertise as one. Only professionally

trained individuals who have met state licensing requirements are certified as psychiatrists, psychologists, or social workers. Before selecting any of these mental health professionals, be sure to check the person's background and credentials.

The most common types of mental health professionals are psychiatrists, psychologists, social workers, psychiatric nurses, and marriage and family therapists. **Psychiatrists** are licensed medical doctors (M.D.) who complete medical school; a year-long internship (including at least four months of internal medicine and usually two months of neurology); and a three-year residency that provides training in various forms of psychotherapy (including couples, family, and group therapy), psychopharmacology (the study of drugs that affect the mind), and both outpatient and inpatient treatment of mental disorders. They can prescribe medications and make medical decisions. *Board-certified* psychiatrists have passed oral and written examinations following completion of residency training. Child psychiatrists undergo additional academic and clinical training to work with children and adolescents; geriatric psychiatrists have special expertise in the problems of older men and women.

Psychologists complete a graduate program (including clinical training and internships) in human psychology but do not study medicine and cannot prescribe medication. They must be licensed in most states in order to practice independently. An increasing number have a doctorate (either a Ph.D. or Psy.D.) plus postdoctoral training, and are trained in a variety of psychotherapeutic techniques rather than in one particular school or theory. Some have additional training in working with children and families.

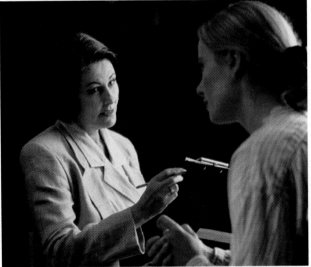
© 2000 Tony Latham/Stone

▲ When choosing a therapist, you should always consider the individual's education, title, and qualifications. Also important are the qualities of compassion and caring.

Certified social workers or **licensed clinical social workers (LCSWs)** usually complete a two-year graduate program and have specialized training in helping people with mental problems in addition to conventional social work. Some have doctoral degrees. Most states certify or license social workers as an independent profession and require two years of supervised postgraduate clinical work and a qualifying examination.

Psychiatric nurses have nursing degrees and have passed a state examination. They usually have special training and experience in mental health care, although no specialty licensing or certification is required.

Marriage and family therapists, licensed in some but not all states, usually have a graduate degree, often in psychology, and at least two years of supervised clinical training in dealing with relationship problems. Psychiatrists, psychologists, and clinical social workers may specialize in marriage and family counseling or devote much of their practices to helping couples and families.

Other therapists include pastoral counselors, members of the clergy who offer psychological counseling; hypnotherapists, who use hypnosis for problems such as smoking and obesity; stress-management counselors, who teach relaxation methods; and alcohol and drug counselors, who help individuals with substance abuse problems. Anyone can use these terms to describe themselves professionally, and there are no licensing requirements.

Options for Treatment

The term **psychotherapy** refers to any type of counseling based on the exchange of words in the context of the unique relationship that develops between a mental health professional and a person seeking help. The process of talking and listening can lead to new insight, relief from distressing psychological symptoms, changes in unhealthy or maladaptive behaviors, and more effective ways of dealing with the world.

Most mental health professionals today are trained in a variety of psychotherapeutic techniques and tailor their approach to the problem, personality, and needs of each person seeking their help. Because skilled therapists may combine different techniques in the course of therapy, the lines between the various approaches often blur.

Because insurance companies and health-care plans often limit the duration of psychotherapy, many mental health professionals are adopting a *time-limited* format in order to make the most of every session, regardless of the length of treatment. Brief or short-term psychotherapy typically focuses on a central theme, problem, or topic and may continue for several weeks to several months. The individuals most likely to benefit are those who are interested in solving immediate problems rather than changing their characters, who can think in psychological terms, and who are motivated to change.

Psychodynamic Psychotherapy

For the most part, today's mental health professionals base their assessment of individuals on a **psychodynamic** understanding that takes into account the role of early experiences and unconscious influences in *actively* shaping behavior. (This is the *dynamic* in psychodynamic.) Psychodynamic treatments work toward the goal of providing greater insight into problems and bringing about behavioral change. Therapy may be brief, consisting of 12 to 25 sessions, or may continue for several years. According to current thinking, psychotherapy can actually rewire the network of neurons within the brain in ways that ease distress and improve functioning in many areas of daily life. Classical psychoanalysis, developed by Sigmund Freud, is a complex, lengthy process that deals with long-repressed feelings and issues. Less widely used than briefer forms of psychotherapy, it remains an option best suited for mentally healthy, high-functioning individuals who want to explore distressing patterns in their lives, such as a series of failed relationships.

Interpersonal Therapy (IPT)

Interpersonal therapy (IPT), originally developed for research into the treatment of major depression, focuses on relationships in order to help individuals deal with unrecognized feelings and needs and improve their communication skills. IPT does not deal with the psychological origins of symptoms but rather concentrates on current problems of getting along with others. The supportive, empathic relationship that is developed with the therapist, who takes an even more active role than in psychodynamic psychotherapy, is the most crucial component of this therapy. The emphasis is on the here and now and on interpersonal—rather than intrapsychic—issues. Individuals with major depression, chronic difficulties developing relationships, chronic mild depression, or bulimia (see Chapter 6 on eating disorders) are most likely to benefit. IPT usually consists of 12 to 16 sessions.

Cognitive-Behavioral Therapy

This approach, which focuses on inappropriate or inaccurate thoughts or beliefs, aims to help individuals break out of a distorted way of thinking. The techniques of **cognitive therapy** include identification of an individual's beliefs and attitudes, recognition of negative thought patterns, and education in alternative ways of thinking. Individuals with major depression or anxiety disorders are most likely to benefit, usually in 15 to 25 sessions. However, many of the positive messages used in cognitive therapy can help anyone improve a bad mood or negative outlook.

Behavior therapy strives to substitute healthier ways of behaving for maladaptive patterns used in the past. Its premise is that distressing psychological symptoms, like all

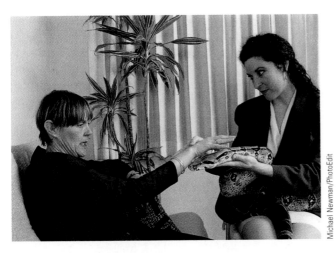

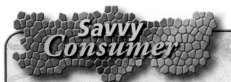

▲ Systematic desensitization is one of the behavior therapies used to treat phobias.

behaviors, are learned responses that can be modified or unlearned. Some therapists believe that changing behavior also changes how people think and feel. As they put it, "Change the behavior, and the feelings will follow." Behavior therapies work best for disorders characterized by specific, abnormal patterns of acting—such as alcohol and drug abuse, anxiety disorders, and phobias—and for individuals who want to change bad habits.

Psychiatric Drug Therapy

Medications that alter brain chemistry and relieve psychiatric symptoms have brought great hope and help to mil-

lions of people. Thanks to the recent development of a new generation of more precise and effective **psychiatric drugs,** success rates for treating many common and disabling disorders—depression, panic disorder, schizophrenia, and others—have soared. Often used in conjunction with psychotherapy, sometimes used as the primary treatment, these medications have revolutionized mental health care.[84]

At some point in their lives, about half of all Americans will take a psychiatric drug. The reason may be depression, anxiety, a sleep difficulty, an eating disorder, alcohol or drug dependence, impaired memory, or another disorder that disrupts the intricate chemistry of the brain. (See Savvy Consumer: "What You Need to Know about Mind-Mood Medications.")

Psychiatric drugs are now among the most widely prescribed drugs in the United States. Three of the top ten prescription drugs sold in this country are serotonin-boosting antidepressants—best known by their trade names Prozac, Paxil, and Zoloft—that are used to treat a variety of problems, including obsessive-compulsive disorder, premenstrual syndrome, and attention deficits, as well as depression.[85]

Psychiatric medications affect every aspect of a person's physical, mental, and emotional functioning. Some take effect immediately; others take several weeks to relieve symptoms; a few continue to exert their effects even after an individual discontinues their use. When taken appropriately, psychiatric agents can alleviate tremendous suffering and reduce the financial and personal costs of mental illness by lessening the need for hospitalization and by restoring an individual's ability to function normally, to work, and to contribute to society. But they do have side effects and must be used with care. This is especially true

---

Savvy Consumer

What You Need to Know About Mind-Mood Medications

Before taking any "psychoactive" drug (one that affects the brain), talk to a qualified health professional. Here are some points to raise:

- What can this medication do for me? What specific symptoms will it relieve? Are there other possible benefits?

- Are there any risks? What about side effects? Do I have to take it before or after eating? Will it affect my ability to study, work, drive, or operate machinery?

- When will I notice a difference? How long does it take for the medicine to have an effect?

- How will I be able to tell if the medication is working? What are the odds that it will help me?

- How long will I have to take medication? Is there any danger that I'll become addicted?

- What if it doesn't help?

- Is there an herbal or natural alternative? If so, has it been studied? What do you know about its possible risks and side effects?

Source: Hales, Robert E., and Dianne Hales. *The Mind-Mood Pill Book.* New York: Bantam, 2001.

for their use in children. More than 500,000 serotonin-boosting drugs are written for children and adolescents each year, even though the FDA approved these medications only for patients over age 18. Although researchers note that these drugs are potentially helpful, their safety and effectiveness have not been assessed in young people, and there are no clear age and dosage guidelines.[86]

Alternative Mind-Mood Products

Increasingly consumers are trying "natural" products, such as herbs and enzymes, that claim to have psychological effects. However, because they are not classified as drugs, they have not undergone the rigorous scientific testing required of psychiatric medications, and little is known about their safety or efficacy. "Natural" doesn't mean risk-free. Opium and cocaine are "natural" substances that have dramatic and potentially deadly effects on the mind.[87]

St. John's wort (named after St. John the Baptist because the yellow flowers of the *Hypericum perforatum* plant bloom in June, the anniversary month of his execution) has been used to treat anxiety and depression in Europe for many years. Although more than 24 clinical trials have investigated St. John's wort, many researchers feel that most had significant flaws in design. In a scientifically rigorous study of 200 hundred patients with major depression, St. John's wort did not prove effective. Using various measures to gauge the severity of depression, the researchers found almost no significant differences between those taking St. John's wort and those taking sugar pills during an eight-week period.[88] Side effects include dizziness, abdominal pain and bloating, constipation, nausea, fatigue, and dry mouth. St. John's wort should not be taken in combination with other prescription antidepressants.[89]

Other substances are widely used despite little or no scientific evaluation of their risks and benefits. Valerian, derived from the root of *Valeriana officinalis,* is taken primarily for insomnia and may help induce sleepiness. Kava, from a pepper tree native to the South Pacific, is thought to have a naturally soothing effect that can relieve anxiety and tension. Gingko biloba, long used in Chinese medicine, is considered a natural brain booster that may improve memory and concentration. However, excessive bleeding and, in rare cases, stroke have been reported with the use of gingko.[90]

Researchers have found a correlation between low levels of S-adenosylmethionine (SAM-e), a naturally occurring compound in human cells that boosts mood-influencing brain chemicals like serotonin, and depression. According to a limited number of small studies, dietary supplements containing SAM-e may enhance the effectiveness of conventional antidepressants.[91] In seven of eight controlled studies since the 1980s, SAM-e has been found more effective than a placebo in treating depression, but its effects are modest, and the methodology used in the studies has been criticized. In some controlled studies in Europe, SAM-e has been shown to be effective as a treatment for arthritic pain and inflammation. Sold as an unregulated dietary supplement, there are no guarantees of the actual contents of SAM-e as purchased in retail stores or on the Internet, nor has it been proven safe for children, nursing or pregnant women, or people with serious medical problems.[92]

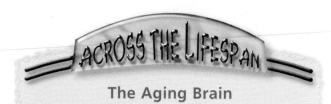

The Aging Brain

Scientists used to think that the aging brain, once worn out, could never be fixed. Now they know that the brain can and does repair itself. When neurons (brain cells) die, the surrounding cells develop "fingers" to fill the gaps and establish new connections, or synapses, between surviving neurons. Although self-repair occurs more quickly in young brains, the process continues in older brains. Even victims of Alzheimer's disease, the most devastating form of senility, have enough healthy cells in the diseased brain to regrow synapses. Scientists hope to develop drugs that someday may help the brain repair itself.

Mental ability does not decline along with physical vigor. Researchers have been able to reverse the supposedly normal intellectual declines of 60- to 80-year-olds by tutoring them in problem solving. Reaction time, intellectual speed and efficiency, nonverbal intelligence, and maximum work rate for short periods may diminish by age 75. However, understanding, vocabulary, ability to remember key information, and verbal intelligence remain about the same.

Memory

Some memory skills, particularly the ability to retrieve names and process information quickly, inevitably diminish over time. What normal changes should you expect? Here is a preview:

- **Recalling information takes longer.** As individuals reach their mid- to late sixties, the brain slows down, but usually just by a matter of milliseconds. As long as they're not rushed, older adults eventually adapt and perform just as well as younger ones.

- **Distractions become more disruptive.** Teenagers can study and listen to the stereo at the same time. Thirty-something moms can soothe the baby, field questions about homework, and put together a dinner all at once. But as individuals pass age 50, they find it much more difficult to divide their attention or to remember details of a story after having switched their attention to something else.

- **"Accessing" names gets harder.** The ability to remember names—especially those that you don't use frequently—diminishes by as much as 50 percent between ages 25 and 65. Preventive strategies can help, such as repeating a person's name when introduced, writing down the name as soon as possible, and making obvious associations (the Golden Gate for a man named Bridges).

- **Learning new information is harder.** The quality of memory doesn't change, just the speed at which we receive, absorb, and react to information. That's why strategies like taking notes or outlining material become critical for older students, especially when learning brand-new skills. However, adding to existing knowledge remains as easy as ever.

- **Wisdom matters.** In any memory test involving knowledge of the world, vocabulary or judgment, older people outperform younger ones.

Alzheimer's Disease

About 15 percent of older Americans lose previous mental capabilities, a brain disorder called **dementia.** Sixty percent of these—a total of 4 million men and women over age 65—suffer from the type of dementia called **Alzheimer's disease,** a progressive deterioration of brain cells and mental capacity.

 Women are more likely to develop Alzheimer's than men. By age 85, as many as 28 to 30 percent of women suffer from Alzheimer's, and women with this form of dementia perform significantly worse than men in various visual, spatial, and memory tests. African Americans have higher rates of Alzheimer's disease than Africans living in Africa, according to the first study to find differences in

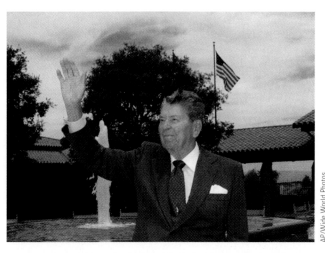

▲ Former President Ronald Reagan was diagnosed with Alzheimer's disease just a few years after leaving office. He suffered a progressive loss of mental abilities.

the incidence of this illness in an industrial and a nonindustrial country.[93]

The American Academy of Neurology has developed new guidelines, based on a review of 1,000 peer-reviewed papers, for diagnosing Alzheimer's. Based on clinical criteria, these guidelines should allow doctors to diagnose this form of dementia with 90 to 95 percent accuracy.[94] The early signs of dementia—insomnia, irritability, increased sensitivity to alcohol and other drugs, and decreased energy and tolerance of frustration—are usually subtle and insidious. Diagnosis requires a comprehensive assessment of an individual's medical history, physical health, and mental status, often involving brain scans and a variety of other tests.

Even though no one can restore a brain that is in the process of being destroyed by an organic brain disease like Alzheimer's, medications can control difficult behavioral symptoms and enhance or partially restore cognitive ability. Often physicians find other medical or psychiatric problems, such as depression, in these patients; recognizing and treating these conditions can have a dramatic impact.

Depression and the Elderly

Depression is a serious problem among the elderly. According to the National Institute of Mental Health, 6 percent of Americans aged 65 or older experience some form of depression. Older people face many challenges, including declining health, the loss of loved ones, social isolation, and physical limitations. However, depression is not inevitable, and the elderly are as likely to benefit from psychotherapy and medications as are younger individuals.

The consequences of not recognizing and treating depression late in life can be tragic. Older Americans have the highest suicide rates in our society, with some 8,500 elderly persons killing themselves every year. The suicide rate is five times higher for those aged 65 than for younger individuals. And depressed older men and women are also more likely to die of other causes. However, late-life depression can be overcome. With treatment, more than 70 percent of the depressed elderly improve dramatically. Since loneliness and loss are often important contributing factors, psychiatrists often combine counseling, such as brief psychotherapy, with medication. Because of various physiological differences in the elderly, they usually respond more slowly to antidepressants than younger persons, and the benefits thus may not be apparent for 6 to 12 weeks.

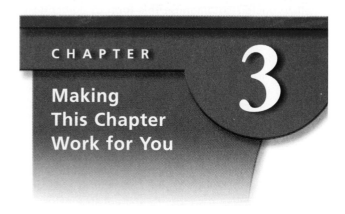

CHAPTER

Making This Chapter Work for You

3

1. Psychological health is influenced by all of the following except
   a. spiritual health.
   b. physical agility.
   c. culture.
   d. a firm grasp on reality.

2. Emotional intelligence encompasses which of the following components?
   a. creativity, sense of humor, scholastic achievement
   b. integrity, honesty, and perseverance
   c. piety, tolerance, and self-esteem
   d. empathy, self-awareness, and altruism

3. Which of the following activities can contribute to a lasting sense of personal fulfillment?
   a. becoming a Big Sister or Big Brother to a child from an inner city single-parent home
   b. volunteering at a local soup kitchen on Thanksgiving
   c. being a regular participant in an Internet chat room
   d. going on a shopping spree

4. Individuals who have developed a sense of mastery over their lives are
   a. skilled at controlling the actions of others.
   b. usually passive and silent when faced with a situation they don't like.
   c. aware that their locus of control is internal, not external.
   d. aware that their locus of control is external, not internal.

5. Mental illness can be described as
   a. a condition associated with migraine headaches and narcolepsy.
   b. a condition that is usually caused by severe trauma to the brain.
   c. a behavioral or psychological disorder that impairs an individual's ability to conduct one or more important activities of daily life.
   d. a psychological disorder that is easily controlled with medication and a change in diet.

6. Neurons
   a. transmit information within the brain and throughout the body by means of electrical impulses and chemical messengers.
   b. are specialized support cells that travel through the spinal cord, carrying signals related to movement.
   c. are protein molecules designed to bind with neurotransmitters.
   d. consist of nuclei, dendrites, and glia.

7. Which of the following statements about anxiety disorders is true?
   a. Anxiety disorders are the least prevalent type of mental illness.
   b. An individual suffering from a panic attack may mistake her symptoms for a heart attack.
   c. The primary symptom of obsessive-compulsive disorder is irrational, intense, and persistent fear of a specific object or situation.
   d. Generalized anxiety disorders respond to systematic desensitization behavior therapy.

8. Some characteristic symptoms of major depression are
   a. difficulty concentrating, lack of energy, and eating more than usual.
   b. exaggerated sense of euphoria and energy.

c. palpitations, sweating, numbness, and tingling sensations.

d. talking in rambling ways, inability to think in a logical manner, and delusions.

9. A person may be at higher risk of committing suicide if
   a. he is taking antidepressant medication.
   b. he lives in a rural environment and is married.
   c. he has been diagnosed with hyperactivity disorder.
   d. he has lost his job because of alcoholism.

10. Which of the following statements is true?
    a. Individuals with schizophrenia are most likely to benefit from psychodynamic therapy in combination with nutritional supplements.
    b. The antidepressants Prozac, Paxil, and Zoloft can also be used to treat premenstrual syndrome and attention deficit disorder.
    c. Psychologists are usually trained in a variety of psychotherapeutic techniques and are licensed to prescribe psychiatric medications.
    d. Interpersonal therapy focuses on the role of early experiences and unconscious influences in shaping patterns of behavior, such as repeated failed relationships.

Answers to these questions can be found on page 640.

 What is known about biofeedback in the treatment of Attention Deficit Disorder?

Critical Thinking

1. Would you say that you view life positively or negatively? Would your friends and family agree with your assessment? Ask two of your closest friends for feedback about what they perceive are your typical responses to a problematic situation. Are these indicative of positive attitudes? If not, what could you do to become more psychologically positive?

2. Paula went to a therapist when she was feeling depressed and was given a prescription for an antidepressant called fluoxetine (trade name Prozac). Her therapist recommended the drug because it causes fewer side effects than other medications. However, Paula later read in a news magazine that some patients, claiming that Prozac had made them violent or suicidal, had sued the drug's manufacturers. Their suits didn't win in court, but Paula was less certain about taking the prescribed medication. What do you think she should do? How would you weigh the risks and benefits of taking a psychiatric drug?

3. Research has indicated that many homeless men and women are in need of outpatient psychiatric care, often because they suffer from chronic mental illnesses or alcoholism. Yet government funding for the mentally ill is inadequate, and homelessness itself can make it difficult, if not impossible, for people to gain access to the care they need. How do you feel when you pass homeless individuals who seem disoriented or out of touch with reality? Who should take responsibility for their welfare? Should they be forced to undergo treatment at psychiatric institutions?

4. Everyone experiences memory lapses on occasion, but the frequency of these may increase with age. How would you respond if you noticed that one of your parents appeared to be growing more forgetful? What could you do to determine whether this forgetfulness was a symptom of a more serious mental disorder?

SITES & BYTES

National Institute of Mental Health
http://www.nimh.nih.gov
This professional site features information for the public as well as health practitioners on a variety of mental health topics, including depression, anxiety, ADHD, eating disorders, learning disabilities, posttraumatic stress disorder, and suicide.

American Psychological Association
http://www.apa.org
This site has information for mental health professionals, students, and the public on a variety of mental health topics, including mind-body medicine. This site also features a help center that provides advice on how to access psychological services and an online literature search.

Psych Central
http://www.psychcentral.com
Dr. John Grohol's Mental Health Page is a comprehensive site for psychology, support, and mental health issues, with an FAQ section and online mental health resources. The site also features interactive quizzes on eating disorders, depression, mania, obsessive-compulsive disorder, and attention disorders. During free, weekly live chats Dr. Grohol answers mental health and relationship questions online.

Please note that links are subject to change. If you find a broken link, use a search engine such as http://www.yahoo.com and search for the website by typing in key words.

InfoTrac Activity Peter M. Lewinsohn, Paul Rohde, John R. Seeley, Carol L. Baldwin. "Gender Differences in Suicide Attempts from Adolescence to Young Adulthood." *Journal of the American Academy of Child and Adolescent Psychiatry,* Vol. 40, No. 4, April 2001, p. 427.

(1) What is the strongest predictor of both future suicide attempts and completions?

(2) What are some of the reasons proposed to explain why the rates of suicide attempts are two to three times greater for female adolescents when compared with male adolescents?

(3) What is the association between suicidal behavior during childhood and adolescence and the incidence of suicide attempts during young adulthood? According to the researchers, why is there a gender difference?

You can find additional readings related to psychological health with InfoTrac College Edition, an online library of more than 900 journals and publications. Follow the instructions for accessing InfoTrac that were packaged with your textbook; then search for articles using a key word search.

For additional links, resources, and suggested readings on InfoTrac, visit our Health & Wellness Resource Center at http://health.wadsworth.com.

Key Terms

The terms listed here are used within the chapter on the page indicated. Definitions of the terms are in the Glossary at the end of the book.

altruism 75
Alzheimer's disease 97
antidepressant 82
anxiety 79
anxiety disorders 83
assertive 76
attention deficit/hyperactivity disorder (ADHD) 90
autonomy 75
axon 81
axon terminal 81
behavior therapy 94
bipolar disorder 87
certified social worker 94
cognitive therapy 94
culture 69
dementia 97
dendrites 81
depression 79
depressive disorders 85
emotional health 68

emotional intelligence 69
generalized anxiety disorder (GAD) 83
glia 81
interpersonal therapy (IPT) 94
licensed clinical social worker (LCSW) 94
locus of control 76
major depression 86
marriage and family therapist 94
mental disorder 78
mental health 68
mood 72
neuron 81
neuropsychiatry 81
neurotransmitters 82
nucleus 81
obsessive-compulsive disorder (OCD) 83
optimism 74
panic attack 83

panic disorder 83
phobia 83
psychiatric drugs 95
psychiatric nurse 94
psychiatrists 93
psychodynamic 94
psychologists 93
psychotherapy 94
receptors 82
reuptake 82
schizophrenia 91
self-actualization 70
self-esteem 71
social isolation 76
social phobia 77
spiritual health 68
spiritual intelligence 69
synapse 82
values 71

References

1. Satcher, David. "Executive Summary: A Report of the Surgeon General on Mental Health." *Public Health Reports*, Vol. 115, No. 1, January 2000.

2. Diener, Ed, et al. "Subjective Well-being: Three Decades of Progress." *Psychological Bulletin*, Vol. 125, No. 2, March 1999.

3. Shapiro, Deane, and Roger Walsh. *Beyond Health and Normalcy.* New York: Van Nostrand Reinhold, 1983.

4. Satcher, "Executive Summary: A Report of the Surgeon General on Mental Health."

5. Moore, Thomas. *Care of the Soul.* New York: Harper Perennial, 1994.

6. Goleman, Daniel. *Emotional Intelligence.* New York: Bantam Books, 1997.

7. Chatterjee, Camille. "Emotional Ignorance." *Psychology Today*, Vol. 33, No. 6, November 2000, p. 12.

8. Sloan, R. P., et al. "Religion, Spirituality, and Medicine." *Lancet*, Vol. 353, No. 9153, February 20, 1999.

9. Harris, T. George. "Spiritual Intelligence." Symposium at American Psychological Association, Annual Meeting, San Francisco, August 1998.

10. Ornish, Dean. Personal interview.

11. Danner, Deborah, et al. "Positive Emotions in Early Life and Longevity: Findings from the Nun Study." *Journal of Personality & Social Psychology*, Vol. 80, No. 5, May 2001, p. 804.

12. Robins, Richard, and Jennifer Beer. "Positive Illusions about the Self: Short-term Benefits and Long-term Costs." *Journal of Personality & Social Psychology*, Vol. 80, No. 2, February 2001, p. 340.

13. Larsen, Randy. Personal interview.

14. Ibid.

15. Myers, David. *The Pursuit of Happiness: Who Is Happy—and Why.* New York: William Morrow, 1992.

16. Reiss, Steven. "Secrets of Happiness." *Psychology Today*, January–February 2001, p. 58.

17. Freeman, Leslie, et al. "The Relationship Between Adult Happiness and Self-Appraised Childhood Happiness and Events." *Journal of Genetic Psychology*, Vol. 160, No. 1, March 1999.

18. Ibid.

19. Chamberlin, Jamie. "People Need Help Finding What Makes Them Happy." *APA Monitor*, Vol. 29, No. 10, October 1998.

20. Freeman, "The Relationship Between Adult Happiness and Self-Appraised Childhood Happiness and Events."

21. Lane, Richard, et al. "Neuroanatomical Correlates of Happiness, Sadness, and Disgust." *American Journal of Psychiatry*, Vol. 154, No. 7, July 1997.

22. Niedenthal, Paula, et al. "Being Happy and Seeing 'Happy': Emotional State Mediates Visual Word Recognition." *Cognition & Emotion*, Vol. 11, No. 4, July 1997.

23. McIntosh, William, et al. "Goal Beliefs, Life Events, and the Malleability of People's Judgments of Their Happiness." *Journal of Social Behavior & Personality*, Vol. 12, No. 2, June 1997.

24. Provine, Robert. "The Science of Laughter." *Psychology Today*, November–December 2000, p. 58.

25. Ornish, Dean. *Love & Survival: The Scientific Basis for the Healing Power of Intimacy.* New York: HarperCollins, 1999.

26. Larsen, Randy. Personal interview.

27. "What Is the Psychiatric Significance of Loneliness?" *Harvard Mental Health Letter*, Vol. 16, No. 10, April 2000.

28. Schwartz, Richard. "Loneliness." *Harvard Review of Psychiatry*, Vol. 5, No. 2, July–August 1997.

29. "What Is the Psychiatric Significance of Loneliness?"

30. Preboth, Monica, and Shyla Wright. "Does the Internet Make People Unhappy?" *American Family Physician*, Vol. 59, No. 6, March 15, 1999.

31. Clinton, Monique, and Lynn Anderson. "Social and Emotional Loneliness: Gender Differences and Relationships with Self-Monitoring and Perceived Control." *Journal of Black Psychology*, Vol. 25, No. 1, February 1999.

32. Cramer, Kenneth, and Kimberley Neyedley. "Sex Differences in Loneliness: The Role of Masculinity and Femininity." *Sex Roles: A Journal of Research*, Vol. 38, No. 7–8, April 1998.

33. Stack, Stephen. "Marriage, Family, and Loneliness: A Cross-National Study." *Sociological Perspectives*, Vol. 41, No. 2, Summer 1998.

34. Koropeckyj-Cox, Tanya. "Loneliness and Depression in Middle and Old Age: Are the Childless More Vulnerable?" *Journals of Gerontology*, Vol. 53, No. 6, November 1998.

35. Stein, Murray, et al. "Social Phobia Symptoms, Subtypes, and Severity." *Archives of General Psychiatry*, Vol. 57, No. 11, November 2000.

36. Lang, Ariel, and Murray Stein. "Social Phobia: Prevalence and Diagnostic Threshold." *Journal of Clinical Psychiatry*, Vol. 62, Suppl. 1, 2001, pp. 5–10.

37. "This Year's International Mental Health Agenda: Erasing the Stigma of Mental Illness." May 2001, p. 24.

38. Satcher, David. "Heads Up." *Psychology Today*, May–June 2001, p. 13.

39. Ibid.

40. American Psychiatric Association. *Diagnostic and Statistical Manual of Mental Disorders.* 4th ed. Washington, DC: American Psychiatric Association, 1994.

41. "Depression and Heart Disease." *Harvard Heart Letter*, Vol. 11, No. 8, April 2001.

42. "Wound Healing and Depression." Short Takes, *UCSF Today*, April 20, 2001.

43. "Depression Can Hasten HIV Progression in Women." *AIDS Weekly*, May 7, 2001.

44. Andrews, Gavin. "Should Depression Be Managed as a Chronic Disease?" *British Medical Journal*, Vol. 322, No. 7283, Feburary 17, 2001, p. 419.

45. Rosenthal, Beth, et al. "Prevalence of Psychological Symptoms Among Undergraduate Students in an Ethnically Diverse Urban Public College," *Journal of American College Health*, Vol. 49, No. 1, July 2000.

46. Stein, "Social Phobia Symptoms, Subtypes, and Severity."

47. "What Are the Current Treatments for Panic Disorder?" *Harvard Mental Health Letter*, Vol. 16, No. 11, May 2000.

48. "What You Should Know About Generalized Anxiety Disorders." *American Family Physician*, Vol. 62, No. 7, October 1, 2000.

49. "Obsessive-Compulsive Disorder: What It Is and How to Treat It." *American Family Physician*, Vol. 61, No. 5, March 1, 2000.

50. "Depressing." Short Takes, *UCSF Today*, November 9, 2000.

51. Pullen, Lisa, et al. "Adolescent Depression: Important Facts That Matter." *Journal of Child and Adolescent Psychiatric Nursing*, Vol. 13, No. 2, April 2000.

52. Walling, Anne. "Depression in Young Adults." *American Family Physician*, Vol. 62, No. 1, July 1, 2000.

53. "Exercise Against Depression." *Harvard Mental Health Letter*, Vol. 17, No. 19, March 2001.

54. Babyak, Michael, et al. "Exercise Treatment for Major Depression: Maintenance of Therapeutic Benefit at 10 Months." *Psychosomatic Medicine*, Vol. 62, No. 5, September–October 2000, pp. 633–638.

55. LeTourneau, Melanie. "Pump Up to Cheer Up." *Psychology Today,* May–June 2001, p. 27.

56. Dubin, Julie Weingarden. "More Than a Mood." *Psychology Today,* May–June 2001, p. 26.

57. Jensen, Peter. Personal interview.

58. March, John. Personal interview.

59. "Teenage Depression Shows Family Ties." *Science News,* Vol. 159, No. 1, February 3, 2001, p. 72.

60. Hughes, Alice, et al. "Depressive Symptoms and Cigarette Smoking Among Teens." *Journal of the American Medical Association,* Vol. 284, No. 23, December 20, 2000, p. 2980.

61. Zito, Julia. "Antidepressant Use in Youth." Presentation, American Psychiatric Association Annual Meeting, New Orleans, May 2001.

62. Babyak, "Exercise Treatment for Major Depression."

63. Hales, Robert E., and Dianne Hales. *The Mind-Mood Pill Book.* New York: Bantam, 2001.

64. Ibid.

65. Wetzstein, Cheryl. "Preventing Suicide." *Insight on the News,* Vol. 16, No. 16, May 1, 2000.

66. "In Brief—Depression and Suicide: What Is the True Risk?" *Harvard Mental Health Letter,* Vol. 17, No. 10, April 2001.

67. Gould, Madelyn. Personal interview.

68. "Suicide in Women." *The Lancet,* Vol. 355, No. 9211, April 8, 2000.

69. Borowsky, Iris, et al. "Adolescent Suicide Attempts: Risks and Protectors." *Pediatrics,* Vol. 107, No. 3, March 2001, p. 485.

70. Barrios, Lisa, et al. "Suicide Ideation Among US College Students." *Journal of American College Health,* Vol. 48, No. 5, March 2000.

71. "Suicide and Suicide Attempts in Adolescents." *Pediatrics,* Vol. 105, No. 4, April 2000.

72. "The Seasons of Suicide." *Harvard Mental Health Letter,* Vol. 16, No. 11, May 2000.

73. Walling, Anne. "Which Patients Are at Greatest Risk of Committing Suicide?" *American Family Physician,* Vol. 61, No. 8, April 15, 2000, p. 2487.

74. "Analysis of Suicide Risk Factors and Suicidal Self-Injury and Concurrent Health Risk Behaviors Among Adolescents." *Research Quarterly for Exercise and Sport,* Vol. 71, March 2000.

75. Bostwick, J. M., et al. "Affective Disorders and Suicide Risk: A Re-examination." *American Journal of Psychiatry,* Vol. 157, No. 12, December 2000, p. 1925.

76. Popper, Charles, and Scott West. "Disorders Usually Diagnosed in Infancy, Childhood or Adolescence." *American Psychiatric Press Textbook of Psychiatry,* 3rd ed. Washington, DC: American Psychiatric Press, 1999.

77. Mostofsky, Stewart. "Brain Abnormalities in Children with ADHD." American Academy of Neurology, Annual Meeting, Toronto, April 1999.

78. "Harbingers of Schizophrenia." *Harvard Mental Health Letter,* Vol. 17, No. 5, November 2000.

79. Walling, Anne. "Update on Schizophrenia." *American Family Physician,* Vol. 61, No. 12, June 15, 2000.

80. "How Schizophrenia Develops: New Evidence and New Ideas." *Harvard Mental Health Letter,* Vol. 17, No. 8, February 2001.

81. Das, Pam. "Retroviruses May Contribute to the Development of Schizophrenia." *Lancet,* Vol. 357, No. 9263, April 14, 2001, p. 1184.

82. "What Is the Relationship Between Schizophrenia and Substance Abuse?" *Harvard Mental Health Letter,* Vol. 17, No. 4, October 2000.

83. "Atypical Antipsychotic Drugs: How Much Better Are They?" *Harvard Mental Health Letter,* Vol. 17, No. 10, April 2001.

84. Hart, Valerie. "The Balance of Psychotherapy and Pharmacotherapy." *Perspectives in Psychiatric Care,* Vol. 36, No. 2, April–June 2000.

85. Hales and Hales, *The Mind-Mood Pill Book.*

86. Ibid.

87. Ibid.

88. Shelton, Richard, et al. "Effectiveness of St. John's Wort in Major Depression: A Randomized Controlled Trial." *Journal of the American Medical Association,* Vol. 285, No. 15, April 18, 2001, p. 1978.

89. Dickstein, Leah. "Nature's Pharmacy Is Full of Surprises." *Psychology Today,* March–April 1999.

90. "Alternative Therapies for Depression, Diabetes and Obesity." *Journal of the American Dietetic Association,* Vol. 101, No. 3, March 2001, p. 364.

91. "SAM-e: The Natural Mood Enhancer." *Psychology Today,* March 2001, p. 46.

92. "SAM-e for Depression." *Harvard Mental Health Letter,* Vol. 17, No. 7, January 2001, p. 1.

93. Josefson, Deborah. "African Americans More at Risk than Africans from Alzheimer's Disease." *British Medical Journal,* Vol. 322, No. 7286, March 10, 2001, p. 574.

94. Larkin, Marilynn. "New U.S. Guidelines for Alzheimer's Disease Released." *Lancet,* Vol. 357, No. 927, May 12, 2001, p. 1505.

HEALTHY LIFESTYLES

You have enormous influence over your health and vitality. This section provides information about the tools you have at hand to become healthier and feel stronger and more energetic throughout your lifetime. By learning how to eat a balanced and varied diet, how to manage your weight, and how to become physically fit, you can get started on a lifelong journey of becoming all you can be. And as you take better care of your body today, you'll build the foundation for feeling your best for many tomorrows to come.

4

The Joy of Fitness

As a boy, Derek never thought about doing anything special to stay physically fit. He loved sports so much that he spent every free moment on a softball field or basketball court. He could sprint faster, jump higher, and hit a ball harder than any of his friends. In high school Derek's life revolved around practices and games. He was a varsity athlete and an all-school star in his hometown.

Early in his first year in college, an injury sidelined Derek. Frustrated that he had to sit out the season, he gave up his rigorous training routine. As he became immersed in academics and other activities, Derek stopped going to the gym or working out on his own. Yet he continued to think of himself as an athlete in excellent physical condition. When Derek went home for spring break, he joined his younger brothers on a neighborhood basketball court. While he

wasn't surprised that his long shots were off, Derek was amazed by how quickly he got winded. In fifteen minutes, he was panting for breath. "Getting old," one of his brothers joked. "Getting soft," the other teased.

Often the college years represent a turning point in physical fitness. Like Derek, many students, busy with classes and other commitments, devote less time to physical activity. About half of college freshmen exercise fewer than six hours a week (See Student Snapshot).[1] Physical activity drops off even more after graduation. In one survey of recent college graduates, 47 percent reported that they were exercising less than they had as students.[2]

The choices you make and the habits you develop now can affect how long and how well you'll live. As you'll see in this chapter, exercise can help you reduce stress, boost your spirits, feel better, live longer, and lower your risk of serious disease. To get these benefits, you don't have to turn into a jock or fitness fanatic. All you have to do is get moving. This chapter can help. It presents the latest activity recommendations, documents the benefits of exercise, describes types of exercise, and provides guidelines for getting into shape and exercising safely.

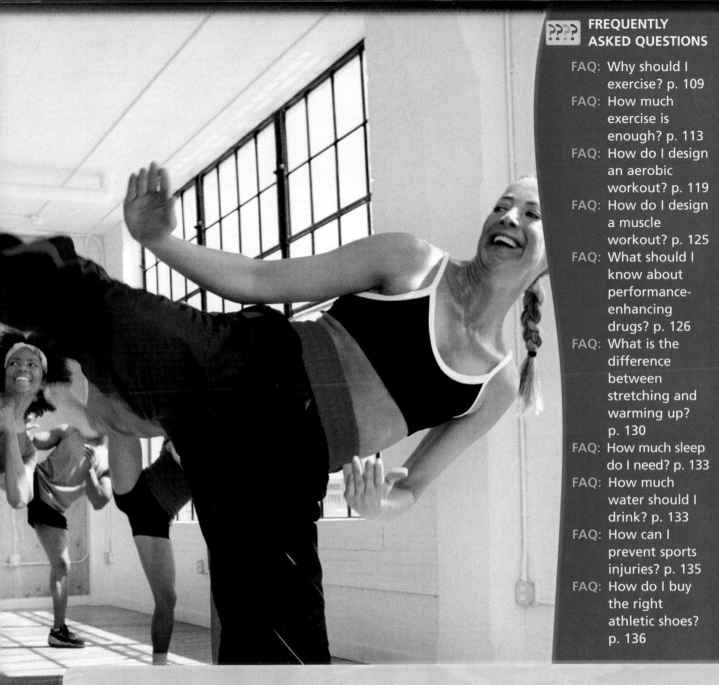

After studying the material in this chapter, you should be able to:

- **Describe** the components of physical fitness.
- **Discuss** the differences between sedentary and active lifestyles and develop strategies to become more active.
- **Describe** the health benefits of regular physical activity.
- **List** the different forms of cardiorespiratory activities and **describe** their potential health benefits and risks.
- **Explain** the benefits of a muscle training program and **describe** how to design a workout.
- **List** the potential health risks of strength-enhancing drugs and supplements.
- **Define** flexibility and describe the different types of stretching exercises.
- **Explain** the process of sleeping and the value of sleep in maintaining health.
- **List** nutritional and safety strategies for physically active individuals.

What Is Physical Fitness?

The simplest, most practical definition of **physical fitness** is the ability to respond to routine physical demands, with enough reserve energy to cope with a sudden challenge. You can consider yourself fit if you meet your daily energy needs, can handle unexpected extra demands, have a realistic but positive self-image, and are protecting yourself against potential health problems, such as heart disease.

Fitness is important both for health and for athletic performance. The health-related components of physical fitness, which this chapter emphasizes, include aerobic or cardiorespiratory endurance, muscular strength and endurance, body composition (the ratio of fat and lean body tissue) and flexibility. Athletic performance depends on additional skills, such as agility, coordination, balance, and speed, which vary with specific sports. While many amateur and professional athletes are in superb overall condition, you do not need athletic skills to keep your body operating at maximum capacity throughout life.

Cardiorespiratory fitness refers to the ability of the body to sustain prolonged rhythmic activity. It is achieved through **aerobic exercise**—any activity, such as brisk walking or swimming, in which the amount of oxygen taken into the body is slightly more than, or equal to, the amount of oxygen used by the body. In other words, aerobic exercise involves working out strenuously without pushing to the point of breathlessness.

Muscular fitness has two components: strength and endurance. **Strength** refers to the force within muscles; it is measured by the absolute maximum weight that we can lift, push, or press in one effort. **Endurance** is the ability to perform repeated muscular effort; it is measured by counting how many times you lift, push, or press a given weight. Both are equally important. It's not enough to be able to hoist a shovelful of snow; you've got to be able to keep shoveling until the entire driveway is clear.

Body composition refers to the relative amounts of fat and of lean tissue (bone, muscle, organs, water) in the body. A high proportion of body fat has serious health implications, including increased incidence of heart disease, high blood pressure, diabetes, stroke, gallbladder problems, back and joint problems, and some forms of cancer.

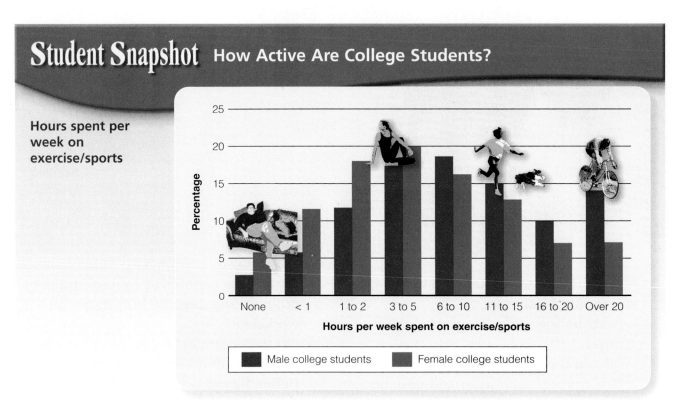

Student Snapshot How Active Are College Students?

Hours spent per week on exercise/sports

Source: Sax, Linda, et al. *The American Freshman: National Forms for Fall 2000.* Los Angeles: Higher Education Research Institute, UCLA, 2000.

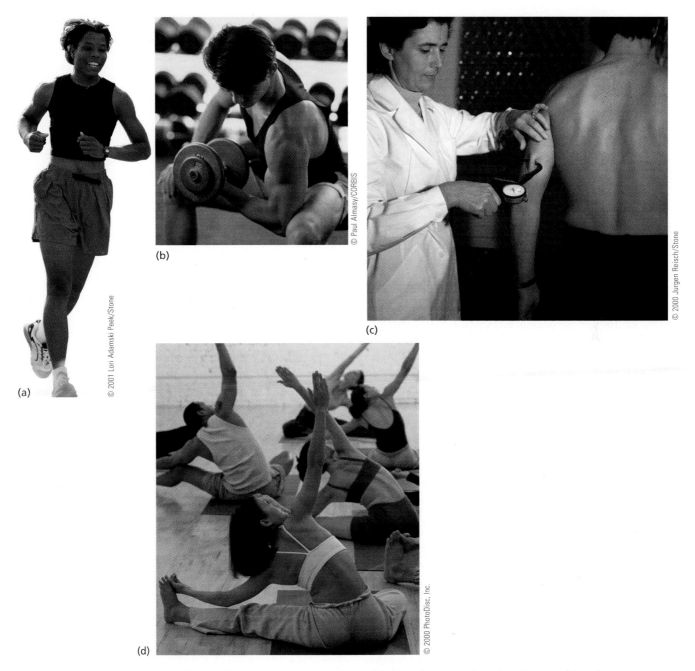

(a)

(b)

(c)

(d)

© 2001 Lori Adamski Peek/Stone

© Paul Almasy/CORBIS

© 2000 Jurgen Reisch/Stone

© 2000 PhotoDisc, Inc.

▲ Four components of physical fitness. (a) Cardiorespiratory fitness. (b) Muscular strength and endurance. (c) Body composition. (d) Flexibility.

College-age men average 15 percent body fat; college-age women, 23 percent. Men with a body fat level higher than 25 percent and women with 32 percent or higher body fat are considered obese.

A combination of regular exercise and good nutrition is the best way to maintain a healthy body composition. Aerobic exercise helps by burning calories and increasing metabolic rate (the rate at which the body uses calories) for several hours after a workout. Strength training increases the proportion of lean body tissue by building muscle mass, which also increases the metabolic rate.

Flexibility is the range of motion around specific joints—for example, the stretching you do to touch your toes or twist your torso. Flexibility depends on many factors: your age, gender, and posture; bone spurs; and how fat or muscular you are. As children develop, their flexibility increases until adolescence. Then a gradual loss of joint mobility begins and continues throughout adult life. Both muscles and connective tissue, such as tendons and ligaments, shorten and become tighter if not used at all or not used through their full range of motion.

Physical **conditioning** (or training) refers to the gradual building up of the body to enhance cardiorespiratory or aerobic fitness, muscular strength and endurance, or flexibility.

The Couch Potato Crisis

A silent epidemic is killing 250,000 Americans a year. "Sedentary death syndrome," or SeDS, refers to the lack of physical activity that is expected to lead to 2.5 million premature deaths in the next decade—a greater toll than alcohol, guns, motor vehicles, illicit drug use, and sexually transmitted diseases combined.[3] The economic impact of SeDS is equally staggering: an estimated $1 trillion in health care bills a year.[4]

Despite extensive research documenting the perils of physical inactivity, Americans remain as sedentary as they were in 1990.[5] According to the National Center for Chronic Disease Prevention and Health Promotion, as many as 60 percent do not exercise regularly; an estimated 150 million do not exercise at all. Only one in four adults meets the levels of physical activity recommended by federal health officials.[6] Women, older adults, ethnic and racial minorities, and those with fewer than twelve years of education are the least active.[7]

Sedentary living is disabling as well as deadly. It increases the likelihood or severity of dozens of serious conditions, including arthritis, arrhythmias, breast cancer, colon cancer, congestive heart failure, depression, gallstone disease, heart attack, hypertension, obesity, osteoporosis, respiratory problems, type 2 diabetes, sleep apnea, and stroke. As a risk factor for heart disease, physical inactivity ranks as high as elevated cholesterol, high blood pressure, or cigarette smoking.

The good news: SeDS is not inevitable. If sedentary men and women were to burn up just 150 additional calories a day walking, gardening, vacuuming, or dancing, they would actually lower their relative heart attack risk more than veteran exercisers who increase the duration or intensity of their regular workouts (see Table 4-1).

Who Exercises, Who Doesn't

According to a (CDC) survey, 29.4 percent of Americans report no leisure-time physical activity at all. City-dwellers tend to be more active than country folks; Westerners are more active than residents of other regions.[8] Yet overall, despite ongoing public health efforts to promote increased physical activity, the number of Americans who choose to take the stairs instead of riding the escalator is similar today to what it was almost 20 years ago.

Education and income both have a dramatic impact on activity levels. Almost half (47 percent) of those who did

▼ Table 4-1	How to Burn 150 Extra Calories a Day
Activity	**Approximate Time* (minutes)**
Bicycling (6 mph)	38
Canoeing	50
Gardening	30–45
Golfing (carrying bag and walking)	26
Hiking (40-pound pack)	22
Jogging (5.5 mph)	12
Running (7.5 mph)	11
Raking leaves	35
Skating (ice or roller)	30
Swimming (slow crawl)	17
Tennis (singles)	23
Walking (3–4 mph)	30
Weight training	20

*These exercise times are calculated for a 150-pound person. If you weigh less than 150 pounds, you'll burn fewer calories per minute and will have to work out longer. If you weigh more than 150 pounds, you'll burn 150 calories in a shorter time.

Source: "Physical Activity, Part I—Start With a Walk," *Harvard Women's Health Watch,* Vol. 8, No. 10, June 2001.

not graduate from high school are inactive, compared with just 26 percent of college graduates. Almost half of those earning less than $10,000 a year are inactive, compared with a third of those earning $35,000 or more a year.[9]

 Ethnicity also correlates with activity levels: 40 percent of the Mexican Americans surveyed did not engage in any physical activity in their leisure time, compared with 35 percent of blacks and 18 percent of whites. African-American and Mexican-American men and women reported less activity than their white counterparts, even when their income and education were similar.

Gender also correlates with activity, with men getting more exercise than women. According to the Surgeon General's office, more than 60 percent of women do not engage in the recommended amount of physical activity. An estimated 30 percent of all women are not active at all.[10] Yet women have every reason to get moving. In addition to exercise's unisex benefits, such as lowering the risk of dying from coronary heart disease and of developing high blood pressure, colon cancer, and diabetes, physical activity helps women keep their bones healthy and strong, controls weight, builds lean muscle, reduces body fat, helps control joint swelling and pain associated with arthritis, eases symptoms of menopause, fosters improvements in mood and feelings of well-being, and can help reduce

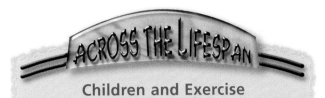

Children and Exercise

The children of the couch potato generation—"small fries," as some call them—are more sedentary than youngsters in the past. More than one-third of all young people between the ages of 12 and 21 do not regularly participate in vigorous physical activity. About one in four, according to the CDC, does not participate in daily physical education at school. What American kids do most is sit—often in front of a television or computer. The average child in the United States spends more than a thousand hours a year watching TV, and the more youngsters watch, the fatter they are likely to be.[12]

Today's youngsters not only move less; they weigh more. Obesity in American children has increased 100 percent in the last twenty years. An estimated 11 percent of children ages six to eleven are overweight, as are 14 percent of adolescents ages twelve to nineteen.[13] (Chapter 6 discusses weight problems in the young.)

As noted in Chapter 1, one of the objectives of *Healthy People 2010* is to get more kids moving. The ideal is for each youngster to accumulate at least an hour of physical activity every day. Studies have shown that once children begin a program of regular exercise, they can lower their health risks dramatically within eight weeks. If you're a parent, experts advise increasing your own activity level. Children of parents who exercise and make fitness a priority are more active and continue to be so throughout life.

Like adults, children benefit from aerobic activities such as swimming and bicycling as well as strength training. Muscle conditioning enhances motor skills and sports performance, helps strengthen bone, controls weight, boosts psychosocial well-being, and improves cardiorespiratory fitness. A stronger musculoskeletal system also may reduce children's risk of sports-related injuries.[14]

Shaping up is good for families as well as kids. Teenagers who exercise regularly report better relationships with their parents (including greater intimacy and more frequent touching), are less depressed, get more involved in sports, use drugs less frequently, and have higher grade point averages than students with a low level of exercise.[15]

The correlation between fitness and academic success does not seem to hold true for college undergraduates. A study at two Texas universities found

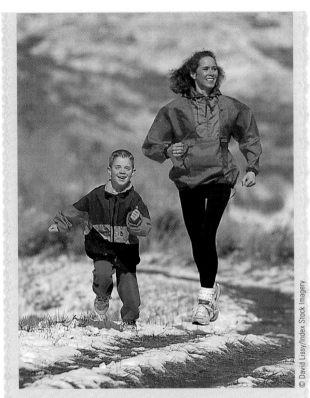

▲ Parents have a powerful influence over their childrens' attitudes toward physical fitness.

 that the fittest students didn't necessarily have higher GPAs. However, increasing their level of physical fitness did have a positive impact on the GPAs of the female students.[16]

blood pressure in some women with hypertension.[11] (For more on gender and exercise, see The X & Y Files: "Gender Differences and Physical Fitness.")

???? Why Should I Exercise?

If exercise could be packed into a pill, it would be the single most widely prescribed and beneficial medicine in the nation. Why? Because nothing can do more to help your body function at its best (Figure 4-1). With regular activity, your heart muscles become stronger and pump blood more efficiently. Your heart rate and resting pulse slow down. Your blood pressure may drop slightly from its normal level.

Regular physical activity thickens the bones and can slow the loss of calcium that normally occurs with age. Exercise increases flexibility in the joints and improves

The X&Y Files — Gender Differences and Physical Fitness

Men and women benefit equally from physical activity and exercise. Nevertheless, the components of physical fitness do have gender differences. Many are related to size. On average, men are 10 to 15 percent bigger than women, with roughly twice the percentage of muscle mass and half the percentage of body fat of women. Overall, men are about 30 percent stronger, particularly above the waist. They have more sweat glands and a greater maximum oxygen uptake. A man's bigger heart pumps more blood with each beat. His larger lungs take in 10 to 20 percent more oxygen. His longer legs cover more distance with each stride. If a man jogs along at 50 percent of his capacity, a woman has to push to 73 percent of hers to keep up.

Women have a higher percentage of body fat than men, and more is distributed around the hips and thighs; men carry more body fat around the waist and stomach. The average woman has a smaller heart, a lower percentage of slow twitch muscle fibers, and a smaller blood volume than a man. Because women have a lower concentration of red blood cells, their bodies are less effective at transporting oxygen to their working muscles during exercise.

Even though training produces the same relative increases for both genders, a woman's maximum oxygen intake remains about 25 to 30 percent lower than that of an equally well-conditioned man. In elite athletes, the gender difference is smaller: 8 to 12 percent. Because the angle of the upper leg bone (femur) to the pelvis is greater in a woman, her legs are less efficient at running.

In some endurance events, such as ultramarathon running and long-distance swimming, female anatomy and physiology may have some aerobic advantages. The longer a race—on land, water, or ice—the better women perform. In an analysis of world-record times in running, swimming, and speed skating, researchers at Northeastern University observed that in all three sports the superiority of men's performances diminished with increasing distance.

	Women	Men
Percent fat	27%	15%
Lean body mass	107.8 pounds	134.2 pounds
Blood volume	4.5–5 liters	5–6 liters
Maximum oxygen consumption	3–3.5 liters per minute	5.5–9 liters per minute

digestion and elimination. It speeds up metabolism, so the body burns up more calories and body fat decreases. It heightens sensitivity to insulin (a great benefit for diabetics) and may lower the risk of developing diabetes. In addition, exercise enhances clot-dissolving substances in the blood, helping to prevent strokes, heart attacks, and pulmonary embolisms (clots in the lungs). Regular, vigorous exercise can actually extend the lifespan. (See Pulse Points: "Ten Reasons to Get Moving" on page 112.)

Here is a summary of the benefits of getting in shape:

Longer Life

Longevity has more to do with one's level of physical activity than with genetics. In a 19-year study tracking the health and lifestyles of twins, the risk of death was 56 percent lower for those who exercised at least 30 minutes, six or more times per month, and 34 percent lower for occasional exercisers.

Protection Against Heart Disease and Certain Cancers

Sedentary people are about twice as likely to die of a heart attack as people who are physically active. (See Chapter 12 for a discussion of heart disease.) In addition to its effects on the heart, exercise makes the lungs more efficient. They take in more oxygen, and their vital capacity (ability to take in and expel air) is increased, providing more energy for you to use.

As recent studies have shown, exercise reduces the risk of colon and rectal cancers, possibly by enhancing digestion and elimination. In women, exercise also may help reduce the risk of cancer of the breast and reproductive organs. Fitter men are less likely to die of prostate and colon cancer than others.[17]

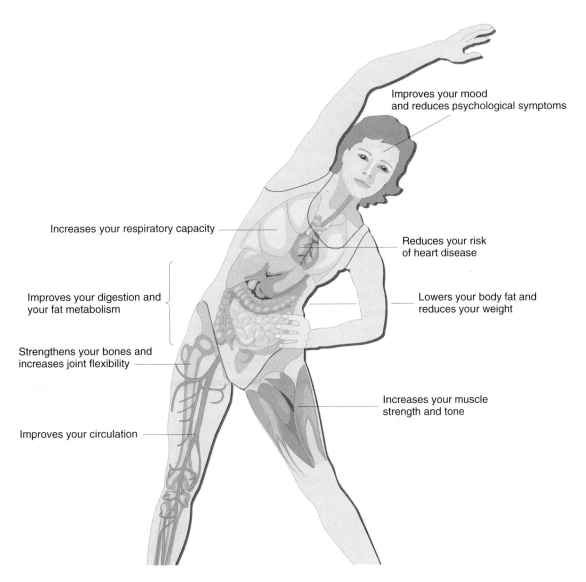

Improves your mood
and reduces psychological symptoms

Increases your respiratory capacity

Reduces your risk
of heart disease

Improves your digestion and
your fat metabolism

Lowers your body fat and
reduces your weight

Strengthens your bones and
increases joint flexibility

Increases your muscle
strength and tone

Improves your circulation

▲ **Figure 4-1** The benefits of exercise.
Regular physical activity enhances your overall health and helps prevent disease.

Better Bones

Weak and brittle bones are common among people who don't exercise. **Osteoporosis,** a condition in which bones lose their mineral density and become increasingly soft and susceptible to injury, affects a great many older people. Women, in particular, are more vulnerable because their bones are less dense to begin with.

Enhanced Immunity

Moderate exercise correlates with a reduced number of sick days. Researchers speculate that exercise may enhance immune function by reducing stress hormones like cortisol that can dampen resistance to disease. In the elderly, exercise has proven more beneficial than additional nutrients in boosting immune response.[18]

Brighter Mood

Exercise makes people feel good from the inside out. Exercise boosts mood, increases energy, reduces anxiety, improves concentration and alertness, and enables people to handle stress better. During long workouts, some people experience what is called "runner's high," which may be the result of increased levels of mood-elevating brain chemicals called **endorphins.**

PULSE POINTS

Ten Reasons to Get Moving

1. **Improve cardiorespiratory fitness.** Regular activity strengthens the heart so it pumps blood more efficiently.

2. **Tone muscles.** With exercise, muscles become firmer, function more smoothly, and are capable of withstanding much more strain.

3. **Reduce stress.** Working out releases tensions and enhances your ability to deal with daily challenges.

4. **Improve mood.** Exercise may be the single most effective strategy for changing a bad mood. It also works wonders for reducing anxiety and depression.

5. **Burn calories.** Exercise speeds up metabolism, so the body uses more calories during and after a workout.

6. **Increase flexibility.** Exercise stretches and lengthens muscles and increases flexibility in the joints.

7. **Enhance strength and stamina.** Muscle workouts improve the circulation of blood in the tissues and increase the body's ability to do sustained work.

8. **Keep bones strong.** Regular physical activity (especially weight-bearing activities) thickens the bones, possibly preventing the slow loss of calcium that normally occurs with age.

9. **Lower the risk of disease.** Exercise helps prevent many serious health problems, including high blood pressure, strokes, heart attacks, and certain cancers.

10. **Put more life in your years, and possibly more years in your life.** Physical activity slows the aging process, so you remain healthier and more active for a longer time. And if you work out often and vigorously enough, you can actually extend your lifespan.

Better Mental Health

Exercise is an effective—but underused—treatment for mild to moderate depression and may help in treating other mental disorders.[19] Regular, moderate exercise, such as walking, running, or lifting weights, three times a week, has proven helpful for depression and anxiety disorders, including panic attacks.[20] It also eases certain symptoms, such as agitation and hallucinations, in schizophrenic patients.[21] In a recent study of people with major depression, exercise proved as effective as medication in improving mood and also helped prevent relapse.[22]

Lower Weight

Aerobic exercise burns off calories during your workout, because as your body responds to the increased demand from your muscles for nutrients, your metabolic rate rises. Moreover, this surge persists for as long as 12 hours after exercise, so you continue to use up more calories than usual even after you've stopped sweating. In addition, aerobic exercise suppresses appetite, so you aren't as tempted to eat. It also helps dieters lose fat rather than lean muscle tissue when they cut back on calories. (See Chapter 6 for information on exercise and weight control.)

A More Active Old Age

Exercise slows the changes that are associated with advancing age: loss of lean muscle tissue, increase in body fat, and decrease in work capacity. In addition to lowering the risk of heart disease and stroke, exercise also helps older men and women retain the strength and mobility needed to live independently. Even in old age, exercise boosts strength and stamina, lessens time in wheelchairs, and improves outlook and sense of control.[23]

Physical Activity and Health

Alarmed by Americans' sedentary ways, health officials have shifted their emphasis from promoting regular and rigorous exercise to urging people to become more active in any way possible. As they point out, all forms of physical activity—any bodily movement that requires energy and is carried out by the muscles—can produce some health benefits. Recent studies have confirmed that "lifestyle" activities, such as walking, housecleaning, and gardening, are as effective as a structured exercise program in improving heart function, lowering blood pressure, and maintaining or losing weight.[24]

While lifestyle activity can improve health, exercise—the structured movement of the body for the purpose of improving or maintaining physical fitness—offers more benefits. Light exercise—activities that increase oxygen consumption no more than three times the level burned by the body at rest—can produce cardiorespiratory benefits.[25] Though light activity is good, moderate is better, and health experts encourage everyone to accumulate at least 30 minutes of moderate physical activity a day.

Exercise may seem to be just what a doctor would order—but physicians seldom advise their patients about physical activity, especially sedentary and low-income individuals at highest risk for weight gain and poorer health. Even when doctors recommend physical activity, patients don't necessarily heed their advice—especially men. In one recent study, female patients followed their doctors' orders and exercised to improve their cardiorespiratory fitness. Men did not, regardless of the type of counseling and follow-up offered.[26]

The Physical Activity Pyramid

Just as the U.S. Department of Agriculture has developed the Food Guide Pyramid to summarize recommendations for a healthy diet, medical experts have developed a similar graphic for appropriate "portions" of exercise (see Figure 4-2). Lifestyle physical activity forms the base of the pyramid. As federal experts have noted, these activities provide

some health benefits for those who have been inactive. Because these are low-intensity activities, they should be performed most frequently.

The next level of the pyramid consists of moderate-intensity activities, such as jogging, biking, tennis, or swimming, that should be performed three to five days a week for a total of 20 or more minutes.

The next level includes exercises for flexibility, strength, and muscular endurance, which should be performed two to three days a week.

At the top of the pyramid is rest or inactivity. Although rest can be important, particularly if you're ill or injured, too much inactivity leads to low fitness as well as poor health.

How Much Exercise Is Enough?

If you're not active at all, any physical exercise will produce some benefits. In the beginning, don't worry about frequency or intensity. You're better off starting slow and small, with just a 10-minute walk or bike ride a few days a week, than pushing to do too much and giving up because of injury or discomfort.[27] (See Self-Survey: "What's Your Physical Activity IQ".)

Although exercising just once or twice a week is not enough to improve cardiorespiratory or aerobic fitness, it does produce benefits: In a study of 45 healthy office workers, even those who exercised just once a week had lower body weights and lower body fat than those who didn't work out at all.[28] Simply walking one hour a week proved to reduce the risk of heart disease for

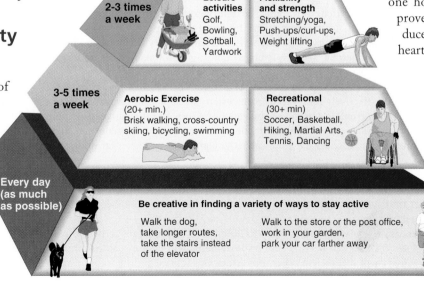
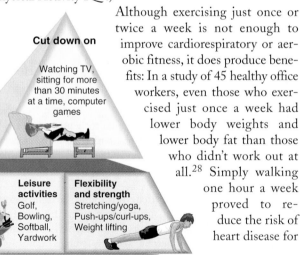

▲ **Figure 4-2** The activity pyramid. Use the pyramid to create a physical activity plan for your life.

SELF SURVEY

1. In general, what percentage of the calories you eat should come from carbohydrate if you are physically active?
   60–65 percent
   40 percent
   50 percent
2. The most effective physical activity plan is:
   strength (resistance) training.
   aerobic workouts at moderate intensity three or more times a week.
   a combination of strength training, flexibility exercises, and aerobic activity.
3. True or False? Certain activities can help you to selectively remove fat from your waist, thighs, or other specific areas of your body.
4. True or False? Women tend to have a lower metabolic rate than men.
5. How long does it take to see improvements in fitness level if you are doing moderate-intensity (somewhat hard) aerobic activity for 30 minutes three times a week?
   a day or two
   a week or two
   a month or two
6. What type of workout maximizes fat burning?
   low-intensity workouts
   moderate-intensity workouts
   high-intensity workouts
7. True or False? A person who weighs more burns more calories doing the same exercise as someone who weighs less.
8. True or False? Because we start losing muscle mass every year after about 30 years of age, physical activity has only a small benefit for older individuals.
9. What are the key components of physical activity that are important for improving your fitness?
   frequency, intensity, duration
   calorie intake, altitude, humidity
   temperature, time, type of activity
10. True or False? People who want bigger muscles should take protein supplements.

Answers:

1. 60–65 percent
   Carbohydrate is the chief fuel for your muscles. The American Dietetic Association recommends that for physically active adults, 60–65 percent of total calories come from carbohydrate. Examples of carbohydrate sources include breads, cereals, pasta, vegetables, and fruits. Athletes who train exhaustively on successive days or who compete in prolonged endurance events (like a marathon) should consume a diet that provides 65–70 percent of calories from carbohydrate.
2. A combination of strength training, flexibility exercises, and aerobic activity
   Strength or resistance training (working out against moderate resistance provided by free weights or your body) increases your muscle size and strength. Aerobic activity (walking, biking) has a beneficial effect on your heart. A combination of aerobic activity, strength training, and flexibility exercises is considered to be the most effective and well-rounded plan.
3. False
   You cannot selectively remove fat from certain areas of your body. Much of the way you look, including the size of different body parts, is determined by genetic factors. But don't give up—there are things you can do! Although activities for specific areas won't burn fat there, the activities will strengthen the underlying muscles and make the muscles more firm. Also, regular physical activity and diet will keep fat under control.
4. True
   Women usually have a greater percentage of body fat than men, and fat burns fewer calories than muscle. This makes women's metabolic rate 5–10 percent slower than men's. Because men have more muscle mass, they usually have an easier time losing weight than women; in fact, they burn more calories than women do just sitting around!
5. A week or two
   In general, if you work your way up to 30 minutes of moderate activity three days a week, you will see improvements in fitness on a regular basis. These improvements will be noticeable within a week or two. As your fitness improves, the activity will feel easier. When this happens, increase your workout until it feels somewhat hard again, and you'll continue to improve your fitness level.

6. Moderate-intensity workouts

   The percentage of fat calories burned is higher for low-intensity workouts, but this can be misleading. A greater absolute number of fat calories are burned during a moderate-intensity workout.

7. True

   The calories burned during an activity are directly related to how much you weigh. A smaller person would have to do an activity for a longer time to use the same amount of energy as a larger person because it takes more calories to move a large arm versus a small arm.

8. False

   It is never too late to include physical activity in your life. Frail and very old people (80+ years) can still participate in a regular physical activity program, improving the capacity of their hearts, decreasing the risk of falling, and improving their psychological outlook.

9. Frequency, intensity, duration

   The hallmarks of an effective physical activity program to improve your fitness level are frequency, intensity, and duration. Frequency means the number of times per week an activity is performed; intensity is how hard you work; duration is the time spent doing the activity. The current recommendations for these components from the American College of Sports Medicine for fitness are: perform physical activity 3–5 days per week (frequency) at 60–90 percent maximum heart rate for 20–60 minutes.

10. False

    There is no evidence that excess protein will lead to bigger muscles. Eating more protein than you need is a waste, since the excess will be converted to fat or burned for energy. If you want to increase the size and strength of your muscles, try strength training.

Source: U.S. Government, Shape Up America.

sedentary middle-aged women, even those who were overweight, smoked, or had high cholesterol.[29]

While some exercise is better than none, more is better. Federal health guidelines call for at least 30 minutes of brisk walking on most days of the week. The American College of Sports Medicine recommends the following weekly minimums (see Table 4-2):

▶ Three to five days of aerobic workouts of 20- to 60-minute duration, either in a single session or in several 10-minute sessions.

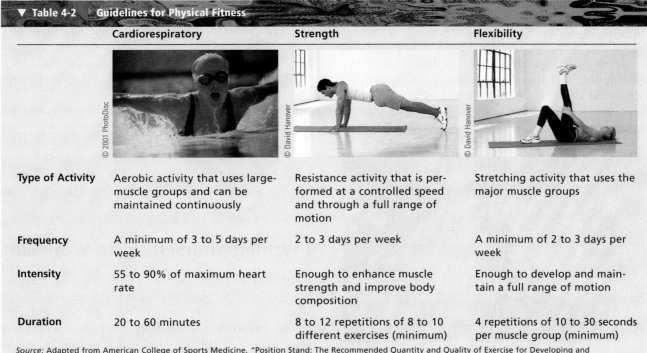

▼ Table 4-2   Guidelines for Physical Fitness

	Cardiorespiratory	Strength	Flexibility
Type of Activity	Aerobic activity that uses large-muscle groups and can be maintained continuously	Resistance activity that is performed at a controlled speed and through a full range of motion	Stretching activity that uses the major muscle groups
Frequency	A minimum of 3 to 5 days per week	2 to 3 days per week	A minimum of 2 to 3 days per week
Intensity	55 to 90% of maximum heart rate	Enough to enhance muscle strength and improve body composition	Enough to develop and maintain a full range of motion
Duration	20 to 60 minutes	8 to 12 repetitions of 8 to 10 different exercises (minimum)	4 repetitions of 10 to 30 seconds per muscle group (minimum)

Source: Adapted from American College of Sports Medicine, "Position Stand: The Recommended Quantity and Quality of Exercise for Developing and Maintaining Cardiorespiratory and Muscular Fitness, and Flexibility in Healthy Adults." *Medicine and Science in Sports and Exercise,* Vol. 30, 1998, pp. 975–991.

▶ Two to three strength training sessions that involve at least one set of eight to twelve repetitions of eight to ten exercises that work all major muscle groups.

▶ Two to three flexibility workouts that stretch the major muscles throughout the body.

Motivation

Before you set your body in motion, you have to make a mental commitment. Sit down and develop a plan of action. The more motivated you are, the more likely you are to stick with an exercise program.

Student Strategies

You know exercise is good for you—but do you work out regularly? As Student Snapshot—"How Active Are College Students?" indicates, most students don't. Men are more likely than women to exercise on college campuses, and more white and Hispanic students work out than do African-American undergraduates. According to an Ohio State University survey, the "buddy system" gets college men moving. If their friends exercise, they do too. This isn't true for college women, who rely more on family support and encouragement and have fewer friends who exercise.[30]

Looking better and feeling better are two of the strongest motivators that pull college students to their feet. However, there are some gender differences. In a study of 258 college freshmen enrolled in a personal health course, the women were significantly more fit than the men and more health- and appearance-conscious. However, the men placed more value on fitness and expressed greater satisfaction with their appearance.[31] As in other studies,

the students—male and female—with a greater sense of self-efficacy and an internal locus of control placed greater value on health and fitness, were more conscious about living a healthy lifestyle, and were more likely to be actively involved in activities that maintain or enhance fitness.[32]

What keeps you from working out? When that question was posted on a national chat board, students listed a variety of excuses: "Gym membership is too expensive." "I'm not going to run in the snow!" "I don't have enough time." "I don't like the school gym—it stinks, people are trying too hard, and it takes too long to get a machine." "The workout room in my dorm is always crowded." Others revealed ways they had managed to overcome these barriers and motivate themselves, including:

▶ Signs up for a fitness class, such as spinning or step-aerobics, so that exercise is built into your weekly schedule.

▶ Go to the gym with friends. "Even if it's rainy and cold, I know they're waiting for me so I go," one woman explained.

▶ Find a fun workout. "I love working out when it's something different—like water aerobics, ice skating, or swing dance," said one student.

▶ Use humor. One student put this sign on the wall: "You think flu season is scary? Wait till bathing suit season hits!"

▶ Build activity into your day. Many students walk to classes or always take the stairs rather than the elevator.

▶ Do double-duty. Some students read class notes while on a Stairmaster or stationary bicycle. Others listen to audiocassettes of required reading books as they work out.

The course in which you're using this text may help you get motivated and moving. In a study that compared college alumni who had taken a health and physical education course with others who had not, those who'd taken the course were more likely to engage in aerobic exercise. Not coincidentally, they also were less likely to smoke and had lower intakes of dietary fat and cholesterol. In another study at a Colorado university, students enrolled in a fitness and wellness course were more likely to participate in regular physical activity when tired, in a bad mood, in bad weather, time-pressured, or unsure of their ability to perform an activity.[33]

Psyching Yourself Up to Work Out

About half of the people who begin an exercise program drop out within the first three to six months.[34] Various strategies, such as telephone reminders from a health professional or trainer and setting short-term goals, have proven useful in helping people stick with their exercise plan. Here are some specific recommendations that may work for you:

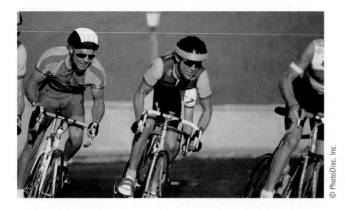

© PhotoDisc, Inc.

▲ Find a group of friends who are as interested in physical fitness as you are to help keep your motivation high.

Visualizing Success

Focus on the person you want to become. Try to visualize both how you'd look and how you'd live. What would you do differently on a daily basis? Define and write down what you want to accomplish and the actions you plan to take. If possible, find an image—from a magazine advertisement, for instance—and post it where you can see it.

Setting Goals

Set long-term goals to achieve in one year and short-term goals to achieve approximately every three months. For example, you could set a short-term goal of completing three 30-minute aerobic workouts and two strength and flexibility sessions a week. Your long-term goal could be to lose weight or lower your blood pressure.

Overcoming Obstacles

Anticipate the barriers you are likely to encounter and devise constructive ways of dealing with them by developing new personal skills, such as stress management and self-motivation. Make exercise easy for yourself. Think through the situations that sidetrack you. Do you have trouble getting to the gym if you go home first? Do you always hit the snooze button when you plan to work out in the morning? Do you often forget your gym clothes? Once you identify what gets in your way, try to reduce or eliminate each obstacle. Pack your gym bag the night before. Go straight to the gym after class.

Monitoring Your Progress

Keep a detailed record of your workouts, noting the types of exercises you do, the intensity you work at, the duration of each session, and the number of repetitions and sets. Determine a reasonable amount of time in which to meet your goals, but be willing to modify your plan.

Following the Hard/Easy Principle

Many serious exercisers and athletes train every day. Some coaches, however, concerned that such intensive training can wear out the body, advocate alternating a day of hard-intensity training with an easy day of more moderate exercise. The lower intensity allows the body time to recover and prepare for the next day of training.

Beating Boredom

Boredom is a common complaint, especially for beginning exercisers. To overcome it, try varying the types of exercise you do. (See Figure 4-3.) In a study of sedentary male and female university students between the ages of 18 to 35,

STRATEGIES FOR CHANGE

How to Bust Through Barriers

✔ Aim to do half a workout. Once you get started, you may find you want to keep going.

✔ Show up. Once you're at the gym, you're more likely to be in the mood to exercise.

✔ If you're embarrassed about your body, remind yourself that you're more concerned about your appearance than anyone else is. Look around: people come in all different shapes and sizes.

✔ If you're easily bored, try to learn at least two new exercises a month.

✔ If you're easily winded, decrease intensity and increase duration. For example, slow your pace as you walk but extend the distance you cover.

those who were able to change their aerobic exercise regimen reported enjoying their workouts more and were most likely to keep up regular physical activity.[35]

Preventing Relapse

 Setbacks are part of the process of behavior change. Why do some people stick with an exercise program while others quit? Researchers recently studied a group of Brown University undergraduates, all of whom had been exercising for at least 20 minutes three times a week. Two months later 87 percent were still exercising, but 13 percent had relapsed. The relapsers had scored lower on measures of self-efficacy, the feelings of competence and control discussed in Chapter 1. They also listed significantly fewer "pros" or advantages of exercising than those who stuck with the program. In time, the "cons" or negatives outweighed their positive motivators. The researchers concluded that one way to prevent relapse might be to reduce the number of "cons" (such as inconvenience, cost, or lack of competence) so that people have less reason to drop out of an exercise program.[36]

Cardiorespiratory or Aerobic Fitness

Since physical activity requires more energy, the heart, lungs, and blood vessels have to work harder to deliver

Monday	Tuesday	Wednesday	Thursday	Friday	Saturday or Sunday
5 minutes warm-up	5 minutes warm-up	5 minutes warm-up	5 minutes warm-up	5 minutes warm-up	Sports, walking, hiking, biking, or swimming
30 minutes of aerobic exercise	30 minutes of weight training	30 minutes of aerobic exercise	30 minutes of weight training	30 minutes of aerobic exercise	
10 minutes cool-down and stretching	10 minutes cool-down and stretching	10 minutes cool-down and stretching	10 minutes cool-down and stretching	10 minutes cool-down and stretching	

▲ **Figure 4-3** A sample balanced fitness program. If you exercise 45 minutes a day and alternate aerobic activities and weight training, you can enjoy both physical and psychological health benefits.

more oxygen to the cells. A person with good cardiorespiratory endurance can engage in a physical activity for a long time without becoming fatigued. The heart of a person who isn't in good condition has to pump more often; as a result, it becomes fatigued more easily.

Unlike muscular endurance, which is specific to individual muscles, cardiorespiratory endurance involves the entire body. The exercises that improve cardiorespiratory endurance are referred to as aerobic because the body uses slightly more, or as much, oxygen than it takes in. Aerobic exercise can take many forms, as noted later in this chapter, but all involve working strenuously without pushing to the point of breathlessness.

In **anaerobic exercise,** the amount of oxygen taken in by the body cannot meet the demands of the activity. This quickly creates an oxygen deficit that must be made up later. Anaerobic activities are high in intensity but short in duration, usually lasting only about ten seconds to two minutes. An example is sprinting the quarter-mile, which leaves even the best-trained athletes gasping for air. In nonaerobic exercise, such as bowling, softball, or doubles tennis, there is frequent rest between activities. Because the body can take in all the oxygen it needs, the heart and lungs really don't get much of a workout.

Your Target Heart Rate

The best way you can be sure you're working hard enough to condition your heart and lungs but not overdoing it is to use your pulse, or heart rate, as a guide. One of the easiest places to feel your pulse is in the carotid artery in your neck. Tilt your head back slightly and to one side. Use your middle finger or forefinger, or both, to feel for your pulse. (Do not use your thumb; it has a beat of its own.) To determine your heart rate, count the number of pulses you feel for 10 seconds and multiply that number by six, or count for 30 seconds and multiply that number by two. Learn to recognize the pulsing of your heart when you're lying or sitting down. On your fitness record, make note of your **resting heart rate.**

Start taking your pulse during, or immediately after, exercise, when it's much more pronounced than when you're at rest. Three minutes after heavy exercise, take your pulse again. The closer that reading is to your resting heart rate, the better your condition. If it takes a long time for your pulse to recover and return to its resting level, your body's ability to handle physical stress is poor. As you continue working out, however, your pulse will return to normal much more quickly.

You don't want to push yourself to your maximum heart rate; yet you must exercise at about 60 to 85 percent of that maximum to get cardiovascular benefits from your training. This range is called your **target heart rate.** If you don't exercise intensely enough to raise your heart rate at least this high, your heart and lungs won't benefit from the workout. If you push too hard, on the other hand, and exercise at or near your absolute maximum heart rate, you run the risk of placing too great a burden on your heart.

Table 4-3 lists target heart rates for various ages. The following formulas can also be used to calculate your maximum and target heart rates (in beats per minute).

For men, the formula is as follows:

$$220 - \text{Age} = \begin{array}{c}\text{Maximum}\\\text{Heart}\\\text{Rate}\end{array} \times .60 \begin{array}{c}\text{(Target}\\\text{Zone for}\\\text{Beginners)}\end{array} = \begin{array}{c}\text{Target}\\\text{Heart}\\\text{Rate}\end{array}$$

Example for a 20-year-old man:

$$220 - 20 = 200 \begin{array}{c}\text{Maximum}\\\text{Heart}\\\text{Rate}\end{array} \times .60 = 120 \begin{array}{c}\text{Target}\\\text{Heart}\\\text{Rate}\end{array}$$

For women, the formula is as follows:

$$225 - \text{Age} = \begin{array}{c}\text{Maximum}\\\text{Heart}\\\text{Rate}\end{array} \times .60 \begin{array}{c}\text{(Target}\\\text{Zone for}\\\text{Beginners)}\end{array} = \begin{array}{c}\text{Target}\\\text{Heart}\\\text{Rate}\end{array}$$

Example for a 20-year-old woman:

$$225 - 20 = 205 \begin{array}{c}\text{Maximum}\\\text{Heart}\\\text{Rate}\end{array} \times .60 = 123 \begin{array}{c}\text{Target}\\\text{Heart}\\\text{Rate}\end{array}$$

In the initial stages of training, aim for the lower end of your target zone (the 60 percent calculated above), and gradually build up to 75 percent of your maximum heart rate. After six months or more of regular exercise, you can push up to 85 percent of your maximum heart rate if you wish, though you don't have to work that hard just to stay in shape. As long as you use your target heart rate as your guide, your exercise intensity should be just right.

How Do I Design an Aerobic Workout?

Whatever activity you choose, your aerobic workout should consist of several stages:

Warm-Up

Just as you don't get in your car and gun your engine to 60 miles per hour, you shouldn't do the same with your body. You need to prepare your cardiorespiratory system for a workout, speed up the blood flow to your lungs, and increase the temperature and elasticity of your muscles and connective tissue to avoid injury.

Start by walking briskly for about 5 minutes. This helps your body make the transition from inactivity to exertion. Follow this general warm-up with about 5 minutes of simple stretches of the muscles you'll be exercising most. Before a jog, for instance, you can stretch the muscles in your ankle and the back of your leg by leaning against a wall, with one leg bent and tilted forward and the other straight. Lean forward until you feel the stretch and hold.

Aerobic Activity

The two key components of this part of your workout are intensity and duration. As described above, you can use your target heart rate to make sure you are working at the proper intensity. The current recommendation is to keep

▼ Table 4-3 Target Heart Rate

	Men			Women		
Age	Average Maximum Heart Rate (100%)	Target Heart Rate (60–85%)		Average Maximum Heart Rate (100%)	Target Heart Rate (60–85%)	
20	200	120	170	205	123	174
25	195	117	166	200	120	170
30	190	114	162	195	117	166
35	185	111	157	190	114	162
40	180	108	153	185	111	157
45	175	105	149	180	108	153
50	170	102	145	175	105	149
55	165	99	140	170	102	145
60	160	96	136	165	99	140
65	155	93	132	160	96	136
70	150	90	128	155	93	132

moving for at least 30 minutes, either in one session or several briefer sessions, each lasting at least 10 minutes.

Cool-Down

After you've pushed your heart rate up to its target level and kept it there for a while, the worst thing you can do is slam on the brakes. If you come to a sudden stop, you put your heart at risk. When you stand or sit immediately after vigorous exercise, blood can pool in your legs. You need to keep moving—though at a slower pace—to ensure an adequate supply of blood to your heart. Ideally, you should walk for 5 to 10 minutes at a comfortable pace before you end your workout session.

Your Long-Term Plan

One of the most common mistakes people make is to push too hard too fast. Often they end up injured or discouraged and quit entirely. If you are just starting an aerobic program, think of it as a series of phases: beginning, progression, and maintenance:

- **Beginning (4–6 weeks).** Start slow and low (in intensity). If you're walking, monitor your heart rate and aim for 55 percent of your maximal heart rate. Another good way to make sure you're moving at the right pace is this rule of thumb: If you can sing as you walk, you're going too slow; if you can't talk, you're going too fast.
- **Progression (16–20 weeks).** Gradually increase the duration and/or intensity of your workouts. For instance, you might add 5 minutes every two weeks to your walking time. You also gradually can pick up your pace, using your target heart rate as your guide. Keep a log of your workouts so you can chart your progress until you reach your goal.
- **Maintenance (lifelong).** Once you've reached the stage of exercising at your target heart rate for at least 30 minutes most days of the week, there's little added benefit—and increased risk of injury—if you push harder or farther. You may want to develop a repertoire of aerobic activities you enjoy and combine or alternate to avoid monotony and keep up your enthusiasm. This is called cross-training.

Walking

More men and women are taking to their feet. Some, casualties of high-intensity sports, can no longer withstand the wear-and-tear of rigorous workouts. Others want to shape up, slim down, or ward off heart disease and other health problems. The good news for all is that walking may well be the perfect exercise.

Recent research has demonstrated the health benefits of walking for both men and women and for both healthy individuals and those with heart disease. One major study of women, the Nurses' Health Study, found that women who walk briskly three hours a week are as well protected from heart disease as women who spend an hour and a half a week in more vigorous activities, such as aerobics or running. Women engaged in either form of exercise had a rate of heart attacks 30 to 40 percent lower than that of sedentary women.[37] The Women's Health Study, a randomized, controlled trial of aspirin and heart disease, found that even walking one hour per week can lower heart disease risk among relatively sedentary women.[38] Walking also protects men's hearts, whether they're healthy or have had heart problems. In a recent British study of 772 men, those who regularly engaged in light exercise, including walking, had a risk of death that was 58 percent lower than that of their sedentary counterparts.[39]

Walking is good for the brain as well as the body. In a study that followed almost 6,000 women age 65 or older for up to eight years, those who walked regularly were less likely to experience memory loss and other age-related declines in mental function.[40] Another bonus is stress reduction. Since you can do it during a break or at lunchtime, walking builds relaxation into your day.

Treadmills are a good alternative to outdoor walks—and not just in bad weather. They keep you moving at a certain pace, they're easier on the knees, and they allow you to exercise in a climate-controlled, pollution-free environment—a definite plus for many city dwellers. Holding onto the handrails while walking on a treadmill reduces both heart rate and oxygen consumption, so you burn fewer calories. Experts advise slowing the pace if necessary so you can let go of the handrails while working out.[41]

Waterwalking in a pool or at a lake or beach is another alternative—and an excellent exercise. Because of water's resistance, you don't have to walk as fast in water as you would on land to burn the same number of calories. Walking two miles per hour in thigh-high water is equivalent to three miles per hour on land.

In race-walking, or striding (as its noncompetitive form is called), you must keep your lead foot on the ground as your trailing leg pushes off, and your knee remains straight as your body passes over that leg. As a result, one foot is always supporting the body, so the maximum impact per step is much lower than when you run and the injury rate is low.

Because their stride is shorter, race-walkers have to stretch their hips forward and backward, which is good for flexibility. Because of the extra effort, they get an added bonus: They burn up more calories than they would running at the same speed over the same distance.

Here are some guidelines for putting your best foot forward:

- Walk very slowly for 5 minutes, and then do some simple stretches.
- Maintain good posture. Focus your eyes ahead of you, stand erect, and pull in your stomach.
- Use the heel-to-toe method of walking. The heel of your leading foot should touch the ground before the ball or toes of that foot do. When you push off with your trailing foot, bend your knee as you raise your heel. You should be able to feel the action in your calf muscles.
- Pump your arms back and forth to burn 5 to 10 percent more calories and get an upper-body workout as well.
- End your walk the way you started it—let your pace become more leisurely for the last 5 minutes.

Jogging and Running

The difference between jogging and running is speed. You should be able to carry on a conversation with someone on a long jog or run; if you're too breathless to talk, you're pushing too hard.

If your goal is to enhance aerobic fitness, long, slow, distance running is best. If you want to improve your speed, try *interval training,* which consists of repeated hard runs over a certain distance, with intervals of relaxed jogging in between. Depending on what suits you and what your training goals are, you can vary the distance, duration, and number of fast runs, as well as the time and activity between them. Interval training is usually done on a track and should not be attempted unless you're in top shape.

If you have been sedentary, it's best to launch a walking program before attempting to jog or run. Start by walking for 15 to 20 minutes three times a week at a comfortable pace. Continue at this same level until you no longer feel sore or unduly fatigued the day after exercising. Then increase your walking time to 20 to 25 minutes, speeding up your pace as well.

When you can handle a brisk 25-minute walk, alternate fast walking with slow jogging. Begin each session walking, and gradually increase the amount of time you spend jogging. If you feel breathless while jogging, slow down and walk. Continue to alternate in this manner until you can jog for 10 minutes without stopping. If you gradually increase your jogging time by 1 or 2 minutes with each workout, you'll slowly build up from 10 to 20 or 25 minutes per session. For optimal fitness, you should jog at least three times a week.

Here's how to be sure you're running right:

- Always take time both to warm up and to stretch. Warm up with jumping jacks or running in place for 3 to 5 minutes. Spend at least one-fourth of the time that you plan to run on stretching exercises.[42]
- As you run, keep your back straight and your head up. Run tall, with your buttocks tucked in. Look straight ahead. Hold your arms slightly away from your body. Your elbows should be bent slightly so that your forearms are almost parallel to the ground. Move your arms rhythmically to propel yourself along.
- Have your heels hit the ground first. Land on your heel, rock forward, and push off the ball of your foot. If this is difficult, try a more flat-footed style.
- Avoid running on the balls of your feet; this produces soreness in the calves because the muscles must contract for a longer time. To avoid shin splints (a dull ache in the lower shins), stretch regularly to strengthen the shin muscles and to develop greater flexibility in your ankles.
- Avoid running on hard surfaces and making sudden stops or turns.
- Breathe through your nose and mouth to get more volume. Learn to "belly breathe": When you breathe in, your belly should expand; when you breathe out, it should flatten. If your breathing becomes labored, try exhaling with resistance through pursed lips so that your body utilizes more oxygen per breath.
- When you approach a hill, shorten your stride. Lift your knees higher; pump your arms more. If the hill is really steep, lean forward. When you start downhill, lean forward, and run as if you were on a flat surface. Don't lean back, because doing so could strain your knees and the muscles in your legs.

Swimming

More than 100 million Americans dive into the water every year. What matters for our heart's health, however, is getting a good workout, not just getting wet. Swimming is an excellent exercise for cardiovascular fitness and also

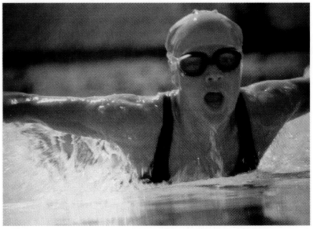

▲ Swimming is good exercise for people of all ages—particularly for cardiovascular fitness and flexibility.

rates fairly high for weight control, muscular function, and flexibility. However, it's not as effective as activities such as walking and running for building strong bones and preventing osteoporosis.

For aerobic conditioning, you have to swim laps, using a freestyle, butterfly, breast-, or backstroke. (The sidestroke is too easy.) You've also got to be a good enough swimmer to keep churning through the water for at least 20 minutes. Your heart will beat more slowly in water than on land, so your heart rate while swimming is not an accurate guide to exercise intensity. You should try to keep up a steady pace that's fast enough to make you feel pleasantly tired, but not completely exhausted, by the time you get out of the pool.

Swimming is good for people of all ages, particularly those over 50 or with physical handicaps. Swimming facilities are available in nearly all communities. Check your college gym; your local YWCA, YMCA, or JCC; your city recreation department; and other schools in your area.

Here are some guidelines for smart swimming:

▷ Start by swimming 50 yards and rest when you feel breathless.
▷ Try to swim 100 yards, rest for a minute, and then swim another 100 yards.
▷ Increase your distance slowly. See if you can work up to 700 yards in 18 minutes.
▷ Stick to the crawl, the butterfly, the breaststroke, or the backstroke.

Cycling

Bicycling, indoors and out, can be an excellent cardiovascular conditioner, as well as an effective way to control weight—provided you aren't just along for the ride. If you coast down too many hills, you'll have to ride longer up hills or on level ground in order to get a good workout. Half of all bikes now sold in the United States are mountain bikes, sturdy cycles with knobby tires that allow bikers to climb up and zoom down dirt trails and explore places traditional racing bikes couldn't go. However, an 18-speed bike can make pedaling too easy, unless you choose gears carefully. To gain aerobic benefits, mountain bikers have to work hard enough to raise their heart rates to their target zone and keep up that intensity for at least 20 minutes.

Using a one-wheel stationary cycle with a tension-control knob, you can adjust the amount of effort required; start with low resistance, then increase the tension until you're working at your target heart rate. You can put the cycle in front of a television set or look out the window if you feel the need for some scenery—or you can read or simply meditate while pedaling.

Bicycle crashes rank second only to riding animals as a sports- or recreation-associated cause of injury. Rider errors (losing control, inexperience, speed), environmental hazards (loose gravel), and bicycle mechanical failure all contribute to crashes.[43]

Here's a guide to smart cycling:

▷ If you're not used to cycling, start slowly. Work up from 5 minutes of steady pedaling (interrupted by rest periods if necessary) to 10, 15, 20, and 25 minutes. Limit your rides to 5–10 minutes the first week. Increase your time and speed gradually to avoid sore thigh muscles. Rest when you feel breathless.
▷ Keep your elbows slightly bent to allow for a more relaxed upper body. Change your hand positions periodically to avoid numbness.
▷ Monitor your heart rate to make sure you're working within your target range.
▷ When riding outdoors, be sure to wear a helmet. Helmets reduce the risk of head injuries by 74 to 85 percent.[44] Look for proof that it conforms to either the Snell or ANSI standard for head protection.
▷ Make yourself visible. Wear reflective clothing if you can. If you cannot, remember that drivers see bright pink, yellow, and orange most easily.
▷ Always follow the rules of the road—stick to the right, stop at stop signs, heed one-way signs, and so on.
▷ Expect the unexpected. A flat tire or broken spoke can occur without warning. Be prepared.[45]

Cross-country Skiing

One of the most effective forms of aerobic exercise, cross-country or Nordic skiing, has become an increasingly popular winter sport. Thanks to machines that simulate the moves of Nordic skiing, it's now possible to "ski" in any season. Because almost every muscle in the body gets a workout, cross-country skiing is excellent for all-around conditioning. Using the poles works the arms, shoulders, back, and abdomen, while the kick-and-glide action of skiing involves virtually all the muscles of the legs, thighs, and abdomen. Also, as exercisers breathe faster and more deeply, their rib, abdominal, and shoulder muscles get a workout. Another plus: The risk of joint and ligament injury while cross-country skiing is lower than for many other impact-aerobic activities (and much lower than for downhill skiing).

Other Aerobic Activities

Because variety is the spice of an active life, many people prefer different forms of aerobic exercise. All can provide many health benefits. Among the popular options:

▷ **Spinning.**™ Spinning is a cardiovascular workout for the whole body that utilizes a special stationary bicycle. Led by an instructor, a group of bikers listen to music and modify their bikes' resistance and their own pace according to the rhythm. An average spinning class lasts 45 minutes and has between 20 and 40 participants.

Unlike an ordinary stationary bike, a spinning bike has a larger saddle area and a heavier flywheel to create greater resistance; the rider, rather than a built-in computer, monitors performance. Introduced in 1987, this indoor cycling program has grown in appeal because it is time efficient and nonimpact and because people of all ages, skills, and fitness levels can participate in the same class.

▶ **Skipping rope.** Essentially a form of stationary jogging with some extra arm action thrown in, skipping rope is excellent both as a heart conditioner and as a way of losing weight. Always warm up before starting and cool down afterward. To alleviate boredom, try skipping to music, and vary the steps: both feet together, alternating left and right feet, or jumping up and down on one leg.

▶ **Aerobic dancing.** This activity combines music with kicking, bending, and jumping. A typical class (you can also dance at home to a video or TV program) consists of stretching exercises and sit-ups, followed by aerobic dances and cool-down exercises. A particular benefit of aerobic dance is that people get enjoyment and stimulation from the music; they're also able to move their bodies without worrying about skill and technique. "Soft," or low-impact, aerobic dancing doesn't put as much strain on the joints as "hard," or high-impact, routines.

▶ **Step training or bench aerobics.** "Stepping" combines step, or bench, climbing with music and choreographed

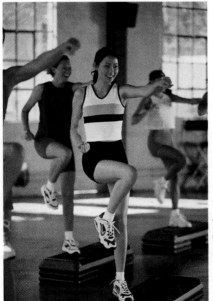

▲ Step workouts can be a fun way of enhancing your cardiorespiratory endurance.

movements. Basic equipment consists of a bench 4 to 12 inches high. The fitter you are, the higher the bench—but the higher the bench, the greater the risk of knee injury. Injuries have skyrocketed in recent years as movements and choreography have become more complex and the pace of the music has picked up.[46]

Tugging on supersized rubber "stretch" cords, which has the same effect as weight training, can increase the benefits of a step workout. In a controlled study, exercisers who added resistance exercises with stretch cords to their step routines showed improvements in aerobic capacity as well as muscle strength and size.[47] A 40-minute step workout is equivalent to running at seven miles an hour in terms of oxygen uptake and calories burned.

▶ **Stair-climbing.** An estimated 4 million Americans are stepping up to fitness, according to the American Sports Data Institute. You could run up the stairs in an office building or dormitory, but most people use stair-climbing machines available in home models and at gyms and health clubs. On most versions of these machines, exercisers push a pair of pedals up and down—much easier on the feet and legs than many other activities.

▶ **In-line skating.** In-line skating can increase aerobic endurance and muscular strength and is less stressful on joints and bones than running or high-impact aerobics. Skaters can adjust the intensity of their workout by varying the terrain. (Obviously, they'll have to work harder while going up hills, and less so on the slide down.) They can also buy special training wheels and weights to increase resistance and make muscles work harder. One caution: Protective gear, including a helmet, knee and elbow pads, and wrist guards, is essential.

Muscular Strength and Endurance

Although aerobic workouts condition your insides (heart, blood vessels, and lungs), they don't exercise many of the muscles that shape your outsides and provide power when you need it. Strength workouts are important because they enable muscles to work efficiently and reliably. Conditioned muscles function more smoothly and contract somewhat more vigorously and with less effort. With exercise, muscle tissue becomes firmer and can withstand much more strain—the result of toughening the sheath protecting the muscle and developing more connective tissue within it (see Figure 4-4).

Muscular strength and endurance are critical for handling everyday burdens, such as cramming a 20-pound suitcase into an overhead luggage bin or hauling a

Strength workouts increase circulation

The heart's right half pumps oxygen-poor blood to capillary beds in lungs. There, O_2 diffuses into blood and CO_2 diffuses out. The oxygenated blood flows into the heart's left half where it is then pumped to capillary beds throughout the body

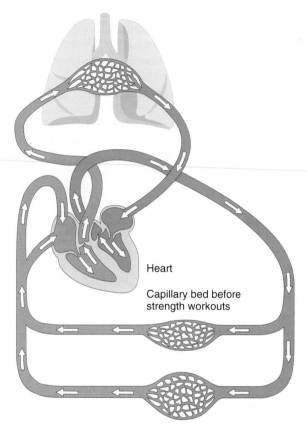

Heart

Capillary bed before strength workouts

Capillary bed after 8–12 weeks of strength workouts (extra capillaries develop, circulation increases)

Strength workouts build muscles

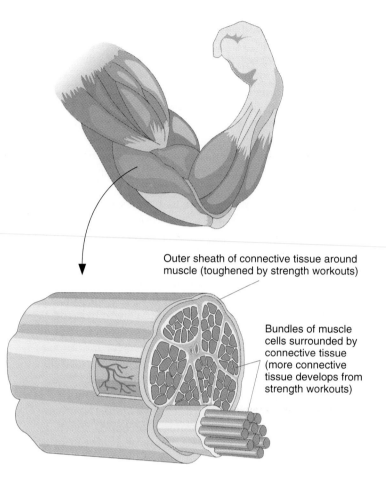

Outer sheath of connective tissue around muscle (toughened by strength workouts)

Bundles of muscle cells surrounded by connective tissue (more connective tissue develops from strength workouts)

▲ **Figure 4-4** The benefits of strength training on the body. Strength training in combination with aerobic exercise increases blood circulation and oxygen supply to body tissues and develops muscles.

trunk down from the attic. Prolonged exercise prepares the muscles for sustained work by improving the circulation of blood in the tissue. The number of tiny blood vessels, called capillaries, increases by as much as 50 percent in regularly exercised muscles; and existing capillaries open wider so that the total circulation increases by as much as 400 percent, thus providing the muscles with a much greater supply of nutrients. This increase occurs after about 8 to 12 weeks in young persons, but takes longer in older individuals. Inactivity reverses the process, gradually shutting down the extra capillaries that have developed.

The latest research on fat-burning shows that the best way to reduce your body fat is to add muscle-strengthening exercise to your workouts. Muscle tissue is your very best calorie-burning tissue, and the more you have, the more calories you burn, even when you are resting. You don't have to become a serious body builder. Using handheld weights (also called free weights) two or three times a week is enough. Just be sure you learn how to use them properly because you can tear or strain muscles if you don't practice the proper weight-lifting techniques. As more people have begun to lift weights, injuries have soared.[48]

A balanced workout regimen of muscle-building and aerobic exercise does more for you than just burn fat. It gives you more endurance by promoting better distribution of oxygen to your tissues and increasing the blood flow to your heart.

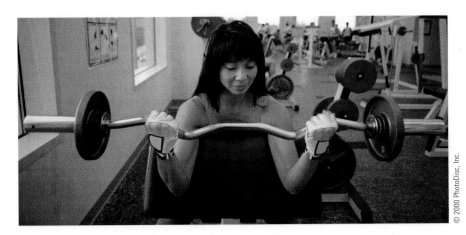

© 2000 PhotoDisc, Inc.

▲ Build up muscular strength and endurance through weight training.

Exercise and Muscles

Your muscles never stay the same. If you don't use them, they atrophy, weaken, or break down. If you use them rigorously and regularly, they grow stronger. The only way to develop muscles is by demanding more of them than you usually do. This is called **overloading.** As you train, you have to increase the number of repetitions or the amount of resistance gradually and work the muscle to temporary fatigue. That's why it's important not to quit when your muscles start to tire. Some exercise enthusiasts believe that the experience of pain—the "burn"—signals that exercise is paying off; however, others contend that it means you're pushing too hard and risking injury.

You need to exercise differently for strength than for endurance. To develop strength, you do a few repetitions with heavy loads. As you increase the load, object, or weight your muscles must move, you increase your strength. To increase endurance, you do many more repetitions with lighter loads. If your muscles are weak and you need to gain strength in your upper body, you may have to work for weeks to do a half-dozen regular push-ups. Then you can start building endurance by doing as many push-ups as you can before collapsing in exhaustion.

Muscles can do only two things: contract or relax. As they do so, skeletal muscles either pull on bones or stop pulling on bones. All exercise involves muscles pulling on bones across a joint. The movement that takes place depends upon the structure of the joint and the position of the muscle attachments involved.

An **isometric** contraction is one in which the muscle applies force while maintaining an equal length. The muscle contracts and tries to shorten but cannot overcome the resistance. An isometric exercise is one in which you push or pull against an immovable object, with each muscle contraction held for five to eight seconds and repeated five to ten times daily. An example is pushing against an immovable object, like a wall, or tightening an abdominal muscle while sitting. The muscle contracts but there is no movement.

An **isotonic** contraction involves movement, but the muscle tension remains the same. Isotonic exercises are those in which the muscle moves a moderate load several times, as in weight lifting or calisthenics. The kind of isotonic exercise best for producing muscular strength involve high resistance and a low number of repetitions. On the other hand, you can develop the greatest flexibility, coordination, and endurance with isotonic exercises that incorporate lower resistance and frequent repetitions.

True **isokinetic** contraction is a constant speed contraction. Isokinetic exercises require special machines that provide resistance to overload muscles throughout the entire range of motion.

How Do I Design a Muscle Workout?

A workout with weights should exercise your body's primary muscle groups: the *deltoids* (shoulders), *pectorals* (chest), *triceps* and *biceps* (back and front of upper arms), *quadriceps* and *hamstrings* (front and back of thighs), *gluteus maximus* (buttocks), and *abdomen* (see Figure 4-5). Various machines and free-weight routines focus on each muscle group, but the principle is always the same: Muscles contract as you raise and lower a weight, and you repeat the lift-and-lower routine until the muscle group is tired.

A weight-training program is made up of both **sets** (set numbers of repetitions of the same movement) and **reps** (the single performance of exercises, such as lifting 75 pounds once). You should allow your breath to return to normal before moving on to each new set. Pushing yourself to the limit builds strength.

Maintaining proper breathing techniques during weight training is crucial. To breathe correctly, inhale when muscles are relaxed, and exhale when you push or lift. Don't ever hold your breath because oxygen flow helps prevent muscle fatigue and injury.

Remember that your muscles need sufficient time to recover from a weight-training session. Allow no less than 48 hours, but no more than 96 hours, between training sessions, so that your body can recover from the workout and so that you'll avoid overtraining. Workouts on consecutive days do more harm than good, because the body can't

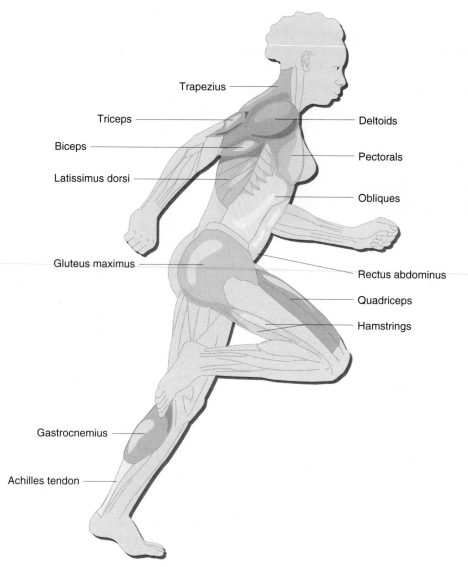

Trapezius

Triceps

Biceps

Latissimus dorsi

Gluteus maximus

Gastrocnemius

Achilles tendon

Deltoids

Pectorals

Obliques

Rectus abdominus

Quadriceps

Hamstrings

▲ **Figure 4-5** The body's primary muscle groups. Different exercises can strengthen and stretch different muscle groups.

recover that quickly. Two or three 30-minute training sessions a week should be sufficient for building strength and endurance. Strength training twice a week at greater intensity and for a longer duration can be as effective as working out three times a week. However, your muscles will begin to atrophy if you let more than three or four days pass without exercising them. For total fitness, you may want to schedule aerobic workouts for your days off from weight training.

What Should I Know About Performance-Enhancing Drugs?

They sound too good to be true: dietary supplements or drugs that boost strength and enhance athletic performance.

Teenage boys and men in their twenties are the heaviest users. Do these aids work? Or are users endangering their health for an unproven benefit? Here's what we know—and don't know—about the most widely used performance boosters.[49]

Androstenedione

Androstenedione ("andro") is a testosterone precursor normally produced by the adrenal glands and gonads. After home-run hitter Mark McGwire admitted that he used this over-the-counter supplement, androstenedione use increased five-fold among young people.[50] Seen as a natural alternative to anabolic steroids, androstenedione has not been proved safe or effective. In a study of its effects on men between the ages of 19 and 29, androstenedione did not show any effect on muscle strength but did increase concentrations of estrogen, which is associated with breast enlargement and increased risk of cardiovascular disease and pancreatic cancer in men. Androstenedione also raises testosterone above normal levels, which can lead to acne, male pattern baldness, and a decrease in "good" cholesterol. In women, high testosterone levels can also cause increased body hair, deepening of the voice, and other male characteristics.[51]

Androstenedione is banned by the Olympics, the National College Athletic Association, the National Football League, and the men's and women's tennis tours.[52]

Steroids

Anabolic steroids are synthetic derivatives of the male hormone testosterone that promote the growth of skeletal muscle and increase lean body mass. Some athletes and others use anabolic steroids to enhance performance and improve physical appearance.

Taken orally or injected, anabolic steroids are typically used in cycles of weeks or months, rather than continuously. Users take multiple doses over a specific period of time, stop for a period, and start again. In addition, users frequently combine several different types of steroids to maximize their effectiveness while minimizing their negative effects. This practice is known as stacking.

Working with Weights

If you plan to work with free weights, here are some guidelines for using them safely and effectively:

✔ Don't train alone—for safety's sake. Work with a partner so you can serve as spotters for each other and help motivate each other as well.

✔ Always warm up and stretch before weight training; also be sure to stretch after training.

✔ Begin with relatively light weights (50 percent of the maximum you can lift), and increase the load slowly until you find the weight that will cause muscle failure at anywhere from eight to twelve repetitions. (Muscle failure is the point during a workout at which you can no longer perform or complete a repetition through the entire range of motion.)

✔ In the beginning, don't work at maximum intensity. Increase your level of exertion gradually over two to six weeks to allow your body to adapt to new stress without soreness.

✔ Always train your entire body, starting with the larger muscle groups. Don't focus only on specific areas, although you may want to concentrate on your weakest muscles.

✔ Always use proper form. Unnecessary twisting, lurching, lunging, or arching can cause serious injury. Remember, quality matters more than quantity. One properly performed set of lifts can produce a greater increase in strength and muscle mass than many sets of improperly performed lifts.

Anabolic steroids have been reported to increase lean muscle mass, strength, and ability to train longer and harder,[53] but they pose serious health hazards, including liver tumors, jaundice (yellowish pigmentation of skin, tissues, and body fluids), fluid retention, high blood pressure, and severe acne. Men may experience shrinking of the testicles, reduced sperm count, infertility, baldness, and development of breasts. Women may experience growth of facial hair, changes in or cessation of the menstrual cycle, enlargement of the clitoris, and deepened voice. In adolescents, steroids may bring about a premature halt in skeletal maturation.

Anabolic steroid abuse may lead to aggression and other psychiatric side effects. Many users report feeling good about themselves while on anabolic steroids, but researchers report that anabolic steroid abuse can cause wild mood swings including manic-like symptoms leading to violent, even homicidal, episodes. Researchers have reported that users may suffer from paranoid jealousy, extreme irritability, delusions, and impaired judgment stemming from feelings of invincibility. Stopping the drugs abruptly can lead to depression.

Creatine

Creatine is an amino acid made by the body and stored predominantly in skeletal muscle. Creatine serves as a reservoir to replenish adenosine triphosphate (ATP), a substance involved in energy production. While some studies show creatine may increase strength and endurance, other effects on the body remain unknown.[54]

Creatine supplements increase muscle stores of the compound, which theoretically allows athletes to work out harder and longer. Athletes typically load up with 20 grams a day for five days and then keep taking 2 grams daily. Some studies have shown that creatine supplements do enhance sports performance and anaerobic power, but only in activities that require repeated short bursts of high-intensity energy, such as sprints and weight lifting, rather than long-distance running or swimming.[55]

 Studies of college football players randomly assigned to placebo or creatine treatment groups have produced inconsistent results.[56] Creatine has not shown any usefulness for lower-intensity, longer-duration exercises, and the water retention and weight gain associated with creatine supplementation may actually hamper performance. Some researchers have observed that only those subjects whose own creatine levels were at the lower end of the normal range benefited from supplementation. It's not known if creatine can benefit the average recreational athlete.

Commercially marketed creatine supplements do not meet the same rigid quality control standards as prescription drugs, so it is difficult to apply efficacy and safety results from published trials to general practice. The dose delivered by a commercially available product may be more or less than that suggested by the labeling. This could influence the effectiveness of the supplement and could lead to unexpected adverse effects.

Muscle cramping, diarrhea, and dehydration have been reported in creatine users, as well as a few cases of kidney dysfunction. Some experts are concerned that creatine may damage internal organs, but there is no evidence of this so far. The Food and Drug Administration has warned consumers to consult a physician before taking creatine supplements. The Association of Professional Team Physicians cautions that creatine may cause dehydration and heat-related illnesses, reduced blood volume, and electrolyte imbalances. Some athletes drink large quantities of water hoping to avoid such effects. However, many coaches forbid or discourage creatine use because its long-term effects remain unknown.

Other Ergogenic Aids

Ergogenic aids are substances used to enhance energy and provide athletes with a competitive advantage. By some estimates, more than three of four athletes in some sports use some sort of supplements to enhance their performance and boost energy.[57] These include everyday substances. Caffeine, for instance, may boost alertness in some people but cause jitteriness in others. Baking soda (sodium bicarbonate) is believed to delay fatigue by neutralizing lactic acid in the muscles, but its potential drawbacks include explosive diarrhea, abdominal cramps, bloating, and nausea.[58]

GBL (gamma butyrolactone) is an unapproved drug that is being studied as a treatment for narcolepsy, a disabling sleep disorder. Nevertheless, it is marketed on the Internet and in some professional gyms as a muscle-builder and performance-enhancer. The Food and Drug Administration has warned consumers to avoid any products containing GBL, noting that they have been associated with at least one death and several incidents in which users became comatose or unconscious.

Glycerol is a natural element derived from fats. Some sports-drink manufacturers are testing formulations that include glycerol, which they claim can lower heart rate and stave off exhaustion in marathon events. Glycerol-induced hyperhydration (holding too much water in the blood) can have a negative impact on performance, however, and may be hazardous to health.

Flexibility

Flexibility is the characteristic of body tissues that determines the range of motion achievable without injury at a joint or group of joints. There are two types of flexibility: static and dynamic. **Static flexibility**—the type most people think of as flexibility—refers to the ability to assume and maintain an extended position at one end point in a joint's range of motion. **Dynamic flexibility,** by comparison, involves movement. It is the ability to move a joint quickly and fluidly through its entire range of motion with little resistance. The static flexibility in the hip joint determines whether you can do a split; dynamic flexibility is what would enable you to perform a split leap.

Static flexibility depends on many factors, including the structure of a joint and the tightness of the muscles, tendons, and ligaments attached to it. Dynamic flexibility is influenced by static flexibility, but also depends on additional factors, such as strength, coordination, and resistance to movement.

Genetics, age, gender, and body composition all influence how flexible you are. Girls and women tend to be more flexible than boys and men, to a certain extent because of hormonal and anatomical differences. The way females and males use their muscles and the activities they engage in can also have an effect. Over time, the natural elasticity of muscles, tendons, and joints decreases in both genders, resulting in stiffness.

The Benefits of Flexibility

Just as cardiorespiratory fitness benefits the heart and lungs and muscular fitness builds endurance and strength, a stretching program produces unique benefits, including enhancement of the ability of the respiratory, circulatory, and neuromuscular systems to cope with the stress and pressures of our high-pressure world. Among the other benefits of flexibility are:

▶ **Prevention of injuries.** Flexibility training stretches muscles and increases the elasticity of joints. Strong, flexible muscles resist stress better than weak or inflexible ones. Adding flexibility to a training program for sports such as soccer, football, or tennis can reduce the rate of injuries by as much as 75 percent. In one study of competitive runners, weekly stretching sessions significantly reduced the incidence of low back pain.

▶ **Relief of muscle strain.** Muscles tighten as a result of stress or prolonged sitting. If you study or work in one position for several hours, you'll often feel stiffness in your back or neck. Stretching helps relieve this tension and enables you to work more effectively.

▶ **Relaxation.** Flexibility exercises are great stress-busters that reduce mental strain, slow the rate of breathing, and reduce blood pressure.

▶ **Relief of soreness after exercise.** Many people develop delayed-onset muscle soreness (DOMS) one or two days after they work out. This may be the result of damage to the muscle fibers and supporting connective tissue. Some researchers theorize that stretching after exercise can decrease this aftereffect, although others contend that it produces only short-term benefits.

▶ **Improved posture.** Bad posture can create tight, stressed muscles. If you slump in your chair, for instance, the muscles in the front of your chest may tighten, causing those in the upper spine to overstretch and become loose.

▶ **Better athletic performance.** Good flexibility allows for more efficient movement and exertion of more force through a greater range of motion, a special benefit for any activity, from gymnastics to golf, where positions beyond the normal range of motion are necessary to perform certain skills.

Flexibility can make everyday tasks, like bending over to tie a shoe or reaching up to a high shelf, easier and safer.

It can also prevent and relieve the ankle, knee, back, and shoulder pain that many people feel as they get older. If you do other forms of exercise, flexibility lowers your risk of injury and may improve your performance.

Types of Stretching

You should stretch a minimum of two or three times a week. Unlike strength training, flexibility exercises do not require time off between sessions. Ideally you should try to incorporate some stretches into your daily routine. The basic types of stretching include static, passive, active, and ballistic stretching. (See Figure 4-6.)

Static stretching involves a gradual stretch held for a short time (10 to 30 seconds). A shorter stretch provides little benefit; a longer stretch does not provide additional benefits. Since a slow stretch provokes less of a reaction from the stretch receptors, the muscles can safely stretch farther than usual. Fitness experts most often recommend static stretching because it is both safe and effective. An

example of such a stretch is letting your hands slowly slide down the front of your legs (keeping your knees in a soft, unlocked position) until you reach your toes and holding this final position for several seconds before slowly straightening up. You should feel a pull, but not pain, during this stretch.

In **passive stretching,** your own body, a partner, gravity, or a weight serves as an external force or resistance to help your joints move through their range of motion. You can achieve a more intense stretch and a greater range of motion with passive stretching. There is a greater risk of injury, however, because the muscles themselves are not controlling the stretch. If working with a partner, it's very important that you communicate clearly so as not to force a joint outside its normal functional range of motion.

Research on stretching demonstrates a 5 to 20 percent increase in static flexibility within four to six weeks of stretching. Much of this long-term increase in range of motion is due to an increased "stretch tolerance," or ability to tolerate the discomfort of a stretched position.

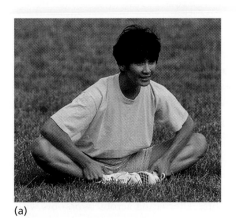
(a)

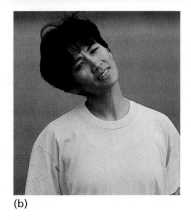
(b)

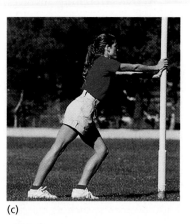
(c)

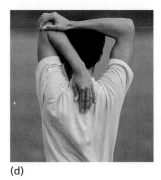
(d)

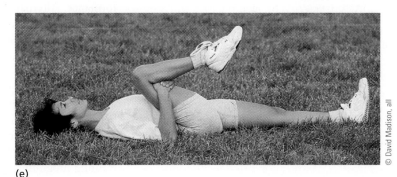
(e)

© David Madison, all

▲ **Figure 4-6** Some simple stretching exercises. (a) *Foot pull for the groin and thigh muscles.* Sit on the ground and bend your legs so that the soles of your feet touch. Pull your feet closer as you press on your knees with your elbows. Hold for 10 seconds; repeat. (b) *Lateral head tilt.* Gently tilt your head to each side. Repeat several times. (c) *Wall stretch for the Achilles tendon.* Stand 3 feet from a wall or post with your feet slightly apart. Keeping your heels on the ground, lean into the wall. Hold for 10 seconds; repeat. (d) *Triceps stretch for the upper arm and shoulder.* Place your right hand behind your neck and grasp it above the elbow with your left hand. Gently pull the elbow back. Repeat with the left elbow. (e) *Knee-chest pull for lower back muscles.* Lying on your back, clasp one knee and pull it toward your chest. Hold for 15–30 seconds; repeat with the other knee.

STRATEGIES FOR PREVENTION

How to Avoid Stretching Injuries

✔ Never stretch to the point of pain.

✔ Don't attempt a ballistic stretch on a weak or injured muscle.

✔ Start small. Work the muscles of the smaller joints in the arms and legs first and then work the larger joints like the shoulders and hips.

✔ Stretch individual muscles before you stretch a group of muscles, for instance, the ankle, knee, and hip before a stretch that works all three.

✔ Don't make any quick, jerky movements while stretching. Even ballistic stretches should be gentle and smooth.

Active stretching involves stretching a muscle by contracting the opposing muscle (the muscle on the opposite side of the limb). In an active seated hamstring stretch, for example, the stretch occurs by actively contracting the muscles on top of the shin, which produces a reflex that relaxes the hamstring. This method allows the muscle to be stretched farther with a low risk of injury.

The disadvantage of active stretching is that a person may not be able to produce enough of a stretch to increase flexibility only by means of contracting opposing muscle groups. Although active stretching is the safest and most convenient approach, an occasional passive assist can be helpful.

Ballistic stretching is characterized by rapid bouncing movements, such as a series of up-and-down bobs as you try again and again to touch your toes with your hands. These bounces can stretch the muscle fibers too far, causing the muscle to contract rather than stretch. They also can tear ligaments and weaken or rupture tendons, the strong fibrous cords that connect muscles to bones. The heightened activity to stretch receptors caused by the rapid stretches can continue for some time, possibly causing injuries during any physical activities that follow. Because of its potential dangers, fitness experts generally recommend against ballistic stretching.

What Is the Difference Between Stretching and Warming Up?

Many people assume that warming up—crucial before all forms of exercise—is the same as stretching, but the two are not interchangeable. Warming up means getting the heart beating, breaking a sweat, and readying the body for more vigorous activity. Stretching is a specific activity intended to elongate the muscles and keep joints limber, not simply a prelude to a game of tennis or a three-mile run.

Although people are often told to stretch during a warm-up, there is little scientific evidence to support its usefulness as a means of preventing injury or enhancing performance.[59] Increasing the temperature of the muscle is what protects against injury. Light to moderate activity, such as walking at gradually increasing intensity, is a better warm-up than stretching for most sports. Stretching for activities such as dance or gymnastics, which push beyond the normal range of motion for joints, should follow several minutes of light activity to raise muscle temperature.

One of the best times to stretch is after an aerobic workout. Your muscles will be warm, more flexible, and less prone to injury. In addition, stretching after aerobic activity can help a fatigued muscle return to its normal resting length and possibly helps reduce delayed muscle soreness.

Total Fitness

No one single exercise can stretch and strengthen your muscles and also enhance your cardiorespiratory fitness. That's why **cross-training** (alternating two or more different types of fitness activities) and **aerobic circuit training** (combining aerobic and strength exercises to build both cardiorespiratory fitness and muscular strength and endurance) have become increasingly popular:

▸ **Cross-training.** The pioneers of contemporary cross-training were triathletes who run, swim, and cycle. Depending on the specific sports, cross-training can yield various benefits. Alternating aerobic workouts with weight lifting, for example, can increase speed and performance. Alternating running with a low-impact aerobic exercise, such as swimming, lessens the risk of knee, ankle, or shin injuries. Cross-training also helps exercisers avoid boredom and offers the pleasures of variety.

No one cross-training combination is right for everyone. To plan a program, first identify your fitness goals: Do you want to control your weight, get stronger, feel better about yourself, improve your general health, and improve your performance in a particular competitive sport? Your unique fitness goals will dictate the cross-training program that's right for you.

▸ **Aerobic circuit training.** Done individually or in a group at a gym or health club, aerobic circuit training generally involves weight-training equipment (such as free weights or exercise machines) and aerobic stations (treadmills, stationary bikes, stair-climbing machines, or cross-country skiing machines). By alternating weight and aerobic stations and moving quickly from one station to the next, exercisers can get a total-body workout. Some aerobic circuit trainers have reported significant improvements in aerobic capacity as well as enhanced toning and shaping of muscles.

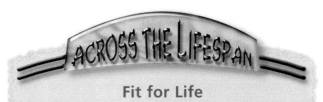

Fit for Life

At one time, everyone, even the medical experts, thought that aging meant weakness, frailty, and declining strength. Now we know better: No one is ever too old to get in shape. Rather than telling seniors to take it easy, the American College of Sports Medicine encourages them to engage in the full range of physical activities, including aerobic conditioning. As much as 50 percent of the physiologic declines commonly attributed to aging are due to sedentary living and can be dramatically reversed. With regular conditioning, 60-year-olds can regain the fitness they had at age 40 to 45.

Exercise is so effective in preserving well-being that gerontologists describe it as "the closest thing

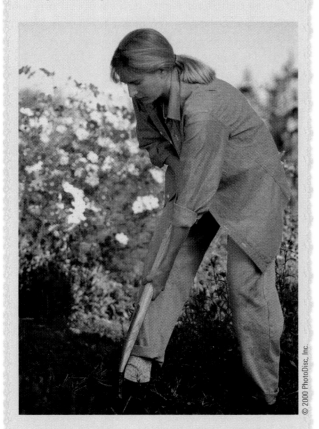

▲ Physical fitness can be enhanced at any age by routine activities such as gardening.

to an anti-aging pill." It slows many changes associated with advancing age, such as loss of lean muscle tissue, increase in body fat, and decreased work capacity. It lowers the risk of heart disease and stroke in the elderly—and greatly improves general health. Male and female runners over age 50 have much lower rates of disability and much lower health-care expenses than less active seniors. Even less intense activities, such as gardening, dancing, and brisk walking, can delay chronic disability.[60] Walking has proven helpful in delaying cognitive decline in older women.[61]

According to the Surgeon General, physical activity offers older Americans additional benefits including the following:

▷ Greater ability to live independently.
▷ Reduced risk of falling and fracturing bones.
▷ Lower risk of dying from coronary heart disease and of developing high blood pressure, colon cancer, and diabetes.
▷ Reduced blood pressure in some people with hypertension.
▷ Fewer symptoms of anxiety and depression.
▷ Improvements in mood and feelings of well-being.

Despite these potential benefits, many seniors are not active. By age 75, about one in three men and one in two women engage in no physical activity. Yet, even sedentary individuals in their eighties and nineties can participate in an exercise program—and gain significant benefits.

Federal health officials recommend a moderate amount of physical activity, either in longer sessions of moderately intense activities (such as walking) or in shorter sessions of more vigorous activities (such as fast walking or stair-climbing). Seniors can gain additional health benefits by increasing the duration, intensity, or frequency of their workouts, but should avoid overdoing their training because of the risk of injury. Older adults should always consult with a physician before beginning a new physical activity program.

The Role of Sleep

You stay up late cramming for a final. You drive through the night to visit a friend at another campus. You get up for an early class during the week but stay in bed until noon on weekends. And you wonder: "Why am I so tired?" The answer: You're not getting enough sleep—and you're not alone. According to the National Commission on Sleep Disorders Research, one of every three Americans has problems sleeping. And even those who aren't having difficulty don't log as much sleep time as they'd like. Over the last century, we have cut our average nightly sleep time by more than 20 percent.

Whenever we fail to get adequate sleep, we accumulate what researchers call a *sleep debit*. With each night of too little rest, our body's need for sleep grows until it becomes irresistible. The only solution to sleep debt is the obvious one: paying it back. Individuals who add an hour or two to their nightly sleep time are more alert, more productive, and less likely to have accidents. And because sleepy people tend to be irritable and edgy, those who get more rest also tend to be happier, healthier, and easier to get along with.

Sleep Basics

We spend a third of our lives sleeping—more time than we spend working, loving, or playing. Although sleepers may look quiet and seem unresponsive to the world around them, their brains and bodies are going through a series of profound changes. Scientists differentiate between certain periods of the night when the eyes dart rapidly back and forth beneath closed lids, called **rapid-eye-movement (REM) sleep,** and quieter, non-REM sleep stages. Most adults spend 20 to 25 percent of the night in REM sleep, when our most vivid dreaming takes place.

Each night as you fall asleep, you go through the same sequence of sleep stages: Your body begins to slow down, and muscular tension decreases. As you enter stage 1 of non-REM sleep, your brain waves become smaller, pinched, and irregular. Mundane thoughts flit through your mind; if awakened from this twilight zone, you might deny having slept at all. As you enter stage 2, your brain waves become larger, with occasional bursts of activity. Your eyes become unresponsive, so that even if your eyelids were gently lifted, you wouldn't see. In stage 3, your brain waves are much slower and about five times larger than in stage 1. In stage 4, the most profound state of unconsciousness, your brain waves form a slow, jagged pattern; and you would be very difficult to arouse. (See Figure 4-7.)

The full journey to the depths of tranquility takes more than an hour. Then you begin your ascent—not to consciousness but to REM sleep. The muscles of your middle ear vibrate. Your brain waves resemble the patterns of waking more than of deep sleep. The muscles of your face, limbs, and trunk are slack. Your pulse and breathing quicken, and your brain temperature and blood flow increase. Your eyes dart back and forth. If wakened, you're likely to report a fantasylike dream.

Your body repeats this sequence four or five times a night. In an eight-hour night's rest, you spend two hours

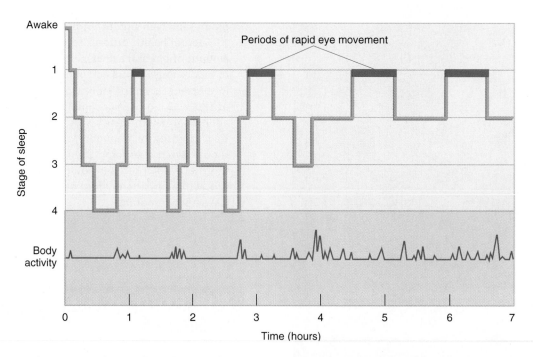

▲ **Figure 4-7** A sleep cycle. During the first hour or so, sleep becomes deeper; then the level ascends to a period of REM sleep (indicated by thick bars). The sleep cycle is repeated, with some variations, throughout the night.

in REM sleep; over the course of a lifetime, you'll spend five or six years dreaming and three times that amount in the quieter stages of sleep.

??? How Much Sleep Do I Need?

No formula can say how long a good night's sleep should be. Normal sleep times range from five to ten hours; the average is seven and a half. About one or two people in a hundred can get by with just five hours; another small minority needs twice that amount. Each of us seems to have an innate sleep *appetite* that is as much a part of our genetic programming as hair color and skin tone.

To figure out your sleep needs, keep your wake-up time the same every morning and vary your bedtime. Are you groggy after six hours of shut-eye? Does an extra hour give you more stamina? What about an extra two hours? Since too much sleep can make you feel sluggish, don't assume that more is always better. Listen to your body's signals, and adjust your sleep schedule to suit them.

Getting Enough Sleep

Although sleep needs vary from person to person, physicians have recognized "problem sleepiness" as a threat to health and safety. Its effects are insidious, however, and often neither the individuals nor their doctors realize that problem sleepiness is undermining emotional and physical health.[62]

STRATEGIES FOR CHANGE

How to Sleep Like a Baby

✔ Keep regular hours for going to bed and getting up in the morning. Stay as close as possible to this schedule on weekends as well as weekdays.

✔ Develop a sleep ritual—such as stretching, meditation, yoga, prayer, or reading a not-too-thrilling novel—to ease the transition from wakefulness to sleep.

✔ Don't drink coffee late in the day. The effects of caffeine can linger for up to eight hours. And don't smoke. Nicotine is an even more powerful stimulant—and sleep saboteur—than caffeine.

✔ Don't rely on alcohol to get to sleep. Alcohol disrupts normal sleep stages, so you won't sleep as deeply or as restfully as you normally would.

✔ Don't nap during the day if you're having problems sleeping through the night.

About 5 percent of Americans suffer from persistent insomnia. Medications can help in the short run but lose their effectiveness over time and interfere, to varying degrees, with the normal stages of sleep. One of the most promising alternatives is cognitive behavioral training (CBT), which combines cognitive therapy with specific strategies to improve sleep habits, such as avoiding daytime naps and limiting time in bed.[63]

Nutrition for an Active Life

The food you eat provides the fuel you use to move through life. Nutrition and physical activity are interrelated. Your level of activity influences your calorie needs, and the foods you eat affect your energy and performance.

 Many people assume that individuals with active lifestyles eat more nutritiously, but that's not necessarily so—at least among college students. A study of 109 undergraduates at a Texas state university found no correlation between fitness levels and healthy eating habits. The fittest students were not more likely to eat a nutritious diet, nor were those consuming the most nutrients more likely to rate highly on fitness tests.[64]

In general, active people need the same basic nutrients as others and should follow the Food Guide Pyramid and other recommendations in Chapter 5. However, athletes in competitive sports—amateur as well as professional—may have increased energy requirements.

??? How Much Water Should I Drink?

Water, which we need more than any other nutrient, is even more important during exercise and exertion. Thirst, the body's way of telling you to replace lost fluids, is not a good way for athletes to monitor their fluid needs. Rather than waiting until you're already somewhat dehydrated, you should be fully hydrated when you begin your activity or exercise and, depending on the duration and intensity of your workout, continue to replace fluids both during and afterward.

Here are the American Dietetic Association's guidelines for fluid intake for active individuals:

▶ Consume at least two cups (16 to 20 ounces) of fluid about two hours before exertion.

▶ Drink another two cups of fluid approximately 15 to 20 minutes before endurance exercise.

▶ If the climate is hot and humid, take small servings (4 to 6 ounces) every 15 minutes of plain cool water (40

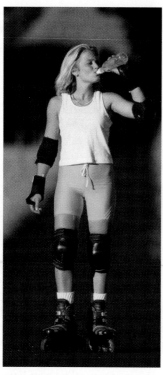

▲ Plain water before and during a workout is the best way to prevent dehydration.

to 50 degrees Fahrenheit) or another rehydration beverage. (Think of an ounce as approximately one "gulp.") Depending on your sport or activity, you may need to drink whenever the opportunity arises (e.g., during breaks or time-outs).

▶ After an activity, drink at least two cups (16 ounces) per pound of body weight lost during the activity. Some exercise physiologists recommend an additional 8 ounces (24 ounces total per pound) to compensate for urine losses as you rehydrate.

Loss of more than 2 percent of body weight during an activity indicates that a person is becoming dehydrated. Any degree of dehydration impairs physical performance; extreme dehydration can lead to heat exhaustion or heat stroke, two serious conditions discussed in on page 579.

Nutrition and Athletic Performance

Most people, even if physically active, do not require special diets, although they may need more servings in each group of the Food Guide Pyramid. Contrary to a common misconception, athletes generally do not need more protein; the exception may be those engaged in intense strength training. Like most Americans, athletes typically consume more than the Recommended Daily Allowance for protein and do not need increased protein. As discussed in Chapter 6, a high-protein diet can be high in fat and low in the nutrients supplied by fruits, vegetables, and grains and can put a strain on the liver and kidneys.

Although complex carbohydrates are essential in an athlete's diet, fat also plays a role. Trained runners who severely limited their fat intake suppressed their immune system and increased their susceptibility to infections and inflammation.[65] Other research has shown that including the right types of fat in the daily diet can actually improve athletic performance—not just by providing calories, but by replenishing intramuscular fat stores (fat stored within the muscle and used to fuel extended exercise).[66]

Energy Bars

Sold as snacks, meal substitutes, or performance enhancers, energy bars come in different forms. High-carbohydrate bars derive more than 70 percent of their calories from carbohydrates (such as corn syrup, grape and pear juice concentrate, oat bran, and brown rice) and are low in protein and fat. Another type gets 40 percent of its energy from carbohydrate, 30 percent from protein, and 30 percent from fat.

Little scientific research has studied the actual benefits of the various types of energy bars, including their effects on blood glucose levels and athletic performance. According to one nutritional analysis, high-carbohydrate energy bars are similar to candy bars in their impact on glucose—even though sugars composed 31 percent of the high-carbohydrate energy bar and 86 percent of the candy bar. In fact, the high-carbohydrate energy bar caused a more rapid peak in blood glucose followed by a sharper decline than did the candy bar. This effect may be desirable for athletes involved in short-duration events who want a quick increase in blood glucose.

Energy bars with a lower carbohydrate level produce a more moderate, sustained increase in blood glucose level, possibly because the protein and fat in a 40–30–30 bar diminish blood glucose response. These bars would be a better choice for athletes involved in endurance events.[67]

For others, energy bars are of dubious value. Even Americans who eat poorly rarely need additional protein. Despite their marketing claims, energy bars don't build muscle or boost energy more than any other food; they just provide extra and often unneeded calories.[68]

Sport and Protein Drinks

Protein shakes and prepackaged drinks also have become popular. However, many sports nutritionists consider them of dubious value.[69] As explained in Chapter 5, most people obtain adequate protein from their daily diet, and dietary protein is just as beneficial as the "high-quality" proteins advertised as ingredients of sports drinks.

Sports Safety

Whenever you work out, you don't want to risk becoming sore or injured. Starting slowly when you begin any new fitness activity is the smartest strategy. Keep a simple diary to record the time and duration of each workout. Get accustomed to an activity first and then begin to work harder or longer. In this way, you strengthen your musculoskeletal system so you're less likely to be injured, you lower the cardiovascular risk, and you build the exercise habit into your schedule.

Even seasoned athletes should "listen to their bodies." If you develop aches and pains beyond what you might expect from an activity, stop. Never push to the point of fatigue. If you do, you could end up with sprained or torn muscles.

How Can I Prevent Sports Injuries?

According to the American Physical Therapy Association, the most common exercise-related injury sites are the knees, feet, back, and shoulders, followed by the ankles and hips. **Acute injuries**—sprains, bruises, and pulled muscles—are the result of sudden trauma, such as a fall or collision. **Overuse injuries,** on the other hand, are the result of overdoing a repetitive activity, such as running. When one particular joint is overstressed—such as a tennis player's elbow or a swimmer's shoulder—tendinitis, an inflammation at the point where the tendon meets the bone, can develop. Other overuse injuries include muscle strains and aches and stress fractures, which are hairline breaks in a bone, usually in the leg or foot.

To prevent injuries and other exercise-related problems before they happen, use common sense and take appropriate precautions, including the following:

- Get proper instruction and, if necessary, advanced training from knowledgeable instructors.
- Make sure you have good equipment and keep it in good condition. Know how to check and do at least basic maintenance on the equipment yourself. Always check your equipment prior to each use (especially if you're renting it).
- Always make sure that stretching and exercises are preventing, not causing, injuries.
- Use reasonable protective measures, including wearing a helmet when cycling or skating.
- For some sports, such as boating, always go with a buddy.

- Take each outing seriously—even if you've dived into this river a hundred times before, even if you know this mountain like you know your own backyard. Avoid the unknown under adverse conditions (for example, hiking unfamiliar terrain during poor weather or kayaking a new river when water levels are unusually high or low) or when accompanied by a beginner whose skills may not be as strong as yours.
- Never combine alcohol or drugs with any sport.

Out of the Gym

Many people are trying exhilarating sports that, by their very nature, entail some risk. If you choose these activities, you're responsible for learning how to stay safe as you push to the limit. Here are some sport-specific guidelines:

- **Inline skating.** Although it may seem easy and safe, inline skating requires good aerobic fitness and strong leg and back muscles. The most common injuries are to the wrists. Skaters should always wear protective gear, including a helmet, wrist guards, and knee pads, and should warm up before strapping on their skates. Learn how to fall: Relax, go down to your knees, and roll to one side.
- **Mountain biking.** Off-road biking requires skills that go beyond biking, including knowing how to shift your weight to keep a bike stable on rough trails. Know the limits of your endurance and of your equipment. Wear a helmet, bicycle gloves, and glasses or goggles to protect your eyes from dirt and overhanging branches. Carry a bike repair kit and a first aid kit if you head for a remote area.
- **Rock climbing.** In addition to overall fitness, rock climbing takes strength, balance, and hand-eye coordination. Training with a qualified instructor is essential to learn proper technique. The best place to learn is indoors, with supervised instruction and controlled conditions.
- **Snowboarding.** This winter sport requires aerobic fitness, muscular strength, and excellent flexibility. Well-fitted snowboarding boots are essential, as is training in how to fall. The most common injuries are to the wrist or thumb, which can fracture if snowboarders put out their palms to break a fall. Sunburn and frostbite are both risks, and snowboarders should wear sunscreen and monitor weather conditions closely.

Thinking of Temperature

Prevention is the wisest approach to heat problems. Always dress appropriately for the weather and be aware of the health risks associated with temperature extremes.

Heeding Heat

Always wear as little as possible when exercising in hot weather. Choose loose-fitting, lightweight, white or light-colored clothes. Cotton is good because it absorbs perspiration. Never wear rubberized or plastic pants and jackets to sweat off pounds. These sauna suits will cause you to lose water only—not fat—and, because they don't allow your body heat to dissipate, they can be dangerous. On humid days, carry a damp washcloth to wipe off perspiration and cool yourself down. Be sure to drink plenty of fluids while exercising (especially water), and watch for the earliest signs of heat problems, including cramps, stress, exhaustion, and heatstroke. (See Chapter 17 for a further discussion of safety precautions.)

Coping with Cold

Protect yourself in cold weather (or cold indoor gyms) by covering as much of your body as possible, but don't over-dress. Wear one layer less than you would if you were outside but not exercising. Don't use warm-up clothes of waterproof material because they tend to trap heat and keep perspiration from evaporating. Make sure your clothes are loose enough to allow movement and exercise of the hands, feet, and other body parts, thereby maintaining proper circulation. Choose dark colors that absorb heat. And because 40 percent or more of your body heat is lost through your head and neck, wear a hat, turtleneck, or scarf. Make sure you cover your hands and feet as well; mittens provide more warmth and protection than gloves.

Toxic Workouts

If you live in a large city, you may have to consider the risks of exercising in polluted air. On smoggy days, avoid a noontime workout. Exposure to ground-level ozone, produced as sunlight reacts with exhaust fumes, can irritate the lungs and constrict bronchial tubes. An ozone level of 0.12 part per million causes, on the average, a 13 percent decline in lung capacity. This level is the maximum considered safe under the Clean Air Act, but it is often surpassed in New York, Los Angeles, and other urban areas.

Overtraining

About half of all people who start an exercise program drop out within six months. One common reason is that they **overtrain,** pushing themselves to work too intensely too frequently. Signs of overdoing it include persistent muscle soreness, frequent injuries, unintended weight loss, nervousness, and an inability to relax. Overtraining for endurance sports like marathon running can damage the lungs and intensify asthma symptoms.[70] If you're pushing too hard, you may find yourself unable to complete a normal workout or have difficulty recovering afterward.

If you develop any of the symptoms of overtraining, reduce or stop your workout sessions temporarily. Make gradual increases in the intensity of your workouts. Allow 24 to 48 hours for recovery between workouts. Make sure you get adequate rest. Check with a physical education instructor, coach, or trainer to make sure your exercise program fits your individual needs.

Evaluating Fitness Products and Programs

As fitness has become a major industry in the United States, consumers have been bombarded with pitches for products that promise to do everything from whittle a waistline to build up biceps. As always, you have to ask questions and do your own research—whether you're buying basic exercise aids (See Savvy Consumer: "Do Low-Tech, Low-Cost, Fitness Aids Work?") or joining a health club. Beware of any promise that sounds too good to be true. And keep in mind that nothing matters more than your own commitment.

How Do I Buy the Right Athletic Shoes?

For many aerobic activities, good shoes are the most important purchase you'll make. Take the time to choose well. Here are some basic guidelines:

- Shop for shoes in the late afternoon, when your feet are most likely to be somewhat swollen—just as they will be after a workout.
- For walking shoes, look for a shoe that's lightweight, flexible, and roomy enough for your toes to wiggle, with a well-cushioned, curved sole; one that has good support at the heel; and one with an upper that is made of a material that breathes (allows air in and out).
- For running shoes (see Figure 4-8), look for good cushioning, support, and stability. You should be able to wiggle your toes easily, but the front of your foot shouldn't slide from side to side, which could cause blisters. Your toes should not touch the end of the shoe because your feet will swell with activity. Allow about half an inch from the longest toe to the tip of the shoe. If you run up to 10 miles a week, replace your shoes every 9 to 12 months.[71]
- For racquetball shoes, look for reinforcement at the toe for protection during foot drag. The sole should allow minimal slippage. There should be some heel elevation to lessen strain on the back of the leg and Achilles ten-

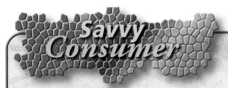

Savvy Consumer

Do Low-Tech, Low-Cost Fitness Aids Work?

Not all fitness equipment comes with a big price tag. Here are some affordable ways to expand and enhance a home workout:

- Dumbbells. You can purchase light weights to carry when walking and jogging to build and firm arm muscles. Training with heavier weights increases muscle strength and endurance, improves balance and body composition, and may reverse some bone loss. An adjustable dumbbell set allows you to add more weight as you build strength.

- Stretchy bands. Low in cost, lightweight, and highly portable, elastic exercise bands allow you to create resistance as you exercise. Available in different strengths, they can also provide for progressive overload. Some trainers believe they work best for novice exercisers, since well-conditioned athletes may need more challenge.

- Exercise balls. Popular in group classes, exercise balls come in various sizes. Heavy, weighted balls can be lifted or tossed to tone the upper body. The larger, inflatable balls are mainly used for balance and back workouts. Some trainers think they add fun and variety to a workout; others question their value. Crunches performed on a ball may be somewhat more effective.

---

don. The shoe should have a long "throat" to ensure greater control by the laces.

For tennis shoes, look for reinforcement at the toe. The sole at the ball of the foot should be well padded, because that's where most pressure is exerted. The sides of the shoe should be sturdy, for stability during continuous lateral movements. The toe box should allow ample room and some cushioning at the tips. A long throat ensures greater control by the laces.

Don't wear wet shoes for training. Let wet shoes air-dry, because a heater will cause them to stiffen or shrink.

Use powder in your shoes to absorb moisture, lessen friction, and prevent fungal infections. Break in new shoes for several days before wearing them for a long-distance run or during competition.

Exercise Equipment

Always try out equipment before buying it. If you decide to purchase a stationary bicycle, for instance, read all the product information. Ask someone in your physical education department or at a local gym for recommendations. Try out a bicycle at the gym. Make sure any equipment you purchase is safe and durable.

Think about your fitness goals. If you're primarily interested in aerobic fitness, try out stationary bicycles, stair-climbing machines, rowing machines, treadmills, and cross-country skiing machines. Spend 5 to 10 minutes working at moderate intensity. How do your movements on this particular piece of equipment feel to you—awkward or fluid, extremely difficult or surprisingly easy?

If you're considering strength-training equipment, remember that free weights are your least expensive option. The best resistance machines are also the most expensive, with prices over $1,000. Would you use

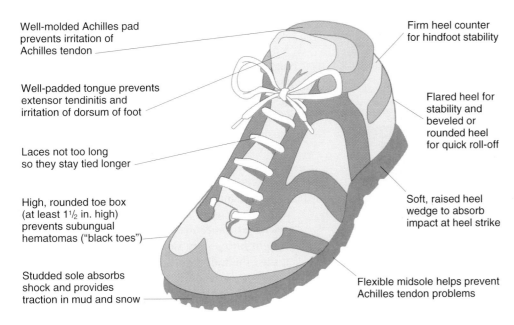

Well-molded Achilles pad prevents irritation of Achilles tendon

Well-padded tongue prevents extensor tendinitis and irritation of dorsum of foot

Laces not too long so they stay tied longer

High, rounded toe box (at least 1½ in. high) prevents subungual hematomas ("black toes")

Studded sole absorbs shock and provides traction in mud and snow

Firm heel counter for hindfoot stability

Flared heel for stability and beveled or rounded heel for quick roll-off

Soft, raised heel wedge to absorb impact at heel strike

Flexible midsole helps prevent Achilles tendon problems

Source: Canadian Podiatric Sports Medicine Academy.

▲ **Figure 4-8** What to Look for When You Buy Running Shoes.

Source: Canadian Podiatric Sports Medicine Academy.

one often enough to justify that cost? Or would an annual health-club membership be more cost-effective?

Your exercise style is also an important consideration. Are you going to find sitting at a stationary bicycle for 30 minutes too boring? Are you motivated enough to hoist free weights on your own several times a week? The best home exercise equipment will do you no good unless you use it.

Fitness Centers and Trainers

If you decide to join a gym or health club, find out exactly what facilities and programs it offers. The club should be located close to home, campus, or work and should be open at convenient hours. Think about your schedule and when you'll have time to work out. Visit the club at the times you're most likely to use it: During peak hours, you might have to wait half an hour for a turn on the machines.

A club should have facilities for a complete workout, including both aerobic and muscle workouts: exercycles, rowing machines, treadmills, stair-climbing machines, stationary bicycles, a running track, aerobics classes, a swimming pool, strength-training equipment, and, if that's what you're looking for, racquetball and squash courts and a large gym for basketball and volleyball.

Find out whether all facilities are available to all members at all times. Some clubs reserve the pool for families only or kids' lessons at certain times. Ask if you can try out the club before joining. Find out what the membership includes. Will you end up paying extra for lockers, towels, classes, and the like? Are student discounts offered? Beware of long-term memberships; many clubs go out of business or change ownership often. Pay attention to cleanliness and to the atmosphere and people. Do the members seem to be significantly older or younger, or in much better or worse shape, than you are? You're more likely to work out regularly in a place, and with people, you like.

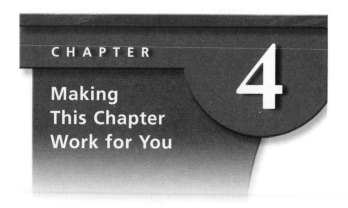

CHAPTER

**Making
This Chapter
Work for You**

4

1. Mary Ann takes a step aerobics class three times a week. Which component of physical fitness does her exercise routine emphasize?

   a. muscular strength and endurance
   b. flexibility
   c. cardiorespiratory fitness
   d. body composition

2. The benefits of regular physical activity include:
   a. decreased bone mass.
   b. lowered risk of shin splints.
   c. enhanced immune response.
   d. altered sleep patterns.

3. To motivate yourself to stick to an exercise program:
   a. Watch professional athletic competitions.
   b. Set a long-term goal, then break it down into short-term goals that can be achieved in a few months.
   c. Keep a detailed record of all the times that you avoided working out.
   d. Join an expensive health club so that you feel pressured to get your money's worth.

4. Which of the following best describes the primary benefit of aerobic exercise?
   a. It improves cardiorespiratory endurance.
   b. It helps condition your muscles, enabling them to work efficiently and reliably.
   c. It can enhance weight loss.
   d. It increases the range of motion of your joints.

5. An aerobic workout may consist of
   a. 5 minutes of brisk walking, 30 minutes of flexibility exercises, 5 minutes of brisk walking.
   b. 15 minutes of resistance exercises followed by 10 minutes of stretching.
   c. 10 minutes of sprints, 5 minutes of slow jogging, 5 minutes of stretching, and 10 minutes of sprints.
   d. 5 minutes of stretching, 5 minutes of brisk walking, 45 minutes of jogging, 5 minutes of slow walking, 5 minutes of stretching.

6. Which statement is true about isometric, isotonic, and isokinetic exercises?
   a. Isokinetic exercises usually involves pushing on an object, isotonic exercises involve pulling on an object, and isotonic exercises involve lifting an object.
   b. Isometric and isokinetic exercises can be done with free weights, but isotonic exercises require special resistance machines.
   c. Weight lifting is an isotonic exercise, pushing against the wall is an isometric exercise, and isokinetic exercises require special machines that move muscles through their range of motion.
   d. Isotonic exercises are much more effective at contracting muscles than isometric or isokinetic.

7. A regular flexibility program provides which of the following benefits?
   a. stronger heart and lungs

b. relief of muscle strain and soreness

c. increased strength and endurance

d. increased bone mass and leaner muscles

8. The sleep cycle refers to

a. the alternating pattern of insomnia, which creates sleep debt, and daytime sleepiness, which affects our mood and productivity.

b. the physical and mental discomfort you feel if you have not gotten enough sleep.

c. the amount of sleep that your body requires to function optimally.

d. alternating periods of deep sleep and periods of active dreaming.

9. Which nutrient is the most important during exercise and exertion?

a. water

b. carbohydrates

c. fat

d. protein

10. Which of the following precautions could help prevent a serious sports injury from occurring?

a. Wearing swimming goggles when doing laps to decrease the irritating effects of chlorine.

b. Wear knee pads when cycling to prevent knee gashes if you fall off your bicycle.

c. To eliminate persistent muscle soreness, increase the frequency and/or time period of your workout.

d. Wear a helmet, wrist guards, and knee pads when inline skating to help prevent fractures and head injuries.

Answers to these questions can be found on page 640.

 What are the behavioral strategies for getting a good nights sleep?

Critical Thinking

1. Allison knows that exercise is good for her health, but she figures she can keep her weight down by dieting, and worry about her heart and health when she gets older. "I look good. I feel okay. Why should I bother exercising?" she asks. What would you reply?

2. When he started working out, Jeff simply wanted to stay in shape. But he felt so pleased with the way his body looked and responded that he kept doing more. Now he runs 10 miles a day (longer on weekends), lifts weights, works out on exercise equipment almost every day, and plays racquetball or squash whenever he gets a chance. Is Jeff getting too much of a good thing? Is there any danger in his fitness program? What would be a more reasonable approach?

3. Your younger brother Andre is hoping to get a starting position on his high school football team. Practices began in July. You are aware that a couple of other players have suffered heat-related incidences, but according to Andre, these players just weren't tough enough. What can you do to help your brother protect his health?

4. Although anabolic steroids have been banned for use by athletes in certain competitions, other performance-enhancing supplements are used routinely to provide a competitive advantage. Do you believe that most athletes use such substances routinely? Do you think that athletes should be able to use these substances without intervention or regulation? Why or why not?

SITES & BYTES

Shape Up America Fitness Assessment

http://www.shapeup.org/fitness/assess/fset2.htm

A battery of physical fitness assessments includes activity level, strength, flexibility, and an aerobic fitness test. You start by entering your weight, height, age, and gender and then taking a quick screen test to assess your physical readiness for physical activity. Your final results in each of these areas will be based on your personal data.

Cooper Fitness Interactive—What Kind of Shape Are You In?

http://www.cooperfitness.com/content/Fitness/FitnessInventory/FitnessInventory.asp

This comprehensive site features personalized fitness assessments in each of the following: cardiorespiratory , body fat, heart rate, strength, flexibility, and basal metabolic rate.

Aerobics and Fitness Association of America
http://www.afaa.com
This interactive site features "Exercise Gets Personal™" where you can create a customized exercise program that includes activities you select, geared to your current level of fitness activity. Exercises include aerobics, muscular conditioning, and flexibility with descriptions and precautions for each activity.

Please note that links are subject to change. If you find a broken link, use a search engine such as **http://www.yahoo.com** and search for the website by typing in key words.

InfoTrac Activity Frank Booth et al. "Physiologists Claim 'Sedentary Death Syndrome (SeDS)' Is Second Greatest Threat to U.S. Public Health." *Medical Letter on the CDC & FDA,* June 24, 2001.

(1) What percentage of Americans are currently at risk for Sedentary Death Syndrome? What percent of Americans are overweight? What percent of children are clinically obese?
(2) Name at least ten of the thirty-five medical conditions exacerbated by physical inactivity.
(3) Describe the four steps outlined by Booth and his colleagues in this article that are necessary for the prevention of Sedentary Death Syndrome.

You can find additional readings related to fitness with InfoTrac College Edition, an online library of more than 900 journals and publications. Follow the instructions for accessing InfoTrac that were packaged with your textbook; then search for articles using a key word search.

For additional links, resources, and suggested readings on InfoTrac, visit our Health & Wellness Resource Center at **http://health.wadsworth.com**.

Key Terms

The terms listed here are used within the chapter on the page indicated. Definitions of the terms are in the Glossary at the end of this book.

active stretching 130	**endorphins** 111	**passive stretching** 129
acute injuries 135	**endurance** 106	**physical fitness** 106
aerobic circuit training 130	**ergogenic aids** 128	**rapid-eye movement (REM) sleep** 132
aerobic exercise 106	**flexibility** 107	**rep (or repetition)** 125
anabolic steroids 126	**isokinetic** 125	**resting heart rate** 118
anaerobic exercise 118	**isometric** 125	**sets** 125
ballistic stretching 130	**isotonic** 125	**static flexibility** 128
body composition 106	**muscular fitness** 106	**static stretching** 129
cardiorespiratory fitness 106	**osteoporosis** 111	**strength** 106
conditioning 108	**overloading** 125	**target heart rate** 119
cross-training 130	**overtrain** 136	
dynamic flexbility 128	**overuse injuries** 135	

References

1. Sax, Linda, et al. *The American Freshman: National Norms for Fall 2000.* Los Angeles: Higher Education Research Institute, UCLA, 2000.
2. Sallis, James, et al. "Evaluation of a University Course to Promote Physical Activity: Project GRAD (Graduate Ready for Activity Daily)." *Research Quarterly for Exercise and Sport,* Vol. 70, No. 1, March 1999.
3. Booth, Frank, et al. "Physiologists Claim 'SeDS' Is Second Greatest Threat to U.S. Public Health." *Medical Letter on the CDC & FDA,* June 24, 2001.
4. Booth, Frank, et al. "Waging War on Modern Chronic Diseases: Primary Prevention Through Exercise Biology." *Journal of Applied Physiology,* Vol. 88, No. 2, February 2000.
5. "Physical Activity Trends in the United States, 1990–1998." *Morbidity and Mortality Weekly Report,* March 9, 2001.
6. "CDC Reports Levels of Physical Activity In the 1990s Remained Unchanged." *Medical Letter on the CDC & FDA,* April 1, 2001.
7. Lindstrom, Martin, et al. "Socioeconomic Differences in Leisure-time Physical Activity." *Social Science & Medicine,* Vol. 52, No. 3, Feburary 2001, p. 441.

8. Rose, Verna. "CDC Report on Physical Inactivity." *American Family Physician,* Vol. 59, Issue 6, March 15, 1999.

9. Dreyfuss, Ira. "Study Made of Who Exercises." *Associated Press,* January 23, 2000.

10. "Physical Activity, Part I—Start With a Walk." *Harvard Women's Health Watch,* Vol. 8, No. 10, June 2001.

11. Krucoff, Carol, and Mitchell Krucoff. "Turbulent Transition: How Exercise Can Relieve Many of the Symptoms Associated with Menopause." *American Fitness,* Vol. 19, No. 2, March 2001, p. 22.

12. Booth, "Waging War on Modern Chronic Diseases: Primary Prevention Through Exercise Biology."

13. "More American Children and Teens Are Overweight." Press release, CDC, March 12, 2001.

14. Faigenbaum, Avery, et al. "Strength Training and Children's Health." *Journal of Physical Education, Recreation & Dance,* Vol. 72, No. 3, March 2001, p. 24.

15. Field, Tiffany, et al. "Exercise Is Positively Related to Adolescents' Relationships and Academics." *Adolescence,* Vol. 36, No. 141, Spring 2001, p. 105.

16. Plunk, Jamey, et al. "The Relationship Between Fitness Level and Academic Success Among College Students." *Research Quarterly for Exercise and Sport,* Vol. 72, No. 1, March 2001, p. A-34.

17. "Regular Physical Exertion May Fight Cancer as Well as Heart Disease." *Tufts University Health & Nutrition Letter,* Vol. 18, No. 7, September 2000.

18. "Defensive Moves." *American Fitness,* Vol. 19, No. 4, July 2001, p. 48.

19. "Exercise Against Depression." *Harvard Mental Health Letter,* Vol. 17, No. 19, March 2001.

20. LeTourneau, Melanie. "Pump Up to Cheer Up." *Psychology Today,* May–June 2001, p. 27.

21. "Exercise as Psychotherapy." *Harvard Mental Health Letter,* Vol. 17, No. 3, September 2000.

22. Babyak, Michael, et al. "Exercise Treatment for Major Depression: Maintenance of Therapeutic Benefit at 10 Months." *Psychosomatic Medicine,* Vol. 62, No. 5, September–October 2000, pp. 633–638.

23. National Blueprint: Increasing Physical Activity Among Adults Age 50 and Older. National Center for Chronic Disease Prevention and Health Promotion. Washington, DC: May 1, 2001.

24. "Heart Lines—Walking and Gardening Beneficial for Heart Disease Patients." *Harvard Heart Letter,* Vol. 11, No. 8, April 2001.

25. "Easy Ways to Reduce the Risk of Heart Disease." *HealthFacts,* April 2001.

26. Wee, C., et al. " Physical Activity Counseling in Primary Care." *Journal of the American Medical Association,* Vol. 286, No. 6, August 8, 2001.

27. "Don't Sweat Over How Much or What Type of Exercise . . . Just Do It." *American Family Physician,* Vol. 63, No. 10, May 15, 2001, p. 1899.

28. Ramadan, J., et al. "Low-frequency Physical Activity Insufficient for Aerobic Conditioning is Associated with Lower Body Fat than Sedentary Conditions." *Nutrition,* Vol. 17, 2001, p. 225.

29. Lee, I-Min, et al. "Physical Activity and Coronary Heart Disease in Women: Is 'No Pain, No Gain' Passé?" *Journal of the American Medical Association,* Vol. 285, No. 11, March 21, 2001.

30. Wallace, Lorraine, et al. "Characteristics of Exercise Behavior Among College Students." *Preventive Medicine,* Vol. 31, No. 5, November 1, 2000.

31. Adams, Daniel, et al. "Body Image and Physical Fitness as a Function of Locus of Control and Gender in College Women and Men." *Research Quarterly for Exercise and Sport,* Vol. 72, No. 1, March 2001, p. A-18.

32. Wallace, "Characteristics of Exercise Behavior Among College Students."

33. DeVoe, Dale, and Cathy Kennedy. "Physical Activity Stages-of-Change and Activity Self-Efficacy of College Students Enrolled in a University-Required Fitness and Wellness Course." *Research Quarterly for Exercise and Sport,* Vol. 72, No. 1, March 2001, p. A-28.

34. Glaros, Nicole, et al. "Varying the Mode of Cardiovascular Exercise to Increase Adherence." *Journal of Sport Behavior,* Vol. 24, No. 1, March 2001, p. 42.

35. Ibid.

36. Sullum, Julie, et al. "Predictors of Exercise Relapse in a College Population." *Journal of American College Health,* Vol. 48, No. 4, January 2000.

37. "Physical Activity, Part I—Start With a Walk."

38. Lee, "Physical Activity and Coronary Heart Disease in Women: Is 'No Pain, No Gain' Passé?"

39. "Heart Lines—Walking and Gardening Beneficial for Heart Disease Patients."

40. Yaffe, Kristin, et al. "A Prospective Study of Physical Activity and Cognitive Decline in Elderly Women." *Archives of Internal Medicine,* Vol. 161, No. 14, July 23, 2001, p. 1703.

41. Welch, Gregory. "Learning to Let Go." *American Fitness,* Vol. 19, No. 4, July 2001, p. 61.

42. "Orthopaedic Surgeons Offer Tips on How Not to 'Run' into Trouble This Spring." News release, American Academy of Orthopaedic Surgeons, May 5, 2001, http://orthoinfo.aaos.org.

43. Thompson, Matthew, and Frederic Rivara. "Bicycle-Related Injuries." *American Family Physician,* Vol. 63, No. 10, May 15, 2001, p. 2071.

44. Ibid.

45. Seabourne, Tom. "Training Tips." *American Fitness,* Vol. 19, No. 3, May 2001.

46. Dibene, Julieanne. "10 Steps to Better Stepping." *American Fitness,* Vol. 19, No. 3, May 2001, p. 28.

47. Kraemer, William, et al. "Resistance Training Combined with Bench-Step Aerobics Enhances Women's Health Profile." *Medicine and Science in Sports and Exercise,* Vol. 33, No. 2, February 2001, p. 259.

48. "Buffed-Up Numbers." Daybreak, University of California, San Francisco, August 23, 2000. www.ucsf.edu/daybreak.

49. Mark, Stephen. "Ergogenic Aids: Powders, Pills, and Potions to Enhance Performance." *American Family Physician,* Vol. 63, No. 5, March 1, 2001, p. 842.

50. King, Douglas, et al. "Effect of Oral Androstenedione on Serum Testosterone and Adaptations to Resistance Training in Young Men." *Journal of the American Medical Association,* Vol. 281, No. 21, June 2, 1999.

51. "Performance Boosters: Science vs. Hype." *Berkeley Wellness Letter,* December 2000.

52. Ahrendt, Dale. "Ergogenic Aids: Counseling the Athlete." *American Family Physician,* Vol. 63, No. 5, March 1, 2001, p. 913.

53. Tamaki, Tetsuro, et al. "Anabolic Steroids Increase Exercise Tolerance." *American Journal of Physiology,* Vol. 280, No. 6, June 2001, p. 973.

54. Schilling, Brian, et al. "Creatine Supplementation and Health Variables: A Retrospective Study." *Medicine and Science in Sports and Exercise,* Vol. 33, No. 2, February 2001, p. 183.

55. Cho, Hunchul, et al. "The Effect of Creatine Supplementation in Anaerobic Power and Blood Fatigue Factors." *Research Quarterly for Exercise and Sport,* Vol. 72, No. 1, March 2001, p. 19.

56. Wilder, Nathan, et al. "The Effects of Low-Dose Creatine Supplementation Versus Creatine Loading in Collegiate Football Players." *Journal of Athletic Training,* Vol. 36, No. 2, April–June 2001, p. 124.

57. Ahrendt, "Ergogenic Aids: Counseling the Athlete."

58. "Performance Boosters: Science vs. Hype."

59. Shrier, Ian. "Should People Stretch Before Exercise?" *Western Journal of Medicine,* Vol. 174, No. 4, April 2001, p. 282.

60. Andrews, Gary. "Care of Older People: Promoting Health and Function in an Ageing Population." *British Medical Journal,* Vol. 322, No. 7288, March 24, 2001, p. 728.

61. Yaffe, "A Prospective Study of Physical Activity and Cognitive Decline in Elderly Women."

62. Kuritzky, Louis. "Sleep Debt on Metabolic and Endocrine Function." *Infectious Disease Alert,* Vol. 19, No. 9, February 1, 2000.

63. Edinger, Jack, et al. "Cognitive Behavioral Therapy for Treatment of Chronic Primary Insomnia." *Journal of the American Medical Association,* Vol. 285, No. 14, April 11, 2001, p. 1856.

64. Bowden, Rodney, and Jamey Plunk. "The Relationship Between Fitness Level and Nutrition Habits." *Research Quarterly for Exercise and Sport,* Vol. 72, No. 1, March 2001, p. A-25.

65. Vankatraman, Jaya. "Very-Low-Fat Diet May Compromise Immunity." International Society for Exercise and Immunology Symposium, Rome, May 20, 1999.

66. Clark, Nancy. "Fat Facts and Fads." *American Fitness,* Vol. 17, No. 3, May 1999.

67. Hertzler, Steve. "Glycemic Index of 'Energy' Snack Bars in Normal Volunteers." *Journal of the American Dietetic Association,* Vol. 100, No. 1, January 2000.

68. "Why Most Energy Bars Should Not Go Home with Most People." *Tufts University Health & Nutrition Letter,* Vol. 19, No. 5, July 2001, p. 6.

69. Clark, Nancy. "Muscle Mix." *American Fitness,* Vol. 19, No. 3, May 2001, p. 48.

70. "Catch a Breather." Daybreak, University of California, San Francisco, September 11, 2000. www.ucsf.edu/daybreak.

71. Kraemer, "Resistance Training Combined with Bench-Step Aerobics Enhances Women's Health Profile."

5

Personal Nutrition

The freshmen on the fifth floor of a university dormitory decided to test a dubious premise: that man—and woman—can live on pizza alone. For a month, they vowed to eat nothing but pizza in all its savory varieties—mushroom, pepperoni, sausage, anchovies, extra cheese, thin crust, double crust. In less than a week, most cringed at the very sight of yet another cardboard delivery box. It wasn't just the boredom of having the same meal that got to them. Some felt bloated. Others had stomachaches. A few complained of headaches and fatigue. One was convinced she had scurvy, a vitamin deficiency disease caused by a lack of fruit and vegetables. None of them managed to stick with pizza for an entire month.

As these students discovered, the foods we choose to eat have an enormous impact on how we feel—and not just in the short term. As demonstrated by the science of **nutrition,** the field that explores the connections between our bodies and the foods we eat, our daily diet affects how long and how well we live. Sensible eating can provide energy for our daily tasks, protect us from many chronic illnesses, and may even extend longevity.

Healthful diets can take many forms—and don't have to be dull. "Eating is one of life's great pleasures," affirms the federal government's most recent *Dietary Guidelines for Americans.* Rather than issuing a list of do's and don'ts or banning specific foods, these recommendations emphasize three key messages, dubbed the "ABCs":

> *Aim for fitness.
> *Build a healthy base.
> *Choose sensibly.[1]

Since many foods can build a healthy lifestyle, you have lots of room for choice. However, making good food choices isn't easy. Faced with a bewildering array of products in stores and restaurants and a blitz of advertising claims, you may well find it hard to select the foods that not only taste good but also are good for you. This chapter can help. It translates the latest information on good nutrition into specific advice that you can use to nourish yourself as well as enjoy the pleasure of eating well.

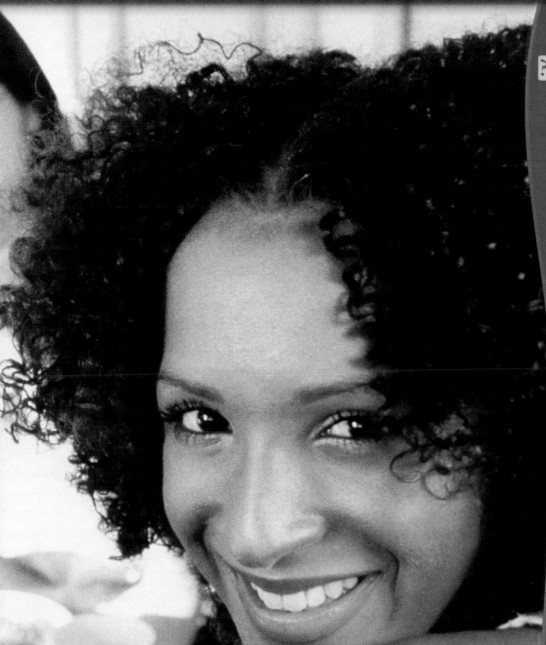

After studying the material in this chapter, you should be able to:

- **List** the basic nutrients necessary for a healthy body and **describe** their functions.
- **Describe** the Food Guide Pyramid and explain its significance.
- **Explain** current recommendations for food portions and servings.
- **Discuss** the purpose of the Dietary Reference Intakes and **explain** how to interpret the nutritional information provided on the food labels.
- **Explain** how nutritional needs change throughout the lifespan.
- **Compare** the advantages and disadvantages of various alternative diets and ethnic foods.
- **List** the food safety hazards and describe prevention measures.

What You Need to Know about Nutrients

Every day your body needs certain **essential nutrients** that it cannot manufacture for itself. They provide energy, build and repair body tissues, and regulate body functions. The six classes of essential nutrients, which are discussed below, are water, protein, carbohydrates, fats, vitamins, and minerals (see Table 5-1).

Calories are the measure of the amount of energy that can be derived from food. Proteins, carbohydrates, and fats are our primary sources of energy. Fats provide 9 calories per gram; protein and carbohydrates, 4 calories per gram. Other **nutrients** serve other functions. Water, for instance, makes up about 60 percent of the body and is essential for health and survival. We need much smaller amounts of vitamins and minerals, yet they are critical for our well-being.

Digestion is the process that releases nutrients into the body by breaking them down into compounds that are absorbed through the gastrointestinal tract (see Figure 5-1). Most foods provide a combination of nutrients, and a healthy diet contains a variety of foods supplying the entire range of essential nutrients.

Water

Water, which makes up 85 percent of blood, 70 percent of muscles, and about 75 percent of the brain, performs many essential functions: It carries nutrients, maintains temperature, lubricates joints, helps with digestion, rids the body of waste through urine, and contributes to the production of sweat, which evaporates from the skin to cool the body. Research has correlated high fluid intake with a lower risk of kidney stones, colon cancer, and bladder cancer. Although you can live for several weeks without food, you would die after a few days without water.

You lose about 64 to 80 ounces of water a day—the equivalent of eight to ten 8-ounce glasses—through perspiration, urine, bowel movements, and normal exhalation. You lose water more rapidly if you exercise, live in a dry climate or at a high altitude, drink a lot of caffeine or alcohol (which increase urination), skip a meal, or become ill. To assure adequate water intake, nutritionists advise drinking enough so that your urine is not dark in color. Particularly in hot and humid weather, anyone can become dehydrated. Early symptoms, include fatigue, weakness, lethargy, dizziness, and headaches.

▼ Table 5-1   The Essential Nutrients

	Functions	Sources
Water	Carries nutrients and removes waste; dissolves amino acids, glucose, and minerals; cleans body by removing toxins; regulates body temperature	Liquids, fruits, and vegetables
Proteins	Help build new tissue to keep hair, skin, and eyesight healthy; build antibodies, enzymes, hormones, and other compounds; provide fuel for body	Meat, poultry, fish, eggs, beans, nuts, cheese, tofu, vegetables, some fruits, pastas, breads, cereal, and rice
Carbohydrates	Provide energy	Grains, cereal, pasta, fruits and vegetables, nuts, milk, and sugars
Fats		
Saturated Fats	Provide energy; trigger production of cholesterol and LDL	Red meat, dairy products, egg yolks, and coconut and palm oils
Unsaturated Fats	Also provide energy, but trigger more HDL production and less cholesterol and LDL production	Some fish; avocados; olive, canola, and peanut oils; shortening; stick margarine; baked goods
Vitamins	Facilitate use of other nutrients; involved in regulating growth, maintaining tissue, and manufacturing blood cells, hormones, and other body components	Fruits, vegetables, grains, some meat and dairy products (see Table 5-6)
Minerals	Help build bones and teeth; aid in muscle function and nervous system activity; assist in various body functions including growth and energy production	Many foods (see Table 5-7)

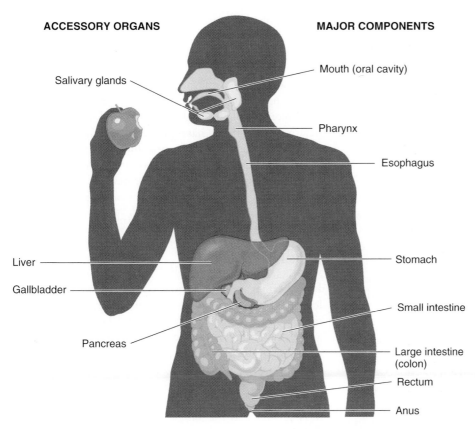

ACCESSORY ORGANS   **MAJOR COMPONENTS**

- Salivary glands
- Liver
- Gallbladder
- Pancreas

- Mouth (oral cavity)
- Pharynx
- Esophagus
- Stomach
- Small intestine
- Large intestine (colon)
- Rectum
- Anus

▲ **Figure 5-1** The digestive system.
The organs of the digestive system break down food into nutrients that the body can use.

Protein

Critical for growth and repair, **proteins** form the basic framework for our muscles, bones, blood, hair, and fingernails. Supplying 4 calories per gram, they are made of combinations of 20 **amino acids,** 9 of which we must get from our diet because the human body cannot produce them. These are called *essential amino acids.*

Animal proteins—meat, fish, poultry, and dairy products—are **complete proteins** that provide the nine essential amino acids. Grains, dry beans, and nuts are **incomplete proteins** that may have relatively low levels of one or two essential amino acids but fairly high levels of others. Combining incomplete proteins, such as beans and rice, ensures that the body gets sufficient protein.

???? Should I Switch to Soy?

Unlike other proteins derived from plants, soy is complete, which makes it an important nutrient for vegetarians (vegetarian diets are discussed later in this chapter). But meat-eaters are also trying the vast new array of soy products and supplements on the market because of claims that soy can relieve hot flashes, strengthen bones, lower cholesterol, and reduce the risk of certain cancers. For now, however, no

strong scientific proof backs up these promises, especially for soy supplements rather than foods.

In Asia, where soybeans are a dietary staple, people do have lower rates of breast and prostate cancers, heart disease, and osteoporosis. Researchers have speculated that the reason may be that compounds in soy, called isoflavones, modulate the effects of certain hormones, such as estrogen and progesterone.[2]

Foods made with the whole soybean, such as tofu and soy milk, have been shown to lower high cholesterol, and the FDA has given manufacturers permission to tout soy protein as an effective means of lowering heart disease risk.[3] However, the amounts used in research studies have been high—25 grams of soy protein a day—and only people with cholesterol levels of 240 or lower have benefited (usually modestly).[4] A recent study did find that soy protein can lower levels of harmful blood fats in individuals with type 2 diabetes (discussed in Chapter 12), who face a higher risk of heart disease than others.[5]

The link between breast cancer and soy intake is not well understood. Most Asian women have eaten at least one serving of soy (the equivalent of 2 to 3 ounces of tofu) daily throughout their lives, and some believe that this early consumption may be more important in explaining

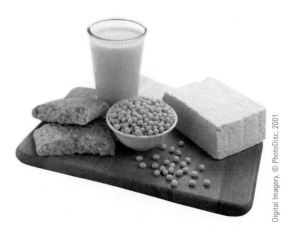

▲ Soybeans contain isoflavones, which appear to inhibit cancer and may also lower blood cholesterol and protect cardiac arteries.

Digital Imagery, © PhotoDisc, 2001

their low breast cancer risk than soy eaten in adulthood.[6] Experts are particularly wary of isoflavone supplements. At least in theory, these weak estrogens could act in conjunction with human estrogen and actually increase a woman's risk of breast cancer.

Scientists are currently investigating the link between soy and a newly discovered type of estrogen receptor in prostate tissue that may influence cancer growth. While they are hoping to determine whether soy protein can reduce high prostate specific antigen (PSA) levels, it is too early to tell if this might lower the risk of prostate cancer.[7] (Prostate cancer is discussed in Chapter 13.)

There is some evidence that soy products may slow bone loss and lower the risk of osteoporosis.[8] In a study of 50 postmenopausal women who consumed three glasses of soy milk daily (providing about 60 milligrams of isoflavones) for 12 weeks, their levels of bone-building cells increased. More studies are needed to confirm this link and determine a recommended dose.

Japanese women consuming a diet high in soy protein have reported fewer hot flashes, but scientific trials have found a very small effect—if any—particularly among breast cancer survivors. In a six month study (the longest time period soy has been studied for hot flashes), perimenopausal women reported improvements whether they took soy protein low in isoflavones, soy protein high in isoflavones, or whey protein. Only more research can fully determine whether soy is effective against hot flashes.[9] The bottom line: As part of a balanced diet, soy remains an excellent low-fat protein source. However, at this time, many of the claims for its health benefits remain unsubstantiated. If you'd like to add soy to your diet, choose whole soy foods rather than isoflavone supplements.

Carbohydrates

Carbohydrates are organic compounds that provide our brains and bodies with glucose, their basic fuel. The major sources of carbohydrates are plants, including grains, vegetables, fruits, and beans, and milk. There are three types: simple carbohydrates (sugars), complex carbohydrates (starches), and fiber. All provide 4 calories per gram.

Forms of Carbohydrates

Simple carbohydrates, or sugars, provide little more than a quick spurt of energy. Nevertheless, they comprise 16 percent of the average American's daily caloric intake and 20 percent of a teenager's calories.[10] Foods rich in added sugars, such as cakes, cookies, candies, and other sweets, may contribute to obesity and heart disease.

Complex carbohydrates are the foundation of a healthy diet. Americans, however, get most of their complex carbohydrates from refined grains, which have been stripped of fiber and many nutrients. Far more nutritious are whole grains, which are made up of all components of the grain: the bran (or fiber-rich outer layer), the endosperm (middle layer), and the germ (the nutrient-packed inner layer). Increasing whole-grain consumption has become a public health priority, and several national health organizations have joined in recommending that Americans increase their consumption of whole-grain foods to at least three servings every day. Individuals who eat whole-grain products each day have about a 15 to 25 percent reduction in death from all causes, including heart disease and cancer.[11]

Fiber

Dietary **fiber** is the indigestible material in food, such as leaves, stems, skins, seeds, and hulls of grains and plants, that can lower blood cholesterol and facilitate digestion and elimination. **Insoluble fibers**—cellulose, lignin, and some hemicellulose—increase bulk in feces, prevent constipation and diverticulosis (a painful inflammation of the bowel), and may lower the risks of heart disease and stroke. Good sources are wheat and corn bran (the outer layer), leafy greens, and the skins of fruits and root vegetables. **Soluble fibers**—such as pectin and gums—lower blood cholesterol and may help control blood sugar levels. Good sources are oats, beans, barley, and the pulp of many fruits and vegetables, such as apples. Table 5-2 offers suggestions for adding fiber to your diet.

Contrary to a long-held assumption, dietary fiber does not appear to protect against the development of colorectal cancer. A study of almost 90,000 women found that those who ate the most dietary fiber had the same risk of developing colorectal cancer as women who ate the least. The link between fiber and colon cancer is complex, however, and researchers have yet to sort it out conclusively. In the meantime, nutritionists continue to urge people to add fiber to their diets because of its other proven health benefits. The National Cancer Institute recommends consuming 20 to 35 grams of fiber a day—much higher than the average intake of about 11 to 13 grams.

Fats

Fats carry the fat-soluble vitamins A, D, E, and K; aid in their absorption in the intestine; protect organs from injury; regulate body temperature; and play an important role in growth and development. They provide 9 calories per gram—more than twice the amount in carbohydrates or proteins. The predominant type of fatty acid a fat contains determines whether the fat is solid or liquid and whether it is characterized as saturated or unsaturated.

▼ Table 5-2 Putting the Fiber into Meals and Snacks

High-Fiber Options for Breakfast

Whole-grain toast		2 g per slice
Bran cereal:		
Bran flakes	1 cup	7 g
All Bran	⅓ cup	10 g
Raisin bran	¾ cup	5 g
Oat bran	⅓ cup	5 g
Bran muffin, with fruit	1 small	3 g
Strawberries	10	2 g
Raspberries	½ cup	3 g
Banana	1 medium	2 g

Lunches That Include Fiber

Whole-grain bread		2 g per slice
Baked beans	½ cup	10 g
Carrot	1 medium	2 g
Raisins	¼ cup	2 g
Peas	½ cup	6 g
Peanut butter	2 tablespoons	2 g

Fiber on the Menu for Supper

Brown rice	½ cup	2 g
Potato	1 medium	3 g
Dried cooked beans	½ cup	8 g
Broccoli	½ cup	3 g
Corn	½ cup	5 g
Tomato	1 medium	2 g
Green beans	½ cup	3 g

Fiber-Filled Snacks

Peanuts	¼ cup	3 g
Apple	1 medium	2 g
Pear	1 medium	4 g
Orange	1 medium	3 g
Prunes*	3	2 g
Sunflower seeds	¼ cup	2 g
Popcorn	2 cups	2 g

*Prunes contain fiber, but their laxative effect is primarily due to a naturally occurring chemical substance that causes an uptake of fluid into the intestines and the contraction of muscles that line the intestines.

Source: Brown, Judith E. *Nutrition Now.* 3rd ed. Belmont, CA: Wadsworth, 2002.

Forms of Fat

Oils such as olive, soybean, canola, cottonseed, corn, and other vegetable oils, which are liquid at room temperature, contain higher levels of unsaturated fatty acids and are considered **unsaturated fats.** Unsaturated fats can be monounsaturated or polyunsaturated (see Table 5-3). Olive oil, which is high in monounsaturated fats, is considered a "good" fat and one of the best vegetable oils for salads and cooking. Used for thousands of years, this staple of the "Mediterranean diet" has been correlated with a lower incidence of heart disease, including strokes and heart attacks. The omega-3 polyunsaturated fatty acids in deep-water fish like salmon may also help lower the risk of cardiovascular disease.

Saturated fats such as lard and butter, which are harder at room temperature, contain higher levels of saturated fatty acids. They are considered dangerous to the heart's health. In response to consumer and health professionals' demand for less saturated fat in the food supply, manufacturers switched to partially hydrogenated oils. However, the process of hydrogenation creates unsaturated fatty acids called **trans fats.** They are found in most foods made with partially hydrogenated oils, such as baked goods and fried foods and some margarine products. Even though trans fats are unsaturated, they appear similar to saturated fats in terms of raising **cholesterol** levels. Epidemiological studies have suggested a possible link between cardiovascular disease risk and high intakes of trans fats, and researchers have concluded that they are, gram for gram, twice as damaging as saturated fat.

Although fats are most notorious as threats to a healthy heart, they also have an effect on our eyes and vision. A recent study found that a higher intake of specific types of fat commonly found in processed, store-bought snack foods, including vegetable, monounsaturated, and polyunsaturated fats, may be associated with a greater risk for advanced age-related macular degeneration (AMD), the leading cause of blindness and vision impairment in the United States. Diets high in omega-3 fatty acids, primarily found in certain types of fish such as albacore tuna and salmon, have the opposite effect and are linked with a lower risk of AMD.[12]

To cut down on both saturated and trans fats, choose soybean, canola, corn, olive, safflower, and sunflower oils, which are naturally trans-fat–free and lower in saturated fats. Look for reduced-fat, low-fat, fat-free, and trans-fat–free versions of baked goods, snacks, and other foods that would otherwise be made with saturated or trans fats. Table 5-4 on page 151 can help you select foods with a lower percentage of calories from fat.

???? Should I Use Butter or Margarine?

The debate over what to spread on bread has been raging for years. First, butter was targeted as an unhealthy choice because it is high in saturated fats. (See Table 5-5 on page 152). Then margarines came under fire because they contain harmful trans fatty acids, which can raise bad LDL cholesterol at least as much as saturated fat. Baffled consumers haven't been sure which to choose. Margarine consumption has fallen since 1993, while butter sales have held steady or spiked upward.[13]

Although butter still has its backers, the healthier choice actually is margarine—particularly tub margarine.[14] A tablespoon of butter contains about 7 grams of saturated fat, while the same amount of stick margarine has, at most,

▼ Table 5-3	Forms of Dietary Fats	
Fat	**Sources**	**What It Does**
Saturated Fat	Red meat, dairy products, egg yolks, coconut and palm oils	Provides energy; triggers production of LDL cholesterol
Unsaturated Fats		
Monounsaturated Fats	Some fish; avocados; olive, canola, and peanut oils	Also provides energy, but triggers more HDL production and less LDL cholesterol production
Polyunsaturated Fats	Some fish; corn, sesame, soybean, and safflower oils	Similar to monounsaturated fats
Omega-3 Fatty Acids	Fish (tuna, salmon, sardines, bluefish, trout)	Reduce the risk of clotting by thinning the blood; may protect against hardening of arteries
Trans fats	Shortening, stick margarine, baked goods	Promote production of harmful LDL cholesterol
Triglycerides	Any food that contains fat	Not fully broken down by the liver, they have effects similar to those of saturated fats

5 grams of saturated fat and trans fatty acids combined. The soft margarines in tubs and tubes have much less because trans fats are formed when the liquid oils used to make margarine are hardened. The harder the margarine, the more trans fatty acids it contains.[15]

In a recent study at the University of Texas Southwestern Medical Center, 46 families followed two diet regimens—one with butter, the other with tub margarine—for five weeks. Compared to the butter diet, the margarine diet lowered the adults' low-density lipoprotein (LDL), the bad form of cholesterol, by 11 percent. The children's LDL levels fell by 9 percent.[16] But switching from butter or stick margarine to a tub variety is not a cure-all for high cholesterol. In the study, LDL changes varied from family to family, suggesting that genetics also plays a role. Overweight individuals also had a smaller response to the diet than those of normal weight.[17]

When looking for a margarine, try to choose one in which the trans fatty acids and the saturated fat content are the lowest. Trans-free margarines are available, but even so, check labels to make sure you're not getting more than 2 grams of saturated fat per serving. If you like the taste of butter, choose a tub margarine that contains whey protein for a close-to-the-real-thing buttery taste.

Some margarines are being marketed as medicines. Benecol, for instance, is a canola-oil based, margarine-like spread that contains phytochemicals from pine trees, soy, corn, and wheat known to inhibit the body's ability to absorb cholesterol—be it cholesterol in foods or cholesterol produced by the liver.[18] Three servings a day may lower LDL by as much as 10 percent.[19]

 How Much Fat Is Okay?

The current Dietary Guidelines advise Americans to limit total fat consumption to 30 percent or less of total caloric intake and saturated fat to less than 10 percent of total caloric intake. Americans haven't quite reached that goal, but they've gotten closer. In the last three decades, they've reduced the percentage of calories from total fat consumption from about 45 percent to about 34 percent.

Some health experts, such as Dean Ornish, M.D., who first demonstrated that a combination of a very-low-fat diet, exercise, and psychological change could reverse atherosclerotic plaque, advocate cutting dietary fat down to 10 percent of daily calories.[20] However, their success with reversing atherosclerosis may have depended on maintaining an integrated program combining exercise and dietary and behavioral change, rather than on eating more low-fat foods.

Others have questioned the benefits of a drastic reduction in dietary fats. Although high-fat diets have long been linked with various cancers, this association does not seem valid for breast cancer. An analysis of the diets of almost 90,000 women participating in the Nurses' Health Study over a 14-year period found that those eating diets with 20 percent fat or less were just as likely to get breast cancer as those eating diets with 30 to 35 percent fat. It made no difference whether the dietary fat was saturated, polyunsaturated, or monounsaturated or animal or vegetable in origin.[21]

High-fat diets are associated with a higher risk of heart disease, but it is not clear whether an extreme reduction in dietary fat invariably lowers this risk. At least in some individuals, a low-fat diet can lead to an increase in a particularly

▼ Table 5-4   Percentage of Fat Calories in Foods

Type of Food	Less Than 15% of Calories from Fat	15%–30% of Calories from Fat	30%–50% of Calories from Fat	More Than 50% of Calories from Fat
Fruits and Vegetables	Fruits, plain vegetables, juices, pickles, sauerkraut		French fries, hash browns	Avocados, coconuts, olives
Bread and Cereals	Grains and flours, most breads, most cereals, corn tortillas, pita, matzoh, bagels, noodles, and pasta	Corn bread, flour tortillas, oatmeal, soft rolls and buns, wheat germ	Breakfast bars, biscuits and muffins, granola, pancakes and waffles, donuts, taco shells, pastries, croissants	
Dairy Products	Nonfat milk, dry curd cottage cheese, nonfat cottage cheese, nonfat yogurt	Buttermilk, low-fat yogurt, 1% milk, low-fat cottage cheese	Whole milk, 2% milk, creamed cottage cheese	Butter, cream, sour cream, half & half, most cheeses (including part-skim and lite cheeses)
Meats		Beef round; veal loin, round, and shoulder; pork tenderloin	Beef and veal, lamb, fresh and picnic hams	All ground beef, spareribs, cold cuts, beef, hot dogs, pastrami
Poultry	Egg whites	Chicken and turkey (light meat without skin)	Chicken and turkey (light meat with skin, dark meat without skin), duck and goose (without skin)	Chicken/turkey (dark meat with skin), chicken-turkey hot dogs and bologna, egg yolks, whole eggs
Seafood	Clams, cod, crab, crawfish, flounder, haddock, lobster, perch, sole, scallops, shrimp, tuna (in water)	Bass and sea bass, halibut, mussels, oysters, tuna (fresh)	Anchovies, catfish, salmon, sturgeon, trout, tuna (in oil, drained)	Herring, mackerel, sardines
Beans and Nuts	Dried beans and peas, chestnuts, water chestnuts		Soybeans	Tofu, most nuts and seeds, peanut butter
Fats and Oils	Oil-free and some lite salad dressings			Butter, margarine, all mayonnaise (including reduced-calorie), most salad dressings, all oils
Soups	Bouillons, broths, consommé	Most soups	Cream soups, bean soups, "just add water" noodle soups	Cheddar cheese soup, New England clam chowder
Desserts	Angel food cake, gelatin, some fat-free cakes	Pudding, tapioca	Most cakes, most pies	
Frozen Desserts	Sherbet, low-fat frozen yogurt, sorbet, fruit ices	Ice milk	Frozen yogurt	All ice cream
Snack Foods	Popcorn (air popped), pretzels, rye crackers, rice cakes, fig bars, raisin biscuit cookies, marshmallows, most hard candy, fruit rolls	Lite microwave popcorn, Scandinavian "crisps," plain crackers, caramels, fudge, gingersnaps, graham crackers	Snack crackers, popcorn (popped in oil), cookies, candy bars, granola bars	Most microwave popcorn, corn and potato chips, chocolate, buttery crackers

Sources: American Heart Association/USDA.

▼ Table 5-5	Butter vs. Margarine			
Product (per Tablespoon)	Total Fat (grams)	Saturated Fat (grams)	Trans Fatty Acids (grams)	Fatty Acids (grams)
Butter	10.8	7.2	0.3	7.5
Margarine, stick (82% fat)	11.4	2.3	2.4	4.7
Margarine, tub (80% fat)	11.2	1.9	1.1	3.0
Margarine, stick (68% fat)	9.5	1.6	1.8	3.4
Margarine, tub (40% fat)	5.6	1.1	0.6	1.7

Sources: U.S. Food and Drug Administration and the U.S. Department of Agriculture.

dangerous form of heart-harming LDL-cholesterol. A one-year study of men with high cholesterol examined the cholesterol-lowering effects of diets that ranged from 30 to 18 percent fat. The men who aggressively restricted their dietary fat intake incurred two worrisome changes: higher triglycerides, fats that circulate in the bloodstream and provide energy, and a reduction of "good" high-density-lipoprotein (HDL) cholesterol. People who eat a high-carbohydrate diet—including excessive hard candies, fat-free cookies, and fat-free frozen yogurt—often have high triglyceride levels even if their fat intake is low.

???? Why Should I Eat Fish?

Polyunsaturated fats known as omega-3 fatty acids make more molecules such as the prostaglandins that have proven beneficial for heart health. Because they are rich in omega-3 fatty acids, fish oils improve healthy blood lipids (fats), prevent blood clots, ward off age-related macular degeneration, and may lower blood pressure, especially in people with hypertension or atherosclerosis.

The American Heart Association recommends two 3-ounce servings of fatty fish, such as salmon, tuna, and sardines, every week. However, nutritionists do not recommend the use of fish oil supplements, which carry risks of their own: They can increase bleeding time, interfere with wound healing, worsen diabetes, and impair immune function. Since they are made from fish skins and livers, the supplements also may contain environmental contaminants.

Vitamins and Minerals

Vitamins, which help put proteins, fats, and carbohydrates to use, are essential to regulating growth, maintaining tissue, and releasing energy from foods. Together with the enzymes in the body, they help produce the right chemical reactions at the right times. They're also involved in the manufacture of blood cells, hormones, and other compounds.

The body produces some vitamins, such as vitamin D, which is manufactured in the skin after exposure to sunlight. Other vitamins must be ingested. Vitamins A, D, E, and K are fat-soluble; they are absorbed through the intestinal membranes and stored in the body. The B vitamins and vitamin C are water-soluble; they are absorbed directly into the blood and then used up or washed out of the body in urine and sweat. They must be replaced daily. Table 5-6 summarizes key information about vitamins.

Carbon, oxygen, hydrogen, and nitrogen make up 96 percent of our body weight. The other 4 percent consists of **minerals** that help build bones and teeth, aid in muscle function, and help our nervous system transmit messages. Every day we need about a tenth of a gram (100 milligrams) or more of the major minerals: sodium, potassium, chloride, calcium, phosphorus, and magnesium. We also need about a hundredth of a gram (10 milligrams) or less of each of the trace minerals: iron (although premenopausal women need more), zinc, selenium, molybdenum, iodine, copper, manganese, fluoride, and chromium. See Table 5-7 on page 155 for a summary of mineral information.

How Antioxidants Work

Antioxidants are substances that prevent the harmful effects caused by oxidation within the body. They include vitamins C, E, and beta-carotene (a form of vitamin A) as well as compounds like carotenoids and flavonoids. All share a common enemy: renegade oxygen cells called free radicals released by normal metabolism, as well as by pollution, smoking, radiation, and stress.

▼ Table 5-6   Key Information about Vitamins

Vitamin	Significant Sources	Chief Functions	Signs of Severe, Prolonged Deficiency	Signs of Extreme Excess
Fat-Soluble				
Vitamin A	Fortified milk, cheese, cream, butter, fortified margarine, eggs, liver; spinach and other dark, leafy greens, broccoli, deep orange fruits (apricots, cantaloupes) and vegetables (squash, carrots, sweet potatoes, pumpkins)	Antioxidant, needed for vision, health of cornea, epithelial cells, mucous membranes, skin health, bone and tooth growth, hormone synthesis and regulation, immunity	Anemia, painful joints, cracks in teeth, tendency toward tooth decay, diarrhea, depression, frequent infections, night blindness, keratinization, corneal degeneration, rashes, kidney stones	Nosebleeds, bone pain, growth retardation, headaches, abdominal cramps and pain, nausea, vomiting, diarrhea, weight loss, overreactive immune system, blurred vision, pain in calves, fatigue, irritability, loss of appetite, dry skin, rashes, loss of hair, cessation of menstruation
Vitamin D	Fortified milk or margarine, eggs, liver, sardines; exposure to sunlight	Promotes calcium and phosphorus absorption	Abnormal growth, misshapen bones (bowing of legs), soft bones, joint pain, malformed teeth	Raised blood calcium, excessive thirst, headaches, irritability, loss of appetite, weakness, nausea, kidney stones, stones in arteries, mental and physical retardation
Vitamin E	Margarine, salad dressings, shortenings, green and leafy vegetables, wheat germ, whole-grain products, nuts, seeds	Antioxidant, needed for stabilization of cell membranes, regulation of oxidation reactions	Red blood cell breakage, anemia, muscle degeneration, weakness, difficulty walking, leg cramps, fibrocystic breast disease	Augments the effects of anticlotting medication; general discomfort
Vitamin K	Liver, green leafy vegetables, cabbage-type vegetables, milk	Needed for synthesis of blood-clotting proteins and a blood protein that regulates blood calcium	Hemorrhage	Interference with anticlotting medication; jaundice
Water-Soluble				
Vitamin B$_6$	Green and leafy vegetables, meats, fish, poultry, shellfish, legumes, fruits, whole grains	Part of a coenzyme needed for amino acid and fatty acid metabolism, helps make red blood cells	Anemia, smooth tongue, abnormal brain wave pattern, irritability, muscle twitching, convulsions	Depression, fatigue, impaired memory, irritability, headaches, numbness, damage to nerves, difficulty walking, loss of reflexes, weakness, restlessness
Vitamin B$_{12}$	Animal products (meat, fish, poultry, milk, cheese, eggs)	Part of a coenzyme used in new cell synthesis, helps maintain nerve cells	Anemia, smooth tongue, fatigue, nervous system degeneration progressing to paralysis, hypersensitivity	None reported

(continued on next page)

▼ **Table 5-6   Key Information about Vitamins—continued**

Vitamin	Significant Sources	Chief Functions	Signs of Severe, Prolonged Deficiency	Signs of Extreme Excess
Vitamin C	Citrus fruits, cabbage-type vegetables, dark green vegetables, cantaloupe, strawberries, peppers, lettuce, tomatoes, potatoes, papayas, mangoes	Antioxidant, collagen synthesis (strengthens blood vessel walls, forms scar tissue, matrix for bone growth), amino acid metabolism, strengthens resistance to infection, aids iron absorption	Anemia, pinpoint hemorrhages, frequent infections, bleeding gums, loosened teeth, muscle degeneration and pain, hysteria, depression, bone fragility, joint pain, rough skin, blotchy bruises, failure of wounds to heal	Nausea, abdominal cramps, diarrhea, excessive urination, headache, fatigue, insomnia, rashes, aggravation of gout symptoms; deficiency symptoms may appear at first on withdrawal of high doses
Thiamin	Pork, ham, bacon, liver, whole grains, legumes, nuts; occurs in all nutritious foods in moderate amounts	Part of a coenzyme needed for energy metabolism, normal appetite function, and nervous system	Edema, enlarged heart, abnormal heart rhythms, heart failure, nervous/muscular system degeneration, wasting, weakness, pain, low morale, difficulty walking, loss of reflexes, mental confusion, paralysis	None reported
Riboflavin	Milk, yogurt, cottage cheese, meat, leafy green vegetables, whole-grain or enriched breads and cereals	Part of a coenzyme needed for energy metabolism, supports normal vision and skin health	Cracks at corner of mouth, magenta tongue, hypersensitivity to light, reddening of cornea, skin rash	None reported
Niacin	Milk, eggs, meat, poultry, fish, whole-grain and enriched breads and cereals, nuts, and all protein-containing foods	Part of a coenzyme needed for energy metabolism, supports skin health, nervous system, and digestive system	Diarrhea, black smooth tongue, irritability, loss of appetite, weakness, dizziness, mental confusion, flaky skin rash on areas exposed to sun	Diarrhea, heartburn, nausea, ulcer irritation, vomiting, fainting, dizziness, painful flush and rash, sweating, abnormal liver function, low blood pressure
Folate	Leafy green vegetables, legumes, seeds, liver, enriched bread, cereal, pasta, and grains	Part of a coenzyme needed for new cell synthesis	Anemia, heartburn, diarrhea, constipation, frequent infections, smooth red tongue, depression, mental confusion, fainting	Masks vitamin B_{12} deficiency
Panothenic acid	Widespread in foods	Part of a coenzyme used in energy metabolism	Vomiting, intestinal distress, insomnia, fatigue	Water retention (rare)
Biotin	Widespread in foods	Used in energy metabolism, fat synthesis, amino acid metabolism, and glycogen synthesis	Abnormal heart action, loss of appetite, nausea, depression, muscle pain, weakness, fatigue, drying, rash, loss of hair	None reported

Source: Adapted from Sizer, Frances, and Eleanor Whitney. *Nutrition: Concepts and Controversies,* 8th ed. Belmont, CA: Wadsworth, 2000.

▼ Table 5-7 **Key Information about Essential Minerals**

Mineral	Significant Sources	Chief Functions	Signs of Severe, Prolonged Deficiency	Signs of Extreme Excess
Major Minerals				
Sodium	Foods processed with salt, cured foods (corned beef, ham, bacon, pickles, sauerkraut), table and sea salt, bread, milk, cheese, salad dressing	Needed to maintain acid-base balance in body fluids, helps regulate water in blood and body tissues, needed for muscle and nerve activity	Weakness, apathy, poor appetite, muscle cramps, headache, swelling	High blood pressure, kidney disease, heart problems
Potassium	Plant foods (potatoes, squash, lima beans, tomatoes, bananas, oranges, avocados), meats, milk and milk products, coffee	Needed to maintain acid-base balance in body fluids, helps regulate water in blood and body tissues, needed for muscle and nerve activity	Weakness, irritability, mental confusion, irregular heartbeat, paralysis	Irregular heartbeat, heart attack
Chloride	Foods processed with salt, cured foods (corned beef, ham, bacon, pickles, sauerkraut), table and sea salt, bread, milk, cheese, salad dressing	Aids in digestion, needed to maintain acid-base balance in body fluids, helps regulate water in the body	Muscle cramps, apathy, poor appetite, long-term mental retardation in infants	Vomiting
Calcium	Milk and milk products, broccoli, dried beans	Component of bones and teeth, needed for muscle and nerve activity, blood clotting	Weak bones, rickets, stunted growth in children, convulsions, muscle spasms, osteoporosis	Drowsiness, calcium deposits in kidneys, liver, and other tissues, suppression of bone remodeling, decreased zinc absorption
Phosphorus	Milk and milk products, meats, seeds, nuts	Component of bones and teeth, energy formation, needed to maintain the right acid-base balance of body fluids	Loss of appetite, nausea, vomiting, weakness, confusion, loss of calcium from bones	Loss of calcium from bones, muscle spasms
Magnesium	Plant foods (dried beans, tofu, peanuts, potatoes, green vegetables)	Component of bones and teeth, nerve activity, energy and protein formation	Stunted growth in children, weakness, muscle spasms, personality changes	Diarrhea, dehydration, impaired nerve activity
Trace Minerals				
Iron	Liver, beef, pork, dried beans, iron-fortified cereals, prunes, apricots, raisins, spinach, bread, pasta	Aids in transport of oxygen, component of myoglobin, energy formation	Anemia, weakness, fatigue, pale appearance, reduced attention span, resistance to infection, developmental delays in children	"Iron poisoning," vomiting, abdominal pain, blue coloration of skin, shock, heart failure, diabetes, decreased zinc absorption
Zinc	Meats, grains, nuts, milk and milk products, cereals, bread	Protein reproduction, component of insulin	Growth failure, delayed sexual maturation, slow wound healing, loss of taste and appetite; in pregnant women, low-birth-weight infants and preterm delivery	Nausea, vomiting, weakness, fatigue, susceptibility to infection, copper deficiency, metallic taste in mouth

(continued on next page)

▼ Table 5-7 **Key Information about Essential Minerals—continued**

Mineral	Significant Sources	Chief Functions	Signs of Severe, Prolonged Deficiency	Signs of Extreme Excess
Selenium	Meats and seafood, eggs, grains	Acts as an antioxidant in conjunction with vitamin E	Anemia, muscle pain and tenderness, Keshar disease, heart failure	Hair and fingernail loss, weakness, liver damage, irritability, "garlic" or "metallic" breath
Molybdenum	Dried beans, grains, dark green vegetables, liver, milk and milk products	Aids in oxygen transfer from one molecule to another	Rapid heartbeat and breathing, nausea, vomiting, coma	Loss of copper from the body, joint pain, growth failure, anemia, gout
Iodine	Iodized salt, milk and milk products, seaweed, seafood, bread	Component of thyroid hormones that help regulate energy prduction and growth	Goiter, cretinism in newborns (mental retardation, hearing loss, growth failure)	Pimples, goiter, decreased thyroid function
Copper	Bread, potatoes, grains, dried beans, nuts and seeds, seafood, cereals	Component of enzymes involved in the body's utilization of iron and oxygen; functions in growth, immunity, cholesterol, and glucose utilization; brain development	Anemia, seizures, nerve and bone abnormalities in children, growth retardation	Wilson's disease (excessive accumulation of copper in the liver and kidneys); vomiting, diarrhea, tremors, liver disease
Manganese	Whole grains, coffee, tea, dried beans, nuts	Formation of body fat and bone	Weight loss, rash, nausea and vomiting	Infertility in men, disruptions in the nervous system, muscle spasms
Fluoride	Fluoridated water, foods, and beverages; tea; shrimp; crab	Component of bones and teeth (enamel)	Tooth decay and other dental diseases	Fluorosis, brittle bones, mottled teeth, nerve abnormalities
Chromium	Whole grains, liver, meat, beer, wine	Glucose utilization	Poor blood glucose control, weight loss	Kidney and skin damage

Source: Adapted from Brown, Judith E. *Nutrition Now,* 3rd ed. Belmont, CA: Wadsworth, 2002.

Like tiny thugs, free radicals constantly roam through the body and attack cells in the brain, heart, bloodstream, and immune system. Antioxidants rush to the rescue, limit damage, and help repair any harm that's been done. Like bouncers in a nightclub, they wrap up the troublemakers and carry them away.

In the cardiovascular system, free radicals combine with cholesterol and dangerous LDL to damage the inner lining of blood vessels. In clinical studies, vitamin E has generally lowered the risk of heart attacks and strokes by 40 to 60 percent.

Other antioxidants, particularly supplements of vitamin C and beta-carotene, have not proved as helpful in protecting the heart. In epidemiological studies, however, individuals eating lots of dark green, yellow, and orange fruits and vegetables (good sources of vitamin C and beta-carotene) consistently have lower rates of coronary disease.

Diets high in antioxidant-rich fruits and vegetables have been linked with lower rates of esophageal, lung, colon, and stomach cancer. Nevertheless, scientific studies

STRATEGIES FOR CHANGE

Getting Enough Antioxidants

What can you do to ensure that you get the antioxidants you need? Here are some guidelines:

✔ Eat a rainbow. The highest concentrations of antioxidants are found in the most deeply or brightly colored vegetables and fruits (spinach, carrots, red bell peppers, tomatoes).

✔ Purchase "grab and eat" fruits and vegetables like apples, plums, pears, and carrots. Keep dried fruit in your briefcase or car.

✔ Take a multivitamin and multimineral supplement. Think of it as insurance for the days when you don't eat the way you should.

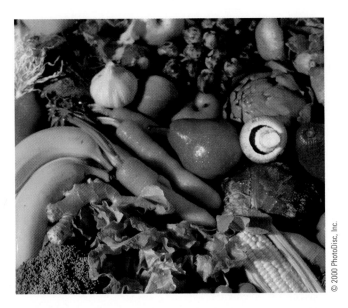

▲ Antioxidants are found in vegetables and fruit. By eating an orange at breakfast and half a carrot for lunch, you will have all the antioxidants you need for the day.

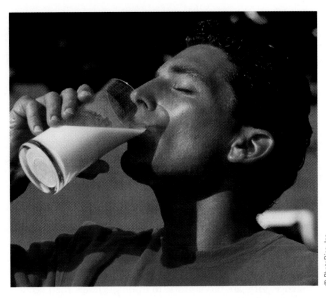

▲ Calcium-rich foods such as milk can help prevent bone loss and osteoporosis.

have not proved conclusively that any specific antioxidant, particularly in supplement form, can prevent cancer. In studies of beta-carotene, this carotenoid did not reduce overall cancer rates or mortality. In two studies of smokers, beta-carotene was actually associated with increased mortality from lung cancer.

In theory, though, antioxidants may slow the cumulative effect of free radicals in diseases associated with age, including memory impairment, cataracts, and arthritis. In laboratory and animal studies, vitamin E has shown particular promise in slowing neurological aging and improving cognitive function. Although there is no evidence that vitamin E can prevent Alzheimer's disease, high doses have modestly slowed progression of this form of dementia. Certain antioxidants, such as vitamin E, vitamin C, and beta-carotene, may also provide protection against age-related macular degeneration.[22]

Folic Acid

Folate is the generic term used to refer to various chemical forms of a water-soluble B vitamin that can be obtained from a diet high in vegetables and citrus fruit. **Folic acid** is the form used in vitamin supplements and fortified foods. Food manufacturers add folic acid to foods, primarily because insufficient levels increase the risk of neural tube defects (abnormalities of the brain and spinal cord), such as spina bifida, in which a piece of the spinal cord protrudes from the spinal column.[23] Folic acid also reduces blood levels of homocysteine, a chemical associated with increased risk of cardiovascular disease,[24] and reduces the excess risk of breast cancer associated with alcohol consumption.

Calcium

Calcium, the most abundant mineral in the body, builds strong bone tissue throughout life and plays a vital role in heart and brain functioning. Pregnant or nursing women need more calcium to meet the additional needs of their babies' bodies. (See The X & Y Files: "Do Men and Women Have Different Nutritional Needs?") Calcium may also help control high blood pressure and prevent colon cancer in adults.

Adequate calcium intake during childhood, adolescence, and young adulthood is crucial to prevent **osteoporosis,** the bone-weakening disease that strikes one of every four women over the age of 60.[25] National health organizations are promoting greater calcium consumption among college students, particularly women, to increase bone density and safeguard against osteoporosis.[26]

 In a study of college athletes, the most common food sources of calcium for both European-American and African-American students were mixed dishes and dairy products. There were no racial differences in calcium consumption levels, but male athletes consumed significantly more calcium than females.[27]

In both men and women, bone mass peaks between the ages of 25 and 35. Over the next 10 to 15 years, bone mass remains fairly stable. At about age 40, bone loss equivalent to 0.3 to 0.5 percent per year begins in both men and women. Women may experience greater bone loss, at a rate of 3 to 5 percent, at the time of menopause. This decline continues for approximately five to seven years and is the primary factor leading to postmenopausal osteoporosis.

The X & Y Files

Do Men and Women Have Different Nutritional Needs?

Men and women do not need to eat different foods, but their nutritional needs are different. Because most men are bigger and taller than most women, they consume more calories. Eating more means it's easier for them to get the nutrients they need, even though many don't make the wisest food choices.

Women, particularly those who restrict their caloric intake or are chronically dieting, are more likely to develop specific deficiencies. Calcium is one example. Women drink less milk than men, and many do not consume the recommended 800 to 1,200 milligrams of calcium daily. This deficiency increases the risk of bone-weakening osteoporosis.

Many women also get too little iron. Even in adolescence, girls are more prone to iron deficiency than boys; some suffer memory and learning impairments as a result. In adult women, menstrual blood loss and poor eating habits can lead to low iron stores, which puts them at risk for anemia. According to U.S. Department of Agriculture research, most women consume only 60 percent of the recommended 15 milligrams of iron per day. (The recommendation for men is 10 milligrams.) Regular blood tests can monitor a woman's iron status.

Here are some gender-specific strategies for better nutrition:

- Men should cut back on fat and meat in their diets—two things they tend to get too much of.
- Women should increase their iron intake by eating meat (iron from animal sources is absorbed better than that from vegetable sources) or a combination of meat and vegetable iron sources together (for example, a meat and bean burrito). Those low in iron should consult a physician. Because large doses of iron can be toxic, iron supplements should be taken only with medical supervision.
- Women should consume more calcium-rich foods, including low-fat and nonfat dairy products, leafy greens, and tofu. Women who cannot get adequate amounts of calcium from their daily diet should take calcium supplements.
- Women who could become pregnant should take a multivitamin with 400 micrograms of folic acid, which helps prevent neural tube defects such as spina bifida. Folic acid is also useful to men because it may cut the risk of heart disease, stroke, and colon cancer.
- Both genders should increase their fruit and vegetable intake to ensure that they are getting adequate amounts of vitamins and fiber in their daily diet.

STRATEGIES FOR CHANGE

Building Stronger Bones

✔ Make calcium-rich foods part of your daily diet. These include dairy products, leafy green vegetables, canned fish, and tofu. Also look for products fortified with calcium and vitamin D, which aids in calcium absorption.

✔ Avoid cigarette smoking, which has been linked with bone loss.

✔ Drink alcohol only in moderation. Prolonged or heavy use of alcohol may decrease bone metabolism.

✔ Be wary of high-protein diets. Excess protein intake may increase the rate of calcium loss from the body.

✔ Do weight-bearing exercises. Activities such as walking, running, doing push-ups and sit-ups, and lifting weights all contribute to the development and maintenance of bone mass.

The higher an individual's peak bone mass, the longer it takes for age- and menopause-related bone losses to increase the risk of fractures. Osteoporosis is less common in groups with higher peak bone mass—men versus women, blacks versus whites. Calcium intake is linked with greater bone mass at all ages, and calcium supplements can prevent or slow bone loss.

Calcium alone cannot protect the bones of most postmenopausal women, however. Other bone-saving treatments include hormone replacement therapy, or HRT; raloxifene (Evista), a "designer" estrogen that targets the bones but does not stimulate estrogen receptors in the breast; the bisphosphonates alendronate (Fosamax) and risedronate; and calcitonin-salmon, a synthetic version of a natural hormone administered as a nasal spray.

Iron

Iron is an essential ingredient of **hemoglobin,** the protein that makes the blood red and carries oxygen to all our tissues. Because oxygen is needed to convert food into energy, too little iron—and thus too little hemoglobin—can trigger an internal energy crisis. Getting enough iron can be a big problem for women, whose iron stores are drained by menstruation, pregnancy, and nursing. Half of all women of childbearing age get less than the recommended 15 milligrams of iron, and 5 percent suffer from iron-deficiency anemia.

The symptoms of iron deficiency are sensitivity to cold, chronic fatigue, edginess, depression, sleeplessness, and susceptibility to colds and infections. To boost your iron, see the Strategies for Change. Don't take supplements unless you've had a blood test that indicates you should. Excess iron can cause severe constipation and other complications.

Phytochemicals and Other Substances in Food

Phytochemicals, compounds that exist naturally in plants, serve many functions, including helping a plant protect itself from bacteria and disease. Some phytochemicals such as solanine, an insect-repelling chemical found in the leaves and stalks of potato plants, are natural toxins, but many are beneficial to humans. Phytochemicals are associated with a reduced risk of heart disease, certain cancers, age-related macular degeneration, adult-onset diabetes, stroke, and other diseases. Research has yet to show a cause-and-effect relationship between consumption of phytochemicals and prevention of a specific disease, however.

Some phytochemicals act as antioxidants and limit and repair damage caused by free radicals. Others act as hormonelike substances to prevent cancer or block the enzymes that promote the development of cancer and other diseases. Flavonoids, found in apples, strawberries, grapes, onions, green and black tea, and red wine, may decrease atherosclerotic plaque and DNA damage related to cancer developments. Carotenoids (beta-carotene, lutein, zeaxanthin, cryptoxanthin, and lycopene) protect the eye from harmful oxidation reactions. Lignans, found in flaxseed, seaweed,

soybeans, bran, and dried beans, are "phytoestrogens" that interfere with the action of the sex hormone estrogen and may help prevent hormone-related cancers, slow the growth of cancer cells, and lower the risk for heart disease.

Phytochemicals appear to work together to enhance health and prevent disease. Studies of supplements of individual phytochemicals, such as beta-carotene, have proved disappointing. There is no solid evidence that specific phytochemicals extracted from foods can benefit health.

Eating for Good Health

No one food can provide all the nutrients we need. To make sure you consume a healthful variety, the federal Dietary Guidelines suggest that you "let the Pyramid guide your food choices." The USDA's Food Guide Pyramid (see Figure 5-2), adopted in 1992, replaced the traditional basic four food groups—meats, milk products, fruits and vegetables, breads and cereals—with five categories. These categories are not considered nutritional equals. For the sake of good health, you need some food from all the groups every day, but in different amounts. (See Self-Survey: "Rate Your Diet.")

"The idea of the pyramid is to get people to eat more of the foods at its base (grains, fruits, and vegetables) and fewer of those toward the top (meat, milk products, sugars, and fats)," says Ann Shaw, a nutritionist with the USDA's Agriculture Research Service.[28] Foods in one group cannot substitute for those in another. Although the new guide doesn't ban any foods from plates or palates, the pyramid clearly advises less of some favorites, including meat. "Your maximum daily protein intake should be 5 to 7 ounces, with no more than half of that coming from red meat," says Shaw. "We're trying to get people to eat fewer servings of meat and to eat smaller ones—the size of a deck of cards, not half the dinner plate."

Although following the pyramid may seem complicated at first, it doesn't have to be. Simple changes in what you eat can transform a lopsided eating plan into a well-balanced one.

Following the Food Guide Pyramid

About one-third of the U.S. population eats at least some food from all the Food Guide Pyramid food groups, but only 1 to 3 percent eat the recommended number of servings from all the food groups on a given day. Fruits are the foods Americans generally skimp on most. Adults do best in eating the recommended amounts of vegetables and meat; children and teens, of dairy products. People of all ages tend not to eat enough dark green and deep yellow vegetables and whole grains, while loading up on fat and added sugars.[29]

STRATEGIES FOR CHANGE

Getting More Iron in Your Diet

✔ Eat vegetables and starches high in iron: whole-grain cereals (such as bran flakes), broccoli, soybeans, and red kidney beans.

✔ To increase the amount of iron your body absorbs from these plant foods, eat foods high in vitamin C at the same meal.

✔ Eat iron-rich lean red meats two or three times a week. Oysters are also a good iron source.

✔ Don't drink tea with your meal, because the tannin in it may interfere with iron absorption.

Bread, Cereal, Rice, and Pasta Group (Grains Group)—whole grain and refined
· 1 slice of bread
· About 1 cup of ready-to-eat cereal
· 1/2 cup of cooked cereal, rice, or pasta

Vegetable Group
· 1 cup of raw leafy vegetables
· 1/2 cup of other vegetables—cooked or raw
· 3/4 cup of vegetable juice

Fruit Group
· 1 medium apple, banana, orange, pear
· 1/2 cup of chopped, cooked, or canned fruit
· 3/4 cup of fruit juice

Milk, Yogurt, and Cheese Group (Milk Group)[1]
· 1 cup of milk[2] or yogurt[2]
· 1 1/2 ounces of a natural cheese[2] (such as Cheddar)
· 2 ounces of processed cheese[2] (such as American)

Meat, Poultry, Fish, Dry Beans, Eggs, and Nuts Group (Meat and Beans Group)
· 2–3 ounces of cooked lean meat, poultry, or fish
· 1/2 cup of cooked dry beans[3] or 1/2 cup of tofu counts as 1 ounce of lean meat
· 2 1/2-ounce soyburger or 1 egg counts as 1 ounce of lean meat
· 2 tablespoons of peanut butter or 1/3 cup of nuts counts as 1 ounce of meat

Fats, Oils & Sweets
USE SPARINGLY

Milk, Yogurt &
Cheese Group
2–3 SERVINGS

Vegetable Group
3–5 SERVINGS

■ Fat (naturally occurring and added)
■ Sugars (added)
These symbols show fat and added sugars in foods

Meat, Poultry, Fish, Dry Beans, Eggs, & Nuts Group
2–3 SERVINGS

Fruit Group
2–4 SERVINGS

Bread, Cereal, Rice, & Pasta Group
6–11 SERVINGS

NOTE: Many of the serving sizes given above are smaller than those on the Nutritional Facts Label. For example, 1 serving of cooked cereal, rice, or pasta is 1 cup for the label but only 1/2 cup for the Pyramid.
[1] This includes lactose-free and lactose-reduced milk products. One cup of soy-based beverage with added calcium is an option for those who prefer a non-dairy source of calcium.
[2] Choose fat-free or reduced-fat dairy products most often.
[3] Dry beans, peas, and lentils can be counted as servings in either the meat and beans group or the vegetable group. As a vegetable, 1/2 cup of cooked, dry beans counts as 1 serving. As a meat substitute, 1 cup of cooked, dry beans counts as 1 serving (2 ounces of meat).

▲ **Figure 5-2** The USDA's Food Guide Pyramid.
This graphic demonstrates the daily food choices that make up a healthy diet. A healthy diet requires only modest amounts of meat, dairy products, and fats, and a larger number of servings of foods containing grains and cereals.

Source: Dietary Guidelines for Americans, 2000.

 College students fall short in following the Food Guide Pyramid (see Student Snapshot: "The Food Guide Pyramid Goes to College" on page 163). In one study, female undergraduates ate adequate servings of meat but failed to consume the minimum recommended number of servings for breads and grains, fruits and vegetables, and dairy products. Two-thirds exceeded the recommended levels of saturated fat.[30] In a study of 162 Mexican-American students at a university in the southern United States, the majority consumed far fewer fruits and vegetables than recommended; their daily average was 2.5 or fewer servings per day.[31]

Food Portions and Servings

Consumers often are confused by what a "serving" actually is, especially since many American restaurants have "super-sized" the amount of food they put on their customers' plates. The average bagel has doubled in size in the last ten to fifteen years.[32] A standard fast-food serving of french fries is larger in the United States than in the United Kingdom. Very often a "serving" at a restaurant, in a cafeteria, or at home is much larger than those referred to in the Food Guide Pyramid and on Nutrition Facts labels on packaged foods—and higher in calories.

 Most college students do not calculate portion sizes accurately.[33] One of the best ways to improve such estimates is by using three-dimensional food models. In a study of 380 undergraduates enrolled in an introductory nutrition course, students first estimated the amount of food in three dinners, each with varying portions of five foods (starchy food, cooked vegetables, salad, milk, and meat). After correcting their own estimates, students were asked to estimate portions sizes on a new display with different foods and amounts after one week, and then again after four weeks. Each day between these two tests, different food models were passed around in class. The accuracy of the students' estimates improved significantly afterward.[34]

A Food Guide Pyramid "serving" describes the total amount of foods recommended *daily* from each of the food groups. It does not describe the size of an individual portion. The size of the daily serving is determined by four criteria:

▶ The amount of foods from a food group typically reported in surveys as consumed on one eating occasion.

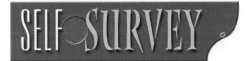

Rate Your Diet

Step 1

For a week, write down everything you eat and drink for meals and snacks. Include the approximate amount eaten (for example, ½ cup, 1 large, 12 oz. can, and so on).

	Mon	Tues	Wed	Thurs	Fri	Sat	Sun
Grains							
Vegetables							
Fruits							
Milk, yogurt, cheese							
Meat, poultry, dry beans, eggs, nuts							
Fats, oil, sweets, cheese							

Step 2: Are You Getting Enough Vegetables, Fruits, and Grains?

How often do you eat:	Seldom/never	1–2 times a week	3–5 times a week	Almost daily
At least three servings of vegetables a day?				
Starchy vegetables like potatoes, corn, or peas?				
Foods made with dry beans, lentils, or peas?				
Dark green or deep yellow vegetables (broccoli, spinach, collards, carrots, sweet potatoes, squash)?				
At least two servings of fruit a day?				
Citrus fruits and 100% fruit juices (oranges, grapefruit, tangerines)?				
Whole fruit with skin or seeds (berries, apples, pears)?				
At least six servings of breads, cereals, pasta, or rice a day?				

The best answer for each of the above is "almost daily." Use your food diary to see which foods you should be eating more often.

Step 3: Are You Getting Too Much Fat?

How often do you eat:	Seldom/never	1–2 times a week	3–5 times a week	Almost daily
Fried, deep-fat fried, or breaded food?				
Fatty meats, such as sausages, luncheon meat, fatty steaks or roasts?				
Whole milk, high-fat cheeses, ice cream?				
Pies, pastries, rich cakes?				
Rich cream sauces and gravies?				
Oily salad dressings or mayonnaise?				
Butter or margarine on vegetables, rolls, bread, or toast?				

Ideally, you should be eating these foods no more than one or two times a week. If your food diary indicates that you're eating them more frequently, your fat intake may well be too high.

(continued on next page)

SELF SURVEY

Step 4: Are You Getting Too Much Sodium?

How often do you eat:	Seldom/never	1–2 times a week	3–5 times a week	Almost daily
Cured or processed meats, such as ham, sausage, frankfurters, or luncheon meats?				
Canned vegetables or frozen vegetables with sauce?				
Frozen TV dinners, entrees, or canned or dehydrated soups?				
Salted nuts, popcorn, pretzels, corn chips, or potato chips?				
Seasoning mixes or sauces containing salt?				
Processed cheese?				
Salt added to table foods before you taste them?				

Ideally, you should be eating these high-sodium items no more than one or two times a week. If your food diary indicates that you're eating them more frequently, your sodium intake may well be too high.

Making Changes

How to Improve Your Diet

- Follow the Food Guide Pyramid in planning your daily meals.
- Read food nutritional labels carefully. Always check fat and sodium content.
- Rethink your meal choices. Have cereal or whole-grain toast instead of eggs for breakfast, salad in place of a burger for lunch, rice or pasta dishes rather than meats as a main course for dinner.
- Include a green or orange food at both lunch and dinner. Add extra vegetables to every recipe that calls for them.
- Serve fresh fruit or vegetable salsas instead of sauces for meat, poultry, or fish.
- Peel and slice fruit at home and take it along to work in a plastic bag for a snack.
- Rather than sipping a soda at your desk or having a sports drink after working out, choose water or 100% fruit juice instead.
- Use herbs and spices as seasonings for vegetables and meats instead of salt.

Source: Adapted from materials prepared by the USDA Human Nutrition Information Service.

- The amount of food that provides a comparable amount of key nutrients from that food group; for example, the amount of cheese that provides the same amount of calcium as a cup of milk.
- The amount of food recognized by most consumers or easily multiplied or divided to describe how much food is actually consumed.
- The amount traditionally used in previous food guides to describe servings.

A food label "serving" is a specific amount of food that contains the quantity of nutrients described on the Nutrition Facts label.

For many foods, the serving size in the Food Guide Pyramid and on the food label are the same (for exam-

ple, half a cup of canned fruit or one slice of bread), but in other cases they differ. The Pyramid describes serving units for each food group in ways that consumers find easy to remember (for example, a cup of leafy raw vegetables), while the food label is meant to help consumers compare nutrient information on a number of food products within a category (for example, frozen dinner entrees containing foods from several food groups).

A "portion" is the amount of a specific food that an individual eats at one time. Portions can be bigger or smaller than the servings on food labels or in the Food Guide Pyramid. According to research by the USDA, portion sizes tend to be bigger for men than women, but to decrease for both genders with age. Particularly if you are trying to balance your diet or control your weight, it's

Student Snapshot   The Food Guide Pyramid Goes to College

Comparison of Participating Students' Nutritional Intakes with Recommended Daily Servings

In a recent study of 103 undergraduates, students fell short. They reported eating adequate servings in only one category: meat, poultry, fish, dry beans, eggs, and nuts. They failed to consume the minimum recommended number of servings for breads and grains, fruits, vegetables, and dairy products but exceeded recommended levels of saturated fat and sodium.

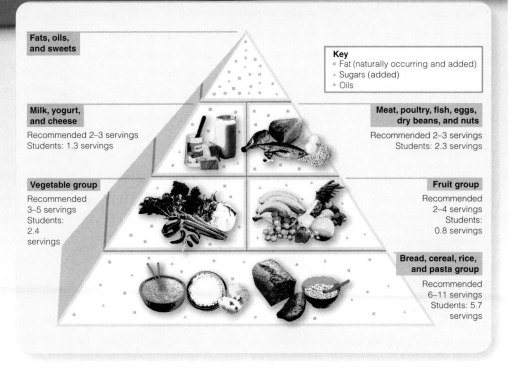

Fats, oils, and sweets

Key
- Fat (naturally occurring and added)
- Sugars (added)
- Oils

Milk, yogurt, and cheese
Recommended 2–3 servings
Students: 1.3 servings

Meat, poultry, fish, eggs, dry beans, and nuts
Recommended 2–3 servings
Students: 2.3 servings

Vegetable group
Recommended 3–5 servings
Students: 2.4 servings

Fruit group
Recommended 2–4 servings
Students: 0.8 servings

Bread, cereal, rice, and pasta group
Recommended 6–11 servings
Students: 5.7 servings

Source: Anding, Jenna, et al. "Dietary Intake, Body Mass Index, Exercise, and Alcohol: Are College Women Following the Dietary Guidelines for Americans?" *Journal of American College Health,* Vol. 49, January 2001, p. 167.

important to keep track of the size of your portions so that you do not exceed the recommended serving. For instance, a 3-ounce serving of meat is about the size of a pack of cards or a computer mouse. If you eat a larger amount, count it as more than one serving. (See Table 5-8.)

Breads, Cereals, Rice, and Pasta (6–11 servings a day)

These foods are the foundation of a healthy diet because they are a good source of complex carbohydrates. Both simple and complex carbohydrates (starches) have 4 calories per gram. Sugars provide little more than a quick spurt of energy, whereas complex carbohydrates are rich in vitamins, minerals, and other nutrients. Less than 25 percent of the daily calories in a typical American diet comes from complex carbohydrates; ideally, they should account for 50 to 60 percent.

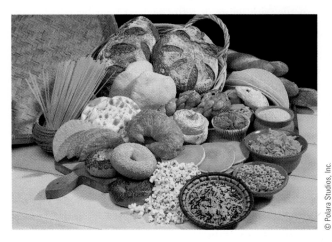

© Polara Studios, Inc.

▲ Eat 6 to 11 servings daily of bread, cereals, and other grain products.

▼ Table 5-8   How Many Servings Do You Need Each Day?

Food group	Children ages 2 to 6 years, women, some older adults (about 1,600 calories)	Older children, teen girls, active women, most men (about 2,200 calories)	Teen boys, active men (about 2,800 calories)
Bread, Cereal, Rice, and Pasta Group (Grains Group)—especially whole grain	6	9	11
Vegetable Group	3	4	5
Fruit Group	2	3	4
Milk, Yogurt, and Cheese Group (Milk Group)—preferably fat free or low fat	2 or 3*	2 or 3*	2 or 3*
Meat, Poultry, Fish, Dry Beans, Eggs, and Nuts Group (Meat and Beans Group)—preferably lean or low fat	2, for a total of 5 ounces	2, for a total of 6 ounces	3, for a total of 7 ounces

*The number of servings depends on your age. Older children and teenagers (ages 9 to 18 years) and adults over the age of 50 need 3 servings daily. Others need 2 servings daily. During pregnancy and lactation, the recommended number of milk group servings is the same as for nonpregnant women.

Source: Adapted from U.S. Department of Agriculture, Center for Nutrition Policy and Promotion. The Food Guide Pyramid, Home and Garden Bulletin Number 252, 1996.

A typical serving in this category might be one slice of bread, and 1 ounce of ready-to-eat cereal (or one-half cup of cooked cereal, rice, or pasta). Although many people think of these foods as fattening, it's actually what you put on them, such as butter on a roll or cream sauce on pasta, that adds extra calories.

Here are suggestions for getting more grains in your diet:

▶ Add brown rice or barley to soups.
▶ Check labels of rolls and bread, and choose those with at least 2 to 3 grams of fiber per slice. Grain products made with white or refined wheat flour have had most of their fiber-rich bran mechanically removed. However, if fiber has been added, some white breads may actually have more fiber than multigrain breads.
▶ Go for pasta power. Pasta has 210 calories per cooked cup and only 9 calories from fat. Like whole-grain breads, whole-grain pastas may provide more nutrients than those made with refined flour.

Vegetables (3–5 servings a day)

Naturally low in fat and high in fiber, vegetables provide crucial vitamins (such as A and C) and minerals (such as iron and magnesium). A serving in this category consists of one cup of raw leafy vegetables, one-half cup of other vegetables (either cooked or raw), three-quarters cup of

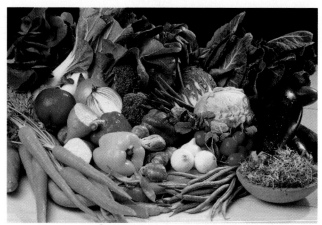

▲ Three to five servings daily of vegetables are recommended.

vegetable juice, or one potato or ear of corn. Since different types of vegetables provide different nutrients, it's best to eat a variety. Dark green vegetables are especially good sources of vitamins and minerals; certain greens (such as collards, kale, turnip, and mustard) provide calcium and iron. Winter squash, carrots, and the plant family that includes broccoli, cabbage, kohlrabi, and cauliflower (the **crucifers**) are high in fiber, rich in vitamins, and excellent sources of **indoles,** chemicals that help lower cancer risk.

Polara Studios, Inc.

Here are ways to increase your vegetable intake:

▶ Make or order sandwiches with extra tomatoes or other vegetable toppings.
▶ Add extra vegetables whenever you're preparing soups, sauces, and so on.
▶ If you can't find fresh vegetables, use frozen. They contain less salt than canned veggies.
▶ Use raw vegetables for dipping, instead of chips.

Fruit (2–4 servings a day)

Like whole grains and vegetables, fruits are excellent sources of vitamins, minerals, and fiber. Along with vegetables, fruits may protect against cancer; those who eat little produce have a cancer rate twice that of people who eat the most fruits and vegetables. A serving consists of a medium apple, banana, or orange; a half-cup of chopped, cooked, or canned fruit; or three-quarters of a cup of fruit juice.

Try the following suggestions to get more fruit into your daily diet:

▶ Carry a banana, apple, or package of dried fruit with you as a healthy snack.
▶ Eat fruit for dessert or a snack. Try poached pears, baked apples, or fresh berries.
▶ Start the day with a daily double: a glass of juice and a banana or other fruit on cereal.
▶ Add citrus fruits (such as slices of grapefruit, oranges, or apples) to green salads, rice, grains, and chicken, pork, or fish dishes.
▶ Squeeze fresh lemon or lime juice over seafood, fruit salads, or vegetable dishes.

Meat, Poultry, Fish, Dry Beans, Eggs, and Nuts (2–3 servings a day)

A serving in this category consists of 2 or 3 ounces of lean, cooked meat, fish, or poultry (roughly the size of an aver-

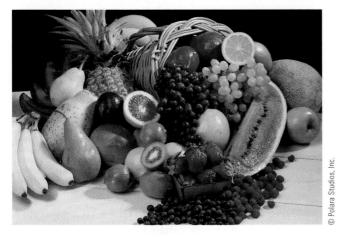

▲ Eat two to four servings daily of fruits to follow the Food Guide Pyramid.

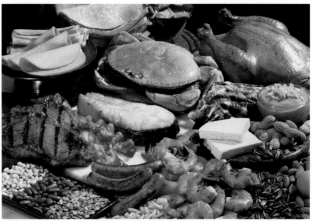

▲ Only two to three servings daily of meat, poultry, fish, protein alternatives are recommended.

age hamburger or the amount of meat on half a medium chicken breast). An egg or one-half cup of cooked dry beans can substitute for 1 ounce of lean meat. Thus, one day's total protein intake might include an egg at breakfast, a serving of beans or 2 ounces of sliced chicken in a sandwich at lunch, and 3 ounces of fish for dinner.

To pick the best protein, follow these recommendations:

▶ Choose the leanest meats, such as beef round or sirloin, pork tenderloin, or veal. Broil or roast instead of fry. Trim fat before cooking, which can lower the fat content of the meat you eat by more than 10 percent. Marinate low-fat cuts to increase tenderness.
▶ Cook stews, boiled meat, or soup stock ahead of time; refrigerate; and remove the hardened fat before using. Drain fat from ground beef after cooking.
▶ Watch out for processed chicken and turkey products; for example, bolognas and salamis made from turkey can contain 45 to 90 percent fat.
▶ Select small chickens when you shop: They're leaner than large ones. Broiler-fryers are lowest in fat, followed by roasters. Remove skin before eating poultry.
▶ Choose fish as a leaner alternative to meat. It's high in protein and packed with vitamins and minerals.
▶ Substitute bean-based dishes, such as chili or lentil stew, for meat entrees.

?? ?? Are Eggs Good or Bad for Me?

Eggs, once America's favorite breakfast food, fell out of favor several years ago. The reason: A single egg yolk contains about 200 mg of cholesterol, the maximum amount that federal guidelines say you should eat in a day. (Egg whites, rich in protein, have no cholesterol.)

However, some scientists came to the egg's defense. In an analysis of two long-term epidemiologic studies, they argued that eating up to one egg per day would not appreciably heighten the risk for heart disease or stroke. Eating eggs, they speculated, might actually increase "good" HDL cholesterol sufficiently to offset any elevation in "bad" LDL cholesterol.

Now eggs are under fire again. In a recent analysis of 17 cholesterol studies conducted over the last quarter century, Dutch researchers showed that cholesterol in the diet did increase harmful LDL levels far more than beneficial HDL. Using a standard equation that computes heart-disease risk for a given cholesterol level, they estimated that adding an egg a day to the diet would, on average, increase heart-attack risk by 2.1 percent. That isn't a big jump for most people but could be significant for individuals at high risk of heart disease.[35]

The bottom line: You don't have to ban eggs from the breakfast table, but limit how often you eat them—and avoid high-fat preparations like frying them in butter. If your diet is low in saturated fat, the kind found in meat and dairy products, the cholesterol in any eggs you eat will have less impact on your blood cholesterol levels than if you're eating a lot of high-fat foods.

Milk, Yogurt, and Cheese (2–3 servings a day)

Most milk products are high in calcium, riboflavin, protein, and vitamins A and B$_{12}$. The Food Guide Pyramid recommends two servings of milk, yogurt, or cheese for most adults and three for women who are pregnant or breast-feeding. In addition, teenagers and young adults up to age 24 should also get three servings of milk products a day. Dairy products, such as milk and yogurt, are the best calcium sources, but be sure you choose products that are low-fat, or preferably nonfat. A serving in this category consists of an 8-ounce cup of milk, one cup of plain yogurt, 1$^1/_2$ ounces of hard cheese, or 1 tablespoon of cheese spread. An 8-ounce glass of nonfat milk is a more nutritious choice than a tablespoon of a high-fat cheese spread.

A growing concern is the problem of lactose intolerance, or inability to digest milk products, which is particularly common in nonwhite minority groups. In individuals who do not produce adequate amounts of the intestinal enzyme lactase, milk products travel through the stomach undigested and ferment in the small bowel, causing gas, cramps, and diarrhea. Overall, 25 percent of Americans have trouble digesting dairy products. Over-the-counter medicines can help, and many dairy products are available in special forms for the lactose-intolerant.

To make sure you get more milk with less fat, try the following:

▶ Gradually switch from whole milk to 2%-fat (reduced fat) milk, then to 1%-fat (low-fat) milk, then to nonfat (skim) milk.
▶ Substitute fat-free sour cream or nonfat plain yogurt for sour cream.

▶ Use part-skim or low-fat cheeses whenever possible.
▶ Note that cottage cheese is lower in calcium than most cheeses. Thus, one cup of cottage cheese counts as only one-half serving of milk.

Fats, Oils, and Sweets (small amounts each day)

The Food Guide Pyramid places fats, oils, and sweets at the very top so that Americans will realize they should use them only in very small amounts. These foods supply calories but little or no vitamins or minerals.

Added sugars include sweeteners used in processing or at the table (such as jams, jellies, syrups, corn sweetener, molasses, fruit-juice concentrate, and the sugar in candy, cake, and cookies). These foods often are hidden in favorites—such as soft drinks (9 teaspoons of sugar per can), low-fat fruit yogurt (7 teaspoons per cup), fruit pie (6 teaspoons per serving), and catsup (a teaspoon in every tablespoon).

Try the following:

▶ Avoid temptation by not keeping a stash of cookies or candies.
▶ Put a small, child-sized spoon in the sugar bowl.
▶ When you crave a sweet, reach for nature's candy: fruit.
▶ If you want a daily sweet, have it as dessert, when you'll eat less of it, rather than as a snack.
▶ Drink fruit juices and water instead of sugar-laden soft drinks.

DRIs, RDAs, and Daily Values

Set by the Food and Nutrition Board of the National Academy of Sciences, the **Recommended Dietary Allowances (RDAs)** were developed fifty years ago to establish suggested levels of intake of essential nutrients. The RDAs are being replaced by **Dietary Reference Intakes (DRIs)**. Informed by the most current scientific knowledge, DRIs reflect a new approach to establishing suggested nutrient intake levels. DRIs include:

▶ **Estimated Average Requirements (EAR)**—These are population-wide average nutrient requirements for nutrition research and policymaking. They are the basis upon which RDA values are set.
▶ **Recommended Daily Allowances (RDA)**—These are the nutrient intake goals for individuals, derived from EARs.
▶ **Adequate Intakes (AI)**—These are nutrient intake goals for individuals, set when there is not enough scientific data to establish EAR or RDA values.
▶ **Tolerable Upper Intake Levels (UL)**—ULs suggest the upper limits of safe intake for nutrients that have the potential to be toxic if taken in too large dosages.

PULSE POINTS

Ten Ways to Eat Smart

1. **Eat five servings of fruits and vegetables per day.** For breakfast, have 100 percent juice or add raisins, berries, or sliced fruit to cereal, pancakes, or waffles. For lunch, have vegetable soup or salad with your meal or pile vegetables on your sandwich. For dinner, choose vegetables that are green, orange (such as carrots or squash), and red (such as tomatoes or bell peppers).

2. **Include three servings of whole-grain foods every day.** To identify whole-grain products, check the ingredient list. The first ingredient should be a whole grain, such as "whole-grain oats," "whole-grain wheat," or "whole wheat."

3. **Consume a calcium-rich food at each meal.** Good options

include low-fat and nonfat milk, cheese, or yogurt; tofu; broccoli; dried beans; spinach; and fortified soy milk.

4. **Eat less meat.** Rather than making meat the heart of a meal, think of it as a flavoring ingredient.

5. **Avoid high-fat fast foods.** Hot dogs, fried foods, packaged snack foods, and pastries are most likely to be laden with fat.

6. **Check the numbers.** When buying prepared foods, choose items that contain no more than 3 grams of fat per 100 calories.

7. **Think small.** Remember that a dinner-size serving of meat should be about the size of a deck of cards; half a cup is the size of a woman's fist; a pancake is the diameter of a CD.

8. **Read labels carefully.** Remember that "cholesterol-free" doesn't necessarily mean fat-free. Avoid products that contain saturated coconut oil, palm oil, lard, or hydrogenated fats.

9. **Switch to low-fat and no-fat dairy products.** Rather than buying whole-fat dairy products, choose skim milk, fat-free sour cream, and low- or nonfat yogurt.

10. **The brighter the better.** When selecting fruits and vegetables, choose the most intense color. A bright orange carrot has more beta-carotene than a pale one. Dark green lettuce leaves have more vitamins than lighter ones. Orange sweet potatoes pack more vitamin A than yellow ones.

The Food and Nutrition Board has set DRIs and ULs for 19 nutrients, including vitamins C and E and selenium.[36] (See Table 5-9 and Table 5-10.)

Daily Values (DV) are the values you will find on food labels at grocery stores. Daily Values differ from DRIs in that they provide one set of general recommendations for everyone, whereas DRIs provide more individualized recommendations based on factors like age and gender. For more on Daily Values, see "What Should I Look for on Nutrition Labels?" in the next section.

Dietary Supplements

Would you take an unproven pill that promises to make you stronger, smarter, younger, healthier? More than half of Americans regularly use nutritional and dietary supplements—vitamins, minerals, and botanical and biological substances that have not been approved for sale as drugs. There are serious questions about the safety and efficacy of these products. (See Chapter 4 for a discussion of strength-building and performance-enhancing supplements, such as creatine.)

Marketed as foods, supplements do not have to undergo the same rigorous testing required of drugs. They can carry "structure/function" claims—claims that a product may affect the structure or functioning of the body—but not claims that they can treat, diagnose, cure, or prevent a disease. For example, statements such as "helps maintain a healthy cholesterol level" are acceptable, while statements as "lowers cholesterol levels" are not.

The FDA has issued rules for dietary supplement labeling. Labels must now include an information panel titled "Supplement Facts," similar to the "Nutrition Facts" panel that appears on processed foods), a clear identity statement, and a complete list of ingredients. Specifically, the "Supplement Facts" panel must show the manufacturer's suggested dose/serving size; information on nutrients when they are present in significant levels (such as vitamins A and C, calcium, iron, and sodium) and the percent Daily Value where a reference has been established; and all other dietary ingredients present in the product, including botanicals and amino acids. Herbal products are identified by the common or usual name and the part of the plant used (such as root, stem, or leaf).

▼ Table 5-9   Dietary Reference Intakes: Recommended Intakes for Individuals: Minerals*

Life Stage Group	Calcium (mg/d)	Chromium (µg/d)	Copper (µg/d)	Fluoride (mg/d)	Iodine (µg/d)	Iron (mg/d)	Magnesium (mg/d)	Manganese (mg/d)	Molybdenum (µg/d)	Phosphorus (mg/d)	Selenium (µg/d)	Zinc (mg/d)
Infants												
0–6 mo	210*	0.2*	200*	0.01*	110*	0.27*	30*	0.003*	2*	100*	15*	2*
7–12 mo	270*	5.5*	220*	0.5*	130*	11	75*	0.6*	3*	275*	20*	3
Children												
1–3 y	500*	11*	340	0.7*	90	7	80	1.2*	17	460	20	3
4–8 y	800*	15*	440	1*	90	10	130	1.5*	22	500	30	5
Males												
9–13 y	1,300*	25*	700	2*	120	8	240	1.9*	34	1,250	40	8
14–18 y	1,300*	35*	890	3*	150	11	410	2.2*	43	1,250	55	11
19–30 y	1,000*	35*	900	4*	150	8	400	2.3*	45	700	55	11
31–50 y	1,000*	35*	900	4*	150	8	420	2.3*	45	700	55	11
51–70 y	1,200*	30*	900	4*	150	8	420	2.3*	45	700	55	11
>70 y	1,200*	30*	900	4*	150	8	420	2.3*	45	700	55	11
Females												
9–13 y	1,300*	21*	700	2*	120	8	240	1.6*	34	1,250	40	8
14–18 y	1,300*	24*	890	3*	150	15	360	1.6*	43	1,250	55	9
19–30 y	1,000*	25*	900	3*	150	18	310	1.8*	45	700	55	8
31–50 y	1,000*	25*	900	3*	150	18	320	1.8*	45	700	55	8
51–70 y	1,200*	20*	900	3*	150	8	320	1.8*	45	700	55	8
<70 y	1,200*	20*	900	3*	150	8	320	1.8*	45	700	55	8
Pregnancy												
≤ 18 y	1,300*	29*	1,000	3*	220	27	400	2.0*	50	1,250	60	13
19–30 y	1,000*	30*	1,000	3*	220	27	350	2.0*	50	700	60	11
31–50 y	1,000*	30*	1,000	3*	220	27	360	2.0*	50	700	60	11
Lactation												
≤ 18 y	1,300*	44*	1,300	3*	290	10	360	2.6*	50	1,250	70	14
19–30 y	1,000*	45*	1,300	3*	290	9	310	2.6*	50	700	70	12
31–50 y	1,000•	45*	1,300	3*	290	9	320	2.6*	50	700	70	12

*This table presents Recommended Dietary Allowances (RDAs) in **bold type** and Adequate Intakes (AIs) in ordinary type followed by an asterisk(*). RDAs and AIs may both be used as goals for individual intake. RDAs are set to meet the needs of almost all (97 to 98%) individuals in a group. For healthy breast-fed infants, the AI is the mean intake. The AI for other life stage and gender groups is believed to cover needs of all individuals in the group, but lack of data or uncertainty in the data prevent being able to specify with confidence the percentage of individuals covered by this intake.

Source: Trumbo, P., S. Schlicker, and M. Poos. *Dietary Reference Intakes: Vitamin A, Vitamin K, arsenic, boron, chromium, copper, iodine, manganese, molybdenum, nickel, silicon, vanadium, and zinc. Journal of the American Dietetic Association,* Vol. 101, 2001, pp. 294–301. Copyright 2001 by The National Academies of Sciences. All rights reserved.

???? Should I Take Vitamin Supplements?

Many health experts feel that the best way to make sure your body gets the vitamins and minerals it needs is to eat a wide variety of foods. If you rely on vitamin/mineral pills and fortified foods to make up for poor nutrition, you may shortchange yourself.

Even though there's little proof that multivitamin supplements can help them, many people figure that taking them certainly can't hurt. As they see it, supplements serve as a nutritional insurance policy, something to fall back on in case they don't get everything they need from whole foods. For the most part, this is true. "If you have a good diet and you take a multivitamin supplement, there's probably no danger," says USDA nutritionist Ann Shaw. "But if you take megadoses of a single vitamin or several different vitamins, you could run into problems."[37] See

Table 5-11 for a summary of what we know about different supplements.

As scientists note, most health benefits and dangers stem from more than one source, so it's unlikely that changing any one nutrient will in itself produce great benefits—and may, by interfering with the complex balance of nutrients, do harm. In particular, the fat-soluble vitamins, primarily A and D, can build up in our bodies and cause serious complications, such as damage to the kidneys, liver, or bones. Large doses of water-soluble vitamins, including the B vitamins, may also be harmful. Excessive intake of vitamin B_6 (pyridoxine), often used to relieve premenstrual bloating, can cause neurological damage, such as numbness in the mouth and tingling in the hands. (An excessive amount in this case is 250 to 300 times the recommended dose.) High doses of vitamin C can produce stomachaches and diarrhea. Niacin, often taken in high doses to lower cholesterol, can cause jaundice, liver damage, and irregular

▼ Table 5-10 Dietary Reference Intakes: Recommended Intakes for Individuals: Vitamins*

Life Stage Group	Vitamin A (µg/d)ᵃ	Vitamin D (µg/d)ᵇ,ᶜ	Vitamin E (mg/d)ᵈ	Vitamin K (µg/d)	Vitamin C (mg/d)	Thiamin (mg/d)	Riboflavin (mg/d)	Niacin (mg/d)ᵉ	Vitamin B_6 (mg/d)	Folate (µg/d)ᶠ	Vitamin B_{12} (µg/d)	Pantothenic Acid (mg/d)	Biotin (µg/d)	Choline⁹ (mg/d)
Infants														
0–6 mo	400*	5*	4*	2.0*	40*	0.2*	0.3*	2*	0.1*	65*	0.4*	1.7*	5*	125*
7–12 mo	500*	5*	5*	2.5*	50*	0.3*	0.4*	4*	0.3*	80*	0.5*	1.8*	6*	150*
Children														
1–3 y	**300**	5*	**6**	30*	**15**	**0.5**	**0.5**	**6**	**0.5**	**150**	**0.9**	2*	8*	200*
4–8 y	**400**	5*	**7**	55*	**25**	**0.6**	**0.6**	**8**	**0.6**	**200**	**1.2**	3*	12*	250*
Males														
9–13 y	**600**	5*	**11**	60*	**45**	**0.9**	**0.9**	**12**	**1.0**	**300**	**1.8**	4*	20*	375*
14–18 y	**900**	5*	**15**	75*	**75**	**1.2**	**1.3**	**16**	**1.3**	**400**	**2.4**	5*	25*	550*
19–30 y	**900**	5*	**15**	120*	**90**	**1.2**	**1.3**	**16**	**1.3**	**400**	**2.4**	5*	30*	550*
31–50 y	**900**	5*	**15**	120*	**90**	**1.2**	**1.3**	**16**	**1.3**	**400**	**2.4**	5*	30*	550*
51–70 y	**900**	10*	**15**	120*	**90**	**1.2**	**1.3**	**16**	**1.7**	**400**	**2.4ʰ**	5*	30*	550*
>70 y	**900**	15*	**15**	120*	**90**	**1.2**	**1.3**	**16**	**1.7**	**400**	**2.4ʰ**	5*	30*	550*
Females														
9–13 y	**600**	5*	**11**	60*	**45**	**0.9**	**0.9**	**12**	**1.0**	**300**	**1.8**	4*	20*	375*
14–18 y	**700**	5*	**15**	75*	**65**	**1.0**	**1.0**	**14**	**1.2**	**400ⁱ**	**2.4**	5*	25*	400*
19–30 y	**700**	5*	**15**	90*	**75**	**1.1**	**1.1**	**14**	**1.3**	**400ⁱ**	**2.4**	5*	30*	425*
31–50 y	**700**	5*	**15**	90*	**75**	**1.1**	**1.1**	**14**	**1.3**	**400ⁱ**	**2.4**	5*	30*	425*
51–70 y	**700**	10*	**15**	90*	**75**	**1.1**	**1.1**	**14**	**1.5**	**400**	**2.4ʰ**	5*	30*	425*
>70 y	**700**	15*	**15**	90*	**75**	**1.1**	**1.1**	**14**	**1.5**	**400**	**2.4ʰ**	5*	30*	425*
Pregnancy														
≤18 y	**750**	5*	**15**	75*	**80**	**1.4**	**1.4**	**18**	**1.9**	**600ʲ**	**2.6**	6*	30*	450*
19–30 y	**770**	5*	**15**	90*	**85**	**1.4**	**1.4**	**18**	**1.9**	**600ʲ**	**2.6**	6*	30*	450*
31–50 y	**770**	5*	**15**	90*	**85**	**1.4**	**1.4**	**18**	**1.9**	**600ʲ**	**2.6**	6*	30*	450*
Lactation														
≤18 y	**1,200**	5*	**19**	75*	**115**	**1.4**	**1.6**	**17**	**2.0**	**500**	**2.8**	7*	35*	550*
19–30 y	**1,300**	5*	**19**	90*	**120**	**1.4**	**1.6**	**17**	**2.0**	**500**	**2.8**	7*	35*	550*
31–50 y	**1,300**	5*	**19**	90*	**120**	**1.4**	**1.6**	**17**	**2.0**	**500**	**2.8**	7*	35*	550*

*This table (taken from the DRI reports, see www.nap.edu) presents Recommended Dietary Allowances (RDAs) in **bold type** and Adequate Intakes (AIs) in ordinary type followed by an asterisk (*). RDAs and AIs may both be used as goals for individual intake. RDAs are set to meet the needs of almost all (97 to 98%) individuals in a group. For healthy breast-fed infants, the AI is the mean intake. The AI for other life stage and gender groups is believed to cover needs of all individuals in the group, but lack of data or uncertainty in the data prevent being able to specify with confidence the percentage of individuals covered by this intake.

ᵃAs retinol activity equivalents (RAEs). 1 RAE = 1 µg retinol, 12 µg β-carotene, 24 µg α-carotene, or 24 µg β-cryptoxanthin in foods. To calculate RAEs from REs of provitamin A carotenoids in foods, divide the REs by 2. For preformed vitamin A in foods or supplements and for provitamin A carotenoids in supplements, 1 RE = 1 RAE.

ᵇCholecalciferol. 1 µg cholecalciferol = 40 IU vitamin D.

ᶜIn the absence of adequate exposure to sunlight.

ᵈAs α-tocopherol. α-Tocopherol includes RRR-α-tocopherol, the only form of α-tocopherol that occurs naturally in foods, and the 2R-stereoisomeric forms of α-tocopherol (RRR-, RSR-, RRS-, and RSS-α-tocopherol) that occur in fortified foods and supplements. It does not include the 2S-stereoisomeric forms of α-tocopherol (SRR-, SSR-, SRS-, and SSS-α-tocopherol), also found in fortified foods and supplements.

ᵉAs niacin equivalents (NE). 1 mg of niacin = 60 mg of tryptophan; 0–6 months = preformed niacin (not NE).

ᶠAs dietary folate equivalents (DFE). 1 DFE = 1 µg food folate = 0.6 µg of folic acid from fortified food or as a supplement consumed with food = 0.5 µg of a supplement taken on an empty stomach.

⁹Although AIs have been set for choline, there are few data to assess whether a dietary supply of choline is needed at all stages of the lifecycle, and it may be that the choline requirement can be met by endogenous synthesis at some of these stages.

ʰBecause 10 to 30% of older people may malabsorb food-bound B_{12} it is advisable for those older than 50 years to meet their RDA mainly by consuming foods fortified with B_{12} or a supplement containing B_{12}.

ⁱIn view of evidence linking folate intake with neural tube defects in the fetus, it is recommended that all women capable of becoming pregnant consume 400 µg from supplements or fortified foods in addition to intake of food folate from a varied diet.

ʲIt is assumed that women will continue consuming 400 µg from supplements or fortified foods until their pregnancy is confirmed and they enter prenatal care, which ordinarily occurs after the end of the periconceptional period—the critical time for formation of the neural tube.

Source: Trumbo, P., S. Schlicker, and M. Poos. Dietary Reference Intakes: Vitamin A, Vitamin K, arsenic, boron, chromium, copper, iodine, manganese, molybdenum, nickel, silicon, vanadium, and zinc. *Journal of the American Dietetic Association*, Vol. 101, 2001, pp. 294–301. Copyright 2001 by The National Academies of Sciences. All rights reserved.

▼ **Table 5-11** **Do Dietary Supplements Work?**

Supplement	Claims	What We Know
Amino acids	Increase muscle mass.	No solid evidence that amino acid supplements promote muscle building. Little is known about the side effects of high doses of single or combination amino acid supplements.
Beta-carotene (converted into vitamin A in the body)	Reduces your risk of cancer.	No evidence that beta-carotene supplements reduce cancer risk.
B complex vitamins	Provide energy; help relieve stress and may help reduce heart disease risk.	No evidence that B vitamins relieve stress. Long thought to be nontoxic, but some B vitamins such as B_6 and niacin may have serious side effects when taken in very high doses.
Vitamin C	Prevents colds, certain cancers, and heart disease.	Vitamin C supplements can lessen the severity of colds but not prevent them. Observational studies have shown that vitamin C may help prevent cancer and heart disease, but too few clinical trials have been conducted to substantiate those results.
Calcium	Prevents osteoporosis and colon cancer and reduces high blood pressure.	Calcium plays a critical role in preventing osteoporosis if taken with vitamin D. Results of research on calcium's role in preventing colon cancer are still preliminary. It may help regulate blood pressure in some people, but there is no way of knowing who might benefit.
Chromium picolinate	Reduces body fat, builds muscle, and improves overall fitness.	Scientists have found that this popular nutritional and dietary supplement causes DNA breakage and may be a cancer risk.
Vitamin E	Reduces the risk of heart disease and cancer.	Supplements of 400–800 IU may protect against heart disease. Very few side effects have been reported, but high doses of vitamin E supplements should not be used by anyone taking anticoagulation medication.
Niacin	Helps lower cholesterol.	Niacin, in the form of nicotinic acid, is an inexpensive alternative to cholesterol-lowering drugs but should be prescribed by a doctor. Side effects include flushing and itching and gastrointestinal distress. Time-released niacin can be toxic to the liver.
Zinc	Boosts immunity, wards off colds, and improves sex drive.	Zinc taken at the onset of a cold can lessen its severity. High doses of zinc, however, may *suppress* immune function. No evidence that zinc supplements affect sexual performance.

heartbeats as well as severe, uncomfortable flushing of the skin. Table 5-6 provides more information about the effects of vitamin excess.

Large doses of vitamins can be especially dangerous for certain individuals. Excessive intake of vitamin C or D may precipitate the formation of kidney stones in the urinary tract. Too much vitamin B_6 may inhibit milk production in breast-feeding mothers. In individuals suffering from epilepsy, folate may interfere with their drug therapy. However, if you belong to any of the following groups, check with your doctor about the potential pluses of adding vitamins or vitamin-rich foods to your daily diet:

▷ Pregnant, breast-feeding, and menopausal women.
▷ People at risk for heart attack, especially smokers.
▷ Strict vegetarians.

▷ People with chronic illnesses that may interfere with appetite or the body's use of nutrients.
▷ Individuals taking medications that affect appetite or digestion.
▷ The elderly.

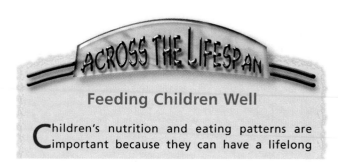

Feeding Children Well

Children's nutrition and eating patterns are important because they can have a lifelong effect on health. According to one study, children who gain a lot of weight as youngsters develop more risk factors for heart disease as adults. Other research has shown that, as a group, Hispanic and African-American children eat significantly more fat than white youngsters, which may contribute to the higher percentage of heart disease in adults in these minority groups.

Like adults, children should base their diet on whole grains, fruits, and vegetables and should limit fats and sweets, including soda. (See Figure 5-3.) According to the USDA, 37 percent of children ages 3 to 5 drink carbonated beverages, which account for about 40 percent of their fluid intake. Because soda contains few if any nutrients, this may mean they drink fewer healthier drinks. Incidentally, the USDA guidelines include a whole-hearted endorsement of physical activity. Kids who play hard not only get strong but also develop an appetite for a wider variety of foods.

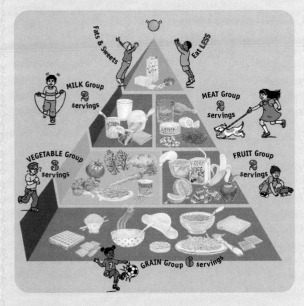

▲ **Figure 5-3** Food Pyramid for Kids. The Pyramid shows the USDA-recommended daily servings for children 2 to 6 years old.

Knowing What You Eat

For years, many manufacturers advertised products as "nutritious," "healthy," or otherwise good for you, but offered little or no proof to back up such claims. Today, thanks to the Nutrition Labeling and Education Act, enacted in 1994, food manufacturers must provide information about fat, calories, and ingredients in large type on packaged food labels that must show how a food item fits into a daily diet of 2,000 calories. The law also restricts nutritional claims for terms such as *healthy, low-fat,* or *high-fiber.*

In evaluating food labels and claims, keep in mind that, while individual foods vary in their nutritional value, what matters is your total diet. If you eat too much of any one food—regardless of what its label states—you may not be getting the variety and balance of nutrients that you need.

What Should I Look For on Nutrition Labels?

As Figure 5-4 on the next page shows, the "Nutrition Facts" on food labels present a wealth of information—if you know what to look for. The label focuses on those nutrients most clearly associated with disease risk and health: total fat, saturated fat, cholesterol, sodium, total carbohydrate, dietary fiber, sugar, and protein.

▸ **Calories.** Calories are the measure of the amount of energy that can be derived from food. Science defines a calorie as the amount of energy required to raise the temperature of 1 gram of water by one degree Celsius. In the laboratory, the caloric content of food is measured in 1,000-calorie units called *kilocalories.* The "calorie" referred to in everyday usage is actually the equivalent of the laboratory kilocalorie.

The label lists two numbers for calories: calories per serving and calories from fat per serving. This allows consumers to calculate how many calories they'll consume and to determine the percentage of fat in an item.

▸ **Serving size.** Rather than the tiny portions manufacturers sometimes used in the past to keep down the number of calories per serving, the new labels reflect more realistic portions. Serving sizes, which have been defined for approximately 150 food categories, must be the same for similar products (for example, different brands of potato chips) and for similar products within a category (for example, snack foods such as pretzels, potato chips, and popcorn). This makes it easier to compare the nutritional content of foods.

▸ **Daily Values (DVs).** DVs refer to the total amount of a nutrient that the average adult should aim to get or not exceed on a daily basis. The DVs for cholesterol, sodium, vitamins, and minerals are the same for all adults. The DVs for total fat, saturated fat, carbohydrate, fiber, and protein are based on a 2,000-calorie daily diet—the amount of food ingested by many American men and active women.

▸ **Percent Daily Values (%DV).** The goal for a full day's diet is to select foods that together add up to 100 percent of the DVs. The %DVs show how a particular food's nutrient content fits into a 2,000-calorie diet. Individuals who consume (or should consume) fewer

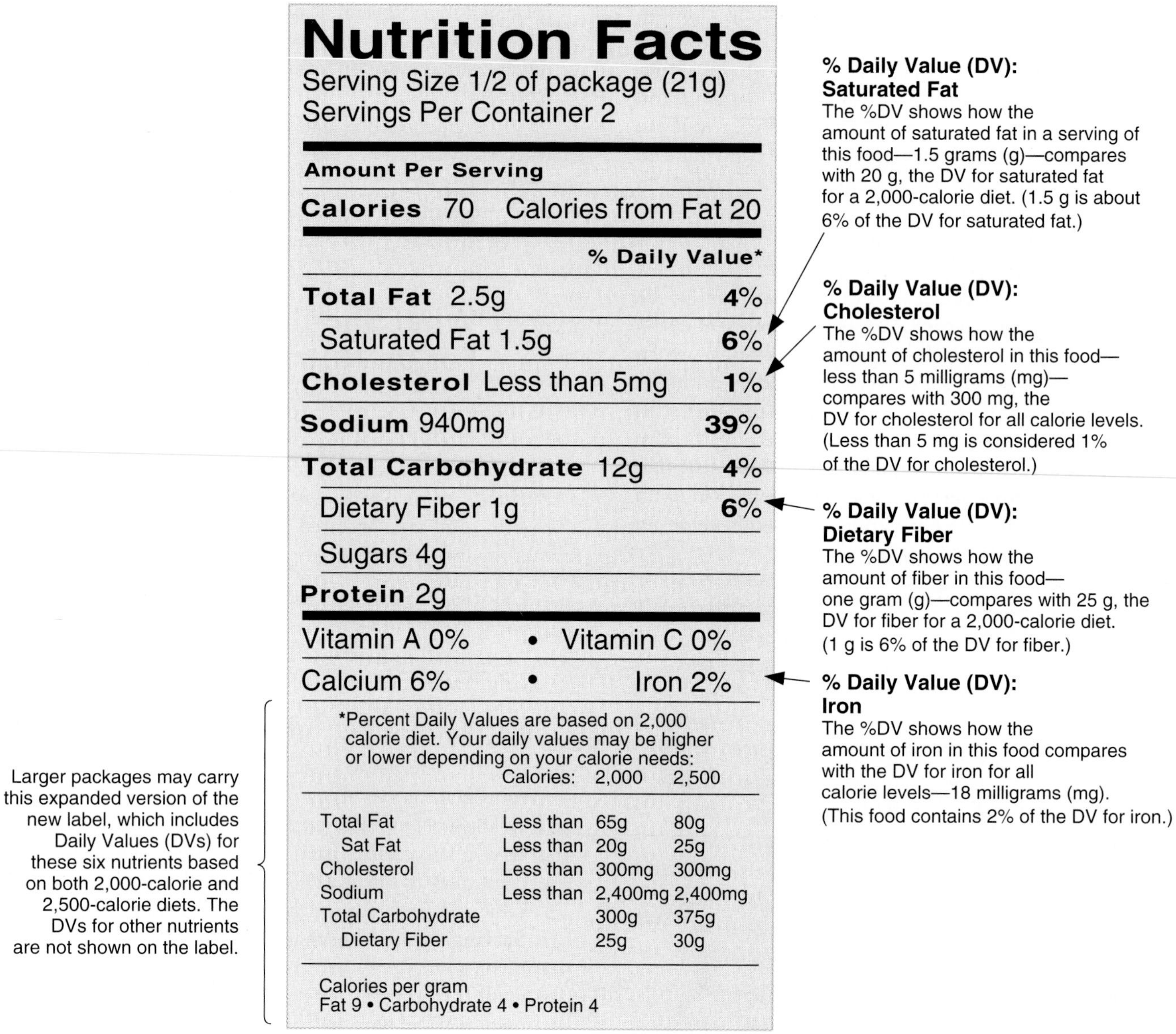

Nutrition Facts

Serving Size 1/2 of package (21g)
Servings Per Container 2

Amount Per Serving

Calories 70   Calories from Fat 20

% Daily Value*

Total Fat 2.5g	**4%**
Saturated Fat 1.5g	**6%**
Cholesterol Less than 5mg	**1%**
Sodium 940mg	**39%**
Total Carbohydrate 12g	**4%**
Dietary Fiber 1g	**6%**
Sugars 4g	
Protein 2g	

Vitamin A 0%   •   Vitamin C 0%

Calcium 6%   •   Iron 2%

*Percent Daily Values are based on 2,000 calorie diet. Your daily values may be higher or lower depending on your calorie needs:

		Calories:	2,000	2,500
Total Fat	Less than		65g	80g
Sat Fat	Less than		20g	25g
Cholesterol	Less than		300mg	300mg
Sodium	Less than		2,400mg	2,400mg
Total Carbohydrate			300g	375g
Dietary Fiber			25g	30g

Calories per gram
Fat 9 • Carbohydrate 4 • Protein 4

% Daily Value (DV): Saturated Fat
The %DV shows how the amount of saturated fat in a serving of this food—1.5 grams (g)—compares with 20 g, the DV for saturated fat for a 2,000-calorie diet. (1.5 g is about 6% of the DV for saturated fat.)

% Daily Value (DV): Cholesterol
The %DV shows how the amount of cholesterol in this food—less than 5 milligrams (mg)—compares with 300 mg, the DV for cholesterol for all calorie levels. (Less than 5 mg is considered 1% of the DV for cholesterol.)

% Daily Value (DV): Dietary Fiber
The %DV shows how the amount of fiber in this food—one gram (g)—compares with 25 g, the DV for fiber for a 2,000-calorie diet. (1 g is 6% of the DV for fiber.)

% Daily Value (DV): Iron
The %DV shows how the amount of iron in this food compares with the DV for iron for all calorie levels—18 milligrams (mg). (This food contains 2% of the DV for iron.)

Larger packages may carry this expanded version of the new label, which includes Daily Values (DVs) for these six nutrients based on both 2,000-calorie and 2,500-calorie diets. The DVs for other nutrients are not shown on the label.

▲ **Figure 5-4** Understanding nutrition labels.
The Nutrition Facts label lists the essential nutrient content of packaged food as well as the amount of potentially harmful substances such as fat and sodium.

than 2,000 total calories a day have to lower their DVs for total fat, saturated fat, and carbohydrates—for example, if their caloric intake is 10 percent less than 2,000 calories, they would lower the DV by 10 percent. Similarly, those who consume more than 2,000 calories should adjust the DVs upward.

▶ **Calories per gram.** The bottom of the food label lists the number of calories per gram for fat, carbohydrates, and protein.

According to national surveys, consumers most often look at nutrition labels for information on fat. Only one-third of them read the other information on the label. More than 72 percent said they would purchase a product with a health claim on the label rather than a product with no such claim. Yet even though 95 percent of students say that nutrition labels are useful, the information they get from them plays only a minor role in their daily diet planning.[38]

People zero in on different figures on the food label—for example, calories if they're watching their weight, specific ingredients if they have **food allergies.** Among the useful items to check are the following:

▶ **Calories from fat.** Get into the habit of calculating the percentage of fat calories in a food before buying or eating it.

▶ **Total fat.** Since the average person munches on 15 to 20 food items a day, it's easy to overload on fat. Saturated fat is a figure worthy of special attention because of its reported link to several diseases.

▶ **Cholesterol.** Cholesterol is made by and contained in products of animal origin only. Many high-fat products, such as potato chips, contain 0 percent cholesterol because they're made from plants and are cooked in vegetable fats. However, the vegetable fats they contain can be processed and made into saturated fats that are more harmful to the heart than cholesterol itself.

▶ **Sugars.** There is no DV for sugars because health experts have yet to agree on a daily limit. The figure on the label includes naturally present sugars, such as lactose in milk and fructose in fruit, as well as those added to the food, such as table sugar, corn syrup, or dextrose.

▶ **Fiber.** A "high-fiber" food has 5 or more grams of fiber per serving. A "good" source of fiber provides at least 2.5 grams. "More or added" fiber means at least 2.5 grams more per serving than similar foods—10 percent more of the DV for fiber.

▶ **Calcium.** "High" equals 200 milligrams (mg) or more per serving. "Good" means at least 100 mg, while "more" indicates that the food contains at least 100 mg more calcium—10 percent more of the DV—than the item usually would have.

▶ **Sodium.** Since many foods contain sodium, most of us routinely get more than we need. Read labels carefully to avoid excess sodium, which can be a health threat.

▶ **Vitamins.** A DV of 10 percent of any vitamin makes a food a "good" source; 20 percent qualifies it as "high" in a certain vitamin.

Nutrition labeling for fresh produce, fish, meat, and poultry remains voluntary. Packages too small for a full-sized label must provide an address or phone number so that consumers can obtain information from the manufacturer. Table 5-12 provides a guide to the required meaning of "front of the package" nutrition terms.

Functional Foods

As the American Dietetic Association has noted, all foods are functional at some physiological level. However, the term generally applies to a food specifically created to have health-promoting benefits. The International Food Information Council defines functional foods as those "that provide health benefits beyond basic nutrition."[39]

Some manufacturers are adding herbs, such as the cold-fighter echinacea, to food products and promoting them as functional foods. However, the amounts added often are too low to have any effect, and many herb-sprinkled foods are high-sugared drinks and snack foods. These products have other dangers, including the use of low-quality or contaminated herbs and adverse drug and food interactions.[40]

The Way We Eat

For centuries, Native Americans ate a diet of corn, beans, fish, game, wild greens, wild fruits, squash, and tomatoes. Over time the United States—a nation of immigrants—has imported a wide variety of ethnic cuisines. Although many people think of foods such as hamburgers, steak, potatoes, and cheesecake or ice cream as "all-American" favorites, in most cities across the country, it is possible to taste dozens of different cultural cuisines.

Dietary Diversity

 Whatever your cultural heritage, you have probably sampled Chinese, Mexican, Indian, Italian, and Japanese foods. If you belong to any of these ethnic groups, you may eat these cuisines regularly. Each type of ethnic cooking has its own nutritional benefits and potential drawbacks.

The African-American Diet

African-American cuisine traces some of its roots to food preferences from West Africa (for example, peanuts, okra, and black-eyed peas), as well as to traditional American foods, such as fish, game, greens, and sweet potatoes. Cajun cuisine, most closely associated with New Orleans, blends both African and French traditions in dishes such as gumbos (thick spicy soups), sausage, red beans, and seafood. African-American cooking uses many nutritious vegetables, such as collard greens and sweet potatoes, as well as legumes. However, some dishes include high-fat food products such as peanuts and pecans or involve frying, sometimes in saturated fat.

The Chinese Diet

The mainland Chinese diet, which is plant-based, high in carbohydrates, and low in fats and animal protein, is considered one of the healthiest in the world. The "food pagoda," developed for Chinese residents, is similar to the USDA food pyramid and recommends plenty of cereals, vegetables, fruits, and beans, with physical activity balancing food intake.[41] However, Chinese food is prepared differently in America. Chinese restaurants here serve more meat and sauces than are generally eaten in China.

▼ **Table 5-12 What Food Labels Really Mean**

Term	Examples	Means That a Serving of the Product Contains
Extra-lean	Extra-lean pork, extra-lean hamburger	Fewer than 5 g of fat, fewer than 2 g of saturated fat *and* fewer than 95 mg of cholesterol per serving (applies to meats only).
Extra, More	Bread with added fiber, fortified foods	At least 10% more of the Daily Value of a nutrient per serving than in a similar food.
Fat-free	Skim milk, no-fat salad dressing	Less than 0.5 g of fat per serving.
Free	Sugar-free, sodium-free	No or negligible amounts of sugars, sodium, or fat.
Good source	Good source of fiber, good source of calcium	10 to 19% of the Daily Value for a particular nutrient.
Healthy	Healthy burritos, canned vegetables	No more than 60 mg of cholesterol, 3 grams of fat, and 1 gram of saturated fat per serving; and more than 10% of the Daily Value of vitamin A, vitamin C, iron, calcium, protein, or fiber per serving. "Healthy" foods must also contain 360 mg or less sodium per serving.
High	High in iron, high in vitamin C	20% or more of the Daily Value for a particular nutrient.
Lean	Lean beef, lean turkey	Fewer than 10 g of fat, fewer than 4 g of saturated fat, *and* fewer than 95 mg of cholesterol per serving (applies to meats only).
Less	Less saturated fat, less cholesterol	25% less of a nutrient than a comparable food.
Light or lite	Light in sodium, lite in fat, light brown sugar, light and fluffy	33% fewer calories or half the fat as the regular product, or 50% or less sodium than usual in a low-calorie, low-fat food. "Light" can also be used on labels to describe the texture or color of a food.
Low-calorie	Low-calorie cookies, low-calorie fruit drink	40 calories or fewer per serving.
Low-fat	Low-fat cheese, low-fat ice cream	3 g or less fat per serving.
Low-saturated fat	Low-saturated fat pancake mix, low-saturated fat eggnog	1 g or less saturated fat per serving.
Low-sodium	Low-sodium soup, low-sodium hot dogs	140 mg or less sodium per serving.
Percent fat-free	95% fat-free; 98% fat-free	The specified percentage of fat on a weight basis (only low-fat foods can use this label).
Reduced	Reduced calories, reduced cholesterol	25% less of a nutrient or calories than the regular product.

According to laboratory tests of typical take-out dishes from Chinese restaurants, many have more fats and cholesterol than hamburger or egg dishes from fast-food outlets.

To eat healthfully when you choose Chinese cuisine, select boiled, steamed, or stir-fried dishes, mix entrees with steamed rice, and lift food out of a container with chopsticks or a fork and transfer it to serving bowls to leave excess sauce behind. Order wonton soup rather than egg rolls or pork spareribs. To avoid the cholesterol in egg yolks, steer away from items made with lobster or egg foo yung sauces. If you are prone to high blood pressure, watch out for the high sodium content of soy and other sauces, and of a seasoner called MSG (monosodium glutamate). Some people are sensitive to MSG, and most restaurants offer some MSG-free dishes or will leave out MSG on request.

The French Diet

Traditional French cuisine, which includes rich, high-fat sauces and dishes, has never been considered healthful. Yet nutritionists have been stumped to explain the so-called French paradox. Despite a diet high in saturated fats, the French have had one of the lowest rates of coronary artery disease in the world.

Recent reports indicate that the French diet is changing. Until 1990 the French ate much less animal fat and had significantly lower blood cholesterol levels than Americans and Britons. Fat consumption in France has since risen as the French have begun eating more meat and fast foods, snacking more, eating fewer relaxed meals, exercising less, and drinking less wine.[42] They've also been getting fatter, and some researchers contend that their rates of heart disease will inevitably rise in the coming decades. The French diet increasingly resembles the American diet, but French portions tend to be one-third to one-half the size of American portions.

The Indian Diet

Many Indian dishes highlight healthful ingredients such as vegetables and legumes (beans and peas). However, many also use "ghee" (a form of butter) or coconut oil, which is rich in harmful saturated fats. The best advice in an Indian restaurant is to ask how each dish is prepared. Good choices include daal or dal (lentils), karbi or karni (chickpea soup), and chapati (tortilla-like bread). Hold back on bhatura (fried bread), coconut milk, and samosas (fried meat or vegetables in dough).

The Japanese Diet

The traditional Japanese diet is very low in fat, which may be why the incidence of heart disease is low in Japan. Dietary staples include soybean products, fish, vegetables, noodles, and rice. A variety of fruits and vegetables are also included in many dishes. However, Japanese cuisine is high in salted, smoked, and pickled foods. Watch out for deep-fried dishes such as tempura, and salty soups and sauces (which you can ask for on the side). Ask for broiled entrees in a restaurant or nonfried dishes made with tofu, which has no cholesterol.

The Mediterranean Diet

Several years ago epidemiologists noticed something unexpected in the residents of regions along the Mediterranean: a lower incidence of deaths from heart disease. They speculated that the plant-based "Mediterranean diet," which is rich in fruits, vegetables, legumes, cereal, wine, and olive oil, may be the reason.

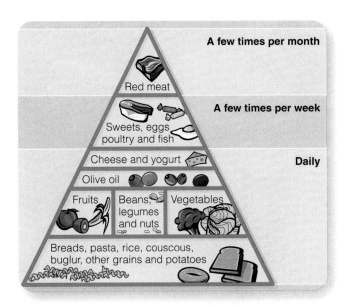

▲ **Figure 5-5** The Mediterranean Diet Pyramid. The Mediterranean diet relies heavily on fruits, vegetables, grain, and potatoes and includes considerable olive oil.

Source: Oldways Preservation & Exchange Trust. Reprinted by permission of *The New York Times.*

Subsequent research has confirmed that heart disease is much less common in countries along the Mediterranean than in other Western nations. In one four-year study of more than 400 men and women in France who had already suffered one heart attack, about half switched to a Mediterranean diet while the others ate a more traditional Western diet relatively low in fat, saturated fat, and cholesterol. Those following the Mediterranean diet were 50 to 70 percent less likely to experience a recurrence of heart disease, including strokes and fatal and nonfatal heart attacks.

No one knows exactly what makes the Mediterranean diet so heart-healthy. As illustrated by the Mediterranean Food Pyramid (see Figure 5-5), the diet features lots of fruits and vegetables, legumes, nuts, and grains. Meat is used mainly as a condiment rather than as a main course, and fish, yogurt, and low-fat feta cheese are the predominant animal foods. The diet is relatively high in fat, but the main source is olive oil, an unsaturated fat. Wine, an essential component of the Mediterranean diet, may be one of the factors responsible for the lower incidence of heart disease. Some researchers have found that wine's effect on blood platelets in men with heart disease differs according to whether they are eating a Mediterranean or a Western diet.[43]

The Mexican Diet

The cuisine served in Mexico features rice, corn, and beans, which are low in fat and high in nutrients. However,

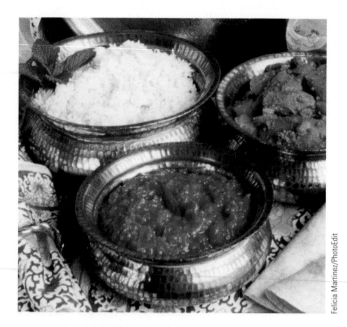

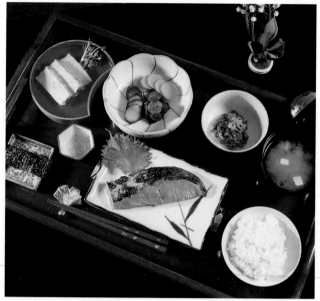

Felicia Martinez/PhotoEdit

© Allan Montaine

▲ In today's ethnically diverse United States, all-American food ranges from Mexican to Japanese. The rice and beans in the Mexican diet are healthy and high in protein, but too much cheese can cancel some of the benefits. The Japanese diet is high in seafood and rice and low in fats, cheese, and meat.

the dishes Americans think of as Mexican are far less healthful. Burritos, especially when topped with cheese and sour cream, are very high in fat. Although guacamole has a high fat content, it contains mostly monounsaturated fatty acids, a better form of fat.

When eating at Mexican restaurants, ask that cheese and sour cream be served on the side. Avoid refried beans, which are usually cooked in lard. Hold back on guacamole, quesadillas, and enchiladas. Nutritious choices include rice, beans, and shrimp or chicken tostadas on unfried cornmeal tortillas.

The Southeast Asian Diet

A rich variety of fruits and vegetables—bamboo shoots, bok choy, cabbage, mangoes, papayas, cucumbers—provides a sound nutritional basis for this diet. In addition, most foods are broiled or stir-fried, which keeps fat low. However, coconut oil and milk, used in many sauces, are high in fat. The use of MSG and pickled foods means the sodium content is high. At Thai or Vietnamese restaurants, choose salads (larb is a chicken salad with mint) or seafood soup (po tak).

What Should I Know About Vegetarian Diets?

Not all vegetarians avoid all meats. Some, who call themselves "lact-ovo-pesco-vegetarians," eat dairy products,

eggs, chicken, and fish, but not red meat. **Lacto-vegetarians** eat dairy products as well as grains, fruits, and vegetables; **ovo-lacto-vegetarians** also eat eggs. Pure vegetarians, called **vegans,** eat only plant foods; often they take vitamin B_{12} supplements, because that vitamin is normally found only in animal products. If they select their food with care, vegetarians can get sufficient amounts of protein, vitamin B_{12}, iron, and calcium without supplements (see Figure 5-6).

The key to getting sufficient protein from a vegetarian diet is understanding the concept of **complementary proteins.** Meat, poultry, fish, eggs, and dairy products are complete proteins that provide the nine essential amino acids—substances that the human body cannot produce itself. Incomplete proteins, such as legumes or nuts, may have relatively low levels of one or two essential amino acids, but fairly high levels of others. By combining complementary protein sources, you can make sure that your body makes the most of the nonanimal proteins you eat. (See Figure 5-7). Many cultures rely heavily on complementary foods for protein. In Middle Eastern cooking, sesame seeds and chickpeas are a popular combination; in Latin American dishes, beans and rice, or beans and tortillas; in Chinese cuisine, soy and rice.

Vegetarian diets have proven health benefits. Studies show that vegetarians' cholesterol levels are low, and vegetarians are seldom overweight. As a result, they're less apt to be candidates for heart disease than those who consume large quantities of meat. Vegetarians also have lower incidences of breast, colon, and prostate cancer; high blood

New York Medical College Vegetarian Pyramid

Vegans Must Consume Daily
Blackstrap Molasses, Vegetable Oil, Brewer's Yeast

Milk and Milk Substitutes Group
Milk, Yogurt, Cheese and Fortified Soy Milk
2–4 Servings

Meat/Fish Substitutes Group
Dry beans, Nuts, Seeds, Peanut butter, Tofu, and Eggs
2–3 Servings

Vegetable Group
3+ Servings

Fruit Group
2–4 Servings

Grains and Starchy Vegetables Group
Bread, Cereal, Rice, Pasta, Potatoes, Corn, and Green Peas
6–11 Servings

▲ **Figure 5-6** Vegetarian Food Guide Pyramid.
This version of the Food Guide Pyramid has been modified for use by vegetarians. Compare it to the Pyramid shown in Figure 5-2 on page 160.

pressure; and osteoporosis. When combined with exercise and stress reduction, vegetarian diets have led to reductions in the buildup of harmful plaque within the blood vessels of the heart. (See Chapter 12 for a further discussion of the connections between diet and heart disease.)

Fast Food: Nutrition on the Run

On any given day, about 25 percent of adults in the United States go to a fast-food restaurant. The typical American consumes three hamburgers and four orders of french fries every week.[44] Not all fast foods are junk foods—that is, high in calories, sugar, salt, and fat, and low in nutrients. But while it's not all bad, fast food has definite disadvantages. A meal in a fast-food restaurant may cost twice as much as the same meal prepared at home and may provide half your daily calorie needs. The fat content of many items is extremely high. A Burger King Whopper with cheese contains 723 calories and 48 grams of fat, 18 grams from saturated fat. A McDonald's Sausage McMuffin with egg has 517 calories and 33 grams of fat, 13 grams from saturated fat. Many fast-food chains have switched from beef tallow or lard to unsaturated vegetable oils for frying, but the total fat content of the foods remains the same.

At regular restaurants or cafeterias, with a little extra

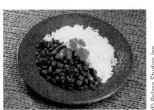
Rice and black beans.

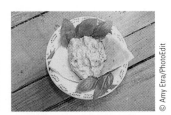
Hummus and bread.

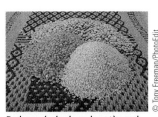
Corn and black-eyed peas.

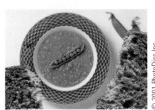
Bulgur (whole wheat) and lentils.

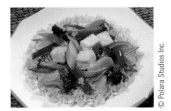
Tofu and rice.

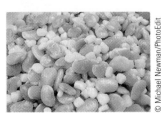
Corn and lima beans (succotash).

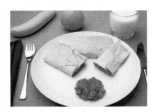
Tortilla with refried beans (e.g., a bean burrito).

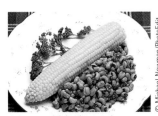
Pea soup and bread.

▲ **Figure 5-7** Vegetarian food combinations that supply complete proteins.

STRATEGIES FOR PREVENTION

A Guide to Fast Foods

✔ For breakfast, avoid croissants or muffins stuffed with eggs or meat; they pack as many as 700 calories. Better options include plain scrambled eggs (150–180 calories), pancakes without butter or syrup (400 calories), and English muffins (185 calories each).

✔ For lunch or dinner, if you want meat, go for plain hamburgers (no cheese), which average 275 to 350 calories. An even better choice is roast beef, which is lower in fat and calories.

✔ Be wary of fast-food fish. With frying oil trapped in the breading and creamy tartar sauce on top, fried-fish sandwiches supply more calories (425–500) and fat than regular hamburgers.

✔ Avoid fried chicken; the coatings tend to retain grease. If you want bite-sized chicken, select bites made of chicken breast, not processed chicken (which contains fatty, ground-up skin).

✔ Ask for unsalted items; they are available. (Many chains have also reduced the amount of sodium used in cooking.)

✔ If you sample the salad bar, steer clear of mayonnaise, bacon bits, oily vegetable salads, and rich dressings.

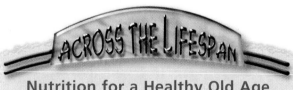

Nutrition for a Healthy Old Age

As many as 40 percent of elderly people who live independently do not get adequate amounts of one or more essential nutrients.[45] The reasons are many: limited income, difficulty getting to stores, chronic illnesses, medications that interfere with the metabolism of nutrients, problems chewing or digesting, poor appetite, inactivity, illness, depression. Among the nutrients often lacking in older Americans are folate, vitamin D, calcium, vitamin E, magnesium, vitamin B_6, vitamin C, and zinc.

While nutritionists urge the elderly—like other Americans—to concentrate on eating healthful foods, many also recommend daily nutritional supplements, which may provide the added benefit of improving cognitive function in healthy people over 65. In a study of 86 older people living independently who took either a supplement or a placebo, those taking the supplement showed significant improvements in short-term memory, problem-solving ability, abstract thinking, and attention. Vitamin supplements may help cognitive function by bolstering the immune system, thereby warding off brain changes associated with Alzheimer's and other forms of dementia.[46]

The Food Pyramid for Older Americans was designed specifically for adults over age 70, but the USDA urges anyone age 50 or older to heed its recommendations. (See Figure 5-8). The new guidelines advise eight or more 8-ounce glasses of water daily to reduce the risk of dehydration and constipation, which become increasing risks because of decreased thirst sensation in the elderly. The pyramid also calls for dietary supplements of calcium and vitamins B_{12} and D.[47]

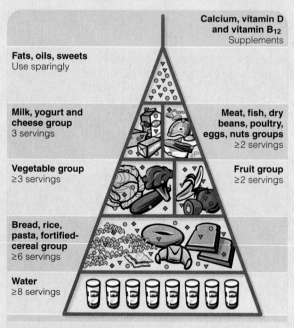

▲ **Figure 5-8** Food Pyramid for older adults. The pyramid shows the USDA-recommended daily servings for adults 70 or older.

attention, you can usually get a better nutritional value for the calories you consume. For example, you can request that your entree be baked or broiled without fat. You can also ask that fresh vegetables be steamed without salt or butter. When possible, ask for luncheon rather than dinner-sized portions.

Food Safety

Increasingly, Americans are concerned not just with whether the food they eat is nutritious, but whether it's safe. Many unsuspected safety hazards have been identified by **food toxicologists,** specialists who detect toxins (potentially harmful substances) and treat the conditions they produce.

Pesticides, Processing, and Irradiation

Plants and animals naturally produce compounds that act as pesticides to aid in their survival. The vast majority of the pesticides we consume are therefore natural, not added by farmers or food processors. As discussed in depth in Chapter 19, *commercial* pesticides save billions of dollars of valuable crops from pests, but they also may endanger human health and life.

Fearful of potential risks in pesticides, many consumers are purchasing **organic** foods. The term organic refers to foods produced without the use of commercial chemicals at any stage. Independent groups now certify foods before they can be labeled organic. Foods that are truly organic are cleaner and have much lower levels of residues than standard commercial produce. There's no guarantee that the organic produce you buy at a grocery or health-food store is more nutritious than other produce. However, buying organic foods is one way in which you can work toward a healthier environment.

Irradiation is the use of radiation, either from radioactive substances or from devices that produce X rays, on food. It doesn't make the food radioactive. Its primary benefit is to prolong the shelf life of food. Like the heat in canning, irradiation can kill all the microorganisms that might grow in a food, and the sterilized food can then be stored for years in sealed containers at room temperature without spoiling. Are irradiated foods safe to eat? The best available answer is a qualified yes, because we don't have complete data yet. Most of the research conducted so far has focused on low-dose irradiation to delay ripening and destroy insects. In 1997 the FDA approved the irradiation of red meat as a means of eliminating dangerous bacteria that could cause food poisoning. Irradiation had previously been approved for poultry, where it was used to kill disease-causing bacteria like salmonella, and fruits and vegetables, where it is used in low doses to kill funguses and molds.

Genetically engineered foods—custom built to improve quality or remove unwanted traits—may become an important part of our diets in the future. By modifying the genetic makeup of plants, engineers will be able to produce apples that resist insects, raspberries that last longer, and potatoes that absorb less fat in cooking. Will these items be as tasty and healthful as foods grown the old-fashioned way? And will they have unforeseen health hazards? That's yet to be seen.

Additives: Risks Versus Benefits

Additives are substances added to foods to lengthen storage time, change taste in a way the manufacturer thinks is better, alter color, or otherwise modify them to make them more appealing. The average American takes in approximately 160 pounds of food additives per year: more than 140 pounds of sweeteners, 15 pounds of table salt, and 5 to 10 pounds of all others.

Additives provide numerous benefits. Sodium and calcium propionate, sodium benzoate, potassium sorbate, and sulfur dioxide prevent the growth of bacteria, yeast, and mold in baked goods. BHA (butylated hydroxyanisole),

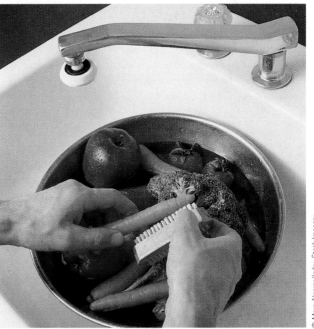

▲ Wash produce thoroughly in fresh water to remove dirt and any pesticide residue, scrubbing when necessary to clean off soil.

STRATEGIES FOR PREVENTION

Protecting Yourself from Food Poisoning

✔ Clean food thoroughly. Wash produce thoroughly. Wash utensils, plates, cutting boards, knives, blenders, and other cooking equipment with very hot water and soap after preparing raw meat, poultry, or fish to avoid contaminating other foods or the cooked meat.

✔ Drink only pasteurized milk. Raw or unpasteurized milk increases the danger of microbial infections.

✔ Don't eat raw eggs. Since raw eggs can be contaminated with salmonella, don't use them in salad dressings, eggnog, or other dishes.

✔ Cook chicken thoroughly. About a third of all poultry sold contains harmful organisms. Thorough cooking eliminates any danger. (See Figure 5-9.)

✔ Cook pork to an internal temperature of 170°F to kill a parasite called trichina occasionally found in the muscles of pigs.

✔ Keep foods hotter than 140°F or colder than 40°F. The temperatures in between are a danger zone. If you must leave foods out—perhaps at a buffet or picnic—don't let them stay in the temperature danger zone for more than two hours. After that time, throw the food away.

✔ Refrigerate leftovers as soon as possible and use them within three days. If frozen, use leftovers within two to three months.

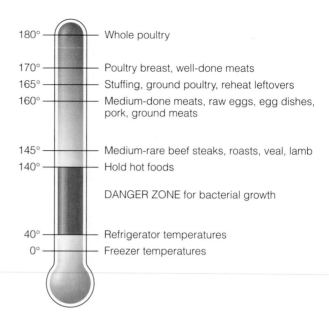

▲ **Figure 5-9** Recommended safe cooking temperatures. Use a food thermometer when cooking to ensure that the temperature recommendations shown here are met.

Source: Dietary Guidelines for Americans, 2000.

BHT (butylated hydroxytoluene), propyl gallate, and vitamin E protect against the oxidation of fats (rancidity). Other additives include leavening agents, emulsifiers, stabilizers, thickeners, dough conditioners, and bleaching agents.

Some additives can pose a risk to eaters. For example, nitrites—used in bacon, sausages, and lunch meats to inhibit spoilage, prevent botulism, and add color—can react with other substances in your body or in food to form potentially cancer-causing agents called *nitrosamines.* In the last decade, the food industry has reduced the amount of nitrite used to cure foods, so there should be less danger than in the past. Sulfites, used to prevent browning, can produce severe, even fatal, allergic reactions in sensitive individuals. The FDA has required the labeling of sulfites in packaged foods and has banned the use of sulfites on fresh fruits and vegetables, including those in salad bars.

Foodborne Illnesses

Americans may be more likely to get sick from what they eat today than they were half a century ago. According to the Centers for Disease Control and Prevention (CDC), the frequency of serious gastrointestinal illness—one indicator of food poisoning—is significantly higher than it was in 1948. Every year food poisoning causes 5,000 deaths, 325,000 hospitalizations, and 76 million illnesses. Cases of potentially deadly E. coli infection more than doubled in the last five years of the twentieth century.

According to the Government Accounting Office, 85 percent of food poisoning comes from fruits, vegetables, cheeses, and seafood. People aren't washing fruits thoroughly or cooking vegetables before eating, increasing the chance of infection with viruses or bacteria. They're also eating more precooked foods rather than sit-down meals served right out of the oven. And the sheer number and types of products on the market far exceed the government's ability to monitor them.

Foodborne infections generally produce nausea, vomiting, and diarrhea from twelve hours to five days after infection. The symptoms and severity depend on the specific microorganism and the victim's overall health. Although the illnesses tend to be short-term and not usually severe, they can be fatal to those whose immune systems are impaired or whose general health is poor. (See Table 5-13).

⁇⁇⁇ What Causes Food Poisoning?

Salmonella is a bacterium that contaminates many foods, particularly undercooked chicken, eggs, and sometimes processed meat. Eating contaminated food can result in salmonella poisoning, which causes diarrhea and vomiting. The CDC estimates 40,000 reported cases of salmonella poisoning a year; the actual number of cases could be anywhere from 400,000 to 4 million. Another bacterium, *Campylobacter jejuni*, may cause even more stomach infections than salmonella. Found in water, milk, and some foods, *Campylobacter* poisoning causes severe diarrhea and has been implicated in causing stomach ulcers.

▼ Table 5-13 Food Poisoning: Common Culprits

	Source	Symptoms	Onset	Prevention
Bacterial				
Campylobacter Jejuni	Bacteria on poultry, cattle, and sheep that can contaminate the meat or milk of these animals.	Diarrhea, abdominal cramping, fever and/or bloody stools.	2 to 5 days	Cook foods thoroughly; drink pasteurized milk.
Escherichia coli (E.coli)	Water, raw or under-cooked meat and cross-contaminated foods.	Watery or bloody diarrhea, abdominal cramps, or vomiting.	10 to 72 hours	Cook foods thoroughly; wash hands well.
Listeria	Deli meats, hot dogs, soft cheese, raw meat, unpasteurized milk.	Headache, fever, and nausea.	24 hours to 12 days	Cook meats thoroughly; buy pasteurized milk; wash hands well.
Salmonella	Raw or undercooked meat, poultry or eggs, and unpasteurized milk.	Fever, muscle aches, nausea, abdominal cramps, diarrhea, fever, and/or headache.	5 hours to 4 days	Cook meats and leftovers thoroughly; wash hands well.
Staphylococcus aureus	Food left too long at room temperature, including meat, poultry, or egg products, tuna, potato salad, and cream-filled pastries. Unlike other bacteria, staphylococci grow well in foods that are high in sugar or salt; any food can be contaminated by infected food handlers.	Vomiting, nausea, diarrhea, abdominal pain, and/or cramps.	30 minutes to 8 hours	Cook foods thoroughly; refrigerate leftovers immediately; wash your hands before and after handling food.
Nonbacterial				
Hepatitis A virus	Oysters, clams, mussels, or scallops that come from waters polluted with untreated sewage, and improper food handling with unwashed hands.	Weakness, appetite loss, nausea, vomiting, and fever; jaundice may develop.	15 to 50 days	Buy seafood from reputable markets; wash hands well.
Trichinella spiralis	(causes trichinosis) A parasite found in raw or undercooked pork or carnivorous animals.	Muscle pain, swollen eyelids, and/or fever; can be fatal.	8 to 15 days	Cook meat thoroughly.

Source: USDA.

Bacteria can also cause illness by producing toxins in food. *Staphylococcus aureus,* the most common cause of foodborne intoxication, occurs when cooked foods are cross-contaminated with the bacteria from raw foods and not stored properly. Staph infections cause nausea and abdominal pain anywhere from thirty minutes to eight hours after ingestion.

Even many "healthy" foods can pose dangers. The FDA has urged consumers to avoid eating raw sprouts because of the risk of getting sick. Sprouts, particularly alfalfa and clover, can be contaminated by salmonella or *E. coli* bacteria, which can cause nausea, diarrhea, and cramping in healthy adults. Children and senior citizens can experience effects that can lead to kidney failure and compromised immune systems. The FDA advises people to either cook sprouts before eating them or request that they be left off sandwiches and other food ordered in restaurants. Homegrown sprouts can also present a risk if they come from contaminated seeds. The FDA also has warned consumers about the dangers of unpasteurized orange juice because of the risk of salmonella contamination.

An uncommon but sometimes fatal form of food poisoning is **botulism,** caused by the *Clostridium botulinum* organism. Improper home-canning procedures are the most common cause of this potentially fatal problem.

There have been several outbreaks of listeriosis, caused by the bacteria **listeria,** commonly found in deli meats, hot dogs, soft cheeses, raw meat, and unpastuerized milk. At greatest risk are pregnant women, infants, and those with weakened immune systems. You can reduce your risk by cooking meats and leftovers thoroughly and by washing everything that may come into contact with raw meat.

Mad Cow Disease

A foodborne illness that has generated international alarm is mad cow disease, the popular term for deadly bovine spongiform encephalopathy (BSE). After first attacking British cattle, BSE crossed species to kill dozens of people in the United Kingdom, Ireland, and France. Caused by eating beef containing brain or spinal tissue from infected cows, BSE seems to be transmitted by a misshapen protein called a prion that cannot be detected by testing blood or tissue. In humans, BSE causes mood swings, hallucinations, uncontrollable body movements, progressive dementia, and eventual death.[48]

Europeans responded to the BSE outbreak of 2001 by destroying thousands of cattle and banning the sale of certain types of beef. Because of a U.S. ban on imports of British livestock, BSE did not spread across the Atlantic. As an added precaution, the FDA recommended that anyone who had lived in England, France, Portugal, or Ireland for a total of ten years since 1980 be prohibited from donating blood in the United States. Nonetheless, 70 percent of

Americans are concerned that mad cow or another problem in European herds, foot-and-mouth disease (which does not affect humans), could cause problems in the United States.[49]

Food Allergies

A woman nibbles on a strawberry and collapses. A boy develops hives immediately after eating a peanut butter sandwich. A baby vomits after swallowing some regular milk. In each case, the body has responded as if the food being consumed were a threatening invader and has mobilized its internal forces to fight against it.

Physicians disagree as to which foods are the most common triggers of food allergies. Cow's milk, eggs, seafood, wheat, soybeans, nuts, seeds, and chocolate have all been identified as culprits. The symptoms they provoke vary. One person might sneeze if exposed to an irritating food; another might vomit or develop diarrhea; others might suffer headaches, dizziness, hives, or a rapid heartbeat. Symptoms may not develop for up to 72 hours, making it hard to pinpoint which food was responsible. (See Chapter 11 for a further discussion of allergies.)

If you suspect that you have a food allergy, see a physician with specialized training in allergy diagnosis. Medical opinion about the merits of many treatments for food allergies is divided. Once you've identified the culprit, the wisest and sometimes simplest course is to avoid it.

Nutritional Quackery

The American Dietetic Association describes nutritional quackery as a growing problem for unsuspecting consumers. Because so much nutritional nonsense is garbed in scientific-sounding terms, it can be hard to recognize bad advice when you get it. One basic rule: If the promises of a nutritional claim sound too good to be true—they probably are. (See Savvy Consumer: "Spotting Nutrition Misinformation.")

If you seek the advice of a nutrition consultant, check his or her credentials and professional associations carefully. Because licensing isn't required in all states, almost anyone can call him- or herself a nutritionist, regardless of qualifications. Be wary of diplomas from obscure schools and organizations that allow anyone who pays dues to join. (One physician obtained a membership for his dog!) Registered dietitians (R.D.s), who have bachelor's degrees from approved programs and specialized training (including an internship), and who pass a certification examination, are usually members of the American Dietetic Association (ADA), which sets the standard for quality in diets. Nutrition experts with M.D.s or Ph.D.s generally belong to the ADA, the American Institute of Nutrition, or the American Society of Clinical Nutrition; all have stringent membership requirements.

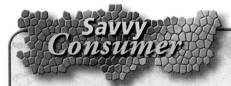

Spotting Nutrition Misinformation

- Don't believe everything you read. A quick way to spot a bad nutrition self-help book is to look in the index for a diet to prevent or treat rheumatoid arthritis (none exists). If you find one, don't buy the book.

- Before you try any new nutritional approach, check with your doctor or a registered dietitian or call the ADA consumer hot line.

- Don't believe ads or advisers basing their nutritional recommendations on hair analysis, which is not accurate in detecting nutritional deficiencies.

- Be wary of anyone who recommends megadoses of vitamins or nutritional supplements, which can be dangerous. High doses of vitamin A, which some people take to clear up acne, can be toxic.

- Question personal testimonies about the powers of some magical-seeming pill or powder, and be wary of "scientific articles" in journals that aren't reviewed by health professionals.

- Be wary of any nutritional supplements sold in health stores or through health and bodybuilding magazines that contain ingredients that have not been tested and proven safe.

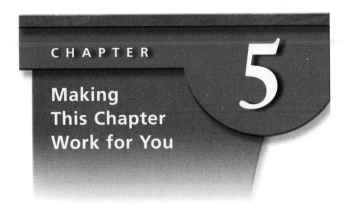

CHAPTER 5
Making This Chapter Work for You

1. The classes of essential nutrients include which of the following?
   a. amino acids, antioxidants, fiber and cholesterol
   b. proteins, calcium, calories, and folic acid
   c. carbohydrates, minerals, fat, and water
   d. iron, whole grains, fruits, and vegetables

2. Which type of fat is not considered a threat to heart health?
   a. omega-3 fatty acids
   b. trans fat
   c. triglycerides
   d. saturated fats

3. Antioxidants
   a. are nutrients important in the production of hemoglobin.
   b. are substances added to foods to make them more flavorful or physically appealing.
   c. are suspected triggers of food allergies.
   d. may help prevent cellular damage that can result in heart attacks, cancer, and other diseases.

4. Which of the following is true about the Food Guide Pyramid?
   a. It advises that, on a daily basis, you eat the same amounts of food from each of the food groups represented in the Pyramid.
   b. The foods at the top of the pyramid are considered to be the most nutritionally essential.
   c. According to the Pyramid, one should eat six to eleven servings of bread, cereals, rice, and pasta every week
   d. The Pyramid advises no more than two to three servings daily of both dairy foods and meat and other high-protein foods.

5. The Dietary Reference Intakes
   a. are the values on food labels.
   b. replace the Recommended Dietary Allowances, which established suggested levels of intake of essential nutrients.
   c. correspond to the five food groups in the Food Guide Pyramid.
   d. are nutrient-intake estimates for those nutrients for which RDAs cannot be scientifically established.

6. Food labels on packaged food include all of the following except
   a. total weight of the package.
   b. total amount of nutrients contained in the food.
   c. the percent of nutrient Daily Values provided in the food.
   d. serving size.

7. Which of the following statements are true?
   a. The Chinese diet, which is high in fats and low in carbohydrates, leads to high incidence of obesity and heart disease.

b. The French diet is considered to be healthful because the food is high in saturated fats.

c. The Mediterranean diet is rich in fruits, vegetables, wine, and olive oil and may help prevent heart disease.

d. Mexican and African-American recipes often include MSG, which is unhealthy for people with high blood pressure.

8. Some vegetarians may
   a. include chicken and fish in their diets.
   b. avoid vitamin B_{12} supplements if they eat only plant foods.
   c. eat only legumes or nuts because these provide complete proteins.
   d. have high cholesterol levels because of the saturated fats in fruits and vegetables.

9. Food hazards include all the following except
   a. nitrites
   b. raw eggs
   c. pesticides
   d. refrigerated leftovers used within 3 days.

10. Common causes of foodborne infections include which of the following?
    a. the influenza virus
    b. salmonella and *E. coli* bacteria
    c. additives
    d. irradiation

Answers to these questions can be found on page 640.

 How can eating fish twice a week help reduce cardiovascular disease?

Critical Thinking

1. Joel's grandparents seem to eat a fairly balanced diet, but he knows that elderly adults are more susceptible to disease. What recommendations could he make to them to ensure that they are getting all the nutrients they need to enhance their health?

2. Scientists are using genetic engineering to develop foods, such as tomatoes that won't bruise easily, cows that will produce more milk, or corn that will grow larger ears. Some consumer advocates argue that these items shouldn't be put on the market because they haven't been studied carefully enough. What do you think of these foods? Would you eat them?

3. Which alternative or ethnic diet do you think has the best-tasting food? Which is the most healthy? Why?

4. Is it possible to meet nutritional requirements on a limited budget? Have you ever been in this situation? What would you recommend to someone who wanted to eat healthfully on $30 a week?

5. Consider the number of times a week you eat fast food. How much money would you have saved it you had eaten home-prepared meals. Which fast foods could you have selected that would have provided more nutritional value?

SITES & BYTES

The Cyberkitchen
http://www.shapeup.org/kitchen/frameset1.htm
This interactive site, sponsored by Shape Up America, will show you how to balance your dietary intake with your physical activity to maintain healthy weight. You provide personal information regarding your age, gender, height, weight, and activity level, and the Cyberkitchen provides you with a healthy diet plan to meet your goals (weight loss or weight gain). It's fun and educational.

Mayo Clinic Food and Nutrition
http://www.mayoclinic.com/home?id=4.1.5
This site features a wealth of reliable nutrition information, including current news, feature articles, interactive tools, nutrition basics, diet planning, nutrition and disease management, dietary supplements, "What's for Dinner" page featuring serving sizes and shopping lists, as well as a virtual cookbook featuring healthy recipes.

Nutrition Analysis Tool

http://www.ag.uiuc.edu/~food-lab/nat

This interactive site, sponsored by the University of Illinois–Urbana/Champaign, consists of a free web-based program that allows you to analyze the foods you eat for a variety of nutrients.

Please note that links are subject to change. If you find a broken link, use a search engine such as **http://www.yahooo.com** and search for the website by typing in key words.

InfoTrac Activity Debra Palmer Keenan and Rayane Abusabha. "The Fifth Edition of the Dietary Guidelines for Americans: Lessons Learned Along the Way." *Journal of the American Dietetic Association,* Vol. 101, Issue 6, June 2001, p. 631.

(1) Name at least five significant changes in the guidelines listed in the new fifth edition compared to previous editions.

(2) What is one of the new guidelines to the fifth edition?

(3) What are two content changes that reflect recent dietary market trends and why were the changes made?

You can find additional readings related to nutrition with InfoTrac College Edition, an online library of more than 900 journals and publications. Follow the instructions for accessing InfoTrac that were packaged with your textbook; then search for articles using a key word search.

For additional links, resources, and suggested readings on InfoTrac, visit our Health & Wellness Resource Center at **http://health.wadsworth.com**.

Key Terms

The terms listed here are used within the chapter on the page indicated. Definitions of the terms are in the Glossary at the end of this book.

additives 179
amino acids 147
antioxidants 152
botulism 182
calorie 146
carbohydates 148
cholesterol 149
complementary proteins 176
complete proteins 147
complex carbohydrates 148
cruicifers 164
Daily Values (DV) 167
Dietary References Intakes (DRIs) 166
essential nutrients 146
fiber 148

folate 157
folic acid 157
food allergies 172
food toxicologists 179
hemoglobin 158
incomplete protein 147
indoles 164
insoluble fibers 148
irradiation 179
lacto-vegetarians 176
listeria 182
minerals 152
nutrients 146
nutrition 144
organic 179

osteoporosis 157
ovo-lacto-vegetarians 176
phytochemicals 159
protein 147
Recommended Dietary Allowances (RDAs) 166
saturated fat 149
simple carbohydrates 148
soluble fiber 148
trans fat 149
unsaturated fat 149
vegans 176
vitamins 152

References

1. *Nutrition and Health: Dietary Guidelines for Americans,* 2000. Washington, DC: United States Department of Agriculture and Department of Health and Human Services, 2000.
2. Goodman-Gruen, Deborah, and Donna Kritz-Silverstein. "Usual Dietary Isoflavone Intake Is Associated with Cardiovascular Disease Risk Factors in Postmenopausal Women." *Journal of Nutrition,* Vol. 131, No. 4, April 2001, p. 1202.
3. "Cardiovascular Benefits of Soy." *Consultant,* Vol. 41, No. 6, May 2001, p. 797.
4. Preboth, Monica. "Cardiovascular Benefits of Soy Protein." *American Family Physician,* Vol. 63, No. 9, May 1, 2001, p. 1862.
5. Wangen, K. E., et. al. "Soy Isoflavones Improve Plasma Lipids in Normocholesterolemic and Mildly Hypercholesterolemic Postmenopausal Women." *Alternative Medicine Review,* Vol. 6, No. 2, April 2001, p. 224.
6. Fleischauer, A.T., et al. "A Meta Analysis of Soy Food Consumption and Risk of Breast Cancer." American Journal of Epidemiology, Vol. 153, No. 11, June 1, 2001, p. S32.

7. Goff, Karen Goldberg. "Better Soy Than Sorry." *Insight on the News,* Vol. 17, No. 16, April 30, 2001, p. 28.

8. Somekawa, Y., et al. "Soy Intake Related to Menopausal Symptoms, Serum Lipids, and Bone Mineral Density in Postmenopausal Japanese Women." *Alternative Medicine Review,* Vol. 6, No. 2, April 2001, p. 223.

9. Nagata, Chisato. "Soy Product Intake and Hot Flashes in Japanese Women: Results from a Community-Based Prospective Study." *Journal of the American Medical Association,* Vol. 285, No. 23, June 20, 2001, p. 2954.

10. Guthrie, Joan. "Food Sources of Added Sweeteners in the Diets of Americans." *Journal of the American Dietetic Association,* Vol. 100, Issue 1, January 2000.

11. Webb, Densie. "Whole Grains Boast Phytochemicals (Not Just Fiber) to Fight Diseases." Environmental Nutrition, Vol. 24, No. 2, February 2001, p. 1.

12. Seddon, Johanna, et al. "Dietary Fat and Risk for Advanced Age-Related Macular Degeneration." Archives of Ophthalmology, Vol. 119, August 2001, p. 1191.

13. "Uncertain, Consumers Still Ooze Toward Butter over Margarine." *Tufts University Health & Nutrition Letter,* Vol. 18, No. 12, February 2001, p. 8.

14. "Butter Versus Margarine: New Study Sheds Light on Best Spread." *Environmental Nutrition,* Vol. 24, No. 2, February 2001, p. 3.

15. "The Butter-vs.-Margarine Debate; Latest Study Shows Margarine Is Better." *American Journal of Nursing,* Vol. 101, No. 3, March 2001, p. 19.

16. Denke, Margo, et al. "Individual Cholesterol Variation in Response to a Margarine- or Butter-Based Diet: A Study in Families." *Journal of the American Medical Association,* Vol. 284, No. 21, December 6, 2000, p. 2740.

17. Kuritzky, Louis. "Individual Cholesterol Variation in Response to a Margarine or Butter-Based Diet." *Neurology Alert,* Vol. 19, No. 6, February 2001, p. 6.

18. Hollingsworth, Pierce. "Margarine: The Over-the-Top Functional Food: Cholesterol-Fighting Foods." *Food Technology,* Vol. 55, No. 1, January 2001, p. 59.

19. Cerrato, Paul. "A 'Medicinal Food' That Lowers LDL Cholesterol." *Contemporary OB/GYN,* Vol. 46, No. 5, May 2001, p. 127.

20. Ornish, Dean. Personal interview.

21. Holmes, Michelle, et al. "Association of Dietary Intake of Fat and Fatty Acids with Risk of Breast Cancer." *Journal of the American Medical Association,* Vol. 281, No. 10, March 10, 1999.

22. Klipstein-Grobusch, Kerstin, et al. "Dietary Antioxidants and Peripheral Arterial Disease: The Rotterdam Study." *American Journal of Epidemiology,* Vol. 154, No. 2, July 15, 2001, p. 145.

23. Moyers, Susan, and Lynn Bailey. "Fetal Malformations and Folate Metabolism: Review of Recent Evidence." *Nutrition Reviews,* Vol. 59, No. 7, July 2001, p. 215.

24. Tice, Jeffrey, et al. "Cost-effectiveness of Vitamin Therapy to Lower Plasma Homocysteine Levels for the Prevention of Coronary Heart Disease: Effect of Grain Fortification and Beyond." *Journal of the American Medical Association,* Vol. 284, No. 21, December 6, 2000, p. 2740.

25. "Calcium Intake Is Low in Child and Adolescent Diets." *Brown University Child and Adolescent Behavior Letter,* Vol. 16, Issue 1, January 2000.

26. Leslie, Maryann, and Richard St. Pierre. "Osteoporosis: Implications for Risk Reduction in the College Setting." *Journal of American College Health,* Vol. 48, Issue 2, September 1999.

27. Slawson, Deborah, et al. "Food Sources of Calcium in a Sample of African-American and Euro-American Collegiate Athletes." *International Journal of Sport Nutrition and Exercise Metabolism,* Vol. 11, No. 2, June 2001.

28. Shaw, Ann. Personal interview.

29. Dixon, Lori Beth, et al. "Let the Pyramid Guide Your Food Choices: Capturing the Total Diet Concept." *Journal of Nutrition,* Vol. 131, No. 2, February 2001, p. 461S.

30. Anding, Jenna, et al. "Dietary Intake, Body Mass Index, Exercise, and Alcohol: Are College Women Following the Dietary Guidelines for Americans?" *Journal of American College Health,* Vol. 49, January 2001, p. 167.

31. Evans, Alexandra, et al. "Fruit and Vegetable Consumption Among Mexican-American College Students." *Journal of the American Dietetic Association.* Vol. 100, No. 11, November 2000, p. 1399.

32. Glanz, Karen. "Reducing Chronic Diseases Risk Through Nutrition." *Facts of Life: Issue Briefing for Health Reporters,* Vol. 5, No. 9, November 2000, p. 2.

33. Knaust, Gretchen, and Irene Foster. "Estimation of Food Guide Pyramid Serving Sizes by College Students." *Family and Consumer Sciences Research Journal,* Vol. 29, No. 2, December 2000, p. 101.

34. Brown, C. Hsing-Kuan. "A Food Display Assignment and Handling Food Models Improves Accuracy of College Students' Estimates of Food Portions." *Journal of The American Dietetic Association,* Vol. 100, No. 9, September 2000, pp. 1063–1064.

35. Weggemans, Rianne, et al. "Dietary Cholesterol from Eggs Increases the Ratio of Total Cholesterol to High-Density Lipoprotein Cholesterol in Humans: A Meta-Analysis." *American Journal of Clinical Nutrition,* Vol. 73, No. 5, May 2001, p. 885.

36. Dietary Reference Intakes: Applications in Dietary Assessment, A Report of the Subcommittees on Interpretation and Uses of Dietary Reference Intakes and Upper Reference Levels of Nutrients, and the Standing Committee on the Scientific Evaluation of Dietary Reference Intakes, Food and Nutrition Board. Washington, DC: National Academy of Sciences, 2001.

37. Shaw, Ann. Personal interview.

38. Marietta, Anne, et al. "Knowledge, Attitudes, and Behaviors of College Students Regarding the 1990 Nutrition Labeling Education Act Food Labels." *Journal of the American Dietetic Association,* Vol. 99, No. 4, April 1999.

39. Reyes, Sonia. "Fast, Functional Fare Fills the Bill." *Brandweek,* Vol. 42, No. 23.

40. McCaffree, Jim. "Herbal Foods: Health and Happiness on a Corn Flake?" Journal of the American Dietetic Association, Vol. 101, No. 4, April 2001, p. 398.

41. "Dietary Guidelines and the Food Guide Pagoda." *Journal of the American Dietetic Association,* Vol. 100, No. 8, August 2000.

42. de Lorgeril, Michel, and Patricia Salen. "Wine, Ethanol, Platelets, and Mediterranean Diet." *Lancet,* Vol. 353, No. 9158, March 27, 1999.

43. Jaret, Peter. "The Perfect Diet." Health, Vol. 15, No. 2, March 2001, p. 142.

44. Schlosser, Eric. *Fast Food Nation.* New York: Simon & Schuster, 2001.

45. Brody, Jane. "Nutrition a Key to Better Health for Elderly." *New York Times,* August 21, 2001.

46. Sato, R., et al. "A Prospective Study of Vitamin C and Cognitive Function in Older Adults." *Gerontologist,* October 15, 2000, p. 218.

47. "Modified Food Guide Pyramid for Adults Age 70+." *Geriatrics,* Vol. 56, No. 1, January 2001, p. 16.

48. Guterl, Fred and William Underhill. "Behind the Science of Mad-Cow Disease." *Bulletin with Newsweek,* Vol. 118, No. 6253, December 2000, p. 88.

49. Moore, David. "Seven in 10 Americans Concerned About Mad Cow and Foot-and-Mouth Diseases Becoming Problem in U.S." *Gallup Poll Monthly,* No. 426, March 2001, p. 63.

6

Eating Patterns and Problems

By the time she went away to college, Gia had lost and gained 10 pounds again and again. During her frantic first semester, Gia never seemed to stop eating. Come spring, she was 12 pounds heavier—and determined to slim down by summer. Gia tried every diet she heard of. For a while, she ate no fat, although she couldn't resist wolfing down entire boxes of no-fat cookies. She started counting carbohydrates and wouldn't eat a single slice of bread or strand of spaghetti. Her favorite was the high-protein diet that allowed her to load up on eggs, bacon, hamburgers, and steak.

Even though Gia began every diet with enthusiasm, she invariably fell off each one. Sooner or later, she started craving the foods she'd been forcing herself to live without. And once she went back to her old eating habits, she felt out of control. When she stepped onto the scale, she weighed more than she did before she went on the diet.

Like Gia, many Americans struggle with their weight. According to federal estimates, 55 percent of Americans aged 20 and older are overweight. In the last thirty years, the prevalence of obesity in adults has increased from nearly 13 percent to 22.5 percent of the population.[1]

Ironically, as average weights have increased, the quest for thinness has become a national obsession. In a society in which slimmer is seen as better, anyone who is less than lean may feel like a failure. Individuals who are overweight or embarrassed by their appearance often assume that they would be happier, sexier, or more successful in thinner bodies. And so they diet. Each year, 15 to 35 percent of Americans go on diets, but no matter how much they lose, 90 to 95 percent regain extra pounds within five years.

This chapter explores our national preoccupation with slimness; explains body mass index (BMI); examines unhealthy eating patterns and eating disorders; tells what obesity is and why excess pounds are dangerous; shows why fad diets don't work; and offers guidelines for how to control weight safely, sensibly, and permanently.

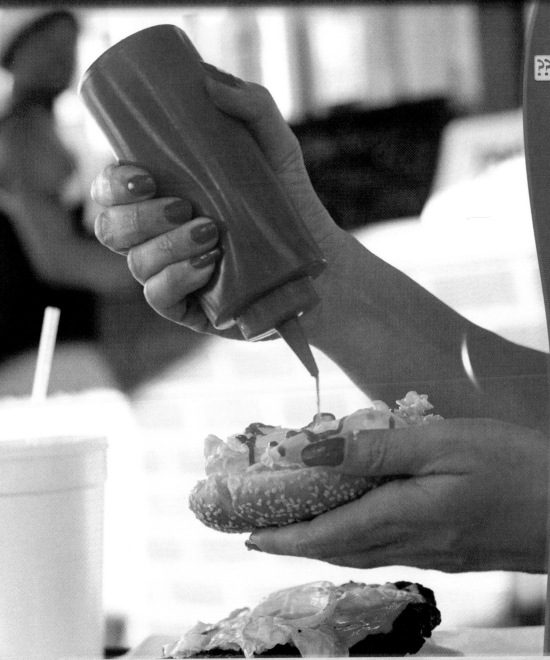

After studying the material in this chapter, you should be able to:

- **Define** body mass index (BMI) and **describe** the different methods of estimating body mass.
- **Identify** several factors that influence food consumption.
- **Discuss** types of unhealthy eating behavior.
- **Identify** and **describe** the symptoms and dangers associated with eating disorders.
- **Define** obesity and **describe** its relationship to genetics, lifestyle, and major health problems.
- **Assess** various approaches to weight loss.
- **Design** a personal plan for sensible weight management.

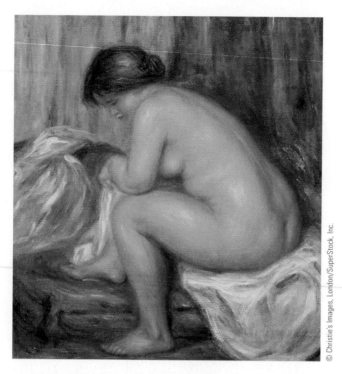

© Christie's Images, London/SuperStock, Inc.

▲ "Thinner is better" is not the global standard, and in past centuries, the fuller figure was considered healthy and beautiful. This painting by Renoir from the late 1880s shows the femnine ideal of the time.

Body Image

Throughout most of history, bigger was better. The great beauties of centuries past, as painted by such artistic masters as Rubens and Renoir, were soft and fleshy, with rounded bellies and dimpled thighs. Culture often shapes views of beauty and health.[2]

 Many developing countries still regard a full figure, rather than a thin one, as the ideal. "Fattening huts," in which brides-to-be eat extra food to plump up before marriage, still exist in some African cultures. Among certain Native Americans of the Southwest, if a girl is thin at puberty, a fat woman places her foot on the girl's back so she will magically gain weight and become more attractive.

Influenced by the media, Americans are paying more attention to their body images than ever before—and at younger ages. In a study of high school girls, those who regularly read women's health and fitness magazines, which may present unrealistic physical "ideals," were more likely to go on low-calorie diets, take pills to suppress their appetites, use laxatives, or force themselves to vomit after eating.[3] In other research, girls who watched a lot of television and expressed concern about slimness and popularity were more dissatisfied with their bodies than girls

involved in sports.[4] Boys' body images also are influenced by media images depicting superstrong, highly muscular males.[5]

African-American women often have more positive attitudes toward their bodies, feeling more satisfied with their weight and seeing themselves as more attractive. However, there are no significant differences between African-American and white women *dieters* in terms of self-esteem and body dissatisfaction.

 College students of different ethnic and racial backgrounds, including Asians, express as much—and sometimes more—concern about their body shape and weight as whites.[6] Men and women are prone to different distortions in body image. Women tend to see themselves as overweight, whether or not they are; men perceive themselves as underweight, even when their weights are normal or above normal.[7]

As men and women age, their attitudes about their bodies change. In a study comparing college students, parents, and grandparents, older men and women were more dissatisfied with their appearance than younger people. Women were more concerned with aging than men, but there were no gender differences in overall body dissatisfaction.[8]

What Should I Weigh?

Many factors determine what you weigh: heredity, eating behavior, food selection, amount of daily exercise. For any individual of a given height, there is no single best weight, but a range of healthy weights. The federal government and medical experts have replaced "ideal weight tables" with a better measure—body mass index (BMI).

Body Mass Index (BMI)

Body mass index (BMI), a ratio between weight and height, is a mathematical formula that correlates with body fat. The BMI numbers apply to both men and women. (See Figure 6-1.) In general, BMI is a better predictor of disease risk than body weight alone.[9] However, certain people should not rely on BMI to estimate their body fat. These include competitive athletes and body builders, whose BMI is high because of a relatively larger amount of muscle, and women who are pregnant or nursing. BMI also is not intended for use in growing children or in frail and sedentary elderly individuals.

If your BMI is high, you may be at increased risk of developing certain diseases, including hypertension, cardiovascular disease, adult-onset diabetes (Type 2), sleep apnea, osteoarthritis, and other conditions. (The section

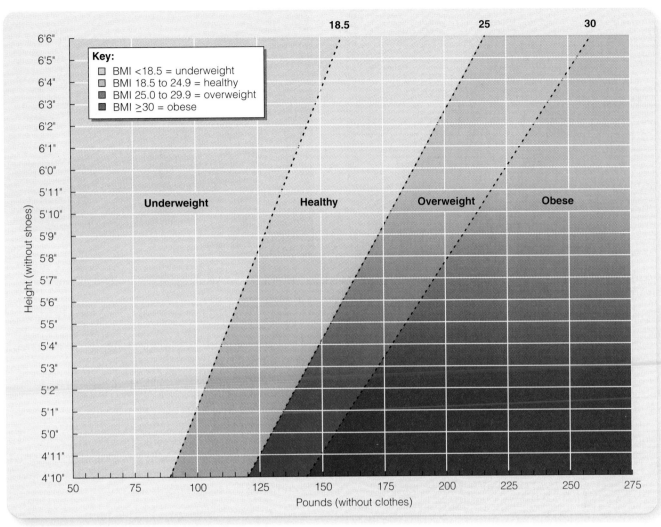

▲ **Figure 6-1** BMI values used to assess weight for adults.

on Being Overweight or Obese discusses the health risks associated with a high BMI.)

You can also calculate your body mass index by following these three simple steps:

1. Multiply your weight in pounds by 703.
2. Multiply your height in inches by itself.
3. Divide the first number by the second and then round up to the nearest whole number. This is your body mass index.

Body Composition Assessment

Tape measurements of various parts of the body, particularly the waist and hips, can provide useful information about body fat and health. Among those with BMIs over 25, men with waists wider than 40 inches and women with

waists wider than 30 inches are at greater risk of heart disease. The danger increases along with the waistline. According to one study, women with waists of 30 inches run twice the risk of heart disease as slimmer women. At 38 inches, the risk is three times higher compared to women with waists of 28 inches or less.[10]

Other methods of assessing body composition include:

❱ *Skinfold fat measurement*, relatively simple and low cost, is a popular method of estimating body composition. The usual sites include the chest, abdomen, and thigh for men, and the triceps, suprailium (hip), and thigh for women. Various equations determine body fat percentage, including calculations that take into account age, gender, race, and other factors. Many types of calipers are available, ranging from research calipers that cost more than $200 to less expensive (but not necessarily

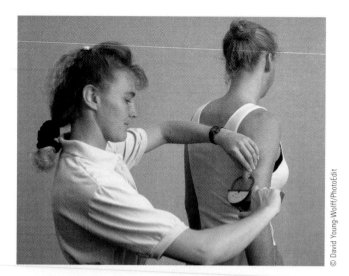 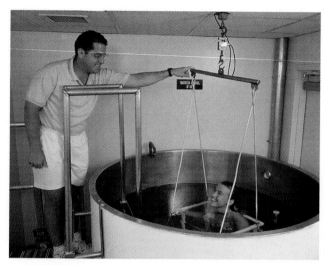

▲ The skinfold test (left) gives a fair approximation of total body fat. Hydrostatic or underwater weighing (right) gives a more accurate measurement.

less accurate) ones that sell for $10 to $50. The skinfold method requires considerable technical skill and precision, and different technicians also may get somewhat different readings from the same person.

▶ *Bioelectrical Impedance Analysis (BIA)* is a noninvasive method for estimating body composition based on the principle that electrical current applied to the body meets greater resistance with different types of tissue. Lean tissue, which contains large amounts of water and electrolytes, is a good electrical conductor; fat, which does not, is a poor conductor. In theory, the easier the electrical conduction, the greater an individual's lean body mass. Although BIA is quick, painless, and safe, some have questioned its accuracy, largely because being overhydrated or underhydrated can throw off the results.

▶ *Hydrostatic (underwater) weighing,* or hydrodensitometry, is a complex and challenging technique based on the Archimedes Principle that a body immersed in a fluid is buoyed by a force equal to the weight of the displaced fluid. Since muscle has a higher density than water and fat has a lower density, fat people tend to displace less water than lean people. The technique is expensive and complex, requiring three underwater weigh-ins to get an accurate reading.

▶ *Dual-energy X-ray absorptiometry (DXA)* uses X rays to quantify the skeletal and soft tissue components of body mass. Whereas other methods are based on variables indirectly related to body composition (such as water content of tissues), DXA provides a direct measurement of body composition. The test itself is simple and quick, usually requiring just 10 to 20 minutes, and radiation dosage is low (800 to 2,000 times lower than a typical chest X ray). Some researchers believe that

DXA will supplant hydrostatic testing as the gold standard for body composition assessment.

▶ *Home body fat analyzers,* hand-held devices and stand-on monitors sold online and in specialty stores, promise to make "reading" your body fat percentage as easy as finding your weight. Prices run as high as several hundred dollars. None has been extensively tested, but those based on bioelectrical impedance analysis may be the most precise The accuracy of devices that use near-infrared (NIR) technology is less certain.

Other approaches used in laboratories and health facilities include the BodPod®, a large, egg-shaped fiberglass chamber that uses an approach based on air displacement plethysmography, that is, the calculation of the relationship between pressure and volume to derive body volume. Computed tomography (CT), magnetic resonance imaging (MRI), and ultrasonography also have been used to evaluate body composition.

ACROSS THE LIFESPAN

Body Composition and Age

According to estimates from the Centers for Disease Control and Prevention, 10 to 15 percent of American children are overweight and overfat. In one study of more than 18,000 children aged 10 to 14, boys and girls of all ethnic backgrounds had higher weights and BMIs than their counterparts did a decade before. They also had higher blood pressures, a troubling trend because elevated pressure often continues into adulthood, increasing the risk of hypertension and heart disease. Accumulation of excess abdominal fat in childhood and adolescence increases the risk of this dangerous pattern of fat storage later in life.[11]

Both weight and body fat percentage typically increase in adulthood. (See Figure 6-2.) Starting in

Age (years)		
20–29	**30–39**	**40–49**
Male 7–17	12–21	14–23

| **Female** 16–24 | 17–25 | 19–28 |

50–59	**60+**
Male 16–24	17–25

| **Female** 22–31 | 22–33 |

▲ **Figure 6-2** Ideal body fat percentages. As we grow older, body fat percentages tend to increase about 5 to 10 percent every decade. An individual whose body fat percentages are outside the ideal range may have a weight problem.

Source: American College of Sports Medicine.

their twenties, American men and women put on an average of 1 pound of weight a year. By age 65, they have gained about 40 pounds. Because activity levels decline with age, the average individual also loses half a pound of fat-free or lean body mass a

year. The result is a dramatic change in body composition over time: a 20-pound loss of lean tissue and a 40-pound gain in body fat.

Body composition can affect how well older individuals function. In a study of women between the ages of 68 and 75, muscle strength was related to fat-free mass. The women with the greatest level of disability had higher BMIs and a higher percentage of body fat. Changes in body composition over time are not inevitable. Researchers have documented that physical activity—both aerobic workouts and resistance exercise—can increase and maintain lean body tissue.

???? How Many Calories Do I Need?

Calories are the measure of the amount of energy that can be derived from food. How many calories you need depends on your gender, age, body-frame size, weight, percentage of body fat, and your **basal metabolic rate (BMR)**—the number of calories needed to sustain your body at rest. An "average" adult woman—with a median height of 5 feet 4 inches and a weight of 138 pounds—generally needs 1,900 to 2,200 calories. An average man—with a median height of 5 feet 10 inches and a weight of 174 pounds—generally consumes 2,300 to 2,900 calories.

Your activity level also affects your calorie requirements. Regardless of whether you consume fat, protein, or carbohydrates, if you take in more calories than required to maintain your size and don't work them off in some sort of physical activity, your body will convert the excess to fat (See Table 6-1).

Hunger, Satiety, and Set Point

Why do you wake up starving or feel your stomach rumbling during a late afternoon lecture? The simple answer is **hunger:** the physiological drive to consume food. More than a dozen different signals may influence and control our desire for food. Researchers at the National Institutes of Health have discovered appetite receptors within the hypothalamus region of the brain that specifically respond to hunger messages carried by chemicals. Hormones, including insulin and stress-related epinephrine (adrenaline), may also stimulate or suppress hunger. Hunger, recent studies show, activates parts of the brain involved with emotions, thinking, and feeling. Even the size of our fat cells may affect how hungry we feel. (Many overweight people have fat cells two to two-and-a-half times larger than normal.)

▼ Body Mass Index (BMI)

Find your height along the lefthand column and look across the row until you find the number that is closest to your weight. The number at the top of that column identifies your BMI. The area shaded in green represents healthy weight ranges. The figure below presents silhouettes of various BMI.

Height	18	19	20	21	22	23	24	25	26	27	28	29	30	31	32	33	34	35	36	37	38	39	40
												Body Weight (pounds)											
4'10"	86	91	96	100	105	110	115	119	124	129	134	138	143	148	153	158	162	167	172	177	181	186	191
4'11"	89	94	99	104	109	114	119	124	128	133	138	143	148	153	158	163	168	173	178	183	188	193	198
5'0"	92	97	102	107	112	118	123	128	133	138	143	148	153	158	163	168	174	179	184	189	194	199	204
5'1"	95	100	106	111	116	122	127	132	137	143	148	153	158	164	169	174	180	185	190	195	201	206	211
5'2"	98	104	109	115	120	126	131	136	142	147	153	158	164	169	175	180	186	191	196	202	207	213	218
5'3"	102	107	113	118	124	130	135	141	146	152	158	163	169	175	180	186	191	197	203	208	214	220	225
5'4"	105	110	116	122	128	134	140	145	151	157	163	169	174	180	186	192	197	204	209	215	221	227	232
5'5"	108	114	120	126	132	138	144	150	156	162	168	174	180	186	192	198	204	210	216	222	228	234	240
5'6"	112	118	124	130	136	142	148	155	161	167	173	179	186	192	198	204	210	216	223	229	235	241	247
5'7"	115	121	127	134	140	146	153	159	166	172	178	185	191	198	204	211	217	223	230	236	242	249	255
5'8"	118	125	131	138	144	151	158	164	171	177	184	190	197	203	210	216	223	230	236	243	249	256	262
5'9"	122	128	135	142	149	155	162	169	176	182	189	196	203	209	216	223	230	236	243	250	257	263	270
5'10"	126	132	139	146	153	160	167	174	181	188	195	202	209	216	222	229	236	243	250	257	264	271	278
5'11"	129	136	143	150	157	165	172	179	186	193	200	208	215	222	229	236	243	250	257	265	272	279	286
6'0"	132	140	147	154	162	169	177	184	191	199	206	213	221	228	235	242	250	258	265	272	279	287	294
6'1"	136	144	151	159	166	174	182	189	197	204	212	219	227	235	242	250	257	265	272	280	288	295	302
6'2"	141	148	155	163	171	179	186	194	202	210	218	225	233	241	249	256	264	272	280	287	295	303	311
6'3"	144	152	160	168	176	184	192	200	208	216	224	232	240	248	256	264	272	279	287	295	303	311	319
6'4"	148	156	164	172	180	189	197	205	213	221	230	238	246	254	263	271	279	287	295	304	312	320	328
6'5"	151	160	168	176	185	193	202	210	218	227	235	244	252	261	269	277	286	294	303	311	319	328	336
6'6"	155	164	172	181	190	198	207	216	224	233	241	250	259	267	276	284	293	302	310	319	328	336	345

Under-weight (<18.5) **Healthy Weight** (18.5–24.9) **Overweight** (25–29.9) **Obese** (≥30)

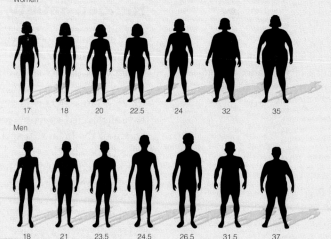

Women
17 18 20 22.5 24 32 35

Men
18 21 23.5 24.5 26.5 31.5 37

Source: Reprinted from "The Body Test" (1988). © Dietitians of Canada.

▼ Table 6-1	How Many Calories Do You Need Daily?		
Desirable Weight (lb)	High Activity	Medium Activity	Low Activity
Women			
99	1700	1500	1300
110	1850	1650	1400
121	2000	1750	1550
128	2100	1900	1600
132	2150	1950	1650
143	2300	2050	1800
154	2400	2150	1850
165	2550	2300	1950
Men			
121	2400	2150	1850
132	2550	2300	1950
143	2700	2400	2050
154	2900	2600	2200
165	3100	2800	2400
176	3250	2950	2500
187	3300	3100	2600

Appetite—the psychological desire to eat—usually begins with the fear of the unpleasant sensation of hunger. We learn to avoid hunger by eating a certain amount of food at certain times of the day, just as dogs in the laboratory learn to avoid electric shocks by jumping at the sound of a warning bell. But appetite is easily led into temptation. In one famous experiment, psychologists bought bags of high-calorie goodies—peanut butter, marshmallows, chocolate-chip cookies, and salami—for their test rats. The animals ate so much on this "supermarket diet" that they gained more weight than any laboratory rats ever had before. The snack-food diet that fattened up these rats was particularly high in fats. Biologists speculate that creamy, buttery, or greasy foods may cause internal changes that increase appetite and, consequently, weight.

We stop eating when we feel satisfied; this is called **satiety,** a feeling of fullness and relief from hunger. According to the **set-point theory,** each individual has an unconscious control system for regulating appetite and satiety to keep body fat at a predetermined level, or *set point*. If our fat stores fall too low, our appetite gnaws at us, so we eat more. Conversely, appetite subsides if we overeat.

From this perspective, diets are doomed to fail because they pit the dieter against tireless internal enemies: the set point and its enforcer, appetite. The only effective alternative is lowering, or resetting, the set point. And the safest, most effective way to do so is through physical activity, which dampens appetite in the short run and lowers the set point for the long term. As discussed later in this chapter, moderate activity not only works up an appetite but also helps work it off.

Unhealthy Eating Behavior

Unhealthy eating behavior can take many forms, from not eating enough to eating too much too quickly. Its roots are complex. In addition to media and external pressures, a family history can play a role. Researchers have linked a specific gene to some cases of anorexia nervosa, but most believe that a variety of factors, including stress and culture, combine to cause disordered eating.[12]

About a third of female athletes in every sport show symptoms of disordered eating or eating disorders.[13] Girls and adolescent females who participate regularly in sports are at risk for disordered eating, menstrual dysfunction, and decreased bone mineral density, according to the American Academy of Pediatrics. The combination of these three disorders is known as the "female athlete triad."[14]

Sooner or later many people *don't* eat the way they should. They may skip meals, thereby increasing the likelihood that they'll end up with more body fat, a higher weight, and a higher blood cholesterol level. Others live on "diet" foods, but consume so much of them that they gain weight anyway. Yet others engage in more extreme eating behavior—dissatisfied with almost all aspects of their appearance, they continuously go on and off diets, eat compulsively, or binge on high-fat treats.[15] Such behaviors can be warning signs of potentially serious eating disorders that should not be ignored.

Disordered Eating in College Students

College students—particularly women, including varsity athletes—are at risk for unhealthy eating behaviors. The prevalence of disordered eating symptoms and eating disorders has increased dramatically in the last 20 years. One reason may be the pressure some young women feel to attain what some have called the "Superwoman" ideal. As they try to excel in multiple roles, they diet, induce vomiting, or restrict food intake for the sake of meeting their idealized standards for appearance.

 The unique demands and stressors of the transition to college do not increase the likelihood of disordered eating for all freshmen. One study that followed more than 100 undergraduate women through their freshman year found that those who reported the most body dissatisfaction and unhealthy eating patterns at the beginning of the first semester were most likely to experience more eating problems, such as losing control of their eating when feeling strong emotions. The strongest predictor that eating symptoms would get worse over the freshman year was not BMI or weight, but body dissatisfaction.[16]

The most common weight-related problem on campuses may be gaining weight, particularly in the first year away from home. Students of both sexes and all racial and ethnic groups are susceptible. According to one study, even international students gain weight and body fat after arriving on American campuses. Ohio University researchers found that after 20 weeks, foreign students, who had incorporated foods high in fat, salt, and sugar into their diets, gained about 3 pounds on average and their percentage of body fat rose by about 5 percent.[17] (See Student Snapshot: "The Freshman 4.5.")

Extreme Dieting

About half of girls attempt to control their weight by dieting.[18] In a year-long study of teenagers, both parents and the media had the most influence on the development of weight concerns and weight control practices, including dieting, among adolescents and preadolescents.[19]

"Extreme" dieters go beyond cutting back on calories or increasing physical activity and become preoccupied with what they eat and weigh. Although their weight never falls below 85 percent of normal, their weight loss is severe enough to cause uncomfortable physical consequences, such as weakness and sensitivity to cold. Technically, these dieters do not have *anorexia nervosa* (discussed later in the chapter), but they are at increased risk for it.

Extreme dieters may think they know a great deal about nutrition, yet many of their beliefs about food and weight are misconceptions or myths. For instance, they may eat only protein because they believe complex carbohydrates, including fruits and breads, are fattening. When they're anxious, angry, or bored, they focus on food and their fear of fatness. Dieting and exercise become ways of coping with any stress in their lives.

Sometimes nutritional education alone can help change this eating pattern. However, many avid dieters who deny that they have a problem with food may need counseling (which they usually agree to only at their family's insistence) to correct dangerous eating behavior and prevent further complications.

Compulsive Overeating

Individuals who eat compulsively cannot stop putting food in their mouths. They eat fast; they eat a lot; they eat even when they're full; and they may eat round the clock rather than at set meal times—often in private because of embarrassment over how much they consume.

Some mental health professionals describe compulsive eating as a food addiction that is much more likely to develop

Student Snapshot The Freshman 4.5

Eating on their own for the first time, many first-year undergraduates put on weight—often dubbed the infamous "Freshman Fifteen." How common are changes in weight and eating habits among freshmen? These findings are from a recent study that followed more than 100 women, who began the year at normal weights, for seven months.

Mean BMI at the beginning of freshman year	22.8
Percent who said they would like to weigh less	94%
Difference in actual and ideal weights	14.56 pounds
Mean weight gain after seven months	4.5 pounds

Source: Cooley, Eric, Tamina Toray. "Disordered Eating in College Freshman Women: A Prospective Study." *Journal of American College Health,* Vol. 49, No. 5, March, 2001, p. 229.

in women. According to Overeaters Anonymous (OA), an international support agency, many women who eat compulsively view food as a source of comfort against feelings of inner emptiness, low self-esteem, and fear of abandonment.

The following behaviors may signal a potential problem:

▶ Turning to food when depressed or lonely, when feeling rejected, or as a reward.

▶ A history of failed diets and anxiety when dieting.

▶ Thinking about food throughout the day.

▶ Eating quickly and without pleasure.

▶ Frequent talking about food, or refusing to talk about food.

▶ Fear of not being able to stop eating once you start. Continuing to eat even when you're no longer hungry.

Recovery from compulsive eating can be challenging because people with this problem cannot give up entirely the "substance" they abuse. Like everyone else, they must eat. However, they can learn new eating habits and ways of dealing with underlying emotional problems. An OA survey found that most of its members joined to lose weight but later felt the most important effect was their improved emotional, mental, and physical health. As one woman put it, "I came for vanity but stayed for sanity."

Binge Eating and Binge Eating Disorder

Binge eating—the rapid consumption of an abnormally large amount of food in a relatively short time—often occurs in compulsive eaters. Individuals with a binge-eating disorder typically eat a larger-than-ordinary amount of food during a relatively brief period, feel a lack of control over eating, and binge at least twice a week for at least a six-month period.[20] During most of these episodes, individuals experience at least three of the following:

▶ Eating much more rapidly than usual.

▶ Eating until they feel uncomfortably full.

▶ Eating large amounts of food when not feeling physically hungry.

▶ Eating large amounts of food throughout the day with no planned mealtimes.

▶ Eating alone because they are embarrassed by how much they eat and by their eating habits.

In a review of the research on dieting, eating disorders, and weight problems, the National Task Force on the Prevention and Treatment of Obesity found that moderate restriction of calories, combined with behavioral approaches, does not cause binge eating in overweight adults who do not already have a binge eating problem. In adults, dieting does not seem to induce bingeing or eating disorders.[21]

Binge eaters may spend up to several hours eating, and consume 2,000 or more calories worth of food in a single binge—more than many people eat in a day. After such binges, they usually do not induce vomiting, use laxatives, or rely on other means (such as exercise) to control weight. They simply get fatter. As their weight climbs, they become depressed, anxious, or troubled by other psychological symptoms to a much greater extent than others of comparable weight.[22]

About 2 percent of Americans—some 5 million in all—may have binge-eating disorder. It is most common among young women in college and, increasingly, in high school. There is a strong connection between women with binge-eating disorder—characterized by episodes of bingeing without purging—and feelings of marked rejection from their fathers.[23] Persons who binge-eat may require professional help to change their behavior. Treatment includes education, behavioral approaches, cognitive therapy, and psychotherapy. As they recognize the reasons for their behavior and begin to confront the underlying issues, individuals usually are able to resume normal eating patterns.

Eating Disorders

According to the American Psychiatric Association, patients with **eating disorders** display a broad range of

---

STRATEGIES FOR PREVENTION

Do You Have an Eating Disorder?

Physicians have developed a simple screening test for eating disorders, consisting of the following questions:

✔ Do you make yourself sick because you feel uncomfortably full?

✔ Do you worry you have lost control over how much you eat?

✔ Have you recently lost more than 14 pounds in a three-month period?

✔ Do you believe yourself to be fat when others say you are too thin?

✔ Would you say that food dominates your life?

Score one point for every "yes"—a score of two or more is a likely indication of anorexia nervosa or bulimia.[24]

symptoms that occur along a continuum between those of anorexia nervosa and those of bulimia nervosa.[25] The best known are anorexia nervosa, which affects fewer than 1 percent of adolescent women, and bulimia nervosa, which strikes 2 to 3 percent. Many more young women do not have the characteristic symptoms of these disorders but are preoccupied with their weight or experiment with unhealthy forms of dieting. (See Table 6-2 for major risk factors.)

The American Psychiatric Association has developed practice guidelines for the treatment of patients with eating disorders, which include medical, psychological, and behavioral approaches. One of the most scientifically supported is cognitive-behavioral therapy, described in Chapter 3.[26]

Who Develops Eating Disorders?

Eating disorders affect an estimated 5 to 10 million women and 1 million men. Most people with these problems are young (from ages 14 to 25), white, and affluent,

▼ Table 6-2 Major Risk Factors for Eating Disorders
Biological
Dieting
Obesity/overweight/pubertal weight gain
Psychological
Body image/dissatisfaction/distortions
Low self-esteem
Obsessive-compulsive symptoms
Childhood sexual abuse
Family
Parental attitudes and behaviors
Parental comments regarding appearance
Eating-disordered mothers
Misinformation about ideal weight
Sociocultural
Peer pressure regarding weight/eating
Media: TV, magazines
Distorted images: toys
Elite athletes as at-risk groups

Source: White, Jane. "The Prevention of Eating Disorders: A Review of the Research on Risk Factors with Implications for Practice." *Journal of Child and Adolescent Psychiatric Nursing,* Vol. 13, No. 2, April 2000.

with perfectionistic personalities. According to the Eating Disorders Awareness and Prevention Group of Seattle, 5 to 7 percent of American undergraduates suffer from eating disorders.[27]

 Despite past evidence that eating disorders were primarily problems for white women, they are increasing among men and members of different ethnic and racial groups.[28] (See The X&Y Files: "Men, Women, and Weight.") In the few studies of eating disorders in minority college students that have been completed, African-American female undergraduates had a slightly lower prevalence of eating disorders than whites. Asian Americans reported fewer symptoms of eating disorders but more body dissatisfaction, concerns about shape, and more intense efforts to lose weight.

In one recent study, researchers analyzed the importance of BMI in evaluating eating disorders in different ethnic groups. The BMIs of Hispanics are generally higher than those of whites, and more Hispanics are categorized as overweight. Asians, as a group, weigh less than whites. In the study, college women with higher BMIs were most concerned about their weights and shapes—regardless of their ethnic backgrounds. Data on Hispanics, Asians, and whites of similar weights show equivalent concern about their weight.[29]

 In a survey of health care professionals at the country's largest colleges and universities, 70 percent said that eating disorders are common among their undergraduates; 11 percent said they were widespread; 19 percent described them as rare. Almost half (45 percent) felt that the incidence of eating disorders on their campuses had increased over the last five years; just 2 percent felt that the incidence had decreased. While 99 percent of the schools surveyed provide general mental health services, 69 percent have professionals on staff who specialize in diagnosing and treating eating disorders. Of all the hurdles to helping students with eating disorders, 39 percent said denial is the biggest, while 24 percent felt it was unwillingness to seek treatment, and 20 percent blamed pressure from peers and the media to stay thin.[30]

Eating disorders affect every aspect of college students' lives, including dating. Both men and women tend to avoid dating individuals with eating disorders, but men are far less accepting of obesity than women. In one study, 74 percent of men and 60 percent of women reported being uncomfortable dating someone who is obese. A smaller percentage—53 percent of the men and 59 percent of the women—said they wouldn't want to date a person with an eating disorder.[31]

Male and female athletes are vulnerable to eating disorders, either because of the pressure to maintain ideal body weight or to achieve a weight that might enhance their performance. Many female athletes, particularly those participating in sports or activities that emphasize

The X&Y Files — Men, Women, and Weight

Women have long been bombarded by the media with idealized images of female bodies that bear little resemblance to the way most women look. Increasingly, more advertisements and men's magazines are featuring idealized male bodies. Sleek, strong, and sculpted, they too do not resemble the bodies most men inhabit. The gap between reality and ideal is getting bigger for both genders.

In the last decade, numerous studies have shown that women in *Playboy* centerfolds and Miss America pageants weigh less than they did in the 1970s. In one analysis, 29 percent of *Playboy* centerfolds and 17 percent of Miss America pageant winners had BMIs below 17.5, one of the criteria for anorexia nervosa and a definite indication of being severely underweight.

As beauty pageant queens and female models have been shrinking, the men featured in *Playgirl* centerfolds have been bulking up. Their BMIs are higher than in the past—as are the BMIs of a sample of Canadian and American men between the ages of 18 and 24. Researchers do not know if the higher BMIs are the result of an increase in lean body mass or body fat. Their theory: The models have gotten more muscular over time, accounting for their high BMIs, while real guys may simply have gotten fatter.

When college men and women step on a scale or look in a mirror, they react in different ways. In a study of 525 undergraduates, the women failed to see themselves as underweight, even when they were, and perceived themselves as overweight, even when when they were not. Many of the women who considered themselves normal weight nonetheless desired to be thinner. Men in the study generally saw themselves as underweight, even when they were not. Most desired to be heavier, though not obese. Both women yearning to be thinner and men wanting to be heavier were equally likely to experience what the researchers dubbed "social physique anxiety."

Both genders are prone to eating disorders, which are increasing in men and in various racial and ethnic groups. Men and women with these problems share many psychological similarities and experience similar symptoms. However, the men are more likely to have other psychiatric disorders and are less likely to seek professional treatment. Some feel that eating disorders fall under the category of "women's diseases." Others may not recognize the symptoms because eating disorders have long been assumed to plague women only.

Sources: Hales, Dianne. *Just Like a Woman.* New York: Bantam Books, 2000. Lofton, Stacy, and Tim Bungum. "Attitudes and Behaviors Toward Weight, Body Shape,and Eating in Male and Female College Students." *Research Quarterly for Exercise and Sport,* Vol. 72, No. 1, March 2001, p. A-32. Emslie, C, et al. "Perceptions of Body Image Among Working Men and Women." *Journal of Epidemiology & Community Health* Vol. 55, No. 6, June 2001, p. 406.

leanness (such as gymnastics, distance running, diving, figure skating, and classical ballet) have "subclinical" eating disorders that could undermine their nutritional status and energy levels. However, there is often little awareness or recognition of their disordered eating.

If someone you know has an eating disorder, let your friend know you're concerned and that you care. Don't criticize or make fun of his or her eating habits. Encourage your friend to talk about other problems and feelings, and suggest that he or she talk to the school counselor or someone at the mental health center, the family doctor, or another trusted adult. Offer to go along if you think that will make a difference.

Anorexia Nervosa

Although anorexia means loss of appetite, most individuals with **anorexia nervosa** are, in fact, hungry all the time. For them, food is an enemy—a threat to their sense of self, identity, and autonomy. In the distorted mirror of their mind's eye, they see themselves as fat or flabby even at a normal or below-normal body weight. Some simply feel fat; others think that they are thin in some places and too fat in others, such as the abdomen, buttocks, or thighs.

The incidence of anorexia nervosa has increased in the last three decades in most developed countries. An estimated 0.5 to 1 percent of young women in their late teens and early twenties develop anorexia. According to the American Psychiatric Association (APA)'s Work Group on Eating Disorders, cases are increasing among males, minorities, women of all ages, and possibly preteens.

In the *restricting* type of anorexia, individuals lose weight by avoiding any fatty foods, and by dieting, fasting, and exercising. Some start smoking as a way of controlling their weight. In the *binge eating/purging* type, they engage in binge eating, purging (through self-induced vomiting, laxatives, diuretics, or enemas), or both. Obsessed with an intense fear of fatness, they may weigh themselves several times a day, measure various parts of their body, check mirrors to see if they look fat, and try on different items of clothing to see if they feel tight.

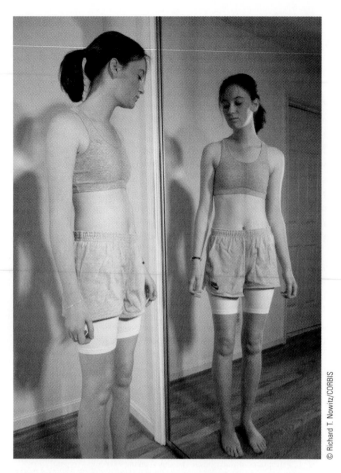

Richard T. Nowitz/CORBIS

▲ Anorexia nervosa is complex in its cause and in its treatment, which usually requires medical, nutritional, and behavioral therapies.

What Causes Anorexia Nervosa?

Many complex factors interact and contribute to this disorder, including biological, psychological, and social ones. Anorexia is more common among close relatives, particularly sisters, than it is in the general population. The relatives of anorexics also have a higher than expected frequency of depressive disorders.

Anorexia is associated with changes within the brain, including abnormalities in the stress-hormone cortisol, the neurotransmitters dopamine, serotonin, and norepinephrine—all of which influence appetite and satiety—and the peptide cholecystokinin, which affects feelings of fullness. It is not clear whether these changes are a cause or a consequence of this disorder.

Anorexia also may be a response to a personal loss or a sign of a driven, perfectionist personality. Often young anorexics have above-average grades and an unwarranted fear of failure. Some theorists speculate that young teenage girls may starve themselves because of fear of their bud-

ding sexuality. By drastically reducing their weight, they can prevent or stop menstruation and breast development.

Girls who develop anorexia often have little insight or awareness of their feelings, needs, and wants. After years of reacting to the expectations of others, they may feel inadequate as they approach the age of independence. In some ways, starvation may serve as a way of creating an identity and asserting independence.

 In one study that followed 21 college women with eating disorders for six years, 11 got better during their post-college years, while 10 continued to struggle with disordered eating. The major difference between the two groups revolved around issues of autonomy and relation. These who could better negotiate the tension between being independent and relating to others had higher self-esteem, a more positive self-concept, and a healthier relationship with food.

About one-third of those with anorexia initially were mildly overweight and cut back on food just to lose a few pounds. Others had normal weights but began to diet to look more attractive or, in the case of male and female athletes and dancers, to gain a performance advantage. Sometimes, illness, stress, or surgery triggers weight loss. Often the initial response to their weight loss—from parents, coaches, or friends—is positive. However, starvation seems to take on a life of its own, and anorexics cannot return to a healthy eating pattern. In time, they may place so much value on thinness that they cannot recognize the dangers to their health.

Recognizing and Treating Anorexia Nervosa

The characteristics of anorexia nervosa include:

▷ A refusal to maintain normal body weight.
▷ An intense fear of gaining weight or becoming fat, even though underweight.
▷ A distorted body image, so that the person feels fat even when emaciated.
▷ In women, the absence of at least three menstrual cycles.

The medical consequences of anorexia nervosa are serious (See Table 6-3). Menstrual periods stop in women; testosterone levels decline in men. Adolescents with this disorder do not undergo normal sexual maturation, such as breast development, and may not reach their anticipated height. Even individuals who look and feel reasonably healthy may have subtle or hidden abnormalities, including heart irregularities and arrhythmias that can increase their risk of sudden death. Women who do not menstruate for six months or more may develop osteoporosis and suffer irreversible weakening and thinning of their bones as a result.

▼ **Table 6-3** **Medical Complications of Eating Disorders**

Related to Weight Loss

Loss of fat and muscle mass, including heart muscle
Increased sensitivity to cold
Irregular heartbeats
Bloating, constipation, abdominal pain
Amenorrhea (absence of menstruation)
Growth of fine babylike hair over body
Abnormal taste sensations
Osteoporosis
Depression
Sudden death

Related to Purging

Abnormal levels of crucial chemicals
Inflammation of the salivary glands and pancreas
Erosion of the esophagus and stomach
Severe abdominal pain
Erosion and decay of dental enamel, particularly of
    front teeth
Fatigue and weakness
Seizures

Even when they realize that they are jeopardizing their health, people with anorexia tend to fear that treatment will make them worse—that is, fatter. They need repeated reassurance that they will not become overweight and that they can and will find healthier ways of coping with life.

According to current practice guidelines, treatment of anorexia nervosa includes medical therapy (such as "refeeding" to overcome malnutrition) and behavioral, cognitive, psychodynamic, and family therapy.[32] Antidepressant medication sometimes can help, particularly when there is a personal or family history of depression. Most people who get help do return to normal weight, but it can take a long time for their eating behaviors to become normal and for them to deal with troubling body image issues. In a study that followed 95 patients with anorexia, about half—56 percent—had no symptoms of an eating disorder after five years; three had died.[33]

Bulimia Nervosa

Individuals with **bulimia nervosa** go on repeated eating binges and rapidly consume large amounts of food, usually sweets, stopping only because of severe abdominal pain or sleep, or because they are interrupted. Those with *purging* bulimia induce vomiting or take large doses of laxatives to relieve guilt and control their weight. In *nonpurging* bulimia, individuals use other means, such as fasting or excessive exercise, to compensate for binges.

According to the DSM-IV, 1 to 3 percent of adolescent and young American women develop bulimia. Some experiment with bingeing and purging for a few months and then stop when they change their social or living situation. Others develop longer-term bulimia. Among males, this disorder is about one-tenth as common. The average age for developing bulimia is 18.

What Causes Bulimia Nervosa?

Bulimia usually begins after a rigid diet that lasted from several weeks to a year or more. Strict dieting may affect brain chemistry in such a way as to disrupt the normal mechanisms for appetite and satiety. Semi-starvation eventually sets off a binge; bingeing leads to purging. Once dieters realize that vomiting reduces the anxiety triggered by gorging, they no longer fear overeating. When this happens, bingeing may become more frequent and severe until, in time, it becomes an all-purpose way of coping with stress. However, the driving force in this disorder may not be the overeating but the vomiting or laxative use. If individuals felt they couldn't get rid of food, they might not overeat.[34]

Obesity in adolescence may increase the likelihood of bulimia in adulthood. Extremely obese individuals may lose weight by vomiting and not want to stop because they fear regaining it. Sometimes bulimia develops after recovery from anorexia. Purging becomes an alternative way of staying thin.

As with anorexia, bulimia is associated with changes in brain chemistry, particularly low levels of the peptide cholescystokinin, which produces feelings of satiety. The cycle of bingeing and purging seems to wreak havoc on the biological controls that keep weight at a certain level.

Family conflicts, life stresses such as going away to school, and struggles with the transition to independent adulthood also may play a role. Bulimia also may be a symptom of depression. About 20 to 30 percent of those with this problem are chronically depressed; others have a history of depressive episodes. Bulimic individuals also are more likely to experience other problems, including anxiety disorders, substance abuse, and impulse disorders, such as shoplifting (kleptomania) and cutting themselves. A significant percentage of bulimics—from a quarter to a half, by some estimates—may have been victims of incest, sexual molestation, or rape, but this correlation is controversial.

Recognizing and Treating Bulimia Nervosa

The characteristics of bulimia nervosa include:

▶ Repeated binge eating.
▶ A feeling of lack of control over eating behavior.

▶ Regular reliance on self-induced vomiting, laxatives, or diuretics.

▶ Strict dieting or fasting, or vigorous exercise, to prevent weight gain.

▶ A minimum average of two bingeing episodes a week for at least three months.

▶ A preoccupation with body shape and weight.

Bulimia may continue for many years, with binges alternating with periods of normal eating. Often dentists are the first to detect bulimia because they notice damage to teeth and gums, including erosion of the enamel from the stomach acids in vomit. Repeated vomiting can lead to other complications as it robs the body of essential nutrients and fluids, causes dehydration and electrolyte imbalances, and impairs the ability of the heart and other muscles to function. Bulimia can trigger cardiac arrhythmias and, occasionally, sudden death.

Most mental health professionals treat bulimia with a combination of nutritional counseling, psychodynamic, cognitive-behavioral therapy, individual or group psychotherapy, and medication. The drug most often prescribed is an antidepressant medication such as fluoxetine (Prozac), which increases levels of the neurotransmitter serotonin. About 70 percent of those who complete treatment programs reduce their bingeing and purging, although flareups are common in times of stress.

Being Overweight or Obese

The federal government has developed clinical guidelines that have changed the definition of what it means to be overweight or obese by focusing on body composition. Based on the most extensive review ever of the scientific evidence, the guidelines shift focus away from body weight—the numbers on the scale—to body mass index (BMI), waist circumference, and individual risk factors for diseases and conditions associated with obesity.

The guidelines define **overweight** as a BMI of 25 to 29.9 and **obese** as a BMI of 30 and above (see Figure 6-1). As noted earlier, very muscular individuals may have a high BMI yet not be overweight or obese.

The risk for cardiovascular and other disease rises significantly in individuals with BMIs above 25; the risk of premature death increases when BMI reaches 30 or above. As BMI levels rise, average blood pressure and total cholesterol levels increase, and average "good" or HDL cholesterol declines. Men in the highest **obesity** category have more than twice the risk of hypertension, high blood cholesterol, or both compared with men whose BMIs are in the healthy range. Women in the highest obesity category have four times the risk.

In addition to BMI, individuals also should be aware of any other risk factors, such as a family history of obesity-related disease, and discuss them with a physician. These additional risks may require more vigilance about weight and more intensive efforts to keep BMI in a healthy range.

 Although more people in certain regions of the country are likely to be heavy, obesity affects all racial and ethnic groups. A third of white American women are obese—as are nearly 50 percent of African-American and Hispanic/Latino women. In some Native American communities, up to 70 percent of all adults are dangerously overweight. Differences in metabolic rates may be one factor.[35]

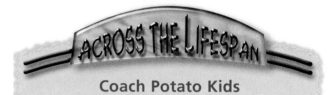

Coach Potato Kids

Not only are there more overweight children, but they're more likely to be severely obese. Many have ominously high blood pressures and cholesterol levels. Sometimes their legs are bowing or their hips require pinning because of the weight they have to carry.

What's supersizing America's children? "There's a snowball effect," says Dr. Deborah Rotenstein, director of pediatric endocrinology at Allegheny Medical Center in Pittsburgh. "Kids have what I call 'automobile feet'; they don't walk anywhere. They spend more time in front of televisions and computers. Foods are fast, instantly available, and high in calories."[36]

A substantial number of children are prone to gaining weight because their mothers developed gestational diabetes during their pregnancies. "Gestational diabetes is a sleeping giant that sets up abnormal glucose (blood sugar) regulation and greatly increases a child's risk of being obese," says Dr. Rotenstein, noting there are always individual differences in rate of metabolism. "Two kids may eat the exact same amount yet only one will be chubby. You can't change genes, but you can change habits."

Change is exactly what doctors, alarmed by the present and future perils of childhood obesity, are prescribing for the most sedentary generation in history. According to federal data, today's children consume about 200 calories more than youngsters did a decade ago—the equivalent of a large soda or juice drink. "That may not seem like much," observes Dr. Christine Williams, director of the Children's Cardiovascular Health Center at Columbia University, "but it takes a lot of exercise—about 40 minutes of brisk walking—to burn up 200 calories." And today's kids are more likely to be on their seats than their feet. On average, grade-schoolers watch five hours of television a day; many spend additional time playing video games and computer games.[37]

The Centers for Disease Control and Prevention recommend that children engage in a minimum of 30 to 60 minutes of physical activity every day, including at least 10 to 15 minutes of exercise rigorous enough to speed up the heart beat.

Waist-Hip Ratio: Apples Versus Pears

The **waist-hip ratio,** which considers the distribution of weight and the location of excess fat, also is important. Excess weight around the abdominal area, creating an "apple shaped" silhouette, is associated with increased cardiovascular risk for both men and women.[38] (See Figure 6-3.) A waist circumference of more than 40 inches in men and more than 35 inches in women signifies an increased risk in those with BMIs over 25.

Many women accumulate excess pounds in their hips and thighs, giving them a "pear" shape. This fat, stored primarily for special purposes such as pregnancy and nursing, is more difficult to lose. When men and women diet, men lose more visceral fat located around the abdominal area. This weight loss produces more cardiovascular benefits for men,

including a decrease in triglycerides (fats circulating in the blood) and an increase in the "good" form of cholesterol, high-density lipoprotein (HDL).[39]

???? What Causes Obesity?

Are some people fated to be fat? Scientists have identified a gene for a protein that signals the brain to halt food intake or to step up metabolic rate to make use of extra calories. If this gene is defective or malfunctions, it could contribute to weight problems. The discovery of a genetic predisposition to excess weight could explain, at least in part, why children with obese parents tend to be obese themselves, especially if both parents are obese.[40] (See Genes in Focus: "The Genetics of Obesity.")

A protein named leptin also may play a role. When laboratory mice are injected with high doses of leptin, they initially decrease their food intake, increase their metabolic rate, and become much thinner. Eventually, the body adapts to the high levels of leptin and becomes resistant to its effects. However, human studies have had contradictory results.[41] Some suggest that increased leptin does not cause, but is caused by, obesity.

Scientists now realize that obesity is a complex and serious disorder with multiple causes, including:

▶ **Developmental factors.** Some obese people have a high number of fat cells, others have large fat cells, and the most severely obese have both more and larger fat cells. Whereas the size of fat cells can increase at any time in life, the number is set during childhood, possibly as the result of genetics or overfeeding at a young age.

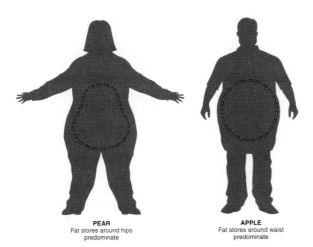

PEAR
Fat stores around hips predominate

APPLE
Fat stores around waist predominate

▲ **Figure 6-3** Pear- versus Apple-Shaped Bodies

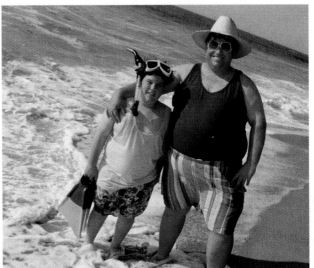

▲ Heredity plays a role in the tendency toward obesity, but so do environment and behavior.

GENES IN FOCUS

The Genetics of Obesity

Are some children fated to be fat? To find the answer, pediatrician Robert Whitaker, M.D., of the University of Cincinnati Medical Center tracked the weights of 854 individuals from birth into young adulthood and of their parents. "Parents and children share genes and the same environment, and both have an impact," says Dr. Whitaker, who found that having one obese parent doubles the likelihood that a child under age ten will be obese. (See Table 6-4.)

▼ Table 6-4	Risk of Adult Obesity (age 21–29) Based on Childhood or Parent Obesity	
Age of child (years)	**Risk of adult obesity**	
Child not obese	**Parents not obese**	**Parents obese**
1–2	10%	28%
3–5	8%	23%
6–9	7%	17%
10–14	8%	15%
15–17	5%	14%
Age of child (years)	**Risk of adult obesity**	
Child obese	**Parents not obese**	**Parents obese**
1–2	8%	40%
3–5	24%	62%
6–9	37%	71%
10–14	64%	79%
15–17	54%	73%

A child's age also affects the likelihood that fatness will persist. A chubby-cheeked baby is not at greater risk of becoming an obese adult than a leaner one. After age three, the odds change. "The older that overweight kids are, the more likely they are to remain heavy as adults," says Dr. Whitaker. Children who are obese at ages 10 to 14 have a 64 percent chance of being obese as adults—six times the risk of their thinner peers. If at least one parent is fat, the chance of these youngsters continuing to be heavy rises to 73 percent.

"What's critical is the interaction between genes and environment," says Dr. Steve Gitelman, a pediatric endocrinologist at the University of California, San Francisco, who explains that most people have genes that make them susceptible to putting on pounds in the wrong environment. "And we are def-initely living in the wrong environment. We spend less energy and burn up fewer calories to obtain our foods. At any age, people gain weight whenever there's an energy imbalance between the calories they take in and the calories they use."

Sources: Whitaker, Robert. Personel interview. Gitelman, Steve. Personal interview. Hales, Dianne. "When Children Are Too Fat." *Parade*, January 7, 2001, p. 14. Kolata, Gina. "As Children Grow Fatter, Researchers Try to Find Solutions." *New York Times*, October 19, 2000.

▶ **Social determinants.** In affluent countries, people in lower socioeconomic classes tend to be more obese. For reasons unknown, those in the upper classes, who can afford as much food as they want, tend to be leaner. Education may be a factor.

▶ **Physical activity.** Obesity tends to go with a sedentary lifestyle. In those countries where many people tend to work at physically demanding jobs, obesity is rare. Physical activity prevents obesity by increasing caloric expenditure, decreasing food intake, and increasing metabolic rate.

▶ **Emotional influences.** Obese people are neither more nor less psychologically troubled than others. Psychological problems, such as irritability, depression, and anxiety, are more likely to be the result of obesity than the cause. However, emotions do play some role in weight problems. Just as some people reach for a drink or a drug when they're upset, others cope by overeating, bingeing, or purging.

▶ **Lifestyle.** People who watch more than three hours of TV a day are twice as likely to be obese as those who watch less than an hour. Even those who log between one and two hours are fatter than those who watch just one. Researchers don't know if TV watching causes obesity or if obese people watch more TV, but they have found that the more TV that viewers watch, the less physically active and fit they are.

The Dangers of Obesity

Obesity has long been singled out as a major health threat that increases the risk of many chronic diseases. During ten years of follow-up of middle-aged men and women, the incidence of diabetes, gallstones, hypertension, heart disease, and colon cancer increased with the degree of overweight in both sexes. Overweight men also were more likely to suffer strokes. Those with BMIs of 35 or more were approximately 20 times more likely to develop diabetes. Individuals who were overweight but not obese, with BMIs between 25 and 29.9, were significantly more likely than leaner women to develop gallstones, high blood pressure, high cholesterol, and heart disease.[42]

If overweight individuals have surgery, they're more likely to develop complications. Even relatively small amounts of excess fat—as little as 5 pounds—can add to the dangers in those already at risk for hypertension and diabetes. Obesity also causes alterations in various measures of immune function.[43]

Obesity now is considered a greater threat to a healthy heart than smoking. People who both smoke and are obese are at especially high risk of cardiovascular disease. While some smokers have felt that they couldn't lose weight until they stopped smoking, researchers have found that weight loss among smokers is possible and beneficial, leading to a reduction in other risk factors, such as lower blood pressure and cholesterol.[44] Health educators also are targeting teenage dieters, who are more likely to begin smoking, often to help control their weight.[45]

In our calorie-conscious and thinness-obsessed society, obesity also affects quality of life, including sense of vitality and pain.[46] Many see it as a heavy psychological burden, a sign of failure, laziness, or inadequate willpower. Overweight men and women often blame themselves for becoming heavy and feel guilty and depressed as a result. In fact, the psychological problems once considered the cause of obesity may be its consequence.

Does obesity lead to a shorter life? The answer is far from clear—and intensely controversial. Studies have shown that overweight middle-aged men and women have a higher risk of dying from all causes, especially from heart disease and certain cancers, than those who are normal weight or underweight. The risk rises if they develop diabetes.[47] Among men who have smoked, the risk of dying is almost two times higher for those with the highest body weight than for those with the lowest body weight. Researchers have found an association between greater Body Mass Index and higher death rates.[48]

How Can I Overcome a Weight Problem?

Each year an estimated 15 to 35 percent of Americans go on a diet, but no matter how much weight they lose, 95 percent gain it back within five years. Most dieters cut back on food, not because they want to *feel* better, but because they want to *look* better. Individuals who drastically reduce their food intake and make weight loss a major part of their lives may be jeopardizing their physical and psychological well-being.

The best approach to a weight problem depends on how overweight a person is. For extreme obesity, medical treatments, including surgery, may be necessary to overcome the danger to a person's health and life. People who are moderately or mildly obese can lose weight through different approaches, including behavioral modification (monitoring food intake, altering eating style, avoiding eating "triggers," and similar strategies); cognitive therapy (changing thoughts or beliefs that lead to overeating); and social support (participating in groups such as Overeaters Anonymous). The keys to overcoming obesity are acknowledging biological limits, addressing individual differences, altering unrealistic expectations, setting limits, and learning coping skills to provide self-nurturing without relying on food.[49]

Severe Obesity

A BMI higher than 40 (or higher than 35 for those with other conditions) indicates a life-threatening condition. Because of the medical dangers they face, some severely obese men and women, as a last resort, may undergo surgery to reduce the volume of their stomachs and to tighten the passageway from the stomach to the intestine. Others opt for a "gastric bubble," a soft, polyurethane sac placed in the stomach to make the person feel full while following a low-calorie diet. It is not yet clear whether people who lose weight with this bubble will be able to keep it off. Diet pills, discussed later in this chapter, are another treatment approach.

Mild to Moderate Obesity

For individuals with a BMI of 30 to 39, doctors recommend a six-month trial of "lifestyle therapy," including a supervised diet and exercise. The initial goal should be a 10 percent reduction in weight, an amount that reduces obesity-related risks. With success and if warranted, individuals can attempt to lose more weight.

Weight loss drugs approved by the FDA also may be part of a comprehensive weight management program for the moderately obese. However, drug safety and effectiveness beyond one year of total treatment have not been established.

Overweight

Rather than going on low-calorie diets, people with BMIs of 25 to 29 should cut back moderately on their food intake and concentrate on developing healthy eating and exercise habits. Many moderately to mildly overweight people turn to national organizations such as Weight Watchers or to other commercial weight-loss groups. Most of these programs offer behavior-modification techniques, inspirational lectures, and carefully designed nutritional programs, but dropout rates are high. As many as half the members drop out in six weeks.

A Practical Guide to Weight Management

Even experienced dieters who've tried dozens of ways of losing weight often know little about the most effective ways to shed pounds and keep them off. In studies of successful dieters, those who were highly motivated, monitored their food intake, increased their activity, set realistic goals, and received social support from others were most likely to lose weight. Another key to long-term success is tailoring any weight-loss program to an individual's gender, lifestyle, and cultural, racial, and ethnic values. You also have to do your homework and look into the claims of promoters of diet programs. (See Savvy Consumer: "Weight-Loss Consumer Bill of Rights.")

A Customized Weight-Loss Plan

"If there's one thing we've learned in decades of research into weight management, it's that the one-diet-fits-all approach doesn't work," says clinical psychologist David Schlundt of Vanderbilt University.[50] The key is recognizing the ways you tend to put on weight and developing strategies to overcome them. (See Self-Survey: "Do You Know How to Lose Weight.") Here are some examples:

▷ Do you simply like food and consume lots of it? If so, keep a diary of everything you put in your mouth and tally up your daily total in calories and fat grams. The numbers may stun you. Look for where most of the calories come from—probably high-fat foods such as whole milk, chocolate, cookies, fried foods, potato chips, steaks—and cut down on how much and how often you eat them. Also watch portion sizes. A "cup" of cooked grains or vegetables is the size of a small fist; a teaspoon of butter or margarine, of a thumb print.

▷ Do you eat when you're bored, sad, frustrated, or worried? If so, you may be especially susceptible to "cues" that trigger eating. "People get in the habit of using food to soothe bad feelings or cope with boredom," says Schlundt. "Sometimes the real issue is a self-esteem or body-image problem." Dealing with these concerns is generally more helpful in the long run than dieting.

▷ Do you "graze," nibbling on snacks rather than eating regular meals? If so, limit yourself to low-calorie, low-fat foods, like carrots, celery, grapes, or air-popped popcorn. Take sips of water regularly to freshen your mouth. Even if you're having only a few crackers or carrots, put them on a plate, and try to eat in the same place, preferably while seated. This helps you break the habit of putting food in your mouth without thinking.

Avoiding Diet Traps

Whatever your eating style, there are only two effective strategies for losing weight: eating less and exercising

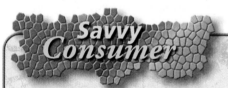

Weight-Loss Consumer Bill of Rights (An Example)

- **Warning:** Rapid weight loss may cause serious health problems. Rapid weight loss is weight loss of more than 1½ to 2 pounds per week or weight loss of more than 1 percent of body weight per week after the second week of participation in a weight-loss program.

- Consult your personal physician before starting any weight-loss program.

- Only permanent lifestyle changes, such as making healthful food choices and increasing physical activity, promote long-term weight loss and successful maintenance.

- Qualifications of the weight-loss provider should be available upon request.

- **You have a right to:**
- Ask questions about the potential health risks of this program and its nutritional content, psychological support, and educational components.

- Receive an itemized statement of the actual or estimated price of the weight-loss program, including extra products, services, supplements, examinations, and laboratory tests.

- Know the actual or estimated duration of the program.

- Know the name, address, and qualifications of the dietitian or nutritionist who has reviewed and approved the weight-loss program.

Source: Whitney, Eleanor, and Sharon Rolfes. *Understanding Nutrition,* 9th ed. Belmont, CA: Wadsworth/Thomson Learning, 2002, p. 277.

SELF SURVEY

Do You Know How to Lose Weight?

When it comes to weight control, willpower isn't enough: A sound knowledge of exercise, nutrition, and healthy eating behavior is essential. To test your weight-loss knowhow, try this quiz, which was developed by Dr. Kelly Brownell, director of the Yale University Center for Eating and Weight Disorders.

Instructions:

In each section, mark the statements True or False.

Section I: Nutrition

1. The calorie is a measure of the amount of fat in a food. _____
2. If you eat an equal number of servings from each of the five food groups in the Food Guide Pyramid, you'll get a balanced diet. _____
3. The recommended daily intake of dietary fat is 30 percent or less of total calories. _____
4. Carbohydrates aren't as important as other nutrients are, and they should make up only about 30 percent of your daily diet. _____
5. One gram of fat contains more than twice the calories of one gram of carbohydrate or protein. _____

Section II: Behavior

1. Keeping a daily record of what you eat is essential for weight loss. _____
2. Ordering à la carte at restaurants is a better idea than ordering package meals. _____
3. It's best to take all of what you'll eat in one serving so that you won't need additional helpings. _____
4. When you're trying to lose weight, it's a good idea to go food shopping when you're hungry so you can test your willpower. _____
5. Controlling how much you eat at a special event is easier if you eat a low-calorie snack before you go. _____

Section III: Exercise

1. Walking 1 mile burns almost as many calories as running 1 mile. _____
2. Exercise can help keep you from losing muscle tissue when you're trying to lose weight. _____
3. Climbing stairs requires more energy per minute—and therefore burns more calories per minute—than many more popular forms of exercise, such as swimming or jogging. _____
4. No exercise can help you lose fat in specific parts of the body. _____
5. Exercise must be done in specific amounts—say, at least 30 minutes at a stretch—to help you lose weight. _____

Section IV: Myths

1. The most important factor in weight reduction is discovering the psychological roots of your weight problem. _____
2. There's no such thing as a slow or underactive metabolism. _____

3. Since excess dietary fat has been linked to heart disease and other health problems, it's best to eliminate all fat from your diet. _____
4. Eating quickly helps you enjoy food more because your taste buds get more stimulation. _____
5. The calorie level necessary to lose weight is the same for all people. _____

Answers

Section I: Nutrition

1. **False.** The calorie is a measure of the energy your body gets from a food. Fat supplies some of the calories in some foods, but so do carbohydrates and protein.
2. **False.** You should eat the following every day: 2 to 3 servings of dairy products; 2 to 3 servings of meat, poultry or other high-protein foods (fish, beans, eggs, and nuts); 2 to 4 servings of fruit; 3 to 5 servings of vegetables; and 6 to 11 servings of breads and cereals (including rice and pasta).
3. **True.** If you follow the Food Guide Pyramid, you should be able to keep your fat calories under 30 percent.
4. **False.** Carbohydrates should make up the largest portion of your daily diet (between 55 and 60 percent of total calories).
5. **True.** One gram of fat contains 9 calories, while one gram of carbohydrate or protein contains only 4 calories.

Section II: Behavior

1. **True.** People who have lost weight and kept it off generally report that record keeping was one key to their success.
2. **True.** If you order a package meal—say, a hamburger with french fries and coleslaw—you'll probably end up with more calories than you want or need.
3. **False.** It's best to take one portion at a time, because it interrupts the tendency to eat without thinking and gives you time to consider whether you really need more food.
4. **False.** Shopping on an empty stomach is asking for trouble. You'll do less impulse buying if you shop *after* eating.
5. **True.** Eating a low-calorie food before you go will take the edge off your hunger and help you resist the high-calorie snacks, such as chips and nuts, typically served at parties.

Section III: Exercise

1. **True.** How far you go is more important than how fast you go, so walking helps with weight control.

(continued)

2. **True.** Exercise can prevent muscle loss while maximizing fat loss. For weight loss, exercise combined with dieting is preferable to dieting alone.
3. **True.** Climbing stairs is an excellent way to burn calories.
4. **True.** You can reduce fat in general, but you cannot dictate where it will come off.
5. **False.** Any amount of exercise helps, so do what you can.

Section IV: Myths

1. **False.** Psychological problems are at the root of some, but not all, cases of overweight. And there's no evidence that uncovering these causes helps with weight loss.
2. **False.** There are wide variations in metabolic rate—how fast calories are used by the body for energy—among different people.
3. **False.** Fat plays an important role in the body, including protecting vital organs and preventing excessive heat loss, so it shouldn't be totally eliminated from your diet.
4. **False.** Your taste buds catch nothing but a blur if the food shoots past. If you slow down, the food will taste better, and you may feel more satisfied and therefore eat less.
5. **False.** There are large differences in how much weight people lose when they have the same caloric intake. Some women, for example, lose weight on 2,000 calories a day while others don't lose any on 1,000.

Scoring

Give yourself one point for each correct answer and total the points for each section.

Section I: Nutrition

5 You're a nutrition nabob! With so many food facts at your fingertips, controlling your weight should be no heavy task.

3 or 4 Your food choices could use a dash more nutrition know-how if you want to keep your weight at a palatable level.

1 or 2 You need to be enlightened on food if you want to scale down.

Section II: Behavior

5 You ain't misbehavin': Your eating and food shopping habits are right on target.

3 or 4 You may want to brush up on your p's and q's: Some of your habits may be hindering your efforts.

1 or 2 If you don't break your bad habits, you'll always be fighting the battle of the bulge.

Section III: Exercise

5 You've got a leg up on controlling your weight.

3 or 4 You should work out the kinks in your workout to help keep your weight in check.

1 or 2 Shape up, or you'll never like the shape of things to come!

Section IV: Myths

5 It's no myth that you know what you're talking about.

3 or 4 Watch out: If you don't separate food fact from food fiction, you may be led astray.

1 or 2 When it comes to weight control, don't believe everything you read.

Making Changes

Long-Term Weight Management

If you decide to change your eating habits in order to lower your weight, try following these steps:

- *Establish your goals.* Subtract your target weight from your actual weight and calculate how long it will take you to lose the difference, based on a weekly loss of $1\frac{1}{2}$ pounds.
- *Never say diet.* Going on a diet implies going off a diet sooner or later.
- *Be realistic.* Trying to shrink to an impossibly low weight dooms you to defeat. Start off slowly and make steady progress. If your weight creeps up 5 pounds, go back to the basics of your program. Take into account normal fluctuations, but watch out for an upward trend. If you let your weight continue to creep up, it may not stop until you have a serious weight problem—again.
- *Recognize that there are no quick fixes.* Ultimately, quick-loss diets are very damaging physically and psychologically because when you stop dieting and put the pounds back on you feel like a failure.
- *Note your progress.* Make a graph, with your initial weight as the base, to indicate your progress. View plateaus or occasional gains as temporary setbacks rather than disasters.
- *Adopt the 90 percent rule.* If you practice good eating habits 90 percent of the time, a few indiscretions won't make a difference. In effect, you should allow for occasional cheating, so that you don't have to feel guilty about it.
- *Try, try again.* Remember, dieters don't usually keep weight off on their first attempt. The people who eventually succeed try various methods until they find the plan that works for them.

Source: American Health, November 1994, pp. 29–31.

How to Spot a Dangerous Weight-Loss Program

The National Council Against Health Fraud cautions dieters to watch for these warnings of dangerous or fraudulent programs.

✔ Promises of very rapid weight loss.

✔ Claims that the diet can eliminate "cellulite" (a term used to refer to dimply fatty tissue on the arms and legs).

✔ "Counselors" who are really salespersons pushing a product or program.

✔ No mention of any risks associated with the diet.

✔ Unproven gimmicks, such as body wraps, starch blockers, hormones, diuretics, or "unique" pills or potions.

✔ No maintenance program.

more. Unfortunately, most people search for easier alternatives that almost invariably turn into dietary dead ends. The following are among the most common traps to avoid.

Diet Foods

According to the Calorie Control Council, 90 percent of Americans choose some foods labeled "light." But even though these foods keep growing in popularity, Americans' weight keeps rising. There are several reasons: Many people think choosing a food that's lower in calories, fat-free, or "light" gives them a license to eat as much as they want. What they don't realize is that many foods that are low in fat are still high in sugar and calories. Refined carbohydrates, rapidly absorbed into the bloodstream, raise blood glucose levels. As they fall, appetite increases.

What about the artificial sweeteners and fake fats that appear in many diet products? Nutritionists caution to use them in moderation, and not to substitute them for basic foods, such as grains, fruits, and vegetables. Foods made with fat substitutes may have fewer grams of fat, but they don't necessarily have significantly fewer calories. Many people who add reduced-fat, fat-free or sugar-free sodas, cookies, chips, and other snacks to their diet often cut back on more nutritious foods, such as fruits and vegetables. They also tend to eat more of low- or no-fat foods so that their daily calorie intake either stays the same or actually increases.

The Yo-Yo Syndrome

On-and-off-again dieting, especially by means of very-low-calorie diets (under 800 calories a day), can be self-defeating and dangerous. Some studies have shown that "weight cycling" may make it more difficult to lose weight or keep it off. (See Figure 6-4.) Repeated cycles of rapid weight loss followed by weight gain may even change food preferences. Chronic crash dieters often come to prefer foods that combine sugar and fat, such as cake frosting.

To avoid weight cycling and overcome its negative effects: Exercise. Researchers at the University of Pennsylvania found that when overweight women who also exercised went off a very-low-calorie diet, their metabolisms did not stay slow but bounced back to the appropriate level for their new, lower body weights. The reason may be exercise's ability to preserve muscle tissue. The more muscle tissue you have, the higher your metabolic rate.

Very-Low-Calorie Diets

Any diet that promises to take pounds off fast can be dangerous. For reasons that scientists don't fully understand, rapid weight loss is linked with increased mortality. Most risky are very-low-calorie diets that provide fewer than 800 calories a day. Whenever people cut back drastically on calories, they immediately lose several pounds because of a loss of fluid. As soon as they return to a more normal way of eating, they regain this weight.

On a very-low-calorie diet, as much as 50 percent of the weight you lose may be muscle (so you'll actually look flabbier). Because your heart is a muscle, it may become so weak that it no longer can pump blood through your body. In addition, your blood pressure may plummet, causing dizziness, light-headedness, and fatigue. You may develop nausea and abdominal pain. You may lose hair. If you're a

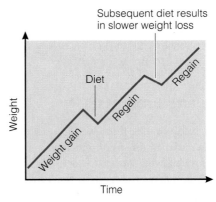

▲ **Figure 6-4** The weight-cycling effect of repeated dieting. Each round of dieting is typically followed by a rebound leading to a greater weight gain.

woman, your menstrual cycle may become irregular, or you may stop menstruating altogether. As you lose more water, you also lose essential vitamins, and your metabolism slows down. Even reaction time slows, and crash dieters may not be able to respond as quickly as usual.

Once you go off an extreme diet—as you inevitably must—your metabolism remains slow, even though you're no longer restricting your food intake. The human body appears to alter its energy use to compensate for weight loss. These metabolic changes may make it harder for people to maintain a reduced body weight after dieting.

Do High-Protein, Low-Carbohydrate Diets Work?

After trying the low-fat diets popular in the 1980s and 1990s, many Americans weighed more than ever. High-protein, low-carbohydrate diets, such as the Atkins diet and "sugar busters," have emerged as the first diet fad of the twenty-first century. These diets appeal to many people because they can eat as much protein as they want, including steaks, eggs, and fatty foods they'd long been told to shun, as long as they strictly limit their carbohydrates.

The American College of Sports Medicine, the American Dietetic Association, and other professional groups have challenged these diets. As they note, there is no scientific evidence that a diet providing more than the 10 to 15 percent protein recommended by federal guidelines enhances health or athletic performance. Although it is possible to lose weight on a high-protein diet, the reason is the same as with other quick weight-loss diets: low calorie count.

Because protein-rich foods tend to be more nutrient dense, dieters usually consume about 1,200 to 1,500 calories a day. They also have a diuretic effect, so individuals lose fluid—and pounds—almost immediately. The American Dietetic Association has noted that these diets tend to be low in calcium, fiber, and healthy phytochemicals. Short-term side effects include fatigue, constipation, nausea, and vomiting as a result of ketosis, an abnormal body process caused by a lack of carbohydrates. The long-term effects of such diets include increased risk of heart disease, breast cancer, and colon cancer.[51]

Diet Pills and Products

In their search for a quick fix to weight problems, millions of people have tried often-risky remedies.[52] In the 1920s, some women swallowed patented weight-loss capsules that turned out to be tapeworm eggs. In the 1960s and 1970s, addictive amphetamines were common diet aids. In the 1990s, appetite suppressants known as fen-phen ("fen" referring to fenfluramine [Pondimin] or dexfenfluramine

[Redux], appetite depressants, and "phen" referring to phentermine, a type of amphetamine) became popular. They were taken off the market after being linked to heart valve problems. Follow-up studies have shown that the problems caused by these drugs do not worsen over time.

Many people rely on meal replacements, usually shakes or snack bars, to lose or keep off weight. If used appropriately—as actual replacements rather than supplements to regular meals and snacks—they can be a useful strategy for weight loss.

In one recent study, the use of liquid meal replacements for one or two meals a day proved as effective in controlling weight over a one-year time span as traditional lifestyle interventions.[53] Liquid meal replacements may be particularly useful for overweight individuals who find it difficult to maintain changes in their eating and lifestyle habits.[54]

More weight-loss drugs have won FDA approval, including Meridia (sibutramine) and Xenical (orlistat). Both are intended only for people with a BMI of at least 30 or a BMI of 27 and additional risk factors.

Unlike fen-phen, which fooled patients into feeling full by boosting production of the brain chemical serotonin, Meridia slows the body's dissipation of the serotonin it naturally produces. The FDA describes Meridia as "moderately effective" at helping obese people shed pounds—in studies, they lost about 7 to 11 more pounds than mere dieters—but it can cause increases in blood pressure and pulse rate that may endanger certain patients.[55] No one who has poorly controlled hypertension, heart disease, or an irregular heartbeat or who has survived a stroke should use the drug. Meridia users should not only see a doctor for regular blood pressure checks but should also check themselves regularly with an at-home blood pressure monitor.

Xenical is the first drug in a new class known as lipase inhibitors, which work by preventing gastrointestinal and pancreatic enzymes from breaking down fat for absorption by the body. Combined with a supervised diet, it has proven effective in promoting weight loss, lessening weight regain, and improving some obesity-related risk factors.[56] Its long-term effects are unknown.[57] Wellbutrin (bupropion), an antidepressant and antismoking drug, also has shown potential for weight loss. In one study women who took the drug and followed a moderate-calorie diet lost four times more weight than women taking a placebo and following the same diet.

Although available only by prescription, Xenical and Meridia are being marketed over the Internet to anyone who fills out a computerized form reviewed by a company doctor. As a result, many people are taking this medication without medical supervision. Such misuse could cause health risks. Xenical causes side effects, including bloating, flatulence, diarrhea, and fecal incontinence. Because it blocks absorption of the fat-soluble vitamins A, D, E, and

K, a daily vitamin supplement is necessary. And there may be additional risks for individuals with eating disorders.

Herbal diet aids, many containing ephedra or ma huang, often combined with caffeine, are potentially dangerous.[58] Among the reported adverse effects are cardiac arrest, arrhythmias, bleeding in the brain, severe hypertension, stroke, and death. Other reactions include anxiety, tremulousness, insomnia, palpitations, and personality changes.[59]

The search for the perfect diet drug continues—with plenty of economic incentives for drug makers. By some estimates, the potential market for weight-loss pills totals at least $5 billion. Other diet products, including diet sodas and low-fat foods, also are a very big business. Yet people who use these products aren't necessarily sure to slim down. In fact, people who consume such products often gain weight because they think that they can afford to add high-calorie treats to their diet.

Liquid Diets

Liquid diets, such as Optifast, Medifast, and other programs, supply 420 to 800 calories a day and include sufficient protein to preserve muscle tissue. For several months, dieters on these plans eat no solid food, consuming only the special liquid formula and water. These extreme diets, generally reserved for those at least 40 percent or more overweight, do result in rapid loss, but they can be hazardous.

Today's liquid diets contain more protein, carbohydrates, vitamins, and minerals than the formulas that led to at least 58 deaths in the late 1970s. However, programs that rely solely on liquid formulas should be supervised by a doctor or hospital that provides weekly screening of blood pressure, heart function, electrolyte levels, urine content, and potassium—all indicators of how the body is coping without real food. The side effects of liquid diets include dry skin, hair loss, constipation, gum disease, sensitivity to cold, and mood swings. Only 10 to 20 percent of those who enroll in liquid-diet programs manage to stay within 10 pounds of their target weight a year and a half after entering the program.

Exercise: The Best Solution

You may think that exercise will make you want to eat more. Actually, it has the opposite effect. The combination of exercise and cutting back on calories may be the most effective way of taking weight off and keeping it off. As research has shown, exercise keeps your metabolic rate up while you're dieting—and afterward. Exercise, along with a healthy diet, can lead to weight losses of up to 10 pounds. However, even though many overweight adults recognize

STRATEGIES FOR PREVENTION

Evaluating a Diet

If you hear about a new diet that promises to melt away fat, don't try it until you get answers to the following questions:

✔ Does it include a wide variety of nutritious foods?

✔ Does it provide at least 1,200 calories a day?

✔ Is it designed to reduce your weight by one-half to two pounds per week?

✔ Does it emphasize moderate portions?

✔ Does it use foods that are easy to find and prepare?

✔ Can you follow it wherever you eat—at home, work, restaurants, or parties?

✔ Is its cost reasonable?

If the answer to any of these questions is no, don't try the diet; then ask yourself one more question: Is losing weight worth losing your well-being?

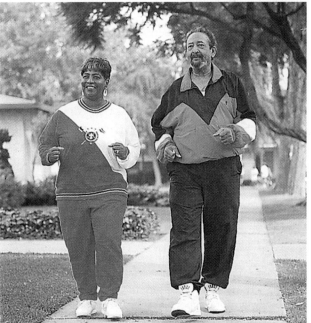

▲ The most effective and healthful way to manage your weight is to combine dietary changes with regular physical exercise.

STRATEGIES FOR CHANGE

Working Off Weight

✔ *Get moving.* Take the stairs instead of the elevator. Get off the bus a few blocks from your home and walk the rest of the way.

✔ *Walk.* Most people find it hard to make excuses for not walking 15 minutes every day. Once you start, increase gradually so that you go farther and faster.

✔ *Exercise daily.* You're more likely to lose and keep weight off if you exercise regularly. Try to burn 1,800 to 2,000 calories a week through exercise—the equivalent of 18 to 20 miles of walking or jogging.

✔ *Get physical.* There are more ways to burn calories than traditional exercise activities: Dancing, hiking, gardening can all help you get in shape. Check your campus bulletin boards and newspapers for information on rock-climbing, kayaking, skiing, and other fun forms of working out.

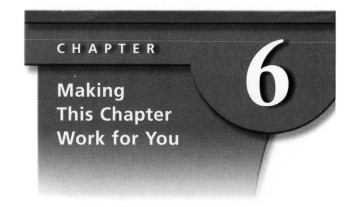

CHAPTER

Making This Chapter Work for You

6

1. The best way to determine whether you are a healthy weight is to
   a. measure your waist and hips.
   b. calculate your body muscle percentage.
   c. check ideal weight tables.
   d. calculate your body fat percentage.

2. Body composition estimates can be obtained with which of the following methods?
   a. skinfold fat weighing
   b. bioelectrical impedance analysis
   c. biofeedback analysis
   d. basal metabolic rate measurement

3. According to the set-point theory:
   a. the physiological drive to consume food is stimulated by hormones
   b. body fat is maintained at a predetermined level by an unconscious control system.
   c. the psychological desire to eat is determined by the size of the hypothalamus.
   d. fat cells cannot increase in number beyond a genetically determined point.

4. Which of the following eating behaviors may be a warning sign of a serious eating disorder?
   a. vegetarianism
   b. compulsive food washing
   c. binge eating
   d. weight gain during the first year of college

5. Individuals with anorexia nervosa
   a. believe they are overweight even if they are extremely thin.
   b. typically feel full all the time, which limits their food intake.
   c. usually look overweight even though their body mass index is normal.
   d. have a reduced risk for heart-related abnormalities.

6. Bulimia nervosa is
   a. characterized by excessive sleeping followed by periods of insomnia.
   b. found primarily in older women who are concerned with the aging process.

the benefits of exercise, few exercise often or intensely enough to lose excess pounds.

Exercise has other benefits: It increases energy expenditure, builds up muscle tissue, burns off fat stores, and stimulates the immune system. Exercise also may reprogram metabolism so that individuals burn up more calories during and after a workout. (See Chapter 4 for a complete discussion of exercise.)

Moderate physical activity also can help control weight. Recent studies have found that everyday activities, such as walking, gardening, and heavy household chores, are as effective as a structured exercise program in maintaining or losing weight. Scientists use the acronym **NEAT**—for **non-exercise activity thermogenesis**—to describe such "nonvolitional" movements and have verified that it can be an effective way of burning calories. In a study of 16 nonobese adults, "intentional" exercise and metabolic rate had little effect on variations in weight gain, whereas NEAT did. One form of NEAT, fidgeting, turns out to play a more important role in daily energy expenditure—and may be particularly useful in preventing weight gain after overeating.

Once you start an exercise program, keep it up. Individuals who've started an exercise program during or after a weight-loss program are consistently more successful in keeping off most of the pounds they've shed.

c. associated with the use of laxatives or excessive exercise to control weight.

d. does not have serious health consequences.

7. Which of the following statements is not true?
   a. Obesity is a greater threat to heart health than smoking.
   b. Men who accumulate fat around their waist are at increased risk for cardiovascular risk.
   c. Individuals who are obese are neither more nor less psychologically troubled than people of normal weight.
   d. Children with an obese parent are more likely to be thin because of their embarrassment about the parent's appearance.

8. Weight management strategies that work include which of the following?
   a. Increase your activity level and eat less, aiming for a weekly weight loss of about 1½ pounds.
   b. Ask friends for recommendations for diet that helped them lose weight quickly.
   c. Practice good eating habits about 50 percent of the time so that you can balance your cravings with healthy food.

   d. Try a number of weight-loss diets to find the one that works best for you.

9. Which of the following statements is true?
   a. Very low-calorie diets increase metabolism, which helps burn calories more quickly.
   b. An individual eating low-calorie or fat-free foods can increase the serving sizes.
   c. High-protein, low-carbohydrate diets tend to be deficient in calcium and fiber.
   d. Yo-yo dieting works best for long-term weight loss.

10. Which of the following nonprescription diet products that have been shown to have dangerous health effects?
    a. Meridia and Xenical
    b. ephedra
    c. liquid meal replacements
    d. diet snack bars

Answers to these questions can be found on page 640.

 How do nutrients fuel the bodies of active teens?

Critical Thinking

1. Do you think that you have a weight problem? If so, what makes you think so? Is your perception based on your actual BMI measurement or on how you believe you look? If you found out that your BMI was within the ideal range, would that change your opinion about your body? Why or why not?

2. Different cultures have different standards for body weight and attractiveness. Within our society, even men and women often seem to follow different standards. What influences have shaped your personal feelings about desired weight?

3. Suppose one of your roommates appears to have symptoms of an eating disorder. You have told her of your concerns, but she has denied having a problem and brushed off your fears. What can you do to help this individual? Should you go contact his or her parent? Why of why not?

SITES & BYTES

Count Your Calories Because Your Calories Count
http://www.bgsm.edu/nutrition/in.html
This interactive site sponsored by Wake Forest University Baptist Medical Center features a four-step assessment of your diet, including "How's Your Diet," "Fit or Not Quiz," "Calorie Counter," and "Drive Through Diet." There is also an "Eating Disorders" quiz.

Something Fishy Website on Eating Disorders
http://www.something-fishy.org
This comprehensive site features a wealth of information on all aspects of eating disorders, including facts, prevention, causes, symptoms, information on helping others, resources, treatment, cultural issues, recovery, chat rooms, and an online support center featuring bulletin boards and an e-mail newsletter.

MIrror-Mirror Eating Disorders

http://www.mirror-mirror.org/eatdis.htm

This site features information on all types of disordered eating, including compulsive eating, binge eating, and how eating disorders affect society, college students, children, teenagers, athletes, women, and men. The site also features information on recovery, getting help, resources, and a survivor's wall created to acknowledge the many people who are fighting to free themselves from their eating disorder and those who have recovered.

Please note that links are subject to change. If you find a broken link, use a search engine such as **http://www.yahoo.com** and search for the website by typing in key words.

InfoTrac Activity
Tanya R. Berry and Bruce L. Howe. "Risk Factors for Disordered Eating in Female University Athletes." *Journal of Sport Behavior,* Vol. 23, No. 3, September 2000, p. 207.

(1) What four risk factors for the development of disordered eating were studied in college student athletes?

(2) Female athletes who participate in what three basic types of physical activities are most likely to develop disordered eating patterns?

(3) What roles do self-esteem, social pressure from peers and coaches, the media, and body image play in predicting who is most likely to develop disordered eating patterns?

You can find additional readings related to eating patterns with InfoTrac College Edition, an online library of more than 900 journals and publications. Follow the instructions for accessing InfoTrac that were packaged with your textbook; then search for articles using a key word search.

For additional links, resources, and suggested readings on InfoTrac, visit our Health & Wellness Resource Center at **http://health.wadsworth.com**.

Key Terms

The terms listed here are used within the chapter on the page indicated. Definition of the terms are in the Glossary at the end of the book.

anorexia nervosa 199
appetite 195
basal metabolic rate (BMR) 193
binge eating 197
body mass index (BMI) 190
bulimia nervosa 201

calorie 193
eating disorders 197
hunger 193
**non-exercise activity thermogenesis
  (NEAT)** 212
obese 202

obesity 202
overweight 202
satiety 195
set-point theory 195
waist-hip ratio 203

References

1. White, Jane. "National Nutrition Summit." *Journal of the American Dietetic Association,* Vol. 100, No. 7, July 2000.
2. Lake, Amelia, et al. "Effects of Western Culture on Eating Attitudes and Body Image." *Nutrition Research Newsletter,* Vol. 19, No. 2, January–April 2000.
3. "Magazine Ideals Wrong." *Journal of the American Medical Association,* Vol. 286, No. 4, July 25, 2001, p. 409.
4. Tiggeman, Marika. "The Impact of Adolescent Girls' Life Concerns and Leisure Activities on Body Dissatisfaction, Disordered Eating, and Self-Esteem." *Journal of Genetic Psychology,* Vol. 162, No. 2, June 2001, p. 133.
5. Cohane, Geoffrey, and Harrison Pope. "Body Image in Boys: A Review of the Literature." *International Journal of Eating Disorders,* Vol. 29, No. 4, May 2001.
6. Arriaza, Ceceilia, and Traci Mann. "Ethnic Differences in Eating Disorders Among College Students: The Confounding Role of

Body Mass Index." *Journal of American College Health,* Vol. 49, No. 6, May 2001, p. 309.
7. Lofton, Stacy, and Tim Bungum. "Attitudes and Behaviors Toward Weight, Body Shape, and Eating in Male and Female College Students." *Research Quarterly for Exercise and Sport,* Vol. 72, No. 1, March 2001, p. A-32.
8. Cramer, M., and C. Murray. "Body Dissatisfaction Across Age and Gender: Function vs. Appearance." *Gerontologist,* October 15, 2000, p. 202.
9. "Use of Body Mass Index and Waist Circumference to Predict Risk of Chronic Disease." *Journal of the American Dietetic Association,* Vol. 101, No. 6, June 2001, p. 708.
10. Hales, Dianne. *An Invitation to Fitness and Wellness.* Belmont, CA: Wadsworth, 2001.
11. "Overweight Children Risk Coronary Heart Disease and Diabetes as Obese Adults." *Medical Letter on the CDC & FDA,* August 19, 2001.

12. McCaffree, Jim. "Eating Disorders: All in the Family?" *Journal of the American Dietetic Association,* Vol. 101, No. 6, June 2001, p. 622.

13. Nagel, Deborah, et al. "Evaluation of a Screening Test for Female College Athletes with Eating Disorders and Disordered Eating." *Journal of Athletic Training,* Vol. 35, No. 4, October–December 2000, p. 431.

14. "Young Female Athletes at Risk, Say US Experts." *Lancet,* Vol. 356, No. 9234, September 16, 2000.

15. "Body Image Concerns," *Nutrition Research Newsletter,* Vol. 19, No. 5, May 2000.

16. Cooley, Eric, and Tamina Toray. "Disordered Eating in College Freshman Women: A Prospective Study." *Journal of American College Health,* Vol. 49, No. 5, March 2001, p. 229.

17. Holben, David. "International Students Gain Fat and Weight from American Diet." Presentation, American Dietetic Association, October 18, 2000.

18. "Emergence of Dieting," *Nutrition Research Newsletter,* Vol. 19, No. 12, December 2000, p. 3.

19. Field, Alison, et al. "Peer, Parent, and Media Influences on the Development of Weight Concerns and Frequent Dieting Among Preadolescent and Adolescent Girls and Boys." *Pediatrics,* Vol. 107, No. 1, January 2001, p. 54.

20. "Nutrient Intake of Binge Eaters." *Nutrition Research Newsletter,* Vol. 20, No. 3, March 2001, p. 3.

21. "Dieting and Development of Eating Disorders in Overweight and Obese Adults." *Journal of the American Dietetic Association,* Vol. 101, No. 3, March 2001, p. 369.

22. "Attempting to Lose Weight, Restraint, and Binge Eating." *Nutrition Research Newsletter,* Vol. 20, No. 3, March 2001, p. 6.

23. LeTourneau, Melanie. "All in the Family." *Psychology Today,* Vol. 33, No. 4, July 2000.

24. Miller, Karl. "Treatment Guideline for Eating Disorders." *American Family Physician,* Vol. 62, No. 1, July 1, 2000.

25. Walling, Anne. "A New Screening Tool for Patients with Eating Disorders." *American Family Physician,* Vol. 61, No. 7, April 1, 2000.

26. Wilson, G., and Stewart Agras. "Practice Guidelines for Eating Disorders." *Behavior Therapy,* Vol. 32, No. 2, Spring 2001, p. 219.

27. Hubbard, Kim, et al. "Out of Control." People, April 23, 1999.

28. Woodside, D. Blake, et al. "Comparisons of Men with Full or Partial Eating Disorders, Men Without Eating Disorders, and Women with Eating Disorders in the Community." *American Journal of Psychiatry,* Vol. 158, April 2001, p. 570.

29. Arriaza and Mann, "Ethnic Differences in Eating Disorders Among College Students: The Confounding Role of Body Mass Index."

30. Hubbard, "Out of Control."

31. Lang, Susan. "Obesity, Eating Disorders Discourage College Dates." *Human Ecology Forum,* Vol. 26, No. 4, Fall, 1998.

32. Lock, James. "Innovative Family-Based Treatment for Anorexia Nervosa." *Brown University Child and Adolescent Behavior Letter,* Vol 17, No. 4, April 2001, p. 1.

33. Ben-Tovim, David I. "Outcome in Patients with Eating Disorders: A 5-Year Study." *Journal of the American Medical Association,* Vol. 286, No. 1, July 4, 2001, p. 21.

34. Waters, Anne, et al. "Bulimics' Responses to Food Cravings: Is Binge Eating a Product of Hunger or Emotional State?" *Behavior Research and Therapy,* Vol. 39, No. 9, August 2001, p. 877.

35. Weyer, Christian. "Basal Metabolic Rate in African-American Women." *Journal of Clinical Nutrition,* July 1999.

36. Rotenstein, Deborah. Personal interview.

37. Williams, Christine. Personal interview.

38. Seidell, Jacob, et al. "Abdominal Adiposity and Risk of Heart Disease." *Journal of the American Medical Association,* Vol. 281, No. 24, June 23, 1999.

39. "Gender Difference in Weight Reduction." *Nutrition Research Newsletter,* Vol. 18, Issue 2, February 1999.

40. Magid, Barry. "Is Biology Destiny After All?" *Journal of Psychotherapy Practice & Research,* Vol. 4, No. 1, Winter 1995.

41. Heymsfield, Steven, et al. "Recombinant Leptin for Weight Loss in Obese and Lean Adults." *Journal of the American Medical Association,* Vol. 282, No. 16, October 27, 1999.

42. Field, Alison, et al. "Impact of Overweight on the Risk of Developing Common Chronic Diseases During a 10-Year Period." *Archives of Internal Medicine,* Vol. 161, No. 13, July 9, 2001, p. 1581.

43. "Dangers Are Overlooked." *Medical Letter on the CDC & FDA,* August 12, 2001.

44. Wilson, K., et al. "Impact on Smoking Status on Weight Loss and Cardiovascular Risk Factors." *Journal of Epidemiology & Community Health,* Vol. 55, No. 3, March 2001, p. 213.

45. Austin, S. Bryn, and Steven Grotmaker. "Dieting and Smoking Initiation in Early Adolescent Girls and Boys: A Prospective Study." *American Journal of Public Health,* Vol. 91, No. 3, March 2001, p. 446.

46. "Weight Change Affects Quality of Life." JOPERD—The Journal of Physical Education, Recreation & Dance, Vol. 71, No. 2, February 2000.

47. "Keeping Diabetes at Bay." Nutrition Action Healthletter, Vol. 28, No. 6, July 2001, p. 11.

48. "Weight Loss Can Decrease Mortality Risk." *Medical Letter on the CDC & FDA,* November 26, 2000.

49. Murphy, Dee. "Fit or Fad: A Dieting Decision." *Current Health 2,* Vol 27, No. 7, March 2001, p. 16.

50. Schlundt, David. Personal interview.

51. Stein, Karen. "High-protein, Low-Carbohydrate Diets: Do They Work?" *Journal of the American Dietetic Association,* Vol. 100, No. 7, July 2000, p. 760.

52. Chiesi, Michele, et al. "Pharmacotherapy of Obesity: Targets and Perspectives." *Trends in Pharmacological Sciences,* Vol. 22, No. 5, May 2001, p. 247.

53. Ashley, Judith, et al. "Weight Control in the Physician's Office." *Archives of Internal Medicine,* Vol. 161, No. 13, July 9, 2001, p. 1599.

54. "Liquid Meal Replacement vs. Traditional Food." *Nutrition Research Newsletter,* Vol. 20, No. 4, April 2001, p. 7.

55. "Sibutramine Evaluated for Weight Maintenance." *Psychopharmacology Update,* Vol. 12, No. 2, February 2001, p. 3.

56. "Weight Loss Pill Offers Added Health Benefits." *Chemist & Druggist,* June 9, 2001, p. 10.

57. "Update to Orlistat." *Chemist & Druggist,* June 2, 2001, p. 10.

58. Gower, Timothy. "The Scoop on Ephedra." *Health,* Vol. 15, No. 6, July–August 2001, p. 66.

59. Cerrato, Paul, "More Bad News on Herbal Weight-Loss Products." *Contemporary OB/GYN,* Vol. 46, No. 4, April 2001, p. 94.

RESPONSIBLE SEXUALITY

Our most special relationships are those that bring us closer to others—our friends, partners, spouses, parents, and children. Such intimacy is the most rewarding and often the most demanding of human involvements. The giving of ourselves to another—sharing thoughts, feelings, experiences, and sexual pleasure—touches the essence of what it means to be human. This section provides a comprehensive philosophical and practical view of relating to others. Each of the chapters focuses on the unique form of personal responsibility involved in every close relationship: a responsibility that looks beyond the self to those we care for and love.

7

Communication and Relationships

Oona compares the people in her life to threads in a magnificent tapestry. Each brings different tones and textures that complement and contrast with others. Her earliest childhood memories are of loving circles of family and friends that she once thought revolved around only her. Now she sees that she is part of these concentric rings and that the friendship and support she offers others enrich all of their lives.

When she left for a college thousands of miles from her home, Oona worried about the people she was leaving behind and the strangers she would be living among. She wondered if she'd be welcomed or shunned, judged by her looks or her race, invited to join social groups or excluded from them. What she discovered was that the choice was largely hers. She could reach out to others, smile and hope that others would smile in return, communicate clearly and honestly, strive to forge connections. Within months of her arrival, Oona was sure she had made friends she would keep forever.

Whether we are shy or outgoing, reserved or exuberant, we all crave human connection. As individuals and as part of society, we need to care about others and to know that others care about us, to feel for others and have others feel for us, to share what we know and to learn from what others know.

Sending clear messages through words, gestures, expressions, and behaviors is the essence of good communication. The more effectively we communicate, the more likely we are to create good relationships built on honesty, understanding, and mutual trust. Such relationships can infuse our lives with a richness no solitary pleasure can match.

This chapter discusses the social needs we all share, the ways some of us respond to those needs, and the possibilities that exist for coming together from our solitude to warm ourselves in each other's glow.

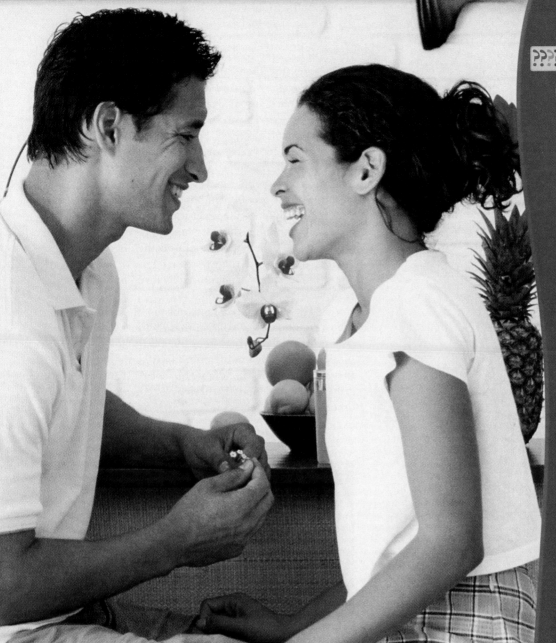

After studying the material in this chapter, you should be able to:

- **Describe** the role verbal and nonverbal communication plays in forming and maintaining relationships, and **discuss** gender differences in communication.
- **Define** friendship and **explain** how friendship grows.
- **Discuss** the behavior and emotional expectations for friendship, dating, and intimate relationships.
- **Compare** and **contrast** romantic love and mature love.

- **List** and **describe** the various living arrangements today's adults might choose.
- **Identify** the problems likely to affect long-term relationships, and **explain** how they can be prevented.
- **Describe** the different types of families and discuss some of the major issues facing them.
- **Identify** the behaviors that may result in dysfunctional relationships.

Personal Communication

Getting to know someone is one of life's greatest challenges and pleasures. When you find another person intriguing—as a friend, as a teacher, as a colleague, as a possible partner—you want to find out as much as you can about him or her and to share more and more information about yourself. Roommates may talk for endless hours. Friends may spend years getting to know each other. Partners in committed relationships may delight in learning new things about each other.

Communication stems from a desire to know and a decision to tell. Each of us chooses what information about ourselves we want to disclose and what we want to conceal or keep private. But in opening up to others, we increase our own self-knowledge and understanding.

Communicating Feelings

A great deal of daily communication focuses on facts: on the who, what, where, when, and how. Information is easy to convey and comprehend. Emotions are not. Some people have great difficulty saying "I appreciate you" or "I care about you," even though they are genuinely appreciative and caring. Others find it hard to know what to say in response and how to accept such expressions of affection.

Some people feel that relationships shouldn't require any effort, that there's no need to talk of responsibility between people who care about each other. Yet responsibility is implicit in our dealings with anyone or anything we value—and what can be more valuable than those with whom we share our lives? Friendships and other intimate relationships always demand an emotional investment, but the rewards they yield are great.

Sometimes people convey strong emotions with a kiss or a hug, a pat or a punch, but such actions aren't precise enough to communicate exact thoughts. Stalking out of a room and slamming the door may be clear signs of anger, but they don't explain what caused the anger or suggest what to do about it. You must learn how to communicate all feelings clearly and appropriately if you hope to become truly close to another person.

As two people build a relationship, they must sharpen their communication skills so that they can discuss all the issues they may confront. They must learn how to communicate anger as well as affection, hurt as well as joy—and they must listen as carefully as they speak. If and when love grows, they will find themselves as concerned with the other as with the self.

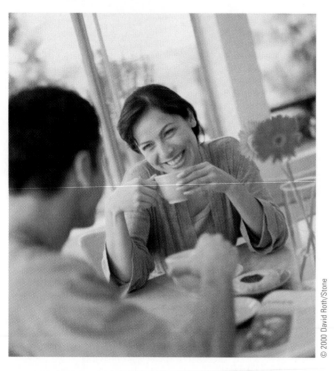

▲ Good communication is essential to a healthy and successful relationship

STRATEGIES FOR CHANGE

How to Enhance Communication

✔ *Use "I" statements.* Describe what's going on with you. Say, "I worry about being liked" or "I get frustrated when I can't put my feelings into words." Avoid generalities such as "You never think about my feelings," or "Nobody understands me."

✔ *Gently ask how the other person feels.* If your friend or partner describes thoughts rather than feelings, ask for more adjectives. Was he or she sad, excited, angry, hurt?

✔ *Become a very good listener.* When another person talks, don't interrupt, ask why, judge, or challenge. Nod your head. Use your body language and facial expression to show you're eager to hear more.

✔ *Respect confidences.* Treat a friend's or partner's secrets with the discretion they deserve. Consider them a special gift entrusted to your care.

?? Do Men and Women Communicate Differently?

Only recently have scientists begun to explore gender differences in the way women and men use language. In ongoing research, psychologist James Pennebaker of the University of Texas developed a computer program to analyze four 450-word essays by more than 900 university students. The preliminary findings suggest that sex differences in written language are huge—larger, in fact, than many other psychological and personality characteristics.

In writing, women use more words overall, more words related to emotion (positive and negative), more idea words, more hearing, feeling, and sensing words, more causal words, such as *because,* and more modal words (*would, should, could*). Men use more numbers, more prepositions, and more articles, such as *an* and *the,* that, Pennebaker notes, "make language more concrete." Women use more question marks, more pronouns (especially *I*), and more references to other people. Men use more body words and, even in an academic assignment, twice as many swear words.[1]

Gender differences also appear online. In general, women tend to write e-mails in much the same way that they talk, using words to build a connection with people. Men's e-mails are briefer and more utilitarian. In chat rooms and online groups, men are more likely to make strong assertions, disagree with others, and to use profanities and sarcasm. Women are more prone to posing questions, making suggestions, and including polite expressions. Communications researchers studying the differences between "he-mails" and "she-mails" have also found that people who are not generally verbally expressive—mainly men—often convey more feelings in e-mails than they do in face-to-face conversations.[2]

When men and women speak, other gender differences emerge. In her insightful studies of language, linguist Deborah Tannen has noted that men speak more often and for longer periods in public, often as a way of putting themselves in a "one-up" situation; women speak more in private, usually to build better connections to others. In a male's hierarchical social order, she explains, conversations "are negotiations in which people try to achieve and maintain the upper hand if they can and protect themselves from others' attempts to put them down and push them around." To women, who see the world as a network of connectedness, conversations are something else entirely: "negotiations for closeness in which people try to seek and give confirmation and support, and to reach consensus." While men use words to preserve independence, women talk to draw others closer.

Perhaps this is why, in public and private, women generally are better listeners, facilitating conversation by nodding, asking questions, and signaling interest by saying "uh-huh," or "yes." Men interrupt more, breaking in on another's monologue if they aren't getting the information they need. Women are more likely to wait for the speaker to finish. "There's more than one interpretation for why a woman is less likely to interrupt," says psychologist Judith Hall. "It could show that she's being submissive and not playing the aggressive role. But it also could mean that she is less of a social blunderer and is more adept at reading the other person's signals."[3]

Beginning in their preteen and teen years, women consistently outsmile men in all sorts of situations—with children, other women, or men—when they're in positions of authority or power. They even manage to grin under stress. "If you put a man and a woman in an equally nerve-wracking situation, the woman will laugh and smile," notes Hall. In hospitals, women physicians smile considerably more than their male colleagues.

 In social interactions, two white women talking together look into each other's eyes far more often than two men; African-American women are less likely to do so. When a man and a woman are together, the man gazes into the woman's eyes more often than he would a man's, while a woman makes eye contact less often than she would if she were with another woman—a nice exercise in reciprocity. "A man talking with a woman will act more like a woman, and a woman will act more like a man," observes Hall. "It's as if they're adjusting to accommodate each other's cultural norm."

Nonverbal Communication

More than 90 percent of communication may be nonverbal. While we speak with our vocal cords, we communicate with our facial expressions, tone of voice, hands, shoulders, legs, torsos, posture. "Body language is a very elementary level of communication that people react to without realizing why," observes Albert Mehrabian, a professor of psychology at the University of California, Los Angeles (UCLA) and author of *Silent Messages.* "It's the building block upon which more advanced verbal forms of communication rest."[4]

Learning to interpret what people *don't* say can reveal more than what they *do* say. "Understanding nonverbal communication is probably the best tool there is for a good life of communicating, be it personally or professionally," says Marilyn Maple, an educator at the University of Florida. "It's one of the most practical skills you can develop. When you can consciously read what others are saying unconsciously, you can deal with issues before they become problems."[5]

Culture has a great deal of influence over body language. In some cultures, for example, establishing eye contact is considered hostile or challenging; in others, it conveys friendliness. A person's sense of personal space—the

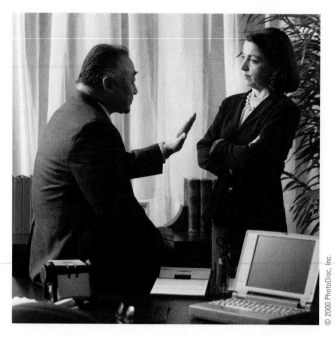

▲ Body language can send powerful nonverbal messages about your true state of mind and feelings.

distance he or she feels most comfortable in keeping from others—varies in different societies. Nonverbal messages also reveal something important about the individual. "Nonverbal messages come from deep inside of you, from your own sense of self-esteem," says Maple. "To improve your body language, you have to start from the inside and work out. If you're comfortable with yourself, it shows. People who have good self-esteem, who give themselves status and respect, who know who they are, have a relaxed way of talking and moving and always come across best."

Forming Relationships

We first learn how to relate in our families, as children. Our relationships with parents and siblings change dramatically as we grow toward independence. In college, students can choose to spend their leisure time socializing or engaging in solitary activities, like watching TV. (See Student Snapshot: "The Social Life of College Students.") Relationships between friends also change as they move or develop different interests; between lovers, as they come to know more about each other; between spouses, as they pass through life together; and between parents and children, as youngsters develop and mature. But throughout life, close relationships, tested and strengthened by time, allow us to explore the depths of our souls and the heights of our emotions.

I, Myself, and Me

The way each of us perceives himself or herself affects all the ways we reach out and relate to others. If we feel unworthy of love, others may share that opinion. Self-esteem (discussed in Chapter 3) provides a positive foundation for our relationships with others. Self-esteem doesn't mean vanity or preoccupation with our own needs; rather, it is a genuine concern and respect for ourselves so that we remain true to our own feelings and beliefs. We can't know or love or accept others until we know and love and accept ourselves, however imperfect we may be.

 If we're lacking in self-esteem, our relationships may suffer. According to research on college students by psychologists at the University of Texas, individuals with negative views of themselves seek out partners (friends, roommates, dates) who are critical and rejecting—and who confirm their low opinions of their own worth.[6]

Friendship

Friendship has been described as "the most holy bond of society." Every culture has prized the ties of respect, tolerance, and loyalty that friendship builds and nurtures. An anonymous writer put it well:

> *A friend is one who knows you as you are,*
> *Understands where you've been,*
> *Accepts who you've become,*
> *And still gently invites you to grow.*

Friends can be a basic source of happiness, a connection to a larger world, a source of solace in times of trouble. Although we have different friends throughout life, often the friendships of adolescence and young adulthood are the closest we ever form. They ease the normal break from parents and the transition from childhood to independence.

Both teenage boys and girls see their same-sex friendships as important. However, girls rate the quality of their friendships more positively, express more positive emotions toward friends, share power more equally, and show less jealousy, particularly in friendships they describe as "satisfying" rather than "unsatisfying." From middle childhood into adulthood, girls and women continue to show more responsive and supportive behavior toward their female friends, disclose more, and disagree less than male friends.[7]

In the past, many people believed that men and women couldn't become close friends without getting romantically involved. But as the genders have worked together and come to share more interests, this belief has changed. Yet unique obstacles arise in male-female friendships, such as distinguishing between friendship

© 2000 PhotoDisc, Inc.

Student Snapshot The Social Life of College Students

Responses are from two-year colleges, four-year colleges, and universities. Statistics are weighted national norms for the Class of 2004.

Source: Sax, Linda, et al. *The American Freshman: National Norms for Fall 2000.* Los Angeles: Higher Education Research Institute, UCLA, 2000.

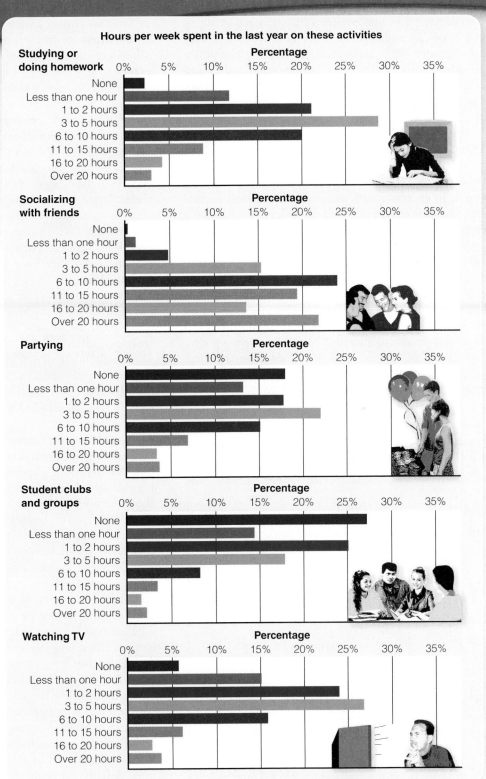

Hours per week spent in the last year on these activities

and romantic attraction and dealing with sexual tension. However, men and women who overcome such barriers and become friends benefit from their relationship—but in different ways. For men, a friendship with a woman offers support and nurturance. What they report liking most is talking and relating to women, something they don't do with their male buddies. Women view their friendships with men as more light-hearted and casual, with more joking and less fear of hurt feelings. They especially like getting insight into what guys really think.[8]

Friendship transcends all boundaries of distance and differences and enhances feelings of warmth, trust, love, and affection between two people. It is a common denominator of human existence that cuts across major social categories: In every country, culture, and language, human beings make friends. Friendship is both a universal and a deeply satisfying experience.

"Wishing to be friends," Aristotle wrote, "is quick work, but friendship is a slowly opening fruit." The qualities that make a good friend include honesty, acceptance, dependability, empathy, and loyalty. In order to sustain a close friendship, both people must be able to see the other's perspective, anticipate each other's needs, and take each other's viewpoint into account.[9] More than anything else, good friends are there when we need them. They see us at our worst but never lose sight of our best. They share our laughter and tears, our triumphs and tragedies.

STRATEGIES FOR CHANGE

Being a Good Friend

✔ *Be willing to open up.* The more you share, the deeper the bond between you and your friend will become.

✔ *Be sensitive to your friend's feelings.* Keep in mind that, like you, your friend has unique needs, desires, and dreams.

✔ *Express appreciation.* Be generous with your compliments. Let your friends know you recognize their kindnesses.

✔ *Know that friends will disappoint you from time to time.* They, too, are only human. Accept them as they are. Admitting their faults need not reduce your respect for them.

✔ *Talk about your friendship.* Evaluate the relationship periodically. If you have any gripes or frustrations, air them.

Dating

A date is any occasion during which two people share their time. It can be a Friday night dance, a bicycle ride, a dinner for two, or a walk in the park. Friends and lovers go on dates; so do complete strangers. Some men date other men; some women date other women. We don't expect to love, or even like, everyone we date. Yet the people you date reveal something about the sort of person you are.

While in school, you may go out with people you meet in class or on campus. However, with more people remaining single longer, the search for a good date has become more complex. Singles bars have become less popular because of the dangers of excessive drinking and casual sex. Cafes, laundromats, health clubs, and bookstores have become more acceptable as places to meet new people. Personal ads and cyberspace—the electronic web linking people through computers—are alternative ways to meet potential dates. (See Savvy Consumer: "Do's and Don'ts of Online Dating.")

Dating can do more than help you meet people. By dating, you can learn how to make conversation, get to know more about others as well as yourself, and share feelings, opinions, and interests. In adolescence and young adulthood, dating also provides an opportunity for exploring your sexual identity. Some people date for months and never share more than a good-night kiss. Others may fall into bed together before they fall in love or even "like."

Separating your emotional feelings about someone you're dating from your sexual desires is often difficult. The first step to making responsible sexual decisions is respecting your sexual values and those of your partner. If you care about the other person—not just his or her body—and the relationship you're creating, sex will be an important, but not the all-important, factor while you're dating. (Chapter 8 discusses sexual decision making and etiquette.)

Dating has potential dangers. As discussed in Chapter 17, approximately one in five female teens is physically and/or sexually abused by a dating partner.[10] Although the roots of such violence are complex, researchers have found a correlation between watching wrestling, with its high levels of vulgar language and physical and verbal abuse, and dating violence.[11]

Most longitudinal studies on dating relationships have shown little change in love over time, although love has been found to increase for individuals who advance to a deeper, more long-lasting commitment. Romantic partners in enduring relationships generally perceive their love, commitment, and satisfaction as increasing over time. A four-year study of romantic couples, all dating as the study began, found that those who remained together perceived that their love, satisfaction, and commitment had grown.[12]

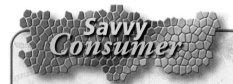

Do's and Don'ts of Online Dating

Forget personal ads or single bars. If you're looking for love in the new millennium, the place more people are turning is cyberspace. Some estimate that thousands, perhaps millions, of people, are using the Internet to find a companion.

E-mail flirtations can be fun, but they also entail some risks, particularly if you decide to go off-line and meet in person. Here are some guidelines:

- Be careful of what you type. Anything you put on the Internet can end up almost anywhere. To avoid embarrassment, don't say anything you wouldn't want to see in newspaper print.

- Don't give out your address, telephone number, or any other identifying information. The people you meet online are strangers, and you should keep your guard up.

- Don't "date" on an office or university computer. You could end up supplying your professors, classmates, or coworkers with unintentional entertainment. Also, many organizations and institutions consider e-mail messages company property.

- Remember that you have no way of verifying if a correspondent is telling the truth about anything—sex, age, occupation, marital status. If your online partner seems insincere or strange in any way, stop corresponding.

- If you do decide to meet, make your first face-to-face encounter a double or group date, and make it somewhere public, like a cafe or museum. Don't plan a full-day outing. Coffee or a drink in a crowded place makes the best transition from e-mails.

- Make sure you tell a friend or family member your plans and have your own way of getting home. It's also a good idea to schedule the first meeting in the afternoon or early in the evening rather than later at night.

- Don't let your expectations run wild. Finding Mr. or Ms. Right is no easier in cyberspace than anywhere else, so be realistic about where your relationship might lead.

- Don't rely on the Internet as your only method of meeting people. Continue to get out in the real world and meet potential dates the old-fashioned ways.

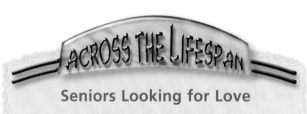

Seniors Looking for Love

Personal advertisements, widely used by young Americans, have gained increasing popularity among seniors interested in romance. Older Americans place ads similar to but somewhat different from those of younger individuals. In a study of 148 personal advertisements placed by men and women over age 55, researchers analyzed the various features mentioned or requested. The men were more likely than women to seek physical attractiveness and an attractive physique, as well as to state a specific ethnic preference. Women were more likely to seek a partner with a good sense of humor and to mention that they are active themselves. More women than men describe their own attractiveness and physique. Older men were more likely to describe themselves as caring and romantic than older women.[13]

 ## What Causes Romantic Attraction?

What draws two people to each other and keeps them together: chemistry or fate, survival instincts or sexual longings? "Probably it's a host of different things," reports sociologist Edward Laumann, coauthor of *Sex in America,* a landmark survey of 3,432 men and women conducted by the National Opinion Research Center at the University of Chicago.[14] "But what's remarkable is that most of us end up with partners much like ourselves—in age, race, ethnicity, socioeconomic class, education."

Why? "You've got to get close for sexual chemistry to occur," says Laumann. "Sparks may fly when you see someone across a crowded room, but you only see a preselected group of people—people enough like you to be in the same room in the first place. This makes sense because initiating a sexual relationship is very uncertain. We all have such trepidations about being too fat, too ugly, too undesirable. We try to lower the risk of rejection by looking for people more or less like us."

 Scientists have tried to analyze the combination of factors that attract two people to each other. In several studies of college students, four predictors ranked as the most important

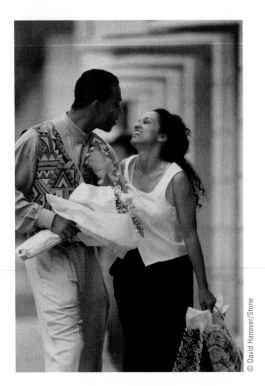

▲ Romantic attraction is characterized by a high-level of emotional arousal, reciprocal liking, and mutual sexual desire.

reasons for attraction: warmth and kindness, desirable personality, something specific about the person, and reciprocal liking.[15]

In his cross-cultural research, psychologist David Buss, author of *The Evolution of Desire,* found that men in 37 sample groups drawn from Africa, Asia, Europe, North and South America, Australia, and New Zealand rated youth and attractiveness as more important in a possible mate than did women. Women placed greater value on potential mates who were somewhat older, had good financial prospects, and were dependable and hardworking.[16]

The reason for this gender difference could be evolutionary. Throughout time, men have sought fertile females of "high reproductive value." Two outward signs of female fertility are youth and a more subtle factor: waist-hip ratio. When researchers analyzed the physical dimensions of the women considered most attractive by men in various studies, those with the slimmest waists and roundest hips were consistently rated as most desirable. Women have had to look for mates who could provide greater security for their offspring. For them, a man's power, wealth, and status—which require more time to assess—mattered more than appearance. (See The X & Y Files: "Men, Women, and Marital Preferences.")

Intimate Relationships

The term **intimacy**—the open, trusting sharing of close, confidential thoughts and feelings—comes from the Latin word for *within.* Intimacy doesn't happen at first sight, or in a day or a week or a number of weeks. Intimacy requires time and nurturing; it is a process of revealing rather than hiding, of wanting to know another and to be known by that other. (See Figure 7-1 for the elements of love.) Although intimacy doesn't require sex, an intimate relationship often includes a sexual relationship, heterosexual or homosexual.

All of our close relationships, whether they're with parents or friends, have a great deal in common. We feel we can count on these people in times of need. We feel that they understand us and we understand them. We give and receive loving emotional support. We care about their happiness and welfare. However, when we choose one person above all others, there is something even deeper and richer—something we call romantic love.

???? How Does Science View Romantic Love?

Falling in love is an intense, dizzying experience. A person not only enters our life but takes possession of it as well.

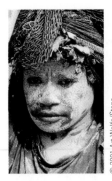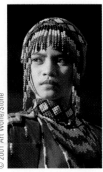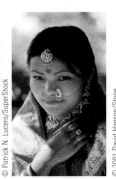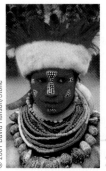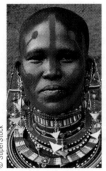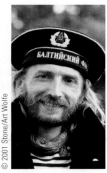

▲ Standards of physical attractiveness vary widely around the world. The women and men in these photos are considered to be attractive in their cultures.

The X&Y Files   Men, Women, and Marital Preferences

In a national survey of more than 13,000 adults in the United States, researchers asked how willing they would be to marry an individual, based on education, income, age, and other factors. As shown in the table below, the women were significantly more willing than men to marry someone who was older, better educated, would earn more, and was not good-looking. The men were more willing than women to marry someone who had less education, was younger, wasn't likely to hold a steady job, and who would earn less. There were minor differences on items related to prior marriages, religion, and already having children.

	Women	Men
How Willing Would You Be to Marry Someone Who. . .		
had more education than you?	5.82	5.22
had less education than you?	4.08	4.67
was older than you by five or more years?	5.29	4.15
was younger than you by five or more years?	2.80	4.54
was not "good-looking"?	4.42	3.41
was not likely to hold a steady job?	1.62	2.73
would earn much less than you?	3.76	4.60
would earn much more than you?	5.93	5.19
had been married before?	3.44	3.35
was of a different religion?	4.31	4.24
already had children?	3.11	2.84

Note: These responses are based on a 7-point scale, ranging from 1 ("not at all") to 7 ("very willing").
Source: Crooks, Robert, and Karla Baur. *Our Sexuality,* 8th ed. Pacific Grove, CA: Wadsworth, 2002, p. 190.

We are intrigued, flattered, delighted—but is this love, or a love of loving? At the time you're experiencing it, you may not care. You're in such a state of giddy elation that it doesn't matter, at least for the moment, whether it stems from a strong sexual attraction, a fear of loneliness, loneliness itself, or a hunger for approval.

We like to think of this powerful force, this source of both danger and delight, as something that defies analysis. However, in recent years, as scientists have attempted to study love objectively, they have provided new perspectives on its nature.

An Anthropological View

 When you first fall in love, you may be sure that no one else has ever known the same dizzying, wonderful feelings. Yet, while every romance may be unique, romantic love is anything but. In a comprehensive study of societies around the world, anthropologists William Jankowiak of the University of Nevada-Las Vegas and Edward Fischer of Tulane University found evidence of romantic love in at least 147 of the 166 cultures they studied. The experience of an "intense attraction that involves the idealization of the other, within an erotic context, with the expectation of enduring for some time in the future," they concluded, "constitutes a human universal, or at the least, a near-universal."

Another anthropologist, Helen Fisher, author of *Anatomy of Love: The Natural History of Monogamy, Adultery and Divorce,* describes romantic love "as a very primitive, basic human emotion, as basic as fear, anger or joy." As she explains, it pulled men and women of prehistoric times into the sort of partnerships that were essential to child rearing. But after about four years—just "long enough to rear one child through infancy," says Fisher—romantic love seemed to wane, and primitive couples tended to break up and find new partners. This "four-year itch" may well have endured through the centuries, contends Fisher, who notes that

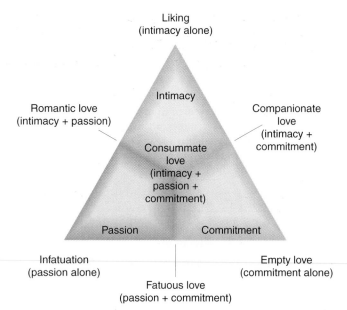

Figure 7-1 Sternberg's love triangle.
The three components of love are intimacy, passion, and commitment. The various kinds of love are composed of different combinations of the three components.

divorce statistics from most of the 62 cultures she has studied still show a pattern of restlessness four years into a marriage.[17]

A Biochemical View

The heart is the organ we associate with love, but the brain may be where the action really is. According to research on **neurotransmitters** (messenger chemicals within the brain), love sets off a chemical chain reaction that causes our skin to flush, our palms to sweat, and our lungs to breathe more deeply and rapidly. The "love chemicals" within the brain—dopamine, norepinephrine, and phenylethylamine (PEA)—have effects similar to those of amphetamines, stimulant drugs that intensify physiological reactions (see Chapter 14).

Infatuation may indeed be a natural high, but like other highs, this rush doesn't last—possibly because the body develops tolerance for love-induced chemicals, just as it does with amphetamines. However, as the initial lovers' high fades, other brain chemicals may come into play: the endorphins, morphinelike chemicals that can help produce feelings of well-being, security, and tranquility. These feel-good molecules may increase in partners who develop a deep attachment.

The hormone **oxytocin,** best known for its role in inducing labor during childbirth (see Chapter 9), seems particularly important in our ability to bond with others. By measuring blood levels of women as they recalled positive and negative relationships, researchers have found that women whose oxytocin levels rose when remembering a positive relationship reported having little difficulty setting appropriate boundaries, being alone, or trying too hard to please others. Women whose oxytocin levels fell in response to remembering a negative emotional relationship reported greater anxiety in close relationships. "It seems that having this hormone 'available' during positive experiences, and not being depleted of it during negative experiences, is associated with well-being in relationships," the researchers concluded.[18]

Mature Love

Social scientists have distinguished between passionate love—characterized by intense feelings of elation, sexual desire, and ecstasy—and companionate love, which is characterized by friendly affection and deep attachment. (See Self-Survey: "How Strong Are the Communication and Affection in Your Relationship?") Often relationships begin with passionate love and evolve into a more companionate love. Sometimes the opposite happens and two people who know each other well discover that their friendship has "caught fire" and the sparks have flamed an unexpected passion.

A romantic relationship shows definite promise if:

▶ You feel at ease with your new partner.
▶ You feel good about your new partner both when you're together and when you're not.
▶ Your partner is open with you about his or her life—past, present, and future.
▶ You can say no to each other without feeling guilty.
▶ You feel cared for, appreciated, and accepted as you are.
▶ Your partner really listens to what you have to say.

Mature love is a complex combination of sexual excitement, tenderness, commitment, and—most of all—an overriding passion that sets it apart from all other love relationships in one's life. This passion isn't simply a matter of orgasm, but also entails a crossing of the psychological boundaries between oneself and one's lover. You feel as if you're becoming one with your partner while simultaneously retaining a sense of yourself. (For other characteristics of mature, healthy love, see Pulse Points: "Ten Characteristics of a Good Relationship.")

When Love Ends

Breaking up is indeed hard to do. Sometimes two people grow apart gradually, and both of them realize that they must go their separate ways. More often, one person falls out of love first. It hurts to be rejected; it also hurts to inflict pain on someone who once meant a great deal to

SELF SURVEY

How Strong Are the Communication and Affection in Your Relationship?

Effective, caring communication and loving affection markedly enhance a couple's relationship. The following self-test may help you to assess the degree of good communication, love, and respect in your intimate relationship.

1.	My partner seeks out my opinion.	Yes	No
2.	My partner cares about my feelings.	Yes	No
3.	I don't feel ignored very often.	Yes	No
4.	We touch each other a lot.	Yes	No
5.	We listen to each other.	Yes	No
6.	We respect each other's ideas.	Yes	No
7.	We are affectionate toward one another.	Yes	No
8.	I feel my partner takes good care of me.	Yes	No
9.	What I say counts.	Yes	No
10.	I am important in our decisions.	Yes	No
11.	There's lots of love in our relationship.	Yes	No
12.	We are genuinely interested in one another.	Yes	No
13.	I love spending time with my partner.	Yes	No
14.	We are very good friends.	Yes	No
15.	Even during rough times, we can be empathetic.	Yes	No
16.	My partner is considerate of my viewpoint.	Yes	No
17.	My partner finds me physically attractive.	Yes	No
18.	My partner expresses warmth toward me.	Yes	No
19.	I feel included in my partner's life.	Yes	No
20.	My partner admires me.	Yes	No

Scoring:

A preponderance of yes answers indicates that you enjoy a strong relationship characterized by good communication

If you agree or mostly agree with a statement, answer yes. If you disagree or mostly disagree, answer no. You may wish to have your partner respond to this assessment as well. If so, mark your answers on a separate sheet.

and loving affection. If you answered yes to fewer than seven items, it is likely that you are not feeling loved and respected and that the communication in your relationship is decidedly lacking.

Source: Gottman, John. *Why Marriages Succeed or Fail.* New York: Simon & Schuster, 1994. See Hyde and DeLameter, 1997, 6th ed., p. 272.

Making Changes

Getting Your Signals Straight

▶ *Tune into your body talk.* Notice details about the way you speak, gesture, and move. If possible, watch yourself on videotape. Analyze the emotions you're feeling at the time and think of how they may be influencing your body language.

▶ *Learn to establish good eye contact, but don't glare or stare.* If you sense that someone feels uncomfortable with an intense eye grip, shift your focus so that your gaze hits somewhere between the eyes and the chin, rather than pupil-to-pupil.

▶ *Avoid putting up barriers.* If you fold your arms across your chest, you'll look defensive or uninterested in contact. Crossing your legs or ankles also can seem like a way of keeping your distance.

▶ *Identify the little things you characteristically do when you're tense.* Some people pat their hair or pick at their ears; others rub their necks, twist a ring or watch, twirl a lock of hair, or play with a pen. Train yourself to become aware of what you're doing (have a friend give you a signal, if necessary) and to control your mannerisms.

you. In surveys, college students say it's more difficult to initiate a breakup than to be rejected. Those who decided to end a relationship reported greater feelings of guilt, uncertainty, discomfort, and awkwardness than those with whom they broke up. However, students with high levels of jealousy are likely to feel a desire for vengeance that can lead to aggressive behavior.[19]

Research suggests that people do not end their relationships because of the disappearance of love. Rather a sense of dissatisfaction or unhappiness develops, which may then cause love to stop growing. The fact that love

does not dissipate completely may be one of the reasons why breakups are so painful. While the pain does ease over time, it can help both parties if they end their relationship in a way that shows kindness and respect. Your basic guideline should be to think of how you would like to be treated if someone were breaking up with you. Would it hurt more to find out from someone else? Would it be more painful if the person you cared for lied to you or deceived you, rather than admitted the truth? Saying, "I don't feel the way I once did about you; I don't want to continue our relationship," is hard, but it's also honest and direct.

PULSE POINTS

Ten Characteristics of a Good Relationship

1. **Trust.** Partners are able to confide in each other openly, knowing their confidences will be respected.

2. **Togetherness.** In a healthy relationship, two people create a sense of both intimacy and autonomy. They enjoy each other's company but also pursue solitary interests.

3. **Expressiveness.** Partners in healthy relationships say what they feel, need, and desire.

4. **Staying power.** Couples in committed relationships keep their bond strong through tough times by proving that they will be there for each other.

5. **Security.** Because a good relationship is strong enough to absorb conflict and anger, partners know they can express their feelings honestly. They also are willing to risk vulnerability for the sake of becoming closer.

6. **Laughter.** Humor keeps things in perspective—always crucial in any sort of ongoing relationship or enterprise.

7. **Support.** Partners in good relationships continually offer each other encouragement, comfort, and acceptance.

8. **Physical affection.** Sexual desire may fluctuate or diminish over the years, but partners in loving, long-term relationships usually retain some physical connection.

9. **Personal growth.** In the best relationships, partners are committed to bringing out the best in each other and have the other's best interests at heart.

10. **Respect.** Caring partners are aware of each other's boundaries, need for personal space, and vulnerabilities. They do not take each other or their relationship for granted.

STRATEGIES FOR CHANGE

Dealing with Rejection

✔ Remind yourself of your own worth. You are no less attractive, intelligent, interesting, or lovable because someone ends his or her relationship with you.

✔ Accept the rejection as a statement of the other person's preference rather than trying to debate or defend yourself.

✔ Think of other people who value or have valued you, who accept and even see as appealing the same characteristics the rejecting person viewed as undesirable.

✔ Don't withdraw from others. Although you may not want to risk further rejection, it's worth the gamble to get involved again. The only individuals who've never been rejected are those who've never reached out to connect with another.

Living Arrangements

Today's adults have many choices to explore regarding how and with whom they might live: returning to one's primary family, staying single, living with one or more friends, living in a long-term relationship with a lover of the same or opposite sex, or getting married. Increasingly, men and women in their twenties are spending more time considering all their options before committing themselves to an exclusive relationship.

Living with Parents

According to the Census Bureau, young adults between the ages of 18 and 24 are more likely to be living in their parents' homes than young people were in the 1970s. Some 18 million Americans between the ages of 18 and 34 are still living with their parents. Of those between ages 19 and 24, 66 percent (including college students) are living at home, compared to 50 percent in 1980.[20] Their reasons include the high cost of housing and the low incomes most men and women earn in their early twenties. People also are getting married later in life. The median age for a first-time groom is 27 years; for a first-time bride, 25 years—significantly older than in decades past.[21]

Single Life

In young adulthood, single men outnumber single women; after age 40, however, there are more single women than single men. Perhaps because there are so many singles, more and more Americans are living alone. (See Figure 7-2). Approximately one-quarter of the households in the nation are one-person homes, and approximately 10 percent of

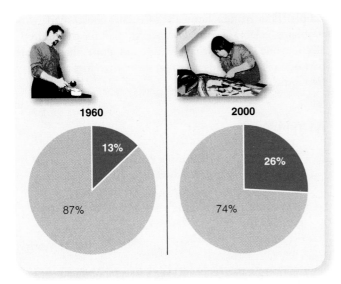

▲ **Figure 7-2** Percent of all households occupied by one person. Between 1960 and 2000, the number of single households doubled.

Source: U.S. Census Bureau.

today's young men and women will never marry. Among Americans between 25 and 34 years old, about 35 percent (14 million) have never been married. Of African Americans in this age group, 53 percent have never been married. Being single no longer marks a transition phase between living with parents and living with a spouse, but is an accepted, appealing lifestyle for millions of men and women.

The number-one reason people remain single is not being able to find the right person, according to psychologist Florence Kaslow, director of the Florida Couples and Family Institute. For women, the next two reasons for

staying single are their careers and independence. For men, independence and resolving personal issues are the second and third reasons for not marrying. Most of the women and all of the men in her study said that they would like to get married—someday.

Only 5 percent of bachelors over age 40 ever marry. Never-married men in this age group tend to avoid emotional intimacy, fear conflict, and shy away from challenges in life, according to a study of 30 lifelong bachelors. In general, the men didn't hate women, but they seemed reluctant to get involved, make demands, or assert their needs in relationships.

Is Living Together a Good Idea?

Although couples have always shared homes in informal relationships without any official ties, "living together," or **cohabitation,** has become more common, increasing by 80 percent in the last two decades. There are about 7 unmarried couples for every 100 married ones. Often young people live together in a trial marriage, getting to know each other better to see whether they're compatible—although this does not necessarily lead to a more successful marriage. People who have been married and divorced may be content just sharing their lives with one another.

More than 4 million unmarried heterosexual couples live together, in contrast to only half a million 40 years ago. (See Figure 7-3.) For many young adults, particularly children of divorced parents, living together seems like a good way to achieve some of the benefits of

STRATEGIES FOR CHANGE

How to Stay Single and Satisfied

✔ Fill your life with meaningful work, experiences, and people.

✔ Build a network of supportive friends who care for and about you.

✔ Be open to new experiences that can expand your feelings about yourself and your world.

✔ Don't miss out on a special event because you don't have someone to accompany you: Go alone.

✔ Volunteer to help others less fortunate, or become involved in church and social organizations.

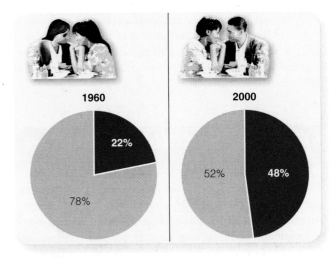

▲ **Figure 7-3** Percent of all households who are unmarried. The number of unmarried couples living together has more than doubled in the last forty years.

Source: U.S. Census Bureau.

marriage as they get to know each other and find out if they're suited to each other. According to surveys, most young people say it is a good idea to live with a person before marrying.

That's not the case, argues a controversial recent report. Researchers for the National Marriage Project of Rutgers University in New Jersey reviewed all available research and concluded that living together is not a good way to prepare for marriage or to avoid divorce. They found that these unions, in comparison to marriages, tend to have more episodes of domestic violence toward women, and more physical and sexual abuse of children. Unmarried couples also report lower levels of happiness and well-being than married couples. Annual rates of depression among unmarried couples are more than three times those of married couples. The divorce rate among couples who eventually marry is also higher.[22]

According to the report, cohabitation is probably least harmful (though not necessarily helpful) when it is prenuptial—when both partners are definitely planning to marry, have formally announced their engagement, and have picked a wedding date. The longer that two people live together, the more likely they are to have problems. The reason, the researchers suggest, is that individuals develop a "low-commitment ethic" that is the opposite of what is required for a successful marriage.[23]

Multiple living-together experiences also have a negative impact, both for an individual's own sense of well-being and for the likelihood of establishing a strong lifelong partnership. Rather than teaching people to have better relationships, repeated cohabiting is a strong predictor of the failure of future relationships.

Cohabitation poses particular risks to children. Since cohabiting parents break up at a much higher rate than married parents, children face a greater likelihood of a potentially devastating breakup.

Unmarried couples are gaining legal recognition. Some U.S. cities have "domestic partnership" laws that grant a variety of spousal rights—such as insurance benefits and bereavement leave—to partners, heterosexual or homosexual, who live together.

Committed Relationships

Even though men and women today may have more sexual partners than in the past, most still yearn for an intense, supportive, exclusive relationship, based on mutual commitment and enduring over time. In our society, most such relationships take the form of heterosexual marriages, but partners of the same sex or heterosexual partners who never marry also may sustain long-lasting, deeply committed relationships. These couples are much like married

people: They make a home, handle daily chores, cope with problems, celebrate special occasions, plan for the future—all the while knowing that they are not alone, that they are part of a pair that adds up to far more than just the sum of two individual souls.

Marriage

Like everything which is not the involuntary result of fleeting emotion but the creation of time and will, any marriage, happy or unhappy, is infinitely more interesting and significant than any romance, however passionate.

W. H. Auden

Contemporary marriage has been described as an institution that everyone on the outside wants to enter and everyone on the inside wants to leave. About 56 percent of all American adults (111 million people) are married and living with their spouses. The marriage rate has dropped dramatically: A lower percentage of couples tied the knot in the 1990s than in previous decades. In fact, the national marriage rate has dropped over the last four decades to its lowest point ever.

Not only are fewer people getting married, but fewer marital partners describe themselves as "very happy" in their relationships. In a recent report on "the social health of marriage in America," researchers at Rutgers University found that more couples are choosing to live together outside of marriage or are putting off vows until later in life.[24] Young people also have grown disenchanted with the prospect of marriage. The percentage of teenagers who thought they would be happier married than not married has fallen over the last two decades.

Not too long ago, marriage was often a business deal, a contract made by parents for economic or political reasons when the spouses-to-be were still very young. Today, in some countries, it is still culturally acceptable to arrange marriages in this manner. Even in America, certain ethnic groups, such as Asians who have recently immigrated to the United States, plan marriages for their children. In such arrangements, the marriage partners are likely to have similar values and expectations. However, the newlyweds also start out as strangers who may not even know whether they like—let alone love—each other. Sometimes arranged marriages do lead to loving unions; sometimes they trap both partners in loneliness and longing.

Most of today's marriages aren't arranged, but even in this day and age, partners often marry because they have to: One of every six brides is pregnant on her wedding day. Other young couples marry as a way to escape from their parents' homes and authority. But most people say they marry for one far-from-simple reason: love.

Preparing for Marriage

With more than half of all marriages ending in divorce, there's little doubt that modern marriages aren't made in heaven. Are some couples doomed to divorce even before they swap "I do's"? Could counseling before a marriage increase its odds of success? According to recent research findings, the answer to both questions is yes.

There have been government attempts to set requirements for couples who want to marry. Some states, such as Arizona and Louisiana, have established "covenant" marriages in which engaged couples are required to get premarital counseling. Utah allows counties to require counseling before issuing marriage licenses to minors and people who have been divorced. Florida requires high school students to take marriage education classes.[25]

Finding Mr. or Ms. Right

Generally, men and women marry people from the geographical area they grew up in and from the same social background. Differences in religion and race can add to the pressures of marriage, but they also can enrich the relationship if they aren't viewed as obstacles. In our culturally diverse society, interracial and crosscultural marriages are becoming more common and widely accepted, although the odds are much greater for partners of the same race to live together or marry.

 In a study of 75,000 couples who lived together and 480,000 married couples in the United States, researchers found that African Americans were 365 times more likely to marry a black than a nonblack spouse and 110 times more likely to live with, or cohabit with, a black partner than someone of another racial group. Asians were 55 times more likely to marry another Asian and 17 times more likely to cohabit with another Asian. Hispanics were 12 times more likely to select a Hispanic spouse and nine times more likely to live with a Hispanic partner. Whites were about eight times more likely to marry another white person and five times more likely to cohabit with someone who is white rather than nonwhite.[26]

Some of the traits that appeal to us in a date become less important when we select a mate; others become key ingredients in the emotional cement holding two people together. According to psychologist Robert Sternberg of Yale University, the crucial ingredients for commitment are the following:

- Shared values.
- A willingness to change in response to each other.
- A willingness to tolerate flaws.
- A match in religious beliefs.
- The ability to communicate effectively.

The single best predictor of how satisfied one will be in a relationship, according to Sternberg, is not how one feels toward a lover, but the difference between how one would like the lover to feel and how the lover actually feels. Feeling that the partner you've chosen loves too little or too much is, as he puts it, "the best predictor of failure."[27]

Premarital Assessments

There are scientific ways of predicting marital happiness. Some premarital assessment inventories identify strengths and weaknesses in many aspects of a relationship: realistic expectations, personality issues, communication, conflict resolution, financial management, leisure activities, sex, children, family and friends, egalitarian roles, and religious orientation. Couples who become aware of potential conflicts by means of such inventories may be able to resolve them through professional counseling. In some cases, they may want to reconsider or postpone their wedding.

Other common predictors of marital discord, unhappiness, and separation are:

- A high level of arousal during a discussion.
- Defensive behaviors such as making excuses and denying responsibility for disagreements.
- A wife's expressions of contempt.
- A husband's stonewalling (showing no response when a wife expresses her concerns).

STRATEGIES FOR PREVENTION

When to Think Twice About Getting Married

Don't get married if:

✔ You or your partner is constantly asking the other such questions as "Are you sure you love me?"

✔ You spend most of your time together disagreeing and quarreling.

✔ You're both still very young (under the age of 20).

✔ Your boyfriend or girlfriend has behaviors (such as nonstop talking), traits (such as bossiness), or problems (such as drinking too much) that really bother you and that you're hoping will change after you're married.

✔ Your partner wants you to stop seeing your friends, quit a job you enjoy, or change your life in some other way that diminishes your overall satisfaction.

By looking for such behaviors, researchers have been able to predict with better than 90 percent accuracy whether a couple will separate within the first few years of marriage.

Types of Marriage

Sociologists have categorized marriages as traditional or companion-oriented. In **traditional marriages,** the couples assume prescribed societal roles. In c**ompanion-oriented marriages,** the partnership and its rewards—rather than the roles of fathering, mothering, and breadwinning—are primary. In addition, there are **romantic marriages,** in which sexual passion never seems to die, and **rescue marriages,** in which one partner suffered a traumatic childhood and sees marriage as a way of healing. About a fifth of all marriages belong to another category that has grown significantly in recent years: marriages of equally dependent spouses (MEDs). Each partner in these unions earns between 40 and 59 percent of the total family income. According to research on these marriages, divorces are more common and occur more often at the wife's initiative. Researchers theorize that wives who are not economically dependent on their spouses may be more likely to leave an emotionally unfulfilling relationship.[28] Regardless of type, a marriage can succeed if it fulfills basic tasks, such as providing a sense of intimacy and autonomy and providing a safe haven that is strong enough to absorb inevitable conflicts.

Issues Couples Confront

No two people can live together in perfect harmony all the time. Some of the issues that crop up in any long-term relationship include expectations, how to disagree, money, sex, and careers.

Unrealistic Expectations

Partners may think that their significant others should always be as attractive, charming, and tolerant as they were when they were dating. They may assume that their partners will always agree with them or will automatically see their point of view; or they may believe that their one true love will always be able to meet all their needs. Because no one could ever live up to such expectations, the partners are doomed to disappointment.

Settling Differences

Contrary to what you may assume, arguments can be good for the health of a relationship. According to the National Institute of Mental Health, couples who learn how to fight fairly and effectively have a 50 percent lower divorce rate than those who haven't mastered the art of disagreeing. Results of a study of 150 couples from premarriage through the first ten years of marriage (the highest risk period for divorce) led researchers to conclude that "nondestructive" arguing lowers the likelihood for physical violence, helps couples stay together longer, and benefits children by preparing them to build good intimate relationships as adults.

Money

Money may make the business world go around, but it has the opposite effect on relationships: It knocks them off their tracks, brings them to a halt, twists them upside down. However, even though almost all couples quarrel about money, they rarely fight over how much they have. What matters more—whether they make $10,000 or $100,000 a year—is what money means to both partners. How does each person use money to meet emotional needs? Who decides how the money is spent? Who keeps track? Until they resolve these issues, couples may quarrel over money as long as they're together.

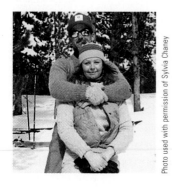
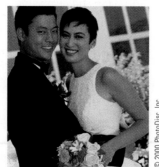
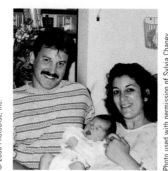
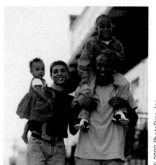

▲ A relationship is just as alive as the individuals who create it. It grows if there is caring; it can blossom if there is emotional nourishment; and it endures if there is commitment.

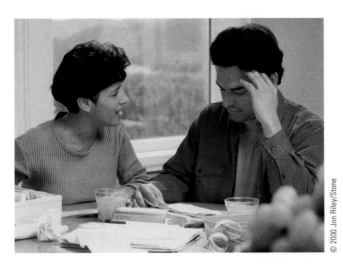

▲ Fight fair. You can learn to argue effectively, without attacking others or damaging relationships.

STRATEGIES FOR CHANGE

How to Fight Fairly

The art of arguing is a skill, like bicycle riding, that anyone can master with time, patience, and plenty of practice. Here are some basic ground rules:

✔ Learn to listen. Rather than thinking about what you're going to say next, tune in to your partner. Think before you open your mouth. Taking a few deep breaths gives you time to weigh your words.

✔ Use the speaker/listener technique. When one person has the floor, the other listens. Start sentences with "I," not "You." Instead of attacking with a statement such as "You're jealous and immature," say, "I feel hurt when you quiz me about my old relationships."

✔ Make sure you're arguing about the right issue. Are you angry simply because your partner is never on time? Or because you don't seem to be the top priority?

✔ Don't embarrass each other by fighting in front of others. Don't attack each other so viciously that one of you is backed into a corner. Be fair. Whenever there's a cheap shot, one of you should stop the fight by crying "Foul!"

✔ If you can't come to terms on a particular issue, agree to disagree, or to keep talking in the future.

To avoid fighting over money, understand that having different money values or expectations doesn't make one of you right and the other wrong. Recognize the value of unpaid work. A partner who's finishing school or taking care of the children is making an important contribution to the family and its future. It also helps to go over your finances together, so you have a firm basis in reality for what you can and can't afford. Talk about the financial goals you hope to attain five years from now. Set priorities to meet them. Also, set aside money for each of you to spend without asking or answering to the other. Even a small amount can make each partner feel more independent.

Sex

Like every other aspect of a relationship, sex evolves and changes over the course of marriage. The redhot sexual chemistry of the early stages of intimacy invariably cools down. Even so, the happiest couples have sex more often than unhappily married pairs do.

What matters most isn't quantity alone, but the quality of sexual activity and intimacy (discussed in Chapter 8). Are both partners satisfied with their sexual relationship? Does one partner always initiate sex? Do the partners talk about their preferences and pleasures? Sexuality, like personality, is dynamic and changes throughout life. Do the partners acknowledge and adapt to these changes? Do they feel sufficiently at ease with each other to discuss anxieties about sex? The answers to these questions can determine how sexually gratifying a marriage is for both spouses.

Extramarital Affairs

How faithful are American mates? The answer depends on the questions researchers ask and whom they ask. In face-to-face interviews with 3,432 Americans, aged 18 to 59, University of Chicago researchers found that 25 percent of men and 15 percent of women had had affairs, and that 94 percent of the married subjects had been monogamous in the last year. Another survey of 1,049 Americans, aged 18 to 65, found that one out of six had had an extramarital relationship—19 percent of the men and 15 percent of the women.[29]

High or low, numbers are little comfort when affairs do occur. A husband or wife who learns about a spouse's affair typically feels a devastating sense of betrayal as well as deep feelings of shame, fear of abandonment, depression, and anger. Two crucial questions determine whether a marriage can survive: Do the spouses still feel a serious commitment to each other? And do they love each other and want to grow old together?

Two-Career Couples

More than 75 percent of women with children work—a dramatic increase from the 1960s, when only 30 percent of

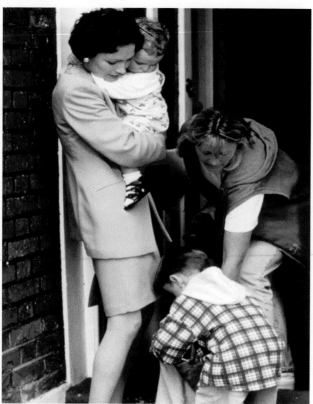

▲ Two-career couples cope with balancing family and work in various and sometimes imperfect ways.

mothers worked outside the home. Two careers can bring pressure to a relationship: Both individuals may come home tired and irritable; both may have to spend a great deal of time on their jobs; both may have to travel or work on weekends. Two-career couples must be able to discuss their problems openly to resolve these pressures.

Couples pursuing individual careers sometimes face difficult choices. What happens, for example, if one of them is offered a promising job in another city? Does the spouse quit his or her job, pack up, and move? Some couples resolve such dilemmas by working in different cities and spending weekends together. Others try to alternate career and home priorities. However imperfect these arrangements may be, they work for some couples.

Do dual careers affect a couple's sex lives? The answers are complex. Some researchers have theorized that long hours and multiple roles would dampen sexual expression in working couples. But that's not necessarily the case. Except for spouses working unusually demanding jobs (more than 54 hours a week), work per se does not cause psychological distress (in women, it actually promotes better mental health) nor does it affect sexual frequency.

In studies comparing homemakers and women working part or full time, there have been no significant differ-

ences in frequency of intercourse, sexual satisfaction, or decreased sexual desire. Fatigue does dampen a woman's sex life—but is just as common in homemakers without paid jobs as in employed women. Wives highly satisfied with their work roles also were more positive about their sex lives.[30]

The working couples most likely to stay together are those who are not tightly tied to traditional gender roles. Because neither spouse has very narrow expectations of what the other should or shouldn't be doing, both are free to pursue individual interests outside the home.

???? Why Has Marriage Endured?

Despite its problems, marriage endures because it is a fulfilling way for two people to live. As researchers have proven, good marriages make people happy and healthy. For years researchers thought that marriage was especially beneficial to men. Married men have lower rates of alcohol and drug abuse, depression, and risk-taking behavior than divorced men. They also earn more money—possibly because they have more incentive to do so.

However, research has shown that marriage also is good for women. Both married men and women live longer than single or divorced individuals. In one national survey, about 90 percent of husbands and wives survived until at least age 65, compared with only about 60 to 70 percent of divorced and never-married men and women. Married people also have healthier behaviors: They drink less alcohol and use fewer illicit drugs. Happily married men and women rate themselves as happier than the divorced or never-married. However, women in unhappy unions—but not their husbands—have higher rates of depression and unhappiness than single women.

Married people, who have sex about twice as often, consistently report greater satisfaction than unmarried partners. Cohabiting couples also have active sex lives, but they get less emotional satisfaction from it than married lovers—especially women. For married men, researchers report, satisfaction stems from sexual frequency, fidelity, and emotional commitment. These factors are equally important to women, but just being married adds an extra kick to their sexual satisfaction.

Although there has not been much research on same-sex committed relationships, most experts believe that gay couples are likely to enjoy similar benefits, as long as they remain together and receive social support for doing so.

Couples Therapy

According to the Association of Family and Marital Therapists, at least one of every five couples in this coun-

STRATEGIES FOR PREVENTION

Making the Most of a Committed Relationship

✔ Focus on what's right with your partner. Be kinder to your partner. Don't take for granted the nice things your spouse does.

✔ Learn to negotiate for what you want. One effective approach is offering your mate what he or she wants in return.

✔ Look for the problem behind the problem. Often an affair or a lack of sexual interest is merely a symptom; the real question is why this problem has developed.

✔ Keep your perspective. Uncapped toothpaste tubes or food not prepared exactly to your taste may be annoying, but are they worth a fight?

✔ Rather than thinking of all the things your partner is or isn't doing, look for things you can do to make your marriage better.

try needs professional counseling—and increasing numbers are seeking help. An estimated five million couples—married or not—now turn to the 50,000 licensed family therapists in the United States, a dramatic increase since 1980. The relationships of about two-thirds of those who get counseling do improve, according to both the couples' own judgments and objective measures of satisfaction.

A well-trained counselor can spot destructive behavior patterns and help couples see their situations in a new light. Therapy often helps stop spouses from hurting each other so badly that they can't stay together. If nothing else, it can help both partners decide whether to continue or end the relationship.

???? What Is the Current Divorce Rate?

About half of all marriages end in divorce, but the odds of a first marriage lasting are slightly better. According to a CDC analysis of the most recent census data, about 43 percent of first marriages end in separation or divorce within 15 years. The older the bride, the better the chance the marriage will last. Nearly 60 percent of brides under age 18 eventually separate or divorce, compared with 36 percent of those age 20 or older. Women who marry and divorce young are more apt to wed again: 81 percent of those

divorced before age 25 remarry within ten years, compared with 68 percent of those divorced at age 25 or older.

 Race also influences marriage and divorce rates. African-American couples are more likely to break up than white couples, and black divorcées are less likely to marry again. Researchers have found that African Americans place an equally high value on marriage. However, there is a smaller "marriageable pool" of black men for a variety of reasons, including a higher mortality rate.[31]

Even after their hopes for happiness with one spouse end, men and women still yearn to mesh two personalities, two life histories, and two persons' dreams into a marriage. Eighty percent of divorced men and women remarry, and the remarriage rate increases with the number of times an individual has been divorced. The remarriage rate after a second divorce is 90 percent; after a third divorce, it's even higher. However, more second, third, and fourth marriages fail than original unions.[32]

Family Ties

America's families are growing—and changing. According to the Census Bureau, the number of households in the United States increased 15 percent from 1990 to 2000, with nonfamily households increasing about twice as much (23 percent) as family households (11 percent).[33] Married couples make up the majority of households, though by a smaller number than in 1990 (see Figure 7-4). Family households headed by women with no husbands outnumber by almost three times households headed by men without wives. Women with children under 18 years head 7.2 percent of all households, up from 6.6 percent in 1990.

Although the number of people and households in the United States increased from 1990 to 2000, both average household size and family size decreased somewhat. Today the average family numbers 3.16 people. People living alone make up one in four households in the United States. One-person households are four times as common as nonfamily households with two or more people.

Utah has the highest proportion of married-couple households (63 percent), followed by Idaho and Iowa. Only 23 percent of households in the District of Columbia are maintained by married couples. Massachusetts, Rhode Island, Louisiana, Mississippi, and Nevada also have less than half of their households maintained by married couples.

The number of households with unmarried partners increased from 3.2 million in 1990 to 5.5 million in 2000 (4.9 million consist of partners of the opposite sex). Unmarried partners account for 5.2 percent of all households, up from 3.5 percent in 1990. California has the largest number of nonmarried-partner households.

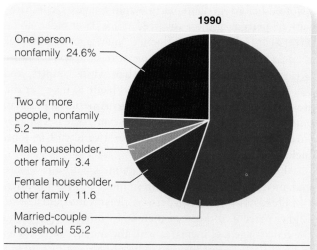

1990

One person, nonfamily 24.6%

Two or more people, nonfamily 5.2

Male householder, other family 3.4

Female householder, other family 11.6

Married-couple household 55.2

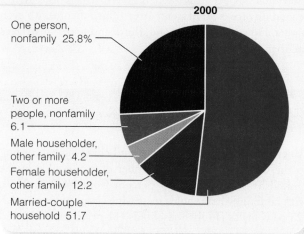

2000

One person, nonfamily 25.8%

Two or more people, nonfamily 6.1

Male householder, other family 4.2

Female householder, other family 12.2

Married-couple household 51.7

▲ **Figure 7-4** A comparison of households by type: 1990 and 2000. The percent of married-couple households has decreased while the number of other types of households have increased.

Source: U.S. Census Bureau.

Diversity Within Families

The "all-American" **family**—as portrayed on television and in movies—is typically white and middle-class. But families of different cultures—Italian to Indian to Indonesian—reflect different traditions, beliefs, and values. Within African-American families, for instance, traditional gender roles are often reversed, with women serving as head of the household, a kinship bond uniting several households, and a strong religious commitment or orientation. In Chinese-American families, both spouses may work and see themselves as breadwinners, but the wife may not have an equal role in decision making. In Latino families, wives and mothers are acknowledged and respected as healers and dispensers of wisdom. At the same time, they are expected to defer to their husbands, who see themselves as the strong, protective, dominant head of the family. As time

passes and families from different cultures become more integrated into American life, traditional gender roles and decision-making patterns often change, particularly among the youngest family members.

American families also are diverse in other ways. Multigenerational families, with children, parents, and grandparents, make up 3.7 percent of households. They occur most often in areas where new immigrants live with relatives, where housing shortages or high costs force families to double up their living arrangements, or where there are high rates of out of wedlock childbearing and unwed mothers live with their children in their parents' home.[34]

Three of every ten households consist of blended families, formed when one or both of the partners getting married bring children from a previous union. In the future, social scientists predict, American families will become even more diverse, or pluralistic. But even as norms or expectations about the configurations of families have changed, values or ideas about the intents and purposes of families have not. American families of every type still support each other and strive toward values such as commitment and caring.

Becoming Parents

Parenting is a 24-hour-a-day, 7-day-a-week, 52-week-a-year job, with no sabbaticals or sick leaves and no opportunity to renegotiate the contract. Having a child is an experience that deeply affects, involves, and changes a man and a woman.

When Baby Makes Three

New parents are likely to feel proud one moment and anxious the next. The infant may fascinate them both, but the adjustment to a baby-centered life can cause resentment. The husband who feels that his wife is more concerned with the baby than with him often feels jealous, which in turn makes him feel guilty. The mother, still recovering from childbirth, may feel overwhelmed by new responsibilities and the daunting physical demands of caring for a newborn.

Experts in family development, who have been studying the changes a baby brings to a marriage, note that marital satisfaction invariably declines, if only slightly, while the number of separations and divorces rises after a baby's arrival. However, couples who stick together as partners through the process of becoming parents can keep their marriages strong.

As Children Grow

A child's greatest need is for love—the feeling of being wanted and cared for, of being special, and of realizing that the parents like the child for him- or herself. According to a study that followed 379 kindergarten-aged children for 36 years, warm, loving parenting—the kind that supplies plenty of hugs, kisses, and cuddles—has more influence on adult social adjustment than any other parental or childhood factor. The individuals whose mothers and fathers were openly affectionate were able to sustain long and relatively happy marriages, raise children, develop close friendships, and enjoy varied activities outside their marriage.

Children have other needs, too. They need security—assurance that their parents will be there when needed most; protection; confidence; and a feeling of belonging. They need role models to learn behavior from and a sense of clear limits and controls. Parents are responsible for establishing values of what is right or wrong and for guiding by example as well as with words.

With each year that passes in a child's life, the conflict between independence and dependence becomes more intense. Children are drawn into the larger world outside the family and home, and their parents are torn between clinging to them and pushing them out of the nest. It's not enough to set rules; parents must also advise a child on how to make decisions within those rules.

The teen years—the transition from childhood to adulthood—are, for parents and children, the best and worst of times. Children becoming teenagers develop more responsibility, a greater sense of self, and more independence. Simultaneously, they may rebel, challenging and testing their parents. Setting limits—such as curfews and dating guidelines—may set off a confrontation instead of being a simple matter of stating policy. A teen's emerging sexuality may be difficult for the parents to acknowledge and accept. (Chapter 8 discusses adolescent sexuality.)

Siblings

The ways in which siblings relate as children often affect their interactions with each other—and with others, including their mates—when they grow up. Sibling rivalry, for instance, though normal, can lead to unhealthy ways of relating to others. For example, siblings who had to compete fiercely for parental attention or affection may remain competitive throughout life, doing anything necessary in order to come out on top. And youngsters who feel that their parents clearly prefer another child in the family may come to think that they're inadequate or somehow unworthy of love.

Siblings typically grow more distant during adolescence, as they focus on developing their own identities. This separation continues during early adulthood. However, in middle age, most adults report positive relationships with siblings. Some are bound by loyalty, even if they don't feel friendly toward a brother or sister. Others socialize with siblings but are closer to friends. In old age, sisters and brother-sister pairs have more positive relationships than brothers; elderly African Americans tend to have more positive relationships with their siblings than do elderly whites.

Working Parents

Throughout the world, mothers have taken on increased economic responsibility for their families. As a result, they are working longer hours at home and on the job. In the United States, nearly half of employed married women contribute half or more of their family's income. Most women with children are working either full- or part-time, including those with very young children.

Marital roles continue to change with the times. The supermoms of the eighties tried to do it all—at home and at work. The "jugglers" of the nineties were always struggling to keep something up in the air. Now trend-watchers have a different term for millennium mates: the new collaborators.

One in four men now does most of the grocery shopping, up from 15 percent of men in 1986. The Family and Work Institute of New York calculates that American husbands put in 75 percent as much time as wives on workday chores—a dramatic rise from 30 percent in 1977. In actual clocktime, the gender difference in domestic "scutwork" amounts to just 45 minutes a day.

Plenty of sociologists—and lots of weary women still doing the lioness share of chores—doubt whether all men in all income groups are doing as much. However, the trend toward greater husbandly involvement is real—and likely to continue. Researchers have actually calculated the exact percentage of shared work that equals a "fair share": Among employed husbands and wives, those who each reported doing less than half—45.8 percent each, to be precise—also reported the highest levels of psychological well-being and lowest levels of distress.[35]

The basis of the new collaboration goes beyond shared chores to shared values. In a study of 300 dual-earner couples in the Boston area, women and men showed remarkable similarities in how they felt about their relationships with each other and with their children. Contrary to the old assumption that family problems were female concerns and work issues male concerns, both spouses showed equal sensitivity to stress at home, problems in the marital relationships, and work concerns. Another study found that gender has virtually no bearing on how parents respond, physically or psychologically, to situations in which work interferes with family life or family life interferes with work. Mothers and fathers care—and care deeply—about both.[36]

Single Parents

Married couples with children account for less than a quarter of all households. About 28 percent of all children under age 18 live with just one parent. Demographers predict that more than half of the youngsters born in the 1990s will spend at least part of their childhood in a single-parent home.

The majority of children who live with just one parent live with their mothers. The number of families headed by single mothers has increased 25 percent since 1990, to more than 7.5 million households. About a third of all babies are born to unmarried women, compared to just 3.8 percent in 1940.

The new breed of single mother doesn't fit the old stereotype of an unwed minority teenager. The median age for unmarried mothers is the late 20s; the fastest growing group is white women. She may be divorced or, like celebrities Calista Flockhart and Rosie O'Donnell, unmarried. Forty percent live with men who may be the fathers of one or more of their children. There has been a 72 percent increase in the number of cohabiting couples, many of whom bring along children from other relationships. This change represents a dramatic transition in the demographic makeup of the United States, although it is not yet clear whether having children outside of marriage will become as widespread as it is in other nations, such as Sweden.[37]

Single fathers head over two millions households. Men now comprise 1 in 6 of the nation's 11.9 million single parents, up from 1 in 7 in 1995 and 1 in 10 in 1980.

The typical single father is 38 years old. One in 9 is under age 25; and 1 in 70 is 60 or older. About 5 of every 6 (83 percent) of the nation's single fathers are white. African Americans and Hispanics together constitute about 13 percent.

Median family income for one-parent families is significantly lower than the median for two-parent families. Twenty percent are poor, compared with 9 percent of two-parent families. Half live in rental housing, compared with one-quarter of two-parent families.

Children of Divorce

Each year divorce separates more than a million children from their parents. The breakup of a marriage has an enormous impact on many aspects of a child's life, including his or her standard of living. Very young children may become more babyish, irritable, and dependent. Preschool or young school-age children may blame themselves, feeling that "Daddy left because I was bad." School-age children may feel lonely, helpless, and depressed; they may develop illnesses or have problems in their friendships. Preteens may experiment with alcohol, drugs, and sex. For teenagers, divorce may make separating from the family and establishing an adult identity even harder.

According to research, children whose parents divorce are more likely to suffer abuse or neglect, to exhibit more physical and emotional problems, to perform less well academically, and to become involved in crime and drug abuse.[38]

Blended Families

Each year about half a million children become part of new, **blended families** when their parents remarry. Over the years many studies have found significant differences in family and relationship processes in these families. However, improved communication and problem solving can help blended families work through their problems.

Children can also be encouraged to spend time with members of the extended family or friends to experience other role models.

Dysfunctional Relationships

Relationships that don't promote healthy communication, honesty, and intimacy are sometimes called **dysfunctional.** Individuals with addictive behaviors or dependence on drugs or alcohol (see Chapters 14 and 15), and the children or partners of such people, are especially likely to find themselves in such relationships.

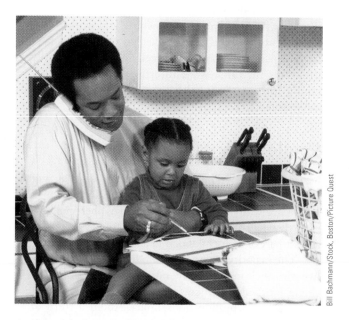

Bill Bachmann/Stock, Boston/Picture Quest

▲ Although the majority of single parents are women, about 17 percent of single-parent families are headed by fathers.

STRATEGIES FOR CHANGE

Helping Children of Divorce

✔ Don't give youngsters everything they want just to get them to like you more than the other parent.

✔ Be honest, but spare your children the gory details. Don't fight in front of them.

✔ Let children know it's okay for them to love both their parents. Give them a chance to talk about how they feel.

✔ Let them know that you love them and that they are not responsible for the breakup.

Often partners have magical, unrealistic expectations (e.g., they expect that a relationship with the right person will make their life okay), and one person uses the other almost as if he or she were a mood-altering drug. The partners may compulsively try to get the other to act the way they want. Both persons may not trust or may deceive each other. Often they isolate themselves from others, thus trapping themselves in a recurring cycle of pain.

Dysfunctional families exist in every economic, social, educational, religious, and racial group. They inflict emotional pain on children through destructive behaviors, such as physical, emotional, verbal, or sexual abuse; physical or emotional neglect; and alcoholism or drug use. Although alcohol or drugs do not in themselves create dysfunctional families, they can push parents over a psychological brink. The results can be emotionally devastating. The children of alcoholics, drug users, and parents with other addictive behaviors are prone to learning disabilities, eating disorders, compulsive achievement, and addiction.

??? What Is Codependence?

Contemporary therapists use the term **codependence** (or coaddiction) for the tendency of the spouses, partners, parents, and friends of individuals with addictive behaviors to allow or *enable* their loved ones to continue their self-destructive habits. Codependent individuals focus on their loved ones, even to the extent of giving up their own lives. They change who they are and what they feel in order to please others, feel responsible for meeting others' needs, have low self-esteem, and frequently have compulsions of their own. However, codependent behaviors need to be evaluated in the context of an individual's culture. For example, the emphasis on family values and support that is part of the value system of many Latinos would not be considered codependent behavior.

Codependents Anonymous, founded in 1986 for men and women whose common problem is an inability to maintain functional relationships, is one of the fastest-growing support programs in the country. Other self-help groups for codependents include Al-Anon (for adult family members of alcoholics), Alateen (for the teenaged children of addicts), Nar-Anon (for people in relationships with individuals who abuse drugs), O-Anon (for those whose family members have eating disorders), and Gam-Anon (for those living with people who have gambling problems). Local chapters of these groups can be found in the white pages of the telephone book. Through such groups, codependent individuals can learn how to leave behind guilt feelings, how to become less judgmental and moralistic, how to understand their powerlessness over their loved one's problem, and how to do what needs to be done for themselves as well as the addict.

If you wonder if you may be codependent, read through the following list of characteristics of codependence and check any that apply to you:

- I find myself covering for another person's alcohol or drug use, eating or work habits, gambling, sexual escapades, or general behavior.
- I spend a great deal of time talking about and worrying about other people's behavior/problems/future instead of living my own life.
- I have marked or counted bottles, searched for a hidden stash, or in other ways monitored someone else's behavior.
- I find myself taking on more responsibility at home or in a relationship, even though I resent it.
- I ignore my own needs in favor of meeting someone else's.
- I'm afraid that if I get angry, the other person will leave or not love me.
- I worry that if I leave a relationship or stop controlling the other person, that person will fall apart.
- I spend less time with friends and more with my partner/parent/child in activities that I wouldn't normally choose.
- My self-esteem depends on what others say and think of me, or on my possessions or job.
- I grew up in a family in which there was little communication, in which expressing feelings wasn't acceptable, and in which there were either rigid rules or none at all.

If you identify with more than three of these statements, you may be codependent. There are many useful books on codependence at libraries and bookstores. You may also wish to visit a support group on campus or in your area or talk with a counselor.

Enabling

Experts on the subject of addiction first identified traits of codependence in spouses of alcoholics, who followed a predictable pattern of behavior: While intensely trying to control the drinkers, the codependent mates would act in ways that allowed the drinkers to keep drinking. For example, if an alcoholic found it hard to get up in the morning, his wife would wake him up, pull him out of bed and into the shower, and drop him off at work. If he was late, she made excuses to his boss. The husband was the one with the substance-abuse problem, but without realizing it, his wife was enabling him to continue drinking. In fact, he might not have been able to keep up his habit without her unintentional cooperation.

The different styles or components of **enabling** include the following:

- **Shielding.** Codependents may cover up for abusers, preventing them from experiencing the full impact of the harmful consequences of their behavior—for example, by dropping off a paper or report so that the addicted person can avoid a missed deadline.

▶ **Controlling.** A codependent may try to control the significant other—for instance, by withholding sex or using sex as a reward for cutting down on an addictive behavior.

▶ **Taking over responsibilities.** The codependent may take over such household chores as shopping or running errands.

▶ **Rationalizing.** Codependents try to rationalize their partners' addiction by telling themselves that a compulsive behavior pattern, like workaholism, is making the person more successful, or that drinking helps him or her relax.

▶ **Cooperating.** Sometimes codependents become involved in the person's compulsion, perhaps placing bets for a gambler or buying alcohol for a drinker.

▶ **Rescuing.** The codependent may become overprotective—for example, by allowing the user to use drugs at home to avoid the risk of an accident or arrest.

Codependence progresses just as an addiction does, and codependents excuse their own behavior with many of the same defense mechanisms used by addicts, such as rationalization ("I cut class so I could catch up on my reading, not to keep an eye on my partner") and denial ("He likes to gamble, but he never loses more than he can afford"). In time, just as an addict's world becomes smaller and smaller, codependents lose sight of everything but their loved one. They feel that if they can only "fix" this person, everything will be fine.

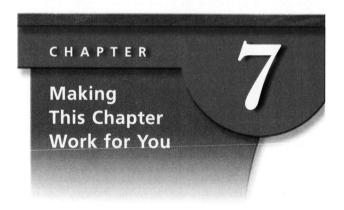

CHAPTER 7

Making This Chapter Work for You

1. Which of the following scenarios demonstrates what might be considered gender differences in verbal and nonverbal communication styles?
   a. While Alyssa and Peter are discussing their vacation plans, Alyssa is gazing at the television and Peter is looking at Alyssa.
   b. Good friends Eva and Julia see each other for the first time after Christmas break and greet each other with a nod and a quick "Hi."
   c. New bank manager Alejandro tells the staff that they should consider him "the team coach and the keeper of the playbook."
   d. During an argument, Tony complains to Nicki, "I don't appreciate your crude jokes and constant swearing."

2. Romantic love
   a. is associated with the depletion of the hormone oxytocin.
   b. is an emotional phenomenon between humans that has its roots in prehistoric times and occurs in almost all cultures.
   c. can only occur between people who share interests and goals.
   d. always result in a committed long-term relationship.

3. The characteristics of a good relationship include which of the following?
   a. trust
   b. financial stability
   c. identical interests
   d. physical attractiveness

4. Which of the following statements is true?
   a. About 25 percent of bachelors over age 40 usually marry by the time they are 50.
   b. Research strongly supports the belief that living with a person before marrying is a good idea.
   c. The number-one reason women remain single is to focus on their career.
   d. Approximately 10 percent of today's young adults will never marry.

5. Partners in successful marital relationships
   a. are generally from the same social and ethnic background.
   b. usually lived together before marrying.
   c. were usually very young at the time of their marriage.
   d. have premarital agreements.

6. Married people
   a. have sex less frequently than unmarried partners.
   b. are more likely to become alcoholics and drug users.
   c. typically have at least one extramarital affair during their marriage.
   d. live longer than single or divorced individuals.

7. When couples have a child,
   a. their marital satisfaction typically increases.
   b. they should resist being openly affectionate to each other to avoid embarrassing situations.
   c. they have a slightly higher risk of divorce.
   d. they are less likely to get divorced for the sake of the child.

8. Single-parent families
   a. account for about one-fourth of all households.

b. exceed the number of married-parent families.

c. are headed by men in about 25 percent of cases.

d. are typically headed by women who were unwed teenagers at the time of the first child's birth.

9. Which of the following statements about divorce is false?

a. The older the bride, the more likely the chance that the marriage will endure.

b. African-American couples are more likely to divorce than white couples.

c. Preschool-aged children are less likely to be affected by the divorce of their parents than older children.

d. The majority of divorced men and women remarry, even after multiple divorces.

10. Which of the following is more likely a sign of a dysfunctional relationship?

a. The partners have frequent disagreements about money.

b. One partner makes all the decisions for the couple and the other partner.

c. Each partner has a demanding career.

d. One partner is much older than the other partner.

Answers to these questions can be found on page 640.

 What important factors should parents consider when blending stepfamilies?

Critical Thinking

1. Reread the section on Personal Communication in this chapter, and think about your own communication skills. How does your communication style compare to the patterns Pennebaker and Tannen have revealed for your gender? Do your personal experiences support or contradict the research results?

2. While our society has become more tolerant, marriages between people of different religious and racial groups still face special pressures. What issues might arise if a Christian marries a Jewish or Muslim man or woman? What about the issues facing partners of different races? How could these issues be resolved? What are your own feelings about mixed marriages? Would you date someone of a different religion or race? Why or why not?

3. What are your personal criteria for a successful relationship? Develop a brief list of factors you consider important, and support your choices with examples or experiences from your own life.

SITES & BYTES

Family and Relationships Information from the American Psychological Association

http://helping.apa.org/family/index.html

This site features information on a variety of parenting topics, including how to handle stress, raising children to resist violence, stepfamilies, and marriage.

Youth.org

http://www.youth.org

This website provides information on gay, lesbian, bisexual, and questioning youth and provides young people with a safe space online to be themselves and to know they are not alone, and to interact with others who have already accepted their sexuality.

Communicating About Sex

http://healthydevil.studentaffairs.duke.edu/info/sex/com.html

Information written specifically for college students, sponsored by the Duke University Student Health Service.

Please note that links are subject to change. If you find a broken link, use a search engine such as http://www.yahoo.com and search for the website by typing in key words.

InfoTrac Activity Susan M. Blake, Linda Simkin, Rebecca Ledsky, Cheryl Perkins, and Joseph M. Calabrese. "Effects of a Parent-Child Communications Intervention on Young Adolescents' Risk for Early Onset of Sexual Intercourse." Family Planning Perspectives, Vol. 33, No. 2, March 2001, p. 52.

(1) How does frequent and positive parent-child communications influence the age of onset of sexual activity in the adolescent child?

(2) What four critical factors and six more general family relationship factors appear to mediate the positive influences of parent-child communications?

(3) What are some of the limitations of the study?

(4) Based on the study results, what are the short-term and long-term observed changes in sexual onset and behavior based on the extent of parent-child communications?

You can find additional readings related to communication and relationships with InfoTrac College Edition, an online library of more than 900 journals and publications. Follow the instructions for accessing InfoTrac that were packaged with your textbook; then search for articles using a key word search.

For additional links, resources, and suggested readings on InfoTrac, visit our Health & Wellness Resource Center at **http://health.wadsworth.com.**

Key Terms

The terms listed here are used within the chapter on the page indicated. Definition of the terms are in the Glossary at the end of the book.

blended family 240
codependence 241
cohabitation 231
companion-oriented marriage 234
dysfunctional 240

enabling 241
family 238
intimacy 226
neurotransmitters 228
oxytocin 228

rescue marriage 234
romantic marriage 234
traditional marriage 234

References

1. Pennebaker, James. Personal interview.
2. Cohen, Joyce. "He-Mails, She-Mails: Where Sender Meets Gender." *New York Times,* May 17, 2001.
3. Hall, Judith. Personal interview.
4. Mehrabian, Albert. Personal interview.
5. Maple, Marilyn. Personal interview.
6. Swann, William, et al. "Socialization Patterns of Depressed and Non-Depressed College Students." *Journal of Abnormal Psychology,* Vol. 104, 1992.
7. Brendgen, Mara, et al. "The Relations Between Friendship Quality, Ranked-Friendship Preference, and Adolescents' Behavior with Their Friends." *Merrill-Palmer Quarterly,* Vol. 47, No. 3, July 2001, p. 395.
8. Chatterjee, Camille. "Can Men and Women Be Friends?" *Psychology Today,* September–October, 2001, p. 61.
9. Gard, Caroline. "The Secrets to Making Lasting Friendships." *Current Health 2,* Vol. 27, No. 2, October 2000.
10. Silverman, Jay, et al. "Dating Violence Against Adolescent Girls and Associated Substance Use, Unhealthy Weight Control, Sexual Risk Behavior, Pregnancy, and Suicidality." *Journal of the American Medical Association,* Vol. 286, No. 5, August 1, 2001, p. 572.
11. DuRant Robert. "Watching Wrestling Positively Associated with Date Fighting." Presentation, American Academy of Pediatrics Meeting, Baltimore, April 2001.

12. Sprecher, Susan. "Insiders' Perspectives on Reasons for Attraction to a Close Other." *Social Psychology Quarterly,* Vol. 61, No. 4, December 1998.
13. Hatala, M. N., et al. "Senior Romance: A Content Analysis of Personal Advertisements Placed by Older Adults." *Gerontologist,* October 15, 2000, p. 51.
14. Laumann, Edward. Personal interview.
15. Sprecher. "Insiders' Perspectives on Reasons for Attraction to a Close Other."
16. Buss, David. *The Evolution of Desire.* New York: Basic Books, 1994.
17. Fisher, Helen. Personal interview.
18. Nowlis, Rebecca Sladek. "Hormone Involved in Reproduction May Have Role in Maintenance of Relationships." News release, UCSF News Service, July 14, 1999.
19. Sommers, Jennifer, and Stephen Vodanovich. "Vengeance Scores Among College Students: Examining the Role of Jealously and Forgiveness." *Education,* Vol. 121, No. 1, Fall 2000.
20. "Households and Families: 2000." U.S. Census Bureau, September 2001.
21. U.S. Census Bureau.
22. Jabusch, Willard. "The Myth of Cohabitation: Cohabiting Couples Lack Both Specialization and Commitment in Their Relationships." *America,* Vol. 183, No. 10, October 7, 2000.
23. Ibid.

24. Popenoe, David. *The State of Our Unions: The Social Health of Marriage in America.* Rutgers, NJ: 2000.

25. Kantrowitz, Barbara, and Pat Wingert. "Unmarried, with Children." *Newsweek,* May 28, 2001, p. 46.

26. Crooks, Robert, and Karla Baur. *Our Sexuality,* 8th ed. Pacific Grove, CA: Wadsworth, 2002.

27. Sternberg, Robert. Personal interview.

28. Nock, Steven. "Marriages of Equally Dependent Spouses." *Journal of Family Issues,* Vol. 22, No. 6, September 2001, p. 755.

29. Crooks and Baur. *Our Sexuality.*

30. Hyde, Janet, et al. "Sexuality and the Dual-earner Couple, Part II: Beyond the Baby Years." *Journal of Sex Research,* Vol. 38, No. 1, February 2001, p. 10.

31. Bramlett, Matthew, and William Mosher. "Love and Marriage." *Forecast,* Vol. 21, No. 10, July 2, 2001, p. 11. Also available at www/cdc.gov/nchs/data/ad/ad323.pdf.

32. Popenoe, *The State of Our Unions.*

33. U.S. Census Bureau.

34. Ibid.

35. Bird, Chloe. "Doing Housework: The 'Ideal' Fair Share." *Journal of Health and Social Behavior,* March 1999.

36. Barnett, Rosalind. Personal interview.

37. Raley, R. Kelly. "Increasing Fertility in Cohabiting Unions: Evidence for the Second Demographic Transition in the United States?" *Demography,* Vol 38, No. 1, February 2001, p. 59.

38. Wetzstein, Cheryl. "Lowering Divorce Rates Urged as National Goal." *Insight on the News,* Vol. 16, No. 30, August 14, 2000.

8

Personal Sexuality

Charles, several years older than the typical college freshman, usually doesn't think much about the age difference—until the conversation turns to sex. He understands his younger classmates' seemingly endless fascination with sex, but his perspective is different. As a teenager, he had plunged recklessly into dangerous territory of every type. Sex—casual and sometimes unprotected—was one of them. Looking back, he feels lucky that he didn't, as he puts it, "end up a statistic." But he still regrets the irresponsible ways he acted.

At 25, Charles is a veteran of military service, a married man, and an expectant father. His enjoyment of sex hasn't faded—in many ways, it's deepened and become more gratifying. He now realizes that there is no such thing as casual sex, that sexual choices have consequences and effects on one's own life and on other people. These are the lessons he hopes someday to pass on to his own children.

As Charles learned with time and experience, you are ultimately responsible for your sexual health and behavior. You make decisions that affect how you express your **sexuality,** how you respond sexually, and how you give and get sexual pleasure. Yet most sexual activity involves another person. Therefore, your decisions about sex—more so than those you make about nutrition, drugs, or exercise—have important effects on other people. Recognizing this fact is the key to responsible sexuality.

Human sexuality—the quality of being sexual—is as rich, varied, and complex as life itself. Along with our **sex,** or biological maleness or femaleness, it is an integral part of who we are, how we see ourselves, and how we relate to others. Of all of our involvements with others, sexual **intimacy,** or physical closeness, can be the most rewarding. But while sexual expression and experience can provide intense joy, they also can involve great emotional turmoil.

Sexual responsibility means learning about your body, your partner's body, your sexual development and preferences, and the health risks associated with sexual activity. This chapter is an introduction to your sexual self and an exploration of sexual issues in today's world. It provides the information and insight you can use in making decisions and choosing behaviors that are responsible for all concerned.

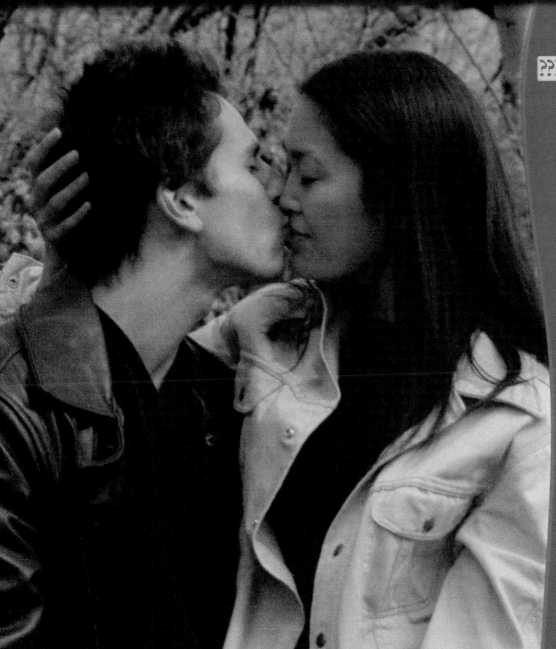

FREQUENTLY ASKED QUESTIONS

FAQ: How do hormones work? p. 248

FAQ: What is the menstrual cycle? p. 251

FAQ: What is circumcision? p. 257

FAQ: How sexually active are college students? p. 264

FAQ: What does it mean to abstain? p. 269

FAQ: What are the most common sexual problems? p. 276

After studying the material in this chapter, you should be able to:

- **Explain** the roles of hormones in sexual development.
- **Describe** the male and female reproductive systems and the functions of the individual structures of each system.
- **Describe** conditions or issues unique to women's and men's sexual health.
- **Define** sexual health and **list** behaviors that can contribute to sexually healthy relationships.
- **Discuss** how sexuality evolves from childhood through older adulthood.
- **Define** sexual orientation and **give examples** of sexual diversity.
- **List** the range of sexual behaviors practiced by adults.
- **Describe** the phases of sexual response.
- **List** the common sexual concerns of men and women.

Becoming Male or Female

Physiological maleness or femaleness, or biological sex, is indicated by the sex chromosomes, hormonal balance, and genital anatomy. **Gender** refers to the psychological and sociological, as well as the physical, aspects of being male or female. You are born with a certain *sexual identity* based on your sexual anatomy and appearance; you, your parents, and society mold your *gender identity.*

Are You an X or a Y?

Biologically, few absolute differences separate the sexes: Males alone can make sperm and contribute the chromosome that causes embryos to develop as males; females alone are born with sex cells (eggs or ova), menstruate, give birth, and breast-feed babies. But the process of becoming male or female is a long and complex one.

In the beginning, all human embryos have undifferentiated sex organs. Only after several weeks do the sex organs differentiate, becoming either male or female **gonads** (testes or ovaries), the structures that produce the future reproductive cells of an individual. This initial differentiation process depends on genetic instructions in the form of the sex chromosomes, referred to as X and Y. (See Figure 8-1.) If a Y (or male) chromosome is present in the embryo, about seven weeks after conception, it signals the sex organs to develop into testes. If a Y chromosome isn't present, an embryo begins developing ovaries in the eighth week. From this point on, the sex hormones pro-

duced by the gonads, not the chromosomes, play the crucial role in making a male or female.

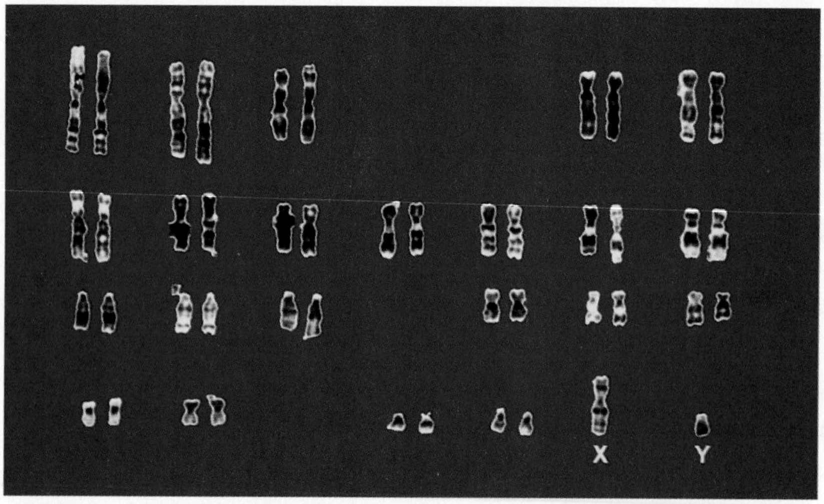

How Do Hormones Work?

In Greek, *hormone* means "set into motion"—and that's exactly what our **hormones** do. These chemical messengers, produced by various organs in the body, including the sex organs, and carried to target structures by the bloodstream, arouse cells and organs to specific activities and influence the way we look, feel, develop, and behave.

The group of organs that produce hormones is referred to as the **endocrine system.** Except for the sex organs, males and females have identical endocrine systems. Directing the endocrine system is the *hypothalamus,* a pea-sized section of the brain. The pituitary gland, directly beneath the hypothalamus, turns the various glands on and off in response to messages from it.

The ovaries produce the sex hormones most crucial to women, **estrogen** and **progesterone.** The primary sex hormone in men is **testosterone,** which is produced by the testes and the adrenal glands. However, both men and women have small amounts of the hormones of the opposite sex. Estrogen, in fact, is crucial to male fertility and gives sperm what researchers describe as their "reproductive punch."

The sex hormones begin their work early in an embryo's development. As soon as the testes are formed, they start releasing testosterone, which stimulates the development of other structures, such as the penis. The absence of testosterone in an embryo causes female genitals to form. (If the testes of a genetic male don't produce testosterone, the fetus will develop female genitals. Similarly, if a genetic female is exposed to excessive testosterone, the fetus will have ovaries but will also develop male genitals.)

As puberty begins, the pituitary gland initiates the changes that transform boys into men and girls into women. When a boy is about 14 years old and a girl about 12, their brains stimulate the hypothalamus to secrete a hormone called *gonadotropin-releasing hormone (GnRH).* This substance causes the pituitary gland to release hormones called **gonadotropins.** These, in turn, stimulate the gonads to make sex hormones. (See Figure 8-2.)

The gonadotropins are *follicle-stimulating hormone (FSH)* and *luteinizing hormone (LH).* In girls, these hormones travel to the ovary and stimulate the production of estrogen. As estrogen increases, a girl's **secondary sex characteristics** develop. Her breasts

▲ **Figure 8-1** Genetic sexual differentiation.
Human cells contain 23 pairs of chromosomes. One of these pairs is the sex chromosomes. A normal female has two X chromosomes and a normal male has an X and a Y chromosome.

© Custom Medical Stock

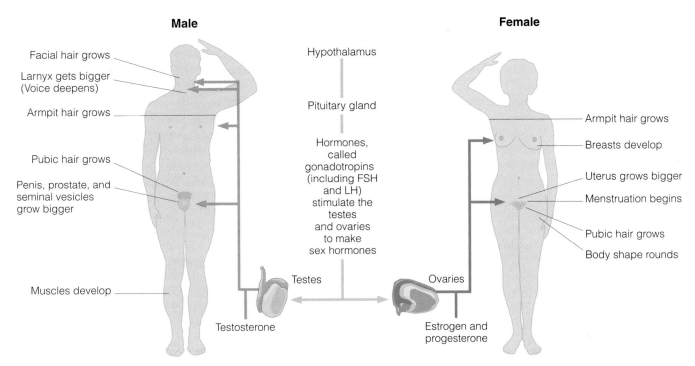

Male   **Female**

Facial hair grows

Larnyx gets bigger
(Voice deepens)

Armpit hair grows

Pubic hair grows

Penis, prostate, and
seminal vesicles
grow bigger

Muscles develop

Hypothalamus

Pituitary gland

Hormones,
called
gonadotropins
(including FSH
and LH)
stimulate the
testes
and ovaries
to make
sex hormones

Testes

Testosterone

Ovaries

Estrogen and
progesterone

Armpit hair grows

Breasts develop

Uterus grows bigger

Menstruation begins

Pubic hair grows

Body shape rounds

▲ **Figure 8-2** Puberty
The body's endocrine system produces hormones that trigger body changes in males and females. Additional body changes include growth spurts and changes to the skeleton.

become fuller, her external genitals enlarge, and fat is deposited on her hips and buttocks. Estrogen keeps her hair thick and skin smooth. She begins menstruating because she has begun ovulating, the process that prepares her body to conceive and carry a baby.

This process seems to be beginning earlier than in the past. "By eight, 15 percent of white girls and 48 percent of African-American girls show signs of sexual development," says Marcia Herman-Giddens, Ph.D., of the University of North Carolina at Chapel Hill, who analyzed 17,077 growth charts from pediatricians around the country. In her study, the mean ages for breast development were 8.87 years for African-American girls and 9.96 years for white girls. African-American girls reach **menarche**—the term for first menstruation—at a mean age of 12.16 years; white girls, at 12.88 years. By comparison, a hundred years ago girls didn't reach menarche until the relatively ripe age of fifteen.[1]

"We don't know precisely why development is starting sooner or why there's a racial discrepancy," notes Herman-Giddens. Improved nutrition and good health seem to be the primary factors. Girls today are bigger, taller, better fed, more sedentary, and have a higher percentage of body fat (one of the triggers of sexual maturation). They also grow up amid a host of environmental influences that may further speed development.

Cultural influences affect a girl's response to menarche. In a cross-cultural study of college students, the most

common emotions expressed by American women at menarche were embarrassment, pride, and anxiety. Malaysian women cited fear, embarrassment, and worry. Lithuanian women described themselves as happy or scared, while Sudanese women cited fear, anxiety, embarrassment, and anger. The Lithuanian women reported feeling more valuable and believing they had entered the world of women. American girls worried about whether they could still play sports, felt superior to friends who had not reached menarche, and became eager to learn about sex. Malaysians described feeling wise, respected, and mature. Sudanese women felt more beautiful and aware that they could now have children.[2]

In boys, the gonadotropins stimulate the testes to produce testosterone, which triggers the development of male secondary sex characteristics. Their voices deepen, hair grows on their faces and bodies, their penises become thicker and longer, and their muscles become stronger.

The sex hormones released during puberty change the growth pattern of childhood, so that a boy or girl may now spurt up 4 to 6 inches in a single year. The skeleton matures very rapidly until, at the end of puberty (usually around age 18), the growth centers at the ends of the bones close off. Estrogen causes girls' bones to stop growing at an earlier age than boys' bones.

Sexual Stereotypes

Being male is not the same as being masculine, and being female is not the same as being feminine. Today more men and women are breaking out of traditional stereotypes. Men are acknowledging their feelings and fears and taking on what were formerly women's jobs—becoming nurses and secretaries at work, and doing the grocery shopping and laundry at home. Although there still aren't any female linebackers in the National Football League (and no one expects that there will be), women have taken their places among astronauts, truck drivers, engineers, pilots, coal miners, physicians, and executives.

An alternative to both male and female sexual typecasting is the concept of **androgyny,** a word that literally translates (from the Greek) as "man woman." Androgynous individuals combine aspects of both masculinity and femininity into their personalities and lifestyles. They act in ways that seem appropriate to a given relationship or situation—instead of in ways that seem appropriately masculine or feminine. Such behaviors can enhance compatibility and satisfaction in a relationship.

Women's Sexual Health

Only recently has medical research devoted major scientific investigations to issues in women's health. Until about a decade ago the National Institutes of Health routinely excluded women from experimental studies because of concerns about menstrual cycles and pregnancy. In clinical settings, women are more likely to have their symptoms dismissed as psychological and not to be referred to a specialist than are men with identical complaints. Some physicians are suggesting the creation of a new medical specialty (distinct from obstetrics and gynecology) that would be devoted to women's health to provide more comprehensive care and overcome the current gender gap in health services. A lack of health insurance, a topic discussed in Chapter 10, is another barrier to adequate health care, particularly for low-income women.[3]

Female Sexual Anatomy

As illustrated in Figure 8-3A, the **mons pubis** is the rounded, fleshy area over the junction of the pubic bones. The folds of skin that form the outer lips of a woman's genital area are called the **labia majora.** They cover soft flaps of skin (inner lips) called the **labia minora.** The inner lips join at the top to form a hood over the **clitoris,** a small elongated erectile organ, and the most sensitive spot in the entire female genital area. Below the clitoris is the **urethral opening,** the outer opening of the thin tube that carries urine from the bladder. Below that is a larger opening, the mouth of the **vagina,** the canal that leads to the primary internal organs of reproduction. The **perineum** is the area

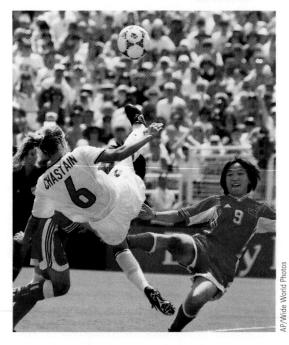

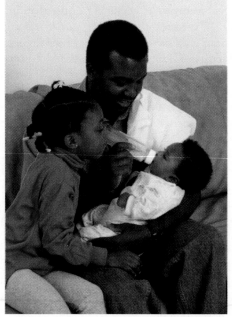

▲ In today's world, many men and women do not allow traditional sexual stereotypes to hinder their career aspirations or personal desires.

between the vagina and the anus (the opening to the rectum and large intestine).

At the back of the vagina is the **cervix,** the opening to the womb, or **uterus** (see Figure 8-3B). The uterine walls are lined by a layer of tissue called the **endometrium.** The **ovaries,** about the size and shape of almonds, are located on either side of the uterus, and contain egg cells called **ova** (singular, **ovum**). Extending outward and back from the upper uterus are the **fallopian tubes,** the canals that transport ova from the ovaries to the uterus. When an egg is

released from an ovary, the fingerlike ends of the adjacent fallopian tube "catch" the egg and direct it into the tube.

??? What Is The Menstrual Cycle?

As shown in Figure 8-4, the hypothalamus monitors hormone levels in the blood and sends messages to the pituitary gland to release follicle-stimulating hormone (FSH) and luteinizing hormone (LH). In the ovary, these

A. External structure

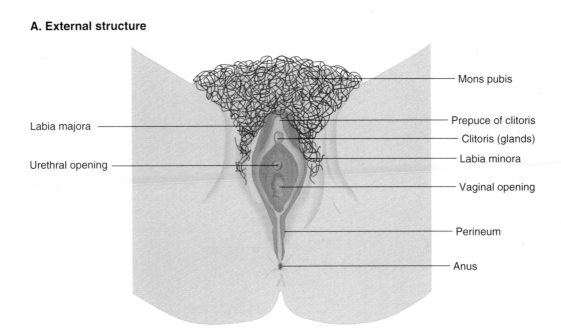

B. Internal structure

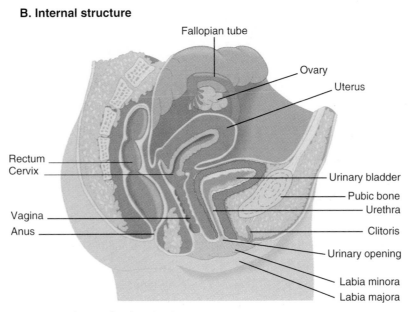

▲ **Figure 8-3** The female sex organs and reproductive structures.

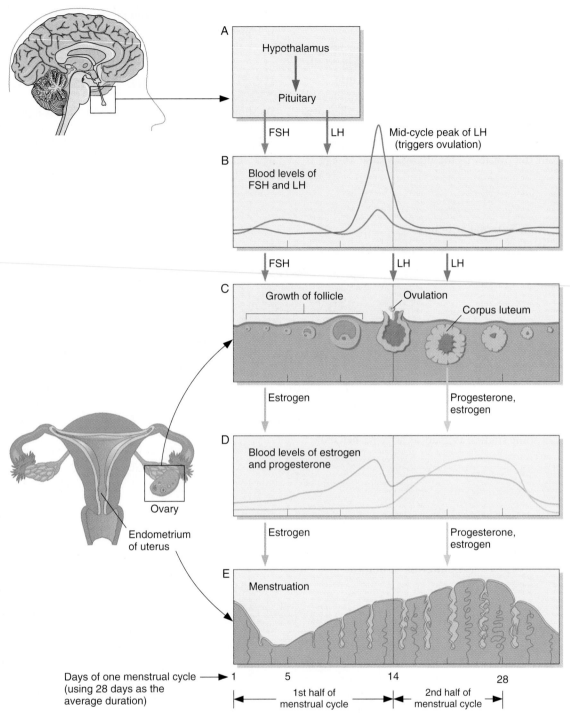

▲ **Figure 8-4** The menstrual cycle.
Levels of the hormones FSH and LH rise and then fall to stimulate the cycle. These changes affect the levels of the hormones estrogen and progesterone, which in turn react with LH and FSH. As a result of the increase in estrogen, the ovarian follicle matures and then ruptures, releasing the ova (eggs) into the fallopian tube. The progesterone helps prepare the lining of the uterus to receive a fertilized egg. If a fertilized egg is deposited into the urerus, pregnancy begins. But if the egg is not fertilized, progesterone production decreases, and the uterine lining is shed (menstruation). At this point, both estrogen and progesterone levels have dropped, so the pituitary responds by producing FSH, and the cycle begins again.

hormones stimulate the growth of a few of the immature eggs, or ova, stored in every woman's body. Usually, only one ovum matures completely during each monthly cycle. As it does, it increases its production of the female sex

hormone estrogen, which in turn triggers the release of a larger surge of LH.

At midcycle, the increased LH hormone levels trigger **ovulation,** the release of the egg cell, or ovum. Estrogen levels drop, and the remaining cells of the follicle then enlarge, change character, and form the corpus luteum, or yellow body. In the second half of the menstrual cycle, the **corpus luteum** secretes estrogen and larger amounts of progesterone. The endometrium (uterine lining) is stimulated by progesterone to thicken and become more engorged with blood in preparation for nourishing an implanted, fertilized ovum.

If the ovum is not fertilized, the corpus luteum disintegrates. As the level of progesterone drops, **menstruation** occurs; the uterine lining is shed during the course of a menstrual period. If the egg is fertilized and pregnancy occurs, the cells that eventually develop into the placenta secrete *human chorionic gonadotropin (HCG),* a messenger hormone that signals the pituitary not to start a new cycle. The corpus luteum then steps up its production of progesterone. Many women experience physical or psychological changes, or both, during their monthly cycles. Usually the changes are minor, but more serious problems can occur.

Premenstrual Syndrome (PMS)

Women with **premenstrual syndrome (PMS)** experience bodily discomfort and emotional distress for up to two weeks, from ovulation until the onset of menstruation. Three to 15 percent of these women develop very severe symptoms. In some studies, as many as 40 to 45 percent of women have reported at least one premenstrual symptom.

Once dismissed as a psychological problem, PMS has been recognized as a very real physiological disorder that may be caused by a hormonal deficiency; abnormal levels of thyroid hormone; an imbalance of estrogen and progesterone; changes in brain chemicals; or social and environmental factors, particularly stress. Because there are no consistent or objective ways of diagnosing premenstrual complaints, it's hard to know precisely how many women are affected.

The most common symptoms of PMS are mood changes, anxiety, irritability, difficulty concentrating, forgetfulness, impaired judgment, tearfulness, digestive symptoms (diarrhea, bloating, constipation), hot flashes, palpitations, dizziness, headache, fatigue, changes in appetite, cravings (usually for sweets or salt), water retention, breast tenderness, and insomnia. For a diagnosis to be made, women—using a self-rating symptom scale or calendar—must report troubling premenstrual symptoms in the period before menstruation in at least two successive menstrual cycles.

Treatments for PMS depend on specific symptoms. Diuretics (drugs that speed up fluid elimination) can relieve water retention and bloating. Relaxation techniques have led to a 60 percent reduction in anxiety symptoms. Sleep deprivation, or the use of bright light to adjust a woman's circadian or daily rhythm, also has proven beneficial. Behavioral approaches, such as exercise

or charting cycles, help by letting women know when they're vulnerable.

Low doses of medications known as selective serotonin-reuptake inhibitors (SSRIs), such as fluoxetine (marketed as Prozac, Sarafem, and in generic forms) provide relief for symptoms such as tension, depression, irritability, and mood swings, even when taken only during the premenstrual phase rather than daily throughout the month.[4] Calcium supplements also may be beneficial.[5] Other treatments with some reported success include vitamins; exercise; less caffeine, alcohol, salt and sugar; acupuncture; and stress management techniques such as meditation or relaxation training.[6]

Premenstrual Dysphoric Disorder (PMDD)

Premenstrual dysphoric disorder, which is not related to PMS, occurs in an estimated 3 to 5 percent of all menstruating women.[7] It is characterized by regular symptoms of depression (depressed mood, anxiety, mood swings, diminished interest or pleasure) during the last week of the menstrual cycles. Women with PMDD cannot function as usual at work, school, or home. They feel better a few days after menstruation begins. The medications known as SSRIs, which are used to treat PMS, also are effective in relieving symptoms of PMDD.[8]

PMDD remains controversial, primarily for political reasons. Some women's advocacy groups oppose labeling women with menstruation-linked symptoms as mentally ill. Others contend that a diagnosis of PMDD simply recognizes the distress some women experience and may make it easier for them to obtain needed help.

Menstrual Cramps

Dysmenorrhea is the medical name for the discomforts—abdominal cramps and pain, back and leg pain, diarrhea, tension, water retention, fatigue, and depression—that can occur during menstruation. About half of all menstruating women suffer from dysmenorrhea. The cause seems to be an overproduction of bodily substances called *prostaglandins,* which typically rise during menstruation.

Women who produce excessive prostaglandins have more severe menstrual cramps. During a cramp, the uterine muscles may contract too strongly or frequently, and temporarily deprive the uterus of oxygen, causing pain. Medications that inhibit prostaglandins can reduce menstrual pain, and exercise can also relieve cramps.

Amenorrhea

Women may stop menstruating—a condition called **amenorrhea**—for a variety of reasons, including a hormonal disorder, drastic weight loss, strenuous exercise, or

STRATEGIES FOR PREVENTION

Preventing Premenstrual Problems

✔ *Get plenty of exercise.* Physically fit women usually have fewer problems both before and during their periods.

✔ *Eat frequently and nutritiously.* In the week before your period, your body doesn't regulate the levels of sugar, or glucose, in your blood as well as it usually does.

✔ *Swear off salt.* If you stop using salt at the table and while cooking, you may gain less weight premenstrually, feel less bloated, and suffer less from headaches and irritability.

✔ *Cut back on caffeine.* Coffee, colas, diet colas, chocolate, and tea can increase breast tenderness and other symptoms.

✔ *Don't drink or smoke.* Some women become so sensitive to alcohol's effects before their periods that a glass of wine hits with the impact of several stiff drinks. Nicotine worsens low blood sugar problems.

✔ *Watch out for sweets.* Premenstrual cravings for sweets are common, but try to resist. Sugar may pick you up, but later you'll feel worse than before.

change in environment. "Boarding-school amenorrhea" is common among young women who leave home for school. Distance running and strenuous exercise also can lead to amenorrhea. The reason may be a drop in body fat from the normal 18 to 22 percent to 9 to 12 percent. To be considered amenorrhea, a woman's menstrual cycle is typically absent for three or more consecutive months. Prolonged amenorrhea can have serious health consequences, including a loss of bone density that may lead to stress fractures or osteoporosis.

In recent years scientists have discovered that the menstrual cycle actually begins in the brain with the production of gonadotropin-releasing hormone (GnRH). Each month a surge of GnRH sets into motion the sequence of steps that lead to ovulation, the potential for conception, and, if conception doesn't occur, menstruation. This understanding has led to the development of chemical mimics, or analogues, of GnRH—usually administered by nasal spray—that trigger ovulation in women who don't ovulate or menstruate normally.

Toxic Shock Syndrome (TSS)

This rare, potentially deadly bacterial infection primarily strikes menstruating women under the age of 30 who use tampons. Both *Staphylococcus aureus* and group A *Streptococcus pyogenes* can produce toxic shock syndrome (TSS). Symptoms include a high fever; a rash that leads to peeling of the skin on the fingers, toes, palms, and soles; dizziness; dangerously low blood pressure; and abnormalities in several organ systems (the digestive tract and the kidneys) and in the muscles and blood. Treatment usually consists of antibiotics and intense supportive care; intravenous administration of immunoglobulins that attack the toxins produced by these bacteria also may be beneficial. (See Chapter 11 for more on TSS.)

Menstruating women should follow these guidelines to reduce their risk of TSS:

▶ Use sanitary napkins instead of tampons.
▶ If you do use tampons, check the labels for information on absorbency (which the FDA has required manufacturers to provide), and avoid superabsorbent brands.
▶ Change tampons every four to eight hours.
▶ Use napkins during the night or for some time during each day of menstrual flow.
▶ As menstrual flow decreases, switch to less-absorbent tampons, which are less likely to cause problems.[9]

Midlife Changes

As the baby-boom generation ages, more people are focusing their attention on the major changes that occur in a woman's middle years. In the next decade, the number of women between the ages of 45 and 54 will increase by half, from 13 million to 19 million. Thus, a large segment of the population will be entering **perimenopause,** the period from a woman's first irregular cycles to her last menstruation.

Perimenopause

During this time, the egg cells, or oocytes, in a woman's ovaries start to "senesce" or die off at a faster rate. Eventually, the number of egg cells drops to a tiny fraction of the estimated 2 million packed into her ovaries at birth. Trying to coax some of the remaining oocytes to ripen, the pituitary gland churns out extra follicle-stimulating hormone (FSH). This surge is the earliest harbinger of menopause, occurring six to ten years before a woman's final periods. Eventually the other menstrual messenger, luteinizing hormone (LH), also increases, but at a slower rate.

These hormonal shifts can trigger an array of symptoms. The most common are night sweats (a subdromal hot flash, in medical terms) that is just intense enough to disrupt sleep. About 10 to 20 percent of perimenopausal women also experience daytime hot flashes—a symptom that becomes more prevalent with the more drastic and enduring hormonal changes of menopause itself.

Even in women who have never suffered from premenstrual syndrome (PMS), perimenopause can trigger its classic symptoms: irritability, tearfulness, fatigue, migraines, mood swings, anxiety. The suspected culprits are changes both in reproductive hormones and in neurochemistry. Some women report headaches, heart palpitations, dizziness, insomnia, tingling sensations in the skin, chills, restlessness, listlessness, headaches, or stress incontinence (release of urine when running, laughing, or sneezing).

While many women feel no need to seek help with such perimenopausal problems, an array of options can ease the way through this physiological prelude to menopause. More and more women are trying herbal and nutritional remedies, such as plant-based estrogens (phytoestrogens), including those found in soy products, and lifestyle changes, like exercise and relaxation, to promote better health. Physicians often suggest low-dose oral contraceptives, which relieve symptoms like night sweats and offer protection from pregnancy—a not insignificant benefit. Among women in their forties, the rate of unplanned pregnancies is almost as high as among teenagers.

Menopause

Menopause, defined as the complete cessation of menstrual periods for 12 consecutive months, generally arrives at age 51 or 52. About 10 to 15 percent of women breeze through this transition with only trivial symptoms. Another 10 to 15 percent are virtually disabled. The majority fall somewhere in between these extremes. Women who undergo surgical or medical menopause (the result of removal of their ovaries or chemotherapy) often experience abrupt symptoms, including flushing, sweating, sleeplessness, early morning awakenings, involuntary urination, changes in libido, mood swings, perception of memory loss, and changes in cognitive function.[10]

Dwindling levels of estrogen subtly affect many aspects of a woman's health, from her mouth (where dryness, unusual tastes, burning, and gum problems can develop) to her skin (which may become drier, itchier, and overly sensitive to touch). The drop in estrogen levels also may cause hot flashes (bursts of perspiration that last from a few seconds to 15 minutes), which often happen at night, disturbing sleep and causing fatigue. With less estrogen to block them, a woman's androgens, or male hormones, may have a greater impact, causing acne, hair loss, and, according to some anecdotal reports, surges in sexual appetite. (Other women, however, report a drop in sexual desire.)

At the same time, a woman's clitoris, vulva, and vaginal lining begin to shrivel, sometimes resulting in pain or bleeding during intercourse. Since the thinner genital tissues are less effective in keeping out bacteria and other pathogens, urinary tract infections may become more common. Some women develop breast or ovarian cysts, which usually go away on their own. Eventually, a woman's ovaries don't respond at all to her pituitary hormones. After the last ovulatory cycle, progesterone is no longer secreted, and estrogen levels decrease rapidly.

Hormone Replacement Therapy

Hormone replacement therapy, or HRT, comes in different combinations, forms, and doses. Many regimens use much lower doses of estrogen than in the past; some use plant-based phytoestrogens or substitute natural progesterone for synthetic progestins; special formulations add testosterone to estrogen and progesterone. Regardless of its form, estrogen has proven far more complex than was once thought, and scientists do not fully understand how various hormonal preparations behave in our bodies.[11]

About 20 million American women take hormone replacement therapy after menopause, but its use remains both confusing and controversial. Because research into the benefits and risks of HRT is ongoing, new findings emerge in bits and pieces, often toppling long-standing assumptions.

HRT entails side effects and risks: Some women who try HRT become depressed (particularly if they had a similar reaction to birth control pills), develop gallstones, or experience a worsening of breast tenderness, migraines, fibroids, or endometriosis.

HRT's primary benefit, medical scientists long believed, is protection from heart disease. Recent studies have challenged this belief. In the first two years of the major longitudinal study called the Women's Health Initiative (WHI), women on HRT experienced a slight increase in heart attacks, strokes, and blood clots in the lungs, as compared to those taking a placebo. The risk for these cardiovascular complications declined in subsequent years. The Heart and Estrogen/Progestin Replacement Study (HERS), which is following postmenopausal women with heart disease, found no cardiovascular benefit from HRT. Yet another report, the three-year Estrogen Replacement and Atherosclerosis (ERA) study, also concluded that postmenopausal women with heart disease did no better on HRT than they did on placebo.[12]

Medical experts are not certain if hormone replacement can prevent heart disease in healthy postmenopausal women, nor are they sure if particular types of HRT may be more beneficial than others. One study using 17 beta-estradiol, a pure form of estrogen that occurs naturally in women, stopped or slowed the process of atherosclerosis in healthy women.

Another possible risk of HRT is stroke. The most recent follow-up of participants in the ongoing Nurses'

Health Study showed a significant increase in stroke risk for women using combined HRT. Estrogen use also increases the likelihood of blood clots, particularly in women already at risk for such problems (for example, because of surgery, hospitalization, or a leg fracture).[13]

The biggest concern for women—and the primary reason they refuse or discontinue HRT—is the threat of breast cancer. The best estimate of risk comes from the Nurses' Health Study, which showed an increased relative risk of breast cancer among women using HRT (estrogen or estrogen plus progestin) for five or more years. Use for less than five years was not associated with increased risk.[14] There also is increased risk of endometrial cancer in women using estrogen without any form of progesterone. In addition, taking estrogen replacement for 10 years or more may double a woman's risk of dying from ovarian cancer, which is small but real (less than 2 percent).[15]

Another touted benefit of HRT—prevention of bone-weakening osteoporosis—also has been challenged. Clinical trials in which healthy women had been randomly assigned to take HRT or a placebo found that HRT preserves bone density but does not necessarily reduce the risk of fractures in women who begin taking the drugs after the age of 60. However, HRT may reduce risk for women who started HRT before age 60.[16]

Questions also remain about HRT's impact on the health of women's brains and memories. Overall, women who had suffered cognitive symptoms prior to menopause appeared to receive more benefits from HRT than those without symptoms. In these women, HRT led to slightly improved verbal memory, vigilance, reasoning, and motor speed, but had no effect on other cognitive functions. The existing research on HRT's ability to prevent dementia remains limited and inconclusive.[17]

HRT does provide short-term "QOL" or quality of life benefits that make living in a menopausal body more comfortable, although many women report that plant-based estrogens and herbal and nutritional remedies, though scientifically untested and unproven, can do the same. NIH-sponsored researchers are testing an herb called black kohosh, widely used to relieve hot flashes in Europe. Sold in capsules and tablets of varying strengths, German studies have shown that it is better at relieving hot flashes than dummy pills.[18]

HRT relieves hot flashes, improves sleep, alleviates sexual symptoms, makes intercourse more enjoyable, and lessens urinary tract problems. Women on HRT report that they think better, remember more, and feel more energetic. They're also less prone to many age-related problems, such as tooth loss and driving accidents (possibly a consequence of improved concentration).

The future should bring more and better choices. A new generation of selective estrogen receptor modulators (SERMS), including the anticancer drug tamoxifen and the osteoporosis drug raloxifene, which target only certain parts of the body, may greatly reduce the cancer risks associated with standard hormone replacement with long-term use. Other SERMS, currently being tested in the United States and Europe, may offer the benefits of estrogen, progesterone, and testosterone with few of their drawbacks. However, SERMS, like all medications, have side effects of their own, and it will take a number of years to sort out which ones may be most helpful to which women. Data from one major trial, for example, showed a 75 percent reduction in invasive breast cancer during three years of raloxifene therapy.[19]

Men's Sexual Health

Because the male reproductive system is simpler in many ways than the female, it's often ignored—especially by healthy young men. However, just like women, men should make regular self-exams (including checking their penises, testes, and breasts, as described in Chapter 13) part of their routine.

Male Sexual Anatomy

The visible parts of the male sexual anatomy are the **penis** and **scrotum**, the pouch that contains the **testes** (see Figure 8-5). The testes manufacture testosterone and **sperm**, the male reproductive cells. Immature sperm are stored in the **epididymis**, a collection of coiled tubes adjacent to each testis.

The penis contains three hollow cylinders loosely covered with skin. The two major cylinders, the *corpora cavernosa*, extend side by side through the length of the penis. The third cylinder, the *corpus spongiosum*, surrounds the **urethra**, the channel for both seminal fluid and urine (see Figure 8-5).

When hanging down loosely, the average penis is about 3¾ inches long. During erection, its internal cylinders fill with so much blood that they become rigid, and the penis stretches to an average length of 6¼ inches. About 90 percent of all men have erect penises measuring between 5 and 7 inches in length. There is no relation, however, between penis size and female sexual satisfaction: A woman's vagina naturally adjusts during intercourse to the size of her partner's penis.

Inside the body are several structures involved in the production of seminal fluid, or **semen**, the liquid in which sperm cells are carried out of the body during ejaculation. The **vas deferens** are two tubes that carry sperm from the epididymis into the urethra. The **seminal vesicles**, which make some of the seminal fluid, join with the vas deferens to form the **ejaculatory ducts**. The **prostate gland** produces some of the seminal fluid, which it secretes into the

A. External structure

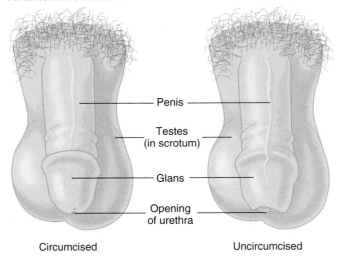

Penis

Testes
(in scrotum)

Glans

Opening
of urethra

Circumcised   Uncircumcised

B. Internal structure

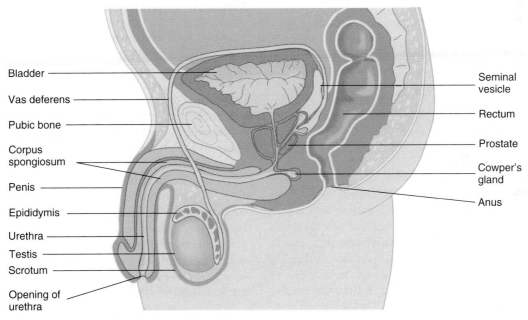

Bladder

Vas deferens

Pubic bone

Corpus
spongiosum

Penis

Epididymis

Urethra

Testis

Scrotum

Opening of
urethra

Seminal
vesicle

Rectum

Prostate

Cowper's
gland

Anus

▲ **Figure 8-5** The male sex organs and reproductive structures.

urethra during ejaculation. The **Cowper's glands** are two pea-sized structures on either side of the urethra (just below where it emerges from the prostate gland) and connected to it via tiny ducts. When a man is sexually aroused, the Cowper's glands often secrete a fluid that appears as a droplet at the tip of the penis. This fluid is not semen, although it occasionally contains sperm.

⁇⁇ What Is Circumcision?

In its natural state, the tip of the penis is covered by a fold of skin called the foreskin. About 60 percent of baby boys

in the United States undergo **circumcision,** the surgical removal of the foreskin. However, increasingly more parents are opting for the natural look.

An estimated 1.2 million newborn males are circumcised in the United States annually for reasons that vary from religious traditions to preventive health measures. Until the last half century, scientific evidence to support or repudiate routine circumcision was limited. The American Academy of Pediatrics reviewed 40 years of data and concluded that, while there are potential medical benefits, the data are not strong enough to recommend routine neonatal circumcision.[20] However, other experts, challenging this controversial view, argue that lack of circumcision increases the risk of sexually transmitted diseases (STDs), including HIV and syphilis.[21]

Boys who are not circumcised are four times as likely to develop urinary tract infections in their first year; however, such infections develop in only 1 percent of circumcised boys. Uncircumcised men are three times as likely to develop penile cancer, but the absolute risk is low. (Only about nine in every million American men ever gets cancer of the penis.) The drawbacks of circumcision include the risk of complications (which tend to be uncommon and minor) and pain. The AAP recommends that, when circumcision is performed, analgesic creams or anesthetic shots be used to minimize discomfort.

Parents who choose not to have their sons circumcised should not attempt to retract the foreskin. This could lead to infection, bleeding, or scarring. As a boy gets older, gradual retraction of the foreskin during bath time helps it dilate, with full retraction possible by age two to four. There is little consensus on what impact the presence or absence of a foreskin has on sexual functioning or satisfaction.

Parents have mixed feelings about the decisions they make. In one study, families who did not have their sons circumcised were less satisfied with their decision. They were more likely to feel that they had not been adequately informed and to reconsider their decision.[22]

Prostate Problems

The chestnut-sized prostate gland, which surrounds the urethra at the base of the bladder, is a common source of concern. The most common problem in younger men is infection, or **prostatitis,** which can cause fever, pain during bowel movements, pain during a rectal exam, and pus in the urine. Infrequent sexual activity is one cause of prostatitis, and occasional bursts of sexual activity between long periods of abstinence are also likely to produce this problem. Prostatitis is usually treated with antibiotics, such as sulfa medications.

After age 40, the prostate enlarges; this condition, called **benign prostatic hypertrophy,** occurs in every man. By age 50, half of all men have some enlargement of the gland; after 70, three-quarters do. As it expands, the prostate tends to pinch the urethra, decreasing urinary flow and creating a sense of urinary urgency, particularly at night. Other warning signs of prostate problems include difficult urination, blood in the urine, painful ejaculation, or constant lower-back pain.

The drug finasteride (brand name Proscar), which shrinks an enlarged prostate, has provided an alternative to corrective surgery for many men. Other drugs and treatments, including nutritional supplements, are being tried experimentally.[23]

The older a man gets, the more likely he is to develop prostate cancer, which now affects one in every six American men and claims 30,000 lives each year (see Chapter 13).[24] Second only to lung cancer in terms of mortality, prostate cancer is more common in African Americans than in white Americans. The risk of prostate cancer in middle-aged men increases directly in relation to the lifetime number of female sexual partners they have had. Those with 30 or more sexual partners have more than twice the risk.[25]

Scientists have developed a screening test that measures levels of a protein called *prostate-specific antigen (PSA)* in the blood. The test, designed to detect prostate cancer at its earliest, most curable stage, is not precise and often indicates cancer where none exists. Men over age 50 should also receive annual rectal examinations, in which a doctor inserts a (gloved) finger into the rectum and feels the prostate for abnormal growths that may indicate cancer.

Midlife Changes

Although men don't experience the dramatic hormonal upheaval that women do at midlife, they do experience a decline by as much as 30 to 40 percent in their primary sex hormone, testosterone, between the ages of 48 and 70. This drop may cause a range of symptoms, including decreased muscle mass, greater body fat, loss of bone density, flagging energy, lowered fertility, and impaired virility. Some researchers are experimenting with testosterone supplements, which, in tests with young men, have been shown to increase lean body mass and decrease body fat—at least temporarily. However, other researchers warn that, particularly in older men, excess testosterone might raise the risk of prostate cancer and heart disease.

While the production of testosterone diminishes with age, sexual ability and enjoyment do not. However, men should expect some differences in their sexual response as they grow older, including the following:

- A need for more time and arousal to achieve erection.
- A longer time before ejaculation.
- A briefer orgasm.
- A decrease in the force of expulsion of the semen at orgasm.
- A smaller volume of ejaculate.
- A more rapid loss of erection after orgasm.
- A lengthening of the time after ejaculation until a man is again capable of intercourse and orgasm.

Responsible Sexuality

The World Health Organization defines **sexual health** as "the integration of the physical, emotional, intellectual, and social aspects of sexual being in ways that are positively enriching, and that enhance personality, communication, and love . . . every person has a right to receive sexual information and to consider sexual relationships for pleasure as well as for procreation."

Characteristics of a Sexually Healthy Adult

The Sexuality Information and Education Council of the United States (SIECUS) has worked with nongovernmental organizations around the world to develop a consensus about the life behaviors of a sexually healthy adult. These include:

- Appreciating one's own body.
- Seeking information about reproduction as needed.
- Affirming that sexual development may or may not include reproduction or genital sexual experience.
- Interacting with both genders in respectful and appropriate ways.
- Affirming one's own sexual orientation and respecting the sexual orientation of others.
- Expressing love and intimacy in appropriate ways.
- Developing and maintaining meaningful relationships.
- Avoiding exploitative or manipulative relationships.
- Making informed choices about family options and lifestyles.
- Enjoying and expressing one's sexuality throughout life.
- Expressing one's sexuality in ways congruent with one's values.
- Discriminating between life-enhancing sexual behaviors and those that are harmful to self and/or others.
- Expressing one's sexuality while respecting the rights of others.
- Seeking new information to enhance one's sexuality.
- Using contraception effectively to avoid unintended pregnancy.
- Preventing sexual abuse.
- Seeking early prenatal care.
- Avoiding contracting or transmitting a sexually transmitted disease, including HIV.
- Practicing health-promoting behaviors, such as regular checkups, breast and testicular self-exam, and early identification of potential problems.
- Demonstrating tolerance for people with different sexual values and lifestyles.
- Exercising democratic responsibility to influence legislation dealing with sexual issues.
- Assessing the impact of family, cultural, religious, media, and societal messages on one's thoughts, feelings, values, and behaviors related to sexuality.
- Promoting the rights of all people to accurate sexuality information.

- Avoiding behaviors that exhibit prejudice and bigotry.
- Rejecting stereotypes about the sexuality of diverse populations.

Sexually Healthy Relationships

A sexually healthy relationship, as defined by SIECUS, is based on shared values and has five characteristics: It is consensual, nonexploitative, honest, mutually pleasurable, and protected against unintended pregnancy and sexuality transmitted diseases (STDs), including HIV/AIDS. All individuals also have sexual rights, which include the right to the information, education, skills, support, and services they need to make responsible decisions about their sexuality consistent with their own values, as well as the right to express one's sexual orientations without violence or discrimination.

Sexual Decision Making

Sexual decision making always takes place within the context of an individual's values and perceptions of right and wrong behavior. Making sexually responsible decisions means considering all the possible consequences of sexual behavior for both yourself and your partner. It must always take into account, not just personal preferences and desires, but the very real risks of unwanted pregnancy, sexually transmitted diseases (STDs), and long-term medical consequences (such as impaired fertility). You also must consider the emotional consequences of a sexual relationship—not just for yourself but also for your partner.

The following sections may help ensure that the sexual decisions you make are responsible ones.

Sexuality Education

Public support for sexuality education has grown. In a national SIECUS poll, 93 percent of Americans said they support teaching about sexuality in high school, while 84 percent support sexuality instruction in middle or junior high schools. More than eight in ten believe young people should be given information to protect themselves from unplanned pregnancies and STDs as well as learning about abstinence.

The CDC estimates that 91.5 percent of American students have been taught about AIDS or HIV infection in school. According to studies of the impact of sexuality programs, learning about sex and protection from STDs does not increase sexual activity and can delay the age of first intercourse, reduce the frequency of intercourse, and decrease the number of sexual partners.[26]

The most effective sexual health education programs for young people combine a dual focus: For younger teens, they emphasize information, attitudes, and skills to delay first intercourse. For older teens, they provide information on contraception and safer sex as well as communications and relationship skills.[27]

Sexuality education is a lifelong process. Your own knowledge about sex may not be as extensive as you might assume. Most people grow up with a lot of myths and misconceptions about sex. (See Self-Survey: "How Much Do You Know About Sex?") Rather than relying on what peers say or what you've always thought was true, find out the facts. This textbook is a good place to start. The student health center and the library can provide additional mate-

SELF-SURVEY

How Much Do You Know About Sex?

Mark each of the following statements True or False:

1. Men and women have completely different sex hormones. _____
2. Premenstrual syndrome (PMS) is primarily a psychological problem. _____
3. Circumcision diminishes a man's sexual pleasure. _____
4. Sexual orientation may have a biological basis. _____
5. Masturbation is a sign of emotional immaturity. _____
6. Only homosexual men engage in anal intercourse. _____
7. Despite their awareness of AIDS, many college students do not practice safe sex. _____
8. After age 60, lovemaking is mainly a fond memory, not a regular pleasure of daily living. _____
9. Doctors advise against having intercourse during a woman's menstrual period. _____
10. Only men ejaculate. _____
11. It is possible to be infected with HIV during a single sexual encounter. _____
12. Impotence is always a sign of emotional or sexual problems in a relationship. _____

Answers:

1. False. Men and women have the same hormones, but in different amounts.
2. False. PMS has been recognized as a physiological disorder that may be caused by a hormonal deficiency, abnormal levels of thyroid hormone, changes in brain chemicals, or social and environmental factors, such as stress.
3. False. Sex therapists have not been able to document differences in sensitivity to stimulation between circumcised and uncircumcised men.
4. True. Researchers documented structural differences in the brains of homosexual men and women.
5. False. Throughout a person's life, masturbation can be a form of sexual release and pleasure.
6. False. As many as one in every four married couples under age 35 have reported that they occasionally engage in anal intercourse.
7. True. In one recent study, more than a third of college students had engaged in vaginal or anal intercourse at least once in the previous year without using effective protection from conception or sexually transmitted diseases (STDs).
8. False. More than a third of American married men and women older than 60 make love at least once a week as do 10% of those older than 70.
9. False. There's no medical reason to avoid intercourse during a woman's menstrual period.
10. False. Stimulation of the Grafenberg spot in a woman's vagina may lead to a release of fluid from her urethra during orgasm.
11. True. Although the risk increases with repeated sexual contact with an infected partner, an individual can contract HIV during a single sexual encounter.
12. False. Many erection difficulties have physical causes.

Making Changes

Informing Yourself About Sex

Your score on this self-survey may indicate that you know a lot more—or less—about sex than you thought you did. Part of sexual responsibility is being informed about sexuality, including reproductive anatomy, sexual orientation, the range of sexual behaviors, and ways of protecting yourself from sexually transmitted diseases.

How can you get good information about sex? If you have questions about sexual biology or behavior, you can usually get accurate and understandable answers from college-level human sexuality textbooks and from authoritative websites. If you're concerned about birth control or protection from sexually transmitted diseases, your college health clinic and your local Planned Parenthood clinic are excellent resources. For questions regarding your own sexual and reproductive health and organs, visit a health care professional for a thorough examination.

Knowledge about sex can help free you from misconceptions that could be dangerous to your health. There's an added psychological benefit as well: The more you know, the less confused you'll feel about your own sexuality.

rials on sexual identity, orientation, behavior, and health, as well as on options for reducing your risk of acquiring sexually transmitted diseases (discussed in Chapter 11) or becoming pregnant.

Talking About Sex

Prior to any sexual activity that involves a risk of sexually transmitted infection or pregnancy, both partners should talk about their prior sexual histories (including number of partners and exposure to STDs) and other high-risk behavior, such as the use of injection drugs. They should also discuss the issue of birth control and which methods might be best for them to use. If you know someone well enough to consider having sex with that person, you should be able to talk about such sensitive subjects. If a potential partner is unwilling to talk or hedges on crucial questions, you shouldn't be engaging in sex. (See Pulse Points: "Top Ten Rules of Sexual Etiquette.")

 Styles of communicating vary among white Americans, African Americans, Hispanic Americans, and Asian Americans. While white and African Americans may openly discuss sex with partners, Hispanic-American couples generally do not discuss their sexual relationship. Asian Americans also are less inclined to discuss sex and to value nonverbal, indirect, and intuitive communication over explicit verbal interaction.[28]

Here are some questions to consider as you think and talk about the significance of becoming sexually intimate with a partner:

▶ What role do we want relationships and sex to have in our life at this time?
▶ What are my values and my potential partner's values as they pertain to sexual relationships? Does each of us believe that intercourse should be reserved for a permanent partnership or committed relationship?
▶ Will a decision to engage in sex enhance my positive feelings about myself or my partner? Does either of us have questions about sexual orientation or the kinds of people we are attracted to?
▶ Do I and my partner both want to have sex? Is my partner pressuring me in any way? Am I pressuring my partner? Am I making this decision for myself or my partner?
▶ Have my partner and I discussed our sexual histories and risk factors? Have I spoken honestly about any

---

PULSE POINTS

Top Ten Rules of Sexual Etiquette

1. **Be sure sexual activity is consensual.** Coercion can take many forms: physical, emotional, and verbal. All cause psychological damage and undermine trust and respect.

2. **No means no.** At any point in a relationship, whether the couple is dating or married, either individual has the right to say no.

3. **In sexual situations, always think ahead.** For the sake of safety, think about potential dangers—parking in an isolated area, going into a bedroom with someone you hardly know, and the like—and options to protect yourself.

4. **Be aware of your own and your partner's alcohol and drug intake.** The use of such substances impairs judgment and

reduces the ability to say no. While under their influence, you may engage in sexual behavior you'll later regret.

5. **Be prepared.** If there's any possibility that you may be engaging in sex, be sure you have the means to protect yourself against unwanted pregnancy and sexually transmitted diseases.

6. **Communicate openly.** If you or your partner cannot talk openly and honestly about your sexual histories and contraception, you should avoid having sex. For the sake of protecting your sexual health, you have to be willing to ask—and answer—questions that may seem embarrassing.

7. **Share responsibility in a sexual relationship.** Both partners should be involved in protecting themselves and each other from

STDs and, if heterosexual, unwanted pregnancy.

8. **Respect sexual privacy.** Revealing sexual activities violates the trust between two partners. Bragging about a sexual conquest demeans everyone involved.

9. **Do not sexually harass others.** Pinches, pats, sexual comments or jokes, and suggestive gestures are offensive and disrespectful. (See Chapter 17 for more on harassment.)

10. **Be considerate.** A public display of sexual affection can be extremely embarrassing to others. Roommates, in particular, should be sensitive and discrete in their sexual behavior.

Source: Adapted from: Hatcher, Robert, et al. *Sexual Etiquette 101.* Atlanta, GA: Emory University School of Medicine.

STDs I've had in the past? Am I sure that neither my partner nor I have a sexually transmitted infection?
▶ Have we taken precautions against unwanted pregnancy and STDs?

Whether couples are on a first date or have been married for years, each partner always has the right not to have sex. Unfortunately, "no" sometimes seems to mean different things to men and women.

 At some campuses, such as Antioch College in Ohio, freshmen must attend workshops on sexual consent and adhere to a campus policy that requires "willing and verbal consent" for each sexual act. (Chapter 17 also discusses sexual coercion.)

Sexual Behavior

From birth to death, we are sexual beings. Our sexual identities, needs, likes, and dislikes emerge in adolescence and become clearer as we enter adulthood, but we continue to change and evolve throughout our lives. In men, sexual interest is most intense at age 18; in women, it reaches a peak in the 30s. (See the X & Y files: "An Evolutionary View of Gender Differences in Attraction.") Although age brings changes in sexual responsiveness, we never outgrow our sexuality.

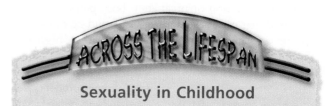

ACROSS THE LIFESPAN

Sexuality in Childhood

For infants, the mouth is the principal source of sensual pleasure, but they are also sensitive to genital and general body contact. By the age of 3 or 4, children recognize the genital differences between males and females and may develop child-

The X & Y Files — An Evolutionary View of Gender Differences in Attraction

What triggers sexual attraction? For heterosexuals, the answer likely depends on gender. These differences may have evolved millions of years ago—and may have helped guarantee the survival of our species.

What attracts a man to a woman? In various surveys in the past decades, men consistently rate one factor as most important: appearance. However, even though men usually report that they notice a woman's bosom or legs, psychologists who carefully measured the proportions of pin-ups of yesteryear, as well as of contemporary *Playboy* centerfolds, homecoming queens, and beauty contestants, found one anatomical feature that most attracted men: the ratio of a woman's waist to her hips. Regardless of the actual measurements, women whose hips were about a third larger than their waists ranked as most desirable.

According to evolutionary theorists, men may have unconsciously learned to assess a woman's waist-hip ratio—or WHR—eons ago. Why? Waist-hip ratio may be a good guarantee of a woman's ability to deliver a healthy infant safely. A slim-hipped woman may be unable to do so; a large-waisted woman may, in fact, already be pregnant with another man's child. As it turns out, WHR also testifies to a woman's health. According to contemporary analyses of apple and pear shapes, women whose hips measure about a third larger than their waists are less likely to develop high blood pressure, diabetes, gallbladder problems, and other diseases. Other features that attract men—shiny hair, white teeth, glowing skin, full lips—also testify to youth, health, and fertility, essentials for guaranteeing their genetic future.

Appearance has never ranked high in determining which men women find attractive. After studying female preferences in various cultures around the world, evolutionary biologist David Buss of the University of Texas concluded that women primarily want good providers of resources for their children. From the perspective of a woman's evolutionary mandate, nothing may have mattered more than finding a mate who would help ensure the survival of her child.

The human baby is born more helpless than any other, explains anthropologist Nina Jablonsky of the California Academy of Sciences. Women must have realized very early on that they would not be able to protect it all by themselves. They needed partners who would provide them and their children with shelter, adequate food, and protection from predators and other dangers.

Do these evolutionary drives still make sense in the modern world? No, say many experts, who note that, nonetheless, knowing about the evolutionary roots of behavior may help contemporary men and women understand each other better.

Source: Hales, Dianne. *Just Like a Woman.* New York: Bantam Books, 2000.

hood romances. Curiosity about adults' and other children's genitals, about where babies come from, and about breasts on women and beards on men continues until age 8 or 9. At that time, interest in sex play becomes less common; but curiosity about sex and where babies come from remains high.

Parents should answer children's questions about sex as honestly as they can. The primary message to convey is simple: Sex is a normal part of life that's done responsibly by two people in a loving relationship. While some awkwardness may be inevitable, parents can master the art of honest, open, and comfortable conversation.

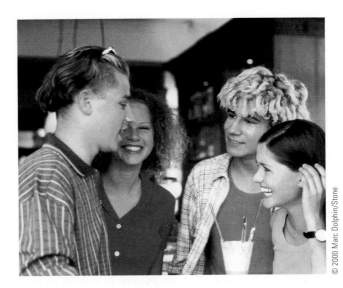

▲ During adolescence, sexuality develops rapidly. Teens explore different social and intimate relationships as they begin to develop a sexual identity.

Adolescent Sexuality

Early in adolescence, sexual curiosity explodes, and sexual exploration—both alone and with a partner—takes on new meaning and intensity. Sexual education programs can make a difference by helping young people become sexually responsible, enable them to form satisfying relationships, help them assess their own attitudes toward sex, and give them information on sexuality. Good programs can clarify values and enhance communication.

It's not unusual for teenage boys to experience frequent erections during the day and night, including **nocturnal emissions,** or wet dreams, during which ejaculation occurs. **Masturbation** (discussed later in this chapter) is the primary form of sexual expression for many teenagers, especially boys. Self-stimulation helps teens learn about their bodies and their sexual potential and serves as an outlet for sexual tension. By the end of adolescence, the majority of teens have masturbated to orgasm.

Other common sexual activities during adolescence include kissing and petting—erotic physical contact that may include holding, touching, manual stimulation of the genitals, and oral sex. As many as 25 percent of teens experience some same-sex attractions. Although many experiment with heterosexual and homosexual sexual experiences, adolescent sexual behavior does not always foretell sexual orientation. Young people, who often feel confused about their sexual identity, may engage in sexual activity with members of the same or the other sex as a way of testing how they really feel.

For the first time since the federal government started keeping statistics in the early 1970s, fewer American teenagers are becoming sexually active. According to the most recent data, half of adolescents aged 15 to 19—55 percent of boys and 49 percent of girls—report having had sexual intercourse at least once. Fewer—38 percent of both

boys and girls—were sexually active in the three months prior to the survey.[29]

Use of contraceptives during first intercourse has risen, with almost eight in ten (77 percent) of teenaged girls reporting that they or their partners had used contraceptives. Fewer girls (71 percent) reported contraceptive use the most recent time they had engaged in intercourse. Although teen pregnancy rates have declined, they remain high compared to other nations, as does the incidence of sexually transmitted diseases among American teens. Every year, an estimated one in four sexually active adolescents—approximately 3 million—acquire an STD.[30]

The teenagers most likely to engage in early sexual activity include those with learning problems or low academic attainment; with other social, behavioral, or emotional problems (including mental health disorders and substance abuse); those from low-income families; victims of physical and sexual abuse; and children in families with marital discord and low levels of parental supervision. Teens who use alcohol or drugs also are more likely to engage in risky sexual behaviors, such as having sex with a stranger or without a condom. Many gay, lesbian, and bisexual youths face special risks because of unsafe sexual practices as well as increased rates of depression, dropping out of school, running away or being thrown out of their homes, and substance abuse.[31]

According to the National Campaign to Prevent Teen Violence, parents exert a greater influence over their child's decision to have sex than any other factor, including friends.[32] In one study, teens who participated in sexuality education programs with parents involved in homework assignments were more likely to avoid risky sexual behavior and were more serious about abstinence than their peers in programs without parental involvement.[33] However, peers definitely exert some influence. Girls say they feel the greatest pressure to engage in sex from boys who want to be their partners. For boys, the pressure comes from male friends.[34]

 ## How Sexually Active Are College Students?

Most unmarried college students are sexually active. In one recent study of college students attending four universities in a southern state, 83 percent reported having had sexual intercourse.[35] Nationwide about 25 percent of female students and 60 percent of males report engaging in casual sex.[36]

College students see sexual activity as normal behavior for their peer group. When researchers at Pennsylvania State University conducted focus groups with undergraduates, most agreed that the majority of college students (80 to 90 percent, in their estimate) are sexually active and that alcohol and drug use make sexual activity more likely.[37]

Yet students' assumptions about their peers' behaviors may be grossly inaccurate. In one study, undergraduates believed that the "average" college student engaged in significantly more frequent HIV-risky sexual activity (such as intercourse without a condom) far more frequently than they did themselves. According to their self-reports, 14 percent of the students engaged in unprotected intercourse, 19 percent in oral sex, and 2 percent had sexual relations with someone they had just met. Yet they believed that much higher percentages of students—more than half in some cases—engaged in these behaviors, particularly if drunk or high.[38]

Students' sexual activity, particularly unsafe practices, often correlate with other risky behaviors. Researchers have found that students who have had multiple sexual partners are more likely to report binge drinking, drinking and driving, physical fighting, thinking about suicide, and marijuana use.[39]

A substantial proportion of college students—male and female—report that they engage in unwanted sexual activity. Sometimes this is the result of sexual coercion (a problem discussed in Chapter 17) or alcohol use.[40] However, some students admit to feigning desire and consenting to an unwanted sexual activity for various reasons, including satisfying a partner's needs, promoting intimacy, and avoiding relationship tension.

College students, even when well informed, do not always take precautions to reduce the risk of STDs. Often they believe that HIV and other infections simply couldn't happen to them, or they use misleading criteria in assessing risk. Some college students, especially men, overrely on a potential partner's physical attractiveness and gave less consideration to sexual history. Women tend to insist on safe-sex practices with a new partner but, as they become more seriously involved, use protection less often—a potentially dangerous practice since knowing someone better doesn't make sex safer.

A study of 61 homosexual college men at a large mid-Atlantic state university found considerable concern about HIV infection. More than a quarter of the men had not engaged in homosexual activity. Of the 72 percent who had had sex with a man, some had made dramatic changes in their sexual behavior because of their fear of HIV: 7 percent had become celibate, and 14 percent no longer engaged in anal intercourse. About half had limited the number of people with whom they had sex and reported being more selective in choosing partners; 36 percent refused to have sex without a condom.

The Sex Life of American Adults

The scientific study of Americans' sexual behavior began in 1938, when Alfred Kinsey, Ph.D., a professor of biology at the University of Indiana, and his colleagues asked some 5,300 white men and 5,940 white women about their sexual practices. In his landmark studies—*Sexual Behavior in the Human Male,* published in 1948, and *Sexual Behavior in the Human Female,* published in 1953—Kinsey reported that 73 percent of men and 20 percent of women had premarital intercourse by age 20, and 37 percent of men and 17 percent of women had some homosexual experience in their lifetime.

Even though Kinsey's research sample was not representative of the population as a whole, for decades his work remained the most definitive and revealing account of the sex lives of ordinary people. In the 1980s, after the emergence and recognition of the AIDS epidemic, researchers and public health officials felt an urgent need for contemporary population-based studies that might help develop strategies to prevent HIV transmission. The last decade has seen several national surveys of sexual behavior.

The Janus Report on Sexual Behavior, published in 1993, was based on a survey of 2,765 individuals across the United States. A larger survey, conducted by researchers at the University of Chicago, was based on face-to-face interviews with 3,432 Americans, aged 18 to 59. It became the basis for two books published in 1994: *Sex in America,* aimed at a lay audience, and *The Social Organization of Sexuality,* a more scholarly work. Since then, the researcher's General Social Survey (GSS) database on sexual activity has grown to nearly 10,000 respondents, about three times larger than the 1992 study.

The GSS data indicate that overall sexual activity in America is relatively infrequent, with an average of 58 episodes per year, or slightly more than one a week. Yet there has been an increase in sexual activity in the 1990s, compared with earlier decades—even though the population is aging, works longer hours, and can choose among a growing number of distractions. About 15 percent of adults engage in half of all sexual activity; 42 percent of adults engage in 85 percent of all sex.[41]

The average adult reports having sex about once a week. However, 1 in 5 Americans has been celibate for at least a year, and 1 in 20 engages in sex at least every other day. Men report more sexual frequency than women—not because men are more boastful about their prowess, the researchers contend, but because the sample of women includes many widows and older women without partners. Among married people, the frequency reports of husbands and wives (not in the same couples) are within one episode per year—58.6 for married men and 57.9 for married women. And if other differences between men and women are statistically controlled (such as sexual preference, age, and educational attainment), married women actually report a slightly higher frequency than men.

People who are married, have children at home, and work long hours report having more sex. Those who work more than 60 hours a week are about 10 percent more sexually active than other workers, and even those who have preschool-aged children report having more sex than average. Even after their answers are controlled for differences in age, gender, and other factors, Americans with the longest work hours report higher sexual frequency.

The main reason why married people have sex more often is the accessibility of a partner. Affluent, well-educated people, those in the top one-tenth of the income distribution, also report above-average sexual frequency. Even then, the rich only report about 5 percent more sex. In fact, adjustment for age and marital status reveals that Americans at the lower rungs of the income ladder may have slightly higher sexual frequency.

Sexual frequency peaks among those with some college education, then decreases among four-year college graduates, and declines even further among those with professional degrees. Americans who have attended graduate school are the least sexually active educational group in the population. These respondents may be more honest than others in reporting sexual activity, or they may be more precise in their definition of what counts as sex.

Sexual frequency increases among those who engage in other pleasurable pursuits, such as attending concerts, sporting events, and active forms of leisure. Yet it also increases along with television viewing. The more TV individuals watch, the more often they have sex. "It is not clear," the researchers observe, "whether the sexual response is stimulated by what is on the screen, or by bore-

dom. And for some reason, watching PBS seems more positively related with increased sexual behavior than watching regular prime-time drama."

Sexual activity is higher among self-defined political liberals than among moderates or conservatives, and it is highest among those who describe themselves as "extreme liberals" and among "extreme conservatives." Catholics are slightly more sexually active than Protestants. But both Christian groups are about 20 percent less active than are Jews or agnostics. Among Protestant groups, Baptists are slightly above average and Presbyterians and Lutherans are slightly below average. Those who attend religious services of any sort at least once a week are less sexually active.

The most sexually active Americans are far more likely than average to approve of premarital or extramarital sex, to see positive benefits in pornography, to watch X-rated movies, and to favor giving birth control pills to teenagers. But those with liberal attitudes aren't the only sexually active individuals. People who own guns also have higher-than-average sexual frequency.

Does sex make people happier or healthier? Based on their analysis, the researchers concluded that the more sex a person has, the more likely he or she is to report having a happy life and a happy marriage. This connection is stronger among women than men. A second and more important predictor of sexual frequency is the feeling that one's life is exciting rather than routine or dull. "Being excited by life is most strongly associated with being happier," the researchers noted. "It seems that increased sexual activity is one of the many benefits of having a positive attitude."

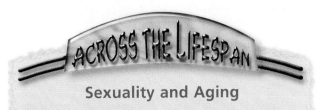

Sexuality and Aging

Health and sexuality interact in various ways as we age. In a review of sexual function in 1,202 aging men, both the men's health status and their partners' perceived responsiveness were key factors in sexual frequency. When they were in good health and had a willing partner, a substantial number of older men continued to be sexually active.[42] A recent study of a group of physically active men and women over age 50 found that the fittest men and women reported more frequent sexual activity; the fittest men (but not women) also showed the greatest sexual satisfaction.

The AARP Modern Maturity Sexual Survey of 1,384 adults, one of the largest national studies of middle-aged and older Americans, found that the number of people who view their partners as romantic and/or physically attractive does not decline with age but may actually increase. Six in ten men aged 45 to 59 gave their partners the highest possible ratings for being "physically attractive," as did 64 percent of 75-year-olds. About half of the women in their forties and fifties gave their partners the highest possible rating as "physically attractive," and 57 percent of those age 75 and over gave the same response.[43]

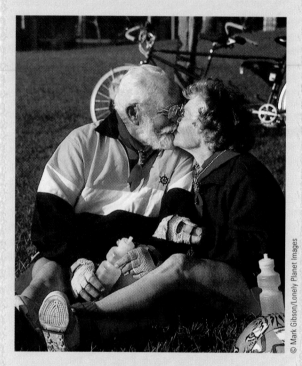

▲ For older couples, sexual desire and pleasure can be enhanced by years of intimacy and affection.

Despite media hype over Viagra, (discussed later in this chapter) few of those with self-reported problems took impotence drugs, and those who did said sexual frequency didn't increase, but the sex was better. Among men, 33 percent reported having sex once a week or more after using Viagra or another treatment, compared to 25 percent reporting weekly intercourse before treatment. However, 62 percent of men and 9 percent of women who used some drug or treatment said it enhanced their satisfaction with their sex life, and 54 percent of men and 57 percent of women said it had a "positive effect."

Other research has found a relationship between sex and longevity. A Swedish study found that men, but not women, who had discontinued intercourse had higher death rates. A study of the entire male population of a small Welsh town found that the sexually active men had half the mortality of the inactive group. In a Duke University study, longevity in women correlated with enjoyment of sexual intercourse, rather than with its frequency.[44]

Aging does cause some changes in sexual response: Women produce less vaginal lubrication, and it takes longer for an older man to achieve an erection or orgasm and longer to attain another erection after ejaculating. Both men and women experience fewer contractions during orgasm. However, none of these changes reduces sexual pleasure or desire.

Sexual Diversity

Human beings are diverse in all ways—including sexual preferences and practices. Physiological, psychological, and social factors attract us to members of a certain sex; this attraction is our **sexual orientation.** Sigmund Freud argued that we all start off **bisexual,** or attracted to both sexes. But by the time they reach adulthood, most males prefer female sexual partners, and most females prefer male partners. **Heterosexual** is the term used for individuals whose primary orientation is toward members of the other sex. In virtually all cultures, some men and women are **homosexuals,** preferring partners of their own sex.

In our society, we tend to view heterosexuality and homosexuality as very different. In reality, these orientations are opposite ends of a spectrum of sexual preferences. Sex researcher Alfred Kinsey devised a seven-point continuum representing sexual orientation in American society. At one end of the continuum are those exclusively attracted to members of the opposite sex; at the other end are people exclusively attracted to members of the same sex. In between are varying degrees of homosexual and heterosexual orientation.

According to Kinsey's original data, 4 percent of men and 2 percent of women are exclusively homosexual. More recent studies have found lower numbers. For instance, in the University of Chicago's national survey, 2.8 percent of the men and 1.4 percent of the women defined themselves as homosexual. However, when asked if they'd had sex with a person of the same gender since age 18, about 5 percent of men and 4 percent of women said yes. If asked if they found members of the same sex sexually attractive, 6 percent of men and 5.5 percent of women said yes.

Bisexuality

Bisexuality—sexual attraction to both males and females—can develop at any point in one's life. In some cultures, bisexual activity is considered part of normal sexual experimentation. Among the Sabmia Highlanders in Papua New Guinea, for instance, boys perform oral sex on one another as part of the rites of passage into manhood.[45]

Some people identify themselves as bisexual even if they don't behave bisexually. Some are "serial" bisexuals—that is, they are sexually involved with same-sex partners for a while and then with partners of the other sex, or vice versa. An estimated 7 to 9 million men, about twice the number thought to be exclusively homosexual, could be described as bisexual during some extended period of their lives. The largest group are married, rarely have sexual relations with women other than their wives, and have secret sexual involvements with men.

Fear of HIV infection has sparked great concern about bisexuality, particularly among heterosexual women who worry about becoming involved with a bisexual man. About 20 to 30 percent of women with AIDS were infected by bisexual partners, and health officials fear that bisexual men who hide their homosexual affairs could transmit HIV to many more women. (See Chapter 11.)

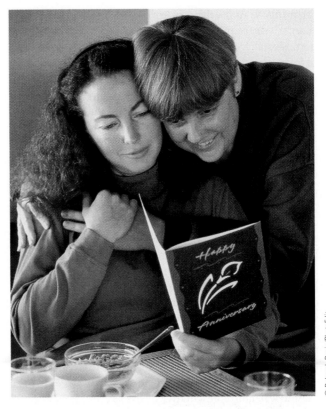

© Deborah Davis/PhotoEdit

▲ Close-couple homosexual relationships are similar to stable heterosexual relationships.

Homosexuality

Homosexuality—social, emotional, and sexual attraction to members of the same sex—exists in almost all cultures. Men and women homosexuals are commonly referred to as *gay;* women homosexuals are also called *lesbians.*

Homosexuality threatens and upsets many people, perhaps because homosexuals are viewed as different, or perhaps because no one understands why some people are heterosexual and others homosexual. Homophobia has led to an increase in "gay bashing" (attacking homosexuals) in many communities, including college campuses. Some blame the emergence of AIDS as a societal danger. However, researchers have found that fear of AIDS has not created new hostility but has simply given bigots an excuse to act out their hatred.

Violations of basic human rights for gays and lesbians remain common around the globe. Amnesty International has documented abuses, ranging from exile to labor camps in China to "social cleansing" death squads in Colombia to the death penalty for homosexual acts in Iran.

According to polls conducted by the Gallup Organization, American attitudes toward homosexuality have become more tolerant over time. In 1977, when pollsters asked Americans, "Do you think homosexual relations between consenting adults should or should not be legal?" 43 percent said they should be legal and 43 percent

said they should not; 14 percent weren't sure. In 2001, 54 percent said yes; 42 percent, no; 4 percent weren't sure. The percentage of those saying that homosexuals should have equal rights in terms of job opportunities rose from 56 percent in 1977 to 85 percent in 2001. About half—52 percent—said that homosexuality should be considered an acceptable alternative lifestyle in 2001, up from 34 percent in 1982.[46]

The Roots of Homosexuality

Most mental health experts agree that nobody knows what causes a person's sexual orientation. Research has discredited theories tracing homosexuality to troubled childhoods or abnormal psychological development. Sexual orientation probably emerges from a complex interaction that includes biological and environmental factors.

For decades, behavioral and medical specialists have debated whether homosexuality is biologically or socially determined. Some say that sexual orientation is genetically determined. However, new research has cast doubt on the existence of a "homosexuality gene." Earlier studies had suggested that male homosexuality might be linked to a set of five DNA sequences located on a specific region of the X chromosome, which is passed down by mothers to their offspring. Gay brothers in earlier studies had tended to share these sequences, suggesting a genetic origin for homosexuality passed through the female line. But a study of 52 gay brothers drawn from 48 families found "no excess sharing for any of the four markers tested" above that which would normally be expected of any two brothers, regardless of sexual orientation. Other studies in families and twins do suggest that sexual orientation may be at least partially linked to genetics.

Others contend that prenatal hormones influence sexual preference. Today, questions and controversies persist about the roots and nature of sexual orientation.

The question of whether so-called reparative therapy can change sexual orientation remains intensely controversial. Some religious groups contend that gays can become heterosexuals through prayer and counseling. In one recent survey of 200 people—143 of them gay men, the others lesbian—psychiatric researchers concluded that 66 percent of the men and 44 percent of the women had arrived at what they called "good heterosexual functioning," as defined by being in a sustained, loving heterosexual relationship, engaging in satisfying heterosexual sex at least monthly, and never or rarely thinking of somebody of the same sex during sex.[47] Critics of this study charge that the sample was not representative of the gay and lesbian community, and there was no way of verifying the truth of their accounts.

Homosexual Lifestyles

Extensive studies of male and female homosexuals have shown that only a minority have problems coping with their homosexuality. The happiest and best adjusted tend to be those in close-couple relationships, the equivalent of stable heterosexual partnerships. An estimated 3 to 5 million gays and lesbians have conceived children in heterosexual relationships; others have become parents through adoption or artificial insemination. These men and women describe their families as much like any other, and studies of lesbian mothers have found that their children are essentially no different from average in self-esteem, gender-related issues and roles, sexual orientation, and general development.[48]

 Different ethnic groups respond to homosexuality in different ways. To a greater extent than white homosexuals, gays and lesbians from ethnic groups tend to stay in the closet longer rather than risk alienation from their families and communities. Often they feel forced to choose between their gay and ethnic identities.

In general, the African-American community has stronger negative views of homosexuals than whites, possibly because of the influence of strong fundamentalist Christian beliefs. Hispanic culture, with its emphasis on machismo, also has a very negative view of male homosexuality. Asian cultures, which tend to view an individual as

a representative of his or her family, tend to view open declarations of sexual orientation as shaming the family and challenging their reputation and future.

Same-sex couples may face more external stressors, but many have communication skills that are superior to straight couples. According to the Family Research Laboratory, same-sex couples use fewer controlling, hostile emotional tactics when arguing and seem better able to calm down during a fight.

Sexual Activity

Part of learning about your own sexuality is having a clear understanding of human sexual behaviors. Understanding frees us from fear and anxiety, so that we may accept ourselves and others as the natural sexual beings we all are.

Celibacy

A celibate person does not engage in sexual activity. Complete **celibacy** means that the person doesn't masturbate (stimulate himself or herself sexually) or engage in sexual activity with a partner. In partial celibacy, the person masturbates but doesn't have sexual contact with others. Many people decide to be celibate at certain times of their lives. Some don't have sex because of concerns about pregnancy or STDs; others haven't found a partner for a permanent, monogamous relationship. Many simply have other priorities, such as finishing school or starting a career and realize that sex outside of a committed relationship is a threat to their physical and psychological well-being.

Abstinence

Increasing numbers of adolescents and young adults are choosing to remain virgins and abstain from sexual intercourse until they enter a permanent, committed, monogamous relationship. About 2.5 million teens have taken pledges to abstain from sex. According to a major study, teens who do so are 34 percent less likely to have premarital sex than others, and are far older when they finally engage in intercourse.[49] The federal government, which has promoted abstinence as a means of preventing pregnancy and sexually transmitted diseases (STDs), funded abstinence education programs for two decades.[50] However, programs receiving no federal funding, such as the "abstinence only" program called Best Friends, also report success by providing teens with moral support and the facts on the real consequences of premarital sex.[51]

Many people who were sexually active in the past also are choosing abstinence rather than getting involved with a new partner, because the risk of medical complications associated with STDs increases with the number of sexual partners a person has.

Abstinence is the safest, healthiest option for many. However, there is confusion about what it means to abstain, and individuals who think they are abstaining may still be engaging in behaviors that put them at risk for HIV and STDs.

 ## What Does It Mean to Abstain?

The CDC defines **abstinence** as "refraining from sexual activities which involve vaginal, anal, and oral intercourse." This is not the same way that many college students think of abstinence. In a survey of more than 1,100 students at a large southeastern university, 10.2 percent of respondents classified engaging in vaginal intercourse as being sexually abstinent. Even larger percentages defined it as engaging in anal intercourse (24.31 percent), having oral contact with another person's genitals (36.93 percent), and having oral-anal contact (47.14 percent).[52]

There also is confusion about virginity. In one study of urban high school students, 47 percent had never engaged in vaginal intercourse. However, more than a third of these "virgins" had engaged in some form of heterosexual genital activity in the preceding year, including masturbation of a partner. About 10 percent had engaged in oral sex.

Sexuality and health educators have expressed concern about these findings, because behaviors such as anal intercourse and oral-anal contact put individuals at risk of HIV transmission.

What Is Sex?

 There is confusion about what it means to "have sex." Past studies have shown that while most American college students think of penile-vaginal intercourse as "having sex," fewer agree that oral sex, manual stimulation of the genitals, and anal intercourse also qualify as "sex." In a survey of 223 undergraduates at a large university in the western United States, more than 90 percent labeled vaginal and anal intercourse as sex. Far fewer—44 percent—thought of oral intercourse as sex.[53]

It's not just Americans whose sexual definitions vary. In a survey of Australian university students, more than 99 percent said that penis-vagina sex with ejaculation was sex; 97 percent thought it was sex even if no ejaculation occurred; 90 percent defined anal intercourse as sex. Far fewer considered other sexual activities as "sex": Only 58 percent regarded oral-sex with orgasm as having sex, while 54 percent thought of oral sex without orgasm as sex; 30 percent regarded touching or stroking as having sex, while 7 percent regarded tongue-kissing as sex.[54]

STRATEGIES FOR CHANGE

How to Say No to Sex

✔ First of all, recognize your own values and feelings. If you believe that sex is something to be shared only by people who've already become close in other ways, be true to that belief.

✔ If you're at a loss for words, try these responses: "I like you a lot, but I'm not ready to have sex." "You're a great person, but sex isn't something I do to prove I like someone." "I'd like to wait until I'm married to have sex."

✔ If you're feeling pressured, let your date know that you're uncomfortable. Be simple and direct. Watch out for emotional blackmail. If your date says, "If you really liked me, you'd want to make love," point out that if he or she really liked you, he or she wouldn't try to force you to do something you don't want to do.

✔ If you're a woman, monitor your sexual signals. Men impute more sexual meaning to gestures (such as casual touching) that women perceive as friendly and innocent.

✔ Communicate your feelings to your date sooner rather than later. It's far easier to say, "I don't want to go to your apartment," than to fight off unwelcome advances once you're there.

✔ Remember that if saying no to sex puts an end to a relationship, it wasn't much of a relationship in the first place.

Fantasy

The mind is the most powerful sex organ in the body, and erotic mental images can be sexually stimulating. Sexual fantasies can accompany sexual activity or be pleasurable in themselves. Fantasies generally enhance sexual arousal, reduce anxiety, and boost sexual desire. They're also a way to anticipate and rehearse new sexual experiences, as well as to bolster a person's self-image and feelings of desirability. Part of what makes fantasies exciting is that they provide an opportunity for expressing forbidden desires, such as sex with a different partner or with a past lover.

In the University of Chicago survey, more than half the men (54 percent)—but only 19 percent of the women—said they thought about sex every day or several times a day. Men and women also have different types of sexy thoughts, with men's fantasies containing more explicit genital images and culminating in sexual acts more quickly than women's. In women's fantasies, emotional feelings play a greater role, and there is more kissing and caressing rather than genital contact. For many women, fantasy helps in reaching orgasm during intercourse; a loss of fantasy often is a sign of low sexual desire.

Sex in Cyberspace

The Internet, designed for communication of very different sorts, has become a new medium for relationships, including those that might be described as sexual. In certain chat rooms, individuals can share explicit sexual fantasies or engage in the cyberspace equivalent of mutual fantasizing. In some ways, the Internet is the perfect venue for a safe form of sexual risk-taking. Individuals can assume any name, gender, race, or personality and can pretend to lead lives entirely different from their actual existences. However, studies of individuals who had sexual intercourse with partners they met through the Internet found a greater risk for sexually transmitted diseases.[55]

Many see cybersex as a harmless way of adding an extra erotic charge to their daily lives. In some cases, individuals who meet in cybersex chat rooms develop what they come to think of as a meaningful relationship and arrange to meet in person. Sometimes these meetings are awkward; sometimes

they do lead to a real-life romance. However, they rarely survive the intrusive reality of everyday existence and sometimes they end disastrously in disappointment and danger.

 In a study of 506 undergraduates at a public university in Texas, 43 percent had logged on to sexually explicit materials through the Internet, although only 2.9 percent said they did so frequently. About one in ten campus computer users logged on to sexually explicit websites from university computers; one in four of home computer users searched for sexually explicit material. Male students were much more likely to have done so; curiosity about sex was their motivation for this behavior. Women were significantly more likely to have experienced sexual harassment while online. Asked about specific behaviors while online, 15 percent of the students reported masturbating and cybersex with an online partner.[56] (See Student Snapshot: "Cybersex on Campus.")

For some individuals, particularly gays and lesbians, the Internet provides the opportunity to join a virtual community. In addition to sexual exchanges, they can find access to information and resources that may not be available elsewhere. For adolescents struggling with gender identity or for closeted homosexuals, going online can be their only opportunity to be open about their sexuality. But they do face an increased risk of syphilis and HIV if they pursue a relationship off-line.[57] (See Savvy Consumer: "X-Rated Online Sites.")

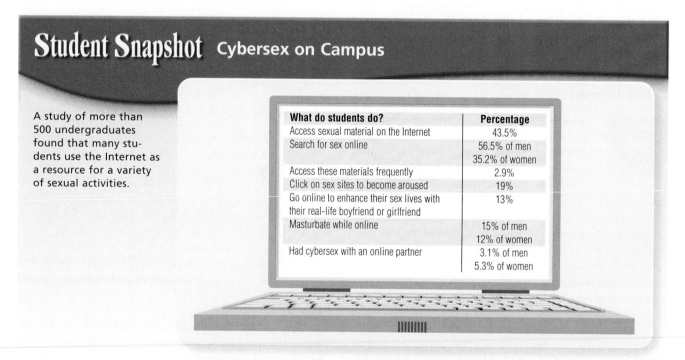

Student Snapshot Cybersex on Campus

A study of more than 500 undergraduates found that many students use the Internet as a resource for a variety of sexual activities.

What do students do?	Percentage
Access sexual material on the Internet	43.5%
Search for sex online	56.5% of men
	35.2% of women
Access these materials frequently	2.9%
Click on sex sites to become aroused	19%
Go online to enhance their sex lives with their real-life boyfriend or girlfriend	13%
Masturbate while online	15% of men
	12% of women
Had cybersex with an online partner	3.1% of men
	5.3% of women

Source: Goodson, Patricia, et al. "Searching for Sexually Explibit Materials on the Internet: An Exploratory Study of College Students' Behavior and Attitudes." *Archives of Sexual Behavior,* Vol. 30, No. 3, April 2001, p. 101.

Masturbation

Not everybody masturbates, but most people do. Kinsey estimated that 7 out of 10 women and 19 out of 20 men masturbate (and admit they do). Their reason is simple: It feels good. Masturbation produces the same physical responses as sexual activity with a partner and can be an enjoyable form of sexual release.

Masturbation has been described as immature; unsocial; tiring; frustrating; and a cause of hairy palms, warts, blemishes, and blindness. None of these myths is true. Even Freud felt that masturbation was normal for children. Sex educators recommend masturbation to adolescents as a means of releasing tension and becoming familiar with their sexual organs. Throughout adulthood, masturbation often is the primary sexual activity of individuals not involved in a sexual relationship and can be particularly useful when illness, absence, divorce, or death deprives a person of a partner. In the University of Chicago survey, about 25 percent of men and 9 percent of women said they masturbate at least once a week.

White men and women have a higher incidence of masturbation than African-American men and women. Latino women have the lowest rate of masturbation, compared with Latino men, white men and women, and black men and women. Individuals with a higher level of education are more likely to masturbate than those with less schooling, and people living with sexual partners masturbate more than those who live alone.

Masturbation helps some people make better decisions about getting sexually involved with others. Self-stimulation also can aid women learning to experience orgasms or men experimenting with ways of delaying ejaculation. Some people find that masturbation enables them to relax and fall asleep more easily at night.

Kissing and Touching

A kiss is a universal sign of affection. A kiss can be just a kiss—a quick press of the lips—or it can lead to much more. Usually kissing is the first sexual activity that couples engage in, and even after years of sexual experimentation and sharing, it remains an enduring pleasure for partners.

Touching is a silent form of communication between friends and lovers. Although a touch to any part of the body can be thrilling, some areas, such as the breasts and genitals, are especially sensitive. Stimulating these **erogenous** regions can lead to orgasm in both men and women. Though such forms of stimulation often accompany intercourse, more couples are gaining an appreciation of these activities as primary sources of sexual fulfillment—and as safer alternatives to intercourse.

Intercourse

Vaginal **intercourse,** or coitus, refers to the penetration of the vagina by the penis (see Figure 8-6). This is the preferred form of sexual intimacy for most heterosexual couples, who may use a wide variety of positions. The most familiar position for intercourse in our society is the so-called missionary position, with the man on top, facing the woman. An alternative is the woman on top, either lying

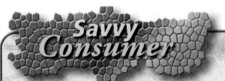

X-Rated Online Sites

Sex is the number-one word searched for online. About 15 percent of Americans logging onto the Internet visit sexually oriented sites. Men are the largest consumers of sexually explicit material and outnumber women by a ratio of six to one. However, while men look for visual erotica, women are more likely to visit chat rooms, which offer more interactions. Most people who check out sex sites on the Internet do not suffer any negative impact, but psychologists warn of some potential risks, including the following:

• *Dependence.* Individuals who spend eleven hours or more a week online in sexual pursuits show signs of psychological distress and admit that their behavior interferes with some areas of their lives.

• *Interference with work and study.* While most individuals use their home computers when surfing the Internet for sex-related sites, one in ten has used a school computer. Some universities have strict policies barring such practices and may take punitive actions against employees who violate the rules.

• *Sexual compulsivity.* A small but significant number of users are at risk of a serious problem as a result of their heavy Internet use.

• *Dishonesty.* Most Internet surfers admit that they occasionally "pretend" about their age on the Internet. Most keep secret how much time they spend on sexual pursuits in cyberspace.

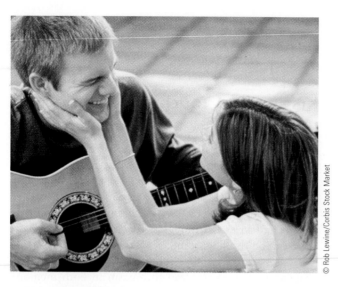

© Rob Lewine/Corbis Stock Market

▲ The magic of touch. Thrilling, soothing, stimulating—touch is a powerful way to communicate affection and sexual pleasure.

Sexual activity, including intercourse, is possible throughout a woman's menstrual cycle. However, some women prefer to avoid sex while menstruating because of uncomfortable physical symptoms, such as cramps, or concern about bleeding or messiness. Others use a diaphragm or cervical cap (see Chapter 9) to hold back menstrual flow. Since different cultures have different views on intercourse during a woman's period, partners should discuss their own feelings and try to respect each other's views. If they choose not to have intercourse, there are other gratifying forms of sexual activity.

Vaginal intercourse, like other forms of sexual activity involving an exchange of bodily fluids, carries a risk of sexually transmitted diseases, including HIV infection. In many other parts of the world, in fact, heterosexual intercourse is the most common means of HIV transmission. (See Chapter 11.)

Oral-Genital Sex

Our mouths and genitals give us some of our most intense pleasures. Though it might seem logical to combine the two, some people are very uncomfortable with it. Some people consider oral-genital sex a perversion; it is against the law in many states and a sin in some religions. However, others find it normal and acceptable. (The same comments apply to anal sex as well—see the next section.)

The formal terms for oral sex are **cunnilingus,** which refers to oral stimulation of the woman's genitals, and

down or sitting upright. Other positions include lying side by side (either face to face or with the man behind the woman, his penis entering her vagina from the rear); lying with the man on top of the woman in a rear-entry position; and kneeling or standing (again, in either a face-to-face or rear-entry position). Many couples move into several different positions for intercourse during a single episode of lovemaking; others may have a personal favorite or may choose different positions at different times.

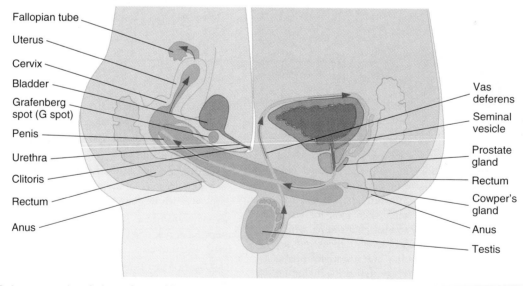

▲ **Figure 8-6** A cross-sectional view of sexual intercourse.

Sperm are formed in each of the testes and stored in the epididymis. When a man ejaculates, sperm traveling in semen travel up the vas deferens. (The prostate gland and seminal vesicles contribute components of the semen.) The semen is expelled from the penis through the urethra and deposited in the vagina, near the cervix. During sexual excitement and orgasm in a woman, the upper end of the vagina enlarges and the uterus elevates. After orgasm, these organs return to their normal states, and the cervix descends into the pool of semen.

fellatio, oral stimulation of the man's genitals. For many couples, oral-genital sex is a regular part of their lovemaking. For others, it's an occasional experiment. Oral sex with a partner carrying a sexually transmitted disease, such as herpes or HIV infection, can lead to infection, so a condom should be used (with cunnilingus, a condom cut in half to lay flat can be used).

 Different groups of the population have diverse views of oral sex. In one survey, more African-American than white men reported never having performed or received oral sex.[58]

Anal Stimulation and Intercourse

Because the anus has many nerve endings, it can produce intense erotic responses. Stimulation of the anus by the fingers or mouth can be a source of sexual arousal; anal intercourse involves penile penetration of the anus. An estimated 25 percent of adults have experienced anal intercourse at least once. However, anal sex involves important health risks, such as damage to sensitive rectal tissues and the transmission of various intestinal infections, hepatitis, and STDs, including HIV.

Cultural Variations

 While the biological mechanisms underlying human sexual arousal and response are essentially universal, the particular sexual stimuli or behaviors that people find arousing are greatly influenced by cultural conditioning. For example, in Western societies, where the emphasis during sexual activity tends to be heavily weighted toward achieving orgasm, genitally focused activities are frequently defined as optimally arousing. In contrast, devotees to Eastern Tantric traditions (where spirituality is interwoven with sexuality) often achieve optimal pleasure by emphasizing the sensual and spiritual aspects of shared intimacy rather than orgasmic release.

Kissing on the mouth, a universal source of sexual arousal in Western society, may be rare or absent in many other parts of the world. Certain North American Eskimo people and inhabitants of the Trobriand Islands would rather rub noses than lips, and among the Thonga of South Africa, kissing is viewed as odious behavior. The Hindu people of India are also disinclined to kiss because they believe such contact symbolically contaminates the act of sexual intercourse. One survey of 190 societies found that mouth kissing was acknowledged in only 21 societies and practiced as a prelude or accompaniment to coitus in only 13.

Oral sex (both cunnilingus and fellatio) is a common source of sexual arousal among island societies of the South Pacific, in industrialized nations of Asia, and in much of the Western world. In contrast, in Africa (with the exception of northern regions), such practices are likely to be viewed as unnatural or disgusting behavior.

Foreplay in general, whether it be oral sex, sensual touching, or passionate kissing, is subject to wide cultural variation. In some societies, most notably those with Eastern traditions, couples may strive to prolong intense states of sexual arousal for several hours. While varied patterns of foreplay are common in Western cultures, these activities often are of short duration as lovers move rapidly toward the "main event" of coitus. In still other societies, foreplay is either sharply curtailed or absent altogether. For example, the Lepcha farmers of the southeastern Himalayas limit foreplay to men briefly caressing their partners' breasts, and among the Irish inhabitants of Inis Beag, precoital sexual activity is reported to be limited to mouth kissing and rough fondling of the woman's lower body by her partner.[59]

Sexual Response

Sexuality involves every part of you: mind and body, muscles and skin, glands and genitals. The pioneers in finding out exactly how human beings respond to sex were William Masters and Virginia Johnson, who first studied more than 800 individuals in their laboratory in the 1950s. They discovered that sexual response is a well-ordered sequence of events, so predictable it could be divided into four phases: excitement, plateau, orgasm, and resolution (see Figure 8-7). In real life, individuals don't necessarily follow this well-ordered pattern. But the responses for both sexes are remarkably similar. And sexual response always follows the same sequence, whatever the means of stimulation.

Excitement

Stimulation is the first step: a touch, a look, a fantasy. In men, sexual stimuli set off a rush of blood to the genitals, filling the blood vessels in the penis. Because these vessels are wrapped in a thick sheath of tissue, the penis becomes erect. The testes lift.

Women respond to stimulation with vaginal lubrication within 10 to 20 seconds of exposure to sexual stimuli. The clitoris becomes larger, as do the vaginal lips (the labia), the nipples, and later the breasts. The vagina lengthens, and its inner two-thirds increase in size. The uterus lifts, further increasing the free space in the vagina.

Plateau

During this stage, the changes begun in the excitement stage continue and intensify. The penis further increases in both length and diameter. The outer one-third of the

Males

Excitement
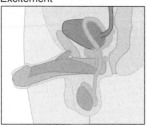
Testes enlarge and elevate, penis becomes partially erect

Plateau
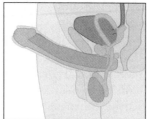
Testes are fully elevated; penis reaches full erection, glans swell, drops of fluid are released

Orgasm
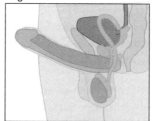
Contractions release semen into urethra; urethral sphincter relaxes, penile contractions occur, semen is ejaculated

Resolution
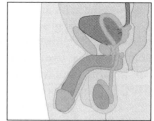
Erection disappears, testes descend

Females

Excitement
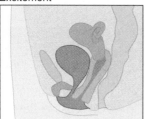
Inner vagina expands, clitoris swells, and labia swell

Plateau
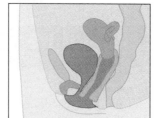
Inner vagina becomes fully expanded, outer vagina swells, and clitoris retracts under hood

Orgasm
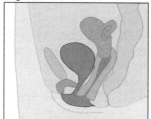
Anal sphincter contracts, uterus contracts, and outer vagina contracts

Resolution
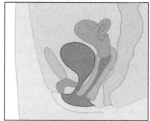
Uterus lowers, vagina returns to normal

▲ **Figure 8-7** Human sexual response.
The four stages of sexual response are excitement, plateau, orgasm, and resolution.

vagina swells. During intercourse, the vaginal muscles grasp the penis to increase stimulation for both partners. The upper two-thirds of the vagina become wider as the uterus moves up; eventually its diameter is 2½ to 3 inches.

Orgasm

Men and women have remarkably similar **orgasm** experiences. Both men and women typically have 3 to 12 pelvic muscle contractions approximately four-fifths of a second apart and lasting up to 60 seconds. Both undergo contractions and spasms of other muscles, as well as increases in breathing and pulse rates, and blood pressure. Both can sometimes have orgasms simply from kisses, stimulation of the breasts or other parts of the body, or fantasy alone.

The process of **ejaculation** (the discharge of semen by a male) requires two separate events. First, the vas deferens, the seminal vesicles, the prostate, and the upper portion of the urethra contract. The man perceives these subtle contractions deep in his pelvis just before the point of no return—which therapists refer to as the point of "ejaculatory inevitability." Then, seconds later, muscle contractions force semen out of the penis via the urethra.

Female orgasms follow several patterns. Some women experience a series of mini-orgasms—a response sometimes described as "skimming." Another pattern consists of rapid excitement and plateau stages, followed by a prolonged orgasm. This is the most frequent response to stimulation by a vibrator.

Female orgasms are primarily triggered by stimulating the clitoris. When stimulation reaches an adequate level, the vagina responds by contracting. Although it sometimes seems that vaginal stimulation alone can set off an orgasm, the clitoris is usually involved—at least indirectly during full penile penetration.

Some researchers have identified what they call the *Grafenberg* (or *G*) *spot* (or *area*) just behind the front wall of the vagina, between the cervix and the back of the pubic bone (see Figure 8-6). When this region is stimulated, women report various sensations, including slight discomfort, a brief feeling that they need to urinate, and increasing pleasure. Continued stimulation may result in an orgasm of great intensity, accompanied by ejaculation of fluid from the urethra. However, other researchers have failed to confirm the existence and importance of the G spot, and sex therapists disagree about its significance for a woman's sexual satisfaction.

Resolution

The sexual organs of men and women return to their normal, nonexcited state during this final phase of sexual response. Heightened skin color quickly fades after orgasm, and the heart rate, blood pressure, and breathing rate soon return to normal. The clitoris also resumes its normal position and appearance very shortly thereafter, whereas the penis may remain somewhat erect for up to 30 minutes.

After orgasm, men typically enter a **refractory period,** during which they are incapable of another orgasm. The duration of this period varies from minutes to days, depending on age and the frequency of previous sexual activity. If either partner doesn't have an orgasm after becoming highly aroused, resolution may be much slower and may be accompanied by a sense of discomfort.

STRATEGIES FOR CHANGE

Improving a Sexual Relationship

✔ Use "I" statements, such as "I really enjoy making love, but I'm so tired right now that I won't be a responsive partner. Why don't we get the kids to bed early tomorrow so we can enjoy ourselves a little earlier?"

✔ If your partner has temporarily lost interest in sex, express concern and ask what the two of you might do to make things better. Don't blame yourself.

✔ Speak up if something hurts during sex. Be specific.

✔ If you would like to try something different, say so. Practice saying the words first if they embarrass you. If your partner feels uncomfortable, don't force the issue, but do try talking it through.

✔ Set aside time for a regular sex talk. Take turns bringing up topics. Mention special pleasures or particular problems.

✔ If you want to request changes or tackle a touchy topic, start with positive statements. Let your partner know how much you enjoy having sex, and then express your desire to enjoy lovemaking more often or in different ways.

✔ Encourage small changes. If you want your partner to be less inhibited, start slowly, perhaps by suggesting sex in a different room or place.

Sexual Concerns

Many sexual concerns stem from myths and misinformation. There is no truth, for instance, behind these misconceptions: men are always capable of erection, sex always involves intercourse, partners should experience simultaneous orgasms, or people who truly love each other always have satisfying sex lives.

Cultural and childhood influences can affect our attitudes toward sex. Even though America's traditionally puritanical values have eased, our society continues to convey mixed messages about sex. Some children, repeatedly warned of the evils of sex, never accept the sexual dimensions of their identity. Others—especially young boys—may be exposed to macho attitudes toward sex and feel a need to prove their virility. Young girls may feel confused by media messages that encourage them to look and act provocatively and a double standard that blames them for leading boys on. In addition, virtually everyone has individual worries. A woman may feel self-conscious about the shape of her breasts; a man may worry about the size of his penis; both partners may fear not pleasing the other.

The concept of sexual normalcy differs greatly in different times, cultures, or racial and ethnic groups. In certain times and places, only sex between a husband and wife has been deemed normal. In other circumstances, "normal"

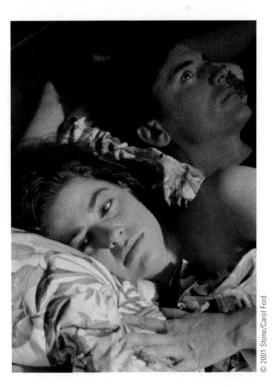

▲ Sexual problems can be difficult for partners to talk about, but lack of communication can create tension and anxiety.

has been applied to any sexual behavior—alone or with others—that does not harm others or produce great anxiety and guilt. The following are some of the most common contemporary sexual concerns.

Safer Sex

Having sex is never completely safe; the only 100 percent risk-free sexual choice is abstinence. If you choose to be sexually active, you can greatly reduce your risk by restricting sexual activity to the context of a mutually exclusive, monogamous relationship in which both partners know, on the basis of laboratory testing, that neither has HIV antibodies or a sexually transmitted disease (STD), sometimes referred to as a sexually transmitted infection (STI).

For centuries, sexually transmitted diseases, such as gonorrhea and syphilis, caused great suffering and many deaths. Modern medicine has developed effective treatments for these health threats, but other STDs, such as herpes and chlamydia, have become serious health problems. The incidence of STDs has been rising, particularly among the young.[60] A quarter of all STDs in the United States occur among adolescents, and a quarter of sexually active adolescents acquire an STD each year. The United States has the highest rate of STDs among all developed countries, yet there is no effective national system of STD prevention. (Chapter 11 provides a complete discussion of the symptoms, diagnosis, and treatment of sexually transmitted diseases, including HIV infection and AIDS.)

Sex with a person who has never been exposed to HIV or to other STDs is safe (for you), regardless of what type of sexual activity you engage in. The only way of knowing for certain that a prospective partner doesn't have an STD or is not infected with HIV is through laboratory testing (see Chapter 11). Sex educators and health professionals strongly encourage couples to abstain from any sexual activity that puts them at risk for STDs until they both undergo medical examinations and testing for STDs. This process greatly reduces the danger of disease transmission and can also help foster a deep sense of mutual trust and commitment. Many campus and public health clinics provide exams or laboratory testing either free of charge or on a sliding scale determined by your income.

⁇⁇⁇ What Are the Most Common Sexual Problems?

A sexual difficulty may occur anywhere in the sexual response sequence. A man's penis may not become erect; a woman's vagina may not become moist. A man may lose his erection while attempting intercourse; the woman's vagina may become dry after penetration. Some men and women become excited, enjoy the plateau stage, but then don't achieve an orgasm; or their sexual cycle may be too long or

too short for one of the partners. Sometimes the cause of the problem is alcohol or drugs, disease, injury, stress, or chronic pain. Often, however, it's fear or ignorance.

One of the most common feelings associated with sex—along with curiosity, desire, and love—is anxiety. No one is born knowing about sex. Most of us learn from our experiences, and—as with most activities, from skiing to speaking French—our first attempts tend to be awkward. A caring, loving relationship can make all the difference.

Sexual Dysfunction

SIECUS defines **sexual dysfunction** as the inability to react emotionally and/or physically to sexual stimulation in a way expected of the average healthy person or according to one's own standards. Sexual dysfunctions, which have a wide range of psychological and physiological origins, can affect different stages in the sexual response cycle. They are not all-or-nothing problems but vary considerably in how severe they are and how frequently they occur. In as many as one-third of people with sexual problems, the partner also has a sexual dysfunction.

Most men and women at one time or another experience some sort of sexual difficulty, but they tend to develop different types. Men are more likely to seek and receive treatment for sexual problems. Nevertheless, they find them very difficult to talk about and may delay or avoid seeking help. In women, the most common sexual dysfunction is loss of desire for sexual activity.

Problems with Arousal

Perfectly healthy couples with no physical impairment sometimes simply become bored with sex, even though they love each other and find each other attractive and enjoyable. Men and women may lose interest in sex, and often neither partner has had previous arousal or orgasm problems. Physical disorders, including neurological and endocrine diseases, can affect sexual desire, as can psychological conditions such as depression and fatigue. Many medications and drugs of abuse also can inhibit desire.

Often stress—perhaps caused by a recent move, a new baby, or a high-pressure job—is the real culprit. Severe stress can short-circuit normal sexual response. Couples who try to unwind by drinking or using tranquilizers usually make the problem worse by further dampening their sexual responses.

Erectile Dysfunction

Erectile dysfunction (ED), or **impotence,** affects many men as they age. Virtually all men are occasionally unable to achieve or maintain an erection because of fatigue, stress, alcohol, or drug use. As clinically defined, impotence means that a man cannot get an erection more often than once in four attempts.

Psychological factors, such as anxiety about performance, may cause impotence. But in as many as 80 percent of cases, the problem has physical origins. Diabetes and reactions to drugs—including an estimated 200 prescription medications—are the most frequent organic causes. Even cigarettes can create erection problems for men sensitive to nicotine. According to the Impotence Information Center, smoking ten or more cigarettes a day increases the likelihood of impotence. Erectile dysfunction increases with advancing age. An estimated 45 percent of men ages 65 and 69 have moderate or complete ED.

Viagra

A little blue pill called Viagra (sildenafil), which delays the breakdown of an enzyme involved in deflating the penis after ejaculation, revolutionized therapy for ED. More than 10 million men worldwide have taken Viagra since its approval by the FDA in 1998. According to its manufacturer, doctors have dispensed more than 300 million tablets in more than 100 countries.

For some men, particularly those with mild cases of impotence, Viagra has lived up to its promise. But Viagra works without side effects in only about one-third of the men who try it; another third benefit but also experience side effects (headache, nasal congestion, facial flushing); the final third do not respond at all.

There are medical risks associated with Viagra use, and more than 130 deaths have been associated with the drug.[61] The FDA requires health labels on bottles of Viagra that warn doctors and patients that men with heart problems and very high or very low blood pressure should be carefully examined before getting a prescription. Interactions with certain drugs, such as heart medications containing nitrate, have proven fatal. Other medications, including antifungal medications and the antibiotic erythromycin, also can affect Viagra's metabolism and excretion. Some users experience visual side effects, but these are temporary and are not considered serious. However, despite the warnings and risks, many men have bought Viagra online after filling out an application reviewed by a medical doctor—a practice condemned by medical societies and by the drug's manufacturer.

Under development is a new potency-enhancing medication that lasts five times longer than Viagra and may extend a man's ability to achieve an improved erection for as long as 24 hours after taking the drug.[62]

Women have tried Viagra to increase their sexual responsiveness, and some studies suggest that it is beneficial.[63] Female interest in Viagra has also spurred new research into treatments that may enhance women's sexual satisfaction.

Other treatments for ED include vacuum devices that increase blood flow to the penis to induce erection; injectable drugs (such as Caverject) that produce an erection within 20 minutes of injection into the base of the penis; vascular reconstruction (grafts of arteries from the lower abdomen are placed around narrowed branches of the main artery leading to the penis to restore blood flow); and penile implants (some inflatable, some permanently rigid) that enable impotent men to have sexual intercourse.

Failure to Respond

Women probably fail to become aroused at least as often as men, but it doesn't seem to be as upsetting to them as the inability to become erect is to men, partly because it isn't as noticeable. Our culture is also more accepting of women who say they simply "don't feel like sex." The myth that a man should become aroused at every opportunity urges many men to have sex—or try to—regardless of how they feel.

Orgasm Problems in Men

About 20 percent of men complain of **premature ejaculation,** which is defined as ejaculating within 30 to 90 seconds of inserting the penis into the vagina, or after 10 to 15 thrusts. Another definition is that a premature ejaculator cannot control or delay his ejaculation long enough to satisfy a responsive partner at least half the time. By this definition, a man may be premature with some women but not with others.

To delay orgasm, men may try to think of baseball or other sports, but this just makes sex boring. Others may masturbate before intercourse, hoping to take advantage of the refractory period, during which they cannot ejaculate again. Others may bite their lips or dig their nails into their palms—although usually this just results in premature ejaculators with bloody lips and scarred palms. Some physicians prescribe drugs, including antidepressants, and androgens (male sex hormones), to cure premature ejaculation. Topical anesthetics used to prevent climax dull pleasurable sensations for the woman as well as for the man.

Men can learn to control their ejaculation by concentrating on their sexual responses, rather than by trying to distract themselves or ignore their reactions. Some men find that they have greater control by lying on their backs with their partner on top, by relaxing during intercourse, and by communicating with their partner about when to stop or slow down movements.

Other techniques for delaying ejaculation include *stop-start,* in which a man learns to sense the feelings that precede ejaculation and stop his movements before the point of ejaculatory inevitability, allowing his arousal to subside slightly before restarting sexual activity. In the *squeeze technique,* a man's partner applies strong pressure with her thumb on the frenum (the thin strip of skin that connects the glans to the shaft on the underside of the penis) and her second and third fingers on the top side of the penis, one above and one below the corona (rim of penile glans), until the man loses the urge to ejaculate.

Intercourse and Orgasm Problems in Women

Some women experience **dyspareunia,** or pain during intercourse. An extreme form of painful intercourse is **vaginismus,** in which involuntary contractions of the muscles of the outer third of the vagina are so intense that they totally or partially close the vaginal opening. This problem often derives from a fear of being penetrated. Relaxation techniques, such as *Kegel exercises* (alternately tightening and relaxing the muscles of the pelvic floor), or the use of fingers or dilators to gradually open the vagina, can make penetration easier.

The female orgasm has long been a controversial sexual topic. According to recent estimates, about 90 percent of sexually active women have experienced orgasm, but only a much smaller percentage achieve orgasm through intercourse alone. Even fewer reach orgasm if intercourse isn't accompanied by direct stimulation of the clitoris. Is intercourse without orgasm a sexual problem? The best answer is that it is a problem if a woman wants to experience orgasm during intercourse but doesn't.

Many counseling programs urge women who have never had orgasms to masturbate. They are then encouraged to share with their partners what they've learned, communicating with words or gestures what is most pleasing to them. Some women regularly want or need more than a single orgasm during intercourse. Partners can help by varying positions and experimenting with sexual techniques. However, in sexual response, more is not necessarily better, and the couple should keep in mind that no one else is counting.

Sex Therapy

Modern sex therapy, pioneered by Masters and Johnson in the 1960s, views sex as a natural, healthy behavior that enhances a couple's relationship. Their approach emphasizes education, communication, reduction of performance anxiety, and sexual exercises that enhance sexual intimacy.

Today most sex therapists, working either alone or with a partner, have modified Masters and Johnson's approach. Most see couples once a week for eight to ten weeks; the focus of therapy is on correcting dysfunctional behavior, not exploring underlying psychodynamics.

Contrary to common misconceptions, sex therapy does not involve conducting sexual activity in front of therapists. The therapist may review psychological and physiological aspects of sexual functioning and evaluate the couple's sexual attitudes and ability to communicate. The core of the program is the couple's "homework"—a series of exercises, carried out in private, that enhances their sensory awareness and improves nonverbal communication. These techniques have proven effective for couples regardless of their age or general health.

You and your partner should consider consulting a sex therapist if any of the following is true for you:

▷ Sex is painful or physically uncomfortable.
▷ You're having sex less and less frequently.
▷ You have a general fear of, or revulsion toward, sex.
▷ Your sexual pleasure is declining.
▷ Your sexual desire is diminishing.
▷ Your sexual problems are increasing in frequency or persisting for longer periods.

Drugs and Sex

Many recreational drugs, such as alcohol and marijuana, are believed to enhance sexual performance. However, none of the popular drugs touted as *aphrodisiac*—including amphetamines, barbiturates, cantharides ("Spanish fly"), cocaine, LSD and other psychedelics, marijuana, amyl nitrite ("poppers"), and L-dopa (a medication used to treat Parkinson's disease)—is truly a sexual stimulant. In fact, these drugs often interfere with normal sexual response. Researchers are studying one drug that may truly enhance sexual performance: yohimbine hydrochloride, which is derived from the sap of the tropical yohimbe tree that grows in West Africa.

Because many psychiatric problems can lower sexual desire and affect sexual functioning, medications appropriate to the specific disorders can help. In addition, psychiatric drugs may be used as part of therapy. Drugs such as certain antidepressants may be used to prolong sexual response in conditions such as premature ejaculation.

Medications can also cause sexual difficulty. In men, drugs that are used to treat high blood pressure, anxiety, allergies, depression, muscle spasms, obesity, ulcers, irritable colon, and prostate cancer can cause impotence, breast enlargement, testicular swelling, priapism (persistent erection), loss of sexual desire, inability to ejaculate, and reduced sperm count. In women, they can diminish sexual desire, inhibit or delay orgasm, and cause breast swelling or secretions.

Atypical Behavior

Although sexual desire and response are universal, some individuals develop sexual appetites or engage in activities that are not typical sexual behaviors.

Sexual Addiction

Some men and women can get relief from their feelings of restlessness and worthlessness only through sex (either masturbation or with a partner). Once the sexual high ends, however, they're overwhelmed by the same negative feelings and driven, once more, to have sex.

Some therapists describe this problem as **sexual addiction;** others, as **sexual compulsion.** Professionals continue to debate exactly what this controversial condition is, how to diagnose it, and how to overcome it. However, most agree that for some people, sex is more than a normal pleasure: It is an overwhelming need that must be met, even at the cost of their careers and marriages.

Sex addicts can be heterosexual or homosexual, male or female. Their behaviors include masturbation, phone sex, reading or viewing pornography, attending strip shows, having affairs, engaging in anonymous sex with strangers or prostitutes, exhibitionism, voyeurism, child molestation, incest, and rape. Many were physically and emotionally abused as children or have family members who abuse drugs or alcohol. They typically feel a loss of control and a compulsion for sexual activity, and they continue their unhealthy sexual behavior despite the dangers, including the risk of contracting STDs. Characteristics exhibited by sex addicts include:

▶ A preoccupation with sex so intense and chronic that it interferes with a normal sexual relationship with a spouse or lover.
▶ A compulsion to have sex again and again within a short period of time, and to engage in sexual behavior that results in feelings of anxiety, depression, guilt, or shame.
▶ A great deal of time spent away from family or work, in order to look for sex partners or engage in sex.
▶ Use of sex to hide from troubles.

With help, sex addicts can deal with the shame that both triggers and follows sexual activity. Professional therapy may begin with a month of complete sexual abstinence, to break the cycle of compulsive sexual behavior. Several organizations, such as Sexaholics Anonymous and Sexual Addicts Anonymous, offer support from people who share the same problem.

Sexual Deviations

Sexual deviations listed by the American Psychiatric Association include the following:

▶ *Fetishism:* Obtaining sexual pleasure from an inanimate object or an asexual part of the body, such as the foot.
▶ *Transvestitism:* Becoming sexually aroused by wearing the clothing of the opposite sex.
▶ *Exhibitionism:* Exposing one's genitals to an unwilling observer.
▶ *Voyeurism:* Obtaining sexual gratification by observing people undressing or involved in sexual activity.
▶ *Sadism:* Becoming sexually aroused by inflicting physical or psychological pain.

▶ *Masochism:* Obtaining sexual gratification by suffering physical or psychological pain.

Another, increasingly common sexual variation, hypoxyphilia, involves attempts to enhance the pleasure of orgasm by reducing oxygen intake. Individuals who do so by tying a noose around the neck have accidentally killed themselves.

Psychiatrists distinguish between passive sexual deviancy, which doesn't involve actual contact with another, and aggressive deviancy. Most voyeurs and obscene phone callers don't seek physical contact with the objects of their sexual desire. These behaviors are performed predominantly, but not exclusively, by males.

Transgenderism

Transgendered individuals, formerly called *transsexuals*, have gender identities opposite their biological sex. Most are males who feel deeply that they are more truly females. More than 3,000 Americans have undergone complex medical procedures to change their genital and secondary sex characteristics. Those who desire *sex-change operations* should be carefully screened and counseled to determine whether such extreme measures would be appropriate and beneficial.

The Business of Sex

Sex, without affection and individuality, becomes a product to be packaged, marketed, traded, bought, and sold. Two of the billion-dollar industries that treat sex as a commodity are prostitution and pornography.

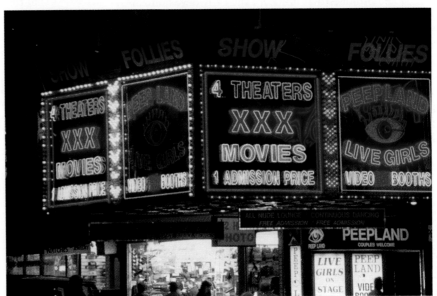

▲ Sex sells. Topless bars and strip clubs are among the businesses that cater to those who enjoy sexual stimulation outside a loving relationship.

Prostitution, described as the world's oldest profession, is a nationwide industry grossing more than $1 billion annually. In every state except Nevada (and in all but a few counties there), prostitution is illegal. Besides the threat of jail and fines, prostitutes and their clients face another danger: sexually transmitted diseases, including HIV infection and hepatitis B.

Pornography is a multimedia industry—books, magazines, movies, the Internet, phone lines, and computer games are available to those who find sexually explicit material entertaining or exciting. Most laws against pornography are based on the assumption that such materials can set off uncontrollable, dangerous sexual urges, ranging from promiscuity to sexual violence. Research indicates that exposure to scenes of rape or other forms of sexual violence against women, or to scenes of degradation of women, does lead to tolerance of these hostile and brutal acts.

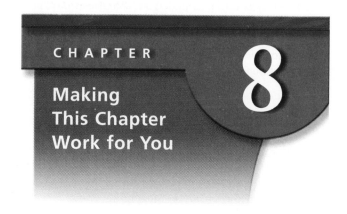

CHAPTER

8

Making
This Chapter
Work for You

1. The hormones that influence the early development of sexual organs
   a. are released by the ovaries in the female and the testes in the male.
   b. begin to work soon after conception during the embryo's development.
   c. begin to work during puberty, when they stimulate the development of secondary male and female sex characteristics.
   d. determine one's biological sex.

2. Which of the following statements about menstruation and the menstrual cycles is true?
   a. During perimenopause, women cannot become pregnant.
   b. Premenstrual syndrome is a physiological disorder that usually results in amenorrhea.
   c. Ovulation occurs at the end of the menstrual cycle.
   d. Premenstrual syndrome is a physiological condition that is unrelated to premenstrual dysphoric disorder.

3. Common midlife changes in men may include which of the following?
   a. gradual enlargement of the prostrate gland
   b. increases in testosterone production, resulting in a longer time before ejaculation
   c. increased muscle mass
   d. a decrease in sexual ability and enjoyment

4. Which of the following behaviors is most likely to be a characteristic of sexually healthy and responsible adults?
   a. engages in frequent sexual encounters with many partners
   b. avoids the use of condoms in order to heighten sexual enjoyment for both partners
   c. uses alcohol sparingly and only to help loosen the inhibitions of a resistant partner
   d. engages in sex that is unquestionably consensual

5. Which of the following statements is true?
   a. More than two-thirds of all teens have sexual intercourse by the time they are 16.
   b. Contrary to popular opinion, the most sexually active teens are from stable families.
   c. Common sexual activities of teens include masturbation and kissing and petting.
   d. Parents have little influence on a teen's decision to have sex.

6. Which of the following statements is true about sexual orientation?
   a. Most individuals who identify themselves as bisexual are really homosexual.
   b. Homosexuality is caused by a poor family environment.
   c. Homosexual behavior is found only in affluent and well-educated cultures.
   d. The African-American, Hispanic, and Asian cultures tend to be less accepting of homosexuality than the white community.

7. According to the Centers for Disease Control, abstinence is defined as
   a. refraining from all sexual behaviors that result in arousal.
   b. refraining from all sexual activities that involve vaginal, anal, and oral intercourse.
   c. having sexual intercourse with only one partner exclusively.
   d. refraining from drinking alcohol before sexual activity.

8. Which of the following statements about erectile dysfunction is false?
   a. ED is usually caused by physical factors.
   b. A popular treatment for ED is Viagra.
   c. ED is usually caused by psychological factors.
   d. Men who are heavy smokers are at risk for developing ED.

9. Women may experience which of the following problems during intercourse?
   a. vaginismus

b. excitement

c. vaginal expansion

d. amenorrhea

10. A typical sexual behaviors include which of the following?

a. masochism

b. sexual desire

c. masturbation

d. celibacy

Answers to these questions can be found on page 640.

 What does research say about the connection between chat rooms and STDs?

Critical Thinking

1. Bill has told his girlfriend, Anita, that he has never taken any sexual risks. But when she suggested that they get tested for STDs, he became furious and refused. Now Anita says she doesn't know what to believe. Could Bill be telling the truth, or is he hiding something? If he is telling the truth, why is Bill so upset? Anita doesn't want to take any risks, but she doesn't want to lose him either. What would you advise her to say or do? What would you advise Bill to say or do?

2. Do you think it is okay to read or look at pornographic books, magazines, websites, and videos? Why or why not?

3. What do you think about the legalization of homosexual marriages? Many gay people feel that they will never be fully accepted in society unless they can legally marry. In addition, without the sanction of marriage, homosexual partners may not be recognized as the legal "next of kin" in medical emergencies or in inheritance situations. Some heterosexuals think that gay marriages would violate the sanctity of marriage. Do you think homosexual marriages should be accepted? Why or why not?

SITES & BYTES

Sexually Transmitted Disease Risk Profiler
http://www.unspeakable.com/truth.jsp
The Naked Truth, a public health outreach project sponsored as an educational service by Pfizer Inc. pharmaceuticals, sponsors this informative website featuring two interactive sections. First, the Risk Profiler can help you determine your risk of acquiring an STD with thirteen questions about your age, gender, sexual history, and behavior, and shows you how these factors play a part in creating your own personal risk profile. The second interactive site is a ten-question STD Quiz that will give you an opportunity to test your knowledge of STDs, and learn more about their symptoms, prevention, and treatment.

National Center for HIV, STD, and TB Prevention
http://www.cdc.gov/hiv/dhap.htm
This site, sponsored by the Centers for Disease Control and Prevention (CDC) features current information, fact sheets, conferences, media campaigns, publications, the 20-year history of HIV/AIDS, information on prevention and treatment, FAQ section, as well as the most current HIV/AIDS statistics.

The Sexuality Information and Education Council of the U.S. (SIECUS)
http://www.siecus.org
This website is sponsored by SIECUS, a national, nonprofit organization that promotes comprehensive education about sexuality and advocates the right of all individuals of all sexual orientations to make responsible sexual choices. The site features a library of facts sheets and articles on a variety of sexuality topics and STDs, designed for educators, adults, teens, parents, media, international audiences, and religious organizations.

Please note that links are subject to change. If you find a broken link, use a search engine such as http://www.yahoo.com and search for the website by typing in key words.

InfoTrac Activity   "New CDC Study Finds High Rates of HIV Infection Among Young Gay and Bisexual Men." *Medical Letter on the CDC & FDA,* July 1, 2001.

(1) Describe the CDC's new HIV prevention strategic plan.

(2) The incidence of HIV infection has increased at the highest rate in what age group? what ethnicity?

You can find additional readings related to sexuality with InfoTrac College Edition, an online library of more than 900 journals and publications. Follow the instructions for accessing InfoTrac that were packaged with your textbook; then search for articles using a key word search.

For additional links, resources, and suggested readings on InfoTrac, visit our Health & Wellness Resource Center at **http://health.wadsworth.com**.

Key Terms

The terms listed here are used within the chapter on the page indicated. Definition of the terms are in the Glossary at the end of the book.

abstinence 269
amenorrhea 253
androgyny 250
benign prostatic hypertrophy 258
bisexual 266
celibacy 268
cervix 251
circumcision 257
clitoris 250
corpus luteum 253
Cowper's glands 257
cunnilingus 272
dysmenorrhea 253
dyspareunia 278
ejaculation 274
ejaculatory duct 256
endocrine system 248
endometrium 251
epididymis 256
erogenous 271
estrogen 248
fallopian tubes 251
fellatio 273
gender 248
gonadotropins 248
gonads 248

heterosexual 266
homosexual 266
hormones 248
hormone replacement therapy 255
impotence 276
intercourse 271
intimacy 246
labia majora 250
labia minora 250
masturbation 263
menarche 249
menopause 255
menstruation 253
mons pubis 250
nocturnal emissions 263
orgasm 274
ovum (ova) 251
ovaries 251
ovulation 252
penis 256
perimenopause 254
perineum 250
premature ejaculation 277
premenstrual dysphoric disorder (PMDD) 253
premenstrual syndrome (PMS) 253

progesterone 248
prostate gland 256
prostatitis 258
refractory period 275
scrotum 256
secondary sex characteristics 248
semen 256
seminal vesicles 256
sex 246
sexual addiction 278
sexual compulsion 278
sexual dysfunction 276
sexual health 258
sexual orientation 266
sexuality 246
sperm 256
testes 256
testosterone 248
transgendered 279
urethra 256
urethral opening 250
uterus 251
vagina 250
vaginismus 278
vas deferens 256

References

1. Herman-Giddens, Marcia. Personal interview.
2. Chrisler, J. C., and C. B. Zitell. "Menarche Stories: Reminiscences of College Students from Lithuania, Malaysia, Sudan and the United States." *Health Care for Women International,* Vol. 19, No. 4, July–August 1998.
3. Wyn, Roberta, et al. "Falling through the Cracks: Health Insurance Coverage of Low-Income Women." Menlo Park, CA: Henry J. Kaiser Family Foundation, February 2001.
4. Dimmock, Paul, et al. "Efficacy of Selective Serotonin-Reuptake Inhibitors in Premenstrual Syndrome: A Systematic Review." *Lancet,* Vol. 356, No. 9236, September 30, 2000.
5. "Calcium for PMS, Bone Health." *Contemporary OB/GYN,* Vol. 46, No. 5, May 2001, p. 151.
6. "New Treatment Approved for Severe Premenstrual Symptoms." *FDA Consumer,* Vol. 34, No. 5, September 2000.
7. Steiner, Meir. "Recognition of Premenstrual Dysphoric Disorder and Its Treatment." *Lancet,* Vol. 356, No. 9236, September 30, 2000.
8. "Premenstrual Mood Disturbance." *Harvard Medical Health Letter,* Vol. 17, No. 12, June 2001.
9. Swayze, Sonia. "Preventing Problems from Tampon Use." *Nursing,* Vol. 31, No. 7, July 2001, p. 28.
10. Ratner, Shari, and Ofri, Danielle. "Menopause and Hormone Replacement: Part 1. Evaluation and Treatment." *Western Journal of Medicine,* Vol. 174, No. 6, June 2001, p. 400.
11. "Hormone Replacement Therapy—Another Chapter in the Heart and Estrogen Story." *Harvard Women's Health Watch,* Vol. 8, No. 8, April 2001.
12. Heckbert, Susan, et al. "Risk of Recurrent Coronary Events in Relation to Use and Recent Initiation of Postmenopausal Hormone

Therapy." *Archives of Internal Medicine,* Vol. 161, No. 14, July 23, 2001, p. 1709.

13. "Heart Lines—Hormone-Replacement Therapy and Stroke Risk." *Harvard Heart Letter,* Vol. 11, No. 11, July 2001.

14. "Hormone Replacement—HRT Forum: Cancer Risk." *Harvard Women's Health Watch,* Vol. 8, No. 10, June 2001.

15. Weiss, Noel, and Mary Anne Rossing. "Oestrogen-Replacement Therapy and Risk of Ovarian Cancer." *Lancet,* Vol. 358, No. 9280, August 11, 2001, p. 438.

16. Villareal, Dennis, et al. "Bone Mineral Density Response to Estrogen Replacement in Frail Elderly Women: A Randomized Controlled Trial." *Journal of the American Medical Association,* Vol. 286, No. 7, August 15, 2001, p. 815.

17. Dunne, Laura, and Terry Seatn. "Does Hormone Replacement Therapy (HRT) Improve Cognitive Function or Either Delay or Prevent Dementia in Postmenopausal Women?" *Journal of Family Practice,* Vol. 50, No. 6, June 2001, p. 547.

18. Stolberg, Sheryl. "The Estrogen Alternative." *New York Times Magazine,* May 6, 2001, p. 108.

19. Lappe, Joan. "Designer Estrogen vs. Hormone Replacement Therapy: The Menopausal Woman's Dilemma." *Orthopaedic Nursing,* Vol. 20, No. 4, July 2001.

20. "Just the Facts . . . Circumcision." American Academy of Pediatrics, http://www.aap.org/mrt/factscir.htm

21. Schoen, Edgar et al. "New Policy on Circumcision—Cause for Concern." *Pediatrics,* Vol. 105, No. 3, March 2000.

22. Adler, Robert, et al. "Circumcision: We Have Heard from the Experts; Now Let's Hear from the Parents." *Pediatrics,* Vol. 107, No. 2, February 2001, p. 395.

23. Walsh, Julie. "Some Prostrate Problems May Benefit from Over-the-Counter Help (overview of medicinal plant products for benign prostatic hyperplasia." *Environmental Nutrition,* Vol. 23, No. 12, December 2001, p. 1.

24. Liebman, Bonnie. "Preventing Prostrate Cancer: So Far, No Clear Answers." *Nutrition Action Healthletter,* Vol. 28, No. 6, July 2001, p. 1.

25. "Risk of Prostate Cancer Rises with Number of Partners." *British Medical Journal,* Vol. 323, No. 7305, July 21, 2001, p. 126.

26. McKay, Alexander. "Postponing Sexual Intercourse Among Urban Junior High School Students—A Randomized Controlled Evaluation (brief article)." *Canadian Journal of Human Sexuality,* Vol. 9, No. 2, Summer 2000, p. 121.

27. Aarons, S. J., et al. "Postponing Sexual Intercourse Among Urban Junior High School Students—A randomized controlled evaluation. *Journal of Adolescent Health,* Vol. 27, 2000, p. 236.

28. Crooks, Robert, and Karla Baur. *Our Sexuality,* 8th ed. Pacific Grove, CA: Wadsworth, 2002.

29. Althaus, F. "Levels of Sexual Experience Among U.S. Teenagers Have Declined for the First Time in Three Decades." *Family Planning Perspectives,* Vol. 33, No. 4, July 2001, p. 180.

30. Ibid.

31. Ibid.

32. National Campaign to Prevent Teen Pregnancy. http://www.teenpregnancy.org

33. Somers, Cheryl, and Sharon Paulson. "Students' Perceptions of Parent-Adolescent Closeness and Communication About Sexuality: Relations with Sexual Knowledge, Attitudes, and Behaviors." *Journal of Adolescence,* Vol. 23, No. 5, October 2000, p. 629.

34. Nahom, Deborah, et al. "Differences by Gender and Sexual Experience in Adolescent Sexual Behavior: Implications for Education and HIV Prevention." *Journal of School Health,* Vol. 71, No. 4, April 2001, p. 153.

35. Kelley, R. Mark. "Sexual Behaviors of College Students Attending Four Universities in a Southern State." *Research Quarterly for Exercise and Sport,* Vol. 72, No. 1, March 2001, p. A-31.

36. Bon, Rebecca, et al. "Normative Perceptions in Relation to Substance Use and HIV-Risky Sexual Behaviors of College Students." *Journal of Psychology,* Vol. 135, No. 2, March 2001, p. 165.

37. Luquis, R., et al. "College Students' Perceptions of Substance Use and Sexual Behaviors." *Research Quarterly for Exercise and Sport,* Vol. 72, No. 1, March 2001, p. A-33.

38. Bon, "Normative Perceptions in Relation to Substance Use and HIV-Risky Sexual Behaviors of College Students."

39. Ogletree, Roberta, et al. "Associations Between Lifetime Sexual Partners and Health Risk Behaviors in a Representative Sample of United States College Students." *Research Quarterly for Exercise and Sport,* Vol. 72, March 2001.

40. Ullman, Sarah, et al. "Alcohol and Sexual Assault in a National Sample of College Women." *Journal of Interpersonal Violence,* Vol. 14, No. 6, June 1999.

41. Robinson, John, and Geoffrey Godbey. "No Sex, Please . . . We're College Graduates." *American Demographics,* February 1998.

42. Bortz, Walter, et al. "Sexual Function in 1,202 Aging Males." *Journal of Gerontology,* Vol. 54, No. 5, May 1999.

43. "AARP's Modern Maturity Reveals Survey Results on Sexual Attitudes, Looks at the Top Issues Affecting Relationships." AARP Press Release, August 3, 1999.

44. Bortz, Walter, et al. "Physical Fitness, Aging and Sexuality." *Western Journal of Medicine,* Vol. 170, Issue 3, March 1999.

45. Crooks and Baur, *Our Sexuality.*

46. McKay, Alexander. "American Attitudes Toward Homosexuality Continue to Become More Tolerant." *Canadian Journal of Human Sexuality,* Vol. 9, No. 3, Fall 2000, p. 212.

47. Spitzer, Robert. American Psychiatric Association, Annual Meeting, New Orleans, May 2001.

48. Baugher, Shirley. "Same Sex Relationships." Journal of Family and Consumer Sciences, Vol. 92, No. 3, May 2000.

49. "Better than Condoms in a Cookie Jar." *American Enterprise,* Vol. 12, No. 3, April 2001, p. 10.

50. Sonfield, Adam, and Rachel Gold. "States' Implementation of the Section 510 Abstinence Education Program." *Family Planning Perspectives,* Vol. 33, No. 4, July 2001, p. 166.

51. Edwards, Catherine. "Teens Really Need 'Best Friends.'" *Insight on the News,* Vol. 17, No. 28, July 30, 2001, p. 18.

52. Horan, P. F., et al. "The Meaning of Abstinence for College Students." *Journal of HIV/AID Prevention and Education for Adolescents and Children,* Vol. 2, No. 2, 1998.

53. Bogart, Laura, et al. "Is it 'Sex'? College Students' Interpretations of Sexual Behavior Terminology." *Journal of Sex Research,* Vol. 39, No. 2, May 2000.

54. Richters, Juliet, and Angela Song. "Australian University Students Agree with Clinton's Definition of Sex." *British Medical Journal,* Vol. 318, No. 7189, April 10, 1999.

55. Toomey, Kathleen, and Richard Rothenberg, "Sex and Cyberspace—Virtual Networks Leading to High-Risk Sex." *Journal of the American Medical Association,* Vol. 284, No. 4, July 26, 2000.

56. Goodson, Patricia, et al. "Searching for Sexually Explicit Materials on the Internet: An Exploratory Study of College Students' Behavior and Attitudes."*Archives of Sexual Behavior,* Vol. 30, p. 2, April 2001, p. 101.

57. McFarlane, M. et al. "The Internet as a Newly Emerging Risk Environment for Sexually Transmitted Diseases. *Journal of the American Medical Association,* Vol. 384, No. 4, July 26, 2000.

58. Crooks and Baur, *Our Sexuality.*

59. Ibid.

60. "Numbers of STI Cases on the Increase." *Chemist & Druggist,* Vol. 10, August 5, 2000.

61. Jackson, G. "Sildenafil (Viagra) and Cardiac Patients: An Open Outpatient Study." *Heart,* Vol. 85, No. 5, May 2001, p. 42.

62. "Viagra Competitor Said to Last Longer." *Chemist & Druggist,* May 12, 2001, p. 10.

63. Caruso, Salvatore. "Premenopausal Women Affected by Sexual Arousal Disorder Treated with Sildenafil: A Double-Blind, Cross-Over, Placebo-Controlled Study." *Journal of the American Medical Association,* Vol. 286, No. 6, August 8, 2001, p. 656.

9

Reproductive Choices

Jess and Sara, juniors at the same community college, can't remember a time when abortion was illegal, when AIDS wasn't a deadly threat, and when safe sex wasn't a concern of every sexually active individual. Yet even though they were aware of the risks and the realities involved, neither used contraception during every single sexual encounter. Then one of Jess's partners had a pregnancy scare. He decided never again to engage in unprotected sex. Sara had a different reality check: At her regular physical, she learned that she had contracted chlamydia, the most common sexually transmitted disease in the United States (see Chapter 11).

When Jess and Sara started dating, both of them felt that something was special about their relationship. Despite their mutual attraction, they decided to take every step toward intimacy slow. Both considered and talked about their personal priorities and concerns. Even though it was awkward, they also discussed their own sexual histories and underwent tests for STDs. Looking toward a continuing committed relationship, they decided on, not one, but two forms of contraception: the birth control pill and a condom. In the future, they realized that they might switch to other forms of birth control—and might well consider different options, including both marriage and parenthood.

As human beings, we have a unique power: the ability to choose to conceive or not to conceive. No other species on Earth can separate sexual activity and pleasure from reproduction. However, simply not wanting to get pregnant is never enough to prevent conception, nor is wanting to have a child always enough to get pregnant. Both desires require individual decisions and actions.

Anyone who engages in vaginal intercourse must be willing to accept the consequences of that activity—the possibility of pregnancy and responsibility for the child who might be conceived—or take action to avoid those consequences. Although many people are concerned about the risks associated with contraception, using birth control is safer and healthier than not using it. According to the Population Reference Bureau, the use of contraceptives, including oral contraceptives, saves millions of lives each year. Some forms of contraception also reduce the risk of sexually transmitted diseases.

This chapter provides information on conception, birth control, abortion, infertility, adoption, and the processes by which a new human life develops and enters the world.

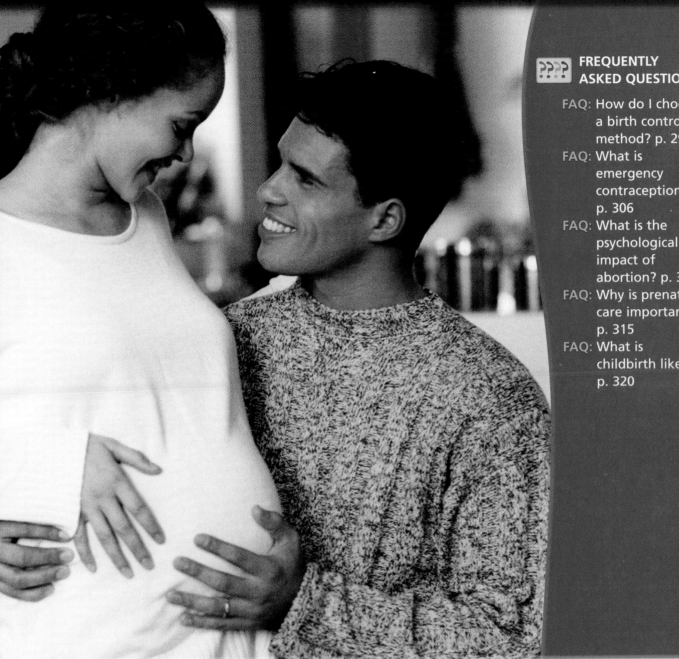

After studying the material in this chapter, you should be able to:

- **Describe** the process of human conception.
- **List** the major options available for contraception, and **identify** the advantages and risks of each.
- **Describe** the commonly used abortion methods.
- **Discuss** the physiological effects of pregnancy on a woman and **describe** fetal development.
- **Give examples** of prenatal care measures.
- **Describe** the three stages of labor and the birth process.
- **Identify** the options available to infertile couples wanting children.

Conception

The equation for making a baby is quite simple: One sperm plus one egg equals one fertilized egg, which can develop into an infant. But the processes that affect or permit **conception** are quite complicated. The creation of sperm, or **spermatogenesis,** starts in the male at puberty, and the production of sperm is regulated by hormones. Sperm cells form in the seminiferous tubules of the testes and are passed into the epididymis, where they are stored until ejaculation (see Figure 9-1); a single male ejaculation may contain 500 million sperm. Each of the sperm released into the vagina during intercourse moves on its own, propelling itself toward its target, an ovum.

To reach its goal, the sperm must move through the acidic secretions of the vagina, enter the uterus, travel up the fallopian tube containing the ovum, then fuse with the nucleus of the egg (**fertilization**). Just about every sperm produced by a man in his lifetime fails to accomplish its mission.

There are far fewer human egg cells than there are sperm cells. Each woman is born with her lifetime supply of ova, and between 300 and 500 eggs eventually mature and leave her ovaries during ovulation. As discussed in Chapter 8, every month, one or the other of the woman's ovaries releases an ovum to the nearby fallopian tube. It travels through the fallopian tube until it reaches the uterus, a journey that takes three to four days. An unfertilized egg lives for about 24 to 36 hours, disintegrates, and, during menstruation, is expelled along with the uterine lining.

Even if a sperm, which can survive in the female reproductive tract for two to five days, meets a ripe egg in a fallopian tube, its success is not assured. It must penetrate the layer of cells and a jellylike substance that surrounds each egg. Every sperm that touches the egg deposits an enzyme that dissolves part of this barrier. When a sperm bumps into a bare spot, it can penetrate the egg membrane and merge with the egg. (See Figure 9-2.) The fertilized egg travels down the fallopian tube, dividing to form a tiny clump of cells called a **zygote.** When it reaches the uterus, about a week after fertilization, it burrows into the endometrium, the lining of the uterus. This process is called **implantation.**

Conception can be prevented by **contraception.** Some contraceptive methods prevent ovulation or implantation, and others block the sperm from reaching the egg. Some methods are temporary; others permanently alter one's fertility.

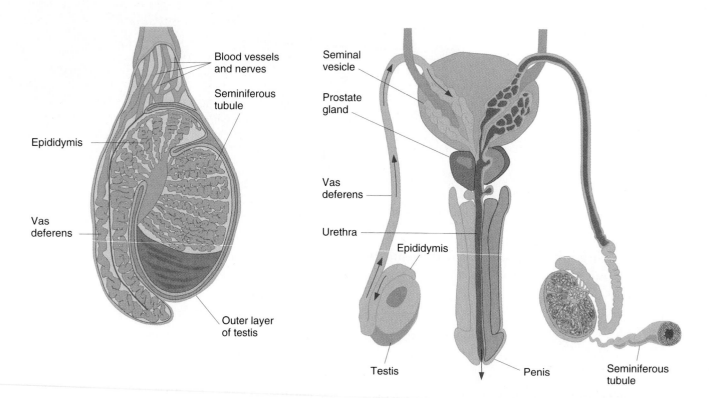

▲ **Figure 9-1 The testes.**
Spermatogenesis takes place in the testes. Sperm cells form in the seminiferous tubules and are stored in the coils of the epididymis. Eventually, the sperm drain into the vas deferens ready for ejaculation.

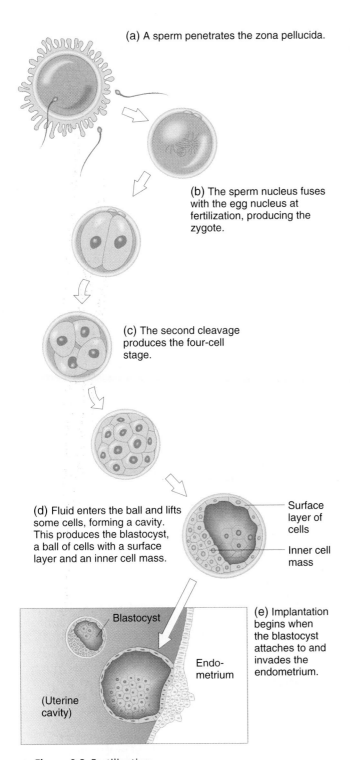

(a) A sperm penetrates the zona pellucida.

(b) The sperm nucleus fuses with the egg nucleus at fertilization, producing the zygote.

(c) The second cleavage produces the four-cell stage.

(d) Fluid enters the ball and lifts some cells, forming a cavity. This produces the blastocyst, a ball of cells with a surface layer and an inner cell mass.

Surface layer of cells

Inner cell mass

Blastocyst

(e) Implantation begins when the blastocyst attaches to and invades the endometrium.

Endo-metrium

(Uterine cavity)

▲ **Figure 9-2** Fertilization
(a) The efforts of hundreds of sperm may allow one to penetrate the ovum's corona radiata, and outer layer of cells, and then the zona pellucida, a thick inner membrane.
(b) The nuclei of the sperm and the egg cells approach. The nuclei merge, and the male and female chromosomes in the nuclei come together, forming a zygote. (c) The zygote divides into two cells, then four cells, and so on. (d) As fluid enters the ball, cells form a ball of cells called a blastocyst. (e) The blastocyst implants itself in the endometrium.

The Basics of Birth Control

A heterosexual woman in Western countries spends 90 percent of her reproductive years trying to prevent prgnancy and 10 percent of these years trying to become or being pregnant. Today birth control is safer, more effective, and more convenient than in the past—yet none of today's contraceptives is 100 percent safe, 100 percent effective, or 100 percent convenient. And even protection that is effective 95 percent of the time (which, some contend, is the best available in real-life use) isn't as good as it may sound. With just a 5 percent failure rate, statistically speaking, seven in ten women who want no more than two children would have to undergo one or more abortions in order to achieve their desired family size. See Table 9-1, which shows the use of contraception around the world.

Ideally, two partners should decide together which form of birth control to use. However, female methods account for 63 percent of all contraceptive methods reported by women between ages 15 and 44.[1] According to a national poll, more than 70 percent of men and women said men were "not responsible enough" to choose a birth control method. Both sexes believed that men were uninvolved because they "don't care" and because they consider birth control the "female's responsibility."[2] Lack of male involvement may account for 40 percent of each year's unwanted pregnancies.

Another barrier to birth control is cost. Although Medicaid contributes one of every two public dollars spent for family planning in the United States, many health insurers have not covered the cost of reversible methods of birth control—a policy that may be changing.[3] However, even when birth control is affordable and available, many college students do not use it consistently. (See Table 9-2.)

If you are engaging in sexual activity that could lead to conception, you have to be realistic about your situation. This may mean assuming full responsibility for your reproductive ability, whether you're a man or a woman. You also have to recognize the risks associated with various methods of contraception. If you're a woman, the risks are chiefly yours. Although most women never experience any serious complications, it's important to be aware of the potential for long-term risks. Risks that are acceptable to others may not be acceptable to you. The more you know about contraception, the more likely you are to use birth control.

 In one recent study at a Western college, undergraduates were more likely to report "almost always" using a reliable, proven method of birth control after completing an introductory health course.[4] (See Pulse Points: "Ten Ways to Avoid Getting Pregnant.")

Table 9-1 Global Use of Contraception		
Method of Contraception	**Regularly Used by (approximate)**	**Most Popular in These Places**
Sterilization	200 million	Asia, Latin America
Intrauterine device (IUD)	110 million	China, Arab states
The Pill	70 million	Latin America, USA, Europe
Injectable methods	10 million	Sub-Saharan Africa
Implants	1.5 million	Indonesia
Condom	>25 million	Worldwide

Unintended Pregnancy

The United States has the highest rate of unintended pregnancies in the world. Many of these occur because couples do not have a method of contraception or do not use their usual form of birth control. Yet 53 percent of the women who unintentionally become pregnant every year are using contraception.

Women between ages 20 and 24 have a higher rate of unintended pregnancy than women in any other age group, including teenagers. They are less likely to report uninterrupted use of an effective birth control method and more likely to use contraception sporadically than women aged 25 to 34. Such high-risk contraceptive behavior is more likely among women in less stable relationships, those having infrequent intercourse, and those who recently experienced nonvoluntary intercourse.[5]

Most pregnancies among contraceptive users are the result of incorrect or inconsistent use. Among the factors that influence the way sexual partners use birth control are the degree of communication and cooperation between them, the predictability and frequency of intercourse, their attitudes about sexuality and fertility, experience or practice with a particular method, and the ease and affordability of

PULSE POINTS

Ten Ways to Avoid Getting Pregnant

1. **Abstain.** The only 100 percent safe and effective way to avoid unwanted pregnancy is not to engage in heterosexual intercourse.

2. **Limit sexual activity to "outercourse."** You can engage in many sexual activities—kissing, hugging, touching, massage, oral-genital sex—without risking pregnancy.

3. **Talk about birth control with any potential sex partner.** If you are considering sexual intimacy with a person, you should feel comfortable enough to talk about contraception.

4. **Know what doesn't work—and don't rely on it.** There are many misconceptions about ways to avoid getting pregnant, such as having sex in a standing posi-

tion or during menstruation. Only the methods described in this chapter are reliable forms of birth control.

5. **Talk with a health-care professional.** A great deal of information and advice is available—in writing, from family planning counselors, from physicians on the Internet. Check it out.

6. **Choose a contraceptive method that matches your personal habits and preferences.** If you can't remember to take a pill every day, oral contraceptives aren't for you. If you're constantly forgetting where you put things, a diaphragm might not be a good choice.

7. **Consider long-term implications.** Since you may well wish to have children in the future, find out about the reversibility of various methods and possible effects on future fertility.

8. **Resist having sex without contraceptive protection "just this once."** It only takes once—even the very first time—to get pregnant. Be wary of drugs and alcohol. They can impair your judgment and make you less conscientious about using birth control—or using it properly.

9. **Use backup methods.** If there's a possibility that a contraceptive method might not offer adequate protection (for instance, if it's been almost three months since your last injection of Depo-Provera), use an additional form of birth control.

10. **Inform yourself about emergency contraception.** Just in case a condom breaks or a diaphragm slips, find out about the availability of forms of after-intercourse contraception.

▼ Table 9-2 Comparison of Contraception Effectiveness: Number of Pregnancies per 100 Women During First Year of Use

Method	Typical Use	Perfect Use	Protection Against Sexually Transmitted Diseases	Cost
Continuous abstinence	0.00	0.00	complete	none
Outercourse	NA	N/A	good	none
Norplant®	0.05	0.05	none	$500–$600 for exam, implants, and insertion $100–$200 for removal
Sterilization				
Men (vasectomy)	0.15	0.1	none	$240–$520 for vasectomy
Women (tubal)	0.5	0.5	none	$1,000–$2,500 for tubal sterilization (Vasectomy costs less because it is a simpler operation that can be done in the clinician's office
Depro-Provera®	0.3	0.3	none	$30–$75 per injection. May be less at clinics. $35–$125 for exam. Some family planning clinics charge according to income. $20–$40 for subsequent visits plus medication.
IUD				
ParaGard® (copper T 380A)	0.8	0.6	none	$150–$300: exam, insertion, and follow-up visit
Progestasert®	2.0	1.5	none	Some family planning clinics charge according to income.
The pill				
Combination	5.0	0.1	none	$15–$25 per monthly pill-pack at drugstores. Often less at clinics.
Progestin-only	5.0	0.5	none	$35–$125 for exam. Some family planning clinics charge according to income.
Male condom	14.0	3.0	good	25 cents and up: dry 50 cents and up: lubricated $2.50 and up: plastic, animal tissue, or textured Some family planning centers given them away or charge very little.
Withdrawal	19.0	4.0	none	none
Diaphragm	20.0	6.0	some	$13–$25 $50–$125 for exam. Often less at family planing clinics $4–$8 for supplies of spermicide jelly or cream
Cervical cap				
Women who have not given birth	20.0	9.0	some	$13–$25 $50–$125 for exam. Often less at family planning clinics
Women who have given birth	40.0	30.0	some	$4–$8 for supplies of spermicide jelly or cream
Female condom	21.0	5.0	good	$2.50
Predicting fertility				
Periodic abstinence	20.0		none	$5–$8 and up for temperature kits (drugstore)
Post-ovulation method		1.0	none	Free classes often available in health and church centers
Symptothermal method		2.0	none	
Cervical mucus (ovulation) method		3.0	none	
Calendar method		9.0	none	
Fertility awareness methods				
With male or female condom	N/A	N/A	none	See costs above
With diaphragm or cap	N/A	N/A	none	See costs above
With withdrawal or other methods	N/A	N/A	none	none
Spermicide	26.0	6.0	none	$8 for applicator kits of foam and gel $4–$8 for refills
No method	85.0	85.0	none	

Emergency Contraception
Emergency Contraception Pills: Treatment initiated within 72 hours after unprotected intercourse reduces the risk of pregnancy by 75–89 percent. (No protection against infection.)
Emergency IUD insertion: Treatment initiated within seven days after unprotected intercourse reduces the risk of pregnancy by more than 99 percent. (No protection against infection.)

Source: www.plannedparenthood.org. © 2001.

contraception. Many women temporarily discontinue birth control, primarily because they're dissatisfied with a particular method.

How Do I Choose a Birth Control Method?

When it comes to deciding which form of birth control to use, there's no one "right" decision. In a study of contraceptive decision-making among African American, Latina, and European-American women ages 18–50, those who were older, single, African-American, used pregnancy prevention, or had histories of sexually transmitted diseases and unintended pregnancies made contraceptive decisions alone. Older African-American women were more likely to choose no contraception. Among contraceptive users, African Americans used effective methods of pregnancy, but not disease, prevention. Women who had a history of sexually transmitted diseases and younger, more educated women were more likely to use methods that prevent both pregnancy and disease.[6] Good decisions are based on sound information. You should consult a physician or family-planning counselor if you have questions or want to know how certain methods might affect existing or familial medical conditions, such as high blood pressure or diabetes.

As Table 9-2 indicates, contraception doesn't always work. As you evaluate any contraceptive, always consider its *effectiveness* (the likelihood that it will indeed prevent pregnancy). Inevitably, theoretical effectiveness, based on statistical estimates, is greater than actual effectiveness. The **failure rate** for a contraceptive refers to the number of pregnancies that occur per year for every 100 women using a particular method of birth control.

The reliability of contraceptives in actual, real-life use is much lower than those reported in national surveys or clinical trials. In general, failure rates are highest among cohabiting and other unmarried women, among very poor families, among black and Hispanic women, among adolescents, and among women in their twenties. Unmarried adolescent women who are living with a partner have an average failure rate of about 31 percent in the first year of contraceptive use, regardless of method of birth control, compared with a failure rate of 7 percent among married women aged 30 and older. The annual failure rate among black women is about 19 percent, regardless of family income. Among Hispanic women, the overall failure rate is 10 percent, but it is higher among poorer women than more affluent ones. Teenagers whose partners are three or more years older are less likely to use contraceptives regularly.

Some couples use withdrawal or **coitus interruptus,** removal of the penis from the vagina before ejaculation, to prevent pregnancy, even though it is not a reliable form of birth control. About half the men who have tried coitus interruptus find it unsatisfactory, either because they don't know when they're going to ejaculate or because they can't withdraw quickly enough. Also, the Cowper's glands, two pea-sized structures located on each side of the urethra, often produce a fluid that appears as drops at the tip of the penis any time from arousal and erection to orgasm. This fluid can contain active sperm and, in infected men, human immunodeficiency virus (HIV).

As many as 3 million unintentional pregnancies each year in the United States are the result of contraceptive failure, either from problems with the drug or device itself or from improper use. Partners can lower the risk of unwanted pregnancy by using backup methods—that is, more than one form of contraception simultaneously. Emergency or after-intercourse contraception (discussed later in this chapter) could prevent as many as 2.3 million unwanted pregnancies each year.[7]

Even college students aware of the risks associated with unprotected sexual intercourse often do not practice safe-sex behaviors. There are many reasons, ranging from the influence of sex and alcohol to embarrassment about buying condoms. Generally, the ability to talk about a desire to use condoms has been found to be associated with a greater use of condoms. However, a recent survey of college students found that a significant percentage of both men and women either tried to dissuade a potential partner from condom use or had a sexual partner who'd tried to discour-

STRATEGIES FOR PREVENTION

Choosing a Contraceptive

Your contraceptive needs may change throughout your life. To decide which method to use now, you need to know:

✔ How well will it fit into your lifestyle?

✔ How convenient will it be?

✔ How effective will it be?

✔ How safe will it be?

✔ How affordable will it be?

✔ How reversible will it be?

✔ Will it protect against sexually transmitted diseases?[8]

See the Self-Survey: "Which Contraceptive Method is Best for You?" on p. 292.

age them from condom use. Both men and women generally used the same arguments against condoms: that sex felt better without them, that the woman wouldn't get pregnant, and that neither would get a sexually transmitted disease.[9] (See Student Snapshot: "Condoms on Campus.")

The bottom line is that it takes two people to conceive a baby, and two people should be involved in deciding *not* to conceive a baby. In the process, they can also enhance their skills in communication, critical thinking, and negotiating.

Abstinence

The contraceptive methods discussed in this chapter are designed to prevent pregnancy as a consequence of vaginal intercourse. Couples who choose abstinence make a very different decision—to abstain from vaginal intercourse and other forms of sexual activity (any in which ejaculation occurs near the vaginal opening) that could result in conception.

For many individuals, abstinence represents a deliberate choice regarding their bodies, minds, spirits, and sexuality. People choose abstinence for various reasons, including waiting until they are ready for a sexual relationship or until they find the "right" partner, respecting religious or moral values, enjoying friendships without sexual

STRATEGIES FOR PREVENTION

Is Abstinence the Right Choice for You?

✔ Think about your values, goals, and priorities. Would abstinence support them?

✔ Realize that drugs and alcohol could affect your ability to make sexual decisions. Are you prepared to avoid their use to be sure to maintain your abstinence?

✔ Talk about your feelings before a relationship gets sexual. Can you put your thoughts and feelings about abstinence into words?

✔ Abstinence does not mean an end to all sexual experiences. What behaviors would you consider? What limits would you set?

involvement, recovering from a breakup, or preventing pregnancy and sexually transmitted disease.

Abstinence is the only form of birth control that is 100 percent effective and risk-free. It is also an important,

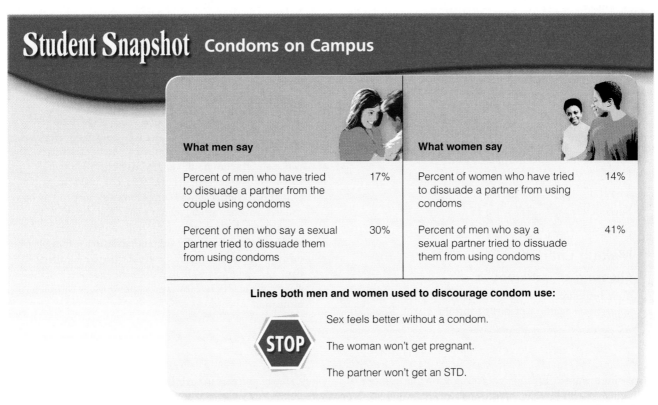

Student Snapshot Condoms on Campus

What men say		What women say	
Percent of men who have tried to dissuade a partner from the couple using condoms	17%	Percent of women who have tried to dissuade a partner from using condoms	14%
Percent of men who say a sexual partner tried to dissuade them from using condoms	30%	Percent of men who say a sexual partner tried to dissuade them from using condoms	41%

Lines both men and women used to discourage condom use:

STOP

Sex feels better without a condom.

The woman won't get pregnant.

The partner won't get an STD.

Sources: Oncale, Renee, and Bruce King. "Comparisons of Men's and Women's Attempts to Dissuade Sexual Partners from the Couple Using Condoms." *Archives of Sexual Behavior,* Vol. 30, No. 4, August 2001, p. 379.

SELF SURVEY

Answer yes or no to each statement as it applies to you and, if appropriate, your partner.

1. You have high blood pressure or cardiovascular disease. _____
2. You smoke cigarettes. _____
3. You have a new sexual partner. _____
4. An unwanted pregnancy would be devastating to you. _____
5. You have a good memory. _____
6. You or your partner have multiple sexual partners. _____
7. You prefer a method with little or no bother. _____
8. You have heavy, crampy periods. _____
9. You need protection against STDs. _____
10. You are concerned about endometrial and ovarian cancer. _____
11. You are forgetful. _____
12. You need a method right away. _____
13. You're comfortable touching your own and your partner's genitals. _____
14. You have a cooperative partner. _____
15. You like a little extra vaginal lubrication. _____
16. You have sex at unpredictable times and places. _____
17. You are in a monogamous relationship and have at least one child. _____

Scoring:

Recommendations are based on Yes answers to the following numbered statements:

The combination pill: 4, 5, 6, 8, 9, 16

The progestin-only pill: 1, 2, 5, 7, 16

Condoms: 1, 2, 3, 6, 9, 12, 13, 14

Norplant and Depo-Provera: 1, 2, 4, 7, 11, 16

Diaphragm or cervical cap: 1, 2, 13, 14

The IUD: 1, 2, 7, 11, 13, 16, 17

Spermicides: 1, 2, 12, 13, 14, 15

Sponge: 1, 2, 12, 13

Making Changes

Choosing a Contraceptive

Your responses may indicate that there's more than one appropriate method of birth control for you. Remember that you may choose different types of birth control at different stages of your life, or switch contraceptives for various reasons. You and your partner should always consider and discuss these factors:

- **Effectiveness.** Keep in mind that your own conscientiousness will play an important role. If you forget to take your daily pill, or if you decide not to use a condom "just this once," you'll increase the odds of pregnancy by interfering with effective birth control.
- **Suitability.** If you don't have sex very often, a contraceptive with many risks and side effects, such as the pill, may be wrong for you. If you have many sexual partners and are at risk of contracting a sexually transmitted disease, a condom may provide protection against pregnancy and infection, especially if used with a diaphragm or cervical cap.
- **Side effects.** Some complications related to contraceptives are serious health threats. Be sure to ask questions and gather as much information as possible about what side effects to expect.
- **Safety.** The risks of certain contraceptives, such as the pill, may be too great to allow their use, if, for example, you have high blood pressure. Be honest in describing your medical history to your physician.
- **Future fertility.** Some women don't return to regular menstrual cycles for six months to a year after discontinuing oral contraceptives. This possibility may or may not be important to you now, but you should try to look ahead.
- **Cost.** The only free contraceptive methods are abstinence and rhythm methods. If you're on a tight budget, you might consider the relative costs of a year's prescription of oral contraceptives compared to a year's supply of condoms or spermicidal foam or jelly. You should also think about the long-term costs and consequences.
- **Reduced risk of sexually transmitted diseases.** Some forms of contraception, in particular barrier contraceptives and spermicides, help reduce the risk of transmission of some STDs. However, none provides complete protection.

increasingly valued lifestyle choice. A growing number of individuals, including some who have been sexually active in the past, are choosing abstinence until they establish a relationship with a long-term partner.

Abstinence offers special health benefits for women. Those who abstain until their twenties and engage in sex with fewer partners in their lifetimes are less likely to get sexually transmitted diseases, to suffer infertility, or to develop cervical cancer. However, some people find it difficult to abstain for long periods of time. There also is a risk that people will abruptly end their abstinence without being prepared to protect themselves against pregnancy or infection.[10]

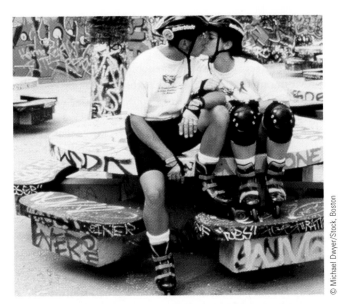

▲ Some couples refrain from intercourse but engage in "outercourse," or intimacy that includes kissing, hugging, and sensual touching.

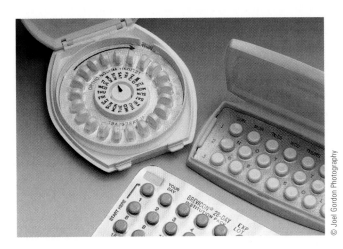

▲ Oral contraceptives. The birth control pill.

"Outercourse"

Individuals who choose abstinence from vaginal intercourse often engage in activities sometimes called "outercourse," such as kissing, hugging, sensual touching, and mutual masturbation. Outercourse is nearly 100 percent effective as a contraceptive measure, but pregnancy is possible if there is genital contact. If the man ejaculates near the vaginal opening, sperm can swim up into the vagina and fallopian tubes to fertilize an egg. Except for oral-genital and anal sex, outercourse also may lower the risk of contracting sexually transmitted diseases. It is an effective form of safe sex as long as no body fluids are exchanged.

Some couples routinely restrict themselves to outercourse; others choose such sexual activities temporarily when it is inadvisable for them to have vaginal intercourse—for example, after childbirth. Other benefits: Outercourse has no medical or hormonal side effects; it may prolong sex play and enhance orgasm, and it can be used when no other methods are available.[11]

Prescription Contraceptives

The most effective and most widely used methods of birth control in the United States include oral contraceptives, hormonal implants and injections, the intrauterine device, the diaphragm, and the cervical cap. All are reversible and available only from health professionals.

The Birth Control Pill

"The pill"—the popular term for **oral contraceptives**—is the method of birth control preferred by unmarried

women and by those under age 30, including college students. Women 18 to 24 years old are most likely to choose oral contraceptives. In use for 30 years, the pill is one of the most researched, tested, and carefully followed medications in medical history—and one of the most controversial. Although many women incorrectly think that the risks of the pill are greater than those of pregnancy and childbirth, long-term studies show that oral contraceptive use does not increase mortality rates. Oral contraceptives significantly reduce the risk of ovarian and endometrial cancer and produce no increase in serious disease, including breast cancer, diabetes, multiple sclerosis, rheumatoid arthritis, and liver disease.[12] There is an increased risk of blood clots and pulmonary embolism for smokers and women who used earlier types of oral contraceptives.[13]

Three types of oral contraceptives are currently widely used in the United States: the constant-dose combination pill, the multiphasic pill, and the progestin-only pill. The **constant-dose combination** or **monophasic pill** releases two hormones, synthetic estrogen and progestin, which play important roles in controlling ovulation and the menstrual cycle, at constant levels throughout the menstrual cycle. The **multiphasic pill** mimics normal hormonal fluctuations of the natural menstrual cycle by providing different levels of estrogen and progesterone at different times of the month. Multiphasic pills reduce total hormonal dose and side effects. Both constant-dose combination and multiphasic pills block the release of hormones that would stimulate the process leading to ovulation. They also thicken and alter the cervical mucus, making it more hostile to sperm, and they make implantation of a fertilized egg in the uterine lining more difficult. Multiphasic pills may heighten a woman's sex drive.

The **progestin-only,** or **minipill,** contains a small amount of progestin and no estrogen. Unlike women who take constant-dose combination pills, those using minipills probably ovulate at least occasionally. The minipills make the mucus in the cervix so thick and tacky, however, that sperm can't enter the uterus. Minipills also may interfere with implantation by altering the uterine lining.

In 2001 the FDA approved a new oral contraceptive, Yasmin, the first birth control pill that contains a type of progestin called drospirenone. As with other oral contraceptives, the most frequent side effects associated with Yasmin are headache, menstrual disorder, breast pain, abdominal pain, and nausea.[14]

Advantages. Birth control pills have several advantages: They are extremely effective. Among women who miss no pills, only 1 in 1,000 becomes pregnant in the first year of use. They are reversible, so a woman can easily stop using them. They do not interrupt sexual activity. Women on the pill have more regular periods, less cramping, and fewer tubal, or ectopic, pregnancies (discussed later in this chapter). After five years of use, the pill halves the risk of endometrial and ovarian cancer. It also reduces the risk of benign breast lumps, ovarian cysts, iron-deficiency anemia, and pelvic inflammatory disease (PID). In actual use, the failure rate is 1 to 5 percent for estrogen/progesterone pills and 3 to 10 percent for minipills. Some physicians suggest that in the future women may use the pill to regulate their menstrual cycle.[15]

Disadvantages. The pill does not protect against HIV infection and other sexually transmitted diseases, so condoms and spermicide should also be used.[16] In addition, the hormones in oral contraceptives may cause various side effects, including spotting between periods, weight gain or loss, nausea and vomiting, breast tenderness, and decreased sex drive. Some women using the pill report emotional changes, such as mood swings and depression. Oral contraceptives can interact with other medications and diminish their effectiveness; women should inform any physician providing medical treatment that they are taking the pill.

Current birth control pills contain much lower levels of estrogen than early pills. As a result, the risk of heart disease and stroke among users is much lower than it once was; the danger may be lowest with the minipill. Yet a risk of cardiovascular problems is still associated with use of the pill, primarily for women over 35 who smoke and those with other health problems, such as high blood pressure. Heart attacks strike an estimated 1 in 14,000 pill users between the ages of 30 and 39, and 1 in 1,500 between the ages of 40 and 44. Strokes occur five times more frequently among women taking oral contraceptives, and clots in the veins develop in 1 of every 500 previously healthy women. (See the Savvy Consumer: "Evaluating the Health Risks of Birth Control Methods.")

Before starting on the pill, you should undergo a thorough physical examination that includes the following tests:

▶ Routine blood pressure test.
▶ Pelvic exam, including a Pap smear.
▶ Breast exam.
▶ Blood test.
▶ Urine sample.

Let your doctor know about any personal or family incidence of high blood pressure or heart disease, diabetes, liver dysfunction, hepatitis, unusual menstrual history, severe depression, sickle-cell anemia, cancer of the breast,

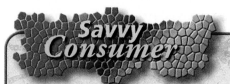

Evaluating the Health Risks of Birth Control Methods

For individuals with certain medical conditions, specific types of birth control can pose a health risk. To be safe, follow these guidelines:

• **High blood pressure** (180/110 mmHg or higher): Avoid birth control pills or injectables containing estrogen, which may increase your risk of a heart attack or stroke.

• **Episodes of depression:** Avoid products that contain progestin, such as Depo-Provera, Norplant, and the minipill. In some women with depression, progestin may worsen depressive symptoms. Also, check with your doctor if you are taking an antidepressant medica-

tion; it may affect or be affected by oral contraceptives and you may require a different dose.

• **Seizure disorder:** Avoid low-dose birth control pills. Some antiseizure medications, such as Dilantin, accelerate liver metabolism of all substances, including oral contraceptives, and make them less effective.

• **Ectopic pregnancy:** Avoid IUDs. Although IUDs do not cause ectopic pregnancies, if your fallopian tubes have been scarred by a previous ectopic gestation, you're more likely to have another ectopic if you use an IUD.

• **Hepatitis** (discussed in Chapter 11): Avoid birth control pills or injectables containing estrogen, which is metabolized in the liver—an organ damaged by hepatitis.

ovaries, or uterus, high cholesterol levels, or migraine headaches.

How to Use Oral Contraceptives. An estimated 2 million women worldwide become unintentionally pregnant every year because they do not use the pill as directed.[17] The pill usually comes in 28-day packets: 21 of the pills contain the hormones, and 7 are "blanks," included so that the woman can take a pill every day, even during her menstrual period. If a woman forgets to take one pill, she should take it as soon as she remembers. However, if she forgets during the first week of her cycle or misses more than one pill, she should rely on another form of birth control until her next menstrual period.

In clinical trials, a transdermal contraceptive patch has proven as effective as oral birth control pills. The patch, which is replaced weekly, may be especially useful for women who find it hard to remember to take a daily pill.[18]

Even if you experience no discomfort or side effects while on the pill, see a physician at least once a year for an examination, which should include a blood pressure test and a pelvic and breast exam. Notify your doctor at once if you develop severe abdominal pain, chest pain, coughing, shortness of breath, pain or tenderness in the calf or thigh, severe headaches, dizziness, faintness, muscle weakness or numbness, speech disturbance, blurred vision, a sensation of flashing lights, a breast lump, severe depression, or yellowing of your skin.

Generally, when a woman stops taking the pill, her menstrual cycle resumes the next month, but it may be irregular for the next couple of months. However, 2 to 4 percent of pill users experience prolonged delays. Women who become pregnant during the first or second cycle after discontinuing use of the pill may be at greater risk of miscarriage; they also are more likely to conceive twins. Most physicians advise women who want to conceive to change to another method of contraception for three months after they stop taking the pill.

Hormonal Implants (Norplant)

About 1 percent of women use hormonal implants, such as Norplant, which prevent pregnancy for up to five years. Six thin silicone rubber capsules release a low, continuous dose of a synthetic form of progestin called levonorgestrel. Other implants are currently being developed.

Norplant works primarily by suppressing ovulation, but it also thickens the cervical mucus (which inhibits sperm migration), inhibits the development and growth of the uterine lining, and limits secretion of progesterone during the second or luteal half of the menstrual cycle. The best candidates for Norplant are women who desire reversible long-term contraception, those who don't want to have to insert or ingest a contraceptive regularly, those who

cannot take estrogen-containing oral contraceptives, those who would face high medical risks if they did become pregnant, and those who are undecided about sterilization.[19] Adolescents using Norplant are considerably less likely than pill users to become pregnant unintentionally, even after one unintended pregancy.[20]

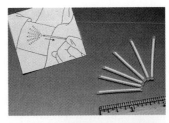
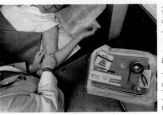

© Joel Gordon Photography (both)

▲ Norplant implants are placed in a woman's arm.

Advantages. A five-year study of some 8,000 users of Norplant in eight developing countries found that this hormonal implant is both safe and effective. Pregnancy rates for Norplant, copper IUD, and sterilization each averaged less than one per 100 woman-years. The report showed no significant increases in cancer or in cardiovascular problems, such as stroke or blood clots in Norplant users compared to women using nonhormonal methods.[21]

Norplant is most effective in women who weigh less than 110 pounds and somewhat less effective in those weighing more than 154 pounds. However, even in heavier women, Norplant is more effective than oral contraceptives. Like the pill, it may reduce the risk of endometrial and ovarian cancer.

For sexually active adolescents and young adults, who often do not use birth control pills and other forms of contraception consistently, Norplant's primary advantage is its long duration of action and the fact that they do not need to remember to use it. However, in clinical studies, teenagers reported more side effects with Norplant than with oral contraceptives.

Disadvantages. Norplant does not protect against STDs, so condoms and spermicides should also be used.

Common side effects of Norplant include menstrual irregularities, spotting, and amenorrhea; these are most likely to occur in the first year of use. Other possible complications include ovarian cysts, headaches, acne, weight changes, breast discharge, nausea, and hair growth. Because Norplant doesn't include estrogen (as birth control pills do), there is no risk of clotting or high blood pressure. However, the FDA advises women with acute liver disease, unexplained vaginal bleeding, breast cancer, or blood clots in the lungs, legs, or eyes to avoid Norplant.

Controversy also arose over the suggestion that women on welfare or convicted of child abuse be ordered or given incentives to use Norplant. The American Medical Association's board of trustees has stated its opposition to the involuntary use of long-acting contraceptives because such a policy inhibits a person's fundamental rights to refuse medical treatment, not to receive cruel and unusual punishment, and to procreate.

How to Use Norplant. You should *not* use Norplant if you are pregnant, have unexplained vaginal bleeding, are breast-feeding or have given birth in the last six weeks, have ever had breast cancer, have had certain rare kinds of headache, or are sensitive to the ingredients in implants.[22]

A qualified health-care professional, using a local anesthetic, implants the Norplant capsules with a needle under the skin of a woman's upper arms. The simple surgical procedure generally takes about five to ten minutes. Once in place, the capsules can be felt and may be visible, particularly in slender women. Removal of the capsules again requires minor surgery, lasting 15 to 20 minutes, with a local anesthetic. Complications can occur during removal; the most common are bruising, slight bleeding, and pain at the removal site. After removal, fertility generally returns with the next menstrual cycle. According to various studies, most former users of Norplant began ovulating again within seven weeks of implant removal, and most of those who wished to conceive did so within one year.

Hormonal Injectables

One injection of Depo-Provera, a synthetic version of the natural hormone progesterone, provides three months of contraceptive protection. This long-acting hormonal contraceptive raises levels of progesterone, thereby simulating pregnancy. The pituitary gland doesn't produce FSH and LH, which normally cause egg ripening and release. The endometrial lining of the uterus thins, preventing implantation of a fertilized egg.

A new monthly injectable contraceptive, the Lunelle Monthly Contraceptive Injection, has proven highly effective and safe in initial studies. Side effects are similar to those of hormonal contraceptives, including weight gain, acne, and irregular bleeding.[23]

Advantages. Because injectable contraceptives contain only progestin, they can be used by women who cannot take oral contraceptives containing estrogen (such as those who've had breast cancer). Their main advantage is that women do not need to take a daily pill. Depo-Provera also may have some protective action against endometrial and ovarian cancer.

Disadvantages. Injectable contraceptives provide no protection against HIV and other STDs. Depo-Provera causes menstrual irregularities in most users, and it causes a delayed return of fertility, excessive endometrial bleeding, and other side effects, including decreased libido, depression, headaches, dizziness, weight gain, frequent urination, and allergic reactions in a small percentage of users. Long-term use may lead to significantly reduced bone density.

How to Use Injectable Contraceptives. Women must receive an injection of Depo-Provera once every 12 weeks, ideally within five days of the beginning of menstruation.

The Intrauterine Device (IUD)

The **intrauterine device (IUD)** is a small piece of molded plastic, with a nylon string attached, that is inserted into the uterus through the cervix. It prevents pregnancy by interfering with implantation. Once widely used, IUDs became less popular after most brands were removed from the market because of serious complications such as pelvic infection and infertility. However, the currently available IUDs have not been shown to increase the risk of such problems for women in mutually monogamous relationships. (See Figure 9-3.)

According to manufacturers' estimates, about 2 percent of American women using contraception currently rely on IUDs. Throughout the world more than 25 million IUDs have been distributed in 70 countries. Progestaser System is a T-shaped device containing progesterone, which prevents implantation; it must be replaced every year.

The Copper T (Paragard) contains copper, which interferes with the growth of a fertilized egg by causing biochemical reactions with the uterine lining. The Copper T remains effective for ten years, making it the longest-acting reversible contraceptive available to women in the United States. Its cumulative failure rate is 2.6.

The newest IUD, Mirena intrauterine system, consists of a polyethylene T-shaped device surrounded by a sleeve containing the progestin levonorgestrel, which is released directly to the lining of the uterus. Mirena, which has been used by more than 1.4 million women in Europe, Asia, and

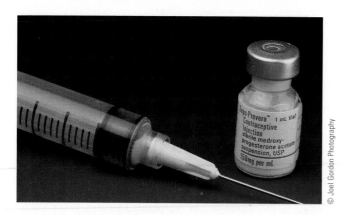

▲ Depo-Provera is given by injection every 12 weeks.

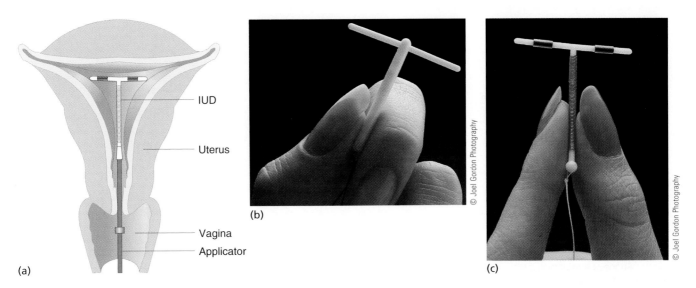

IUD

Uterus

Vagina

Applicator

(a)

(b)

(c)

© Joel Gordon Photography

▲ **Figure 9-3** The IUD.
The intrauterine device is effective and cost-efficient for preventing pregnancy, although some women may expel the device. The IUD does not offer protection against STDs, and there is increased risk of pelvic inflammatory disease (PID). (a) The IUD is placed in uterus. (b) The Progesterset system. (c) The copper T.

Latin America, contains no estrogen and is 99 percent effective in preventing pregnancy for up to five years.[24]

Advantages. The IUD is highly effective and easy to reverse. According to recent analyses, the Copper T is the cheapest and most cost-effective form of birth control. Current models cause fewer complications than the pill. The IUD does not interrupt sexual activity.

IUDs were long believed to increase the risk of pelvic inflammatory disease, which can lead to scarring and infertility. More recent research has shown that, while IUD users are more likely to develop PID than nonusers, it is an uncommon complication.[25] The greatest risk of PID occurs during the first few weeks following insertion; it falls at about 20 days.[26]

Disadvantages. Many gynecologists recommend other forms of birth control for childless women who someday may want to start a family. Women who have never given birth and have used an IUD for an extended period of time may find it more difficult to conceive after discontinuing its use.[27] In addition, women with many sexual partners, who are at highest risk of PID, are not good candidates for this method.

During insertion of an IUD, women may experience discomfort, cramping, bleeding, or pain, which may continue for a few days or longer. The hormonal IUD causes less excess bleeding and cramping than the Copper T. An estimated 2 to 20 percent of users expel an IUD within a year of insertion.

If a woman using an IUD does become pregnant, the IUD is removed to reduce the risk of miscarriage (which can be as high as 50 percent). Physicians generally offer therapeutic abortion to the woman because of the serious risks (including infection, premature delivery, and possibly a higher rate of birth defects) of continuing the pregnancy.

How to Use an IUD. A physician inserts an IUD during the woman's period, when the cervix is slightly softened and dilated. Antibiotics may be prescribed to lower any risk of infection. An IUD can be removed at any time during her cycle. A woman should check regularly, particularly after each menstrual period, for the nylon string attached to the IUD, because she may not otherwise notice if an IUD has been expelled.

The Diaphragm

The **diaphragm** is a bowl-like rubber cup with a flexible rim that is inserted into the vagina to cover the cervix and prevent the passage of sperm into the uterus during sexual intercourse (see Figure 9-4). When used with spermicide, the diaphragm is both a physical and a chemical barrier to sperm. The effectiveness of the diaphragm in preventing pregnancy depends on strong motivation (to use it faithfully) and a precise understanding of its use. If diaphragms with spermicide are used consistently and carefully, they can be 95 to 98 percent effective. Without a spermicide, the diaphragm is not effective.

Advantages. Diaphragms have become increasingly popular, most likely because of concern about the side effects of hormonal contraceptives. Many women feel that using a diaphragm makes them more knowledgeable and comfortable about their bodies.

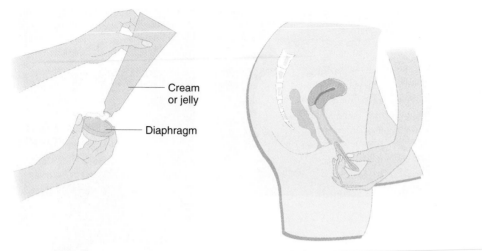
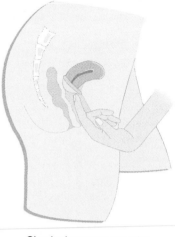

Squeeze spermicide into dome of diaphragm and around the rim.

Squeeze rim together; insert jelly-side up.

Check placement to make certain cervix is covered.

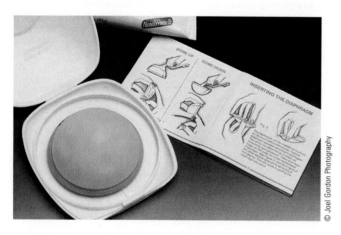

© Joel Gordon Photography

▲ **Figure 9-4** The diaphragm.
When used correctly and consistently and with a spermicide, the diaphragm is effective in preventing pregnancy and STDs. It must be fitted by a health-care professional.

Disadvantages. Some people find that the diaphragm is inconvenient and interferes with sexual spontaneity or that the spermicidal cream or jelly is messy, detracts from oral-genital sex, and can cause irritation. A poorly fitted diaphragm may cause discomfort during sex; some women report bladder discomfort, urethral irritation, or recurrent cystitis as a result of diaphragm use.

How to Use a Diaphragm. Diaphragms are fitted and prescribed by a qualified health-care professional in sizes ranging from 2 to 4 inches (50–105 millimeters) in diameter. The diaphragm's main function is to serve as a container for a spermicidal (sperm-killing) foam or jelly, which is available at pharmacies without a prescription. A diaphragm should remain in the vagina for at least six hours after intercourse to assure that all sperm are killed. If intercourse occurs again during this period, additional spermicide cream or jelly must be inserted with an applicator tube.

The key to proper use of the diaphragm is having it available. A sexually active woman should keep it in the most accessible place—her purse, bedroom, bathroom. Before every use, a diaphragm should be checked for tiny leaks (hold up to the light or place water in the dome). A health-care provider should check its fit and condition every year when the woman has her annual Pap smear.

Oil-based lubricants will deteriorate the latex of the diaphragm and should not be used with one.

The Cervical Cap

Like the diaphragm, the **cervical cap,** combined with spermicide, serves as both a chemical and physical barrier blocking the path of the sperm to the uterus. The rubber or plastic cap is smaller and thicker than a diaphragm and resembles a large thimble that fits snugly around the cervix (see Figure 9-5). It is about as effective as a diaphragm.

Advantages. Women who cannot use a diaphragm because of pelvic-structure problems or loss of vaginal muscle tone can often use the cap. Also, the cervical cap is less messy and does not require additional applications of spermicide if intercourse occurs more than once within several hours.

Disadvantages. Cervical caps are more difficult to insert and remove and may damage the cervix. Some women find it uncomfortable to wear. Because only four sizes of conventional cervical caps were available, about 25 percent of women have had difficulty with getting a proper fit. Newer

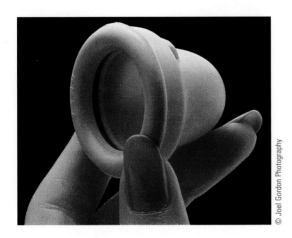

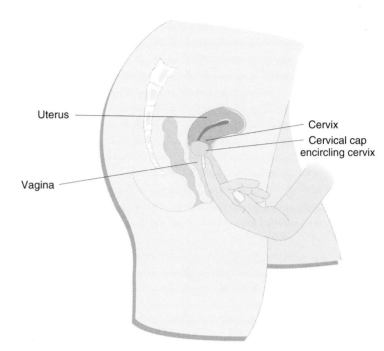

Uterus

Vagina

Cervix
Cervical cap
encircling cervix

▲ **Figure 9-5** The cervical cap
This method is very similar to the diaphragm
and may work better for some women. It is
smaller than the diaphragm and covers only the
cervix.

products, such as Lea's Shield, come in one size and are designed to fit all women.[28]

Some cap users have developed abnormal Pap smears within three months of beginning this birth control method. Doctors recommend a Pap smear before beginning and after three months of cervical cap use.[29]

How to Use a Cervical Cap. Like the diaphragm, the cervical cap is fitted by a qualified health-care professional. For use, the woman fills it one-third to two-thirds full with spermicide and inserts it by holding its edges together and sliding it into the vagina. The cup is then pressed onto the cervix. (Most women find it easiest to do so while squatting or in an upright sitting position.) The cap can be inserted up to 6 hours prior to intercourse and should not be removed for at least 6 hours afterward. It can be left in place up to 24 hours. Pulling on one side of the rim breaks the suction and allows easy removal. Oil-based lubricants should not be used with the cap because they can deteriorate the latex.

Nonprescription Contraceptives

As their name implies, **barrier contraceptives,** available without a prescription, block the meeting of egg and sperm by means of a physical barrier (a condom, diaphragm, or a cervical cap), or a chemical one (vaginal spermicide in jellies, foams, creams, suppositories, or film). These forms of birth control have become increasingly popular because they can do more than prevent conception—they can also help reduce the risk of STDs.

The Male Condom

The male **condom** covers the erect penis and catches the ejaculate, thus preventing sperm from entering the woman's reproductive tract (see Figure 9-6 on p. 300). Most are made of thin surgical latex or sheep membrane; a new type is made of polyurethane, which is thinner, stronger, more heat-sensitive, and more comfortable than latex. Condoms with a spermicidal lubricant (nonoxynol-9) kill most sperm on contact and are thus more effective than other brands.

Although the theoretical effectiveness rate for condoms is 97 percent, the actual rate is only 80 to 85 percent. The condom can be torn during the manufacturing process or during its use; testing by the manufacturer may not be as strenuous as it could or should be. Careless removal can also decrease the effectiveness of condoms. However, the major reason that condoms have such a low actual effectiveness rate is that couples don't use them each and every time they have sex. Users who have little experience with condoms, who are young, single, or childless, or who engage in risky behaviors are more likely to have condoms break.[30]

Condoms are second only to the pill in popularity among college-age adults. Condom use has increased in the last decade. Approximately one in five women, ages 15 to 44 who used contraception, rely on their partner's use of condoms as their primary method of birth control.[31]

More teens also are using condoms but not consistently. (See the X&Y Files: "Sex, Lies, and Condom Use" on p. 301.) From one-third to one-half of sexually active teens report using condoms for every act of intercourse. However,

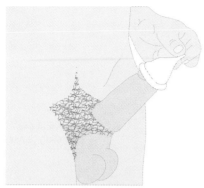

Pinch or twist the tip of the condom, leaving one-half inch at the tip to catch the semen.

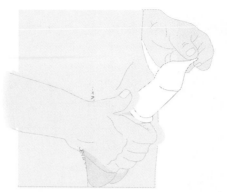

Holding the tip, unroll the condom.

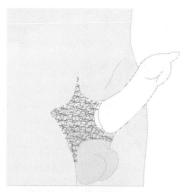

Unroll the condom until it reaches the pubic hairs.

▲ **Figure 9-6** The male condom.
Condoms effectively reduce the risk of pregnancy as well as STDs. Using them consistently and correctly are important factors.

condom use decreases as teens get older, with fewer males ages 18 and 19 using condoms than 15 to 17 year olds. Teenage girls report less frequent use of condoms than males.[32]

For girls, being from an intact family and having a mother with higher educational achievement are associated with greater condom use at first intercourse. Black adolescents, teens with more educated parents, and teens who were older at first intercourse also had greater condom use. The less similar adolescents and their partners are to one another—whether because of a difference in age, grade, or school—the less likely adolescents are to use condoms and other contraceptive methods.[33]

According to the National Longitudinal Study of Adolescent Health, one-fifth to one-half of sexually active adolescents share common misconceptions about condoms.[34] Many believe that there is no space at the tip of a condom or think that Vaseline can be used with condoms; some say that lambskin protects against HIV better than latex. None of these is true.[35] Television advertising of condoms, which has been controversial in the past, may help correct such misinformation. According to a recent study, nine in ten of Americans surveyed endorsed condom advertising on TV, either freely, like any other product, or at restricted times.[36]

Advantages. Condoms made of latex or polyurethane, especially when used with spermicides containing nonoxynol-9, can help reduce the risk of certain STDs, including syphilis, gonorrhea, chlamydia, and herpes. They appear to lower a woman's risk of pelvic inflammatory disease (PID) and may protect against some parasites that cause urinary tract and genital infections. Public health officials view condoms as the best available defense against HIV infection. They are available without a prescription or medical appointment, and their use does not cause harmful side effects. Some men appreciate the slight

blunting of sensation they experience when using a condom because it helps prolong the duration of intercourse before ejaculation.

Disadvantages. Condoms are not 100 percent effective in preventing pregnancy or STDs, including infection with HIV or HPV (human papilloma virus, discussed in Chapter 11). For anyone not in a monogamous relationship with a mutually exclusive, healthy partner—heterosexual or homosexual—condoms can reduce the risks of sexual involvement, but they cannot eliminate them. Condoms may have manufacturing defects, such as pinsize holes, or they may break or slip off during intercourse.

STRATEGIES FOR PREVENTION

Seven Steps to Correct Condom Use

✔ Use a new condom at each act of intercourse.

✔ Handle the condom carefully to avoid damage from fingernails, teeth, or other sharp objects.

✔ Put on condom after penis is erect and before any genital contact with a partner.

✔ Make sure that air is trapped in the tip of the condom.

✔ Ensure adequate lubrication during intercourse.

✔ Use only water-based lubricants with latex condoms.

✔ Withdraw the penis while it is still erect to prevent slippage. Hold the condom firmly against the base of the penis during withdrawal.[37]

The X&Y Files   Sex, Lies, and Condom Use

In a series of focus groups with 92 sexually active, young, ethnically and racially diverse individuals, aged 15 to 20, in five American cities, researchers focused on their views and motivations for sex and for condom use. Most found it difficult to believe that people their age used condoms every single time they had sex. Although they acknowledged that everyone is at risk for sexually transmitted diseases, the young people saw their own risk as minimal.

The genders had very different motives both for engaging in sex and for using condoms. In the interviews, young women said they engaged in sexual relations because of a desire for physical intimacy and a committed relationship. They generally reported having sex only with men they cared for and deeply trusted and expected that these men would be honest and forthright about their sexual history. This trust played a significant role in their decision whether to insist on condom use.

In contrast, few of the young men said "relationships" were an important dimension of their sexual involvements. Their primary motivation was a desire for physical and sexual satisfaction. Most said they were not interested in commitment and viewed emotional expectations as a complication of becoming sexually involved with a woman. The young men also admitted to making judgments about "types" of girls. To them, young women they didn't care about were "sluts" with whom they used a condom for their own protection.

Which partner determined whether a couple would use a condom? In these interviews, the answer was the women—if they chose to do so. Regardless of race or ethnicity, many of the young women were adamant in demanding that their partners use condoms—and many young men said they would not challenge such a demand out of fear of losing the opportunity for sex. Men often expected potential partners to want to use condoms and described themselves as "suspicious" of women who did not.

Both sexes named two primary reasons for using condoms: preventing pregnancy and protecting against sexually transmitted diseases. Young women saw an unwanted pregnancy as an occurrence that would be disruptive, expensive, and could "ruin" their lives and their parents' lives. Young men saw condom use as a way of protecting themselves against emotional entanglements and paternity issues.

The young people were most strongly motivated to use condoms when they did not know a potential sexual partner well or were at the earliest stages of sexual involvement with others. Nearly all said they solicited information about a potential partner's sexual history from this person or from friends. Rather than directly asking about the number of past partners, they more often relied on feelings and visual observations. Some admitted to lying when asked about their own sexual experience in order to avoid being seen as promiscuous. Once a couple had sex without a condom, both partners—but especially women—found it awkward to resume condom use because doing so would imply a lack of trust.

Source: Michaels Opinion Research. *"In the Heat of the Moment."* Menlo Park, CA.: Henry J. Kaiser Family Foundation, June 2001.

The main objections to condoms include odor, lubrication (too much or too little), rips or breaks, access, disposal, feel, taste, and difficulty opening the packages. Some couples feel that putting on a condom interferes with sexual spontaneity; others incorporate it into their sex play. Some men dislike the reduced penile sensitivity or will not use them because they believe they interfere with sexual pleasure. Others cannot sustain an erection while putting on a condom. A small number are allergic to latex condoms.

How to Use a Condom. Most physicians recommend prelubricated, spermicide-treated American-made latex or polyurethane condoms, not membrane condoms ("natural" or "sheepskin"). Before using a condom, check the expiration date, and make sure it's soft and pliable. If it's yellow or sticky, throw it out. Don't check for leaks by blowing up a condom before using it; you may weaken or tear it.

The condom should be put on at the beginning of sexual activity, before genital contact occurs (Figure 9-6).

There should be a little space at the top of the condom to catch the semen. Wait until just before intercourse to apply spermicide. Any vaginal lubricant should be water-based. Petroleum based creams or jellies (such as Vaseline, baby oil, massage oil, vegetable oils, or oil-based hand lotions) can deteriorate the latex. After ejaculation, the condom should be held firmly against the penis so that it doesn't slip off or leak during withdrawal. Couples engaging in anal intercourse should use a water-based lubricant as well as a condom but should never assume the condom will protect them from HIV infection or other STDs.

The Female Condom

The female condom, made of polyurethane, consists of two rings and a polyurethane sheath, and is inserted into the vagina with a tampon-like applicator (see Figure 9-7). Once in place, the device loosely lines the walls of the vagina. Internally, a thickened rubber ring keeps it

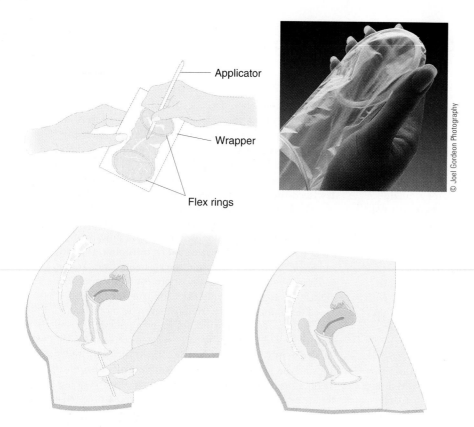

Applicator

Wrapper

Flex rings

© Joel Gordeon Photography

▲ **Figure 9-7** The female condom.
This method is less effective than the male condom for preventing pregnancy and STDs (since no spermicide is used). Like the male condom, this method does not require a prescription.

Women complained that the condom, which retails for $2 to $3, was too expensive, difficult to use, squeaked, and looked odd.

How to Use the Female Condom. As illustrated in Figure 9-7, a woman removes the condom and applicator from the wrapper and inserts the condom slowly by gently pushing the applicator toward the small of the back. When properly inserted, the outer ring should rest on the folds of skin around the vaginal opening, and the inner ring (the closed end) should fit against the cervix. The condom should be used with a spermicide and a water-based lubricant.

The female condom can be washed and reused several times and still meet the standards set by the Food and Drug Administration (FDA), according to the study conducted in South Africa in which a sample of women washed, dried and relubricated female condoms up to seven times.[39]

anchored near the cervix. Externally, another rubber ring, 2 inches in diameter, rests on the labia and resists slippage.

Although not widely used in the West, the female condom is gaining acceptance in Africa, Asia, and Latin America. Properly used, it is believed to be as good or better than the male condom for preventing infections, including HIV, because it is stronger and covers a slightly larger area.[38] However, it is slightly less effective at preventing pregnancy.

Advantages. The female condom gives women more control in reducing their risk of pregnancy and STDs. It does not require a prescription or medical appointment. One size fits all.

Disadvantages. The failure rate for the female condom is higher than for other contraceptives. The statistical failure rate is 12.2 percent, which means that 12 of every 100 women using the device could expect to get pregnant during a six-month period. In clinical trials, the actual failure rate was even higher—20.6 percent. Since it does not have spermicide on it, the female condom does not provide as much risk-reduction against STDs as male condoms with spermicide.

Vaginal Spermicides

The various forms of **vaginal spermicides** include chemical foams, creams, jellies, vaginal suppositories, and gels (see Figure 9-8). Some creams and jellies are made for use with a diaphragm; others can be used alone. Several vaginal suppositories claim high effectiveness, but no American studies have confirmed these claims. In general, failure rates for vaginal suppositories are as high as 10 to 25 percent.

Advantages. Conscientious use of a spermicide together with another method of contraception, such as a condom, can provide safe and effective birth control and reduce the risk of some vaginal infections, pelvic inflammatory disease, and STDs. The side effects of vaginal spermicides are minimal.

Disadvantages. Even though spermicides can be applied in less than a minute, couples may feel that they interfere with sexual spontaneity. Some people are irritated by the chemicals in spermicides, but often a change of brand solves this problem. Others find foam spermicides messy or feel they interfere with oral-genital contact. Spermicidal suppositories that do not dissolve completely can feel gritty.

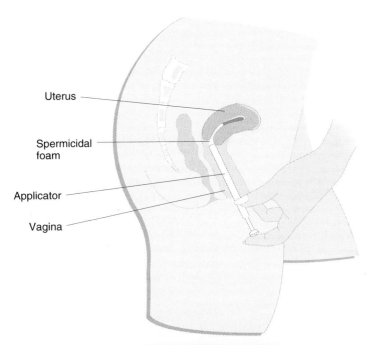

Uterus

Spermicidal foam

Applicator

Vagina

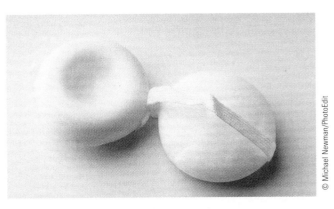

▲ The contraceptive sponge, discontinued in 1995, will be available from a new U.S. manufacturer. A similar sponge is available in Canada.

© Michael Newman/PhotoEdit

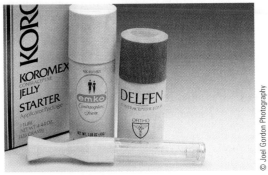

© Joel Gordon Photography

▲ **Figure 9-8** Vaginal spermicides.
These various creams and jellies are available without a prescription and have minimal side effects. They are most effective in preventing pregnancy and STDs when used together with a condom.

How to Use Vaginal Spermicides. The various types of spermicide come with instructions that should be followed carefully for maximum protection. Contraceptive vaginal suppositories take about 20 minutes to dissolve and cover the vaginal walls. Foam, inserted with an applicator, goes into place much more rapidly. You must apply additional spermicide before each additional intercourse. After sex, women should shower rather than bathe to prevent the spermicide from being rinsed out of the vagina and should not douche for at least six hours.

The Contraceptive Sponge

The nonprescription Today Sponge is a soft, disposable polyurethane sponge permeated with a spermicide. On the market from 1983 to 1995, the Today Sponge was one of the most popular contraceptive options for women. It was taken off the market because of problems at the product's sole manufacturing plant, including bacterial contamination of water and sanitizing equipment. Although the original manufacturer sold the manufacturing rights and it was approved by the FDA, the Today Sponge has not become available as expected. A similar device, the Protectaid Sponge, is available in Canada. An estimated 6.4 million women used the sponge at some time.

The sponge is believed to work by inactivating sperm with the spermicide, absorbing semen and thereby preventing sperm from entering the cervix, and acting as a mechanical barrier.

Advantages. The contraceptive sponge does not affect hormonal levels, is easy to use, and is reversible.

Disadvantages. Its failure rate as a contraceptive is fairly high: about 10 percent over a year's use—comparable to that of other barrier methods. If not used properly, the failure rate rises to 15 percent. The sponge does not provide any protection against STDs.

How to Use the Contraceptive Sponge. A woman inserts the sponge, a half-inch-thick rubbery disc with a diameter of about 1¾ inches, into her vagina before sex. It can be left there for 24 hours of protection. She removes the sponge by grasping on a ribbon-like loop attached to it.

Vaginal Contraceptive Film (VCF)

Available from pharmacies without a prescription, the 2-inch-by-2-inch thin film known as **vaginal contraceptive film (VCF)** is laced with spermicide (Figure 9-9). Once folded and inserted into the vagina, it dissolves into a

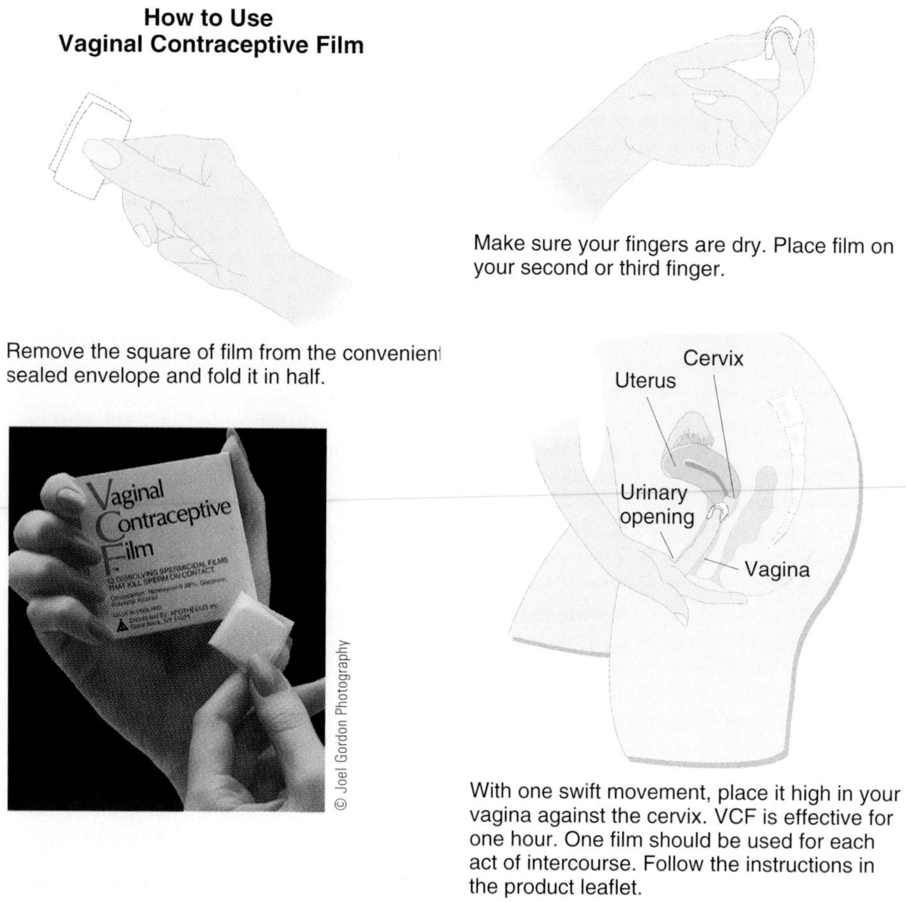

SECTION III / RESPONSIBLE SEXUALITY

**How to Use
Vaginal Contraceptive Film**

Make sure your fingers are dry. Place film on your second or third finger.

Remove the square of film from the convenient sealed envelope and fold it in half.

© Joel Gordon Photography

Cervix
Uterus
Urinary opening
Vagina

With one swift movement, place it high in your vagina against the cervix. VCF is effective for one hour. One film should be used for each act of intercourse. Follow the instructions in the product leaflet.

▲ **Figure 9-9** Vaginal contraceptive film (VCF). This thin film is laced with spermicide. Its effectiveness is similar to other vaginal spermicides, and it is most effective paired with a condom.

stay-in-place gel. Its theoretical effectiveness is similar to that of other forms of spermicide; paired with a condom, it is almost 100 percent effective.

Advantages. VCF film can be used by people allergic to foams and jellies. Unlike foams and jellies, it dissolves gradually and almost unnoticeably.

Disadvantages. Some people feel that insertion, even though it takes only seconds, interrupts sexual spontaneity.

Periodic Abstinence and Fertility Awareness Methods

Awareness of a woman's cyclic fertility can help in both conception and contraception. The different methods of birth control based on a woman's menstrual cycle are sometimes referred to as natural family planning or fertility awareness methods. They include the cervical mucus method, the cal-

endar method, and the basal-body-temperature method (all described below). New fertility monitors that use saliva for testing can improve the accuracy of these methods.

Advantages. Birth control methods based on the menstrual cycle involve no expense, no side effects, and no need for prescriptions or fittings. On the days when the couple can have intercourse, there is nothing to insert, swallow, or check. In addition, abstinence during fertile periods complies with the teachings of the Roman Catholic Church.

Disadvantages. During times of possible fertility (usually eight or nine days a month), couples must abstain from vaginal intercourse or use some form of contraception. Conscientious planning and scheduling are essential. Women with irregular cycles may not be able to rely on the calendar method. Others may find the mucus or temperature methods difficult to use. For all these reasons, this approach to birth control is less reliable than many others. In theory, the overall effectiveness rate for the various fertility awareness —methods is 80 percent. In practice, of every 100 women using one of these methods for a year, 24 become pregnant. However, using a combination of the basal-body-temperature method and the cervical mucus method may be 90 to 95 percent effective in preventing pregnancy (see Figure 9-10).

Cervical Mucus Method

This method, also called the **ovulation method,** is based on the observation of changes in the consistency of the mucus in the vagina. In the first days after menstruation, the vagina feels dry because of a decline in hormone production, indicating a safe period for unprotected intercourse. Within a few days, estrogen levels rise, and the mucus begins to thin out and becomes less cloudy: The fertile period begins. At peak estrogen levels, the mucus is smooth, stretchable, and slippery (like raw egg white), and very clear. Mucus with these characteristics is usually observed within 24 hours of ovulation and lasts one to two

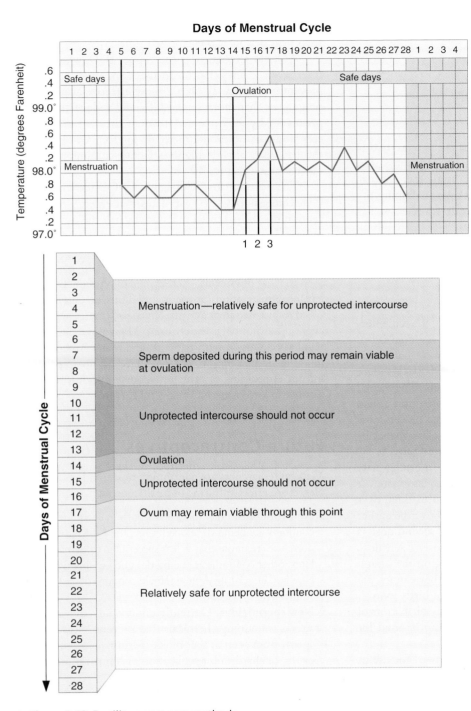

Days of Menstrual Cycle

▲ **Figure 9-10** Fertility awareness methods.
These methods are based on a woman's menstrual cycle and involve charting basal body temperature (top), careful calculation of the menstrual cycle (bottom), or careful observations of cervical mucus. Periods of abstinence are a necessary part of these methods.

Calendar Method

This approach, often called the **rhythm method,** involves counting the days after menstruation begins to calculate the estimated day of ovulation. Ideally, a woman first keeps a chart of her monthly cycles for about a year so she knows the average length of her cycle. The first day of menstruation is day one. She counts the number of days until the last day of her cycle, which is the day before menstrual flow begins. To determine the starting point of the period during which she should avoid unprotected intercourse, she subtracts 18 from the number of days in her shortest cycle. For instance, if her shortest cycle was 28 days, day 10 would be her first high-risk day. To calculate when she can again have unprotected intercourse, she subtracts 10 from the number of days in her longest cycle. If her longest cycle is 31 days, she could resume intercourse on day 21. Other forms of sexual activity can continue from day 10 to day 21. This method requires careful timing to avoid the possible meeting of a ripe egg and active sperm in the woman's fallopian tube.

Basal Body Temperature Method

In this method the woman measures her **basal body temperature,** the body temperature upon waking in the morning, using a specially calibrated rectal thermometer, which is more precise than an oral one. She records her temperature on a chart (see Figure 9-10). The basal body temperature remains relatively constant from the beginning of the menstrual cycle to ovulation. After ovulation, however, basal body temperature rises by more than 0.5 degree F. The woman knows that her safe period has begun when her temperature has been elevated for three consecutive days. After eight to ten months, she should have a sense

days, signaling maximum fertility. The mucus becomes sticky and cloudy again three days thereafter, and the second safe period begins. Most women using this method have to refrain from unprotected intercourse for about 9 days of each 28-day menstrual cycle.

of her ovulatory pattern, in addition to knowing her daily readings.

What Is Emergency Contraception?

Emergency contraception (EC) is the use of a method of contraception to prevent unintended pregnancy after unprotected intercourse or the failure of another form of contraception, such as a condom breaking or slipping off. Medical researchers do not fully understand how EC works. Emergency contraception pills (ECPs) may inhibit or delay ovulation, prevent union of sperm and ovum, or alter the endometrium so a fertilized ovum cannot implant itself. The copper-bearing intrauterine device (IUD) is also an EC option.[40]

There are two types of emergency contraceptive pills. Combined ECPs use estrogen and progestin, the same hormones used in ordinary birth control pills. A brand called Preven is specifically packaged for emergency use, but several other brands can be used as well. Combined ECPs reduce the risk of unintended pregnancy by 75 percent. The second type of ECP contains only the hormone progestin and is packaged under the brand name Plan B. It has proven more effective than the first type, reducing the risk of pregnancy by 89 percent, with a lower risk of nausea and vomiting.

Although ECPs are sometimes called "morning after pills," it is not necessary to wait until the morning after. A woman can start the pills right away or up to three days after unprotected sex. Therapy is more effective the earlier it is initiated, ideally within 24 hours. The second dose is generally taken 12 hours after the first dose. Each dose may consist of 1, 2, 4, or 5 pills, depending on the brand. Most women can safely use them, even if they cannot use birth control pills as their regular method of birth control. Although ECPs use the same hormones as birth control pills, not all brands of birth control pills can be used for emergency contraception.

Although no specific ECPs were approved for use in the United States until 1998, one approach, the "Yuzpe regimen," named for the doctor who developed it, has been used since 1974 in some European countries and was also prescribed for years in the United States by physicians in hospital emergency departments, reproductive health clinics, university health centers, and private practice. However, physicians had to open and repackage oral contraceptives and give the tablets to patients with instructions to take a particular dose, depending on the brand. Once Preven came on the market, repackaging was no longer necessary. The newer progestin-only Plan B kit contains two pills, each containing levonorgestrel. Some women may experience spotting or a full menstrual period a few days after taking ECs, depending on where they were in their cycle when they began therapy. Most women have their next period at the expected time.

Another alternative is the copper IUD, which can be inserted by a physician up to five days after ovulation to prevent pregnancy. IUDs are more effective at preventing pregnancy than hormonal ECPs and reduce the risk of pregnancy by 99 percent. However, they are not used as commonly as hormonal methods for EC. Once inserted, the IUD can provide highly effective continuous contraceptive protection for 10 years.

The American College of Obstetricians and Gynecologists (ACOG) estimates that emergency contraception has the potential to reduce by half the three million unintended pregnancies each year in the United States.[41] Along with other women's health groups, ACOG supports over the counter availability for ECP and has recommended that physicians offer women of reproductive age an advance prescription for use in any future emergency.[42]

Despite its safety and effectiveness, emergency contraception has not been widely used. Many physicians do not regularly discuss it with patients, and many Americans are unaware of this option.[43] There have been campaigns to inform Americans of after-intercourse options, including setting up a website: NOT-2-LATE.com.

Future Contraceptives

Medical researchers are continuing to search for safer, simpler, more effective forms of birth control:

▷ **New condoms.** New models for both male and female condoms are being developed. One, the Kraton male condom, uses material that is less susceptible to damage than latex; other condoms are being designed with a tighter base and larger top. A new female condom described as an "underwear type" also is in development.[44]

▷ **New spermicides.** Currently under study are various agents containing chemicals that prevent release of sperm from semen, that block sperm penetration of an ovum, or that inhibit replication of human immunodeficiency virus (HIV).

▷ **New hormonal injectables.** Longer-acting contraceptives that would last for six to eight months are under study, as are self-administered monthly injectables.

▷ **A vaginal ring.** A woman would insert this device, which contains estrogen and progestin, into the back of her vagina, much like a diaphragm. The ring can be kept in place for three weeks, followed by one ring-free week.

▷ **A contraceptive patch.** This hormonal contraceptive, applied every week, releases a low, daily dose of estrogen and progestin. The side effects are similar to those experienced by users of combined oral contraceptives.

▷ **Male hormonal contraceptives.** Researchers are experimenting with a male contraceptive vaccine using a gonadotropin-releasing hormone inhibitor (LHRH agonist). Daily injections have reduced the number and movement of sperm, but inability to achieve erection was a common side effect. Adding testosterone to the treatment can maintain sexual potency. In another study in Edinburgh and Shanghai, 66 men took female hormones every day for four weeks along with testosterone implants or injections. Within 16 weeks, they completely stopped producing sperm. Once treatment ended, their sperm counts returned to pretreatment levels within 16 weeks.

Even if such research should lead to the development of a male pill, men might not use it for fear that it might cause impotence. Women also have expressed doubt because they would have no way of knowing if a man really is taking his pill. Cultural differences also will influence reactions to a male pill. In a study of more than 1,800 men, those in Cape Town and Edinburgh liked the idea of a daily birth control pill, while Chinese men strongly preferred condoms.[45]

Sterilization

The most popular method of birth control among married couples in the United States is **sterilization** (surgery to end a person's reproductive capability). Each year an estimated 1 million men and women in the United States undergo sterilization procedures. Fewer than 25 percent ever seek reversal.

Advantages. Sterilization has no effect on sex drive in either men or women. Many couples report that their sexual activity increases after sterilization, because they're free from the fear of pregnancy or the need to deal with contraceptives.

Disadvantages. Sterilization should be considered permanent and should be used only if both individuals are sure they want no more children. Although sterilization doesn't usually create psychological or sexual problems, it can worsen existing problems, particularly marital ones. Couples should discuss sterilization, together and with a physician, to understand fully the possible physical and emotional consequences. Although a link between vasectomy and an increased risk of prostate cancer was reported, the most recent research did not find a correlation.

Male Sterilization

In men, the cutting of the *vas deferens*, the tube that carries sperm from one of the testes into the urethra for ejaculation, is called **vasectomy**. During the 15- or 20-minute office procedure, done under a local anesthetic, the doctor makes small incisions in the scrotum, lifts up each vas deferens, cuts them, and ties off the ends to block the flow of sperm (see Figure 9-11). Sperm continue to form, but they are broken down and absorbed by the body.

The man usually experiences some local pain, swelling, and discoloration for about a week after the procedure. More serious complications, including the formation of a blood clot in the scrotum (which usually disappears without treatment), infection, and an inflammatory reaction, occur in a small percentage of cases. The National Institute of Child Health and Human Development, in a 15-year follow-up study of nearly 5,000 men, found that sterilization poses no increased danger of heart disease, even decades after the procedure.

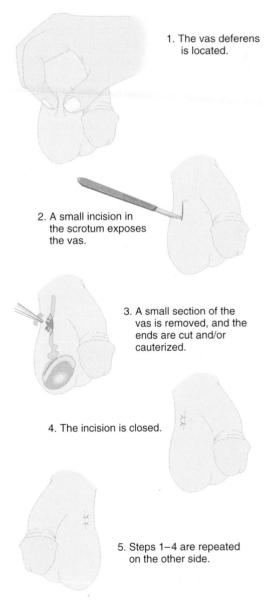

1. The vas deferens is located.

2. A small incision in the scrotum exposes the vas.

3. A small section of the vas is removed, and the ends are cut and/or cauterized.

4. The incision is closed.

5. Steps 1–4 are repeated on the other side.

▲ **Figure 9-11** Male sterilization, or vasectomy.

The pregnancy rate among the wives of men who've had vasectomies is about 15 in 10,000 women per year. Most result from a couple's failure to wait several weeks after the operation, until all sperm stored in each vas deferens have been ejaculated, before having unprotected coitus.

Sometimes men want to reverse their vasectomies, usually because they want to have children with a new spouse. Although anyone who chooses to have a vasectomy should consider it permanent, surgical reversal (*vasovasostomy*)* is sometimes successful. New microsurgical techniques have led to annual pregnancy rates for the wives of men undergoing vasovasostomies of about 50 percent, depending on such factors as the doctor's expertise and the time elapsed since the vasectomy.

Female Sterilization

Female sterilization procedures modify the fallopian tubes, which each month normally carry an egg from the ovaries to the uterus. These operations may soon surpass the pill as the first contraceptive choice among women under, as well as over, age 30. The two terms used to describe female sterilization are **tubal ligation** (the cutting or tying of the fallopian tubes) and **tubal occlusion** (the blocking of the tubes). The tubes may be cut or sealed with thread, a clamp, or a clip, or by coagulation (burning) to prevent the passage of eggs from the ovaries (see Figure 9-12). They can also be blocked with bands of silicone.

The procedures used for sterilization are laparotomy, laparoscopy, and colpotomy. **Laparotomy** involves making an abdominal incision about 2 inches long and cutting the tubes. A laparotomy usually requires a hospital stay and up to several weeks of recovery. It leaves a scar and carries the same risks as all major surgical procedures: the side effects of anesthesia, potential infection, and internal scars. In a **minilaparotomy,** an incision about an inch long is made just above the pubic hairline. Most often the tubes are tied and cut. They can also be sealed by electrical coagulation, which causes extensive damage to the tubes; there is also the risk of burns to nearby organs. The operation can be performed by a skilled physician in 10 to 30 minutes, usually under local anesthesia, and the woman can generally go home the same day. The failure (pregnancy) rate is only 1 in 1,000.

Tubal ligation or occlusion can also be performed with the use of **laparoscopy,** commonly called "belly-button" or "band-aid" surgery. This procedure is done on an outpatient basis and takes 15 to 30 minutes. A lighted tube called a laparoscope is inserted through a half-inch incision made right below the navel, giving the doctor a view of the fallopian tubes. Using surgical instruments that may be inserted through the laparoscope or through other tiny incisions, the doctor then cuts or seals the tubes, most commonly by electrical coagulation. The possible complications are similar to those of minilaparotomy, as is the failure rate.

In a **colpotomy,** the fallopian tubes are reached through the vagina and cervix. This procedure leaves no external scar, but is somewhat more hazardous and less effective. A **hysterectomy** (removal of the uterus) is a major surgical procedure that is too dangerous to be used as a method of sterilization, unless there are other medically urgent reasons for removing the uterus.

Abortion

Each year an estimated 5.4 million pregnancies occur in the United States. More than half of unintended pregnancies end in induced abortions.[46] Abortion rates vary greatly around the world. The U.S. abortion rate, which declined through most of the last decade, still remains higher than that of many Western countries, including Canada, Great Britain, the Netherlands, and Sweden. Although there is no one single or simple explanation for this difference, researchers focus on America's high rate of unintended pregnancies. In many nations with fewer unwanted pregnancies and lower abortion rates, contraceptives are generally easier and cheaper to obtain, and early sex education strongly emphasizes their importance.

No woman in any country ever elects to be in a situation where she has to consider abortion. But if faced with an unwanted pregnancy, many women consider *elective abortion* as an option. Every year 3 out of every 100 American women between the ages of 15 and 44 choose to terminate a pregnancy. According to federal data, 43 percent of American women undergo an abortion by age 45.

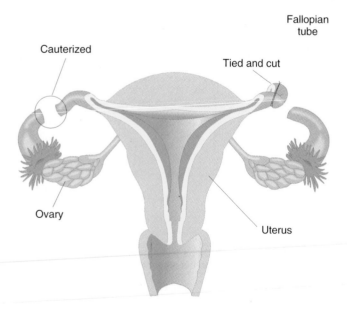

Fallopian tube

Cauterized

Tied and cut

Ovary

Uterus

▲ **Figure 9-12** Female sterilization, or tubal ligation.

These women do not fit neatly into any particular category. About 80 percent are unmarried. Most—70 percent—intend to have children, but not at this point in time. Many cannot afford a baby. Some feel unready for the responsibility; others fear that another child would jeopardize the happiness and security of their existing family.

About 55 percent of women who undergo abortion are under age 25; only 22 percent are older than age 30. Unmarried pregnant women are six times more likely to have abortions than married ones; poor women are three times more likely to abort a pregnancy than women in higher economic groups. White women account for 63 percent of abortions, yet statistically, nonwhite women (who make up a smaller proportion of the population) are twice as likely to have an abortion as white women. Catholic women are more likely than Protestant women to have abortions, but women with no religious affiliations have a higher abortion rate than those who belong to a particular religion.

Thinking Through the Options

A woman faced with an unwanted pregnancy—often alone, unwed, and desperate—can find it extremely difficult to decide what to do. The political debate over the right to life almost always is secondary to practical and emotional matters, such as the quality of her relationship with the baby's father, their capacity to provide for the child, the impact on any children she already has, and other important life issues.

Giving up her child for adoption is an option for women who do not feel abortion is right for them. Because the number of would-be adoptive parents greatly exceeds the number of available newborns, some women considering adoption may feel pressured by offers of money from couples eager to adopt. Others, particularly minority women, may feel cultural pressures to keep a child—regardless of their age, economic situation, or ability to care for an infant. Advocates of adoption reform are pressing for mandatory counseling for all pregnant women considering adoption (available now in agency-arranged, but not private, adoptions) and for extending the period of time during which a new mother can change her mind about giving her child up for adoption.

In deciding whether or not to have an abortion, women report asking themselves many questions, including the following:

▶ How do I feel about the man with whom I conceived this baby? Do I love him? Does he love me? Is this man committed to staying with me?

▶ What sort of relationship, if any, have we had or might we have in the future?

▶ If I continue the pregnancy and give birth, could I love the baby?

▶ Who can help me gain perspective on this problem?

▶ Have I thought about adoption? Do I think I could surrender custody of my baby? Would it make a difference if the adoption process were open and I could know the adoptive parents?

▶ If I keep my child, can I care for him or her properly? How would the birth of another baby affect my other children?

▶ Do I have marketable skills, an education, an adequate income? Would I be able to go to school or keep my job if I have a child? Who would help me?

▶ Would this child be born with serious abnormalities? Would it suffer or thrive?

▶ How does each option fit with what I believe is morally correct? Could I handle each of the options emotionally?

Answering these questions honestly and objectively may help women as they think through the realities of their situation.

Medical Abortion

The term **medical abortion** describes the use of drugs, also called "abortifacients," to terminate a pregnancy. In 2000 the abortion pill mifepristone (Mifeprex)—formerly known as RU-486—became available for use in the United States. Mifepristone, which is 97 percent effective in inducing abortion, blocks progesterone, the hormone that prepares the uterine lining for pregnancy. Two days after taking this compound, a woman takes a prostaglandin to increase uterine contractions. The uterine lining is expelled along with the fertilized egg (see Figure 9-13). Women have compared the discomfort of this experience to severe menstrual cramps. Common side effects include excessive bleeding, nausea, fatigue, abdominal pain, and dizziness. About 1 woman in 100 requires a blood transfusion.

Other agents used in medical abortion are methotrexate, widely used to treat certain cancers and arthritis, and misoprostol (Cytotec), primarily prescribed in the United States to prevent gastrointestinal ulcers. Methotrexate interferes with the ability of cells to multiple and divide, which halts development of an embryo or placenta. Misoprostol causes the uterus to contract, which helps expel a fertilized egg. Although misoprostol has been used in combination with mifespristone, researchers are investigating whether it can be used alone to terminate pregnancy.[47]

Although condemned by right-to-life advocates, abortion medications may in time lower the public profile of pregnancy termination. They are not painless, cheap, or equally available to all, but they do offer women a chance to carry through on their personal choice in greater privacy and safety. In a recent study, women who had a medical abortion reported a significantly higher level of satisfaction than those undergoing surgical abortion.[48]

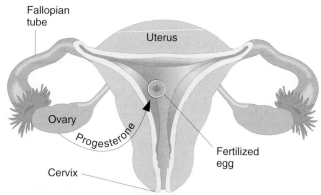

Progesterone, a hormone produced by the ovaries, is necessary for the implantation and development of a fertilized egg.

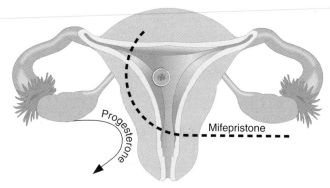

Taken early in pregnancy mifepristone blocks the action of progesterone and makes the body react as if it isn't pregnant.

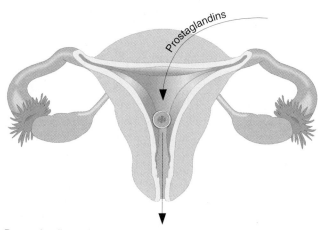

Prostaglandins, taken two days later, cause the uterus to contract and the cervix to soften and dilate. As a result, the fertilized egg is expelled in 97% of the cases.

▲ **Figure 9-13** Medical abortion.
Mifepristone works by blocking the action of progesterone.

Medical abortion does not require anesthesia, can be performed very early in pregnancy, and may feel more private. However, women experience more cramping and bleeding during medical abortion than during surgical abortion, and bleeding lasts for a longer period.[49]

Other Abortion Methods

More than half of all abortions (54 percent) are performed within the first 8 weeks of pregnancy. Only about 1 percent of abortions occur after 20 weeks. Medically, first-trimester abortion is less risky than childbirth. However, the likelihood of complications increases when abortions are performed in the second trimester (that is, the second three-month period) of pregnancy.[50]

The vast majority of abortions performed in the United States today are surgical.[51] **Suction curettage,** usually done from 7 to 13 weeks after the last menstrual period, involves the gradual dilation (opening) of the cervix, often by inserting into the cervix one or more sticks of *laminaria* (a sterilized seaweed that absorbs moisture and expands, thus gradually stretching the cervix). Some women feel pressure or cramping with the laminaria in place. Occasionally, the laminaria itself starts to bring on a miscarriage.

At the time of abortion, the laminaria is removed, and dilators are used to enlarge the cervical opening further, if needed. The physician inserts a suction tip into the cervix, and the uterine contents are drawn out via a vacuum system (see Figure 9-14). A curette (a spoon-shaped surgical instrument used for scraping) is used to check for complete removal of the contents of the uterus. With suction curettage, the risks of complication are low. Major complications, such as perforation of the uterus, occur in fewer than 1 in 100 cases.

For early-second-trimester abortions, physicians generally use a technique called **dilation and evacuation (D and E),** in which they open the cervix and use medical

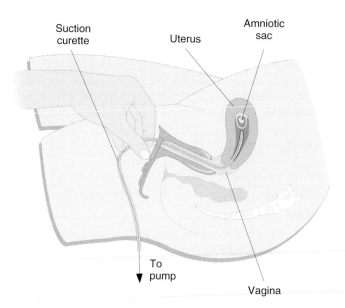

▲ **Figure 9-14** Suction curettage.
The contents of the uterus are extracted through the cervix with a vacuum apparatus.

instruments to remove the fetus from the uterus. D and E procedures are performed under local or general anesthesia.

To induce abortion from week 16 to week 20, prostaglandins (natural substances found in most body tissues) are administered as vaginal suppositories or injected into the amniotic sac by inserting a needle through the abdominal wall. They induce uterine contractions, and the fetus and placenta are expelled within 24 hours. Other methods for second-trimester abortions include injecting saline or urea solutions into the amniotic sac; they terminate the pregnancy by fetus-triggering contractions that expel the fetus and placenta. Sometimes vaginal suppositories or drugs that help the uterus contract are used. Complications from abortion techniques that induce labor include nausea, vomiting, diarrhea, tearing of the cervix, excessive bleeding, and possible shock and death.

Hysterotomy involves surgically opening the uterus and removing the fetus. It is generally done from week 16 to week 24 of the pregnancy, primarily in emergency situations when the woman's life is in danger, or when other methods of abortion are considered too risky. However, late pregnancy abortions increase the risk of spontaneous abortion or premature labor in subsequent pregnancies and should be avoided if possible.

⏭⏭⏭ What is the Psychological Impact of Abortion?

Many assume that abortion must be psychologically devastating, that women who abort a fetus sooner or later develop what some have termed "post-abortion trauma syndrome." In her studies at the University of Chicago, psychiatrist Nada Stotland found that there is no such thing. The primary emotion of women who have just had an abortion, she discovered, is relief. Although many women also express feelings of sadness or guilt, their anxiety levels eventually drop until they are lower than they were immediately before the abortion.

Nonetheless, although psychologists consider the mental health risks "minimal" compared to those of bearing an unwanted child, this does not mean women who have abortions never have regrets. In one recent study, nearly one in five women reported sadness, dissatisfaction, and regret about her abortion two years later.[52] But a feeling—even one as painful as loss, sadness, or guilt—is not a syndrome, and a woman's responses to abortion often change with passing days, weeks, months, or years. Anniversaries—of conception, of the date a woman found out she was pregnant, of the abortion, of the delivery date—can trigger memories and a sense of loss, but most women deal with these and move on with their lives.

The best predictor of psychological well-being after abortion is a woman's emotional well-being prior to pregnancy. At highest risk are women who have had a psychiatric illness, such as an anxiety disorder or clinical depression, prior to an abortion, and those whose abortions occurred among complicated circumstances (such as a rape, or coercion by parents or a partner). The vast majority of women manage to put the abortion into perspective as one of many life events.

The Politics of Abortion

Abortion is one of the most controversial political, religious, and ethical issues of our time. The issues of when life begins, a woman's right to choose, and an unborn child's right to survival are among the most divisive Americans face. Abortions were legal in the United States until the 1860s. For decades after that, women who decided to terminate unwanted pregnancies did so by attempting to abort themselves or by obtaining illegal abortions—often performed by untrained individuals using unsanitary and unsafe procedures. In the late 1960s, some states changed their laws to make abortions legal. In 1973, the U.S. Supreme Court, following a 1970 ruling on the case of *Roe v. Wade* by the New York Supreme Court, said that an abortion in the first trimester of pregnancy was a decision between a woman and her physician and was

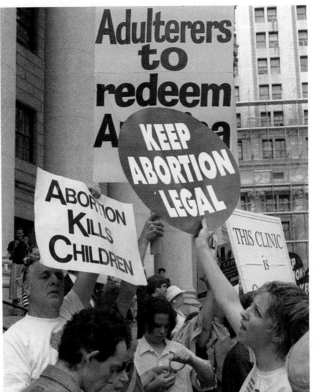

▲ The controversy about abortion has resulted in countless demonstrations and encounters between pro-choice and pro-life supporters.

protected by privacy laws. The Court further ruled that abortion during the second trimester could be performed on the basis of health risks and that abortion during the final trimester could be performed only for the sake of the mother's health.

Since then, several laws have restricted the availability of legal abortions for low-income women. In 1989, the U.S. Supreme Court narrowed the interpretation of *Roe v. Wade* by upholding a law that sharply restricted publicly funded abortions and required doctors to test if a fetus could survive if they suspected a woman was more than 20 weeks pregnant. In 1992, in *Planned Parenthood v. Casey,* the Court upheld the right to legalized abortion but gave states the right to restrict abortion as long as they did not place an "undue burden" on a woman. This limited the availability of abortion to young, rural, or low-income women.

In 2000 in *Sternberg v. Carhart,* the U.S. Supreme Court struck down Nebraska's ban on "partial birth abortions," a term abortion opponents use for dilation and extraction, a second-trimester surgical procedure. Stating that the ban placed an "undue burden" on women's right to end their pregnancies, the Court noted that its broad warning could have been used to ban other abortion methods used after the first trimester, such as dilation and evacuation.[53]

The debate over abortion continues to stir passionate emotion, with pro-life supporters arguing that life begins at conception and that abortion is therefore immoral, and pro-choice advocates countering that an individual woman should have the right to make decisions about her body and health. The controversy over abortion has at times become violent: Physicians who performed abortions have been shot and killed; abortion clinics have been bombed, wounding and killing patients and staff members.

Although the majority of Americans continue to support abortion, many feel that it should be more restricted and difficult to obtain. While 61 percent of Americans say abortion should be permitted during the first three months of pregnancy, only 15 percent support second-trimester abortions and 7 percent feel that abortions in the last trimester should be legal.

A Cross-Cultural Perspective

Throughout the world an estimated 10 to 20 million illegal abortions are performed each year. About 1 in 100 women dies as a result. Women who survive illegal abortions may suffer chronic health problems related to the lack of adequate medical care.

In other countries, abortion laws vary greatly. In Eastern Europe, where abortions were once legal and common, the collapse of communism has led to new restrictions on abortion. By contrast, Spain's supreme court has relaxed legal restrictions on abortions performed on social grounds. In

Pakistan, new, more liberal rules on abortion state that abortion is no longer a crime if carried out to provide "necessary treatment." In Latin America, where anti-abortion laws are very strict, Cuba is the only country in which abortion on request is legal in early pregnancy. In other nations of Central and South America, women obtaining abortions and those performing them face criminal penalties, including imprisonment.

Childfree by Choice

In Europe, fertility rates in many nations are at an all-time low. In the United States, one in five women in the baby boom generation has not given birth—many because of a decision not to. More women and men are deliberately choosing to remain "childfree."

According to the limited data available, single childfree women tend to be better educated, more cosmopolitan, less religious, and more professional than those in the general population. In general, childfree women are high achievers, often in demanding careers, who describe their work as exciting and satisfying. Childless couples are predominantly urban, well-educated, and upper middle class, with egalitarian and long-running marriages.

Their reasons for not having children are diverse: a desire to maintain their freedom, more time with their partners, career ambitions, concern about overpopulation and the fate of the Earth. Some women cite the hostile work environment for mothers and the inadequacy of day care. Others say they're disillusioned with the have-it-all hopes of baby boomers and believe in a have-most-of-it philosophy.

Some observers theorize that childfree women will regret their choice after it's too late to do anything about it. However, this doesn't seem to be the case. In a study of 90 childless women over age 60, a Philadelphia anthropologist found that, while the women who believed that a woman's primary duty is to have children did express some regret, most women had come up with satisfying alternative ways of living. In another study of nearly 700 Canadian women and men over age 55, those who chose childlessness were just as happy as parents who had good relationships with their children—and happier than parents who described their relationships with their children as distant.[54] "Not everybody needs children to have a full life," says Leslie Lafayette, who founded the ChildFree Network (CFN) to create a sense of belonging among people without children.[55]

Pregnancy

In the last half century, pregnancy rates have generally declined, although the absolute number of births has risen.[56] The average age of mothers has risen, but about 70 percent of babies are still born to women in their twenties. Mothers are now averaging slightly fewer than two children each. Not every married couple is opting for parenthood.

Of course, you don't have to be part of a couple to want or to conceive a child. The number of never-married college-educated and career women who are becoming single parents has risen dramatically. They want children—with or without an ongoing relationship with a man—and may feel that, because of their age, they can't delay getting pregnant any longer.

Preconception Care: A Preventive Approach

The time *before* a child is conceived can be crucial in assuring that an infant is born healthy, full-size, and full-term. Women who smoke, drink alcohol, take drugs, eat poorly, are too thin or too heavy, suffer from unrecognized infections or illnesses, or are exposed to toxins at work or home may start pregnancy with one or more strikes against them and their unborn babies. The best chance for lowering the infant mortality rate and preventing birth defects is before pregnancy. **Preconception care**—the enhancement of a woman's health and well-being prior to conception in order to ensure a healthy pregnancy and baby—includes risk assessment (including evaluation of medical, genetic, and lifestyle risks), health promotion (such as teaching good nutrition guidelines), and interventions to reduce risk (such as treatment of infections and other diseases) or assistance in quitting smoking or drug use.

To determine whether you might benefit from preconception counseling, ask yourself the following questions:

- Do you have a major medical problem, such as diabetes, asthma, anemia, or high blood pressure?
- Do you know of any family members who have had a child with a birth defect or mental retardation?
- Have you had a child with a birth defect or mental retardation?
- Are you concerned about inherited diseases, such as Tay-Sachs disease, sickle-cell anemia, hemophilia, or thalassemia?
- Are you 35 years of age or older?
- Do you smoke, drink alcohol, or take illegal drugs?
- Do you take prescription or over-the-counter medications regularly?
- Do you use birth control pills?
- Do you have a cat?
- Are you a strict vegetarian?
- Are you dieting or fasting for any reason?
- Do you run long distances or exercise strenuously?
- Do you work with chemicals, toxic substances, radiation, or anesthesia?

- Do you suspect that you or your partner may have a sexually transmitted disease?
- Have you had German measles (rubella) or a German measles vaccination?
- Have you ever had a miscarriage, ectopic pregnancy, stillbirth, or complicated pregnancy?
- Have you recently traveled outside the United States?

If your answer to any of these questions is yes, you definitely should seek counseling from an obstetrician, nurse-midwife, or family practitioner three to six months before you hope to conceive a child.

How a Woman's Body Changes During Pregnancy

The 40 weeks of pregnancy transform a woman's body. At the beginning of pregnancy, the woman's uterus becomes slightly larger, and the cervix becomes softer and bluish due to increased blood flow. Progesterone and estrogen trigger changes in the milk glands and ducts in the breasts, which increase in size and feel somewhat tender. The pressure of the growing uterus against the bladder causes a more frequent need to urinate. As the pregnancy progresses, the woman's skin stretches as her body shape changes, her center of gravity changes as her abdomen protrudes, and her internal organs shift as the baby grows (see Figure 9-15 on page 314). Pregnancy is typically divided into three-month periods called trimesters.

How a Baby Grows

Silently and invisibly, over a nine-month period, a fertilized egg develops into a human being. When the zygote reaches the uterus, it's still smaller than the head of a pin. Once nestled into the spongy uterine lining, it becomes an **embryo.** The embryo takes on an elongated shape, rounded at one end. A sac called the **amnion** envelops it (see photo, Figure 9-15). As water and other small molecules cross the amniotic membrane, the embryo floats freely in the absorbed fluid, cushioned from shocks and bumps. At nine weeks the embryo is called a **fetus.**

A special organ, the **placenta,** forms. Attached to the embryo by the umbilical cord, it supplies the growing baby with fluid and nutrients from the maternal bloodstream and carries waste back to the mother's body for disposal (see Figure 9-16 on page 315).

Emotional Aspects of Pregnancy

Almost all prospective parents worry about their ability to care for a helpless newborn. By talking openly about their

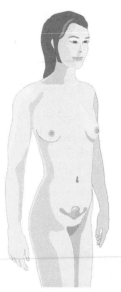

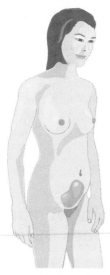

First Trimester

Increased urination because of hormonal changes and the pressure of the enlarging uterus on the bladder.

Enlarged breasts as milk glands develop.

Darkening of the nipples and the area around them.

Nausea or vomiting, particularly in the morning.

Fatigue.

Increased vaginal secretions.

Pinching of the sciatic nerve, which runs from the buttocks down through the back of the legs, as the pelvic bones widen and begin to separate.

Irregular bowel movements.

Before conception   At 4 months

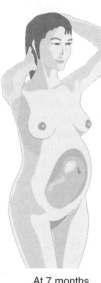

Second Trimester

Thickening of the waist as the uterus grows.

Weight gain.

Increase in total blood volume.

Slight increase in size and change in position of the heart.

Darkening of the pigment around the nipple and from the navel to the pubic region.

Darkening of the face.

Increased salivation and perspiration.

Secretion of colostrum from the breasts.

Indigestion, constipation, and hemorrhoids.

Varicose veins.

At 7 months

At 9 months

Third Trimester

Increased urination because of pressure from the uterus.

Tightening of the uterine muscles (called Braxton-Hicks contractions).

Shortness of breath because of increased pressure by the uterus on the lungs and diaphragm.

Heartburn and indigestion.

Trouble sleeping because of the baby's movements or the need to urinate.

Descending ("dropping") of the baby's head into the pelvis about two to four weeks before birth.

Navel pushed out.

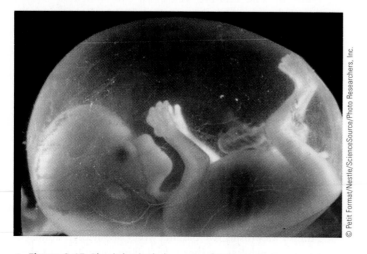

© Petit Format/Nestle/ScienceSource/Photo Researchers, Inc.

▲ **Figure 9-15** Physiological changes of pregnancy.

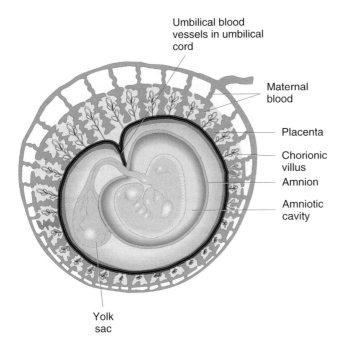

Umbilical blood
vessels in umbilical
cord

Maternal
blood

Placenta

Chorionic
villus

Amnion

Amniotic
cavity

Yolk
sac

▲ **Figure 9-16** The placenta.
The placenta supplies the growing embryo with fluid and
nutrients from the maternal bloodstream and carries waste
back for disposal.

feelings and fears, however, they can strengthen the bonds between them, so that they can work together as parents as well as partners. Psychological problems, such as depression, can occur during pregnancy. The availability of social support and other resources for coping with stress can make a great difference in the potential impact of emotional difficulties.

The physiological changes of pregnancy can affect a woman's mood. In early pregnancy, she may feel weepy, irritable, or emotional. As the pregnancy continues, she may become calmer and more energetic. Men, too, feel a range of intense emotions about the prospect of having a child: pride, anxiety, hope, fears for their unseen child and for the woman they love. Although many men want to be as supportive as possible, they may think that they have to be strong and calm—and may therefore pull away from their wives. The more involved fathers become in preparing for birth, the closer they feel to their partners and babies afterward.

Why Is Prenatal Care Important?

A pregnant woman has to take good care of herself to provide good care for her unborn child. This means regular medical and dental checkups. A woman should have her first prenatal visit as soon as she discovers that she's preg-

nant. A study group of the American College of Obstetricians and Gynecologists (ACOG) has recommended seven or eight prenatal visits for women with low-risk pregnancies; women at higher risk require more frequent checkups. Many teenage and unmarried pregnant women don't get adequate prenatal care, and some don't see a health-care professional until late in their pregnancy, because they can't afford or don't have access to medical services.

Age

The risk of a poor pregnancy outcome increases with age. Women 30 or older face a 40 percent greater risk of late fetal death, compared with women ages 20 to 24. Women over 35 also face an increased risk of very low birthweight, preterm delivery, and small-for-gestational-age (SGA) infants. Preconception and prenatal care, including good nutrition and careful monitoring, increase the chances of a healthy baby for older mothers.

Nutrition

A well-balanced diet throughout pregnancy is critical for a mother and her fetus both before and at birth. If a woman—regardless of her prepregnancy weight—gains too little weight, the risk to the growing fetus is high. ACOG recommends a weight gain of 22 to 27 pounds during pregnancy. The National Academy of Sciences' Food and Nutrition Board advises a maximum weight gain of 35 pounds, based on findings that weight gain aids fetal growth and lowers the risk of infant mortality and mental retardation.

No vitamin supplement can replace a well-balanced diet, but a multivitamin can help reduce or avoid deficiencies. According to the CDC, women who take a simple daily multivitamin containing a B vitamin called folate (or folic acid) before conception can cut in half the risk that their children will suffer neural tube defects, which stem from faulty development of the spinal column. These conditions include spina bifida, a defect in which the bones of the spine, the vertebrae, are incompletely formed.

Activity and Rest

Almost all pregnant women can benefit from exercise throughout pregnancy—as long as they don't push too hard or too far. Regular exercise (three times a week) is better, safer, and more effective than occasional workouts. While women who were athletic prior to pregnancy generally can continue their physical activity, they should be aware of warning signs that could indicate a potential problem, such as faintness, dizziness, pain, or vaginal bleeding. Research has found that regular, sustained exercise during pregnancy

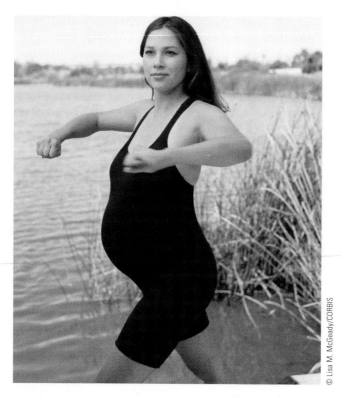

▲ Most pregnant women benefit from regular, moderate exercise. For women who were very active before their pregnancies, a higher level of activity is probably fine, but they should consult with their physician first.

does not affect infants' physical growth or mental development at age 1.

Rest is as important as exercise; the pregnant woman who's not used to taking naps may have to make time in her schedule for rest periods. If insomnia or the frequent need to urinate during the night becomes a problem, she may have to rely on catnaps during the day. She should *not* take sleeping pills.

Substance Use

Smoking endangers two lives: the mother's and the fetus's. The sooner a mother-to-be stops smoking, the better the chances that the fetus will develop normally. Smoking increases the risk of miscarriage, stillbirth, low birthweight, heart defects, and premature birth, and also impairs growth.[57] The fetus's oxygen supply is impaired by the increased levels of carbon monoxide in the smoking mother's bloodstream. Passive smoking (inhaling other people's smoke) can be hazardous for the mother and fetus as well. (See Chapter 16.) Mothers who quit smoking in the first trimester have fewer preterm deliveries and low-birthweight infants than those who continue smoking.

Approximately 16 percent of pregnant women report drinking in the previous month.[58] According to the CDC, more than 8,000 alcohol-damaged babies are born every year. One of every 750 newborns has a cluster of physical and mental defects called **fetal alcohol syndrome (FAS):** low birthweight, smaller-than-normal head circumference, smaller and shorter size, irritability as newborns, and permanent mental impairment as a result of their mothers' alcohol consumption. The milder forms of these problems, particularly impaired intellectual ability and school performance, are called fetal alcohol effects (FAE). (See Chapter 15.)

The risk of fetal alcohol syndrome is greatest if a mother drinks 3 ounces or more of pure alcohol (the equivalent of six or seven cocktails) a day. However, moderate drinking—one or two cocktails daily—may also have an effect. Even one drink a day has been associated with birth defects; binge drinking (five or more drinks on one occasion) is most toxic. The National Institute on Alcohol Abuse and Alcoholism and the Surgeon General advise pregnant women—and those trying to become pregnant—to abstain from drinking alcohol.

Moderate to heavy caffeine users are at greater risk of miscarriage than women who use little or no caffeine. Even more than one cup of coffee a day is linked with low birthweight. The FDA's advice is for pregnant women to "avoid caffeine containing products or use them sparingly."

At least one of every ten newborns is exposed to illegal drugs before birth. The consequences of drug use during pregnancy include severe damage to the child's brain and nervous system and birth defects. Marijuana smokers have smaller, sicker babies and a higher risk of stillbirths, according to some research. Drug use also may lead to "neurochemical" birth defects by disrupting normal development of the brain. Cocaine use increases the risk of premature birth, stillbirths, and malformations.

Environmental Risks

According to a study of more than 23,000 pregnant women, exposure to heat from a hot tub, sauna, or fever during the first trimester of pregnancy increases the risk of neural tube defects. Hot tubs presented the greatest single danger, while exposure to heat from multiple sources led to even greater risk. Electric blankets were not associated with increased risk.

High levels of radiation of the type used for cancer therapy have been associated with birth defects. Diagnostic X rays should be avoided during pregnancy if possible, but they're not a significant threat, particularly after the first trimester. In theory, the rapidly developing fetus is particularly vulnerable to pollutants, toxic wastes, heavy metals, pesticides, gases, and other hazardous compounds in the environment.

© Lisa M. McGeady/CORBIS

Prenatal Testing

All parents worry that their unborn baby might not be normal and healthy. Sophisticated new tests can answer some, but not all, of their questions and can identify more than 250 diseases and defects. Prenatal tests are being performed earlier and with less risk to a fetus than ever before. The most common prenatal tests include the following:

▶ *Ultrasonography* uses high-frequency sound waves to produce an image of the fetus on a video screen and as a photographic picture. Ultrasound can check fetal age and spot certain birth defects.

▶ *Alpha-fetoprotein (AFP) screening,* performed from the 13th to 20th week of pregnancy, measures a substance produced by the baby's kidneys in the mother's blood. Levels that are too high could indicate a neural tube defect; levels that are too low may signal Down syndrome.

▶ *Amniocentesis,* performed from the 14th to 16th week of pregnancy, consists of removing a small amount of the amniotic fluid surrounding the fetus. This fluid contains cells shed by the fetus, which can be grown in tissue culture and then checked for any chromosomal or genetic defects (see Figure 9-17).

▶ *Chorionic villi sampling (CVS),* performed from the eighth to tenth week of pregnancy, involves suctioning a small sample of the chorionic villi, the tissue surrounding the fetus, for laboratory analysis (see Figure 9-17). Results are generally available within a week.

There are no known risks for ultrasonography and AFP screening. For both amniocentesis and CVS, there is about a 1 percent risk of miscarriage. Some testing centers have reported a higher incidence of both limb defects and miscarriage following CVS than others using this technique. Before choosing a facility for testing, pregnant women should inquire about that facility's experience and complication rate. Prenatal tests are usually recommended only if the mother is over age 35, has had a child with a genetic disorder, or is a known carrier of a detectable genetic disorder.

Complications of Pregnancy

In about 10 to 15 percent of all pregnancies, there is increased risk of some problem, such as a baby's failure to grow normally. **Perinatology,** or maternal-fetal medicine, focuses on the special needs of high-risk mothers and their unborn babies. Perinatal centers, with state-of-the-art equipment and 24-hour staffs of specialists in this field, have been set up around the country. Several of the most frequent potential complications of pregnancy are discussed below.

Ectopic Pregnancy

Any woman who is of childbearing age, has had intercourse, and feels abdominal pain with no reasonable cause may have an **ectopic pregnancy.** In this type of pregnancy, the fertilized egg remains in the fallopian tube instead of traveling to the uterus. Ectopic, or tubal, pregnancies have increased dramatically in recent years, now accounting for 2 percent of all reported pregnancies. STDs, particularly chlamydia infections (discussed in Chapter 11), have become a major cause of ectopic pregnancy. Other risk factors include previous pelvic surgery, particularly involving the fallopian tubes; pelvic inflammatory disease; infertility; and use of an IUD.

In an ectopic pregnancy, a misplaced egg develops normally, producing the usual signs of pregnancy, until the cramped amniotic sac bursts, damaging the fallopian tube. The woman will bleed internally and feel lower abdominal

---

STRATEGIES FOR PREVENTION

A Mother-to-Be's Guide to a Healthy Pregnancy

✔ ACOG recommends consuming about 300 more calories a day than before pregnancy and concentrating on eating the right foods, not on watching your weight. Never diet during pregnancy. Don't restrict salt intake either, unless specifically directed to by your doctor.

✔ Drink six to eight glasses of liquids each day, including water, fruit and vegetable juices, and milk.

✔ Don't exercise strenuously for more than 15 minutes, ACOG advises. Avoid vigorous exercise in hot, humid weather. Never let your body temperature rise above 100°F or your heart rate climb above 140 beats per minute.

✔ Stretch and flex carefully because the joints and connective tissue soften and loosen during pregnancy. After the fourth month of pregnancy, don't do any exercises while lying on your back, as this could impair blood flow to the placenta.

✔ Walk, swim, and jog in moderation; play tennis only if you played before pregnancy. Ski only if you're experienced, and stick to low altitudes and safe slopes. Do not water-ski, surf, or ride a horse.

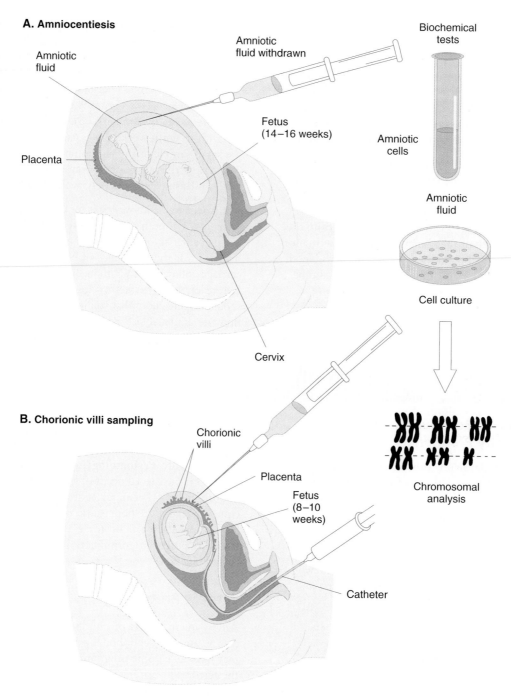

▲ **Figure 9-17** Prenatal testing.
(A) In amniocentesis, a sample of the amniotic fluid is withdrawn; fetal cells found in that fluid can then be grown in tissue culture and checked for chromosomal defects. (B) In chorionic villi sampling (CVS), a tissue sample of the villi is removed from the uterus and analyzed for chromosomal defects.

pains, or she may feel an aching in her shoulders, as the blood flows upward toward the diaphragm. If the bleeding is substantial, the woman can go into shock, with low blood pressure and a high pulse rate. Symptoms are hot and cold flashes, nausea, dizziness, fainting, pelvic pain, and irregular bleeding.

Treatment for the damaged fallopian tube is usually removal, but microsurgery can often repair the damage. About 50 percent of the women who have had an ectopic pregnancy conceive again; 10 percent have another ectopic pregnancy. Ectopic pregnancies can lead to permanent infertility.

Miscarriage

About 10 to 20 percent of pregnancies end in **miscarriage,** or spontaneous abortion, before the 20th week of gestation. Major genetic disorders may be responsible for 33 to 50 percent of pregnancy losses. About 0.5 to 1 percent of women suffer three or more miscarriages, possibly because of genetic, anatomic, hormonal, infectious, or autoimmune factors.[59] An estimated 70 to 90 percent of women who miscarry eventually become pregnant again.

Physicians typically recommend bed rest if a woman begins bleeding or cramping early in pregnancy. In some cases, the cramping stops, and the pregnancy continues normally. In others, the bleeding becomes intense, the cervix widens, and the embryo is expelled. If the miscarriage is complete, the bleeding stops and the uterus returns to its normal state and shape. If it is incomplete, a physician has to remove any bits of tissue remaining in the uterus.

Few medical events are more emotionally devastating than a pregnancy loss. Women often feel the loss in an extremely intense, almost physical way. Many who miscarry had not reached the point in pregnancy where the fetus seems separate from them. Typically, women feel both vulnerable and responsible, as if they did something to cause the loss or should have, could have, done something to prevent it. They try to identify what they did wrong: exercising or not exercising, working or not working; eating too much or not enough. Some women interpret a loss as a punishment for past sins, imagined or real. Such self-inflicted guilt, allowed to fester, can lead to major depression.

Infections

The infectious disease most clearly linked to birth defects is **rubella** (German measles). All women should be vaccinated against this disease at least three months prior to conception, to protect themselves and any children they may bear. (See Chapter 11 for more on immunization.) The most common prenatal infection today is *cytomegalovirus.* This infection produces mild flulike symptoms in adults but can cause brain damage, retardation, liver disease, cerebral palsy, hearing problems, and other malformations in unborn babies.

STDs, such as syphilis, gonorrhea, and genital herpes, can be particularly dangerous during pregnancy if not recognized and treated. If a woman has a herpes outbreak around the date her baby is due, her physician will deliver the baby by caesarean section to prevent infecting the baby. HIV infection endangers both a pregnant woman and her unborn baby, and all pregnant women and new mothers should be aware of the HIV epidemic, the risks to them and their babies, and the availability of anonymous testing.

Premature Labor

Approximately 10 percent of all babies are born too soon (before the 37th week of pregnancy). According to researchers, prematurity is the main underlying cause of stillbirth and infant deaths within the first few weeks after birth. Bed rest, close monitoring, and, if necessary, medications for at-risk women can buy more time in the womb for their babies. But women must recognize the warning signs of **premature labor**—dull, low backache; a feeling of tightness or pressure on the lower abdomen; and intestinal cramps, sometimes with diarrhea—early enough. Low-birthweight premature babies face the highest risks, but comprehensive, enriched programs can reduce developmental and health problems.

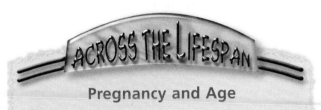

Pregnancy and Age

Although teen pregnancy rates have declined, they remain the highest in the world. Approximately 900,000 adolescents become pregnant each year. About two-thirds of these pregnancies occur in women 18 and 19 years old; a third, in women 17 years and younger. About half of teen pregnancies result in a live birth; 35 percent end with an abortion, and 14 percent end with a miscarriage or stillbirth.[60]

In the past, most teenage mothers married the fathers of their unborn children. Today most do not. Many teenage girls who become pregnant have partners who are aged 20 or older. However, they themselves are generally aged 18 or 19.

As teen births have begun to decline, the number of women deciding to have children later in life has increased. One of every five women in the United States now has her first baby after age 35; first births among women older than 40 have increased 50 percent in the last 15 years.

Risks to the fetus are greater when mothers are older than 35, primarily an increase in fetal birth defects due to chromosomal abnormalities, such as Down syndrome. At age 30, the estimated risk is 2.6 per thousand; the incidence rises to 5.6 per thousand at age 35; 15.8 at age 40; and 53.7 at age 45. However, pregnancy itself for healthy women over age 35 is safe. As discussed later in this chapter, assisted reproductive technologies have enabled women in their forties, fifties, and even sixties to have successful pregnancies.

Childbirth

A generation ago, delivering a baby was something a doctor did in a hospital. Today parents can choose from an almost bewildering array of birthing options. The first decision parents-to-be face is choosing a birth attendant, who can be a physician or a nurse-midwife. Certified nurse-midwives in the United States deliver more than 90,000 babies a year, mostly in hospitals and birth centers. Their approach is based on the belief that the typical pregnant woman can deliver her baby naturally without technological intervention. Lay midwives have a similar orientation but less formal training; only a handful of states permit lay midwives to deliver babies.

When interviewing physicians or midwives, look for the following:

▷ Experience in handling various complications.
▷ Extensive prenatal care.
▷ A commitment to be at the mother's side for the entire labor in order to spot complications quickly and provide assistance.
▷ A compatible philosophy toward childbirth and medical interventions.

Preparing for Childbirth

The most widespread method of childbirth preparation is **psychoprophylaxis,** or the **Lamaze method.** Fernand Lamaze, a French doctor, instructed women to respond to labor contractions with prelearned, controlled breathing techniques. As the intensity of each contraction increases, the laboring woman concentrates on increasing her breathing rate in a prescribed way. Her partner coaches her during each contraction and helps her cope with discomfort.

Women who have had childbirth preparation training tend to have fewer complications and require fewer medications. However, painkillers or anesthesia are always an option if labor is longer or more painful than expected. The lower body can be numbed with an **epidural block,** which involves injecting an anesthetic into the membrane around the spinal cord, or a **spinal block,** in which the injection goes directly into the spinal canal. General anesthesia is usually used only for emergency caesarean births.

???? What Is Childbirth Like?

There are three stages of **labor.** The first starts with *effacement* (thinning) and *dilation* (opening up) of the cervix. Effacement is measured in percentages, and dilation in centimeters (cm) or finger-widths. Around this time, the amniotic sac of fluids usually breaks, a sign that the woman should call her doctor or midwife.

The first contractions of the early, or *latent,* phase of labor are usually not uncomfortable; they last 15 to 30 seconds, occur every 15 to 30 minutes, and gradually increase in intensity and frequency. The most difficult contractions come after the cervix is dilated to about 8 cm, as the woman feels greater pressure from the fetus. The first stage ends when the cervix is completely dilated to a diameter of 10 cm (or five finger-widths) and the baby is ready to come down the birth canal (see Figure 9-18). For women having their first baby, this first stage of labor averages 12 to 13 hours. Women having another child often experience shorter first-stage labor.

When the cervix is completely dilated, the second stage of labor occurs, during which the baby moves into the vagina, or birth canal, and out of the mother's body. As this stage begins, women who have gone through childbirth preparation training often feel a sense of relief from the acute pain of the transition phase and at the prospect of giving birth.

This second stage can take up to an hour or more. Strong contractions may last 60 to 90 seconds and occur every two to three minutes. As the baby's head descends, the mother feels an urge to push. By bearing down, she helps the baby complete its passage to the outside.

As the baby's head appears, or *crowns,* the doctor may perform an *episiotomy*—an incision from the lower end of the vagina toward the anus to enlarge the vaginal opening. The purpose of the episiotomy is to prevent the baby's head from causing an irregular tear in the vagina, but routine episiotomies have been criticized as unnecessary. Women may be able to avoid this procedure by trying different birthing positions or having an attendant massage the perineal tissue.

Usually the baby's head emerges first, then its shoulders, then its body. With each contraction, a new part is born. However, the baby can be in a more difficult position, facing up rather than down, or with the feet or buttocks first (a **breech birth**), and a caesarean birth may then be necessary.

In the third stage of labor, the uterus contracts firmly after the birth of the baby; and, usually within five minutes, the placenta separates from the uterine wall. The woman may bear down to help expel the placenta, or the doctor may exert gentle external pressure. If an episiotomy has been performed, the doctor sews up the incision. To help the uterus contract and return to its normal size, it may be massaged manually, or the baby may be put to the mother's breast to stimulate contraction of the uterus.

Caesarean Birth

In a **caesarean delivery** (also referred to as a caesarean section), the doctor lifts the baby out of the woman's body through an incision made in the lower abdomen and uterus. The most common reason for caesarean birth is

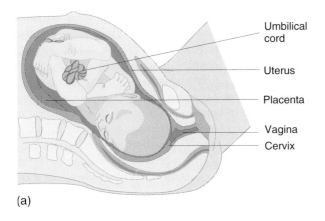

Umbilical
cord

Uterus

Placenta

Vagina

Cervix

(a)

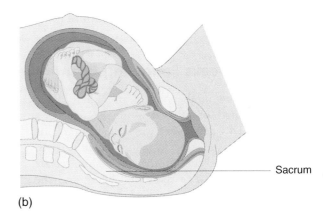

Sacrum

(b)

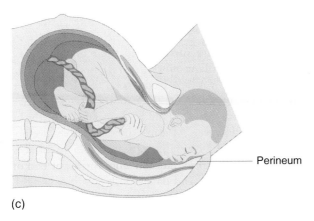

Perineum

(c)

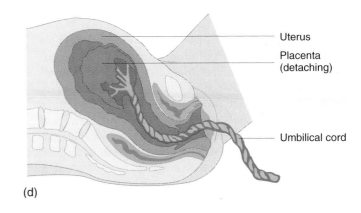

Uterus

Placenta
(detaching)

Umbilical cord

(d)

▲ **Figure 9-18** Birth.
(a) The cervix is partially dilated, and the baby's head has entered the birth canal. (b) The cervix is nearly completely dilated. The baby's head rotates so that it can move through the birth canal. (c) The baby's head extends as it reaches the vaginal opening, and the head and the rest of the body pass through the birth canal. (d) After the baby is born, the placenta detaches from the uterus and is expelled from the woman's body.

"failure to progress," a vague term indicating that labor has gone on too long and may put the baby or mother at risk. Other reasons include the baby's position (if feet or buttocks are first) and signs that the fetus is in danger. Thirty years ago, only 5 percent of babies born in America were delivered by caesarean birth; the current rate is 22.6 percent—substantially higher than in most other industrialized countries.

About 36 percent of caesarean sections are performed because the woman has had a previous caesarean birth. Yet research indicates that more than two-thirds of women who undergo caesarean births because of failure to progress in labor, and approximately four of every five women who have had caesarean births for other reasons, can have successful vaginal deliveries in subsequent pregnancies.

Caesarean birth involves abdominal surgery, so many women feel more physical discomforts after a caesarean than a vaginal birth. These discomforts include nausea, pain, and abdominal gas. Women who have had a caesarean

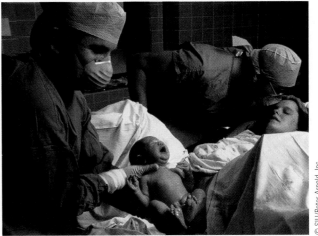

▲ Fathers are routinely present at the birth of their children and often act as birth coaches after both parents train in Lamaze techniques.

section must refrain from strenuous activity, such as heavy lifting, for several weeks.

The Days and Weeks Following Birth

Hospital stays for new mothers are shorter than in the past. The average length of stay is now only 2.6 days for a vaginal delivery and 4.1 days after a caesarean birth. A primary reason has been pressure to reduce medical costs. Obstetricians have voiced concern that the rush to release new mothers may jeopardize their well-being and the health of their babies, who are more likely to require emergency care for problems such as jaundice. The American College of Obstetricians and Gynecologists and the American Academy of Pediatrics recommend that women remain in the hospital two days after a vaginal delivery and four days after a caesarean birth.

For the new mother, the high of delivery may be followed by a low known as **postpartum depression.** This time of fatigue, anxiety, and fluctuating moods is so common that it is listed in obstetrics texts as a normal consequence of delivery. For most women, it is a temporary feeling. For others, the depression, combined with fatigue and the new demands of the newborn, can persist and deepen. If postpartum depression lasts more than three or four weeks, the woman should seek help from a qualified psychotherapist.

It takes a while for the mother's body to return to normal after having given birth. The woman usually loses about 11 pounds at delivery and an additional 4 to 5 pounds in the following weeks. Usually four to eight weeks are required for the woman's reproductive organs, especially the uterus, to return to normal. Breast-feeding hastens this process, and exercises help restore the abdomen's size, shape, and tone. For three to six weeks after birth, there is a vaginal discharge called **lochia,** a mixture of blood from the site in the uterus where the placenta was attached, and tissue from the uterine lining. If the mother doesn't breast-feed her infant, menstruation typically resumes about four to ten weeks after giving birth.

Breast-Feeding Versus Bottle-Feeding

A generation ago, most middle- and upper-class women bottle-fed their babies. Today, an increasing number of medical professionals state that breast milk is best. Breast-fed babies have fewer illnesses, a much lower hospitalization rate, and a lower mortality rate. Breast milk seems not only to prevent disease, but also to help bring infection under control. When breast-fed babies do get sick, they recover more quickly.

Despite the benefits of breast-feeding, there are valid reasons to choose bottle-feeding. According to the American Council on Science and Health, at least 20 percent of women are unable to breast-feed after their first deliveries, and 50 percent of new mothers encounter significant difficulties nursing. Sometimes the woman's breasts become inflamed, or she must take medications that would endanger her infant; sometimes the infant is unable to suckle vigorously enough to get an adequate milk supply. Another problem is that in certain areas of the country, the levels of pesticides and other chemical contaminants in mother's milk can be high.

Babies at Risk

 According to the National Center for Health Statistics, a record percentage of U.S. newborns are surviving to their first birthday. The infant mortality rate, as reported in 1999, is a record low of 7.9 deaths per 1,000 live births—a continued decline that puts the nation on track to reach its goal of no more than 7 infant deaths per 1,000 births by the year 2000. However, African-American babies are not faring as well. Their mortality rate was 16.5 in 1992—making them 2.4 times more likely to die, primarily because of prematurity and dangerously low birthweight, before their first birthday. This gap has widened from just a 60 percent greater risk in 1950. Babies of Chinese and Japanese descent have the lowest mortality rates.

In all, more than 1.3 million newborns each year require special care after birth because of prematurity, low birthweight, birth defects, jaundice, respiratory difficulties, or other problems. About 6 percent of newborns—more than 200,000 babies a year—require immediate intensive care for potentially life-threatening problems that developed before, during, or after birth.

Genetic Disorders

Two to four percent of babies are born with a genetic abnormality. (See Genes in Focus: "Genetic Defects.") While the overall infant mortality rate has declined, the proportion of infant deaths due to birth defects has increased. However, the most common birth defects are not fatal. They include:

▸ **Cystic fibrosis.** The most common genetic problem among white Americans, this is a disabling abnormality of the respiratory system and sweat and mucous glands.
▸ **Down syndrome.** This disorder is caused by an extra number 21 chromosome and occurs in one of every 600 to 1,000 births. Infants are born with varying degrees

of physical and mental retardation. The chances of a woman delivering an infant with Down syndrome increase with her age. At age 25, the chances are 1 in 1,200; at age 35, they rise to 1 in 365; and at age 40, they are 1 in 100.

GENES IN FOCUS

Genetic Defects

In some sense, each of us is a carrier of a genetic problem. Every individual has an estimated four to six defective genes, but the chances of passing them on to a child are slim. Almost all are recessive, which means they are "masked" by a more influential dominant gene. The likelihood of a child inheriting the same faulty recessive gene from both parents is remote—unless the parents are so closely related that they have very similar genetic makeup.

The child of a parent with an abnormal dominant gene has a 50 percent likelihood of inheriting it. The most common of such defects are minor, such as the growth of an extra finger or toe. However, some single-gene defects can be fatal. Huntington's chorea, for example, is a degenerative disease that in the past was usually not diagnosed until midlife. Genetic testing can now predict which individuals will develop this disorder. However, since no preventive measures or treatments are available, many people with a family history of Huntington's prefer not to be tested.

Genetic tests also can identify "carriers" of abnormal recessive genes for diseases such as sickle-cell anemia (the most common genetic disorder among African Americans), beta-thalassemia (found in families of Mediterranean origin), and Tay-Sachs (found in Jews of Eastern European origin). Two carriers of the same abnormal recessive genes can pass such problems on to their children.

Some abnormal recessive genes are found only on the female X chromosome and are a risk only to sons. A boy faces a 50–50 chance of inheriting a defective gene on his mother's sex chromosome. While a daughter may also inherit the gene and become a carrier, she will not develop symptoms because of the matching healthy gene on her other X chromosome. The most common X-linked problems are hemophilia and Duchenne's muscular dystrophy, which impairs muscle tissue.

- **Sickle-cell anemia.** About 8 to 10 percent of North America's 25 million African Americans carry a gene for sickle-cell anemia, a blood disorder that occurs when hemoglobin, the oxygen-carrying protein of red blood cells, is abnormal and causes red blood cells to assume a crescent (sickle) shape. Unable to provide adequate oxygen to vital organs of the body, sickled cells cause fatigue, loss of interest and appetite, pain, and a host of other symptoms. Blood transfusions can prolong a victim's life, but there's no cure for sickle-cell anemia. About half the victims die before age 20.
- **Phenylketonuria (PKU).** This disease occurs when the liver enzyme needed by the body for the metabolism of the amino acid phenylalanine is absent. If both parents are carriers, there's a one-in-four chance that the child will develop phenylketonuria (PKU). In most states, the law requires testing newborns for PKU. If PKU is detected, an immediate, long-term phenylalanine-free diet can reduce the effects of the disorder. If untreated, the victim becomes severely mentally retarded.
- **Tay-Sachs disease.** Occurring almost exclusively among young children of Eastern European Jewish ancestry, Tay-Sachs disease is caused by an enzyme deficiency. Infants with this disorder appear normal for perhaps nine months, but then gradually deteriorate physically and mentally. Death usually occurs before the fifth birthday. Carriers can be identified by a blood test.

The Littlest Addicts

Cocaine and crack babies suffer major complications, including withdrawal and permanent disabilities. (See Chapter 14 for a discussion of these drugs.) They have higher-than-normal incidences of respiratory and kidney troubles, premature birth, and low birthweight, and may be at greater risk of sudden infant death syndrome. Visual problems, lack of coordination, and developmental retardation are also common.

Sudden Infant Death Syndrome (SIDS)

SIDS, or **crib death**—the unexplained death of an apparently healthy baby under one year of age—is the second-leading cause of infant mortality in the United States. About 900 infants die of crib death each year, a significant decrease from the past. Typically, a seemingly healthy infant, usually 1 to 7 months old, is put to bed according to the daily routine. The baby may have some signs of a cold or cough. When the parents return to the crib, they find the child dead. There is no sign of a struggle, nor does the baby suffocate in the blankets. Determining the cause of death often proves impossible. Premature and very small babies are the most vulnerable. A recognized risk factor, based on studies of 20,000 infants during the first week of life, is the "resonance frequency" of each cry—an acoustic measure of a child's cry that cannot be easily determined by listening. Computer analysis found that infants with a high-resonance frequency were more likely to die of SIDS. A screening test based on this factor may be developed to detect newborns at risk.

Based on a review of studies on SIDS from around the world, health professionals have found that sleeping on its stomach increases a baby's risk of SIDS. As a result, pediatricians now recommend that normal, full-term infants be placed on their backs for the first six months. Parents should remove pillows, quilts, comforters, stuffed toys, and other soft products from the crib.

Infertility

The World Health Organization defines infertility as the failure to conceive after one year of unprotected intercourse. About 85 percent of couples will conceive during one year, rising to almost 90 percent by two years. The main causes of infertility are ovulation problems, tubal damage, or sperm dysfunction. Less common causes are endometriosis, cervical factors, or coital difficulties. Even after intensive investigation, 10 to 20 percent of couples have "unexplained infertility" in which no cause can be demonstrated.

Of the couples who marry this year, 1 in 12 won't be able to conceive a child, and 10 percent of couples already married won't be able to have additional children. The percentage of women seeking infertility services rose from 12 to 15 percent since the 1980s.[61] **Infertility** is a problem of the couple, not of the individual man or woman. In 40 percent of cases, infertility is caused by female problems; in 40 percent by male problems; in 10 percent by a combination of male and female problems; and in 10 percent by unexplained causes. A thorough diagnostic workup can reveal a cause for infertility in 90 percent of cases.

In women, the most common causes of subfertility or infertility are age, abnormal menstrual patterns, suppression of ovulation, and blocked fallopian tubes. Other gynecologic disorders that can lead to infertility include endometriosis, in which cells from the endometrium (the lining of the uterus) migrate to other locations within the pelvic cavity; fibroids, benign growths of tissue within the uterus that can interfere with conception; uterine defects; problems with the cervical mucus; and an immunological reaction to a man's sperm. The prevention of STDs can help prevent some cases of infertility in women.

Male subfertility or infertility is usually linked to either the quantity or the quality of sperm, which may be inactive, misshapen, or insufficient (less than 20 million sperm per milliliter of semen in an ejaculation of 3 to 5 mL). Sometimes the problem is hormonal or a blockage of a sperm duct. Some men suffer from the inability to ejaculate normally, or from retrograde ejaculation, in which some of the semen travels in the wrong direction, back into the body of the male. Another problem is a *varicocele,* an enlarged vein that carries too much blood and makes the testicle too warm. An undergarment that uses a small amount of water to cool the testicles may help overcome this problem; some men require surgery to eliminate the varicocele. The use of drugs such as cocaine and marijuana can also interfere with the creation of sperm.

Infertility can have an enormous emotional impact. Often, the wife begins to worry first because infertility touches on a core aspect of femininity. Many women long to experience pregnancy and childbirth and feel great loss if they cannot conceive. Their self-esteem may be diminished, and they may become obsessed with success and outcome. Women in their thirties and forties fear that their "biological clock" is running out of time. Men may be confused and surprised by the intensity of their partners' emotions. Most are more concerned about their wives than about having a baby, but they feel helpless and frustrated in their husbandly role of fixing matters for the wife. Although they both need each other's support more than ever, they may pull away because of their sadness and a sense of losing control over their lives.

The treatment of infertility has become a $2 billion a year enterprise in the United States. The odds of successful pregnancy range from 30 to 70 percent, depending on the specific cause of infertility. One result of successful infertility treatments has been a boom in multiple births, including quintuplets and sextuplets. Some obstetricians have urged less aggressive treatment for infertility to avoid such high-risk multiple births.

There have been complaints about unethical treatment in infertility centers. Fertility specialists and government licensing agencies have been working together to set uniform standards for licensing. Infertile couples should obtain as much information as possible, including the credentials of any fertility specialists, who should be board-certified in obstetrics and gynecology, with additional training in reproductive endocrinology and infertility. Those performing surgery should be members of the Society of Reproductive Surgeons; centers offering in vitro fertilization or alternative techniques should be staffed by members of the Society of Assisted Reproductive Technology.

Artificial Insemination

Since the 1960s, **artificial insemination**—the introduction of viable sperm into the vagina by artificial means—

has led to an estimated 250,000 births in the United States, primarily in couples in which the husband was infertile. However, some states do not recognize such children as legitimate; others do, but only if the woman's husband gave his consent for the insemination.

Assisted Reproductive Technology

New approaches to infertility include microsurgery, sometimes with lasers, to open destroyed or blocked egg and sperm ducts; new hormone preparations to induce ovulation; and the use of balloons, inserted through the cervix and inflated, to open blocked fallopian tubes (a procedure called *balloon tuboplasty*). However, less than 2 percent of infertile women undergo assisted reproductive technologies in order to conceive.

Among the most well-known techniques to overcome fertility problems is *in vitro fertilization (IVF),* which involves removing the ova from a woman's ovary just before normal ovulation would occur. The woman's egg and her mate's sperm are placed in a special fertilization medium (a substance that encourages fertilization) for a specific period of time, and are then transferred to another medium to continue developing. If the fertilized egg cell shows signs of development, within several days it is returned to the woman's uterus by means of a hollow tube placed through the vagina and cervix. The egg cell implants itself in the lining of the uterus, and the pregnancy continues as normal. The success rate varies but is generally less than 20 percent, and the costs are high.

Less time-consuming and less expensive than IVF, *gamete intrafallopian transfer (GIFT)* involves placing sperm and eggs into the fallopian tubes. GIFT mimics nature by allowing fertilized eggs to develop in the fallopian tubes according to a normal timetable. The success rate is about 20 percent. In *zygote intrafallopian transfer (ZIFT),* eggs are collected from the mother-to-be and combined with the father's sperm in a laboratory dish. One day after fertilization occurs, the single-celled zygote that

forms is placed in the fallopian tube. In a variation called *intracytoplasmic sperm injection (ICSI),* several eggs are harvested, and each is injected with a single sperm by means of a fine hollow needle. (This overcomes problems related to the inability of sperm to penetrate the egg.) The fertilized eggs are then placed in the fallopian tube. Fertilization rates are comparable to in vitro fertilization with sperm from normal ejaculation.

In *gestational surrogacy,* an embryo is conceived in a laboratory dish using a woman's egg and her partner's sperm and then implanted into another woman's (the surrogate's) uterus. Alternatively, the fertilized donor egg can later be transferred to the uterus of the infertile woman, who carries and delivers the developing embryo. Embryos can be frozen for later implantation in a process (called *cryopreservation*) that is highly controversial because of legal issues concerning the "ownership" of the unborn. Some women are considering an experimental technique to freeze some of their eggs at a young age for later use.

Older women are just as likely as younger women to have a successful pregnancy after implantation of a donor embryo. In some experimental and controversial cases, donor eggs and embryos have been successfully implanted in women in their forties, fifties, and (in at least two cases) sixties. The use of a donor egg from a younger woman eliminates the risk of increased genetic problems. There are ethical questions about using expensive assisted reproductive technologies for the sake of enabling older women to become mothers or of allowing creation of "designer" babies of a certain racial or ethnic identity or with certain attributes, such as sex, height, or intelligence.

Fertility drugs and assisted reproduction techniques have extended the limits of motherhood. In 1996 a 63-year-old bank teller in southern California, became the oldest mother on record when she gave birth to a baby girl. She had lied about her age to qualify for infertility treatments.

Assisted reproductive techniques involve some problems, including high costs and a low success rate. One attempt at in vitro fertilization ranges from $6,000 to $10,000, and insurance rarely covers these expenses. The overall success rate for any form of assisted pregnancy is about 25 percent.

Of the pregnancies achieved by fertility treatments, 20 to 30 percent result in multiple births. As a result of hormonal stimulation, the woman's ovaries usually release several eggs; often more than one is fertilized. To increase the chances of conception, fertility specialists usually implant more than one embryo. The more that survive, the greater the risk of prematurity, low birth-weight, birth defects, and death in

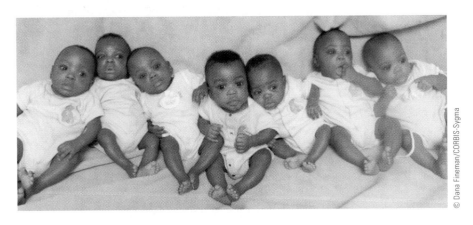

▲ Fertility drugs can increase the chances of multiple births.

© Dana Fineman/CORBIS-Sygma

the womb or after birth. In some cases, one or more fetuses are aborted to increase the likelihood that at least one other will survive.

There also has been controversy over whether the hormones used to stimulate the ovaries in infertility treatment may increase the risk of ovarian cancer. However, an analysis of all the research on this topic concluded that, as currently used, ovarian-stimulating drugs do not increase this risk.

Adoption

Men and women who cannot conceive children biologically can still become parents. **Adoption** matches would-be parents yearning for youngsters to love with infants or children who need loving. Couples interested in adoption can work with either public agencies or private counselors who contact obstetricians directly. Or they can contact organizations that arrange adoptions of children in need from other countries.

Approximately 1 percent of the U.S. population are adopted; among children under age 18, 3 to 4 percent are adopted. Each year some 50,000 U.S. children become available for adoption—far fewer than the number of would-be parents looking for youngsters to adopt. By some estimates, only 1 in 30 couples receive a child—and they spend an average of two years and as much as $100,000 on the adoption process.

Not only are the stakes high, but adoption arrangements often are chaotic. Private adoptions are legal in some states, banned in others. In some places, birth mothers sign over all claims to a child within 72 hours of giving birth; in others they have up to a year to change their minds. Sometimes foster parents are encouraged to adopt—particularly if they're African Americans caring for an African-American child. In others, they face a daunting series of bureaucratic barriers. What's needed most, say experts on every side of the issue, are uniform adoption laws in all fifty states.

An increasing number of people support *open adoptions,* which allow for visiting and communication with the biological parents even though the adoptive parents retain legal custody. Even after a *closed adoption,* the biological (or birth) parents may at some point search for their children, if only to explain why they chose to give them up for adoption.

Although fewer than 2 percent of each year's 50,000 adoptions of American children are contested, adoptive parents are nervous and confused.

"Adoptive or foster parents have no rights whatsoever until the rights of the biological parents are legally terminated," says Mary Beth Style, Vice President for policy and practice for the National Council on Adoption[62]—even when they have nurtured a child for months or years, as often happens in foster care. Although mental health pro-

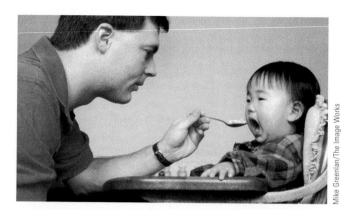

▲ Adoption gives people the option to become parents when they would otherwise not be able to have children.

Mike Greenlar/The Image Works

fessionals contend that the courts should recognize the rights of a child's "psychological" parents, most rulings have placed little importance on such bonds. Political pressure for reform has increased, which makes birthparent support groups fearful. "There's a rush to sever quickly and permanently the biological bonds between parents and their children," says Janet Fenton, President of Concerned United Birthparents. "The focus in adoption is shifting from finding homes for children who need them to finding babies for couples who can't have them."[63]

The best advice for prospective adoptive parents is to learn as much as they can about their state's adoption laws and to prepare for the reality that their plans might not work out.

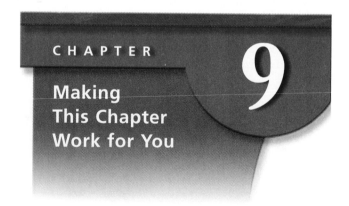

CHAPTER **9**

Making This Chapter Work for You

1. Conception occurs
   a. when a fertilized egg implants in the lining of the uterus.
   b. when sperm is blocked from reaching the egg.
   c. when a sperm fertilizes the egg.
   d. after the uterine lining is discharged during the menstrual cycle.

2. Factors to consider when choosing a contraceptive method include all of the following except
   a. cost
   b. failure rate
   c. effectiveness in preventing sexually transmitted diseases
   d. preferred sexual position

3 When used correctly, the most effective nonhormonal contraceptive methods are
   a. the copper T intrauterine device
   b. condom
   c. spermicide
   d. diaphragm

4. Which of the following contraceptive choices offers the best protection against STDs?
   a. condom alone
   b. condom plus spermicide
   c. abstinence
   d. withdrawal plus spermicide

5. Which of the following statements is true about sterilization?
   a. In women, the most frequently performed sterilization technique is hysterectomy.
   b. Many couples experience an increase in sexual encounters after sterilization.
   c. Vasectomies are easily reversed with surgery.
   d. Sterilization is recommended for single men and women who are unsure about whether they want children.

6. The incidence of abortion is
   a. highest in women older than 30 and who have several children.
   b. lower in the United States than in countries where birth control education begins early and contraceptives are easier and cheaper to obtain.
   c. higher in affluent women, who can afford the procedure, than in poor women.
   d. higher in Catholic women than in Protestant women.

7. In the third trimester of pregnancy,
   a. the woman experiences shortness of breath as the enlarged uterus presses on the lungs and diaphragm.
   b. the embryo is now called a fetus.
   c. the woman should begin regular prenatal checkups.
   d. the woman should increase her activity level to ensure that she is fit for childbirth.

8. During childbirth,
   a. breech birth can be prevented by practicing the Lamaze method.
   b. the cervix thins and dilates so that the baby can exit the uterus.
   c. the intensity of contraction decreases during the second stage of labor.
   d. the placenta is expelled immediately before the baby's head appears.

9. Parents of a new baby
   a. must decide whether to breast-feed or use baby food.
   b. should be tested immediately after the child is born to determine whether they carry genetic diseases.
   c. should seek professional help if the mother experiences depression lasting more than a few weeks after the child is born.
   d. can help prevent SIDS by placing the baby on his side for the first six months.

10. Which of the following statements is true about infertility?
   a. Infertility is most often caused by female problems.
   b. In men, infertility is usually caused by a combination of excess sperm production and an ejaculation problem.
   c. In vitro fertilization involves introducing sperm into the vagina with a long needle.
   d. The success rate of the GIFT technique is usually higher than that of in vitro fertilization.

Answers to these questions can be found on page 640.

 Are emergency contraceptives like "The Morning After Pill" safe and should they be made available over-the-counter?

Critical Thinking

1. After reading about the various methods of contraception, which do you think would be most effective for you? What factors enter into your decision (convenience, risks, effectiveness, etc.)?

2. In Wyoming, a pregnant woman went to the police station to report that here husband had beaten her. Instead of charges being brought against him, she was arrested for intoxication and charged with abusing her

fetus by drinking. Across the country, other women who use hard drugs or alcohol while pregnant or whose newborns test positive for drugs have been arrested and put on trial for abusing their unborn children. Prosecutors argue that they are defending the innocent victims of substance abuse. Some health officials, on the other hand, argue that addicted women need help, not punishment. What do you think? Why?

3. Suppose that you and your partner were told that your only chance of having a child is by using fertility drugs. After taking the drugs, you and your partner are informed that there are seven fetuses. Would you carry them all to term? What if you knew that the chances of them all surviving were very slim and that eliminating some of them would improve the odds for the others? What ethical issues do cases like these raise?

SITES & BYTES

Planned Parenthood
http://www.plannedparenthood.org
This excellent site describes birth control options, emergency contraception, sexually transmitted diseases, safer sex, pregnancy and parenting, abortion, teen issues, and women's health. In addition, links can take you to a variety of research information, including statistics, FAQs, press releases, newsletters, and a sexual health glossary.

National Women's Health Information Center—U.S. Public Health Office on Women's Health
http://www.4woman.org
This site features information for both health professionals and the general public that includes current women's health articles, a newsletter, a calendar of national women's health events, information on pregnancy, body image, and violence prevention.

Reproductive Health Online
http://www.reproline.jhu.edu
This site is sponsored by Johns Hopkins University and features comprehensive information on all types of contraception, including the latest advances. These are also sections on maternal and neonatal health, cervical cancer, and sexually transmitted diseases.

Please note that links are subject to change. If you find a broken link, use a search engine such as http://www.yahoo.com and search for the website by typing in key words.

InfoTrac Activity Donald E. Greydanus, Dilip R. Patel, and Mary Ellen Rimsza. "Contraception in the Adolescent: An Update." *Pediatrics*, Vol. 107, No. 3, March 2001, p. 562.

(1) According to the article, what is the preferred method of contraception?
(2) What is the best way to reduce (not eliminate) the risk of acquiring most types of sexually transmitted diseases?
(3) Name at least three different types of barrier contraceptives and the relative efficacy of each.
(4) What are the major contraindications to the use of oral contraceptives (WHO Category 4)?
(3) List five noncontraceptive benefits of oral contraceptive pills.

You can find additional readings related to reproductive choices with InfoTrac College Edition, an online library of more than 900 journals and publications. Follow the instructions for accessing InfoTrac that were packaged with your textbook; then search for articles using a key word search.

For additional links, resources, and suggested readings on InfoTrac, visit our Health & Wellness Resource Center at http://health.wadsworth.com.

Key Terms

The terms listed here are used within the chapter on the page indicated. Definitions of the terms are in the Glossary at the end of the book.

References

1. Darroch, Jacqueline. "The Pill and Men's Involvement in Contraception." *Family Planning Perspective,* Vol. 32, No. 2, March 2000.
2. Steinhauer, Jennifer. "Men Avoiding Obligation for Birth Control." *New York Times,* May 25, 1995.
3. Gold, Rachel Benson, and Cory Richards. *Medicaid Support for Family Planning in the Managed Care Era.* New York: Alan Guttmacher Institute, 2001, p. 10.
4. Murray, Steven, and Jessica L. Miller. "Birth Control and Condom Usage Among College Students." *Research Quarterly for Exercise and Sport,* Vol. 71, No. 1, March 2000.
5. Glei, Dana. "Measuring Contraceptive Use Patterns Among Teenage and Adult Women." *Family Planning Perspectives,* Vol. 31, No. 2, March 1999.
6. Wyatt, Gail, et al. "Factors Affecting HIV Contraceptive Decision-Making Among Women." *Sex Roles: A Journal of Research,* April 2000.
7. Pennachio, Dorothy. "New Approaches to Emergency Contraception. *Patient Care,* Vol. 35, No. 5, March 15, 2001, p. 19.
8. "Facts About Birth Control." www.plannedparenthood.org
9. Oncale, Renee, and Bruce King. "Comparisons of Men's and Women's Attempts to Dissuade Sexual Partners from the Couple Using Condoms." *Archives of Sexual Behavior,* Vol. 30, No. 4, August 2001, p. 379.
10. "Is Abstinence Right for You?" www.plannedparenthood.org
11. "Facts About Birth Control."
12. Kemmeren, Jeanet, et al. "Third Generation Oral Contraceptives and Risk of Venous Thrombosis: Meta-analysis." *British Medical Journal,* Vol. 323, No. 7305, July 21, 2001.
13. Ibid.
14. Schwetz, Bernard. "New Oral Contraceptive." *Journal of the American Medical Association,* Vol. 286, No. 5, August 1, 2001, p. 527.
15. Nelson, Anita. "Whose Pill Is It Anyway." *Family Planning Perspectives,* Vol. 32, No. 2, March 2000.
16. Guillebaud, John. "Will the Pill Become Obsolete in This Century?" *Family Planning Perspectives,* Vol. 32, No. 2, March 2000.
17. "Helping Women Use the Pill." *Population Reports,* Vol. 28, No. 2, Summer 2000.
18. Audet, Marie-Claude, et al. "Evaluation of Contraceptive Efficacy and Cycle Control of a Transdermal Contraceptive Patch vs. an Oral Contraceptive: A Randomized Controlled Trial." *Journal of the American Medical Association,* Vol. 285, No. 18, May 9, 2001.
19. "Norplant Implant Deemed Safe, Effective." *Contraceptive Technology Update,* Vol. 22, No. 6, June 2001, p. 64.

20. Stevens-Simon, Catherine, et al. "A Village Would Be Nice but . . . It Takes a Long-acting Contraceptive to Prevent Repeat Adolescent Pregnancies." *American Journal of Preventive Medicine,* Vol. 21, No. 1, 2001, pp. 60–65.

21. Meirik, Olav, et al. "Safety and Efficacy of Levonorgestrel Implants, Intrauterine Devices, and Sterilization." *Obstetrics & Gynecology,* Vol. 97, No. 4, April 2001.

22. "Facts About Birth Control."

23. Kupecz, Deborah. "Lunelle: A New Contraceptive Alternative." *Nurse Practitioner,* Vol. 26, No. 6, June 2001, p. 55.

24. Vernarec, Emil. "This Non-Estrogen IUD Is Effective for Five Years." *RN,* Vol. 64, No. 3, March 2001, p. 98.

25. Farley, Timothy, et al. "Intrauterine Devices and Pelvic Inflammatory Disease: An International Perspective." *Lancet,* Vol. 339, No. 8796, March 28, 1992, p. 785.

26. "The IUD and PID: What Are the Risks? *Contraceptive Technology Update,* Vol. 22, No. 6, June 2001, p. 68. "Rediscovering the Benefits of the IUD." *Contraceptive Technology Update,* Vol. 22, No. 1, January 2001, p. 5.

27. Hirozawa, A. "A First Pregnancy May Be Difficult to Achieve After Long-Term Use of an IUD." *Family Planning Perspectives,* Vol. 33, No. 4, July 2001, p. 181.

28. Greydanus, Donald, et al. "Contraception in the Adolescent: An Update." *Pediatrics,* Vol. 107, No. 3, March 2001, p. 562.

29. Ibid.

30. Murray, and Miller, "Birth Control and Condom Usage Among College Students."

31. Michaels Opinion Research. "In the Heat of the Moment." Menlo Park, CA: Henry J. Kaiser Family Foundation, June 2001.

32. "Condom Use by Adolescents." *Pediatrics,* Vol. 107, No. 6, June 2001, p. 463.

33. Ford, Kathleen, et al. "Characteristics of Adolescents' Sexual Partners and Their Association with Use of Condoms and Other Contraceptive Methods." *Family Planning Perspectives,* Vol. 33, No. 3, May 2001, p. 100.

34. "Condom Misconceptions Abound Among Sexually Active Adolescents." *Medical Letter on the CDC and FDA,* May 27, 2001.

35. "Perceived Versus Actual Knowledge About Correct Condom Use Among U.S. Adolescents: Results from a National Study." *Journal of Adolescent Health,* Vol. 28, No. 5, May 2001, p. 415.

36. "Condom Ads on Television: Unwrapping the Controversy." Menlo Park, CA: Henry J. Kaiser Family Foundation, June 2001.

37. "Condoms." Menlo Park, CA: Henry J. Kaiser Family Foundation, May 2001.

38. "Study of Female Condom Aims to Combat AIDS Worldwide." *AIDS Weekly,* November 13, 2000.

39. Hollander, D. "Female Condoms Remain Structurally Sound After Being Washed and Reused as Many as Seven Times." *Family Planning Perspectives,* Vol. 33, No. 4, July 2001, p. 186.

40. Grimes, David, et al. "New Approaches to Emergency Contraception." *Contemporary OB/GYN,* Vol. 46, No. 6, June 2001, p. 89.

41. "Statement Supporting the Availability of Over-the-Counter Emergency Contraception." *American College of Obstetricians and Gynecologists,* March 2001.

42. Gardner, Jacqueline, et al. "Increasing Access to Emergency Contraception Through Community Pharmacies." *Family Planning Perspectives,* Vol. 33, No. 4, July 2001.

43. Golden, Neville, et al. "Emergency Contraception: Pediatricians' Knowledge, Attitudes, and Opinions." *Pediatrics,* Vol. 107, No. 2, February 2001, p. 287.

44. Greydanus. "Contraception in the Adolescent: An Update."

45. Formichelli, Linda. "The Male Pill." *Psychology Today,* January–February 2001, p. 16.

46. "Abortion in the United States." Menlo Park, CA: Henry J. Kaiser Family Foundation, May 2001.

47. "Mifepristone: An Early Abortion Option." Menlo Park, CA: Henry J. Kaiser Family Foundation, May 2001.

48. Hollander, D. "Most Abortion Patients View Their Experience Favorably, But Medical Abortion Gets a Higher Rating Than Surgical." *Family Planning Perspectives,* Vol. 32, No. 5, September 2000.

49. "Mifepristone: An Early Abortion Option."

50. "Chemical Abortion vs. Surgical." *Insight on the News,* Vol. 17, No. 4, January 29, 2001, p. 16.

51. "Abortion Policy and Politics." Menlo Park, CA: Henry J. Kaiser Family Foundation, May 2001.

52. Bower, B. "Study Explores Abortion's Mental Aftermath." *Science News,* Vol. 158, No. 8, August 19, 2000.

53. "Abortion Policy and Politics."

54. Stotland, Nada. *Abortion: Facts and Feelings.* Washington, D.C.: American Psychiatric Press, 1998.

55. Lafayette, Leslie. Personal interview.

56. "Births, Marriages, Divorces, and Deaths." *National Vital Statistics Reports,* Vol. 49, No. 6, August 22, 2001.

57. "Medical Care Expenditures Attributable to Cigarette Smoking During Pregnancy—United States, 1995." *Journal of the American Medical Association,* Vol. 278, No. 23, December 17, 1997.

58. "Drinking in Pregnancy." *Morbidity and Mortality Weekly Report,* U.S. Centers for Disease Control, April 1997.

59. Moore, Peter. "Tackling Autoantibody-linked Pregnancy Loss." *Lancet,* Vol. 350, No. 9073, July 26, 1997. Cowchock, Susan. "Autoantibodies and Pregnancy Loss." *New England Journal of Medicine,* Vol. 337, No. 3, July 17, 1997.

60. Wetzstein, Cheryl. "Teen Pregnancy Rate Reaches Record Low." *Insight on the News,* Vol. 17, No. 28, July 30, 2001, p. 33.

61. Stephen, Elizabeth, and Aniani Chandra. "Use of Infertility Services in the United States." *Family Planning Perspectives,* Vol. 32, No. 3, May 2000.

62. Style, Mary Beth. Personal interview.

63. Fenton, Janet. Personal interview.

IV

PERSONAL HEALTH CARE

Every day you make choices that affect both the quantity and the quality of your life. The right choices aren't always easy to make or to sustain. The chapters in this section can help by providing information you can use in making and implementing healthful decisions. By understanding the risks to your health, you can prepare to overcome them—and not simply live life, but celebrate it every day.

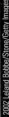

10

Consumerism, Complementary and Alternative Medicine, and the Health-Care System

Long after she immigrated to the United States from India, Tapu's grandmother refused to go to Western doctors. She preferred practitioners who used the herbs and techniques she had relied on in her homeland. Tapu's father, an American-trained physician, would argue with his mother-in-law about what he considered her old-fashioned views. As a doctor's son, Tapu grew up believing in the superiority of Western medicine.

In his sophomore year at college, Tapu found out that he needed oral surgery. To his sur-

prise, the oral surgeon suggested an alternative method of controlling post-operative pain: acupuncture. "My Dad's never going to approve," he said. "And he's the one who's still paying my medical bills." The doctor referred Tapu—and his father—to recent studies conducted by National Institute of Health researchers on acupuncture's efficacy in relieving postsurgical pain. After doing more research online, Tapu agreed to try acupuncture following his operation.

Like Tapu, millions of Americans are turning to complementary and alternative medicine (CAM), a term that includes a broad range of healing philosophies, approaches, and therapies not traditionally taught in medical schools or provided in hospitals. But consumers are learning that they have to be just as savvy—and skeptical—about these therapies and practitioners as they are with any other form of health care.

Because there are so many health-care choices, you face a greater responsibility for your personal well-being. Whether you are monitoring your blood pressure, considering elective surgery, or deciding whether to try an alternative therapy, you need to gather information, ask questions, weigh advantages and disadvantages, and take charge of your health. The reason: No one cares more about your health than you do, and no one will do more to promote your well-being than you.

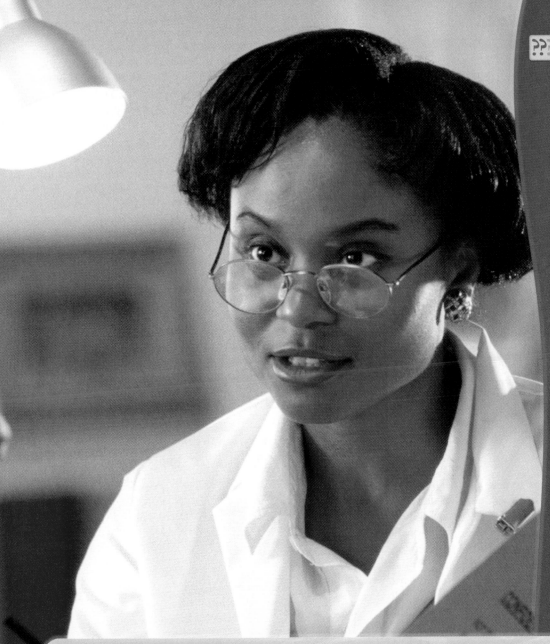

After studying the material in this chapter, you should be able to:

- **List** ways of becoming an informed health-care consumer.
- **Discuss** strategies for self-care, as well as how to get the best possible health care.
- **Describe** common medical exam procedures and medical tests.
- **Identify** strategies for maintaining good oral health.
- **List** your rights as a medical consumer.
- **Describe** the different types of complementary and alternative therapies and **explain** what research has shown about their effectiveness.
- **Compare** and **contrast** the different types of health-care practitioners and health-care facilities.
- **Explain** what managed care is.

Becoming a Savvy Health-Care Consumer

Americans are the world's foremost health-care consumers. We see more health practitioners, undergo more surgery, take more prescription drugs, and spend more time in hospitals than the citizens of any other nation. Not surprisingly, we also spend more money on health care: National health expenditures are expected to reach $2.2 trillion in 2008 and are likely to account for 16.2 percent of the gross domestic product.[1]

Despite such enormous expense, not every American receives good, or even adequate, medical care.[2] Consumers have long complained about insensitive treatment, lack of comprehensive care, and far too little emphasis on the prevention of disease. Because of recent efforts to curb spending, health-care providers may now seem to pay greater attention to cost than caring. And because of a lack of insurance, millions of people have limited access, or no access at all, to needed health services.

Knowing how to spot health problems, how to evaluate health news, what to expect from health-care professionals, and where to turn for appropriate treatment can help you keep your own costs down while ensuring the best possible care.

Informing Yourself

Knowledge is power. In the case of health care, knowledge gives you the power to make the best possible decisions about your well-being. Recognizing this need, government experts have called on colleges and universities to provide health information, particularly on prevention, to the more than 14 million people enrolled in institutions of higher learning. They've carried out this mission, at least in part.

 According to a CDC survey of approximately 4,600 undergraduates at 136 colleges and universities, about three-quarters of undergraduates have received some form of health information.[3] About half of all students surveyed had been given some information on prevention of alcohol and drug use and HIV infection and AIDS. Black students were more likely than white students to say they'd been taught about AIDS and HIV in college classes. African-American, Hispanic, or students of other racial and ethnic groups also were more likely than whites to report receiving information on any health topic. More traditional full-time students between ages 18 and 24 who have never been married and were not working full-time had received health information, compared to part-time, older, nontraditional students. (See Student Snapshot: "How Well Informed Are College Students?")

Self-Care

Most people do treat themselves. You probably prescribe aspirin for a headache, chicken soup or orange juice for a cold, or a weekend trip to unwind from stress. At the very least, you should know what your **vital signs** are and how they compare against normal readings. (See Table 10-1.)

Once a thermometer was the only self-testing equipment found in most American homes. Now an estimated 300 home tests are available to help consumers monitor everything from fertility to blood pressure to cholesterol levels. (See Table 10-2 on page 336.) More convenient and less expensive than a visit to a clinic or doctor's office, the new tests are generally as accurate as those administered by a professional. Always follow directions precisely, and if your concerns persist, see your doctor.

Self-care also can mean getting involved in the self-help movement, which has grown into a major national trend. Initially criticized for implicitly blaming victims rather than changing society, many self-help groups have

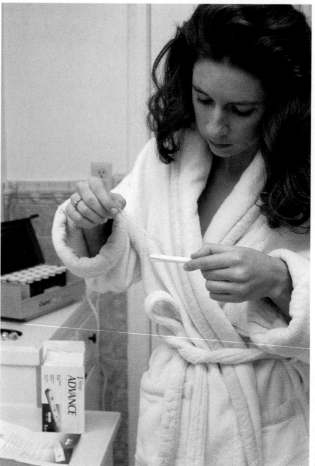

© Michael Newman/PhotoEdit

▲ Home health tests can be more convenient and less expensive than a trip to a clinic or doctor's office.

Student Snapshot How Well Informed Are College Students?

Health topic	Students receiving information from their college or university
Any type of health information	77.4%
Alcohol and drug use prevention	49.2%
HIV and AIDS prevention	49.1%
STD prevention	43%
Physical activities and fitness	35.9%
Dietary behaviors and nutrition	30.4%
Pregnancy prevention	26.8%
Injury prevention	22.5%
Suicide prevention	17.6%
All of the above topics	6%

Source: Data based on a survey conducted by the Centers for Disease Control and Prevention (CDC) of 4,609 undergraduates at 136 colleges and universities. Brener, Nancy, and Vani Gowda. "U.S. College Students' Reports of Receiving Health Information on College Campuses." *Journal of American College Health,* Vol. 49, No. 5, March 2001, p. 223.

▼ Table 10-1 Take your own vital signs.

Vital Sign	Normal Values
Temperature	98.9°F in the morning or 99.9°F later in the day is upper limit of the normal oral tempeature for people 40 years old or younger. • Women's temperatures are slightly higher than men's. • African-Americans' temperatues are slightly higher than white Americans. Measure your temperature with a mercury or digital thermometer.
Blood pressure	120/70 to 140/90, depending on age and gender. You can measure your own blood pressure if you want to invest in blood pressure equipment. Check your local drugstore to purchase a blood pressure cuff or digital blood pressure monitor.
Pulse	72 beats per minute. Take your pulse rate at your wrist or at the carotid artery in your neck.
Respiration rate	15–20 breaths per minute.

▼ Table 10-2 **Home Health Tests: A Consumer's Guide**

Type of Test	What It Does
Pregnancy	Determines if a woman is pregnant by detecting the presence of human chorionic gonadotropin in urine. Considered 99 percent accurate.
Fertility	Measures levels of luteinizing hormone (LH), which rise 24 to 36 hours before a woman conceives. Can help women increase their odds of conceiving.
High blood pressure	Measures blood pressure by means of automatically inflating armbands or cuffs for the finger or wrist; helps people taking hypertension medication or suffering from high blood pressure monitor their condition.
Cholesterol	Checks blood cholesterol in blood from a finger prick; good for anyone concerned about cholesterol.
Colon cancer	Screening test to detect hidden blood in stool; recommended for anyone over 40 or concerned about colorectal disease.
Urinary tract infection	Diagnoses infection by screening for certain white blood cells in urine; advised for women who get frequent UTIs and whose doctors will prescribe antibiotics without a visit.
HIV	Detects antibodies to HIV in a blood sample sent anonymously to a lab. Controversial because no face-to-face counseling is available for those who test positive.

become more politicized and are working not just to address specific needs of individuals, but to transform social structures. The National Self-Help Clearinghouse has an information hotline and a directory of more than 700 self-help groups. (See Your Health Almanac at the back of the book).

The American Medical Association has called for disciplinary action for doctors who prescribe drugs to people they have never met or examined. Other "cyberdocs" offer "virtual house calls" with board-certified physicians who engage in private chat sessions on minor illnesses and prescribe medicine (except controlled drugs like narcotics). In the future, videoconferencing may allow doctors to examine patients in

???? How Can I Evaluate Online Health Advice?

The Internet has become a major source of health information—and misinformation—with more than 10,000 health-related sites. An estimated 41 million Americans go online for medical information every year.[4] Many people want to learn more about medications and treatments; others share experiences with people with similar problems via chat rooms and bulletin boards.

The Internet permits ease of access to cutting-edge medical knowledge and bridges the communication gap created by high-tech medicine. However, it also has serious drawbacks. According to a recent analysis, simple queries for terms such as obesity or depression often lead to irrelevant sites, relevant sites with incomplete information, or sites that are difficult for most consumers to understand.[5] Many sites are used to promote products or people. Some chat rooms can lead to encounters with unpleasant people. Even when information is technically precise, laypeople may not know how to interpret it properly.

Some doctors have set up websites for the sole purpose of selling drugs such as Viagra—a practice that state and federal regulators have deemed unethical, though not illegal.

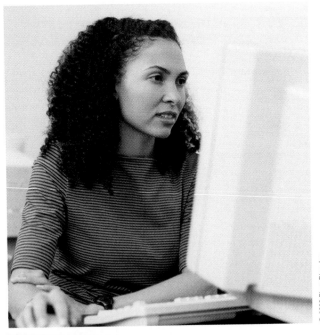

▲ Millions of Americans go online to learn about medical problems and treatments and to chat with others who have similar questions or problems.

cyberspace. However, there are no professional standards for doctors on the Internet, and experts advise caution. The "doctor" who treats your allergies may be a urologist or pathologist who is not up-to-date on new therapies or is unaware of potential side effects.

Here are some specific guidelines for evaluating online health sites:

▶ Check the creator. Websites are produced by health agencies, health support groups, school health programs, health-product advertisers, health educators, and health-education organizations. It is often difficult to distinguish biased commercial advertisements from unbiased sites created by scientists and health agencies. Read site headers and footers carefully.

▶ If you are looking for the most recent research, check the date the page was created and last updated as well as the links. Several nonworking links signal that the site isn't carefully maintained or updated.

▶ Check the references. As with other health-education materials, web documents should provide the reader with references. Unreferenced suggestions may be unwarranted, scientifically unsound, and possibly unsafe.

▶ Consider the author. Is he or she recognized in the field of health education or otherwise qualified to publish a health-information web document? Does the author list his or her occupation, experience, and education?

▶ Look for possible bias. Websites may be attempting to provide healthful information to consumers, but they also may be attempting to sell a product. Many sites are merely disguised advertisements.

Evaluating Health News

Cure! Breakthrough! Medical miracle! These words make headlines. Remember that although medical breakthroughs and cures do occur, most scientific progress is made one small step at a time. Even though medicine is considered a science, some experts estimate that no more than 15 percent of medical interventions can be supported by reliable scientific evidence.

Medical opinions invariably change over time, sometimes going from one extreme to another. For instance, several decades ago the treatment of choice for breast cancer was radical mastectomy—removal of the woman's breast, lymph nodes, and chest wall. Since then much less extensive surgery (lumpectomy), coupled with chemotherapy or radiation, or both, has proven equally effective. Once individuals who'd suffered heart attacks were advised to limit all physical activity. Today a progressive exercise program is a standard component of rehabilitation.

Health researchers are struggling to find better ways of assessing what they know and need to know in order to offer more complete and balanced information to consumers. However, sometimes the only certainty is uncertainty. Rather than putting your faith in the most recent report or the hottest trend, try to gather as much background information and as many opinions as you can. Weigh them carefully—ideally with a trusted physician—and make the decision that seems best for you.

When reading a newspaper or magazine story or listening to a radio or television report about a medical advance, look for answers to the following questions:

▶ Who are the scientists involved? Are they recognized, legitimate health professionals? What are their credentials? Are they affiliated with respected medical or scientific institutions? Be wary of individuals whose degrees or affiliations are from institutions you've never heard of, and be sure that the person's educational background is in a discipline related to the area of research reported.

▶ Where did the scientists report their findings? The best research is published in peer-reviewed professional journals, such as the *New England Journal of Medicine.* Research developments also may be reported at meetings of professional societies.

▶ Is the information based on personal observations? Does the report include testimonials from cured patients or satisfied customers? If the answer to either question is yes, be wary.

▶ Does the article, report, or advertisement include words like *amazing, secret,* or *quick?* Does it claim to be something the public has never seen or been offered before? Such sensationalized language is often a tip-off to a dubious treatment.

▶ Is someone trying to sell you something? Manufacturers who cite studies to sell a product have been known to embellish the truth.

▶ Does the information defy all common sense? Be skeptical. If something sounds too good to be true, it probably is.

Making Sense of Medical Research

Medical research is the only way that anyone, physician or consumer, can assess the quality of diagnostic methods, medications, or surgical treatments. The principal rule of science is that nothing works until it's been proven.

Researchers rely on a variety of studies to determine whether a new approach to prevention, diagnosis, or treatment works. These include:

▶ *Epidemiological studies,* in which scientists assess the health status of a large, defined group of people, such as the population of a country or region. They may look at various health habits, such as alcohol consumption, to determine whether those who practice these habits have a higher likelihood of developing certain diseases.

▶ *Animal studies,* or *preclinical trials,* in which scientists administer a drug or try a procedure on various laboratory animals to assess its safety and determine its effects.

▶ *Clinical trials,* in which volunteers agree to act as test subjects—"human guinea pigs," as it were. Patients must give written permission in order to participate. Clinical trials generate data for the purpose of evaluating one or more diagnostic or therapeutic approaches in a population. Well-designed clinical trials, which must have strict eligibility criteria, a standardized intervention, follow-up, and measures of outcome, set the "gold standard" for new diagnostic tests or medical or surgical treatments.

In *controlled studies,* the group receiving an experimental drug or treatment is compared with a group receiving no treatment or standard therapy. In *single-blind studies,* the subjects don't know whether they're receiving the experimental drug or treatment, or an inactive substance. In *double-blind studies,* neither the subjects nor the researchers have this information. In *prospective studies,* patients are selected, assessed, participate in the trial, and are then followed for a preset period. In *retrospective studies,* investigators look back at their past experiences with a certain group of patients.

The results of even the most careful studies aren't considered conclusive in and of themselves. The FDA reviews every new drug, as well as the research methods used to test it, before it's allowed on the market. And a new therapy is widely accepted (or rejected) only after publication of study results in a *peer-reviewed* journal (one in which scientists in the same field critique the research methods before accepting the paper) and after *replication* (the repetition of the same investigation by other researchers with similar results). In recent years, a technique called **meta-analysis,** which summarizes and reviews research in a particular area, has been used to evaluate the results of several large trials in a uniform manner.

One reason why study results must be confirmed is that, no matter what treatment patients receive, one-third to one-half of all patients improve temporarily. This well-documented but little-understood phenomenon is called the *placebo effect.* Scientific trials of a new treatment must show that the patients receiving the experimental medication or therapy improve *more* than those receiving a sugar pill or mock procedure (the placebo).

As part of the nationwide effort to cut costs while maintaining quality care, more research has focused on **outcomes**—the ultimate impact of treatment. Outcomes research is designed to answer questions such as: Is treatment better or worse than no treatment? Is one treatment better than another? If a treatment is effective, is a little just as good as a lot? Does quality of life change because of treatment? Are the benefits of treatment worth the cost or the risks to the patient?

Studies of outcomes look at how patients fared with or without a specific treatment, the costs involved, and the impact of undergoing or not undergoing treatment on the patients' quality of life. Outcomes research can help determine which of several therapies or approaches provides the best results at the most reasonable costs.

Getting the Best Health Care

Although considered the best in the world, the American health-care system is complex. Simply gaining access to a health-care provider can be difficult, and you may have to struggle through mountains of red tape to get a particular test or treatment. As discussed later in this chapter, many aspects of our health-care system are changing. However, some things remain the same, including the importance of a good doctor-patient relationship and of doing your part to get quality health care. (See Pulse Points: "Ten Ways to Get Good Health Care.")

You and Your Doctor

Once the family doctor was indeed part of the family. The family doctor brought babies into the world, shepherded them through childhood, comforted and counseled them, stood by their bedside in their darkest hours. Patients entrusted the doctor with their cares, their confidences, their very lives. In the twentieth century, dramatic breakthroughs in diagnosing and treating illness shifted the focus in medicine from the family physician to the specialist, from basic caring to high-tech medical care. Patients today are more likely to be cured of a vast array of illnesses than were patients a century ago. However, they often complain of insensitive, uncaring physicians who focus on their diseases rather than on them as individuals.

As more physicians have joined managed-care organizations (discussed later in this chapter), which emphasize efficiency, they sometimes feel pressure to see more patients a day, to spend less time with each, and to discourage expensive tests and treatments. Because physicians have less time and less autonomy, patients today must do more. Your first step should be learning more about your body, any medical conditions or problems you develop, and your options for treatment. You can find a great deal of information via computer online services, patient advocacy

PULSE POINTS

Ten Ways to Get Good Health Care

1. **Trust your instincts.** You know your body better than anyone else. If something is bothering you, it deserves medical attention. Don't let your health-care provider—or your health plan administrator—dismiss it without a thorough evaluation.

2. **Do your homework.** Go to the library or an online information service and find articles that describe what you're experiencing. The more you know about possible causes of your symptoms, the more likely you are to be taken seriously.

3. **Find a good primary care physician who listens carefully and responds to your concerns.** Look for a family doctor or general internist who takes a careful history, performs a thorough exam, and listens and responds to your concerns.

4. **See your doctor regularly.** If you're in your twenties or thir-

ties, you may not need an annual exam, but it's important to get checkups at least every two or three years, not so much for the sake of finding hidden disease, but so you and your doctor can get to know each other and develop a trusting, mutually respectful relationship.

5. **Get a second opinion.** If you are uncertain of whether to undergo treatment or which therapy is best, see another physician and listen carefully for any doubts or hesitation about what you're considering.

6. **Challenge medical judgments based on personal circumstances.** Insist that your doctor base any diagnosis on a thorough medical evaluation, not on a value judgment about you or your lifestyle.

7. **Seek support.** Patient support and advocacy groups can offer emotional support, information on many common problems, and referral to knowledgeable physicians. (See the Hales Health

Almanac at the back of the book for numbers and addresses.)

8. **If your doctor cannot or will not respond to your concerns, get another one.** Regardless of your health coverage, you have the right to replace a physician who is not meeting your health-care needs.

9. **Speak up.** If you don't understand, ask. If you feel that you're not being taken seriously or being treated with respect, say so. Sometimes the only difference between being a patient or becoming a victim is making sure your needs and rights are not forgotten or overlooked.

10. **Bring your own advocate.** If you become intimidated or anxious talking to physicians, ask a friend to accompany you, to ask questions on your behalf, and to take notes.

---

and support organizations (see the Health Almanac at the end of this book for listings), and libraries.

This information can help you know what questions to ask and how to evaluate what your doctor says. But you have to be willing to speak up. Busy doctors give patients less than a minute on average during a routine visit to say what's bothering them before they interrupt. This doesn't mean your doctor isn't interested, but it does mean that you have to develop good communication skills so you can tell physicians what they need to know to help you.

How Should I Choose My Primary Care Physician?

The primary care physicians who are playing increasingly important roles in American health care include family practitioners, general internists, and pediatricians. Obstetrician-gynecologists serve as the primary providers of health care for more than half of all women. If you're a woman and your gynecologist is the only physician you

see, make sure that he or she performs other tests, such as measuring your blood pressure, in addition to a pelvic and breast exam. If you develop other symptoms or health concerns, ask for an appropriate referral.

At college health centers, clinics, and some health-care organizations, consumers may be assigned to a primary physician or restricted to certain doctors. Even if your choices are limited, don't suspend your critical judgment. If your assigned physician does not listen to your concerns or is not providing adequate care, you can—and should—request another physician. Your rapport with your primary physician and the feelings of mutual trust and respect that develop between you can have as much of an impact on your well-being as your doctor's technical expertise.

When consumers can freely choose their physicians, they often do so, not just on the basis of qualifications, but also because of the physician's gender, race, or ethnic background. Frustrated by what they see as insensitive treatment by male physicians, many women have turned to female physicians—especially for gynecologic care. For

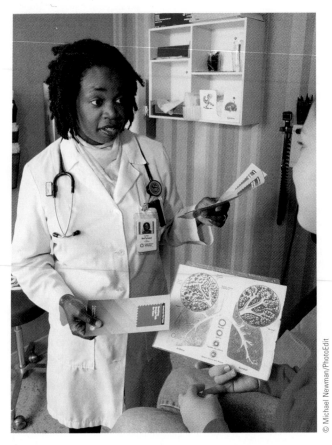

Take charge of your health by educating yourself and asking your doctor questions about your health and treatments.

other health services, women say that what matters most is having a caring physician who makes them feel comfortable and secure and invites them to participate in treatment decisions.

In a study of HMO patients in California, patients who chose doctors of the opposite gender generally were more satisfied with their physicians than patients who selected doctors of the same gender. Fewer women who chose female physicians (74 percent) were satisfied with their doctors than male patients who chose female physicians (85 percent). About 79 percent of female patients of male doctors and male patients of male doctors were satisfied. The reason, the researchers theorized, may be that the women expected female doctors to provide more communication and personalized care—which may not have been possible because they were working part-time and had larger workloads.[6]

 As the number of minority physicians has increased, more racial and ethnic minority group members are seeking out physicians with similar backgrounds. Often they see them as role models for their children. They may also feel that these professionals will have a natural empathy for

---

STRATEGIES FOR CHANGE

How to Talk with Your Doctor

✔ Prepare in advance. Write down your questions, organize them in a logical fashion, and select the top ten queries you want answered. Make a copy of all your questions to review and leave with your doctor.

✔ Ask about a "question hour." Many health-care practitioners set aside a specific time of day for patients with call-in questions. Find out if your college health center offers this service. Does a nurse field all calls? Can you get specific advice?

✔ Go online. Many doctors' offices answer queries by e-mail. Ask your doctor if you can e-mail follow-up questions or progress reports on how you're feeling.

✔ Interrupt the interrupter. If you're having difficulty explaining what's wrong, say so. If your doctor tries to put words in your mouth, say, "Please just listen so I can tell you the whole story without getting sidetracked."

---

their needs and concerns. Language also affects patient choices. Some individuals, such as Mexican-American and Puerto Rican patients, find it easier to communicate with Spanish-speaking physicians.

One key to making the health-care system work for you lies in choosing a good physician. After seeing your primary care physician, ask yourself the following questions to evaluate the quality of care you are getting.

◗ Did your physician take a comprehensive history? Was the physical examination thorough?
◗ Did your physician explain what he or she was doing during the exam?
◗ Did he or she spend enough time with you?
◗ Did you feel free to ask questions? Did your physician give you straight answers? Did he or she reassure you when you were worried?
◗ Does your physician seem willing to admit that he or she doesn't know the answers to some questions?
◗ Does your physician hesitate to refer you to a specialist even when you have a complex problem that warrants such care?

Look back at your answers. If they make you feel uneasy, have a talk with your physician. Or find a physician or a health plan that provides better service. (See X & Y Files: "Men and Women as Health-Care Consumers.")

The X & Y Files — Men and Women as Health-Care Consumers

The genders differ significantly in the way they use health-care services in the United States. Women see more doctors than men, take more prescription drugs, are hospitalized more, and control the spending of three of every four health-care dollars. In a national telephone poll, 76 percent of American women—but only 60 percent of men—said they had had a health exam in the last 12 months.

Many experts believe that the need for birth control and reproductive health services gets women into the habit of making regular visits to health-care professionals, primarily gynecologists. There are no comparable specialists for men, who tend to visit urologists, specialists in male reproductive organs, only when they develop problems. Men also are conditioned to take a stoic, tough-it-out attitude to early symptoms of a disease.

Men feel they are not allowed to manifest illness unless it's overt, says family practitioner Martin Miner, M.D., who has conducted research on men and health care. One reason why men die earlier than women is because of the length of time they wait to go for treatment.

The genders also differ in the symptoms and syndromes they develop. For instance, men are more prone to back problems, muscle sprains and strains, allergies, insomnia, and digestive problems. Men develop heart disease about a decade earlier in life than women. More men develop ulcers and hernias; women are more likely to get gallbladder disease and irritable bowel syndrome. An estimated 3 to 6 percent of men suffer from migraines, compared with 15 to 17 percent of women. Yet women and men spend similar proportions of their lifetimes—about 81 percent—free of disability. For men, whose lifespans are shorter, this translates into an average of 58.8 years; for women, 63.9 years.

The genders also differ in access to health services. Women are more likely than men to lack health insurance, and the lower a woman's income and education, the less her likelihood of getting important preventive services, such as an annual Pap smear or prenatal care. Women and men are about equally likely to use complementary and alternative medicine—but different types. Men outnumber women in use of chiropractic services and acupuncture, while women are more likely to try herbal medicine, mind-body remedies, folk remedies, movement and exercise techniques, and prayer or spiritual practices. However, both sexes turn to alternative treatments for the same reason: a desire for greater control over their health.

Sources: "Is It a Man's World? *Chemist & Druggist,* June 24, 2000. Thomas Richard. "The Feminization of Medicine." *Marketing Health Services,* Vol. 20, No. 3, Fall 2000. "Fact Sheet: Women's Health Insurance Coverage." Menlo Park, CA: Henry J. Kaiser Family Foundation, 2001.

What Should I Expect in a Medical Exam?

Most physicians believe that you don't need annual checkups if you're young and feel well. However, certain types of screening tests should be performed periodically, particularly if you're 45 or older, or if you are at a higher-than-average risk of developing a particular disease, such as high blood pressure (discussed in Chapter 12) or colon cancer (discussed in Chapter 13).

Your physician will want a past **medical history,** including major illnesses, surgery, and treatments. Report any allergies you have, particularly to drugs, and the medications you take, including aspirin, antacids, sleeping pills, oral contraceptives, and recreational drugs, even if illegal. Your physician may also want to know about topics you consider private, such as sexually transmitted diseases. Remember that he or she needs all this information to provide you with comprehensive treatment. Note, too, that a physician must report certain information—for example, certain sexually transmitted diseases—to health authorities.

After the physician has asked you questions about your complaints, medical history, and lifestyle, he or she will probably perform the standard tests described below. (See Figure 10-1.) During the examination, point out any pains, lumps, or skin growths you've noticed. If you feel pain when the physician palpates (feels) any part of your body, say so.

▶ **Head.** Using a flashlightlike instrument called an *ophthalmoscope,* the physician will look at the lens, retina, and blood vessels of your eyes. For patients over 40, he or she may test for a treatable eye disease called *glaucoma* (a disorder characterized by increased pressure within the eye), which can cause blindness if not detected early. The physician presses against the surface of each eye a soft instrument that measures the pressure within the eye and checks to see if the reading is normal. He or she will also examine your ears, mouth, tongue, teeth, and gums.

▶ **Neck.** Feeling around your neck, the physician will check for enlarged lymph glands (a sign of infection), for lumps in the thyroid gland, and for warning signs of stroke in the neck arteries.

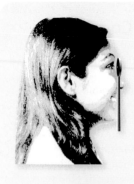

Looking into the eyes. With an opthalmoscope, your doctor will look for changes in eye's blood vessels or the optic nerve. These can signal severe diabetes, high blood pressure, or a tumor in the brain.

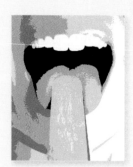

Examining the throat. Your doctor will look for signs of infection and other abnormalities.

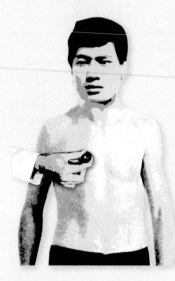

Listening to the heart, lungs, and abdomen. Your doctor will use a stethoscope to listen to the heart sounds to detect heart murmurs and other abnormalities. He or she will listen for wheezing or crackling sounds in your lungs, which could indicate asthma, bronchitis, or pneumonia. Your abdomen should make gurgling sounds. If it doesn't, the bowel may not be working properly.

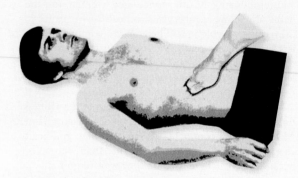

Probing the abdomen. A swelling on the right side may indicate a liver problem. A swelling on the left may mean that the spleen is enlarged, which could be a sign of infection or another condition.

▲ **Figure 10-1** Standard tests performed during a medical checkup.

▶ **Chest.** With a *stethoscope*, the physician will listen to the sounds made by your heart, to detect heart murmurs and irregular contractions, and by your lungs, to detect asthma or emphysema. By tapping on your chest and back with his or her fingers, the physician can tell the size and shape of your heart, which may reveal some forms of heart disease, and whether any fluid has collected in your lungs. The physician will also check for abnormal lumps in a woman's breasts.

▶ **Abdomen.** Here the physician uses his or her fingers to probe for tender spots and malformations of the liver and other organs, which may reveal signs of alcoholism, hepatitis, or hernias.

▶ **Rectum and genitals.** With a gloved hand, the physician can feel in the rectum for growths and hemorrhoids. A rectal examination can also reveal enlargement of the male's prostate gland. The physician will check male testicles and spermatic cords for abnormalities.

▶ **Pelvic examination.** During a pelvic examination, a woman lies on her back, with her heels in stirrups at the end of the examining table and her legs spread out to the sides. The physician inspects the labia, clitoris, and vaginal opening. Using two gloved, lubricated fingers, the physician will check for abnormalities in the vagina, uterus, fallopian tubes, and ovaries. Many physicians will also perform a rectal or rectovaginal (one finger in the rectum and one in the vagina) examination. A nurse or other health-care worker should be present throughout the exam.

The *speculum* is a medical instrument that spreads the walls of the vagina so that the inside can be seen. The physician will gently scrape cells from the cervix for a **Pap smear,** a procedure that identifies abnormal cells that may indicate an infection or, more seriously, cervical cancer, a slow-growing cancer that's usually curable if detected early (see Chapter 13). All women should start having regular Pap smears once they begin having intercourse, or at age 18. While there has been debate about how often women should have Pap smears, many health-care providers recommend Pap

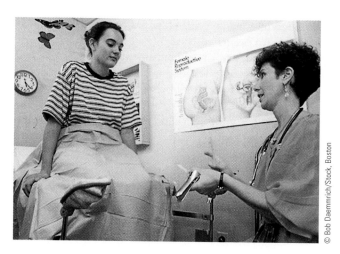

▲ Many women choose female health-care practitioners to provide gynecologic services.

smears every year for women who are sexually active or have other risk factors, such as infection with the human papilloma virus (see Chapter 11).

▷ **Extremities.** The physician may check your knees and other joints for reflexes, which can indicate nerve disorders, and look for tremors in outstretched hands or in the face. The color, elasticity, and wetness or dryness of your skin can alert him or her to nutritional problems, or can indicate diabetes or skin cancer. Hair and nails can give indications of internal health, such as blood disorders. Swelling of the ankles can be an indication of heart, kidney, or liver disease.

▷ **Pulse and blood pressure.** Your physician may check your pulse in various places, looking for signs of poor circulation. The rhythm and speed of the heart may also signal diseases of the heart or thyroid gland. High blood pressure can be an early warning sign of possible heart attack, stroke, or kidney damage.

Medical Tests

Besides the diagnostic tests listed above, the physician may order some laboratory and other tests, including the following:

▷ **Chest X ray.** A chest X ray can reveal abnormalities of the heart and lungs; if you're a smoker, the physician may insist on one.

▷ **Electrocardiogram.** The *electrocardiogram*, performed while you're at rest, records the electrical activity of your heart. It can show irregularities in heart rhythm or muscle damage, as well as hardening of the arteries.

▷ **Urinalysis.** Your urine may be analyzed by a medical laboratory. If sugar (glucose) is found in your urine,

your physician may order a separate blood test to check for diabetes. The presence of blood cells may indicate infection of the bladder or kidneys. Abnormal amounts of albumin (protein) in the urine may also suggest kidney disease.

▷ **Blood tests.** The physician or laboratory technician may draw blood to do a blood cell count. An excess of white blood cells may indicate an infection or, occasionally, leukemia. A deficiency of red blood cells may

STRATEGIES FOR PREVENTION

The Whats, Whys, and Hows of Testing

✔ Before undergoing any test, find out why you need it. Get a specific answer, not a "just in case" or "for your peace of mind." If you've had the test before, could the earlier results be used? Would a follow-up exam be just as helpful?

✔ Get some practical information as well: Should you do specific things before the test (such as not eat for a specified period)? How long will the test take? What will the test feel like? Will you need help getting home afterward?

✔ Check out the risks. Any invasive test—one that penetrates the body with a needle, tube, or viewing instrument—involves some risk of infection, bleeding, or tissue damage. Tests involving radiation also present risks, and some people develop allergic reactions to the materials used in testing.

✔ Get information on the laboratory that will be evaluating the test. Ask how often **false positives** or **false negatives** occur. (False positives are abnormal results indicating that you have a particular condition when you really don't; false negatives indicate that you don't have a particular condition when you really do.) Find out about civil or criminal **negligence** suits filed against the laboratory on charges such as failing to diagnose cervical cancer because of incorrect reading of Pap smears.

✔ You'll also want to know what happens when the test indicates a problem: Will the test be repeated? Will a different test be performed? Will treatment begin immediately? Could any medications you're taking (including nonprescription drugs, like aspirin) affect the testing procedures or results?

indicate anemia. Your blood may also be analyzed to measure the levels of its various components. High levels of glucose can indicate diabetes, and high levels of uric acid may mean gout or kidney stones. A high cholesterol level may indicate cardiac risk (see Chapter 12).

See the Hales Health Almanac at the back of this book for a comprehensive guide to medical tests.

Developing a Treatment Plan

After your exam, the physician will report his or her findings about your health and complaints, and advise you about treatment. Depending on your problem, your physician may recommend an **over-the-counter (OTC)** drug, such as aspirin or an antihistamine; prescribe a medication; or recommend more invasive treatment, such as surgery. Medications are discussed in Chapter 13 on drug use.

Once a treatment recommendation has been made, you face a decision: Do you follow the advice? Be sure you understand fully the consequences of what you do—or don't do. You may be risking harm if, for instance, you don't take the antibiotics prescribed for your strep throat, or if you stop taking them in midtreatment (strep throat can lead to heart damage). For major nonemergency procedures, get more than one physician's opinion. Eight out of ten operations are elective, meaning that they don't have to be performed to save the patient's life.

Elective Treatments

As medical technology has developed new options, millions of Americans are trying elective procedures and products that are not medically necessary but that promise to enhance health or appearance. Some are new alternatives for correcting common problems, such as poor vision, while others offer the promise of looking younger or more attractive.

Laser Vision Surgery

An estimated 1.5 million people in the United States undergo laser surgery to correct their vision every year—more than four times as many as in 1998.

In LASIK (laser-assisted in situ keratomileusis), the most common technique, a surgeon uses a razorlike instrument to lift a flap of the cornea—the clear stiff outer layer over the colored iris—and then reshapes the exposed area using a laser. The surgery alters the way the eye focuses light, correcting nearsightedness, farsightedness, and some astigmatism. Laser surgery cannot make an aging eye's lens flexible again to improve close-up vision in middle-aged adults. Numbing eye drops make the treatment painless,

although burning and scratchiness are normal for a couple of hours. An estimated 10 to 30 percent of patients require additional surgery, or "enhancements," to sharpen their vision. Other complications include glare, sensitivity to bright lights, and poor night vision.

Prices have fallen, but ophthalmologists have warned consumers that some laser surgery centers have cut corners to cut prices, such as hiring inexperienced surgeons or using optometrists or technicians rather than M.D.'s for pre- and post-operative checkups. A qualified eye surgeon should have a record of 100 or more LASIK procedures and at least 25 enhancements—but on no more than 20 percent of his or her patients. Ideally, the surgeon should also be the one doing your pre- and post-procedure checks.

Cosmetic Surgery

In 2000 more than 1.3 million Americans underwent cosmetic surgery (See Table 10-3), a 198 percent increase since 1992.[7] Most are aging baby boomers seeking treatments for wrinkles and sags; an increasing number are men. The most common operations are liposuction, eyelid surgery, breast augmentation, and face-lifts. Also popular are simpler cosmetic procedures, such as chemical peels and injections to combat wrinkles, that can be done quickly and require little "down" time for recovery.[8] Health insurance rarely covers cosmetic procedures, which range from $300 to upward of $10,000.

The most common cosmetic operation is liposuction, the removal of fatty tissue by means of a vacuum device. It can be performed on many areas of the body, from sagging jowls to midsection "love handles." The doctor first flushes the target area with a solution of lidocaine (a local anesthetic with a numbing effect), saline, and epinephrine (a drug that reduces bleeding by constricting blood vessels). Inserting a hollow wand-like cannula under the skin, the doctor breaks up fatty deposits and suctions them, along with other body fluids, with a vacuum device.[9]

Risks and complications include infection, numbness, bleeding, discoloration, lumpiness, and, if too much tissue is removed without proper cautions, potentially fatal complications. The Amercian Society of Plastic and Reconstructive Surgeons estimates the mortality rate is one in 5,000 liposuction patients. Several states are considering legislation to tighten restrictions on training and credentialing doctors who perform liposuction.

Breast augmentation is the second most common cosmetic procedure, and surgeons report a 300 percent increase in demand in the last six years. The Institute of Medicine, after reviewing all available evidence, has reported that there appears to be no link between breast implants and autoimmune disease, connective tissue disorders, or cancer. However, today's surgeons use implants filled with a saltwater solution. Patients still face possible

▼ Table 10-3 The Plastic Surgery Boom			
Type of Surgery	Number in 1992	Number in 2000	Cost
Forehead lift	13,501	41,668	$2,446
Eyelid surgery*	59,461	172,244	$3,055
Breast implants	32,607	187,755	$2,993
Tummy tuck	16,810	58,463	$4,158
Liposuction**	47,212	229,588	$1,960
Buttock lift	291	1,356	$3,509
Thigh lift	1,023	5,096	$3,877

*Upper and lower on both eyes.
**Single site.
Source: American Society of Plastic Surgeons.

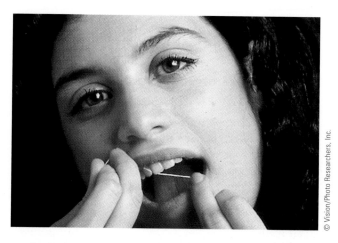

▲ Flossing every day helps prevent gum disease and other health problems. Using a gentle sawing motion, work the fooss down to your gum line. Move the floss up and down to scrape the sides of each tooth. Clean between all your teeth, using a fresh section of floss for each tooth.

complications, including rupture, scarring, infection, and leaking or hardening of their implants.

Oral Health

Oral health involves more than healthy teeth—it refers to the entire mouth, including all the structures that allow us to talk, bite, chew, taste, swallow, smile, scream, or scowl. Oral health is a critical part of overall health. Recent research has revealed links between chronic oral infection and heart and lung diseases, stroke, low birthweight, premature births, and diabetes.[10]

Thanks to fluoridated water and toothpaste, and improved dental care, Americans' oral health is better than in the past. Today's children have far less tooth decay than their parents had, and adults are keeping their teeth longer. However, as many as 32 percent of Americans are left with none of their own teeth by age 70. Without good self-care, you probably will lose some teeth to decay and gum disease. The best way to prevent such problems is through proper and regular brushing and flossing.

Gum, or periodontal, **disease,** is an inflammation that attacks the gum and bone that hold your teeth in place. The culprit is **plaque,** the sticky film of bacteria that forms on teeth. More than 300 species of bacteria live under the gum line, and about half a dozen have been linked to serious gum problems. The early stage of gum disease is called **gingivitis.** If untreated, it develops into a more serious form known as **periodontitis,** in which plaque moves down the tooth to the roots, which then become infected. In advanced periodontitis, the infection destroys the bone and fibers that hold teeth in place.

Symptoms of gum disease include bleeding during brushing or flossing, redness and puffiness of gums, tenderness or pain, persistent bad breath or a bad taste in the mouth, receding gums, shifted or loosened teeth, and changes in the way your teeth fit together when you bite. New treatments, which offer an alternative to traditional gum surgery, include a single antibiotic injection or the implant of a small antibiotic chip in the periodontal pockets to promote healing.

Taking care of your mouth isn't important only for dental health: It may affect how long you live. Gingivitis and periodontitis trigger an inflammatory response that causes the arteries to swell, which leads to a constriction of blood flow that can increase the incidence of cardiovascular disease. Periodontal disease also leads to a higher white blood cell count, an indicator that the immune system is under increased stress. The good news: You can prevent these problems by flossing daily and brushing your teeth and your tongue (to get rid of bacteria that can cause gum disease and bad breath).

Many Americans favor dental implants, artificial teeth attached to full or partial dentures, as an option for replacing missing teeth. According to the American Dental Association (ADA), implant procedures nearly tripled in the last ten years. Tooth brighteners also have grown in popularity, but the ADA cautions against over-the-counter whitening products. Safer and more effective are in-office "power" bleaches, in which an oxidizing agent is painted onto the teeth and activated by a special light, and nightguard bleaching, which uses a bleaching gel placed in a custom-made mold and worn at night for about two weeks. Dentists often combine these two approaches. Some dentists are using lasers to whiten teeth, but the ADA has not yet evaluated or endorsed this new approach.

STRATEGIES FOR PREVENTION

Taking Care of Your Mouth

✔ Brush your teeth every morning and every night. Oral bacteria reach their highest count during sleep because fluids in the mouth accumulate. Nighttime cleaning reduces the bacterial population; morning cleaning lets you reduce the buildup.

✔ Use a toothpaste that has the American Dental Association (ADA) seal of acceptance and a toothbrush with soft, rounded bristles. Replace your toothbrush every three months.

✔ Hold the brush at a 45-degree angle from your gums. Pay particular attention to the space between your teeth and gums, especially on the inside, toward your tongue. Brush for two to five minutes. Don't brush too vigorously. If you scrub as hard as you can, you may damage your teeth and gums. Abrasion—a problem for more than half of American adults—erodes tooth surfaces, weakens teeth, and increases sensitivity to hot and cold foods.

✔ Because brushing can't reach plaque and food trapped between teeth, daily flossing is essential. Using waxed or unwaxed floss, start behind the upper and lower molars at one side of your mouth and work toward the other side.

✔ See your dentist twice a year for routine cleaning and examination. To find a dentist, call a local dental school, which may have a public clinic, or check with your county dental society. Ask for information regarding fees, hours, and after-hour emergency service. Your dentist should take a complete medical history from you and update it every six months, examine your mouth for signs of cancer, and thoroughly outline all treatment options.

✔ Make sure that everyone who works on the inside of your mouth wears a mask and rubber gloves to reduce the risk of disease transmission (that is, bacterial and viral infections, such as hepatitis, herpes, and HIV).

✔ Check your family's dental insurance coverage. Many dental plans cover all costs for regular six-month checkups and cleanings and a percentage of the costs for fillings, gum treatment, root canals, and so on.

Your Medical Rights

As a consumer, you have basic rights that help ensure that you know about any potential dangers, receive competent diagnosis and treatment, and retain control and dignity in your interactions with health-care professionals. Many hospitals publish a patient's bill of rights, including your rights to know whether a procedure is experimental; to refuse to undergo a specific treatment; to designate someone else to make decisions about your care if and when you cannot; and to leave the hospital, even against your physician's advice. (See the Self-Survey: "Are You a Savvy Health-Care Consumer?")

You have the right to be treated with respect and dignity, including being called "Mr." or "Ms." or whatever you wish, rather than by your first name. Make clear your preferences. If you feel that health-care professionals are being condescending or inconsiderate, say so—in the same tone and manner that you would like others to use with you. If you're hospitalized, find out if there's a patient advocate or representative at your hospital. These individuals can help you communicate with physicians, make any special arrangements, and get answers to questions or complaints.

You have the right to give consent to donate an organ while alive, or have your organs removed in the event of an accident, injury, or illness that leaves you brain-dead. However, you cannot agree to donate a body part for money or other compensation. Congress has prohibited the marketing of organs; any attempt to do so is a felony punishable by up to five years in jail and a $50,000 fine.

Your Right to Information

By law, a patient must give consent for hospitalization, surgery, and other major treatments. **Informed consent** is a right, not a privilege. Use this right to its fullest. Ask questions. Seek other opinions. Make sure that your expectations are realistic and that you understand the potential risks, as well as the possible benefits, of a prospective treatment. Informed consent is required for research studies, but patients often don't realize that they have the right not to participate and to get complete information on the purpose and nature of the study.

Your Medical Records

You have a right to know what is in your medical records. Some states have laws assuring patient access to records. Consumer advocates advise that you routinely request records from physicians, hospitals, and laboratories—first

SELF SURVEY

Are You a Savvy Health-Care Consumer?

1. You want a second opinion, but your doctor dismisses your request for other physicians' names as unnecessary. Do you:
   a. Assume that he or she is right and you would merely be wasting time
   b. Suspect that your physician has something to hide and immediately switch doctors
   c. Contact your health plan and request a second opinion

2. As soon as you enter your doctor's office, you get tongue-tied. When you try to find the words to describe what's wrong, your physician keeps interrupting. When giving advice, your doctor uses such technical language that you can't understand what it means. Do you:
   a. Prepare better for your next appointment
   b. Pretend that you understand what your doctor is talking about
   c. Decide you'd be better off with someone who specializes in complementary/alternative therapies and seems less intimidating

3. You feel like you're running on empty, tired all the time, worn to the bone. A friend suggests some herbal supplements that promise to boost energy and restore vitality. Do you:
   a. Immediately start taking them
   b. Say that you think herbs are for cooking
   c. Find out as much as you can about the herbal compounds and ask your doctor if they're safe and effective

4. Your hometown physician's office won't give you a copy of your medical records to take with you to college. Do you:
   a. Hope you won't need them and head off without your records
   b. Threaten to sue
   c. Politely ask the office administrator to tell you the particular law or statute that bars you from your records

5. Your doctor has been treating you for an infection for three weeks, and you don't seem to be getting any better. Do you:
   a. Talk to your doctor, by phone or in person, and say, "This doesn't seem to be working. Is there anything else we can try?"

   b. Stop taking the antibiotic
   c. Try an herbal remedy that your roommate recommends

6. Your doctor suggests a cutting-edge treatment for your condition, but your health plan or HMO refuses to pay for it. Do you:
   a. Try to get a loan to cover the costs
   b. Settle for whatever treatment options are covered
   c. Challenge your health plan

7. You call for an appointment with your doctor and are told nothing is available for four months. Do you:
   a. Take whatever time you can get whenever you can get it
   b. Explain your condition to the nurse or receptionist, detailing any symptoms and pain you're experiencing
   c. Give up and decide you don't need to see a doctor at all

8. Even though you've been doing sit-ups faithfully, your waist still looks flabby. When you see an ad for waist-whittling liposuction, do you:
   a. Call for an appointment
   b. Talk to a health-care professional about a total fitness program that may help you lose excess pounds
   c. Carefully research the risks and costs of the procedure

9. You have a condition that you do not want anyone to know about, including your health insurer and any potential employer. Do you:
   a. Use a false name
   b. Give your physician a written request for confidentiality about this condition
   c. Seek help outside the health-care system

10. Your doctor suggests a biopsy of a funny-looking mole that's sprouted on your nose. Rather than using a laboratory that specializes in skin analysis, your HMO requires that all samples be sent to a general lab, where results may not be as precise. Do you:
    a. Ask your doctor to request that a specialty pathologist at the general lab perform the analysis
    b. Hope that in your case, the general lab will do a good-enough job
    c. Threaten to change HMOs

Answers:

1: c; 2: a; 3: c; 4: c; 5: a; 6: c; 7: b; 8: b and c; 9: b; 10: a

verbally, then in writing. Privacy has become an increasing concern as patients' records have been computerized in large databases. The Medical Information Bureau (MIB) (see the Health Almanac for its address and number) obtains information on individuals' medical claims and conditions from about 750 life insurance companies and combines it into the equivalent of a credit report. Anytime you fill out an application for insurance or file a claim for disability or reimbursement, your insurance company or health-care plan can contact MIB to review every medical claim you've made in the previous seven years.

To protect your privacy, don't routinely fill out medical questionnaires or histories. Always ask the purpose and find out who will have access to it. Specifically ask if your history may be entered into a database. Tell your physician or health-care group that you do not want your records to leave their offices without your approval. Put it in writing. When you do have to authorize the release of your records, limit the information to a specific condition, physician, and hospital rather than authorizing release of all your records. Contact the MIB to find out if there is a file on you and ask to review it. Be sure to correct any inaccuracies.

Your Right to Good, Safe, Care

Concern about **malpractice** suits provides an incentive for physicians to provide high-quality care. The essence of a malpractice suit is the claim that the physician failed to meet the standard of care required of a reasonably skilled and careful medical doctor. Although physicians don't have to guarantee good results to their patients and aren't held liable for unavoidable errors, they are required to use the same care and judgment in treatment that other physicians in the same specialty would use under similar circumstances. To protect themselves financially, physicians, particularly those in surgical specialties who are most likely to be sued, pay tens of thousands of dollars a year in malpractice-insurance premiums. Some of this cost is passed on to patients.

Most lawsuits are based on negligence and assert that a physician failed to render diagnosis and treatment with appropriate professional knowledge and skill. Other cases are brought for failure to provide information, obtain consent, or respect a patient's confidentiality. However, analysis of malpractice cases has shown that, in 70 to 80 percent, a doctor's attitude and inability to communicate effectively—by devaluing patients' views, delivering information poorly, failing to understand patients' perspectives, or displaying an air of superiority—also played a role.

The Public Citizen Health Research Group has compiled a national directory of "questionable physicians," which lists physicians disciplined by state medical boards or the federal government for offenses ranging from overprescribing drugs to sexual misconduct to negligent or substandard care. Some of these physicians committed minor misdeeds, such as failing to complete continuing medical education requirements. Consumer advocates urge patients to find out why a particular name appears on the list by calling the state licensing board. At the federal level, the agencies most involved in ensuring quality health care are the Food and Drug Administration (FDA), which approves the production and labeling of drugs; and the

Federal Trade Commission (FTC), which oversees advertising and prohibits deceptive or false claims.

Quackery

Every year millions of Americans go searching for medical miracles that never happen. In all, they spend more than $10 billion on medical **quackery,** unproven health products and services. Those who lose only money are the lucky ones. Many also waste precious time, during which their conditions worsen. Some suffer needless pain, along with crushed expectations. Far too many risk their lives on a false hope—and lose.

The peddlers of such false hopes are quacks, who, by definition, promote for profit worthless or unproven treatments. The Internet has become a popular method for quacks to promote themselves and their wares." Nations have joined together in Operation Cure All, a law enforcement and public education campaign to stop Internet health fraud. It has targeted various devices, herbal prod-

STRATEGIES FOR PREVENTION

Protecting Yourself Against Quackery

✔ Arm yourself with up-to-date information about your condition or disease from appropriate organizations, such as the American Cancer Society or the Arthritis Foundation, which keep track of unproven and ineffective methods of treatment.

✔ Ask for a written explanation of what a treatment does and why it works, evidence supporting all claims (not just testimonials), and published reports of the studies that have been done, including specifics on numbers treated, doses, and side effects. Be skeptical of self-styled "holistic practitioners," treatments supported by crusading groups, and endorsements from self-proclaimed experts or authorities.

✔ Don't part with your money quickly. Be especially careful because insurance companies won't reimburse for unproven therapies.

✔ Don't discontinue your current treatment without your physician's approval. Many physicians encourage supportive therapies—such as relaxation exercises, meditation, or visualization—as a supplement to standard treatments.

ucts, and other dietary supplements purported to treat or cure cancer, AIDS, arthritis, hepatitis, Alzheimer's disease, diabetes, and other chronic conditions.[11]

Sometimes individuals with certain diseases, such as arthritis or multiple sclerosis, who try unproven remedies do indeed improve. "If someone with arthritis starts feeling better the day after getting a copper bracelet, the bracelet will get the credit," says one physician. "Yet it's just coincidence." This is one reason scientists put little stock in enthusiastic testimonials from people who genuinely believe they have been helped by a new drug or treatment. Their heartfelt stories can be persuasive but are scientifically meaningless. The satisfied patient may not actually have had the disease in the first place, may have gotten other treatments too, or may be responding to a remedy that masks the symptoms without treating the disease.

Complementary and Alternative Medicine

The last decade has seen an enormous increase in the use of a broad range of therapies sometimes called alternative, unconventional, or holistic. The medical research community uses the term **complementary and alternative medicine (CAM)** to apply to all health-care approaches, practices, and treatments not widely taught in medical schools, not generally used in hospitals, and not usually reimbursed by medical insurance companies.[12]

CAM includes many healing philosophies, approaches, and therapies, including preventive techniques designed to delay or prevent serious health problems before they start and **holistic** methods that focus on the whole person and the physical, mental, emotional, and spiritual aspects of well-being. Some approaches are based on the same physiological principles as traditional Western methods; others, such as acupuncture, are based on different healing systems.

According to national surveys, 40 to 45 percent of Americans say they have tried at least one nontraditional treatment.[13] Americans make more visits (an estimated 629 million) to alternative practitioners than they do to primary care physicians and spend about as much in annual out-of-pocket expenditures, including money for practitioners, herbal remedies, megavitamins, diet products, and books, classes, and equipment. Most people use CAM along with their traditional medical care.[14]

Integrative medicine, which combines selected elements of both conventional and alternative medicine in a comprehensive approach to diagnosis and treatment, is gaining greater acceptance within the medical community.[15] Approximately 1,500 articles on CAM are published annually in medical literature; recent international surveys found that the prevalence of CAM use ranges from

9 percent to 65 percent.[16] More medical schools are teaching courses in CAM, and more than 60 percent of physicians say they've recommended alternative therapies to their patients at least once in the preceding year.[17] More than two-thirds of health maintenance organizations cover at least one form of CAM, but the majority of people pay with their own funds.[18]

Why People Use Complementary and Alternative Therapies

People seek out CAM for various reasons, including dissatisfaction with or skepticism about conventional medicine and a desire for greater personal control over their health. Many see alternative therapies as more compatible with their worldview regarding nature and the meaning of health and illness. People who use CAM tend to have more education, an interest in personal and spiritual growth, and a belief that body, mind, and spirit are all involved in health.[19] Compared to those who don't use CAM, users often report poorer health and see alternative health care as more in tune with their own values, beliefs, and philosophies about life. The main benefit they report is relief from symptoms of an illness.[20]

An estimated 10 to 50 percent of cancer patients try alternative treatments, many without their physicians' knowledge.[21] The American Cancer Society and the National Cancer Institute are supporting research into various alternative approaches in cancer care, such as the use of vitamin A derivatives, green tea, melatonin, shark cartilage, and detoxification with coffee enemas.[22]

Cancer patients seek out alternatives as way of taking an active role in their treatment and to be sure that "everything possible is being done," according to one survey. In one study of prostate cancer patients, 37 percent of those undergoing treatment with conventional therapies also turn to one or more complementary practices.[23] Other research suggests that cancer patients in the greatest emotional distress may seek out alternative treatments. For example, women who tried alternative as well as convetional treatments for early-stage breast cancer tended to have more depression, greater fear of recurrence, and less robust mental health.[24]

Many have criticized health-care providers for giving alternative therapies "a free ride" by not demanding the same proof and regulation required of traditional treatments.[25] Under current FDA regulations, testing required for natural health products is the same as required for food, not drugs, which allows them to be marketed without proof of purity, standardization of ingredients, or proof of medicinal efficacy.

Many doctors are calling upon their colleagues not to dismiss or embrace CAM but to consider each approach thoroughly and evaluate its potential to benefit patients.

"In the future, the terms *alternative* and *complementary* may well be passé, and research will have integrated what works into our everyday practices," one primary care physician observes. "Then we won't have to draw a line in the sand, saying that one treatment is **allopathic** or **osteopathic** and another is alternative."

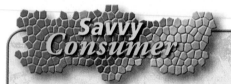

Is Alternative Medicine Effective?

The National Center for Complementary and Alternative Medicine (NCCAM), part of NIH, conducts and supports studies using the same rigorous standards applied to conventional medicine and disseminates information to patients and health-care consumers. Its three goals are evaluating the safety and efficacy of natural products, supporting their scientific study, and evaluating the practices that implement them. Its budget has grown dramatically, jumping from $2 million 1993 to $68.7 million in 2000.[21] Current studies are investigating shark cartilage as a cancer treatment, St. John's wort for depression, and a complex nutritional approach to pancreatic cancer.

As studies are conducted, some alternative therapies are gaining acceptance, while others have shown little or no demonstrable benefits. (See Savvy Consumer: "Evaluating

---

Savvy Consumer

Evaluating Complementary and Alternative Medicine

You should never decide on any treatment—traditional or complementary/alternative medicine (CAM)—without fully evaluating it. Here are some key questions to ask:

- **Is it safe?** The fact that a substance is "natural" or that a treatment does not require hospitalization or surgery doesn't mean it is safe. Talk to your medical doctor so you understand any particular risks to your overall health or any unknown long-term effects. Be particularly wary of unregulated products.

- **Is it effective?** We know far less about the efficacy of many alternative treatments than we do about traditional therapies. You can obtain information on what is known about the effectiveness of specific treatments from the NCCAM through its website and information clearinghouse (http://nccam.nih.gov).

- **Will it interact with other medicines or conventional treatments?** This is an important question to discuss with your doctor and to investigate by doing research online or in the library. Some combinations—such as the use of a prescription sleeping pill and sleep-inducing melatonin—can be dangerous, and some herbal remedies can interfere with hypertension drugs and increase the risks of anesthesia. Many widely used alternative remedies can interact with prescription medications in dangerous ways.

- **Is the practitioner qualified?** Many states license practitioners who provide acupuncture, chiropractic services, naturopathy, herbal medicine, homeopathy, and other treatments. Find out if yours does, and always choose a licensed professional. You also can contact medical regulatory agencies and consumer affairs departments, which provide information about a specific practitioner's license, education, and accreditation and will let you know if any complaints have been filed against him or her. Many organizations of specific types of practitioners have websites. However, remember that they are presenting information from an advocate's point of view.

- **What has been the experience of others?** Talk to people who have used CAM for a similar problem, both recently and in the past. Keep in mind that their perspectives—positive or negative—are subjective and should not be your only criterion for selecting a therapy. Also try to find people who have been cared for by the practitioner you are considering.

- **Can you talk openly and easily with the practitioner?** Your relationship with your CAM practitioner is as important as your relationship with your medical doctor. You should feel comfortable asking questions and confident in the answers you receive. What is his or her educational background, principles, and beliefs?

- **Are you comfortable with the CAM care setting?** Visit the practitioner's office, clinic, or hospital. Does it put you at ease or make you feel out-of-place or anxious? How do conditions such as cleanliness and staff professionalism compare with the health-care settings you are more familiar with? Find out how many clients a practitioner sees every week and how much time is spent with each one.

- **What are the costs?** Many CAM services are not covered by HMOs or health insurers. Find out if your plan will cover any treatments. Also check what other practitioners charge for the same service so you can decide if a fee is appropriate. Regulatory agencies and professional associations often provide cost information.

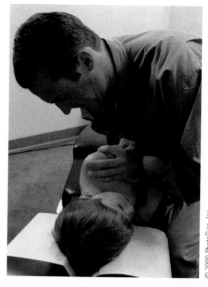

Complementary and Alternative Medicine.") Among the forms of CAM that have proven effective are:

▶ Moxibustion (burning of Chinese herbs) directly over a specific acupuncture point to help breech fetuses turn around in the womb.

▶ Chinese herbs for irritable bowel syndrome. Chinese herbs (including dang shen, huo xiang and wu wei zi) proved more effective than placebo in relieving diarrhea, abdominal pain, and other symptoms.

▶ Saw palmetto for enlarged prostate gland. In 18 studies with a total sample size of nearly 3,000 patients, men with benign prostatic hyperplasia who took this herbal remedy were twice as likely to report improvement as those taking a placebo.[27]

NCCAM has classified CAM practices into five categories (see Table 10-4). The three most widely used approaches are chiropractic, herbal medicine, and acupuncture.

▲ A chiropractor can help relieve lower-back pain.

Chiropractic

Chiropractic is a treatment method based on the theory that many human diseases are caused by misalignment of the bones (subluxation). Chiropractors are licensed in all 50 states, but chiropractic is considered a mainstream therapy by some and a form of CAM by others. Significant research in the last ten years has demonstrated its efficacy for acute lower-back pain. NIH is funding research on other potential benefits, including headaches, asthma, middle ear inflammation, menstrual cramps, and arthritis.

Chiropractors, who emphasize wellness and healing without drugs or surgery, may use X rays and magnetic

▼ **Table 10-4 Complementary and Alternative Medicine Practices**

The National Center for Complementary and Alternative Medicine (NCCAM) developed the following classifications.

1. Alternative Medical Systems
These include acupuncture, Oriental medicine, tai chi, external and internal Qi, Ayurvedic medicine, naturopathy, and unconventional Western systems, such as homeopathy and orthomolecular medicine.

2. Mind-Body Interventions
These approaches include many behavioral medicine techniques, such as journaling, as well as hypnosis, yoga, meditation, biofeedback, imagery, music, art and dance therapy, spiritual healing, and community-based approaches (for example, Alcoholics Anonymous and Native American sweat rituals).

3. Biologically Based Therapies
These include botanical medicine or phytotherapy, the use of individual herbs or combinations; special diet therapies, such as macrobiotics, Ornish, McDougall, and high fiber; Mediterranean orthomolecular medicine (use of nutritional and food supplements for preventive or therapeutic purposes); and use of other products (such as shark cartilage) and procedures applied in an unconventional manner not covered in other categories.

4. Manipulative and Body-Based Methods
These are systems based on manipulation and/or movement of the body, divided into three subcategories: chiropractic medicine; massage and body work (including osteopathic manipulation, Swedish massage, Alexander technique, reflexology, Pilates, acupressure, and rolfing); and unconventional physical therapies (including colonics, hydrotherapy, and light and color therapies).

5. Energy Therapies
These therapies focus either on energy fields originating within the body (biofields) or those from other sources (electromagnetic fields). Biofields include therapeutic touch, SHEN, and biorelax methods.

Source: NCCAM. For more information on complementary/alternative treatment, visit http://nccam.nih.gov

resonance imaging (MRI) as well as orthopedic, neurological, and manual examinations in making diagnoses. However, chiropractic treatment consists solely of the manipulation of misaligned bones that may be putting pressure on nerve tissue and affecting other parts of the body. Many HMOs offer chiropractic services, which are the most widely used alternative treatment among managed care patients.

Herbal or Botanical Medicine

About one in three Americans has tried an herbal remedy at least once.[28] In the last decade the market for **herbal** or botanical **medicines** has grown to an estimated $12 billion.[29]

Herbal medicines can pose serious risks, particularly when taken along with prescription medications. St. John's wort affects the action of drugs like the anticlotting agent warfarin (Coumadin). When taken with dextromethrophan, an ingredient in cough syrup, St. John's wort can cause serotonin syndrome, a potentially fatal condition characterized by rapid pulse, high fever, and convulsions. Ginkgo biloba and ginseng also interact with warfarin; kava, with sedatives and other agents. Because of the potential of dangerous interactions, you should always tell your doctor if you're taking an alternative medicine.

Even when used alone, herbs and natural substances, just like synthetic drugs, can have side effects and risks. (See Table 10-5.) Some users experience allergic reactions.

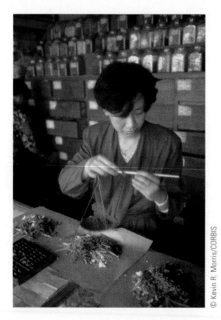

▲ Herbal medicines are a popular form of alternative medicine.

Recent studies have connected some herbs, including St. John's wort, echinacea, and ginkgo, with blocking contraception and, in other cases, with infertility. St. John's wort has also been linked to high blood pressure. Echinacea, used for fighting off cold and flu symptoms, may exacerbate autoimmune disorders, such as lupus, rheumatoid arthritis, and multiple sclerosis. There also are suggestions of genetic damage to sperm with several popular herbs.

Unlike over-the-counter and prescription drugs, "natural" remedies have not been subject to rigorous testing. The FDA categorizes herbs as "dietary supplements," which are not subject to the same efficacy and safety trials that all new drugs must undergo. Under the provisions of the 1994 Dietary Supplement Health and Education Act, herbal medicine manufacturers can advertise the supposed benefits of their wares as long as they don't claim that the products affect a specific illness.

Some botanicals used for weight loss are particularly dangerous. When a Belgian weight loss clinic using a combination of appetite suppressants and Chinese herbs switched to an herb containing aristolochic acid, dozens of patients suffered kidney failure. Belgian researchers have since found that the clinic's patients have high rates of cancer of the lining of the bladder and ureter.[30] The amphetamine-like herb called ephedra, or Ma huang, sold as an energy booster and weight loss aid, can cause dangerous rises in blood pressure and speed up the heart rate. More than 800 injuries and 17 deaths have been linked to this herb.[31] The FDA has proposed a limit on the amount of ephedra that can be added to supplements and has issued warnings on other potentially dangerous herbs, including chaparral, comfrey, yohimbe, *Lobelia*, germander, willow bark, jin bu huan, and products containing magnolia or *Stephania*.

Another problem with using herbal preparations wisely is that potency varies greatly, depending on the form in which they're used. The U.S. Pharmacopeia, a nonprofit organization that sets strength and purity standards for prescription and over-the-counter drugs, has published standards for some popular botanicals. Those that meet these standards have "NF" (National Formulary) on the package. The FDA also now requires a "supplements facts" panel on the label, similar to the nutritional facts panel on most foods. It contains information on which part of the plant was used to make the product and how much is an appropriate amount to use.

The American Dietetic Association has called for further study of a number of dietary alternative treatments, including St. John's wort and SAM-e (discussed in Chapter 3).[32] In a scientifically rigorous study of two hundred patients with major depression, St. John's wort did not prove effective. Using various measures to gauge the severity of depression, the researchers found almost no

▼ **Table 10-5 Popular Herbal Remedies**

Herb	Used For	Does It Work?	Warning
Acidophilus	Diarrhea, digestive problems, upset stomach, or yeast infections caused by use of antibiotics	Acidophilus, either in live lactobacillus acidophilus cultures in yogurt or in capsules, can restore the body's normal bacterial balance.	Refrigerate to preserve potency.
Aloe vera	Sunburn, cuts, burns, eczema, psoriasis	In studies on both humans and animals, aloe vera applied directly to the skin has been shown to speed healing and have antibacterial, anti-inflammatory, and mild anesthetic effects.	Refrigerate gel to extend its shelf life.
Chamomile	Relaxation, better sleep, stomach aches, menstrual cramps	Laboratory and animal studies indicate that chamomile's active compounds have properties that combat inflammation, bacterial infection, and spasms.	People allergic to plants in the daisy family, such as ragweed, may have an allergic reaction.
Echinacea	Colds and flu	Inconsistent findings, although one study found that flu sufferers who used echinacea extract recovered more quickly than others.	Use for more than eight weeks at a time may lessen its effectiveness and suppress immunity. Should not be taken by pregnant women and those with diabetes, tuberculosis, or autoimmune disorders.
Evening primrose oil	PMS, endometriosis, eczema	Although at least one clinical trial found that evening primrose oil does relieve endometriosis symptoms, the research on its effects on PMS and eczema has been inconclusive.	Some users report nausea or headache.
Garlic	Fighting infection, preventing heart disease and cancer, stimulating the immune system	Extensive laboratory and animal studies and a review of clinical trials have shown that the active ingredient in garlic has anti-infective and anti-tumor properties and lowers cholesterol.	Check with your doctor if you take blood-thinning medication, including aspirin or ibuprofen, because garlic also is an anticoagulant.
Ginkgo biloba	Improving memory, cognition, and circulation	There is some evidence that ginkgo biloba can help stabilize mental deterioration in patients with early Alzheimer's disease or stroke-related dementia. One study found that healthy seniors who took ginkgo performed mental tasks better.	Do not take with aspirin because of risk of excessive bleeding. Should not be used during pregnancy. Side effects include upset stomach, headache, and an allergic skin reaction.
Ginseng	Improving mental and physical energy and stamina	Small studies have shown that ginseng can help improve mental performance and respiratory function during exercise.	If used for more than two weeks, ginseng can cause nervousness and heart palpitations, especially in those with high blood pressure.
Goldenseal	Colds, allergies, upper respiratory tract infections	Little research has been done, but some laboratory and animal studies suggest that one of goldenseal's components may have some antibiotic and antihistamine effects.	Goldsenseal should not be used instead of traditional antibiotics and should never be used for more than ten days at a time. Long-term use may interfere with the normal bacterial balance in the digestive system.

significant differences between those taking St. John's wort and those taking sugar pills during an eight-week period.[33] A second major clinical trial of St. John's wort, comparing it to both a placebo and a conventional antidepressant, is in progress.

Acupuncture

An ancient Chinese form of medicine, **acupuncture** is based on the philosophy that a cycle of energy circulating through the body controls health. Pain and disease are the result of a disturbance in the energy flow, which can be corrected by inserting long, thin needles at specific points along longitudinal lines, or *meridians,* throughout the body. Each point controls a different corresponding part of the body. Once inserted, the needles are rotated gently back and forth or charged with a small electric current for a short time. Western scientists aren't sure exactly how acupuncture works, but some believe that the needles alter the functioning of the nervous system.

In *acupressure,* the therapist uses his or her finger and thumb to stimulate certain points, relieve pain, and relax muscles. **Reflexology** is based on the theory that massaging certain points on the foot or hand relieves stress or pain in corresponding parts of the body. These methods seem most effective in easing chronic pain, arthritis, and withdrawal from nicotine, alcohol, or drugs.

An NIH consensus development panel that evaluated current research into acupuncture concluded that there is "clear evidence" that acupuncture can control nausea and vomiting in patients after surgery or while undergoing chemotherapy and relieve postoperative dental pain. The panel said that acupuncture is "probably" also effective in the control of nausea in early pregnancy and that there were "reasonable" studies, some using "sham" needles that make it more difficult for patients to know if they are or are not undergoing acupuncture,[34] showing that the use of acupuncture, by itself or as an adjunct to other therapies, resulted in satisfactory treatment of a number of other conditions, even though there was not "firm evidence of efficacy at this time." These conditions include addiction to illicit drugs and alcohol (but not to tobacco), stroke rehabilitation, headache, menstrual cramps, tennis elbow, general muscle pain, low back pain, carpal tunnel syndrome, and asthma. Ongoing studies are evaluating its efficacy for chronic headaches and migraines.

Other Alternative Treatments

Considered alternative here, **ayurveda** is a traditional form of medical treatment in India, where it has evolved over thousands of years. Its basic premise is that illness stems from incorrect mental attitudes, diet, and posture. Practitioners use a discipline of exercise, meditation, herbal medication, and proper nutrition to cope with such stress-induced conditions as hypertension, the desire to smoke, and obesity. The best known advocate of ayurvedic medicine is Deepak Chopra, M.D., an endocrinologist (specialist in hormone-related disorders) who has written several books on ayurveda and the intimate relationship between consciousness and health.

Biofeedback uses machines that measure temperature or skin responses and then relays this information to the subject. In this way, people can learn to control usually involuntary functions, such as circulation to the hands and feet, tension in the jaws, and heartbeat rates. Biofeedback has been used to treat dozens of ailments, including asthma, epilepsy, pain, and Reynaud's disease (a condition in which the fingers become painful and white when exposed to cold). Many health insurers now cover biofeedback treatments.

Homeopathy is based on three fundamental principles: "like cures like"; treatment must always be individualized; and less is more—the idea that increasing dilution (and lowering the dosage) can increase efficacy. By administering doses of animal, vegetable, or mineral substances to a large number of healthy people to see if they all develop the same symptoms, homeopaths determine which substances may be given, in small quantities, to alleviate the symptoms. Some of these substances are the same as those used in conventional medicine: nitroglycerin for certain heart conditions, for example, although the dose is minuscule.

Naturopathy emphasizes natural remedies, such as sun, water, heat, and air, as the best treatments for disease. Therapies might include dietary changes (such as more

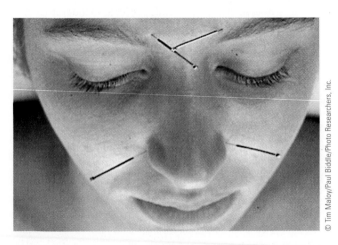

© Tim Maloy/Paul Biddle/Photo Researchers, Inc.

▲ The ancient Chinese practice of acupuncture produces healing through the insertion and manipulation of needles at specific points throughout the body. The procedure is not painful.

vegetables and no salt or stimulants), steam baths, and exercise. Some naturopathic physicians (who are not M.D.s) work closely with medical doctors in helping patients.

Carl Simonton, M.D., a cancer specialist, developed the technique of creative **visualization,** or imaging, to help heal cancer patients, including some diagnosed as terminally ill. On the premise that positive and negative beliefs and attitudes have a great deal to do with whether people get well or die of disease, patients imagine themselves getting well—they "see," for instance, their immune-system cells marching to conquer the cancer cells. Others use visualization in different ways—for example, to create a clear idea of what they want to achieve, whether the goal is weight loss or relaxation.

Massage therapy involves the use of the hands to rub, stroke, or knead the body to "positively affect the health and well being of the individual." Some states have created licensing statutes for massage therapy; others allow local jurisdictions to regulate massage professionals.[35]

The Health-Care System

In the past, getting health care was fairly simple. When people were sick, they went to their family physician and paid in cash. If they didn't have enough money, the physician would still provide care. Today health care involves many more people, places, and processes. As a college student, you can turn to the student health service if you get sick. There, a nurse, nurse practitioner, physician's assistant, or medical doctor may evaluate your symptoms and provide basic care. However, you may rely on a primary care physician in your hometown to perform regular checkups or manage a chronic condition like asthma. If you're injured in an accident, you probably will be treated at the nearest emergency room. If you become seriously ill and require highly specialized care, you may have to go to a university-affiliated medical center to receive a state-of-the-art treatment.

Health-Care Practitioners

Fewer than 10 percent of health-care practitioners are physicians; other types of health professionals are assuming more important roles in delivering primary, or basic, health services. As a consumer, you should be aware of the range and special skills of the most common types of health-care providers.

Physicians

A medical doctor (M.D.) trained in American medical schools usually takes at least three years of premedical col-

lege courses (with an emphasis on biology, chemistry, and physics) and then completes four (but sometimes three or five) years of medical school. The first two years of medical school are devoted to the study of human anatomy, embryology, pharmacology, and similar basic subjects. During the last two years, students work directly with physicians in hospitals. Medical students who pass a series of national board examinations then enter a one-year internship in a hospital, followed by another two to five years of residency (depending on their specialty), which leads to certification in a particular field, or specialty.

About 500,000 of the nation's 700,000 physicians are specialists or subspecialists, who focus on a specific part of the body, organ system, type of disease, or type of treatment. Traditionally, they have had greater status and earned much larger incomes than primary care physicians—family practitioners, pediatricians, and internists—who provide preventive care, regular checkups, and routine treatments of uncomplicated medical conditions. However, in recent years, changes in health policy (such as increases in Medicare payments to primary care physicians) and in the delivery of services have given a more prominent role to primary care physicians. They now often function as "gatekeepers" who decide whether a patient needs to see a medical specialist.

Nurses

A registered nurse (R.N.) graduates from a school of nursing approved by a state board and passes a state board examination. R.N.s may have a bachelor's or an associate degree and may specialize in certain areas, such as intensive care or nurse-midwifery. Nurse practitioners, R.N.s with advanced training and experience, may run community clinics or provide screening and preventive care at group medical practices. Some have independent practices.

Licensed practical nurses (L.P.N.s), also called licensed vocational nurses, are licensed by the state. After graduating from state-approved schools of practical nursing, they must take a board exam. They work under the supervision of R.N.s or physicians. Nursing aides and orderlies assist registered and practical nurses in providing services directly related to the comfort and well-being of hospitalized patients.

Specialized and Allied-Health Practitioners

More than 60 types of health practitioners work with physicians and nurses in providing medical services. Some, such as *occupational therapists,* have at least a bachelor's degree. Allied-health professionals may specialize in a variety of fields. *Clinical psychologists* have graduate degrees and provide a wide range of mental health services but don't prescribe medications—as do *psychiatrists. Optometrists,* trained in special schools of optometry, diagnose visual abnormalities and prescribe lenses or visual aids; however, they don't prescribe drugs, diagnose or treat eye diseases, or perform surgery—functions performed by *ophthalmologists. Podiatrists* are specially trained, licensed health-care professionals who specialize in problems of the feet.

Dentists

Most dental students earn a bachelor's degree and then complete two more years of training in the basic sciences and two years of clinical work before graduating with a degree of D.D.S. or D.M.D. (Doctor of Dental Surgery or Doctor of Medical Dentistry). To qualify for a license, graduates must pass both a written and a clinical examination. Dentists may work in general practice or choose a specialty, such as *orthodontics* (straightening teeth).

Chiropractors

Chiropractors hold the degree of Doctor of Chiropractic (D.C.), which signifies that they have had two years of college-level training, plus four years in a health-care school specializing in chiropractic, described earlier in this chapter.

Health-Care Facilities

As a prospective patient, you can choose from various options: a physician's office, a clinic, an emergency room, or a hospital. Most **primary care**—also referred to as ambulatory or outpatient care—is provided by a physician in an office, emergency room, or clinic. *Secondary care* usually is provided by specialists or subspecialists in either an outpatient or inpatient (hospital) setting. *Tertiary care,* available at university-affiliated hospitals and regional referral centers, includes special procedures such as kidney dialysis, open-heart surgery, and organ transplants.

College Health Centers

 The American College Health Association estimates that 1,500 institutions of higher learning provide direct health services. Student health centers range in size from small dispensaries staffed by nurses to large-scale, multi-specialty clinics that provide both inpatient and outpatient care and are fully accredited by the Joint Commission on Accreditation of Healthcare Organizations. Some serve only students; others provide services for faculty, staff, and family members.

On some campuses, health educators work with the student health centers to provide counseling on such topics as nutrition; tobacco, drug, and alcohol abuse; exercise and fitness; sexuality; and contraception. Some college health centers provide psychological counseling, as well as dental, pharmacy, and optometric services. Some campuses also provide sports-medicine services for student athletes. Services are paid for by various combinations of prepaid health fees, general university funds, fee-for-service charges, and health-insurance reimbursements.

Outpatient Treatment Centers

Increasingly, procedures that once required hospitalization, such as simple surgery, are being performed at outpatient centers, which may be freestanding or affiliated with a medical center. Patients have any necessary tests performed beforehand, undergo surgery or receive treatment, and return home after a few hours to recuperate. Outpatient centers can handle many common surgical procedures, including cataract removal, tonsillectomy, breast biopsy, dilation and curettage (D and C), vasectomy, and face-lifts.

Without the high overhead costs of a hospital, outpatient surgery costs run only about 30 to 50 percent of standard hospital fees. Today, 70 percent of hospitals do outpatient, or "in-and-out," surgery. To cut health-care costs, insurance companies are encouraging, or in some cases requiring, their policyholders to choose outpatient surgery. However, operations requiring prolonged general anesthesia or extensive postoperative care must still be performed on an inpatient basis.

Freestanding emergency centers (those not part of a hospital) claim that they deliver high-quality medical treatment with maximum convenience in minimal time. Critics dismiss them as impersonal and mechanized, and refer to them as "Big Mac" medicine. Nevertheless, many customers seem pleased. Rather than going to crowded hospital emergency rooms when they slice a finger in the kitchen, they can go to a freestanding emergency center and receive prompt attention.

Hospitals and Medical Centers

Different types of hospitals offer different types of care. The most common type of hospital is the *private,* or community, *hospital,* which may be run on a profit or a non-profit basis, generally contains 50 to 400 beds, and provides more personalized care than public hospitals do. The quality of care individual patients receive depends mostly on the physicians themselves. Public *hospitals* include city, county, public health service, military, and Veterans Administration hospitals. The quality of patient care depends on the overall quality of the institution.

Of the more than 6,500 hospitals nationwide, about 300 are major *academic medical centers* or teaching hospitals. Affiliated with medical schools, they generally provide the most up-to-date and experienced care, because staff physicians must stay current in order to teach their students. These centers, with the best equipment, researchers, and resources, offer high-technology care—at a price. The cost of treatment at all teaching hospitals averages approximately 20 percent higher than at nonteaching hospitals. At major teaching hospitals with large graduate training programs for physicians and other health providers, the costs are as much as 45 percent higher than those at nonteaching hospitals. Faced with declining revenues as a result of the advent of managed care (discussed later in this chapter), teaching hospitals have been forced to make major cutbacks in personnel and patient services. Many are forming networks with other hospitals and developing less costly methods (such as home health services) to deliver health care.

The Joint Commission on the Accreditation of Healthcare Organizations (JCAH) reviews all hospitals every three years. Eighty percent of hospitals qualify for JCAH accreditation. If you have to enter a hospital and your health insurance or plan allows a choice, try to find out as much as you can about the alternatives available to you:

▶ Talk to your physician about a hospital and why he or she recommends it.

▶ As a cost-cutting strategy, many hospitals have cut back on the use of registered nurses. Check with the local nursing association about the ratio of patients to nurses, and the ratio of R.N.s to licensed practical, or vocational, nurses.

▶ Find out room rates and charges for ancillary services, including tests, lab work, X rays, and medications. Check with your health plan to see whether you need preapproval for any of these costs and ask what you will be expected to pay.

▶ Ask how many times in the past year the hospital has performed the procedure recommended for you, and what the success and complication rates have been. Ask about the hospital's nosocomial (hospital-caused) infection rate and accident rate. You also have the right to information on the number and types of malpractice claims filed against a hospital.

▶ If possible, go on a tour of the hospital. Does the setting seem comfortable? Is the staff courteous? Does the hospital seem clean and efficiently run?

Emergency Services. Hospital emergency rooms should be used only in a true emergency. Most are overwhelmed, understaffed, and underfinanced—particularly in big cities. Patients usually see a different physician each time; he or she deals with their main complaints but doesn't have time for a full examination. Extensive tests and procedures are difficult to arrange in an emergency room, and patients who don't have truly urgent problems may have to wait for a long time. Emergency-room fees are higher than those for standard office visits and are not always covered by medical insurance.

Inpatient Care. Inpatient hospital care remains the most expensive form of health care. Health-insurance companies and health-care plans (described below) often demand a second opinion or make their own evaluation before approving coverage of an elective, or nonemergency, hospital admission. As another means of controlling costs, health insurers (including Medicare) may limit hospital stays or pay for hospital care on the basis of **diagnostic-related groups, or DRGs.** Under this system, hospitals are paid according to a patient's diagnosis—for example, a set number of dollars for every appendectomy. If the hospital can treat and discharge patients more quickly than the national average for that DRG, it makes money. On the other hand, if a patient develops unexpected complications or is slow to recover, the hospital loses money.

Because hospital stays are shorter than in the past, patients often leave "quicker and sicker"—after a shorter stay and not as far along in their recovery. Nevertheless, the benefits of shorter hospital stays, including reduced complications and more rapid resumption of normal life activities, may outweigh the slightly increased risks associated with early discharge.

The Risks of a Hospital Stay

Hospitals are places where lives are both saved and lost, and the quality of care varies greatly. Large hospitals in big cities tend to provide better care and have lower death rates than small, rural hospitals with fewer than 100 beds.

The risks associated with hospitalization include what health workers call the "terrible I's": infection; inactivity; incorrect actions; and the inherent risks of drugs, X rays, and false lab tests. The simplest method for preventing hospital-acquired infection—handwashing—is often ignored by health-care providers.

Surgical and medication mistakes are another hazard. In highly publicized cases, hospital physicians have amputated a patient's healthy leg, operated on the wrong side of a woman's brain, and administered deadly doses of cancer drugs. As hospitals cut back on staff and services in order to control costs, the likelihood of such errors may increase. In a recent survey conducted by the Robert Wood Johnson Foundation, 95 percent of physicians and 89 percent of nurses said they had witnessed a serious medical error.[36]

Home Health Care

With hospitals discharging patients sooner, **home health care**—the provision of equipment and services to patients in the home to restore or maintain comfort, function, and health—has become a major industry. Advances in technology have made it possible for treatments once administered only in hospitals—such as kidney dialysis, chemotherapy, and traction—to be performed at home at 10 to 40 percent of the cost. The physician's house call, once considered an anachronism, has also come back in fashion. According to various surveys, the majority of primary care physicians see patients in their homes.

Hospital discharge planners usually arrange home health care for patients who've been hospitalized. Families can also contact health aides, nurses, and other needed professionals on their own. According to the Health Insurance Association of America, most private insurance policies offer some coverage for these home health-care costs.

Paying for Health Care

Health insurance did not become common as a standard benefit until World War II, when the government imposed wage controls and businesses offered free health-insurance policies to lure prospective employees. For the next 50 years, patients went to the physicians of their choice, with insurance companies usually paying part or all of their fees.

As technological breakthroughs, such as new imaging techniques and bone-marrow transplants, transformed modern medicine, subspecialists multiplied, and medical costs spiraled upward. Finally, in the 1990s, health policymakers and the employers that had footed the bills agreed that health costs, which had grown to almost 14 percent of the gross domestic product, had to be controlled. This led to the emergence of **managed care,** a new way of delivering and paying for health-care services. Managed-care organizations provide health-care or health-care insurance at lower costs to employers. The tradeoff for such savings is that a third party makes the final decision on when or if a medical visit or treatment is necessary. This differs from traditional *fee-for-service* medicine, in which patients decide when to seek care and choose which physician to see.

Both fee-for-service and managed-care systems have drawbacks. Fee-for-service medicine errs on the side of doing too much and providing unneeded tests and therapies. Managed-care organizations are more likely to do too little so they can keep costs low.

Traditional Health Insurance

In the past, most working Americans relied on conventional **indemnity** insurance policies to pay major medical expenses. Policyholders paid a percentage (generally 20 percent) of hospitalization costs and a deductible (a minimum paid out each year before the insurance company pays anything). While indemnity insurance gave patients

freedom to choose physicians and hospitals, it often failed to cover routine physical exams and screening tests. Individuals with "preexisting" conditions often could not qualify for coverage or were not reimbursed for treatments related to these conditions. In the last decade, as health-care costs skyrocketed, insurers increasingly refused to pay claims, canceled groups with high medical bills, or denied coverage to people in high-risk occupations.

???? What Is Managed Care?

Managed care has become the predominant form of health care in the United States. More than 180 million Americans are enrolled in managed care.[37] Managed-care organizations, which take various forms, deliver care through a network of physicians, hospitals, and other health-care professionals who agree to provide their services at fixed or discounted rates.

Consumers in a managed-care group must follow certain procedures in advance of seeking care (for example, getting prior approval for a test or treatment) and must abide by a limit on reimbursement for certain services. Some procedures may be deemed unnecessary and not be covered at all. Patients who choose to see a physician who is not a participating member of the medical-insurance coverage group may have to pay the entire fee themselves.

Managed-care plans have been criticized for pressuring providers to "undertreat" patients—for example, sending them home from the hospital too soon or denying them costly tests or treatments. Members have complained of long waits, the need to switch primary physicians if their doctor leaves the plan, difficulty getting approval for needed services, and a sense that providers pay more attention to the bottom line than to their health needs.

As dissatisfaction with managed care has grown, consumers have demanded more choice of physicians, direct access to specialists, and the ability to go "out of network." In response to patients' complaints, many states have approved "patient protection acts" or "comprehensive consumer bills of rights." Federal legislators also have debated a national patients' bill of rights for years, but have disagreed over controversial provisions, such as allowing patients to sue their insurers or employers in either state or federal courts if they feel their rights have been violated.[38]

State bills generally have tried to ensure that patients get the care they need when they need it with provisions such as the following:

- Allow any pharmacy to provide medications for enrollees.
- Ban any limit on doctors' ability to inform patients of treatment options, especially if some choices cost more.
- Outlaw rewards to physicians for performing a less costly procedure or prescribing a less costly drug.

▶ Guarantee direct access to women's health specialist without referral from a primary care provider.

▶ Ensure a minimum 48-hour maternity stay.

▶ Establish a "prudent layperson" standard for emergencies. This requires insurance coverage for emergency medical conditions if they are of sufficient severity, in a nonprofessional's judgment, to place the person's health in jeopardy

▶ Require annual report cards on how well plans are complying with state laws and regulations.

Health Maintenance Organizations (HMOs)

Health maintenance organizations, or **HMOs,** are managed-care plans that emphasize routine care and prevention by providing complete medical services in exchange for a predetermined monthly payment. In a *group-model* HMO, physicians provide care in offices at a clinic run by the HMO. In an *individual practice association (IPA),* or network HMO, independent physicians provide services in their own offices. HMOs generally pay a fixed amount per patient to a physician or hospital, regardless of the type and number of services actually provided. This is called *capitation.*[39]

Members of HMOs pay a regular, preset fee that usually includes diagnostic tests, routine physical exams, and vaccinations as well as treatment of illnesses. HMOs usually do not require a deductible, and copayments for medications or services are small. The primary drawback of standard HMOs is that the consumer is limited to a particular health-care facility and staff. Open-ended or point-of-service HMOs charge more but let members seek treatment elsewhere if they prefer. These "hybrid" plans have proven the most popular. Although some large HMOs have earned profits, the HMO industry as a whole consistently lost money in the last decade. Enrollment in HMOs rose steadily in the early 1990s but has declined in more recent years. The total number of HMOs also has dropped.[40]

Although HMOs have been accused of undermining the quality of patient care, recent studies of the outcomes of cancer patients in HMOs and in traditional fee-for-service practices have found little difference. HMOs are, on average, more likely to detect breast cancer early and just as likely to offer breast-saving lumpectomies rather than mastectomy. Prostate cancer patients treated in HMOs also had similar ten-year survival rates as those receiving fee-for-service care.

Preferred Provider Organizations (PPOs)

In a **preferred provider organization (PPO),** a third party—a union, an insurance company, or a self-insured business—contracts with a group of physicians and hospitals to treat members at a discount. PPO members may choose any physician within the network, and usually pay a 10 percent copayment for care within the system and a higher percentage (20 to 30 percent) for care elsewhere. PPOs generally require prior approval for expensive tests or major procedures.

A *point-of-service (POS)* plan is a PPO that permits patients to use physicians outside the network. Consumers pay the difference between the preferred provider's discounted fee and the outside physician's fee. A *gatekeeper* plan requires members to choose a primary physician, as in an HMO, who must approve all referrals to specialists.

Government-Financed Insurance Plans

The government provides two major forms of health financing: Medicare and Medicaid. Under Medicare, the federal government pays 80 percent of most medical bills, after a deductible fee, for people over age 65. Medicare doesn't cover drugs, eyeglasses, or dental work.

Medicaid, a federal and state insurance plan that protects people with very low or no incomes, is the chief source of coverage for the unemployed. However, many unemployed Americans don't qualify because their family incomes are above the poverty line. Publicly insured patients are more likely than those with private insurance to receive inadequate care and to experience adverse health outcomes.

The Uninsured

As many as 33 million Americans lack health insurance (see Figure 10-2). Many others are underinsured, meaning that they don't have adequate coverage and are less likely to receive preventive care or routine checkups. According to the Commonwealth Fund, women, who are more likely to be caring for children or aging parents, are themselves less likely than men to have good access to health care. The number of uninsured women has grown three times faster than the number of uninsured men and, if this trend continues, will exceed that of uninsured men by the year 2005.[41] (See Figure 10-2).

Eleven million children under age 19 do not have insurance coverage. Nearly one in three young adults between ages 18 and 24 has no health insurance—the highest proportion of any age group.[42] Some universities, such as those in the University of California system, are requiring all students to purchase insurance that can be used to cover services beyond those provided in university clinics.[43]

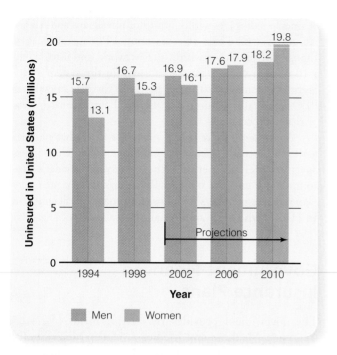

▲ **Figure 10-2** The number of uninsured (in millions) in the United States.

Source: Jeanne M. Lambrew, "Diagnosing Disparities in Health Insurance for Women: A Prescription for Change." The Commonwealth Fund, August 2001.

Uninsured patients have shorter hospital stays, cannot undergo costly therapies, and have a greater risk of dying in the hospital than insured patients. About 85 percent of uninsured Americans are from families in which the head of the family works but can't get insurance through his or her employer.[44] Some of these people work part-time and do not qualify for insurance. Others work for businesses too small to qualify for group insurance. The availability of insurance affects both access to care and the way care is delivered.

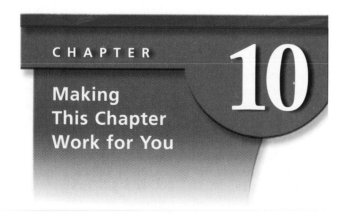

CHAPTER

Making This Chapter Work for You

10

1. Which of the following statements about health information on the Internet is true?
   a. Chat rooms are the most reliable source of accurate medical information.
   b. Physicians who have websites must adhere to a strict set of standards set by the American Medical Association.
   c. Government-sponsored sites such as that of the Centers for Disease Control and Prevention are excellent sources of accurate health-care information.
   d. The internet is safe and cost-effective source of prescription drugs.

2. In a preclinical trial,
   a. researchers examine the cost-effectiveness of a specific treatment.
   b. animals are used to test new medical treatments.
   c. humans are used to test new medical treatments.
   d. the health status of a large group of people who exhibit certain health habits is reviewed.

3. A good primary care physician
   a. appears to know all the answers to your questions.
   b. stays on schedule, never spending more than the allotted time with each patient.
   c. is willing to treat complex problems rather than send you to an expensive specialist.
   d. encourages you to do research about your diagnosis and answers all your questions.

4. During a medical exam, you doctor will
   a. check your cardiovascular system by listening to your heart and feeling your neck arteries.
   b. check your lungs by probing for tender spots and malformations.
   c. look into your eyes to see if you have vision problems that require glasses or contact lenses.
   d. evaluate your joints by tapping on the knees and elbows.

5. Periodontal disease
   a. results from poor eating habits.
   b. can lead to cardiovascular problems.
   c. in its early stage can be prevented by brushing alone.
   d. is caused by a variety of bacteria and viruses.

6. Patients have all the rights below except which of the following?
   a. access to their medical records
   b. medical care that meets accepted standards of quality
   c. to donate a body part for compensation
   d. to leave the hospital against their physician's advice

7. Examples of complementary and alternative therapies include all of the following except
   a. psychiatry
   b. acupuncture
   c. chiropractic
   d. homeopathy

8. Herbal remedies that appear to have positive health effects include

a. ayurveda for controlling asthma.
b. acidophilus for improving memory.
c. aloe vera for diabetes.
d. garlic for preventing infection and tumor growth.

9. Which of the following statements about the health-care system is true?
   a. Primary care is usually provided by specialists in a hospital.
   b. Nurses can perform some surgical procedures once they are board certified.
   c. Most hospitals in the United States are teaching hospitals and affiliated with medical schools.
   d. The length of hospital stays may be determined by a patient's diagnosis rather than the person's pace of recovery.

10. Managed care features all of the following except
   a. health maintenance organizations.
   b. a fee-for-service system of insurance.
   c. preferred provider organizations.
   d. limitations on reimbursement for certain health services.

Answers to these questions can be found on page 640.

 Are patient office visits with physicians getting longer or shorter?

Critical Thinking

1. Think about an experience you've had with a traditional medical practitioner. How did you feel during the physical examination? Did you trust the practitioner? Were you comfortable with the level of communication? Evaluate your experience and give your opinion of the value of the checkup.

2. Have you used any complementary or alternative approaches to health care? If so, were you satisfied with the results? How did your experience with the CAM therapist compare with your most recent experience with a traditional medical practitioner? Do you feel confident that you know the difference between alternative care and quackery?

3. If you're young and healthy, you'll have little problem getting health insurance. However, if you develop a chronic illness, sustain serious injuries in an accident, or simply get older, you may find insurance harder to get and more expensive to keep. What is your insur-

ance coverage? Do you believe insurance companies have the right to turn down applicants with preexisting conditions, such as high blood pressure? Do they have the right to require screening for potentially serious health problems, such as HIV infection, or to cancel the policies of individuals who have run up high medical bills in the past?

4. Jocelyn has been experiencing a great deal of fatigue and frequent headaches for the past couple of months. She doesn't have health insurance and doesn't want to spend money on a doctor visit. So she did some research on the Internet about ways to relieve her symptoms and was considering taking a couple of herbal supplements that were touted as potential treatments. If she asked you for your advice, what would you tell her? Do you think that self-care is appropriate in this situation?

SITES & BYTES

National Institute of Health
http://www.nih.gov
This site from the U.S. Department of Health and Human Services features a wealth of consumer information on a variety of health topics, alternative (complementary) therapy, and health-care services, including publications and fact sheets, clinical trials, health hotlines, A–Z topic index, and current news events and special reports.

MedicineNet
http://www.medicinenet.com/Script/Main/hp.asp
This comprehensive site is written for the consumer by board-certified physicians and contains medical news, directory of procedures, medical dictionary, pharmacy, and first aid information. You can use the information at MedicineNet.com to prepare for a doctor visit and to learn about a diagnosis or understand a prescribed treatment or procedure.

Health Insurance Association of America
http://www.hiaa.org
This site, sponsored by the Health Insurance Association of America (HIAA), the nation's most prominent organization representing the private health-care system, provides comprehensive information about health insurance and managed care for the consumer.

Please note that links are subject to change. If you find a broken link, use a search engine such as http://www.yahoo.com and search for the website by typing in key words.

InfoTrac Activity   "The FDA's Guide to Dietary Supplements." *Nutrition Health Review,* Winter 2001, p. 3.

(1) What is the difference between a drug and a dietary supplement? Answer in two different ways—one in terms of FDA regulation and the other in terms of structure-function claims.

(2) List three different health claims that show a link between the intake of certain dietary supplements and the prevention of neural tube defects, osteoporosis, and heart disease.

You can find additional readings related to CAM and health care with InfoTrac College Edition, an online library of more than 900 journals and publications. Follow the instructions for accessing InfoTrac that were packaged with your textbook; then search for articles using a key word search.

For additional links, resources, and suggested readings on InfoTrac, visit our Health & Wellness Resource Center at http://health.wadsworth.com.

Key Terms

The terms listed here are used within the chapter on the page indicated. Definitions of the terms are in the Glossary at the end of this book.

acupuncture 354
allopathic medicine 350
ayurveda 354
biofeedback 354
chiropractic 351
complementary and alternative medicine (CAM) 349
diagnostic-related group (DRG) 357
false negative 343
false positive 343
gingivitis 345
gum disease 345
health insurance organization (HMO) 359

herbal medicine 352
holistic 349
home health care 357
homeopathy 354
indemnity 358
informed consent 346
integrative medicine 349
malpractice 348
managed care 358
massage therapy 355
medical history 341
meta-analysis 338
naturopathy 354
negligence 343

osteopathy 350
outcomes 338
over-the-counter (OTC) 344
Pap smear 342
periodontitis 345
plaque 345
preferred provider organization (PPO) 359
primary care 356
quackery 348
reflexology 354
visualization 355
vital signs 334

References

1. "Sharp Rise in Healthcare Costs Projected." *Healthcare Financial Management,* Vol. 54, No. 11, November 2000.
2. Starfield, Barbara. "Is U.S. Health Really the Best in the World?" *Journal of the American Medical Association,* Vol. 284, No. 4, July 26, 2000.
3. Brener, Nancy, and Vani, Gowda. "U.S. College Students' Reports of Receiving Health Information on College Campuses." *Journal of American College Health,* Vol. 49, No. 5, March 2001, p. 223.
4. Fischman, Josh, "Play Doctor Online." *U.S. New & World Report,* Vol. 129, No. 22, December 4, 2000.
5. "Good Health Is Hard to Find on the Internet." *Medicine & Health,* Vol. 55, No. 21, May 28, 2001, p. 5.
6. "Patients' Expectations of Physicians Vary by the Gender of Patients and Doctors," *Health Care Strategic Management,* Vol. 19, No. 5, May 2001, p. 7.
7. "Facial Plastic and Reconstructive Surgery Increases 12% since 1997." *Health Care Strategic Management,* Vol. 19, No. 2, February 2001, p. 9.
8. Gottlieb, Scott. "Plastic Surgery Rockets as Baby Boomers Search for Youth and Beauty." *British Medical Journal,* Vol. 322, No. 7286, March 10, 2001, p. 574.

9. Greeley, Alexandra. "Planning To Look Flab-u-less?" *FDA Consumer,* Vol. 34, No. 6, November 2000, p. 31.

10. Satcher, David. "Surgeon General's Report on Oral Health." *Public Health Reports,* Vol. 115, No. 5, September 2000, p. 489.

11. Larkin, Marilynn. "No Cure-alls, Says US FTC." *Lancet,* Vol. 358, No. 9275, July 7, 2001, p. 80.

12. NCCAM website: http://nccam.nih.gov.

13. Silverstein, Daniel, and Allen Spiegel. "Are Physicians Aware of the Risks of Alternative Medicine?" *Journal of Community Health,* Vol. 26, No. 3, June 2001, p. 159.

14. "Alternative Medicine." *Harvard Health Letter,* Vol. 25, No. 11, September 2000.

15. Rees, Lesley, and Andrew Weil. "Integrated Medicine Imbues Orthodox Medicine with the Values of Complementary Medicine." *British Medical Journal,* Vol. 322, No. 7279, January 20, 2001, p. 119.

16. Ernst, E. "Prevalence of Use of Complementary/Alternative Medicine: A Systematic Review." *Bulletin of the World Health Organization,* Vol. 78, No. 2, February 2000.

17. Berman, Brian. "Complementary Medicine and Medical Education: Teaching Complementary Medicine Offers a Way of Making Teaching More Holistic." *British Medical Journal,* Vol. 33, No. 7279, January 20, 2001, p. 121.

18. Ernst E. "The Role of Complementary and Alternative Medicine." *British Medical Journal,* Vol. 321, No. 7269, November 4, 2000.

19. Barrett, Bruce, et al. "Bridging the Gap Between Conventional and Alternative Medicine." *Journal of Family Practice,* Vol. 49, No. 3, March 2000.

20. Lamarine, Roland. "Alternative Medicine: More Than a Harmless Option." *Current Health 2,* Vo. 27, No. 6, February 2001, p. 19.

21. "When Cancer Patients Keep Alternative Medicine Secrets." *Tufts University Health & Nutrition Letter,* Vol. 18, No. 2, April 2000.

22. Josefson, Deborah. "U.S. Cancer Institute Funds Trials of Complementary Therapy." *British Medical Journal,* Vol. 320, No. 7251, June 24, 2000.

23. "Complementary Health Practices Much More Widespread Than Is Suspected by Doctors." *Cancer Weekly,* February 15, 2000.

24. Lamarine. "Alternative Medicine: More Than a Harmless Option."

25. Nahin, Richard, and Stephen Straus. "Research into Complementary and Alternative Medicine: Problems and Potential." *British Medical Journal,* Vol. 33, No. 7279, January 20, 2001, p. 161.

26. Dworkin, Norine. "Doing What Comes Naturally." *Psychology Today,* Vol. 34, No. 2, March 2001, p. 39.

27. Vickers, Andrew. "Complementary Medicine." *British Medical Journal,* Vol. 321, No. 7262, September 16, 2000.

28. Vickers, Andrew, et al. "Herbal Medicine." *Western Journal of Medicine,* Vol. 175, No. 2, August 2001, p. 125.

29. Grant, Michael, et al. "Alternative Pharmacotherapy." *Journal of Family Practice,* Vol. 49, No. 10, October 2000.

30. Kessler, David. "Cancer and Herbs." *New England Journal of Medicine,* Vol. 342, No. 23, June 9, 2000.

31. Haller, Christine, and Neal Benowitz. "Adverse Cardiovascular and Central Nervous System Events Associated with Dietary Supplements Containing Ephedra Alkaloids." *New England Journal of Medicine,* Vol. 343, No. 25, December 21, 2000.

32. "Alternative Therapies for Depression, Diabetes and Obesity." *Journal of the American Dietetic Association,* Vol. 101, No. 3, March 2001, p. 364.

33. Shelton, Richard, et al. "Effectiveness of St. John's Wort in Major Depression: A Randomized Controlled Trial." *Journal of the American Medical Association,* Vol. 285, No. 15, April 18, 2001, p. 1978.

34. Cummings. Mike. "Commentary: Controls for Acupuncture—Can We Finally See the Light?" *British Medical Journal,* Vol. 322, No. 7302, June 30, 2001, p. 1578.

35. Josefek, Kristen. "Alternative Medicine's Roadmap to the Mainstream." *American Journal of Law & Medicine,* Summer–Fall, 2000.

36. Robert Wood Johnson Foundation. www.rwjf.org.

37. Cauchi, Richard. "Making the Best of Managed Care." *State Legislatures,* Vol. 27, No. 6, June 2001, p. 22.

38. Loiacono, Kristin. "Patient's Rights Legislations: What the Senators Said." *Trial,* Vol. 37, No. 8, August 2001, p. 11.

39. Roberts, Shauna. "Health Maintenance Organizations Part 1: Kinds of HMOs." *Diabetes Forecast,* Vol. 53, No. 11, November 2000.

40. "HMO Enrollment Grows Slowly, Steadily." *Healthcare Financial Management,* Vol. 54, No. 7, July 2000.

41. Lambrew, J. "Expanding Health Insurance for Working Americans." *Commonwealth Fund,* August 2001.

42. Siskos, Catherine. "Don't Get Sick." *Kiplinger's Personal Finance Magazine,* Vol. 54, No. 4, July 2000.

43. "UC Set to Require Student Insurance." *Policy & Practice of Public Human Services,* Vol. 58, No. 4, December 2000.

44. Wyn, Roberta, et al. "Falling Through the Cracks." Menlo Park, CA: Henry J. Kaiser Family Foundation, February 2001.

11

Protecting Yourself from Infectious Diseases

"There's something I have to tell you." Jill knew, just by the sound of her boyfriend's voice, that the "something" wasn't good news.

"My herpes is back."

Stunned, Jill tried to absorb all the information packed into this short sentence: She'd had no idea that the man she'd been sleeping with for several months had a sexually transmitted disease (STD). How did he get it? What else hadn't he told her about his past? What did he mean that it was "back"? Could she have caught it? And, finally, she asked the all-too-human question: How could this have happened to me?

By their very nature, infectious diseases take people by surprise. Throughout history, they have claimed more lives than any military conflict or natural disaster. Although modern medicine has won many victories against the agents of infection, we remain vulnerable to a host of infectious illnesses. Drug-resistant strains of tuberculosis and *Staphylococcus* bacteria challenge current therapies. And scientists warn of the potential danger of new "emerging" viruses and of the use of infectious agents as weapons of war and terrorism.

Some of today's most common and dangerous infectious illnesses spread primarily through sexual contact, and their incidence has skyrocketed. The federal government estimates that 65 million Americans have a sexually transmitted disease.[1] These diseases cannot be prevented in the laboratory. Only you, by your behavior, can prevent and control them.

This chapter is a lesson in self-defense against all forms of infection. The information it provides can help you boost your defenses, recognize and avoid enemies, protect yourself from sexually transmitted diseases, and realize when to seek help.

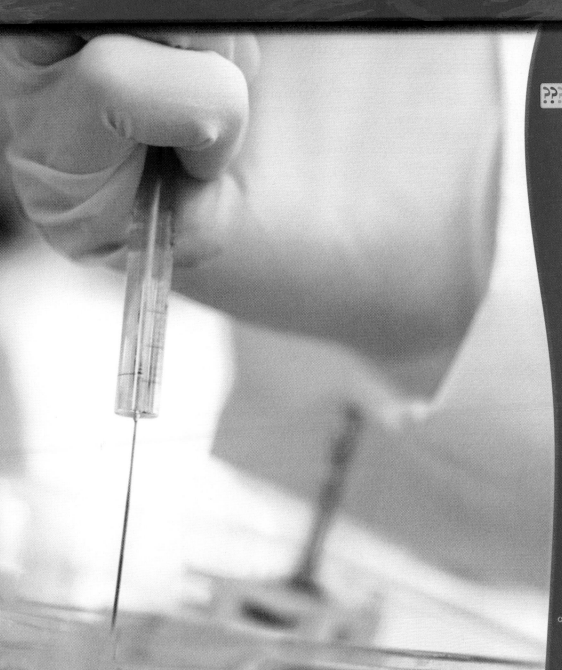

FREQUENTLY ASKED QUESTIONS

FAQ: How do you catch an infection? p. 368

FAQ: Who is at highest risk of infectious diseases? p. 375

FAQ: What do I need to know about biological warfare? p. 383

FAQ: What is herpes? p. 394

FAQ: What progress has been made in treating HIV/AIDS? p. 402

After studying the material in this chapter, you should be able to:

- **Explain** how the different agents of infection spread disease.
- **Describe** how your body protects itself from infectious disease.
- **List** and **describe** some common infectious diseases.
- **Identify** the sexually transmitted diseases and the symptoms and treatment for each.

- **Define** HIV infection and **describe** its symptoms.
- **List** the methods of HIV transmission.
- **Explain** some practical methods for preventing HIV infection and other sexually transmitted diseases.

Understanding Infection

We live in a sea of microbes. Most of them don't threaten our health or survival; some, such as the bacteria that inhabit our intestines, are actually beneficial. Yet in the course of history, disease-causing microorganisms have claimed millions of lives. The twentieth century brought the conquest of infectious killers such as cholera and scarlet fever.[2] However, although modern science has won many victories against the agents of infection, infectious illnesses remain a serious health threat.

Infection is a complex process, triggered by various **pathogens** (disease-causing organisms) and countered by the body's own defenders. Physicians explain infection in terms of a **host** (either a person or a population) that contacts one or more agents in an environment. A **vector**—a biological or physical vehicle that carries the agent to the host—provides the means of transmission.

Agents of Infection

The types of microbes that can cause infection are viruses, bacteria, fungi, protozoa, and helminths (parasitic worms) (see photos below).

Viruses

The tiniest pathogens—**viruses**—are also the toughest; they consist of a bit of nucleic acid (DNA or RNA, but never both) within a protein coat. Unable to reproduce on its own, a virus takes over a body cell's reproductive machinery and instructs it to produce new viral particles, which are then released to enter other cells.

The most common viruses are these types:

▶ Rhinoviruses and adenoviruses, which get into the mucous membranes and cause upper-respiratory tract infections and colds.

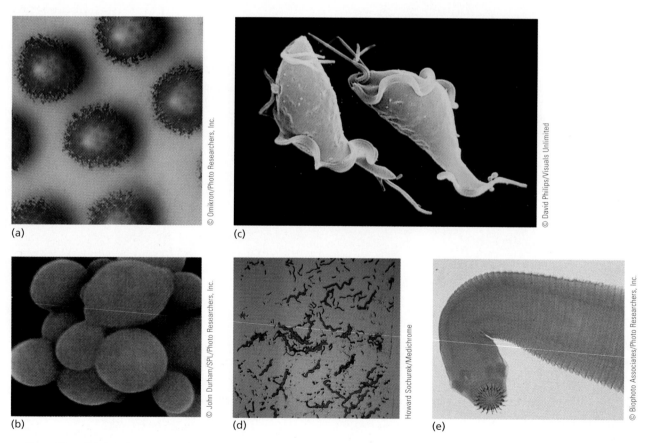

(a) © Omikron/Photo Researchers, Inc.

(c) © David Philips/Visuals Unlimited

(b) © John Durham/SPL/Photo Researchers, Inc.

(d) Howard Sochurek/Medichrome

(e) © Biophoto Associates/Photo Researchers, Inc.

▲ Examples of the major categories of organisms that cause disease in humans. Except for the helminths (parasitic worms), pathogens are microorganisms that can be seen only with the aid of a microscope. (a) Viruses: common cold, (b) Fungi: yeast, (c) Protozoa: trichomonas, (d) Bacteria: syphilis, (e) Helminths: tapeworm.

▶ Influenza viruses, which can change their outer protein coats so dramatically that individuals resistant to one strain cannot fight off a new one.

▶ Herpes viruses, which take up permanent residence in the cells and flare up periodically.

▶ Papilloma viruses, which cause few symptoms in women and almost none in men, but may be responsible, at least in part, for a rise in the incidence of cervical cancer among younger women.

▶ Hepatitis viruses, which cause several forms of liver infection, ranging from mild to life threatening.

▶ Slow viruses, which give no early indication of their presence but can produce fatal illnesses within a few years.

▶ Retroviruses, which are named for their backward ("retro") sequence of genetic replication compared to other viruses. One retrovirus, human immunodeficiency virus (HIV), causes acquired immune deficiency syndrome (AIDS). Scientists have identified retroviruses that have been linked to several diseases, including some forms of leukemia and lymphoma (cancers of the blood and lymph glands, respectively).

▶ Filoviruses, which resemble threads and are extremely lethal. Most of those infected with the two known filoviruses, Marburg and Ebola, develop *viral hemorrhagic fever,* which causes uncontrollable bleeding and usually proves fatal.

The problem in fighting viruses is that it's difficult to find drugs that harm the virus and not the cell it has commandeered. **Antibiotics** (drugs that inhibit or kill bacteria) have no effect on viruses. **Antiviral drugs** (such as amantadine for influenza and acyclovir for herpes simplex) don't completely eradicate a viral infection, although they can decrease its severity and duration. Because viruses multiply very quickly, antiviral drugs are most effective when taken before an infection develops or in its early stages.

Bacteria

Simple one-celled organisms, **bacteria** are the most plentiful microorganisms as well as the most pathogenic. Most kinds of bacteria don't cause disease; some, like *Escherichia coli* that aid in digestion, play important roles within our bodies. Even friendly bacteria, however, can get out of hand and cause acne, urinary tract infections, vaginal infections, and other problems.

Bacteria harm the body by releasing enzymes that digest body cells or toxins that produce the specific effects of such diseases as diphtheria or toxic shock. In self-defense the body produces specific proteins (called *antibodies*) that attack and inactivate the invaders. Tuberculosis, tetanus, gonorrhea, scarlet fever, and diphtheria are examples of bacterial diseases.

Because bacteria are sufficiently different from the cells that make up our bodies, antibiotics can kill them without harming our cells. Some of these drugs are produced by microorganisms; others are synthetic agents. Antibiotics work only against specific types of bacteria. If your doctor thinks you have a bacterial infection, tests of your blood, pus, sputum, urine, or stool can identify the particular bacterial strain. Antibiotic medication is prescribed after determination of the bacteria.

Antibiotics may cause undesirable and sometimes serious side effects, including allergic reactions. Furthermore, frequent exposure of bacteria to a particular antibiotic can cause the bacteria to become resistant to that drug so that the antibiotic loses its effectiveness. As a result, in recent years, more virulent treatment-resistant forms of bacterial infections (discussed later in this chapter) have developed.

Fungi

Single-celled or multicelled organisms, **fungi** consist of threadlike fibers and reproductive spores. These plants, lacking chlorophyll, must obtain their food from organic material, which may include human tissue. Fungi release enzymes that digest cells and are most likely to attack hair-covered areas of the body, including the scalp, beard, groin, and external ear canals. They also cause athlete's foot. Treatment consists of antifungal drugs.

Protozoa

These single-celled, microscopic animals release enzymes and toxins that destroy cells or interfere with their function. Diseases caused by **protozoa** are not a major health problem in this country, primarily because of public health measures. Around the world, however, some 2.24 billion people (more than 40 percent of the world's population) are at risk for acquiring malaria—a one protozoan-caused disease—every year. Up to 3 million die of this disease annually. Many more come down with amoebic dysentery. Treatment for protozoa-caused diseases consists of general medical care to relieve the symptoms, replacement of lost blood or fluids, and drugs that kill the specific protozoan.

The most common disease caused by protozoa in the United States is *giardiasis,* an intestinal infection caused by microorganisms in human and animal feces. It has become a threat at day-care centers, as well as among campers and hikers who drink contaminated water. Once ingested, giardia organisms use an adhesive sucker to stick to the intestinal walls, where they multiply and absorb nutrients from their host. Symptoms include nausea, lack of appetite, gas, diarrhea, fatigue, abdominal cramps, and bloating. Many people recover in a month or two even without treatment. However, in some cases, the microbe causes recurring attacks over many years. Giardiasis can be life-threatening in small children and the elderly, who are especially prone to severe dehydration from diarrhea. Treatment usually consists of antibiotics.

Helminths (Parasitic Worms)

Small parasitic worms that attack specific tissues or organs and compete with the host for nutrients are called **helminths.** One major worldwide health problem is *schistosomiasis,* a disease caused by a parasitic worm, the fluke, that burrows through the skin and enters the circulatory system. Infection with another helminth, the tapeworm, may be contracted from eating undercooked beef, pork, or fish containing larval forms of the tapeworm. Helminthic diseases are treated with appropriate medications.

?!?!? How Do You Catch an Infection?

The major vectors, or means of transmission, for infectious disease are animals/insects, person-to-person, food, water, and air.

Animals/Insects

Disease can be transmitted by house pets, livestock, or wild animals. Insects also spread a variety of diseases. The housefly may spread dysentery, diarrhea, typhoid fever, or trachoma (an eye disease rare in the United States but common in other parts of the world). Other insects, including mosquitoes, ticks, mites, fleas, and lice, can transmit such diseases as malaria, yellow fever, encephalitis, dengue fever (a growing threat in Mexico), and Lyme disease.

A new threat in the United States is West Nile virus, carried by birds and transferred to humans via mosquito bites. Scientists estimate that less than 1 percent of mosquitoes in the United States are infected with West Nile virus, but CDC officials are trying to monitor and control their spread. First identified in metropolitan New York in 1999, West Nile virus has been found in birds in several states. In the year 2000, there were 21 reported cases in humans, 2 of them fatal.[3]

Person-to-Person/Airborne

The people you're closest to can transmit pathogens through the air, through touch, or through sexual contact. To avoid infection, stay out of range of anyone who's coughing, sniffling, or sneezing and don't share food or dishes. Carefully wash your dishes, utensils, and hands, and abstain from sex or make self-protective decisions about sexual partners. (See the sections on STDs later in this chapter.)

Food

Every year foodborne illnesses strike millions of Americans, sometimes with fatal consequences. Bacteria account for two-thirds of foodborne infections, and thousands of suspected cases of infection with *Escherichia coli* bacteria in undercooked or inadequately washed food have been reported.

Every year as many as 4 million Americans have a bout with *Salmonella* bacteria, which have been found in about a third of all poultry sold in the United States. These infections can be serious enough to require hospitalization and can lead to arthritis, neurological problems, and even death. Consumers can greatly reduce the number of salmonella infections by proper handling, cooking, and refrigeration.

A deadly food disease, *botulism,* is caused by certain bacteria that grow in improperly canned foods. Although its occurrence is rare in commercial products, botulism is a danger in home canning. Another uncommon threat is *trichinosis,* caused by the larvae of a parasitic roundworm in uncooked meat. This infection, which causes nausea, vomiting, diarrhea, fever, thirst, profuse sweating, weakness, and pain, can be avoided by thoroughly cooking meat.

Water

Waterborne diseases, such as typhoid fever and cholera, are still widespread in less developed areas of the world. They have been rare in the United States, although outbreaks caused by inadequate water purification have occurred.

The Process of Infection

If someone infected with the flu sits next to you on a bus and coughs or sneezes, tiny viral particles may travel into your nose and mouth. Immediately the virus finds or creates an opening in the wall of a cell, and the process of infection begins. During the **incubation period,** the time between invasion and the first symptom, you're unaware of the pathogen multiplying inside you. In some diseases, incubation may go on for months, even years; for most, it lasts several days or weeks.

The early stage of the battle between your body and the invaders is called the *prodromal* period. As infected cells die, they release chemicals that help block the invasion. Other chemicals, such as *histamines,* cause blood vessels to dilate, thus allowing more blood to reach the battleground. During all of this, you feel mild, generalized symptoms, such as headache, irritability, and discomfort. You're also highly contagious. At the height of the battle—

the typical illness period—you cough, sneeze, sniffle, ache, feel feverish, and lose your appetite.

Recovery begins when the body's forces gain the advantage. With time, the body destroys the last of the invaders and heals itself. However, the body is not able to develop long-lasting immunity to certain viruses, such as colds, flu, or HIV.

How Your Body Protects Itself

Various parts of your body safeguard you against infectious diseases and provide **immunity,** or protection, from these health threats. Your skin, when unbroken, keeps out most potential invaders. Your tears, sweat, skin oils, saliva, and mucus contain chemicals that can kill bacteria. Cilia, the tiny hairs lining your respiratory passages, move mucus, which traps inhaled bacteria, viruses, dust, and foreign matter, to the back of the throat, where it is swallowed; the digestive system then destroys the invaders.

When these protective mechanisms can't keep you infection-free, your body's immune system, which is on constant alert for foreign substances that might threaten the body, swings into action. The immune system includes structures of the lymphatic system, which includes the spleen, thymus gland, lymph nodes, and lymph vessels, that help filter impurities from the body (see Figure 11-1). More than a dozen different types of white blood cells are

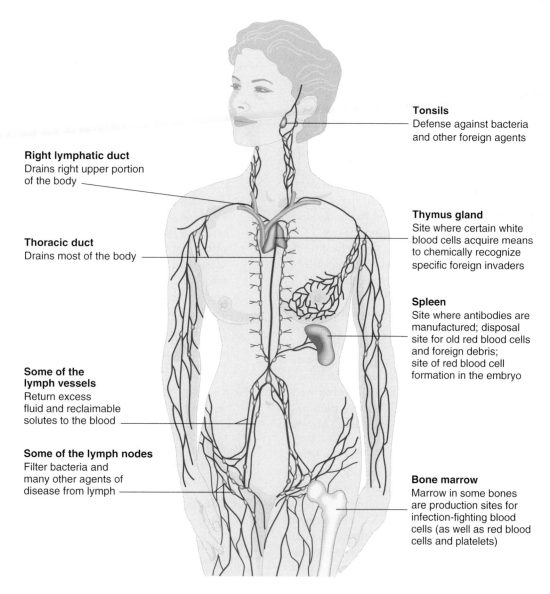

Tonsils
Defense against bacteria and other foreign agents

Right lymphatic duct
Drains right upper portion of the body

Thoracic duct
Drains most of the body

Thymus gland
Site where certain white blood cells acquire means to chemically recognize specific foreign invaders

Spleen
Site where antibodies are manufactured; disposal site for old red blood cells and foreign debris; site of red blood cell formation in the embryo

Some of the lymph vessels
Return excess fluid and reclaimable solutes to the blood

Some of the lymph nodes
Filter bacteria and many other agents of disease from lymph

Bone marrow
Marrow in some bones are production sites for infection-fighting blood cells (as well as red blood cells and platelets)

▲ **Figure 11-1** The human lymphatic system and its functions.

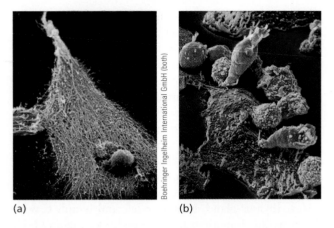

(a)   (b)

Boehringer Ingelheim International GmbH (both)

▲ Types of lymphocytes. (a) B cell covered with bacteria. The B cells function in humoral immunity by producing antibodies. (b) T cells attack a cancer cell. The T cells function in cell-mediated immunity.

concentrated in the organs of the lymphatic system or patrol the entire body by way of the blood and lymph vessels. The two basic types of immune mechanisms are humoral and cell-mediated.

Humoral immunity refers to the protection provided by antibodies, proteins derived from white blood cells called B lymphocytes or B cells. Humoral immunity is most effective during bacterial or viral infections. An *antigen* is any substance that enters the body and triggers production of an antibody. Once the body produces antibodies against a specific antigen—the mumps virus, for instance—you're protected against that antigen for life. If you're again exposed to mumps, the antibodies previously produced prevent another episode of the disease.

But you don't have to suffer through an illness to acquire immunity. Inoculation with a vaccine containing synthetic or weakened antigens can give you the same protection. The type of long-lasting immunity in which the body makes its own antibodies to a pathogen is called *active* immunity. Immunity produced by the injection of **gamma globulin,** the antibody-containing part of the blood, from another person or animal that has developed antibodies to a disease, is called *passive* immunity.

The various types of T cells are responsible for cellular, or **cell-mediated,** immunity. These lymphocytes are manufactured in the bone marrow and carried to the thymus for maturation. Cell-mediated immunity mainly protects against parasites, fungi, cancer cells, and foreign tissue (see photos above). Thousands of different T cells work together to ward off disease. Some T cells activate other immune cells; others help in antibody-mediated responses; and still others suppress lymphocyte activity while others carry out different functions.

Immune Response

Attacked by pathogens, the body musters its forces and fights. Sometimes the invasion is handled like a minor border skirmish; other times a full-scale battle is waged throughout the body. Together, the immune cells work like an internal police force. When an antigen enters the body, the T cells aided by *macrophages* (large scavenger cells with insatiable appetites for foreign cells, diseased and run-down red blood cells, and other biological debris) engage in combat with the invader. Meanwhile, the B cells churn out antibodies, which rush to the scene and join in the fray. Also busy at surveillance are natural killer cells that, like the elite forces of a SWAT team, seek out and destroy viruses and cancer cells.

The **lymph nodes,** or glands, are small tissue masses in which some protective cells are stored. If pathogens invade your body, many of them are carried to the lymph nodes to be destroyed. This is why your lymph nodes often feel swollen when you have a cold or the flu.

STRATEGIES FOR PREVENTION

Natural Ways to Bolster Immunity

✔ *Eat a balanced diet* to be sure you get essential vitamins and minerals. Severe deficiencies in vitamins B_6, B_{12}, and folic acid impair immunity. Keep up your iron and zinc intake. Iron influences the number and vigor of certain immune cells, whereas zinc is crucial for cell repair. Too little vitamin C may also increase susceptibility to infectious diseases.

✔ *Avoid fatty foods.* A low-fat diet can increase the activity of immune cells that hunt down and knock out cells infected with viruses.

✔ *Get enough sleep.* Without adequate rest, your immune system cannot maintain and renew itself.

✔ *Exercise regularly.* Aerobic exercise stimulates the production of an immune-system booster called interleukin-2.

✔ *Don't smoke.* Smoking decreases the levels of some immune cells.

✔ *Control your alcohol intake.* Heavy drinking interferes with normal immune responses and lowers the number of defender cells.

If the microbes establish a foothold, the blood supply to the area increases, bringing oxygen and nutrients to the fighting cells. Tissue fluids, as well as antibacterial and antitoxic proteins, accumulate. You may develop redness, swelling, local warmth, and pain—the signs of **inflammation.** As more tissue is destroyed, a cavity, or **abscess,** forms, and fills with fluid, battling cells, and dead white blood cells (pus). If the invaders aren't killed or inactivated, the pathogens are able to spread into the bloodstream and cause what is known as **systemic disease.** The toxins released by the pathogens cause fever, and the infection becomes more dangerous.

Immunity and Stress

Whenever we confront a crisis, large or small, our bodies produce powerful hormones that provide extra energy. However, this stress response dampens immunity, reducing the number of some key immune cells and the responsiveness of others.

Stress affects the body's immune system in different ways, depending on two factors: the controllability or uncontrollability of the stressor and the mental effort required to cope with the stress. An uncontrollable stressor that lasts longer than 15 minutes may interfere with cytokine interleukin-6, which plays an essential role in activating the immune defenses. Uncontrollable stressors also produce high levels of cortisol, which suppresses immune system functioning. The mental efforts required to cope with high-level stressors produce only brief immune changes that appear to have little consequence for health. However, stress has been shown to slow proinflammatory cytokine production, which is essential for wound-healing.

Immune Disorders

Sometimes our immune system overreacts to certain substances, mistakes the body's own tissues for enemies, or doesn't react adequately. The result is an immune disorder. The most common are **allergies,** which essentially represent a hypersensitivity to a substance in our environment or diet.

According to the American College of Allergy, Asthma and Immunology, allergies affect about 38 percent of all Americans—almost twice as many as allergy experts once believed—and millions of them suffer unnecessarily because they don't know about effective treatment options, such as allergy shots (immunotherapy). Allergy sufferers run annual tabs of up to $2 billion in doctor visits, diagnostic tests, prescriptions, and decreased productivity. Every year they account for more than 10 million workdays missed; every day they keep 10,000 children out of school.

"Allergies may seem trivial to people who don't have them, but they have an enormous effect on a person's quality of life," says Robert Miles, M.D., of the American College of Allergy, Asthma and Immunology.[4] Their symptoms are many and miserable: itching, nasal congestion, eye irritation, coughing, wheezing, hives, vomiting, and diarrhea (from food allergies), even sudden, life-threatening collapse (from anaphylaxis, the most extreme allergic reaction). While victims seldom die of allergies, they just as rarely recover. And when individuals try to outrun allergies by moving away from one region's irritants, they often end up acquiring new sensitivities on their new home ground.

A list of allergic triggers, or allergens, reads like an inventory of creation, including life's pleasures (such as foods and flowers), perils (insect stings and poison ivy), and inescapable realities (like mold and dust). The very air we breathe can be a danger. The symptoms of allergy and of its more sinister sister-disease, asthma, increase along with pollutants, such as diesel fumes, and the number of small particles in the environment.

STRATEGIES FOR PREVENTION

Fighting Hidden Allergens

✔ *Switch to feather pillows.* Researchers in the United Kingdom found significantly higher levels of house dust mite allergens in synthetic pillows.

✔ *Use bleach rather than detergent.* Very low concentrations of bleach are more effective in removing allergens from various surfaces around the house than other common cleaners.

✔ *Cover mattresses and pillows with tightly woven fabrics.* These materials, compared with non-woven or semipermeable synthetic fabrics, effectively block cat and dust allergens even after repeated washings.

✔ *Use multilayer vacuum bags.* To prevent allergens from "leaking" into the air, choose bags that have two to three layers.

✔ *Store clothing in sealed containers with moth-killing products.* Products such as moth balls or crystals and lavandin oil packets also kill house dust mites and their eggs.

✔ *Put comforters in the clothes dryer.* An hour of dry heat in a home dryer dramatically reduces the number of house dust mites in comforters and duvets filled with synthetic materials.

Breakthroughs in treatments are helping many allergy sufferers breathe more easily. "In the past, allergy symptoms and medications both made people so drowsy that they often couldn't concentrate or function at their best," says Miles, who notes that today's allergy sufferers no longer have to choose between feeling better or feeling alert. Treatment options include oral medications, nasal sprays, and **immunotherapy,** which consists of a series of injections of small but increasing doses of an allergen.

Immunotherapy has proven to have long-term, perhaps permanent, benefits. In one study, traditional allergen immunotherapy with a grass-pollen extract, administered for three to four years, induced a clinical remission that persisted for at least three years after treatment. Immunotherapy in patients allergic to insect stings also induces long-lasting immunologic changes and reduces their risk of potentially fatal reactions. Immunotherapy has the greatest benefit, relative to the investment of time and cost, for allergies that persist for more than one season or throughout the year.

Autoimmune disorders result when the immune system fails to recognize body tissue as self and attacks it. Many of these severely disabling diseases, such as myasthenia gravis, rheumatoid arthritis, and systemic lupus erythematosus, primarily strike women systematically in their childbearing years.[5] (See X & Y Files: "Gender Differences in Susceptibility.") These diseases, which often worsen with time, can be treated with drugs that suppress the immune system.

Some people have an **immune deficiency**—either inborn or acquired. A very few children are born without

The X & Y Files   Gender Differences in Susceptibility

When the flu hits a household, the last one left standing is likely to be Mom. The female immune system responds more vigorously to common infections, offering extra protection against viruses, bacteria, and parasites. But this enhanced immunity doesn't apply to sexually transmitted diseases (STDs). A woman who has unprotected sex with an infected man is more likely to contract an STD than a man who has sex with an infected woman. Symptoms of STDs also tend to be more "silent" in women, so they often go undetected and untreated, leading to potentially serious complications.

The genders also differ in their vulnerability to allergic and autoimmune disorders. Although both men and women frequently develop allergies, allergic women are twice as likely to experience potentially fatal anaphylactic shock. A woman's "robust" immune system also is more likely to overreact and turn on her own organs and tissues. On average, three of four people with autoimmune disorders, such as multiple sclerosis, Hashimoto's thyroiditis, and scleroderma, are women. Of the 8.5 million people in the United States with rheumatoid arthritis, about 6.7 million are women. Another autoimmune disease, lupus, affects nine times as many women as men.

Autoimmune disorders often follow a different course in men and women. Women with multiple sclerosis develop symptoms earlier than men, but the disease tends to progress more quickly and be more severe in men. In lupus, women first show symptoms during their childbearing years, while men develop the illness later in life.

Why are there such large gender differences in susceptibility? Scientists believe that the sex hormones have a great impact on immunity. Estrogen, which protects heart, bone, brain, and blood vessels, also bolsters the immune system's response to certain infectious agents. Women produce greater numbers of antibodies when exposed to an antigen; after immunization, they show increased cell-mediated immunity.

In contrast, testosterone may dampen this response—possibly to prevent attacks on sperm cells, which might otherwise be mistaken as alien invaders. When the testes are removed from mice and guinea pigs, their immune systems become more active. Pregnancy dampens a woman's immune response, probably to ensure that her natural protectors don't attack the fetus as a "foreign" invader. This impact is so great that pregnant women with transplanted kidneys may require lower doses of drugs to prevent organ rejection. Pregnant women with multiple sclerosis and rheumatoid arthritis typically experience decreased symptoms during the nine months of gestation, then return to their prepregnancy state after giving birth. Oral contraceptives also can diminish symptoms of multiple sclerosis and rheumatoid arthritis. Neither pregnancy nor birth control pills has such an impact on lupus.

Other hormones, such as prolactin and growth hormone, may affect autoimmune disease. Women have higher levels of these hormones, which may act directly on immune cells through interactions with receptors on the surface of cells. These hormones also may affect the complex interworkings of the hypothalamus, pituitary, and adrenal glands.

Source: Lahita, Robert. "Gender and the Immune System." *Journal of Gender-Specific Medicine,* Vol. 3, No. 7, October 2000. Committee on Understanding the Biology of Sex and Gender Differences. *Exploring the Biological Contributions to Human Health: Does Sex Matter?* Washington, DC: National Academy Press, 2001.

an effective immune system; their lives can be endangered by any infection. Although still experimental, genetic therapy to implant a missing or healthy gene may offer new hope for a normal life.

Immunization: The Key to Prevention

One of the great success stories of American medicine has been the development of vaccines that provide protection against many infectious diseases. Immunization has reduced cases of measles, mumps, tetanus, whooping cough, and other life-threatening illnesses by more than 95 percent.[6] Unfortunately, many Americans, including large numbers of children in urban centers and a proportionately high number of African-American youngsters, haven't been properly immunized.[7] About a quarter of children lack complete protection against polio, tetanus, and other illnesses, according to the National Vaccine Advisory Committee. While there has been progress in protecting most American children against diphtheria, whooping cough, tetanus, *Hemophilus influenzae* type B (HIB), polio,

and measles, some children are going without the booster shots necessary for complete immunization.[8]

As shown in Figure 11-2, the American Academy of Pediatrics recommends that all children be immunized against hepatitis B, diphtheria, tetanus, whooping cough (pertussis); HIB infection; polio; pneumoccal pneumonia; measles, mumps, German measles (rubella); and chickenpox (varicella). Although some vaccines confer lifelong protection, others do not. The protection provided by diphtheria and tetanus vaccinations, for example, diminishes over time, so booster vaccinations are required every ten years. Health officials also recommend measles booster shots for students entering college, and suggest that people born after 1956 be revaccinated for polio, measles, and other infectious diseases before visiting developing countries.

If you're uncertain about your past immunizations, check with family members or your doctor. If you can't find answers, a blood test can show whether you carry antibodies to specific illnesses.

If you're pregnant or planning to get pregnant within the next three months, do not get a measles, mumps, rubella, or oral polio vaccination. If you're allergic to neomycin, consult your doctor before getting a measles, mumps, rubella, or intramuscular polio vaccination. Those with egg allergies should also check with a doctor before

Vaccines are listed under routinely recommended ages.

Bars indicate range of recommended ages for immunization. Any dose not given at the recommended age should be given as a "catch-up" immunization at any subsequent visit when indicated and feasible.

Ovals indicate vaccines to be given if previously recommended doses were missed or given earlier than the recommended minimum age.

Vaccine	Birth	1 month	2 months	4 months	6 months	12 months	15 months	18 months	24 months	4–6 years	11–12 years	14–18 years
Hepatitis B		Hep B #1				Hep B #3					Hep B	
			Hep B #2									
Diphtheria, Tetanus, Pertussis			DTaP	DTaP	DTaP		DTaP			DTaP	Td	
H. influenzae type b			Hib	Hib	Hib	Hib						
Inactivated Polio			IPV	IPV		IPV				IPV		
Pneumococcal Conjugate			PCV	PCV	PCV	PCV						
Measles, Mumps, Rubella						MMR				MMR	MMR	
Varicella						Var					Var	
Hepatitis A										Hep A in selected areas		

Approved by the Advisory Committee on Immunization Practices (ACIP), the American Academy of Pediatrics (AAP), and the American Academy of Family Physicians (AAFP).

▲ **Figure 11-2** Recommended childhood immunization schedule, United States, January–December 2001.

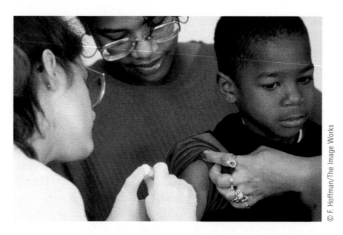

▲ Immunizations are an important protection against childhood diseases. Neighborhood clinics in urban centers offer immunizations to those children at particular risk.

getting a measles, mumps, or flu vaccination. Also, never get a vaccination when you have a high fever.

Hepatitis B

The U.S. Public Health Service recommends immunization against hepatitis B for infants as a way of preventing a disease (discussed later in this chapter) that infects an estimated 200,000 people in the United States and kills 4,000 to 5,000 Americans each year. However, some object to hepatitis B vaccinations for children, because the potential risks associated with the vaccine are greater than the odds of a child contracting what is primarily an adult disease. Public health professionals counter by saying that children under age 5, although they constitute a small minority of those with hepatitis B, face the highest risk of death from cirrhosis and liver cancer.

A problem with delaying immunization until the teen years is a lower compliance rate among some groups of adolescents.[9] A new vaccine against both hepatitis A and hepatitis B has proven to be effective over long periods (at least five years) in both children and adults.[10]

Diphtheria

Diphtheria, a dangerous disease, is rare because of immunization. An average of fewer than three cases per year have been reported in the last decade. Diphtheria and tetanus vaccinations (toxoids) are usually given in combination with the pertussis (whooping cough) vaccine—part of the DTP shot. The schedule for these consists of a basic series and two boosters prior to entering school. Older children and adults receive only diphtheria and tetanus toxoid (DT) in a more dilute form. Adults as well as children should get booster shots every 10 years.

Tetanus (Lockjaw)

Tetanus is an uncommon disease transmitted via a variety of injuries. Since the tetanus germ cannot grow in the presence of air, puncture wounds, such as those caused by stepping on a nail or gardening rake, pose the greatest danger. Tetanus is often called lockjaw, because the characteristic symptom is a stiffening of the jaws so severe that the patient is unable to open his or her mouth. Everyone should get booster inoculations for tetanus at least once every 10 years.

Pertussis

Pertussis (whooping cough), a bacterial infection that can develop into pneumonia, is potentially fatal. Until recently, the pertussis vaccine was made with killed whole pertussis cells and mixed with diphtheria and tetanus vaccines to make the whole cell DTP shot. For years parents have been concerned about its safety because of reports of permanent brain damage and even death. Careful analysis by many investigators found that any increased risk of permanent neurological damage was so small as to be virtually unmeasurable. However, new *acellular* pertussis vaccines, made of only a few parts of the pertussis cell, have proven effective against pertussis and produce fewer side effects. An estimated 95 percent of two-year-olds have been vaccinated against pertussis.[11]

HIB Infection

In the United States, *Hemophilus* influenza type B, or HIB, was once a cause of bacterial *meningitis*, a life-threatening infection of the lining of the brain and spinal cord. A vaccine that protects children has nearly eliminated this potentially deadly disease. The frequency of HIB infection dropped by 99 percent in the 1990s.[12]

Poliomyelitis

Immunization has greatly reduced the incidence of polio in the United States. The American Academy of Pediatrics recommends two doses of inactivated polio virus at 2 months and 4 months, followed by oral polio vaccine at 12 to 18 months and 4 to 6 years.[13] Additional boosters for polio aren't necessary, except when traveling to an area where the disease is common.

Measles

The number of cases of measles has fallen to an all-time low. However, the Centers for Disease Control (CDC) recommends continued vigilance and immunizations.[14]

Symptoms include a rash on the face and body, runny nose, high fever, cough, eye inflammation, and fatigue. Ten to 15 percent of measles patients develop serious complications, such as ear infections, diarrhea, or pneumonia. One out of every 1,000 develops encephalomyelitis, an inflammation of the brain that can be fatal or lead to mental retardation, or to movement, behavioral, or neurological disorders.

CDC officials estimate that 5 to 15 percent of college students are susceptible to measles because they were vaccinated at 12 months of age rather than the currently recommended 15 months, or did not receive a second dose of the vaccine between ages 4 and 12. Others were given immune globulin, which was intended to lower the risk of reaction but which also reduced the vaccine's effectiveness. Many colleges are requiring students to submit proof of measles immunization before allowing them to enroll. In all, some 3 million Americans, aged 20 to 37, are at risk.

Rubella (German Measles)

About 85 percent of adults are immune to rubella, even if they have no history of the disease. The most serious result of this mild disease is the destructive effect it has on an unborn baby—including blindness—if the mother is infected in early pregnancy. All children should be immunized against rubella at 1 year of age or later.[15]

Adults who are not immune may be immunized at any age, but women should not receive the vaccine during pregnancy or during the two to three months immediately preceding pregnancy. All unimmunized children in a pregnant woman's household should be immunized against rubella, for they are the most likely potential carriers. Recent outbreaks of rubella among newborns have been blamed on the lack of routine rubella screening and followup vaccination of susceptible women of childbearing age.

Varicella (Chickenpox)

A vaccine against chickenpox, a common childhood disease that causes itchy red pustules, seems more effective when given alone rather than in combination with MMR vaccine.[16]

Infectious Diseases

An estimated 500 microorganisms cause disease; no effective treatment exists for about 200 of these illnesses. Although infections can be unavoidable at times, the more you know about their causes, the more you can do to protect yourself.

????? Who Is at Highest Risk of Infectious Diseases?

Like human bullies, the viruses responsible for the most common infectious illnesses tend to pick on those least capable of fighting back. Among the most vulnerable are the following groups:

▶ **Children and their families.** Youngsters get up to a dozen colds annually; adults average two a year. When a flu epidemic hits a community, about 40 percent of school-age boys and girls get sick, compared with only 5 to 10 percent of adults. But their parents get up to six times as many colds as other adults.

▶ **The elderly.** Statistically, fewer older men and women are likely to catch a cold or flu, yet when they do, they face greater danger than the rest of the population. People over 65 who get the flu have a one in ten chance of being hospitalized for pneumonia or other respiratory problems, and a one in fifty chance of dying from the disease.

▶ **The chronically ill.** Lifelong diseases, such as diabetes, kidney disease, or sickle-cell anemia, decrease an individual's ability to fend off infections. Individuals taking medications that suppress the immune system, such as steroids, are more vulnerable to infections, as are those with medical conditions that impair immunity, such as infection with HIV.

▶ **Smokers and those with respiratory problems.** Smokers are a high-risk group for respiratory infections and serious complications, such as pneumonia. Chronic breathing disorders, such as asthma and emphysema, also greatly increase the risk of respiratory infections.

▶ **Those who live or work in close contact with someone sick.** Health-care workers who treat high-risk patients, nursing home residents, and others living in close quarters—such as students in dormitories—face greater odds of catching others' colds and flus.

▶ **Residents or workers in poorly ventilated buildings.** Building technology has helped spread certain airborne illnesses, such as tuberculosis, via recirculated air. Indoor air quality can be closely linked with disease transmission in winter, when people spend a great deal of time in tightly sealed rooms.

The Common Cold

There are more than 200 distinct cold viruses, or rhinoviruses. Although in a single season you may develop a temporary immunity to one or two, you may then be hit by a third. Americans come down with 1 billion colds a year. Colds can strike in any season, but different cold viruses are more common at different times of years. Rhinoviruses cause most spring, summer, and early fall colds, and tend to cause more symptoms above the neck (stuffy nose,

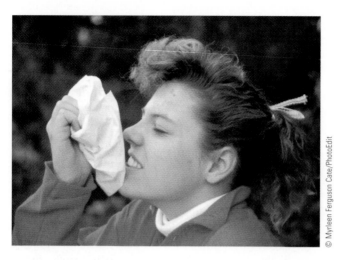

▲ One of the telltale symptoms of a cold is sneezing.

headache, runny eyes). Adenoviruses, parainfluenza viruses, corona viruses, influenza viruses, and others that strike in the winter are more likely to get into the bronchi and trachea (the breathing passages) and cause more fever and bronchitis.

Cold viruses spread by coughs, sneezes, and touch. Cold-sufferers who sneeze and then touch a doorknob or countertop leave a trail of highly contagious viruses behind them. The best preventive tactics are frequent hand-washing, replacing toothbrushes regularly, and avoiding stress overload. High levels of stress increase the risk of becoming infected by respiratory viruses and developing cold symptoms. New research shows that people who feel unable to deal with everyday stresses have an exaggerated immune reaction that may intensify cold or flu symptoms once they've contracted a virus.

Until scientists develop truly effective treatments, experts advise against taking aspirin and acetaminophen (Tylenol), which may suppress the antibodies the body produces to fight cold viruses and increase symptoms such as nasal stuffiness. A better alternative for achiness is ibuprofen (brand names include Motrin, Advil, and Nuprin), which doesn't seem to affect immune response. Children, teenagers, and young adults should never take aspirin for a cold or flu because of the danger of Reye's syndrome, a potentially deadly disorder that can cause convulsions, coma, swelling of the brain, and kidney damage.[17]

The main drawback of antihistamines, the most widely used cold remedy, is drowsiness, which can impair a person's ability to drive or operate machinery safely. Another ingredient, pseudoephedrine, can open and drain sinus passages without drowsiness but can speed up heart rate and cause complications for individuals with high blood pressure, diabetes, heart disease, or thyroid disorders. Nasal sprays can clear a stuffy nose, but they invariably cause a rebound effect.

Fluids (especially chicken soup) help, but dairy products contribute to congestion. Mild exercise boosts immunity, but once you're sick, it's better not to work out strenuously. In general, doctors recommend treating specific symptoms—headache, cough, chest congestion, sore throat, and so on—rather than taking a multisymptom medication.[18]

For a cough, the ingredient to look for in any suppressant is dextromethrophan, which turns down the brain's cough reflex. In expectorants, the only medicine the FDA has deemed effective is guaifenesin, which helps liquefy secretions so you can bring up mucus from the chest. Unless you're coughing up green or foul yellow mucus—signs of a "secondary" bacterial infection—antibiotics won't help. They have no effect against viruses and may make your body more resistant to such medications when you develop a bacterial infection in the future.

Many Americans try alternative remedies for colds. One of the most popular herbal remedies is an extract of the echinacea plant, which is widely used in Europe. Although it is not clear how it works, echinacea is believed to increase the number and efficiency of white blood cells, components of the immune system that battle infection. Although extensive research has not been done, there is some evidence that taking echinacea several times a day at the first sign of sniffles diminishes the symptoms or shortens the duration of an oncoming cold. Most experts recommend only limited use of echinacea, since long-term use can actually suppress the immune system.[19]

Zinc lozenges, another popular alternative treatment in recent years, have not proven to be clearly beneficial. In at least ten studies that have evaluated the benefits of zinc, some have found no benefit, while others have found significant reductions in the severity or duration of cold symptoms. Almost all have been criticized for various reasons, such as the size of the sample or the formulation of zinc used. The compound zinc gluconate does seem to have a modest effect in shortening cold symptoms, but zinc acetate has not been shown to have a benefit.[20]

Although sore throats—a frequent cold symptom—are caused by viruses, many people seek treatment with antibiotics, which are effective only against bacteria. An estimated 5 to 17 percent of sore throats in adults are caused by a bacteria *(Group A streptococci)*. Yet in one recent survey, primary care physicians prescribed antibiotics for almost three-quarters of patients with sore throats. They were more likely to receive more expensive, broad-spectrum antibiotics rather than the recommended antibiotics for strep (penicillin and erythromycin).[21]

 Colds are common among college students, many of whom do not recognize its signs or respond effectively to its symptoms. In a survey of 425 students at three college campuses in Louisiana and Indiana, 10 percent said they would see a physician for a cold; 41 percent believed that antibiotics were an effective treatment. More students said they would

STRATEGIES FOR PREVENTION

Protecting Yourself from Colds and Flus

✔ Wash your hands frequently with hot water and soap. In a public restroom, use a paper towel to turn off the faucet after you wash your hands, and avoid touching the doorknob. Wash objects used by someone with a cold.

✔ Take good care of yourself: Make sure you're getting adequate sleep. Eat a balanced diet. Exercise regularly. Don't share food or drinks.

✔ Spend as little time as possible in crowds, especially in closed places, such as elevators and airplanes. When out, keep your distance from sneezers and coughers. Don't touch your eyes, mouth, and nose after being with someone who has cold symptoms.

✔ Use tissues rather than cloth handkerchiefs, which may harbor viruses for hours or days.

✔ Try to avoid irritating air pollutants. Don't smoke, which destroys protective cells in the airways and worsens any cough. Limit your intake of alcohol, which depresses white blood cells and increases the risk of bacterial pneumonia in flu sufferers.

gious, particularly in the first three days of the disease. The usual incubation period is two days, but symptoms can hit hard and fast.[24] Two varieties of viruses—influenza A and influenza B—cause most flus. In recent years, the deadliest flu epidemics have been caused by various forms of influenza A viruses.[25]

A vaccine against the flu is available, but it is not foolproof. "Because the flu virus is constantly changing, you need a new shot every year," explains Edwin Kilbourne, M.D., of New York Medical College, who decides the components of each year's flu vaccine. "And because it takes the body time to manufacture antibodies to the new viruses, you should get a vaccination at least 10 to 14 days before an outbreak hits your area."[26]

Long recommended for high-risk individuals, such as the elderly or chronically ill, flu shots now are advised for almost everyone.[27] Doctors recommend flu shots for pregnant women, particularly those who will be in the later stages of pregnancy because flu could endanger an unborn child. "The vaccine is well proven to be safe and effective—providing 70 to 80 percent protection against flu," says Kilbourne. The only individuals who should steer clear are those allergic to eggs, since the inactivated flu viruses are grown in chick embryos.

A new alternative to flu shots is an intranasal spray containing a live, attenuated influenza virus (LAIV) vaccine. Researchers have found that the aerosol vaccine significantly reduces flu severity, days lost from work, health-care visits, and the use of over-the-counter medication. The spray

use antibiotics if their symptoms included a fever or discolored nasal discharge.[22]

Your own immune system can do something modern science cannot: cure a cold. All that it needs is time, rest, and plenty of fluids. Warmth also is important, because the aptly named "cold" viruses replicate at lower temperatures. Hot soups and drinks (particularly those with a touch of something pungent, like lemon or ginger) both raise body temperature and help clear the nose. Even more important is getting off your feet. Taking it easy reduces demands on the body, which helps speed recovery.

Influenza

Although similar to a cold, **influenza**—or the flu—causes more severe symptoms that last longer. Every year an estimated 65 million Americans develop influenza, 30 million seek medical care, 300,000 are hospitalized, and 20,000 die.[23] (See Figure 11-3.)

Flu viruses, transmitted by coughs, sneezes, laughs, and even normal conversation, are extraordinarily conta-

Wash hands	70%
Avoid sick people	52%
Get flu shot	41%
Avoid crowds	24%

▲ **Figure 11-3** How Americans try to avoid the flu. Frequent hand washing is the number-one way for most adults. The next most popular technique is avoiding sick people.

Source: Data from Opinion Research Corp. for Kleenex.

represents a particular advantage for children since more than 30 percent of youngsters get the flu, but most don't receive a flu shot. Children who received the vaccine and still got the flu had milder symptoms, were less likely to have a fever, and recovered faster than the children given the placebo.[28]

For those who don't get vaccinated this year, antiviral drugs, such as Relenza (zanamivir) and Tamiflu (oseltamivir), are the next best line of defense.[29] These "neuraminidase inhibitors" are designed to block a protein (neuraminidase) that allows the flu virus to escape from one cell and infect others. A small handheld oral inhaler, used twice a day for five days, delivers Relenza to the surface of the lungs, the primary site of flu infection. Tamiflu, taken twice a day for five days, comes in pill form. These agents act against both influenza A and influenza B viruses and cause few side effects. In research trials, they shortened the duration of flu by up to two days and decreased the likelihood of complications such as bronchitis, sinusitis, and ear infections. However, in order to be effective, treatment with either medication must begin within 36 to 48 hours of the first flu symptom. Although approved only for use as a treatment, antiviral drugs also can prevent flu from spreading through a family, workplace, or school.

Meningitis

Meningitis, or invasive meningococcal disease, attacks the membranes around the brain and spinal cord and can result in hearing loss, kidney failure, and permanent brain damage. An estimated 2,400 to 3,000 cases occur every year; approximately 10 percent are fatal. One of the most common types is caused by the bacterium *Neisseria meningitis,* which is spread through coughing; kissing; sharing drinks, eating utensils, or cigarettes; or prolonged exposure to infected individuals. Viral meningitis is typically less severe.[30]

Most common in the first year of life, the incidence of bacterial meningitis rises in young people between ages 15 and 24.[31] College students are generally not at greater risk—except for freshmen living in dormitories (see Table

11-1). In an analysis of data from 50 state health departments and 231 college health centers, CDC researchers found that the risk of meningitis is three times greater for freshmen in dorms than for other college students.[32]

Early symptoms of meningitis include rash, fever, severe headache, nausea, vomiting, and lethargy. A tell-tale symptom in many, but not all, cases is stiffness of the neck when bending forward. Meningitis progresses rapidly, often in as little time as 12 hours. If untreated, it can lead to permanent hearing loss, brain damage, seizures, or death. If it is caught early and treated with antibiotics, however, it is usually curable.

Meningitis Vaccination

The Advisory Committee on Immunization Practices of the CDC and the American Academy of Pediatrics have recommended that all college freshmen be informed that vaccination is effective against 70 percent of the bacterial strains found on campuses. According to the AAP, vaccination could prevent 60 percent or more of cases among undergraduates.[33] Immunization is recommended primarily for freshmen living in dormitories who make up 4 percent of the total college population but 31 percent of those diagnosed with meningitis.[34] Other factors increasing meningitis risk are smoking and alcohol consumption, especially binge drinking. Smokers, who cough more, and drinkers, who often share glasses, are at higher risk of transmitting and contracting meningitis.[35] Peak incidence for bacterial meningitis is November to March.

Some experts disagree about whether colleges should recommend or require vaccination. According to CDC statistics, only about five deaths as a result of meningitis would be expected annually among the 520,000 freshmen who live in dormitories. By comparison, binge drinking, car accidents, and suicide claim many more lives. Some contend that colleges should devote their limited resources to fighting these threats. Others argue that students should do everything possible to avoid any potential threat to their health.

At most schools, the cost of vaccination ranges from $50 to $75. Research into the success of meningococcal vaccination programs on college campuses has shown that women are more likely than men to be vaccinated and that vaccination rates for all nonwhite ethnic groups are somewhat lower than rates for whites. Students majoring in science-oriented fields have higher vaccination rates than those majoring in the humanities. More younger students living on campus than older ones get vaccinations, possibly because of greater parental influence or because they see themselves as being at higher risk.[36]

The current vaccine protects against the most common strains for the *N. meningitis* bacterium but does not provide complete protection and remains effective for only

▼ Table 11-1 Incidence of Meningitis in College Students	
Population Studied	**Rate of Meningitis**
Students between ages 18 and 23	0.7 per 100,000
Nonstudents between ages 18 and 23	1.4 per 100,000
Freshmen living in dormitories	5.1 per 100,000

Source: Bruce, Michael, et al. "Meningococcal Disease in College Students." *Journal of the American Medical Association,* Vol. 286, No. 6, August 8, 2001.

about three years. More effective vaccines that confer long-lasting immunity and could be administered with other routine infant immunizations have been developed. Some have been introduced in the United Kingdom and other European countries.[37]

Hepatitis

At least five different viruses, referred to as **hepatitis** A, B, C, Delta, and E, can cause this inflammation of the liver. Newly identified viruses also may be responsible for some cases of what is called "non-A, non-B" hepatitis. An estimated 500,000 Americans contract hepatitis each year; about 6,000 people die as a result.

All forms of hepatitis target the liver, the body's largest internal organ. Symptoms include headaches, fever, fatigue, stiff or aching joints, nausea, vomiting, and diarrhea. The liver becomes enlarged and tender to the touch; sometimes the yellowish tinge of jaundice develops. Treatment consists of rest, a high-protein diet, and the avoidance of alcohol and drugs that may stress the liver until the disease runs its course. Alpha interferon, a protein that boosts immunity and prevents viruses from replicating, may be used for some forms.

Most people begin to feel better after two or three weeks of rest, although fatigue and other symptoms can linger. As many as 10 percent of those infected with hepatitis B and up to two-thirds of those with hepatitis C become carriers of the virus for several years or even life. Some have persistent inflammation of the liver, which may cause mild or severe symptoms and increase the risk of liver cancer.

Hepatitis A, a less serious form, is generally transmitted by poor sanitation, primarily fecal contamination of food or water, and is less common in industrialized nations than in developing countries. Among those at highest risk in the United States are children and staff at day-care centers, residents of institutions for the mentally handicapped, sanitation workers, and workers who handle primates such as monkeys. Gamma globulin can provide short-term immunity; vaccines against hepatitis A have been approved by the FDA. The CDC has recommended routine immunization against hepatitis A in 11 Western states with high rates.

Hepatitis B, a potentially fatal disease transmitted through the blood and other bodily fluids, infects an estimated 350,000 people around the world each year. Once spread mainly by contaminated tattoo needles, needles shared by drug addicts, or transfusions of contaminated blood, hepatitis B is now transmitted mostly through sexual contact. It can cause chronic liver infection, cirrhosis, and liver cancer.

Hepatitis B is a particular threat to young people, because 75 percent of new cases are diagnosed in those between ages 15 to 39. They usually contract hepatitis B through high-risk behaviors such as multiple sex partners and use of injected drugs. Individuals who have tattoos or body piercing may also be at risk if procedures are not done under regulated conditions. At highest risk are male homosexuals, heterosexuals with multiple sex partners, health-care workers with frequent contact with blood, IV-drug abusers, and infants born to infected mothers. Vaccination can prevent hepatitis B and is recommended for children, teens, and adults at high risk.

As many as 4 million people in the United States and 200 million people worldwide harbor the hepatitis C virus (HCV). Without effective prevention strategies, the number of cases is expected to triple in the next decade.[38] Hepatitis C, which can lead to chronic liver disease, cirrhosis, and liver cancer, is the leading reason for liver transplantation in the United States. The CDC estimates that HCV is responsible for 8,000 to 10,000 deaths every year. However, long-term studies have shown that the majority of people infected with HCV do not develop severe liver disease.[39]

Mononucleosis

You can get **mononucleosis** through kissing—or any other form of close contact. "Mono" is a viral disease that's most common among people 15 to 24 years old; its symptoms include a sore throat, headache, fever, nausea, and prolonged weakness. The spleen is swollen, and the lymph nodes are enlarged. You may also develop jaundice or a skin rash similar to German measles.

The major symptoms usually disappear within two to three weeks, but weakness, fatigue, and often depression may linger for at least two more weeks. The greatest danger is from physical activity that might rupture the spleen, resulting in internal bleeding. The liver may also become inflamed. A blood test can determine whether you have mono. However, there's no specific treatment for it, other than rest.[40]

Chronic Fatigue Syndrome (CFS)

An estimated 200,000 to 500,000 Americans have the array of symptoms known as **chronic fatigue syndrome (CFS)**. According to the CDC, symptoms of chronic fatigue syndrome include chills or low-grade fever, sore throat, tender lymph nodes, muscle pain, muscle weakness, extreme fatigue that doesn't improve with rest, headaches, joint pain (without swelling), neurological problems (confusion, memory loss, visual disturbances), and sleep disorders. Symptoms may begin suddenly and persist for six months to several years. Depression and anxiety attacks generally develop after ten months of illness.

Once dismissed as the yuppie flu, CFS has long baffled scientists. Some researchers contend that a single agent, perhaps a retrovirus, triggers the collapse of the immune system. Others think that repeated, undetected infections by bacteria, viruses, fungi, and parasites may lead to a gradual decline, while another theory blames symptoms on chronic low blood pressure.

Diagnosis of CFS remains difficult, although numerous studies have found significant immune abnormalities, such as high levels of certain immune cells (B lymphocytes and cytokines) that act as if they were constantly battling a viral infection. Researchers are working to develop a blood test that will definitively diagnose CFS. No specific treatments have proven effective for all patients, although some have responded to nicotinamide adenine dinucleotide (NADH), a coenzyme that plays a role in cellular energy production.

Pneumonia

An inflammation of the lungs, **pneumonia** fills the fine, spongy networks of the lungs' tiny air chambers with fluid. It can be caused by bacteria, viruses (including flu), or foreign material in the lungs (such as smoke). The symptoms of classic bacterial pneumonia are fever, shortness of breath, and general weakness. Along with influenza, pneumonia is the fifth-leading killer of Americans and the most common infectious cause of death.

The typical signs of pneumonia include cough, a fever of more than 101°F, difficulty breathing, chills, and excessive yellow-green phlegm. Symptoms of pneumonia can develop either gradually or else so quickly that a person's life is in danger within hours. Antibiotics can control bacterial pneumonia, but they must be given before microbes erode local tissues and spread through the blood elsewhere in the body, causing a condition known as septicemia, or blood poisoning. Because of the dangers of pneumonia, you should see a doctor if there's any chance you have it. Severe cases may require hospitalization and high doses of antibiotics.

Vaccination against pneumonia is recommended for those who've had pneumonia in the past, those with impaired immune function, and those over age 50. The pneumonia vaccine greatly reduces the risk of this disease, especially for women and those with impaired immunity.

Tuberculosis

A bacterial infection of the lungs that was once the nation's leading killer, **tuberculosis (TB)** claims the lives of more people than any acute infectious disease other than pneumonia (Figure 11-4). One-third of the world's population is infected with the TB organism, although not all develop

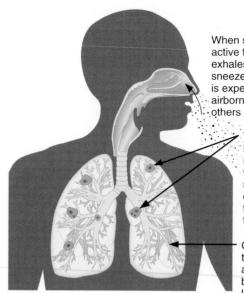

When someone with active tuberculosis exhales, coughs, or sneezes, tuberculosis is expelled in tiny airborne droplets that others may inhale.

The TB bacteria lodge mainly in the lungs, where they slowly multiply, creating patches, then cavities, in the lungs.

Other parts of the lung are affected, including bronchi and the lining of the lung.

If untreated, TB can eventually spread to and damage the brain, bone, eyes, liver and kidneys, spine, and skin.

▲ **Figure 11-4** How tuberculosis spreads.

active disease. Each year the infection spreads to another 8 million people. In the United States, TB cases, after declining for decades, increased from the mid-1980s to the early 1990s. The reasons include immigration from countries where TB is common, poverty, homelessness, alcoholism and drug abuse, the HIV/AIDS epidemic, and the emergence of resistant strains of TB. By the late 1990s, some cities reported a decline in TB, thanks to better infection control and greater monitoring to ensure completion of treatment.

Although TB is most prevalent among high-risk groups, the overall danger increases as more people develop active disease because TB is highly contagious. TB outbreaks have occurred throughout the country in hospitals, nursing homes, prisons, and office buildings, where inadequate ventilation increases the risk of infection.

Most TB patients recover completely after six months of taking a combination of three different medicines. Drug-resistant forms of the tuberculosis microorganism strike mostly patients who start drug treatment but don't follow through with it. Because they don't take enough of the medication to kill all the TB bacteria in their system, those that survive become resistant. Even with full treatment, the risk of dying from drug-resistant tuberculosis is 50 percent. HIV infection greatly increases susceptibility to infection with TB and the risk of dying if infected with treatment-resistant forms.

If you think you may have been exposed to TB or if you develop suspicious symptoms (loss of appetite and weight,

low-grade fever, fatigue, chills, night sweats, coughing), see your doctor for a TB test. This consists of an injection just under the skin. The area of the arm where the test was administered should be checked by a health-care professional to determine the presence of the TB bacteria; further tests confirm the diagnosis. If the skin test is positive, indicating that TB is present, you'll be monitored with yearly chest X rays. You may also require treatment with a drug such as rifampin or isoniazid (also called INH).

Group A and Group B Strep Infection

Sore throats are common winter complaints, but those caused by group A streptococcus bacteria—"strep throats"—are more than a trivial threat. If not treated promptly with antibiotics, strep bacteria can travel to the kidneys, the liver, or the heart, where they can cause rheumatic fever—an inflammation of the heart that can cause weakness, shortness of breath, joint pain, and an abnormal heartbeat. In recent years clusters of rheumatic fever have sprung up in several major cities. Pediatricians are urging parents to consult their doctors if a youngster complains of a sore throat or if strep is widespread in the community. Rapid new diagnostic tests can identify strep within minutes. If the test is positive, treatment with penicillin or a similar antibiotic is indicated. Brief treatment (five days) with Omnicef, a new antibiotic, has proven as effective as ten days of oral penicillin.[41]

Toxic streptococcal shock syndrome, or toxic strep, is an invasive form of the disease in which strep gains access to the blood and causes a drop in blood pressure, a very high fever, and the production of exotoxins (substances that can attack various organs, such as the kidneys, heart or, in rare cases, flesh). Toxic strep is rather rare and usually doesn't occur with strep throats. Prompt treatment is critical.

Group B streptococcus (GBS), the leading cause of life-threatening perinatal infections in the United States, is primarily a threat to newborns. Because some 15 to 40 percent of pregnant women carry GBS but have no symptoms, the American Academy of Pediatrics has called for universal screening of expectant mothers. Each year 12,000 newborns are infected, most of them during childbirth; more than 1,600 die, and another 1,600 suffer permanent brain damage from meningitis. Women at high risk of infecting their newborns with GBS are those who have premature labor, early rupture of their amniotic membranes, fever, and a high group B strep count before or during pregnancy, or who have previously borne an infant infected with GBS. Also at risk are diabetics, poor women, and those under age 20. Treating all high-risk pregnant women could prevent most GBS infections in newborns.

Toxic Shock Syndrome

As discussed in Chapter 8, **toxic shock syndrome (TSS)** is a potentially deadly disease associated with the use of tampons, particularly high-absorbency types. It is caused by *Staphylococcus aureus* and group A *Streptococcus pyogenes* bacteria that release toxins (poisonous waste products) into the bloodstream. Symptoms include a high fever; a rash that leads to peeling of the skin on the fingers, toes, palms, and soles; dizziness; dangerously low blood pressure; and abnormalities in several organ systems (the digestive tract and the kidneys) and in the muscles and blood.

In addition to women who use high-absorbency tampons, or leave their tampons in too long, those who have given birth within the preceding six to eight weeks are at greater risk. Children (including newborns), men, and postmenopausal women also have developed TSS, which usually has been traced to bacteria in skin abscesses, boils, cuts, or postsurgical wounds.

Without prompt treatment, TSS can cause severe and permanent damage, including muscle weakness, partial paralysis, amnesia, disorientation, an inability to concentrate, and impaired lung and kidney function. Sometimes toxic shock weakens the blood vessels, increasing the risk of heart problems. Victims can enter the life-threatening crisis called shock, in which blood flow throughout the body is inadequate to sustain life. Treatment usually consists of immediate hospitalization, intravenous administration of fluids, medications to raise blood pressure, and powerful antibiotics; intravenous administration of immunoglobins that attack the toxins produced by these bacteria may also be beneficial.

Lyme Disease

Lyme disease, a bacterial infection, is spread by ticks carrying a particular bacterium—the spirochete *Borrelia burgdorferi*. An infected person may have various symptoms, including joint inflammation, heart arrhythmias,

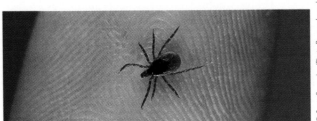

▲ Ticks are responsible for the spread of Lyme disease. If you spot a tick, remove it as soon as possible with tweezers or small forceps. Put it in a plastic bag or sealed bottle and save it. If you develop a rash or other symptoms, take it with you to the doctor.

blinding headaches, and memory lapses. The disease can also cause miscarriages and birth defects. Lyme disease is by far the most commonly reported vector-borne infectious disease in the United States. The vast majority of all reported cases have occurred in just ten states; those leading the list are New York, New Jersey, Connecticut, Pennsylvania, and Wisconsin.[42]

The FDA has licensed a vaccine to prevent Lyme disease in individuals 15 to 70 years old. LYMErix, like most vaccines, stimulates the immune system to produce antibodies, in this case against the bacteria that cause Lyme disease. But the vaccine, administered in three doses over a one-year period, is not 100 percent effective and should not be considered a substitute for protective clothing and tick repellent. Administration must be timed so the second and third doses are given at the beginning of the tick transmission season, usually April in the Northeastern United States. It is not known how long protection against Lyme disease lasts after vaccination. Vaccination is recommended for individuals at very high risk of Lyme disease, such as park rangers, others who spend much time in wooded areas, and people who live where Lyme disease is exceptionally prevalent.[43]

The primary culprit in most cases of Lyme disease is the deer tick, although other ticks, including the Western black-legged tick, the dog tick, and the Lone Star tick, also may transmit the bacterium that causes Lyme disease as well as organisms that transmit other diseases, such as Rocky Mountain spotted fever and babesiosis.

Hunters and campers are more likely to test positive for Lyme disease. Pet owners are not at additional risk. The most important preventive step is to check yourself for ticks whenever you come in from the outdoors. However, detecting some types of ticks can be difficult. In their nymphal stage, when they're most likely to bite, ticks are about the size of a poppyseed. Even as adults, some ticks are no bigger than a sesame seed.

Regardless of whether or not they've spotted a tick, residents of infested areas should check regularly for signs of a bite. About two-thirds of those bitten develop some skin changes from two days to four weeks afterward. The classic skin lesion is a small, clear-centered red doughnut that expands, but most people simply have a red blotch or two blotches. However, the rash always expands, usually to about 2 inches in diameter. In some cases, it may cover a person's entire chest or thigh; others develop rashes far from the bite, caused by spirochetes that travel through the bloodstream. More sensitive diagnostic tests allow detection of extremely low numbers of spirochetes and make earlier diagnosis possible.

According to a recent study of 482 people bitten within the previous three days, a single dose of the antibiotic doxycycline can ward off Lyme disease after a tick bite.[44] Guidelines issued by the Infectious Diseases Society of America do not recommend routine use of blood testing or antibiotics after a tick bite. However, experts do recommend antibiotic treatment if a tick may have been attached for more than 48 hours (which can be determined by the engorgement of the tick with blood) and monitoring of individuals who have removed ticks.[45] However, prolonged antibiotic treatment does not appear to help patients with Lyme disease who do not respond to the initial antibiotic treatment.[46]

STRATEGIES FOR PREVENTION

Protecting Yourself

✔ If you live in the North Atlantic states, the north central Midwest, or along the Pacific coast, wear long pants rather than shorts, and tuck your pants into your socks when walking through woods or fields of high grass.

✔ Stick to the center of trails when hiking, and avoid piles of leaves and branches.

✔ In tick-infested areas, use insect repellents. People who use insect repellents are half as likely to get Lyme disease as those who don't.

✔ After spending time outdoors, examine yourself for ticks or bites every day. Check less obvious places, such as the scalp and behind the ears.

✔ If you do spot a tick, remove it right away. Using tweezers or forceps, grasp the tick firmly as close to its head and as near to your skin as possible. Gently pull backward, without squeezing the tick's body, until its hold is released. Wash your hands thoroughly. Treat the wound with rubbing alcohol.

Future Threats

At times in recent decades scientists have predicted the conquest of agents of infections and the end of the age of infectious illnesses. Despite the progress that has been made, these have proved to be elusive goals. The future is sure to bring dangers of its own—either from new or resurrected infectious illnesses or from the deliberate use of infectious agents to sicken or kill large numbers of people.

Emerging and Re-emerging Infectious Diseases

As defined by the National Institute of Allergy and Infectious Diseases (NIAID), emerging infections are those that have been recently recognized, are increasing in humans, or threaten to spread to new areas in the near future. The most widespread is HIV, which is believed to have emerged from Central Africa less than 30 years ago. Other emerging viruses, such as hantavirus, Ebola, dengue, Lassa, and Marburg, have been responsible for deadly outbreaks around the globe.[47] The most well-known may be Ebola, a particularly virulent virus that is transmitted by direct contact with blood or bodily fluids. In several outbreaks in Africa, this filovirus has resisted all medication and killed up to 90 percent of its victims.

As civilization spreads into previously undeveloped areas, such as the rain forests of Central Africa, and goods and animals are imported from distant lands, more human beings are encountering microbes that were once confined to very remote regions.

Another threat comes from mutated, or changed, forms of familiar microbes (such as those that cause tuberculosis) that have become resistant to standard medications. Why, despite enormous scientific progress, do emerging and resistant microbes remain such a formidable foe? "Viruses and bacteria have the capacity to reinvent themselves rapidly," says John La Montagne of NIAID. "Because they have few genes compared to people, one mutation can change an organism's ability to infect, spread, or cause disease."

??? What Do I Need to Know about Biological Warfare?

In 2001, Americans learned firsthand that certain infectious agents could be used as weapons of terrorism and war. Letters contaminated with anthrax bacteria were sent to several locations around the country, infecting a number of individuals.

Anthrax, which is found naturally in wild and farm animals, can also be produced in a laboratory. The disease is spread through exposure to anthrax spores and not through exposure to an infected person. Another infectious agent, the smallpox virus, is highly contagious, however, and could threaten many millions of people because routine inoculations against smallpox stopped in 1972. Those vaccinated before that year may have lost much of their immunity within 10 years. Smallpox was officially eradicated as a disease in 1980, but stores of the virus exist for research purposes.

Even the deadliest microbes are not designed for deliberate mass murder. While they can be grown in test tubes and stored in various ways, they are difficult to disseminate. Anthrax spores, for instance, tend to clump together in humid conditions. Smallpox is so contagious that it's likely to kill anyone who attempts to handle or release it. Vaccines are available, if only in limited quantities, against agents such as anthrax and smallpox. Certain antibiotics also might be effective against bacterial agents. With the anthrax attack, the United States government began a preparedness initiative which includes working with private companies to research and produce effective vaccines and treatments for potential biological threats. (See Table 11-2 on page 384.)

Reproductive and Urinary Tract Infections

Reproductive and urinary tract infections are very common. Many are not spread exclusively by sexual contact, and so they are not classified as sexually transmitted diseases (STDs), discussed next.

Vaginal Infections

The most common vaginal infections are **trichomoniasis, candidiasis,** and **bacterial vaginosis.**

Protozoa *(Trichomonas vaginalis)* that live in the vagina can multiply rapidly, causing itching, burning, and discharge—all symptoms of trichomoniasis. Male carriers usually have no symptoms, although some may develop urethritis or an inflammation of the prostate and seminal vesicles. All patients with this infection should be screened for syphilis, gonorrhea, chlamydia, and HIV. Sexual partners must be treated with oral medication (metronidazole; trade name Flagyl), even if they have no symptoms, to prevent reinfection.

Populations of a yeast called *Candida albicans*—normal inhabitants of the mouth, digestive tract, and vagina—are usually held in check. Under certain conditions, however (such as poor nutrition, stress, or antibiotic use), the microbes multiply, causing burning, itching, and a whitish discharge, and producing what is commonly known as a yeast infection. Common sites for candidiasis, which is also called moniliasis, are the vagina, vulva, penis, and mouth. The women most likely to test positive for candidiasis have never been pregnant, use condoms for birth control, have sexual intercourse more than four times a month, and have taken antibiotics in the previous 15 to 30 days. Vaginal medications, such as GyneLotrimin and Monistat, are nonprescription drugs that provide effective treatment. Male sexual partners may be advised to wear condoms during outbreaks of candidiasis. Women should keep the genital area dry and wear cotton underwear.

Bacterial vaginosis is characterized by alterations in the microorganisms that live in the vagina, including depletion of certain bacteria and overgrowth of others. It typically causes a white or gray vaginal discharge with a distinctive fishy odor similar to that of trichomoniasis. Its underlying cause is unknown, although it occurs most frequently in women with multiple sex partners. Long-term dangers include pelvic inflammatory disease (PID, discussed later in this chapter) and pregnancy complications. Metronidazole, either in the form of a pill or a vaginal gel,

▼ **Table 11-2 Biological Threats**

Disease	Germ	Symptoms	Mortality	Treatment	What's Needed
Smallpox	Variola virus	Fever, aches, pustules on face and torso	30%	Vaccination up to 4 days after exposure; no treatment later	New vaccine: CDC is accelerating production program for completion in 2002
Inhalation anthrax	*Bacillus anthracis*	Fever, chest pain, difficulty breathing	90%	Cipro and other antibodies work before symptoms emerge	Early diagnosis tests and new drugs for treatment at later stages
Pneumonic plague	*Yersinia pestis*	Fever after 2–4 days, then pneumonialike symptoms	50–90%	Antibiotics such as streptomycin, tetracycline, and doxycycline	Vaccine was discontinued; a new one is in development
Botulism	*Clostridium botulinum*	Progressive paralysis, respiratory failure	5%	Equine antitoxin given early treats the most common botulinum toxins	Rapid diagnostic tests and a vaccine; broader, less risky antitoxins
Tularemia	*Francisella tularensis*	Fever, sore throat, weakness, weight loss	30–60%	Antibiotics such as streptomycin and gentamicin	Simple and reliable diagnostic tests; a vaccine is in development
Hemorrhagic fevers	Several viruses	Vary, but include bleeding, shock, coma	Varies	Some, such as Ebola, have no cure; the antiviral ribavirin helps others	A promising Ebola vaccine is being researched; new antivirals

is the primary treatment. According to CDC guidelines, treatment for male sex partners appears to be of little benefit, but some health practitioners recommend treatment for both partners in cases of recurrent infections.

Urinary Tract Infections (UTIs)

A urinary tract infection (UTI) can be present in any of the three parts of the urinary tract: the urethra, bladder, or kidney. An infection involving the urethra is known as **urethritis.** If the bladder is also infected, it's called **cystitis.** If it reaches the kidneys, it's called **pyelonephritis.**

An estimated 40 percent of women report having had a UTI at some point in their lives. Three times as many women as men develop UTIs, probably for anatomical reasons. A woman's urethra is only 1.5 inches long; a man's is 6 inches. Therefore bacteria, the major cause of UTIs, have a shorter distance to travel to infect a woman's bladder and kidneys. About one-fourth to one-third of all women between ages 20 and 40 develop UTIs, and 80 percent of those who experience one infection develop recurrences.

Conditions that can set the stage for UTIs include irritation and swelling of the urethra or bladder as a result of pregnancy, bike riding, irritants (such as bubble bath, douches, or a diaphragm), urinary stones, enlargement in men of the prostate gland, vaginitis, and stress. Early diagnosis is critical, because infection can spread to the kidneys and, if unchecked, result in kidney failure. Symptoms include frequent burning, painful urination, chills, fever, fatigue, and blood in the urine.

Recurrent UTIs, a frequent problem among young women, have been linked with a genetic predisposition, sexual intercourse, and the use of diaphragms. Post-intercourse treatment with antibiotics can lower the risk. Frequent recurrence of symptoms may not be caused by infection but by interstitial cystitis, a little-understood bladder inflammation that affects an estimated 450,000 Americans, almost all of them women.

Sexually Transmitted Diseases (STDs)

Venereal diseases (from the Latin *venus,* meaning "love" or "lust") are more accurately called **sexually transmitted diseases (STDs)** or sexually transmitted infections (STIs).

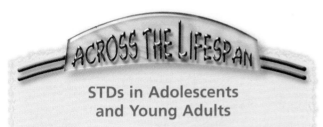

STDs in Adolescents and Young Adults

Nearly two-thirds of the people who acquire STDs in the United States are under age 25. The most common bacterial STD is chlamydia, with two of the highest rates of chlamydia occurring among adolescents in general and among young adult women. Cases of genital herpes among white adolescents have increased five times, and cases among white people in their twenties have doubled over the past few years.

Among college-age women in one study, cases of human papilloma virus (HPV) infections increased from 26 percent to 43 percent over a three-year period. Contracting STDs may increase the risk of being infected with HIV, and as many as half of new HIV infections may be among people under age 25. Because college students have more opportunities to have different sexual partners and may use drugs and alcohol more often before sex, they are at greater risk. More than half of 13- to 24-year-old women with HIV are infected heterosexually.[51]

Even when high school and college students have generally accurate knowledge about STDs, they don't necessarily practice safe sex. According to research, those students with the greatest number of sexual partners are least likely to use condoms. Other studies have shown that proximity to a high-density AIDS epicenter (such as San Francisco) has no impact on HIV/AIDS knowledge and attitudes and that religious affiliation does not decrease risky sexual behavior, at least among religious students who are sexually active. While college students admit to engaging in behaviors that put them at risk of HIV and other STDs, they believe that other students do so much more often. (See Student Snapshot: "Perceived and Actual Risky Sexual Behavior.")

According to a survey of 410 students at a public university in the Southeast, students engaged in more unprotected intercourse and oral sex when they were not under the influence of drugs or alcohol—but were more likely to engage in sexual activity with someone they'd just met when drunk or high. However, the undergraduates perceived that the "average" student engaged in risky behaviors more frequently under any circumstance.[52]

Various factors put young people at risk of STDs, including:

- **Feelings of invulnerability,** which lead to risk-taking behavior. Even when they are well informed of the risks, adolescents may remain unconvinced that anything bad can or will happen to them.
- **Multiple partners.** In surveys of students, a significant minority report having had four or more sexual partners during their lifetime.
- **Failure to use condoms.** Among those who reported having had sexual intercourse in the previous three months, fewer than half reported condom use. Students who'd had four or more sexual partners were significantly less likely to use condoms than those who'd had fewer partners.
- **Substance abuse.** Teenagers who drink or use drugs are more likely to engage in sexually risky behaviors, including sex with partners whose health status and history they do not know, and unprotected intercourse.[53]

The college years are a prime time for contracting STDs. According to the American College Health Association, chlamydia and HPV have reached epidemic levels at many schools—although many of those infected aren't even aware of it.

Although young adulthood is the age of greatest risk for acquiring STDs, the likelihood that men and women will receive information about prevention declines after they graduate from high school. The media, particularly television, are by far the most common sources of health information for young men. In a recent survey, about one-third of young adult men said they received no information about AIDS or STDs from any other source.[54]

Race and ethnicity also affect risk in the young. Young African-American men, who are more likely to be sexually active and to have more partners than young white men, also have higher STD infection rates. While the chlamydia rate for Hispanics is almost three times that of whites, the rate for blacks is ten times that of whites. The gonorrhea rate for African American males aged 20 to 24 is 40 times that of whites. Although HIV infection rates have declined for all men, they are falling at a slower rate for African-American men.

Early communication about AIDS and STDs also affects risk later in life. Several studies have shown that discussing sexual risks with parents or counseling by physicians can promote changes in condom use and sexual behavior.[55] Although parents believe that talking to children about sex is important, adolescents say that their parents do not talk to them early enough about sexual issues.

Student Snapshot Perceived and Actual Risky Sexual Behavior

In a survey of 136 male and 258 female undergraduates, students indicated that they engaged in risky behaviors less frequently than they thought the average student did. The students in the survey ranged in age from 18 to 46 years and attended a public university in the Southeast. For all behaviors, students responded using a 9-point scale, in which 1 = Never and 9 = Everyday.

Type of HIV-risky behavior	Student's personal behavior	Perceived behavior of the "average student"
When not drunk or high		
Genital or anal intercourse without a condom	3.11	4.28
Oral sex	3.6	4.67
Intercourse or oral sex with someone just met	1.25	3.61
When drunk or high		
Genital or anal intercourse without a condom	1.25	3.61
Oral sex	2.14	4.5
Intercourse or oral sex with someone just met	1.32	4.18

Source: Bon, Rebecca, et al. "Normative Perceptions in Relation to Substance Use and HIV-Risky Sexual Behaviors of College Students." *Journal of Psychology,* Vol. 135, No. 2, March 2001, p. 165.

Around the world, some 50 million cases of curable STDs occur each year (not including HIV and herpes).[48] Almost 700,000 people are infected every day with one of the over 20 STDs tracked by world health officials. The highest rates of sexually transmitted infections occur among 16- to 24-year-olds, particularly older teenagers.[49] STDs are much more widespread in developing nations because of lack of adequate health standards, prevention practices, and access to treatment.[50]

More Americans are infected with STDs now than at any other time in history. According to the Institute of Medicine, the odds of acquiring an STD during a lifetime are one in four. STDs are among the top ten most frequently reported diseases in the United States, and their annual economic cost is $17 billion. The major cause of preventable sterility in America, STDs have tripled the rate of ectopic (tubal) pregnancies, which can be fatal if not detected early. STD complications, including miscarriage, premature delivery, and uterine infections after delivery, affect more than 100,000 women annually. Moreover, infection with an STD greatly increases the risk of HIV transmission (discussed later in this chapter). The inci-

dence of STDs is highest in young adults and homosexual men. Others affected by STDs include unborn and newborn children who can "catch" potentially life-threatening infections in the womb or during birth.

Although each STD is a distinct disease, all STD pathogens like dark, warm, moist body surfaces, particularly the mucous membranes that line the reproductive organs; they hate light, cold, and dryness. It is possible to catch or have more than one STD at a time. Curing one doesn't necessarily cure another, and treatments don't prevent another bout with the same STD. (See Table 11-3.)

Many STDs, including early HIV infection and gonorrhea in women, may not cause any symptoms. As a result, infected individuals may continue their usual sexual activity without realizing that they're jeopardizing others' well-being.

Prevention and Protection

Abstinence is the only guarantee of sexual safety—and one that more and more young people are choosing. By

▼ **Table 11-3 Common Sexually Transmitted Diseases (STDs): Mode of Transmission, Symptoms, and Treatment**

STD	Transmission	Symptoms	Treatment
Chlamydial infection	The *Chlamydia trachomatis* bacterium is transmitted primarily through sexual contact. It can also be spread by fingers from one body site to another.	In women, PID (pelvic inflammatory disease) caused by *Chlamydia* may include disrupted menstrual periods, pelvic pain, elevated temperature, nausea, vomiting, headache, infertility, and ectopic pregnancy. In men, chlamydial infection of the urethra may cause a discharge and burning during urination. *Chlamydia*-caused epididymitis may produce a sense of heaviness in the affected testicle(s), inflammation of the scrotal skin, and painful swelling at the bottom of the testicle.	Doxycycline, azithromycin, or ofloxacin
Gonorrhea ("clap")	The *Neisseria gonorrhoeae* bacterium ("gonococcus") is spread through genital, oral–genital, or genital–anal contact.	The most common symptoms in men are a cloudy discharge from the penis and burning sensations during urination. If disease is untreated, complications may include inflammation of scrotal skin and swelling at base of the testicle. In women, some green or yellowish discharge is produced but commonly remains undetected. Later, PID may develop.	Dual therapy of a single dose of ceftriaxone, cefixime, ciprofloxacin, or ofloxacin plus doxycycline for seven days or a single dose of azithromycin
Non-gonococcal urethritis (NGU)	Primary causes are believed to be the bacteria *Chlamydia trachomatis* and *Ureaplasma urealyticum,* most commonly transmitted through coitus. Some NGU may result from allergic reactions or from *Trichomonas* infection.	Inflammation of the urethral tube. A man has a discharge from the penis and irritation during urination. A woman may have a mild discharge of pus from the vagina but often shows no symptoms.	A single dose of azithromycin or doxycycline for seven days
Syphilis	The *Treponema pallidum* bacterium ("spirochete") is transmitted from open lesions during genital, oral–genital, or genital–anal contact.	*Primary stage:* A painless chancre appears at the site where the spirochetes entered the body. *Secondary stage:* The chancre disappears and a generalized skin rash develops. *Latent stage:* There may be no visible symptoms. *Tertiary stage:* Heart failure, blindness, mental disturbance, and many other symptoms occur. Death may result.	Benzathine penicillin G, doxycycline, erythromycin, or ceftriaxone
Herpes	The genital herpes virus (HSV-2) seems to be transmitted primarily by vaginal, anal, or oral–genital intercourse. The oral herpes virus (HSV-1) is transmitted primarily by kissing.	Small, painful red bumps (papules) appear in the genital region (genital herpes) or mouth (oral herpes). The papules become painful blisters that eventually rupture to form wet, open sores.	No known cure; a variety of treatments may reduce symptoms; oral or intravenous acyclovir (Zovirax) promotes healing and suppresses recurrent outbreaks.
Chancroid	The *Haemophilus ducrevi* bacterium is usually transmitted by sexual interaction.	Small bumps (papules) in genital regions eventually rupture and form painful, soft, crater-like ulcers that emit a foul-smelling discharge.	Single doses of either ceftriaxone or azithromycin or seven days of erythromycin
Human papilloma virus (HPV) (genital warts)	The virus is spread primarily through vaginal, anal, or oral–genital sexual interaction.	Hard and yellow-gray on dry skin areas; soft, pinkish-red, and cauliflowerlike on moist areas.	Freezing, application of topical agents like trichloroacetic acid or podofilox, cauterization, surgical removal, or vaporization by carbon dioxide laser

(continued)

▼ **Table 11-3 Common Sexually Transmitted Diseases (STDs): Mode of Transmission, Symptoms, and Treatment (Continued)**

STD	Transmission	Symptoms	Treatment
Pubic lice ("crabs")	*Phthirus pubis,* the pubic louse, is spread easily through body contact or through shared clothing or bedding.	Persistent itching. Lice are visible and may often be located in pubic hair or other body hair.	1% permethrin cream for body areas; 1% Lindane shampoo for hair.
Scabies	*Sarcoptes scabiei* is highly contagious and may be transmitted by close physical contact, sexual and nonsexual.	Small bumps and a red rash that itch intensely, especially at night.	5% permethrin lotion or cream
Acquired immunodeficiency syndrome (AIDS)	Blood and semen are the major vehicles for transmitting HIV, which attacks the immune system. It appears to be passed primarily through sexual contact, or needle sharing among injecting drug users.	Vary with the type of cancer or opportunistic infections that afflict an infected person. Common symptoms include fevers, night sweats, weight loss, chronic fatigue, swollen lymph nodes, diarrhea and/or bloody stools, atypical bruising or bleeding, skin rashes, headache, chronic cough, and a whitish coating on the tongue or throat.	Commence treatment early after a positive HIV test with a combination of three or more antiretroviral drugs (HAART) plus other specific treatment(s), if necessary, of opportunistic infections and tumors.
Viral hepatitis	The hepatitis B virus can be transmitted by blood, semen, vaginal secretions, and saliva. Manual, oral, or penile stimulation of the anus are strongly associated with the spread of this virus. Hepatitis A seems to be primarily spread via the fecal–oral route, but oral–anal sexual contact is a common mode for sexual transmission of hepatitis A.	Vary from nonexistent to mild, flulike symptoms to an incapacitating illness characterized by high fever, vomiting, and severe abdominal pain.	No specific therapy for A and B types; treatment generally consists of bed rest and adequate fluid intake. Combination therapy with interferon and ribavarin may be effective for hepatitis C infections.
Bacterial vaginosis	The most common causative agent, the *Gardnerella vaginalis* bacterium, is sometimes transmitted through coitus.	In women, a fishy- or musty-smelling, thin discharge, like flour paste in consistency and usually gray. Most men are asymptomatic.	Metronidazole (Flagyl) by mouth or intravaginal applications of topical metronidazole gel or clindamycin cream
Candidiasis (yeast infection)	The *Candida albicans* fungus may accelerate growth when the chemical balance of the vagina is disturbed; it may also be transmitted through sexual interaction.	White, "cheesy" discharge; irritation of vaginal and vulval tissues.	Vaginal suppositories or topical cream, such as clotrimazole and miconazole, or oral fluconazole
Trichomoniasis	The protozoan parasite *Trichomonas vaginalis* is usually passed through genital sexual contact.	White or yellow vaginal discharge with an unpleasant odor; vulva is sore and irritated.	Metronidazole (Flagyl) for both women and men

Source: Crooks, Robert L., and Karla Baur. *Our Sexuality,* 8th ed. Pacific Grove, CA: Wadsworth, 2002.

choosing not to be sexually active with a partner, individuals can safeguard their physical health, their fertility, and their future.

For men and women who are sexually active, a mutually faithful sexual relationship with just one healthy partner is the safest option. For those not in such relationships,

safer-sex practices are essential for reducing risks. (See the Self-Survey: "STD Attitude Scale.")

 According to a recent analysis, many factors affect women's decisions about safer-sex practices, including race and ethnicity. African-American women were more likely to make

SELF SURVEY

STD Attitude Scale

Directions: Read each statement carefully: STD means sexually transmitted diseases. Record your first reaction by marking an "X" through the letter that best describes how much you agree or disagree with the idea.

1. How one uses his/her sexuality has nothing to do with STDs.
   SA   A   U   D   SD
2. It is easy to use the prevention methods that reduce one's chances of getting an STD.
   SA   A   U   D   SD
3. Responsible sex is one of the best ways of reducing the risk of STDs.
   SA   A   U   D   SD
4. Getting early medical care is the main key to preventing harmful effects of STDs.
   SA   A   U   D   SD
5. Choosing the right partner is important in reducing the risk of getting an STD.
   SA   A   U   D   SD
6. A high rate of STDs should be a concern for all people.
   SA   A   U   D   SD
7. People with an STD have a duty to get their sex partners to seek medical care.
   SA   A   U   D   SD
8. The best way to get a sex partner to STD treatment is to take him/her to the doctor with you.
   SA   A   U   D   SD
9. Changing one's sex habits is necessary once the presence of an STD is known.
   SA   A   U   D   SD
10. I would dislike having to follow the medical steps for treating an STD.
    SA   A   U   D   SD
11. If I were sexually active, I would feel uneasy doing things before and after sex to prevent getting an STD.
    SA   A   U   D   SD
12. If I were sexually active, it would be insulting if a sex partner suggested we use a condom to avoid STDs.
    SA   A   U   D   SD
13. I dislike talking about STDs with my peers.
    SA   A   U   D   SD
14. I would be uncertain about going to the doctor unless I was sure I really had an STD.
    SA   A   U   D   SD
15. I would feel that I should take my sex partner with me to a clinic if I thought I had an STD.
    SA   A   U   D   SD

Use This Key: SA = Strongly agree; A = Agree; U = Undecided; D = Disagree; SD = Strongly disagree.
Remember: STD means sexually transmitted disease, such as gonorrhea, syphilis, genital herpes, and AIDS.

16. It would be embarrassing to discuss STDs with one's partner if one were sexually active.
    SA   A   U   D   SD
17. If I were to have sex, the chance of getting an STD makes me uneasy about having sex with more than one person.
    SA   A   U   D   SD
18. I like the idea of sexual abstinence (not having sex) as the best way to avoid STDs.
    SA   A   U   D   SD
19. If I had an STD, I would cooperate with public health persons to find the sources of the STD.
    SA   A   U   D   SD
20. If I had an STD, I would avoid exposing others while I was being treated.
    SA   A   U   D   SD
21. I would have regular STD checkups if I were having sex with more than one partner.
    SA   A   U   D   SD
22. I intend to look for STD signs before deciding to have sex with anyone.
    SA   A   U   D   SD
23. I will limit my sex activity to just one partner because of the chances I might get an STD.
    SA   A   U   D   SD
24. I will avoid sex contact anytime I think there is even a slight chance of getting an STD.
    SA   A   U   D   SD
25. The chance of getting an STD would not stop me from having sex.
    SA   A   U   D   SD
26. If I had a chance, I would support community efforts toward controlling STDs.
    SA   A   U   D   SD
27. I would be willing to work with others to make people aware of STD problems in my town.
    SA   A   U   D   SD

Scoring: Calculate total points for each subscale and total scale, using the point values below.

For items 1, 10–14, 16, 25:
Strongly agree = 5 points; Agree = 4 points;
Undecided = 3 points;
Disagree = 2 points; and Strongly disagree = 1 point.

(continued)

For items 2–9, 15, 17–24, 26, 27:
Strongly agree = 1 point; Agree = 2 points;
Undecided = 3 points;
Disagree = 4 points; and Strongly disagree = 5 points.

Total scale: items 1–27
Belief Subscale: items 1–9
Feeling Subscale: items 10–18
Intention to Act Subscale: items 19–27

Interpretation

High score predisposes toward high-risk STD behavior.
Low score predisposes toward low-risk STD behavior.

Yarber, et al. (1989) developed the STD Attitude Scale by administering three experimental forms of 45 items each. Respondents were 2,980 students in six secondary school districts in the Midwest and East. Based on statistical analysis, the scale was reduced to the final 27 items. Reliability coefficients for the entire scale and the three subscales ranged from .48 to .73. The developers reported evidence of construct validity in that the scale was sensitive to positive attitude changes resulting from STD education.

Reference: Yarber, W. L., et al. Development of a Three-Component STD Attitude Scale. *Journal of Sex Education and Therapy,* Vol. 15, 1989, pp. 36–39. Used by permission.

contraceptive decisions without the influence of partners and to focus on pregnancy rather than STD prevention. European-American and Latina women were more likely to be influenced by their partners in making decisions about safer sex and STD protection. Women who'd had an STD were much more vigilant about using methods to prevent disease and pregnancy.[56] In a survey of 123 sexually experienced African-American undergraduate women, 38 percent reported at least one previous diagnosis of an STD, yet only 24 percent said that they always used condoms. Early age at first intercourse and a greater number of sexual partners increased a woman's likelihood of having an STD.[57]

How can you tell if someone you're dating or hope to date has been exposed to an STD? The bad news is, you

can't. But the good news is, it doesn't matter—as long as you avoid sexual activity that could put you at risk of infection. Ideally, before engaging in any such behavior, both of you should talk about your prior sexual history (including number of partners and sexually transmitted

© LWA/Corbis Stock Market

▲ Talking openly about STDs and being tested with your partner protects your health and can foster a sense of trust and commitment.

STRATEGIES FOR PREVENTION

Telling a Partner You Have an STD

Even though the conversation can be awkward and embarrassing, you need to talk honestly about any STDs that you may have been exposed to or contracted. What you don't say can be hazardous to your partner's health. Here are some guidelines:

✔ **Talk before you become intimate.** A good way to start is simply by saying, *"There is something we need to talk over first."*

✔ **Be honest.** Don't downplay any potential risks.

✔ **Don't blame.** Even if you suspect that your partner was the source of your infection, focus on the need for medical attention.

✔ **Be sensitive to your partner's feelings.** Anger and resentment are common reactions when someone feels at risk. Try to listen without becoming defensive.

✔ **Seek medical attention.** Do not engage in sexual intimacies until you obtain a doctor's assurance that you are no longer contagious.[58]

diseases) and other high-risk behavior, such as the use of injection drugs. If you know someone well enough to consider having sex with that person, you should be able to talk about STDs. If the person is unwilling to talk, you shouldn't have sex. People who seek sex partners through the Internet may be at a greater risk for sexually transmitted diseases. In a CDC survey, online seekers were more likely to have had a previous STD and reported a greater number of partners.[59]

Even if you do talk openly, you can't be sure a potential partner is telling you the truth. In various surveys of college students, a significant proportion of the men and women said they would lie to a potential partner about having an STD or testing positive for HIV. The only way of knowing for certain that a prospective partner is safe is through laboratory testing. Sex educators and health professionals strongly encourage couples to abstain from any sexual activity that puts them at risk for STDs until they both undergo medical examinations and laboratory testing to rule out STDs. This process greatly reduces the danger of disease transmission and can also help foster a deep sense of mutual trust and commitment. Many campus and public health clinics provide exams or laboratory testing either free of charge or on a sliding scale determined by your income.

Chlamydia

The most widespread sexually transmitted bacterium in the United States is *Chlamydia trachomatis*, which causes 3 to 5 million **chlamydial infections** each year. *Chlamydia trachomatis* infections are more common in younger than in older women, in African-American than in white women, and in unmarried than in married pregnant women. They also occur more often in both men and women with gonorrhea.

Those at greatest risk of chlamydial infection are individuals 25 years old or younger who engage in sex with more than one new partner within a two-month period and women who use birth control pills or other nonbarrier contraceptive methods. The U.S. Preventive Services Task Forces recommend regular screening for chlamydia for all sexually active women under age 25 and for older women with multiple sexual partners, a history of STDs, or inconsistent use of condoms.[60]

As many as 75 percent of women and 50 percent of men with chlamydia have no symptoms or symptoms so mild that they don't seek medical attention. Without treatment, up to 40 percent of cases of chlamydia can lead to pelvic inflammatory disease, a serious infection of the woman's fallopian tubes that can also damage the ovaries and uterus. Also, women infected with chlamydia may have three to five times the risk of getting infected with HIV if exposed. Babies exposed to chlamydia in the birth canal during delivery can be born with pneumonia or with an eye

infection called conjunctivitis, both of which can be dangerous unless treated early with antibiotics. Symptomless women who are screened and treated for chlamydial infection are almost 60 percent less likely than unscreened women to develop pelvic inflammatory disease.

Traditional methods of screening require a health professional to collect a swab sample of genital secretions. In the past, the sample had to be cultured in a laboratory to look for *C. trachomatis*, and results could take three days or more. Today, a number of tests are available to supplement or sometimes replace the relatively expensive and slow traditional culture. The three major types of nonculture tests are:

- Direct fluorescent antibody test, which uses a scientific method called staining to make chlamydia easier to spot under a microscope. DFA can give quicker results than culture and can be performed on specimens taken from the eye, cervix, or penis.
- Enzyme immunoassays, available in some forms that don't require special lab equipment. Results are more rapid than with culture, and costs can be lower.
- Tests to detect the genes of *C. trachomatis* in urine, as well as genital, samples, which can accurately identify even very small numbers of genes in a specimen. While expensive, they are easy to perform and have a high level of accuracy

According to CDC guidelines, the treatment of choice for uncomplicated chlamydia infections is a seven-day regimen of doxycycline or a single, 1-gram dose of azithromycin (Zithromax). Because chlamydia often occurs along with gonorrhea, some health practitioners prescribe seven days of ofloxacin, a drug effective against both chlamydial and gonorrheal infections. The use of condoms with spermicide can reduce, but not eliminate, the risk of chlamydial infection. Sexual partners should be examined and treated if necessary.

Pelvic Inflammatory Disease (PID)

Infection of a woman's fallopian tubes or uterus, called **pelvic inflammatory disease (PID),** is not actually an STD, but rather a complication of STDs. About one in every seven women of reproductive age has PID; half of all adult women may have had it. Each year, about 1 million new cases are reported.

Ten to 20 percent of initial episodes of PID lead to scarring and obstruction of the fallopian tubes severe enough to cause infertility. Other long-term complications are ectopic pregnancy and chronic pelvic pain. The risk of these complications rises with subsequent PID episodes, bacterial vaginosis (discussed earlier in this chapter), and use of IUDs. Smoking also may increase the likelihood of PID. Two bacteria—gonococcus (the culprit in gonorrhea) and chlamydia—are responsible for one-half to one-third of all cases of PID. Other organisms are responsible for the remaining cases.

Most cases of PID occur among women under age 25 who are sexually active. Gonococcus-caused cases tend to affect poor women; those caused by chlamydia range across all income levels. One-half to one-third of all cases are transmitted sexually, and others have been traced to some IUDs that are no longer on the market. Several studies have shown that women with PID are more likely to have used douches than those without the disease. Consistent condom use may decrease PID risk.[61]

PID is a silent disease that, in half of all cases, often produces no noticeable symptoms as it progresses and causes scarring of the fallopian tubes. Experts are encouraging women with mild symptoms, such as abdominal pain or tenderness, to seek medical evaluation and encouraging physicians to test these patients for infections. Urine testing is a cost-effective method of detecting gonorrhea and chlamydia in young women and can prevent development of PID. For women with symptoms, magnetic resonance imaging (MRI) is highly accurate in establishing a diagnosis of PID and detecting other processes responsible for the symptoms.

Women may learn that they have PID only after discovering that they cannot conceive, or after they develop an ectopic pregnancy (see Chapter 9). PID causes an estimated 15 to 30 percent of all cases of infertility every year, and about half of all cases of ectopic pregnancy. Most women do not experience any symptoms, but some may develop abdominal pain, tenderness in certain sites during pelvic exams, or vaginal discharge. Treatment may require hospitalization and intensive antibiotics therapy.

Gonorrhea

Gonorrhea (sometimes called "the clap" in street language) is one of the most common STDs in the United States and is increasing in occurrence, reversing a downward trend in the previous two decades.[62] By some estimates, there may be approximately 1 million new cases every year. The incidence is highest among teenagers and young adults. Sexual contact, including oral-genital sex, is the primary means of transmission.

Most men who have gonorrhea know it. Thick, yellow-white pus oozes from the penis, and urination causes a burning sensation. These symptoms usually develop two to nine days after the sexual contact that infected them. Men have a good reason to seek help: It hurts too much not to. Women also may experience discharge and burning on urination. However, as many as eight out of ten infected women have no symptoms.

Gonococcus, the bacterium that causes gonorrhea, can live in the vagina, cervix, and fallopian tubes for months, even years, and continue to infect the woman's sexual part-

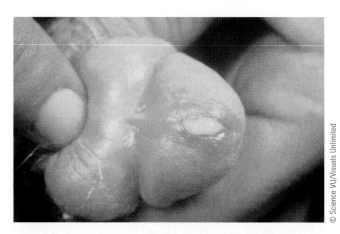

▲ A cloudy discharge is symptomatic of gonorrhea.

ners. Approximately 5 percent of sexually active American women have positive gonorrhea cultures but are unaware that they are silent carriers.

If left untreated in men or women, gonorrhea spreads through the urinary-genital tract. In women, the inflammation travels from the vagina and cervix, through the uterus, to the fallopian tubes and ovaries. The pain and fever are similar to those caused by stomach upset, so a woman may dismiss the symptoms. Eventually these symptoms diminish, even though the disease spreads to the entire pelvis. Pus may ooze from the fallopian tubes or ovaries into the peritoneum (the lining of the abdominal cavity), sometimes causing serious inflammation. However, this, too, can subside in a few weeks. Gonorrhea, the leading cause of sterility in women, can cause PID. In pregnant women, gonorrhea becomes a threat to the newborn. It can infect the infant's external genitals and cause a serious form of conjunctivitis, an inflammation of the eye that may lead to blindness. As a preventive step, newborns may have penicillin dropped into their eyes at birth.

In men, untreated gonorrhea can spread to the prostate gland, testicles, bladder, and kidneys. Among the serious complications are urinary obstruction and sterility caused by blockage of the vas deferens (the excretory duct of the testis). In both sexes, gonorrhea can develop into a serious, even fatal, bloodborne infection that can cause arthritis in the joints, attack the heart muscle and lining, cause meningitis, and attack the skin and other organs.

Although a blood test has been developed for detecting gonorrhea, the tried-and-true method of diagnosis is still a microscopic study and analysis of cultures from the male's urethra, the female's cervix, and the throat and anus of both sexes.

In the last decade, antibiotic-resistant strains of gonorrhea have emerged, and the current CDC treatment guidelines suggest the use of drugs effective against both resistant and nonresistant strains of *Neisseria gonorrhoeae*.

PULSE POINTS

Ten Ways to Prevent Sexually Transmitted Diseases (STDs)

1. **Abstain from sexual intercourse.** You don't have to abstain from all sexual activity. Fantasizing, masturbating, touching, hugging, and petting are all safe and pleasurable.

2. **Don't rush into a sexual relationship.** Get to know a potential partner well over a period of several months or more. Share your sexual histories, and build an honest, mutually caring, and trusting relationship.

3. **Get checked out.** The only accurate way to assess the risks of STDs is a thorough medical examination, including laboratory testing.

4. **Maintain a mutually faithful sexual relationship with just** one uninfected partner. An exclusive sexual relationship with a person who has never been exposed to any STD is safe, regardless of what type of sexual activity you engage in.

5. **Always use condoms and spermicides.** Although their use reduces your risk, keep in mind that doing so does not guarantee protection.

6. **Don't have sex with multiple partners.** The risk of STDs increases along with the number of sexual partners. Also avoid sexual contact with individuals who've had multiple or anonymous sexual partners.

7. **Inspect your partner's genitals before sex.** Although some STDs produce no visible signs, it is possible to see herpes blisters, chancres, rashes, genital warts, and the like.

8. **Wash your own—and your partner's—genitals before and after sex.** Although it's not clear how effective soap and water are, washing—especially of the penis—is generally believed to have some benefits.

9. **Don't have sexual contact with individuals who use injection drugs.** Regardless of the type of drug—anabolic steroids, cocaine, heroin, and so on—users are at higher risk for several STDs, including hepatitis and HIV infection.

10. **Keep a clear head.** Don't make decisions about sexual activity while under the influence of alcohol or drugs that could affect your judgment.

Because gonorrhea often occurs along with chlamydia, practitioners often use an agent effective against both, such as ofloxacin. Antibiotics taken for other reasons may not affect or cure the gonorrhea because of their dosage or type. And you can't develop immunity to gonorrhea; within days of recovering from one case, you can catch another.

Nongonococcal Urethritis (NGU)

The term **nongonococcal urethritis (NGU)** refers to any inflammation of the urethra that is not caused by gonorrhea. NGU is the most common STD in men, accounting for 4 million to 6 million visits to a physician every year. Three microorganisms—*Chlamydia trachomatis*, *Ureaplasma urealyticum*, and *Mycoplasma genitalium*—are the primary causes; the usual means of transmission is sexual intercourse. Other infectious agents, such as fungi or bacteria, allergic reactions to vaginal secretions, or irritation by soaps or contraceptive foams or gels may also lead to NGU.

In the United States, NGU is more common in men than gonoccocal urethritis. The symptoms in men are similar to those of gonorrhea, including discharge from the penis (usually less than with gonorrhea) and mild burning during urination. Women frequently develop no symptoms or very mild itching, burning during urination, or discharge. Symptoms usually disappear after two or three weeks, but the infection may persist and causes cervicitis or PID in women and, in men, may spread to the prostate, epididymis, or both. Treatment usually consists of doxycycline and should be given to both sexual partners after testing. For men, a single oral dose of azithromycin has proven as effective as a standard seven-day course of doxycycline.

Syphilis

A corkscrew-shaped, spiral bacterium called *Treponema pallidum* causes **syphilis.** This frail germ dies in seconds if dried or chilled but grows quickly in the warm, moist tissues of the body, particularly in the mucous membranes of the genital tract. Entering the body through any tiny break in the skin, the germ burrows its way into the bloodstream. Sexual contact, including oral sex or intercourse, is a primary means of transmission. Genital ulcers caused by syphilis may increase the risk of HIV infection, while individuals with HIV may be more likely to develop syphilis.

Public education programs, expanded screening and surveillance, increased tracing of contacts, and condom promotion have helped to control the spread of syphilis in some areas. Syphilis rates have fallen to the lowest ever reported in the United States.[63] The decline has been particularly significant in African Americans.

Syphilis has clearly identifiable stages:

▶ **Primary syphilis.** The first sign of syphilis is a lesion, or chancre (pronounced "shanker"), an open lump or crater the size of a dime or smaller, teeming with bacteria. The incubation period before its appearance ranges from 10 to 90 days; three to four weeks is average. The chancre appears exactly where the bacteria entered the body: in the mouth, throat, vagina, rectum, or penis. Any contact with the chancre is likely to result in infection.

▶ **Secondary syphilis.** Anywhere from one to twelve months after the chancre's appearance, secondary-stage symptoms may appear. Some people have no symptoms. Others develop a skin rash or a small, flat rash in moist regions on the skin; whitish patches on the mucous membranes of the mouth or throat; temporary baldness; low-grade fever; headache; swollen glands; or large, moist sores around the mouth and genitals. These are loaded with bacteria; contact with them, through kissing or intercourse, may transmit the infection. Symptoms may last for several days or several months. Even without treatment, they eventually disappear as the syphilis microbes go into hiding.

▶ **Latent syphilis.** Although there are no signs or symptoms, no sores or rashes at this stage, the bacteria are invading various organs inside the body, including the heart and brain. For two to four years, there may be recurring infectious and highly contagious lesions of the skin or mucous membranes. However, syphilis loses its infectiousness as it progresses: After the first two years, a person rarely transmits syphilis through intercourse.

After four years, even congenital syphilis is rarely transmitted. Until this stage of the disease, however, a pregnant woman can pass syphilis to her unborn child. If the fetus is infected in its fourth month or earlier, it may be disfigured or may even die. If infected late in pregnancy, the child may show no signs of infection for months or years after birth, but may then become disabled with the symptoms of tertiary syphilis.

▶ **Tertiary syphilis.** Ten to twenty years after the beginning of the latent stage, the most serious symptoms of syphilis emerge, generally in the organs in which the bacteria settled during latency. Syphilis that has progressed to this stage has become increasingly rare. Victims of tertiary syphilis may die of a ruptured aorta or of other heart damage, or may have progressive brain or spinal cord damage, eventually leading to blindness, insanity, or paralysis. About a third of those who are not treated during the first three stages of syphilis enter the tertiary stage later in life.

Health experts are urging screening for syphilis for everyone who seeks treatment for an STD, especially adolescents; for everyone using illegal drugs; and for the partners of these two groups. They also recommend that anyone diagnosed with syphilis be screened for other STDs and be counseled about voluntary testing for HIV.

Early diagnosis of syphilis can lead to a complete cure. The most widely used diagnostic techniques are the Venereal Disease Research Laboratory (VDRL) test or the rapid-plasma-reagin (RPR) test. However, these may be positive only during the secondary stage of the disease, when the bacteria have reached the bloodstream. A positive finding always requires additional information, including a physical exam and other laboratory tests, to confirm the diagnosis and help in planning treatment.

Penicillin is the drug of choice for treating primary, secondary, or latent syphilis. The earlier treatment begins, the more effective it is. Those allergic to penicillin may be treated with doxycycline, ceftriaxone, or erythromycin. An added danger of not getting treatment for syphilis is an increased risk of HIV transmission.

???? What Is Herpes?

Herpes (from the Greek word that means "to creep") collectively describes some of the most common viral infections in humans. Characteristically, **herpes simplex** causes blisters on the skin or mucous membranes. Herpes simplex exists in several varieties. Herpes simplex virus 1 (HSV-1) generally causes cold sores and fever blisters around the mouth. Herpes simplex virus 2 (HSV-2) may cause blisters on the penis, inside the vagina, on the cervix, in the pubic area, on the buttocks, or on the thighs. With the increase of oral-genital sex, some doctors report finding type 2 herpes lesions in the mouth and throat.

An estimated 135 million Americans age 12 or over carry HSV-1, the most common herpes virus.[64] The prevalence of HSV-2 has increased 30 percent since the late 1970s. According to the CDC, one in five American adolescents and adults is now infected, but 80 to 90 percent of these individuals do not realize they carry the virus because they never develop genital lesions, or they experience only very subtle symptoms. Men and women ages 20 to 29 have higher rates of infection than other age groups.[65]

Recent research with a new, more sensitive test reveals that individuals without any obvious symptoms shed the virus "subclinically" whether or not they have lesions. Most people with herpes contract it from partners who were not aware of any symptoms or of their own contagiousness. Standard methods of diagnosing genital herpes in women, which rely primarily on physical examination and viral cultures, may miss as many as two-thirds of all cases. Newly developed blood tests are more effective in detecting unrecognized and subclinical infections with HSV-2.

A recent study confirmed that people infected with genital herpes can spread it even between flare-ups when

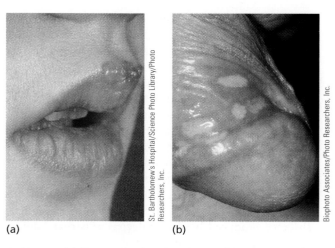

St. Bartholomew's Hospital/Science Photo Library/Photo Researchers, Inc.

Biophoto Associates/Photo Researchers, Inc.

(a)   (b)

▲ Herpes. (a) Herpes simplex virus 1, or HSV-1, as a mouth sore. (b) Herpes simplex virus 2, or HSV-2, usually causes genital sores.

they have no symptoms. In the past, patients and most doctors thought people with herpes could safely have unprotected sex when they had no symptoms. Research shows, however, that the herpes virus is present in genital secretions even when patients do not notice any signs of the disease.[66] There is growing evidence that genital herpes promotes the spread of HIV.

HSV transmission occurs through close contact with mucous membranes or abraded skin. Condoms help prevent infection but aren't foolproof. When herpes sores are present, the infected person is highly contagious and should avoid bringing the lesions into contact with someone else's body through touching, sexual interaction, or kissing. However, HSV also can be transmitted when there are no signs or symptoms of the disease.

A newborn can be infected with genital herpes while passing through the birth canal, and the frequency of mother-to-infant transmission seems to be increasing. Most infected infants develop typical skin sores, which should be cultured to confirm a herpes diagnosis. Some physicians recommend treatment with acyclovir. Because of the risk of severe damage and possible death, caesarean delivery may be advised for a woman with active herpes lesions.

The virus that causes herpes never entirely goes away; it retreats to nerves near the lower spinal cord, where it remains for the life of the host. Herpes sores can return without warning weeks, months, or even years after their first occurrence, often during menstruation or times of stress, or with sudden changes in body temperature. Of those who experience HSV recurrence, 10 to 35 percent do so frequently—that is, about six or more times a year. In most people, attacks diminish in frequency and severity over time. Herpes, like other STDs, can trigger feelings of shame, guilt, and depression.

Antiviral drugs, such as acyclovir (Zovirax), have proven effective in treating and controlling herpes. Available as an ointment, in capsules, and in injection form, acyclovir relieves the symptoms but doesn't kill the virus. Whereas the ointment works only for the initial bout with herpes, acyclovir in injectable and pill form dramatically reduces the length and severity of herpes outbreaks. Continuing daily oral acyclovir can reduce recurrences by about 80 percent. However, its safety in pregnant women has not been established. Infection with herpes viruses resistant to acyclovir is a growing problem, especially in individuals with immune-suppressing disorders.

Various treatments—compresses made with cold water, skim milk, or warm salt water, ice packs, or a mild anesthetic cream—can relieve discomfort. Herpes sufferers should avoid heat, hot baths, or nylon underwear. In recent years physicians have tried a host of therapies, including topical ointments, various vaccines, exposure to light, and ultrasonic waves—all with little success. Some physicians have used laser therapy to vaporize the lesions. Clinical trials of an experimental vaccine to protect people from herpes infections are underway.[67]

Can stress trigger a flare-up of genital herpes? To test this common assumption, researchers followed 58 women, aged 20 to 44, with a history of herpes for six months and assessed stress, mood, life changes, and diary reports of herpes recurrences. The researchers found that single stressful events and temporary bad moods were not related to recurrence of the disease, but long-term stresses (lasting more than seven days) were. The more intense the long-term stress, the greater the likelihood of a herpes flare-up.[68]

Human Papilloma Virus Infection (Genital Warts)

Infection with **human papilloma virus (HPV)**, a pathogen that can cause genital warts, is the most common viral STD. By some estimates, 20 million or more women in the United States are infected with HPV, as are three out of four of their male sexual partners.

College-age women are among those at greatest risk of acquiring HPV infection. In various studies conducted in college health centers, 10 to 46 percent of female students (mean age 20 to 22) had a cervical HPV infection—and increased risk of precancerous cell changes. Risk factors include smoking, use of oral contraceptives, multiple sex partners, anal as well as vaginal intercourse, alcohol consumption at the time of engaging in vaginal intercourse, and sex partners with a history of HPV. Many women often believe they are at low risk for HPV, even if they engage in unprotected sexual activity.

HPV infections in young women tend to be of short duration. In a three-year study, 60 percent of 608 college

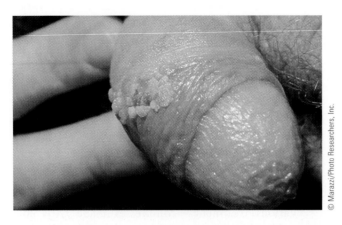

© Marazzi/Photo Researchers, Inc.

▲ Human papilloma virus, which causes genital warts, is the most common viral STD.

may not develop any symptoms, can spread the infection to their partners. People with visible genital warts also may have asymptomatic or subclinical HPV infections that are extremely difficult to treat.

No form of therapy has been shown to eradicate HPV completely, nor has any single treatment been uniformly effective in removing warts or preventing their recurrence. CDC guidelines suggest treatments that focus on the removal of visible warts—cryotherapy (freezing) and topical applications of podofilox, podophyllin, or trichloroacetic acid—and then eradication of the virus. At least 20 to 30 percent of treated individuals experience recurrence. In experimental studies, interferon—a biologic substance produced by virus-infected cells that inhibits viral replication—has proven helpful.

women became infected with the virus; the average duration of infection was eight months. According to the researchers, many young women who get HPV may not require treatment because the condition often regresses on its own.

HPV is transmitted primarily through vaginal, anal, or oral-genital sex. More than half of HPV-infected individuals do not develop any symptoms. Genital warts may appear from three weeks to eighteen months after contact, with an average period of about three months after contact with an infected individual. These are treated by freezing, cauterization, chemicals, or surgical removal. Recurrences are common because the virus remains in the body.

HPV infection may invade the urethra and cause urinary obstruction and bleeding. It greatly increases a woman's risk of developing a precancerous condition called cervical intraepithelial neoplasia, which can lead to cervical cancer. There also is a strong association between HPV infections and cancer of the vagina, vulva, urethra, penis, and anus.

HPV may be the single most important risk factor in 95 percent of all cases of cervical cancer. Adolescent girls infected with HPV appear to be particularly vulnerable to developing cervical cancer. It is not known if HPV itself causes cancer or acts in conjunction with cofactors (such as other infections, smoking, or suppressed immunity). HPV transmission may be the reason women are five to eleven times as likely to get cervical cancer if their steady sexual partner has had 20 or more previous partners.

Women who have had an HPV infection should examine their genitals regularly and get an annual Pap smear. However, this standard diagnostic test for cervical cancer doesn't identify HPV infection. A newer, more specific test can recognize HPV soon after it enters the body. Women who test positive should undergo checkups for cervical changes every six to twelve months. If precancerous cells develop, surgery or laser treatment can prevent further growth. Smoking may interact with HPV to increase the risk of cancer.

HPV may also cause genital warts in men and increase the risk of cancer of the penis. HPV-infected men, who

Chancroid

A **chancroid** is a soft, painful sore or localized infection caused by the bacterium *Haemophilus ducrevi* and usually acquired through sexual contact. Half of the cases heal by themselves. In other cases, the infection may spread to the lymph glands near the chancroid, where large amounts of pus can accumulate and destroy much of the local tissue. The incidence of this STD, widely prevalent in Africa and tropical and semitropical regions, is rapidly increasing in the United States, with outbreaks in several states, including Louisiana, Texas, and New York. Chancroids, which may increase susceptibility to HIV infection, are believed to be a major factor in the heterosexual spread of HIV. This infection is treated with antibiotics (ceftriaxone, azithromycin, or erythromycin) and can be prevented by keeping the genitals clean and washing them with soap and water in case of possible exposure.

Pubic Lice and Scabies

These infections are sometimes, but not always, transmitted sexually. Pubic lice (or "crabs") are usually found in the

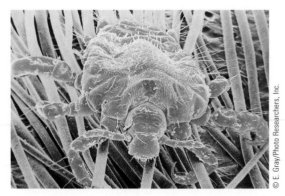

© E. Gray/Photo Researchers, Inc.

Actual size

▲ A pubic louse, or "crab."

pubic hairs, although they can migrate to any hairy areas of the body. Lice lay eggs called nits that attach to the base of the hair shaft. Irritation from the lice may produce intense itching. Scratching to relieve the itching can produce sores. Scabies is caused by a mite that burrows under the skin and lays eggs that hatch and undergo many changes in the course of their life cycle, producing great discomfort, including intense itching.

Lice and scabies are treated with applications of permethrin cream and Lindane shampoo to all the areas of the body where there are concentrations of body hair (genitals, armpits, scalp). You must repeat treatment in seven days to kill any newly developed adults. Wash or dry-clean clothing and bedding.

HIV

Thirty years ago, no one knew what the **human immunodeficiency virus (HIV)** was. No one had ever heard of **acquired immunodeficiency syndrome (AIDS).** Globally, HIV, once seen as an epidemic affecting primarily gay men and injection drug users, has taken on a very different form. Today, heterosexuals in developing countries have the highest rates of infection and mortality. And the HIV epidemic continues to spread, doubling at an estimated rate of every ten years. The United Nations AIDS Program estimates that about 47 million people have been infected with HIV since the start of the global epidemic. (See Figure 11-5 on p. 398.)

STRATEGIES FOR CHANGE

What to Do If You Have an STD

✔ If you suspect that you have an STD, don't feel too embarrassed to get help through a physician's office or a clinic. Treatment relieves discomfort, prevents complications, and halts the spread of the disease.

✔ Following diagnosis, take oral medication (which may be given instead of or in addition to shots) exactly as prescribed.

✔ Try to figure out from whom you got the STD. Be sure to inform that person, who may not be aware of the problem.

✔ If you have an STD, never deceive a prospective partner about it. Tell the truth—simply and clearly. Be sure your partner understands exactly what you have and what the risks are.

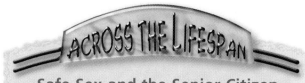

Safe Sex and the Senior Citizen

According to CDC statistics, some of the fastest-growing rates of HIV infection and AIDS are for people age 50 and older. In this age group, AIDS has increased 22 percent since 1991. The most common form of HIV transmission in men and women over age 50 is sexual intercourse.[69]

Why this surge in STDs among seniors? More and more people are beginning new relationships in their sixties and seventies. Viagra has allowed many older men to invigorate their dormant sex lives, and many older women are finding themselves single again after long monogamous relationships. According to a national survey sponsored by the American Association of Retired People, many seniors do not use condoms because they are no longer concerned about pregnancy.

There also have been few efforts to educate seniors about HIV and AIDS. According to researchers, fewer than 11 percent of people over age 50 have talked to their doctor about the risk for HIV or other STDs. In addition, many physicians are reluctant to discuss sex with patients of any age. In one survey, just 57 percent of doctors said they always ask about a patient's sexual history, and only about three in ten cover the patient's STD history and current sexual activity.[70] Primary care physicians are generally much less likely to assess sexual risk behaviors than other harmful habits, such as smoking and alcohol use. They are even less likely to do so when patients are older.

AIDS has surpassed tuberculosis and malaria as the leading infectious cause of death and has become the fourth-largest killer worldwide. The cumulative death toll for AIDS exceeds 22 million. The region that has been hardest hit is sub-Saharan Africa, the site of seven of every ten of the world's cases of HIV infection and nine of every ten deaths due to AIDS. In the two hardest-hit countries, Zimbabwe and Botswana, one of every four adults is infected, and AIDS has cut the average life expectancy by nearly 20 years.[71] In Asia, the total number of people infected is expanding rapidly, even though the rate of new infection remains relatively low.

In the United States, the CDC estimates that between 800,000 and 900,000 people are living with HIV. The

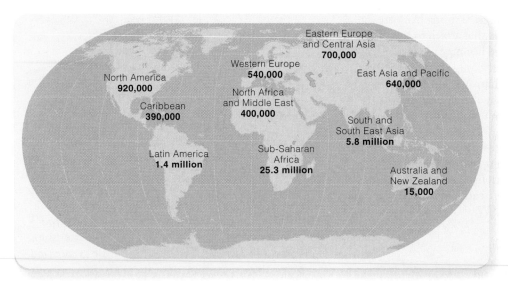

Eastern Europe
and Central Asia
700,000

Western Europe
540,000

North America
920,000

East Asia and Pacific
640,000

North Africa
and Middle East
400,000

Caribbean
390,000

South and
South East Asia
5.8 million

Latin America
1.4 million

Sub-Saharan
Africa
25.3 million

Australia and
New Zealand
15,000

▲ **Figure 11-5** Adults and children with HIV/AIDS worldwide.

Source: Joint United Nations Program on AIDS.

mortality rate for AIDS is declining, but HIV infection rates are increasing in certain groups, including women and racial and ethnic minorities. (See Table 11-4.) Almost two-thirds of new infections occur in blacks and Hispanics, who account for just 24 percent of the population. About 40,000 Americans become infected with HIV every year. HIV infection has continued to climb, but the number of AIDS cases and of deaths has fallen dramatically, thanks to advances in HIV treatments.[72] However, the rate of decline for both cases and deaths has begun to slow.

There has been progress in lowering the rates of HIV transmission through measures such as reducing the incidence of unprotected intercourse and the number of sex partners, delaying sexual initiation, decreasing the incidence of other STDs, directing injection drug users into drug treatment programs, and reducing needle sharing. Screening

the blood supply has reduced the rate of transfusion-associated HIV transmission by 99.9 percent.

Treatment with antiretroviral drugs during pregnancy and birth has reduced transmission by about 90 percent in optimal conditions. Among drug users in some settings, programs that combine addiction treatment and needle exchange reduced the incidence of HIV infection by 30 percent. Even in developing nations, such as Thailand and Uganda, national prevention programs, such as free distribution of condoms and needle-exchange programs, have reduced HIV prevalence by as much as 50 percent.

With the decline in AIDS cases and deaths, there has been an increase in sexually risky behavior.[73] More people at high risk for HIV infection (injection drug users, gay men, heterosexuals diagnosed with STDs) say they are less concerned about HIV/AIDS and more inclined to engage in risky behaviors.[74]

The Spread of HIV

HIV came to the United States in the late 1970s. Several factors—including frequent sexual activity with multiple, anonymous partners and high-risk sexual practices, such as anal intercourse—may have caused its quick spread through gay communities in the 1980s. As more became known about HIV transmission, many homosexual men adopted safer ways of sexual expression, reduced their number of sexual partners, or entered into monogamous relationships. As a result, the spread of HIV among gay men—especially older men in metropolitan areas—slowed. However, the incidence of AIDS in young gay men and homosexual men in rural or suburban areas increased steadily in the 1990s.

In the 1980s, HIV also spread among injecting drug users, who, by sharing contaminated needles, injected the virus directly into their bloodstream. Injection drug use has been the number-one source of HIV infection in heterosexual men and women in this country. Sex with an infected injecting drug user is also a major cause of HIV infection. (See Chapter 14 for further discussion of drug use.) Almost one-third of reported cases of AIDS have been directly or indirectly related to injection drug use. CDC-sponsored studies indicate that needle exchange

▼ Table 11-4 Estimated Annual Rise in New HIV Infections in the United States		
	Men	**Women**
Gender	70%	30%
Risk		
Men who have sex with men	60%	—
Heterosexual sex	15%	75%
Injection drug use	25%	25%
Race		
Black	50%	64%
White	30%	18%
Hispanic	20%	18%

Source: Centers for Disease Control

programs that provide drug users with sterile needles could significantly reduce HIV transmission.

During the period between 1978 and 1985, before testing to identify contaminated blood became routine, HIV also spread through blood transfusions, blood products, and organ transplants from HIV-positive individuals. Today's blood and organ supply is much safer, primarily because of more sophisticated testing of donated blood, blood products used for hemophiliacs, and donated organs, tissues, and sperm. Several cases of HIV infection through artificial insemination performed prior to 1986 have been documented. Even today, women who use semen from men who have not been tested for HIV are at risk of infection.

The percentage of individuals who acquired AIDS through heterosexual contact increased from about 2 percent in 1985 to about 15 percent in 2000. However, many heterosexual adults are not aware of their partners' HIV status and may not see themselves as at risk of HIV. According to the CDC, about a third of the HIV-infected individuals in the United States have not been diagnosed.[75]

 Although HIV/AIDS is often seen as a threat to men, 30 percent of new HIV infections in the United States occur among women. About a quarter of Americans living with HIV/AIDS are women. Women of color, particularly African Americans, have been hardest hit. While African-American women make up just 13 percent of the female population of the United States, they account for 63 percent of newly diagnosed cases. HIV/AIDS is most prevalent among women in their childbearing years. Most women are infected with HIV through heterosexual contact or injection drug use. While treatment advances have reduced AIDS cases and deaths for both sexes, women have not benefitted as much as men. Their rate of new AIDS cases and of AIDS death has declined much less than that of men.[76]

Reducing the Risk of HIV Transmission

HIV/AIDS can be so frightening that some people have exaggerated its dangers, whereas others understate them. The fact is that although no one is immune to HIV, you can reduce the risk if you abstain from sexual activity, remain in a monogamous relationship with an uninfected partner, and do not inject drugs. If you're not in a long-term monogamous relationship with a partner you're sure is safe, and you're not willing to abstain from sex, there are things you can do to lower your risk of HIV infection. Remember that the risk of HIV transmission depends on sexual behavior, not sexual orientation. Among young men, the prevalence and frequency of sexual risk behaviors are similar regardless of sexual orientation, ethnicity, or age.[77] Homosexual, heterosexual, and bisexual individuals all need to know about the kinds of sexual activity that increase their risk.

Here's what you should know about HIV transmission (see Figure 11-6):

▷ Casual contact does *not* spread HIV infection. Compared to other viruses, HIV is extremely difficult to get. HIV can live in blood, semen, vaginal fluids, and breast milk. Many chemicals, including household bleach, alcohol, and hydrogen peroxide, can inactivate it. In studies of family members sharing dishes, food, clothing, and frequent hugs with people with HIV infection or AIDS, those who have contracted the virus have shared razor blades, toothbrushes, or had other means of blood contact.

▷ You cannot tell visually whether a potential sexual partner has HIV. A blood test is needed to detect the antibodies that the body produces to fight HIV, thus indicating infection.

▷ HIV can be spread in semen and vaginal fluids during a single instance of anal, vaginal, or oral sexual contact between heterosexuals, bisexuals, or homosexuals. The risk increases with the number of sexual encounters with an infected partner.

▷ Teenage girls may be particularly vulnerable to HIV infection because the immature cervix is easily infected.

▷ Anal intercourse is an extremely high-risk behavior because HIV can enter the bloodstream through tiny breaks in the lining of the rectum. HIV transmission is much more likely to occur during unprotected anal intercourse than vaginal intercourse.

▷ Other behaviors that increase the risk of HIV infection include having multiple sexual partners, engaging in sex without condoms or virus-killing spermicides, sexual contact with persons known to be at high risk (for example, prostitutes or injection drug users), and sharing injection equipment for drugs.

▷ Individuals are at greater risk if they have an active sexual infection. Sexually transmitted diseases, such as herpes, gonorrhea, and syphilis, facilitate transmission of HIV during vaginal or rectal intercourse.

▷ No cases of HIV transmission by deep kissing have been reported, but it could happen. Studies have found blood in the saliva of healthy people after kissing; other lab studies have found HIV in saliva. Social (dry) kissing is safe.

▷ Oral sex can lead to HIV transmission. The virus in any semen that enters the mouth could make its way into the bloodstream through tiny nicks or sores in the mouth. A man's risk in performing oral sex on a woman is smaller because an infected woman's genital fluids have much lower concentrations of HIV than does semen.

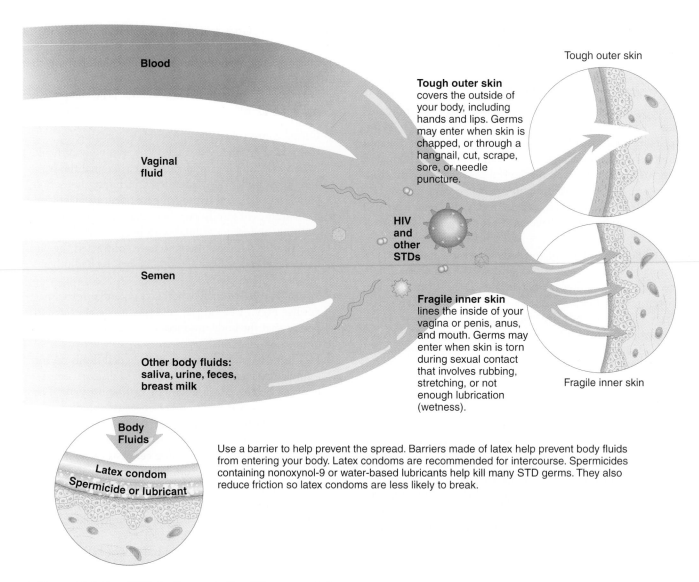

▲ **Figure 11-6** How HIV infection and other STDs are spread. Most STDs are spread by viruses, such as HIV, or bacteria carried in certain body fluids.

❿ HIV infection is not widespread among lesbians, although there have been documented cases of possible female-to-female HIV transmission. In each instance, one partner had had sex with a bisexual man or male injection drug user or had injected drugs herself.

HIV Infection

HIV infection refers to a spectrum of health problems that result from immunologic abnormalities caused by the virus when it enters the bloodstream. In theory, the body may be able to resist infection by HIV. In reality, in almost all cases, HIV destroys the cell-mediated immune system, particularly the CD4+ T-lymphocytes (also called T4

helper cells). The result is greatly increased susceptibility to various cancers and opportunistic infections (infections that take hold because of the reduced effectiveness of the immune system).

According to new insights into the pathogenesis of HIV—the way in which HIV attacks the immune system—researchers now know that HIV triggers a state of all-out war within the immune system. Almost immediately following infection with HIV, the immune system responds aggressively by manufacturing enormous numbers of CD4 cells. It eventually is overwhelmed, however, as the viral particles continue to replicate, or multiply. The intense war between HIV and the immune system indicates that the virus itself, not a breakdown in the immune system, is responsible for disease progression.

Shortly after becoming infected with HIV, individuals may experience a few days of flulike symptoms, which most ignore or attribute to other viruses. Some people develop a more severe mononucleosis-type syndrome. After this stage, individuals may not develop any signs or symptoms of disease for a period ranging from weeks to more than 12 years.

HIV infection can itself be a serious illness and is associated with a variety of HIV-related diseases, including different cancers and dangerous infections. HIV-infected individuals may develop persistent generalized lymphadenopathy, enlargement of the lymph nodes at two or more different sites in the body. This condition typically persists for more than three months without any other illness to explain its occurrence. Diminished mental function may appear before other symptoms. Tests conducted on infected, but apparently healthy, men have revealed impaired coordination, problems in thinking, or abnormal brain scans.

HIV Testing

Every year approximately 25 million people in the United States are tested for HIV. About 10,000 facilities provide publicly funded HIV testing and counseling in the United States; approximately 2.6 million tests are performed annually at these sites. Men and women between the ages of 18 and 29 are most likely to report that they've been tested for HIV.

All HIV tests measure antibodies, cells produced by the body to fight HIV infection. A negative test indicates no exposure to HIV. It can take three to six months for the body to produce the telltale antibodies, however, so a negative result may not be accurate, depending on the timing of the test.

HIV testing can be either confidential or anonymous. In confidential testing, a person's name is recorded along with the test results, which are made available to medical personnel and, in 32 states, the state health department. In anonymous testing, no name is associated with the test results. Anonymous testing is available in 39 states.

 Different groups of individuals at risk prefer different tests. Asian–Pacific Islander and white men who have sex with men are most likely to choose anonymous testing; African-American men who have sex with men are much more likely to choose confidential testing.[78] Consumers must be wary of bogus HIV tests offered via the Internet. (See Savvy Consumer: "Bogus HIV Tests on the Internet.")

The HIV tests currently available in the United States are:

▶ **ELISA** *(Enzyme-Linked ImmunoSorbent Assay)*. This is the most commonly used HIV test. A health-care provider draws a blood sample, which is analyzed for antibodies produced to fight against HIV particles. Results are generally available within a few days to two weeks.

▶ **Oral HIV tests.** These tests have become available in some doctors' offices and health clinics. A health-care worker swabs a tissue sample from the inside of the mouth. The only oral test approved by the Food and Drug Administration (FDA) is the OraSure.

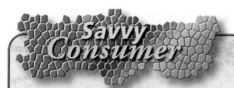

Bogus HIV Tests on the Internet

The Internet has been used as a tool for marketing unscientific HIV self-diagnostic tests. The Federal Trade Commission (FTC) has issued a warning that home test kits for HIV that are advertised and sold over the Internet—some of which claim or imply that they are approved by the Food and Drug Administration (FDA) or the World Health Organization—are unreliable. After testing a variety of such kits, the FTC found that in every case, the kits yielded false negatives. In other words, they showed a negative result when they should have shown a positive one. This means that a person who might be infected with HIV would get the false impression that he or she is HIV-negative.

In several cases, businesspersons have been found guilty of fraud for selling medically useless HIV test kits for home use via the Internet. In one case, the tests were represented as "confidential, safe, accurate, and easy to use," although they lacked any scientific or factual basis. As part of the scheme, the marketer provided bogus test results to purchasers.

The FTC suggests that anyone who has used such a kit be retested for HIV. The only kit approved by the FDA for self-diagnosis is the Home Access Express HIV-1 Test System, which allows a person to collect a blood sample at home and ship it to a laboratory for analysis.

STRATEGIES FOR CHANGE

Lowering Your Risk of Exposure to HIV

✔ Abstain from sexual contact with anyone who is infected with HIV, whether or not he or she has symptoms, or with anyone who is at high risk of HIV infection because of his or her behavior or sexual history.

✔ Avoid sexual contact with anyone who has had sex with people at risk of HIV infection. Avoid multiple or anonymous sexual partners. Avoid sex with anyone who has had multiple or anonymous sexual partners, or with anyone who has had a sexual partner infected with HIV.

✔ Use a condom during every sexual act, including oral sex, from start to finish. Condoms reduce but do not eliminate the risk of infection. Also use a spermicide that provides extra protection against STDs.

✔ Don't have sexual contact with individuals who use injection drugs.

✔ Avoid receptive anal intercourse, as well as the insertion of fingers or objects into your anus, because these acts could tear your rectal tissues, allowing direct access to your bloodstream. Avoid contact with your partner's blood, semen, urine, and feces.

✔ Don't use amyl nitrite (poppers), a sexual stimulant that may be associated with the development of a cancer characteristic of AIDS.

✔ Don't have sex with prostitutes.

✔ Don't share needles (or other injection drug equipment), razor blades, or toothbrushes.

✔ In addition to their partner's use of a condom, women should use a diaphragm with a spermicide for extra protection.

▶ **Home Access.** This test—the only home HIV test approved by the FDA—is available in drug stores for $40–50. An individual draws a blood sample by pricking a finger and sends it to a laboratory along with a personal identification number. Results are given over the phone by a trained counselor, usually within several days.

▶ **Western blot.** This more accurate and expensive test is used to confirm the results of a positive HIV test.

Newly developed blood tests can determine how recently a person was infected with HIV and distinguish between long-standing infections and those contracted within the previous four to six months. Health officials recommend HIV testing for the following individuals:

▶ Men who have had sex with other men, regardless of whether they consider themselves homosexual.
▶ Anyone who uses injection drugs and has shared needles or has had sex with someone who has done so.
▶ Women who have had sex with bisexual men.
▶ Anyone who has had sex with someone from an area with a high incidence of HIV infection.
▶ Individuals who have had sex with people they do not know well.
▶ Anyone who received blood transfusions or blood products between 1978 and 1985. (Their sexual partners or, if they are new mothers, their infants may also be at risk.)

AIDS

A diagnosis of AIDS applies to anyone with HIV whose immune system is severely impaired, as indicated by a CD4 count of less than 200 cells per cubic millimeter of blood, compared to normal CD4 cell counts in healthy people not infected with HIV of 800 to 1,200 per cubic millimeter of blood. In addition, AIDS is diagnosed in persons with HIV infection who experience recurrent pneumonia, invasive cervical cancer, or pulmonary tuberculosis.

People with AIDS also may experience persistent fever, diarrhea that persists for more than one month, or involuntary weight loss of more than 10 percent of normal body weight. Generalized lymphadenopathy may persist. Neurological disease—including dementia (confusion and impaired thinking) and other problems with thinking, speaking, movement, or sensation—may occur. Secondary infectious diseases that may develop in people with AIDS include *Pneumocystis carinii* pneumonia, tuberculosis, or oral candidiasis (thrush). Secondary cancers associated with HIV infection include Kaposi's sarcoma and cancer of the cervix.

What Progress Has Been Made in Treating HIV/AIDS?

More Americans—322,865 in the year 2000—are living with AIDS. New forms of therapy have been remarkably effective in boosting levels of protective T cells and reducing "viral load"—the amount of HIV in the bloodstream. People with high viral loads are more likely to progress rapidly to AIDS than people with low levels of the virus.

The current "gold standard" approach to combating HIV is known as HAART (Highly Active Antiretroviral Therapies), which dramatically reduces viral load even though it does not eradicate the virus. This complex regimen uses one of 250 different combinations of three or more antiretroviral drugs. A year's treatment costs more than $10,000, which is not always covered by health insurance and which has restricted the use of HAART in poor nations. Its success depends on consistent adherence to the drug regimen over a prolonged period of time. However, as many as 30 to 70 percent of patients do not strictly adhere to their schedules.[79] Another drawback are serious side effects, including anemia, mouth ulcers, diarrhea, respiratory difficulties, digestive problems, liver damage, and skin rashes.[80]

Researchers are continuing to work toward development of more effective and less toxic treatments as well as a vaccine against HIV. NIH is testing one vaccine, designed to stimulate an immune system to destroy HIV-infected cells, in volunteers undergoing treatment with HAART.[81] Another type of vaccine uses a protein found on the surface of HIV to trigger an immune response. Despite progress, most scientists believe that it will take many years before a safe, effective vaccine is available.[82]

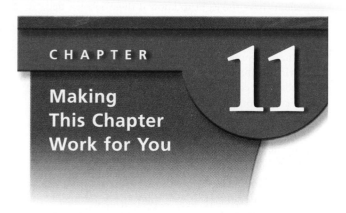

CHAPTER 11

Making This Chapter Work for You

1. Which of the following statements about disease-causing microbes is false?
   a. Helminths cause malaria, one of the major worldwide diseases.
   b. AIDS is caused by a retrovirus.
   c. In the United States, the most common protozoan disease is giardiasis.
   d. Salmonella and botulism are foodborne illnesses caused by bacteria.

2. Which of the following statements about the immune system is false?
   a. The immune system has two types of white blood cells: B cells, which produce antibodies that fight bacteria and viruses, and T-cells, which protect against parasites, fungi, and cancer cells.
   b. Immune system structures include the spleen, tonsils, thymus gland, and lymph nodes located throughout the body.
   c. You can strengthen your immunity by limiting your alcohol intake, exercising occasionally,

cutting down on smoking, and becoming accustomed to high levels of stress.
   d. The immune system may respond to the body's own tissues as pathogens, resulting in severely disabling diseases including rheumatoid arthritis and lupus.

3. Booster immunizations are recommended for all of the following diseases except
   a. diphtheria
   b. tetanus
   c. measles
   d. pertussis

4. Which of the following statements about cold and influenza is true?
   a. Influenza is just a more severe form of the common cold.
   b. Aspirin should be avoided by children and young adults who have a cold or influenza.
   c. The flu vaccine is also effective against most of the viruses that cause the common cold.
   d. Antibiotics are appropriate treatments for colds but not for influenza.

5. Which of the following statements about specific infectious diseases is false?
   a. Group A streptococcus bacteria is responsible for both the frequently occurring strep throat and the more serious and invasive disease called toxic streptococcal shock syndrome.
   b. Symptoms of Lyme disease include a rash, joint pain, and severe headaches.
   c. Hepatitis A is usually transmitted through contaminated needles, transfusions, and sexual contact.
   d. College freshmen are at higher risk for contracting meningitis than the general population of young people between the ages of 18 and 23.

6. Sexually transmitted diseases
   a. are the major cause of preventable sterility in the United States.
   b. can result in a severe kidney disease called pylonephritis.
   c. have declined in incidence in developing nations due to improving health standards.
   d. often cause no symptoms in the early stages.

7. Bacterial agents cause all of the following STDs except for
   a. genital warts
   b. syphilis
   c. chlamydia
   d. gonorrhea

8. Viral agents cause all of the following STDs except for
   a. herpes
   b. genital warts
   c. hepatitis B
   d. candidiasis

9. Which of the following statements about HIV transmission is true?
   a. Individuals are not at risk for HIV if they are being treated for chlamydia or gonorrhea.
   b. HIV can be transmitted between lesbians.
   c. Heterosexual men who do not practice safe sex are at less risk for contracting HIV than homosexual men who do practice safe sex.
   d. HIV cannot be spread in a single instance of sexual intercourse.
10. A person with AIDS
    a. has a low viral load and a high number of T4 helper cells.
    b. can no longer pass HIV to a sexual partner.
    c. may suffer from secondary infectious diseases and cancers.
    d. will not respond to treatment.

Answers to these questions can be found on page 640.

 How large is the threat of emerging or re-emerging infectious diseases?

Critical Thinking

1. Before you read this chapter, describe what you did to avoid contracting infectious disease. Now that you have read the chapter, will you be making any changes in your practices? Briefly explain the convenience, advantages, and disadvantages of each practice that you have and/or will be using to prevent infection.

2. The U.S. military and some employers routinely screen personnel for HIV. Some hospitals test patients and note their HIV status on their charts. Some insurance companies test for HIV before selling a policy. Do you believe that an individual has the right to refuse to be tested for HIV? Should a physician be able to order an HIV test without a patient's consent? Can a surgeon refuse to operate on an HIV-infected patient or one who refuses HIV testing? Do patients have the right to know if their doctors, dentists, or nurses are HIV-positive?

3. A man who developed herpes sued his former girlfriend. A woman who became sterile as a result of pelvic inflammatory disease (PID) took her ex-husband to court. A woman who contracted HIV infection from her dentist, who had died of AIDS, filed suit against his estate. Do you think that anyone who knowingly transmits a sexually transmitted disease should be held legally responsible? Do you think such an act should be a criminal offense?

4. Biological terrorism is now a very real concern in the United States. What do you think the government should do to protect its citizens? Are there measures that you can take to protect yourself?

SITES & BYTES

Understanding the Immune System
http://newscenter.cancer.gov/sciencebehind/uis/uisframe.htm
The site, sponsored by the National Cancer Institute, provides interactive animations and illustrations to illustrate how the immune system works in the human body.

Immunization Action Coalition
http://www.immunize.org
Information for children, adolescents, and adults, including color photographs of people with vaccine-preventable diseases and vaccine information sheets in both English and Spanish. This site features childhood and adult immunization information from the Centers for Disease Control and Prevention and the latest statements from the Advisory Committee on Immunization Practices (ACIP).

National Institute of Allergy and Infectious Diseases
http://www.niaid.nih.gov

This site features information on a variety of infectious diseases, including the common cold, influenza, infectious mononucleosis, chronic fatigue syndrome, foodborne illnesses, Lyme disease, immune disorders, and emerging infectious diseases, tuberculosis, and vaccine research.

Please note that links are subject to change. If you find a broken link, use a search engine such as http://www.yahoo.com and search for the website by typing in key words.

InfoTrac Activity   Michelle Meadows. "Understanding Vaccine Safety: FDA Vaccine Safety Standards." *FDA Consumer,* Vol. 35, No. 4, July 2001, p. 18.

(1) Describe the physiological mechanisms of vaccine action to prevent infectious diseases.

(2) What are the benefits and the shortcomings of the Vaccine Adverse Event Reporting System (VAERS)?

(3) List the benefits of vaccination. List the potential side effects, both mild and potentially serious.

You can find additional readings related to infectious diseases with InfoTrac College Edition, an online library of more than 900 journals and publications. Follow the instructions for accessing InfoTrac that were packaged with your textbook; then search for articles using a key word search.

For additional links, resources, and suggested readings on InfoTrac, visit our Health & Wellness Resource Center at http://health.wadsworth.com.

Key Terms

The terms listed here are used within the chapter on the page indicated. Definitions of the terms are in the Glossary at the end of this book.

abscess 371	helminth 368	nongonococcal urethritis (NGU) 393
acquired immunodeficiency syndrome (AIDS) 397	hepatitis 379	pathogen 366
allergy 371	herpes simplex 394	pelvic inflammatory disease (PID) 391
antibiotics 367	host 366	pneumonia 380
antiviral drug 367	human immunodeficiency virus (HIV) 397	protozoa 367
autoimmune 372	human papilloma virus (HPV) 395	pyelonephritis 384
bacteria 367	humoral 370	sexually transmitted diseases (STDs) 384
bacterial vaginosis 383	immune deficiency 372	syphilis 393
candidiasis 383	immunity 369	systemic disease 371
cell-mediated 370	immunotherapy 372	toxic shock syndrome (TSS) 381
chanchroid 396	incubation period 368	trichomoniasis 383
chlamydial infections 391	inflammation 371	tuberculosis (TB) 380
chronic fatigue syndrome (CFS) 379	influenza 377	urethritis 384
cystitis 384	Lyme disease 381	vector 366
fungi 367	lymph nodes 370	virus 366
gamma globulin 370	meningitis 378	
gonorrhea 392	mononucleosis 379	

References

1. Centers for Disease Control and Prevention. "Tracking the Hidden Epidemics: Trends in STDs in the United States." December 2000.
2. Centers for Disease Control and Prevention. *Morbidity and Mortality Weekly Report,* July 30, 1999.
3. "Between 31 March 2000 and 31 March 2001: Death Statistics of Birds Caused by West Nile Virus, Pesticides and Lead." *Environment,* Vol. 43, No. 7, September 2001, p. 8.
4. Miles, Robert. Personal interview.

5. Committee on Understanding the Biology of Sex and Gender Differences. *Exploring the Biological Contributions to Human Health: Does Sex Matter?* Washington, DC: National Academy Press, 2001.

6. "Understanding Vaccine Safety." *FDA Consumer,* Vol. 35, No. 4, July 2001, p. 18.

7. "African-American Children More Likely Not to Get All Vaccines." *Medical Letter on the CDC & FDA,* June 10, 2001.

8. "One More Visit Could Close Demographic Gaps in Infant Immunization Efforts." Media Release, National Center for HIV, STD, and TB Prevention, Office of Communication, April 20, 2001.

9. Seid, Michael, et al. "Correlates of Vaccination for Hepatitis B Among Adolescents: Results from a Parent Survey." *Archives of Pediatrics & Adolescent Medicine,* Vol. 155, No. 8, August 2001, p. 921.

10. "Combination Hepatitis Vaccine Remains Effective In Long-Term Follow-up." *Vaccine Weekly,* September 5, 2001.

11. "Whooping Cough—Still Around." *Pediatrics for Parents,* Vol. 18, No. 4, April 1999.

12. "Decrease in Incidence of HIB Disease." *American Family Physician,* February 15, 1999.

13. "Polio Vaccination Schedule." *Lancet,* Vol. 353, No. 9160, April 10, 1999.

14. "Measles on the Run." *Pediatrics for Parents,* Vol. 18, No. 3, March 1999.

15. Liesegang, Thomas. "The Ocular Manifestation of Congenital Infection: A Study of the Early Effect and Long-Term Outcome of Maternally Transmitted Rubella and Toxoplasmosis." *American Journal of Ophthalmology,* Vol. 127, No. 4, April 1999.

16. Sadovsky, Richard. "Varicella Vaccine: Alone or with MMR and DTP/HbOC?" *American Family Physician,* Vol. 59, No. 6, March 15, 1999.

17. "Myths and Facts About the Common Cold." *Pediatrics for Parents,* Vol. 19, No. 1, January 2001, p. 7.

18. Goff, Karen. "Cold Facts." *Insight on the News,* Vol. 17, No. 2, January 8, 2001, p. 32.

19. "Cold-Fighting Echinacea." *Psychology Today,* March 2000, p. 40.

20. Kirchner, Jeffrey. "A Final Look at Oral Zinc for the Common Cold." *American Family Physician,* Vol. 63, No. 9, May 1, 2001, p. 1851.

21. Linder, Jeffrey, and Randall Stafford. "Antibiotic Treatment of Adults with Sore Throat by Community Primary Care Physicians." *Journal of the American Medical Association,* Vol. 286, No. 10, September 12, 2001, p. 1181.

22. Zoorob, Roger, et al. "Use and Perceptions of Antibiotics for Upper Respiratory Infections Among College Students." *Journal of Family Practice,* Vol. 50, No. 1, January 2001, p. 32.

23. "WHO Plans New Fight Against Flu." *Medical Letter on the CDC & FDA,* August 26, 2001.

24. "Flu Basics." CDC, Division of Media Relations, June 22, 2000.

25. "Flu Season 2000–01." CDC, Division of Media Relations, June 22, 2000.

26. Kilbourne, Edwin. Personal Interview.

27. *Prevention and Control of Influenza: Recommendations of the Advisory Committee on Immunization Practices,* April 14, 2000. Available at http://www.cdc.gov/mmwr/preview/mmwrhtml/mm5027a3.htm.

28. Luce, Bryan, et al. "Cost-Effectiveness Analysis of an Intranasal Influenza Vaccine for the Prevention of Influenza in Healthy Children." *Pediatrics,* Vol. 108, No. 2, August 2001, p. 456.

29. "Flu Drugs (Antiviral)." CDC, Division of Media Relations, June 22, 2000.

30. Myers, Frank. "Meningitis: The Fears, the Facts." *RN,* Vol. 63, No. 11, November 2000.

31. Harrison, Lee, and Margaret Pass. "Invasive Meningococcal Disease in Adolescents and Young Adults." *Journal of the American Medical Association,* Vol. 286, No. 6, August 8, 2001.

32. Bruce, Michael, et al. "Meningococcal Disease in College Students." *Journal of the American Medical Association,* Vol. 286, No. 6, August 8, 2001.

33. American Academy of Pediatrics Committee on Infectious Diseases. "Meningococcal Disease Prevention and Control Strategies for Practice-Based Physicians (Addendum: Recommendations for College Students)." *Pediatrics,* Vol. 106, No. 6, December 2000.

34. Wenger, Jay. "Toward Control of Meningococcal Disease: Reducing Risk in College Students." *Journal of the American Medical Association,* Vol. 286, No. 6, August 8, 2001.

35. Brody, Jane. "Lowering the Risk of Bacterial Meningitis." *New York Times,* September 4, 2001, p. D8.

36. Paneth, Nigel, et al. "Predictors of Vaccination Rates During a Mass Meningococcal Vaccination Program on a College Campus." *Journal of American College Health,* Vol. 49, No. 1, July 2000.

37. Wenger, "Toward Control of Meningococcal Disease."

38. Dougherty, Augustine, and Heyward Dreher. "Hepatitis C: Current Treatment Strategies for an Emerging Epidemic." *MedSurg Nursing,* Vol. 10, No. 1, February 2001, p. 9.

39. Bren, Linda. "Hepatitis C." *FDA Consumer,* Vol. 35, No. 4, July 2001, p. 24.

40. Riccio, Nina. "When Mono Strikes." *Current Health 2,* Vol. 26, No. 7, March 2000, p. 16.

41. Sagall, Rich. "Short Treatment for Strep Throat." *Pediatrics for Parents,* Vol. 18, No. 3, March 1999.

42. Steere, Allen. "Lyme Disease." *New England Journal of Medicine,* Vol. 345, No. 2, July 12, 2001, p. 115.

43. Hines, Silvia, et al. "Lyme Disease: The Debate Continues." *Patient Care,* Vol. 35, No. 11, June 15, 2001, p. 60.

44. Nadelman, Robert, et al. "Prophylaxis with Single-Dose Doxycycline for the Prevention of Lyme Disease After an *Ixodes scapularis* Tick Bite." *New England Journal of Medicine,* Vol. 345, No. 2, July 12, 2001, p. 79.

45. Preboth, Monica. "IDSA Issues Guidelines on the Treatment of Lyme Disease." *American Family Physician,* Vol. 63, No. 10, May 15, 2001, p. 2065.

46. Klempner, Mark, et al. "Two Controlled Trials of Antibiotic Treatment in Patients with Persistent Symptoms and a History of Lyme Disease." *New England Journal of Medicine,* Vol. 345, No. 2, July 12, 2001, p. 85.

47. CDC Fact Sheet on Viral Hemorrhagic Fevers. http://www.cdc.gov/ncidod/dvrd/sp6/mnpages/factmenu.htm

48. Panchaud, Christine, et al. "Sexually Transmitted Diseases Among Adolescents in Developed Countries." *Family Planning Perspectives,* Vol. 32, No. 1, January 2000.

49. Catchpole, Mike. "Sexually Transmitted Infections: Control Strategies." *British Medical Journal,* Vol. 322, No. 7295, May 12, 2001, p. 1135.

50. Celentano, David, et al. "Preventive Intervention to Reduce Sexually Transmitted Infections." *Archives of Internal Medicine,* Vol. 160, No. 4, February 28, 2000.

51. Bon, Rebecca, et al. "Normative Perceptions in Relation to Substance Use and HIV-Risky Sexual Behaviors of College Students." *Journal of Psychology,* Vol. 135, No. 2, March 2001, p. 165.

52. Ibid.

53. O'Connor, M. L. "Social Factors Play Major Role in Making Young People Sexual Risk-Takers." *Family Planning Perspectives,* Vol. 32, No. 1, January 2000.

54. Bradner, Carolyn, et al. "Older, But Not Wiser: How Men Get Information about AIDS and Sexually Transmitted Diseases After High School." *Family Planning Perspectives,* Vol. 32, No. 1, January 2000.

55. "Counseling Can Help Correct Misconceptions About Sexually Transmitted Diseases." *Medical Letter on the CDC & FDA,* October 8, 2000.

56. Wyatt, Gail. "Factors Affecting HIV Contraceptive Decision-Making Among Women." *Sex Roles: A Journal of Research,* April 2000.

57. Lewis, Lisa, et al. "Factors Influencing Condom Use and STD Acquisition Among African-American College Women." *Journal of American College Health,* Vol. 49, No. 1, July 2000.

58. Crooks, Robert, and Karla Baur. *Our Sexuality,* 8th ed. Pacific Grove, CA: Wadsworth, 2002.

59. Toomey, Kathleen, and Richard Rothenberg. "Sex and Cyberspace—Virtual Networks Leading to High-Risk Sex." *Journal of the American Medical Association,* Vol. 284, No. 4, July 26, 2000.

60. "Chlamydia Screening for Young Women." *American Journal of Preventive Medicine,* Vol. 20, April 2001, p. 90.

61. Ross, Jonathan. "Pelvic Inflammatory Disease." *British Medical Journal,* Vol. 322, No. 7287, March 17, 2001, p. 658.

62. Altman, Lawrence. "Rates of Gonorrhea Rise After a Long Decline." *New York Times,* December 6, 2000.

63. Mitka, Mike. "U.S. Effort to Eliminate Syphilis Moving Forward." *Journal of the American Medical Association,* Vol. 283, No. 12, March 22/29, 2000.

64. "Taming Herpes." Mayo Clinic Women's HealthSource, September 2001.

65. Armstrong, Gregory, et al. "Herpes." *American Journal of Epidemiology,* Vol. 153, May 2001, p. 912.

66. Wald, Ann, et al. "Reactivation of Genital Herpes Simplex Virus Type 2 Infection in Asymptomatic Seropositive Persons." *New England Journal of Medicine,* Vol. 343, No. 12, March 23, 2000.

67. Drake, Susan, et al. "Improving the Care of Patients with Genital Herpes." *British Medical Journal,* Vol. 321, No. 7261, September 9, 2000.

68. Cohen, Frances. "Persistent Stress as a Predictor of Genital Herpes Recurrence." *Archives of Internal Medicine,* Vol. 282, No. 11, March 15, 2000.

69. Davis, Sonia. "Subject: Safe Sex and the Senior Citizen." Baylor News Bureau, February 7, 2000.

70. Hollander, Dore. "Don't Know Much About History." *Family Planning Perspectives,* Vol. 32, No. 1, January 2000.

71. "The 20th Year of AIDS: A Time to Re-energize Prevention." *Morbidity and Mortality Weekly Report,* Vol. 50, No. 21, June 1, 2001, p. 444.

72. "HIV and AIDS—United States, 1981–2000." *Morbidity and Mortality Weekly Report,* Vol. 50, No. 21, June 1, 2001, p. 444.

73. "The 20th Year of AIDS: A Time to Re-energize Prevention."

74. Scheer, S., et al. "Effects of Highly Active Antiretroviral Therapy on Diagnosis of Sexually Transmitted Disease in People with AIDS." *Lancet,* Vol. 357, February 10, 2001, p. 432.

75. Klevens, R. Monina, et al. "Many Heterosexuals Unaware of their HIV Risk." *American Journal of Preventive Medicine,* April 2001.

76. "Women and HIV/AIDS Fact Sheet." Menlo Park, CA: Henry J. Kaiser Family Foundation, May 2001.

77. Rotheram-Borus, Mary Jane, et al. "HIV Risk Among Homosexual, Bisexual, and Heterosexual Male and Female Youths." *Archives of Sexual Behavior,* Vol. 28, No. 2, April 1999.

78. CDC. "Anonymous or Confidential HIV Counseling and Voluntary Testing in Federally Funded Testing Sites." *Journal of the American Medical Association,* Vol. 282, No. 4, July 28, 1999.

79. Murphy, D., et al. "Barriers to Antiretroviral Adherence Among HIV-infected Adults." *AIDS Patient Care and STDs,* Vol. 14, 2000, p. 47.

80. Barreiro, P., et al. "Risks and Benefits of Replacing Protease Inhibitors by Nevirapine in HIV-infected Subjects Under Long-term Successful Triple Combination Therapy." *AIDS 2000,* No. 4, p. 807.

81. Cohen, J. "Debate Begins over New Vaccine Trials," *Science,* Vol. 293, September 14, 2001, p. 5537.

82. Mitchell, Deborah. "NIH Accelerates AIDS Vaccine Research." *AIDS Weekly,* August 6, 2001.

12

Keeping Your Heart Healthy

J amal never forgot the terror he felt when his Dad had his first heart attack. Only ten, he couldn't understand why this towering giant of a man had fallen to the ground, his face twisted in pain, his fist pressed against his chest. His father seemed different when he came home from the hospital, as if something had gone out of him. But his face would still light up with an impish grin, especially when he'd sneak a cigarette and wink at Jamal so he wouldn't tell his mother. The second heart attack came four years later. This time Jamal's Dad didn't come home.

Jamal promised his mother that he'd take better care of his heart. He wouldn't smoke; he'd watch his blood pressure and weight; he'd keep tabs on his diet; he'd exercise regularly. Jamal didn't forget these promises as time passed. But like many college students, he felt invincible. He was shocked when a sports physical revealed that his blood pressure was high and his levels of the most dangerous type of cholesterol were elevated. But he also felt lucky: "I got my wake-up call," he explains. "And I'm not going to ignore it."

As Jamal realizes, it's never too soon, or too late, to start being heart smart. Cardiovascular disease remains the nation's top killer, but death rates have dropped by 60 percent since 1950, one of the major U.S. health achievements of the twentieth century. The medical advances described in this chapter have contributed to this decline, but much of the credit goes to lifestyle changes, such as quitting smoking and making dietary changes that lower blood pressure and cholesterol levels.

Yet we still have a long way to go to keep the hearts of all Americans healthy. One of every two men and one of every three women in the United States will develop some form of cardiovascular illness. Each year an estimated one million Americans suffer a heart attack; nearly half of them die.[1] Heart-related disorders account for almost as many deaths as the *combined* total for cancer, accidents, influenza, pneumonia, AIDS, and all other causes. Globally, heart disease and stroke are responsible for, respectively, 7 million and 5.5 million deaths.[2]

This chapter provides the information you need about risk factors, silent dangers such as high blood pressure and cholesterol, and medical advances that can improve your chances to have a healthier heart and a longer life.

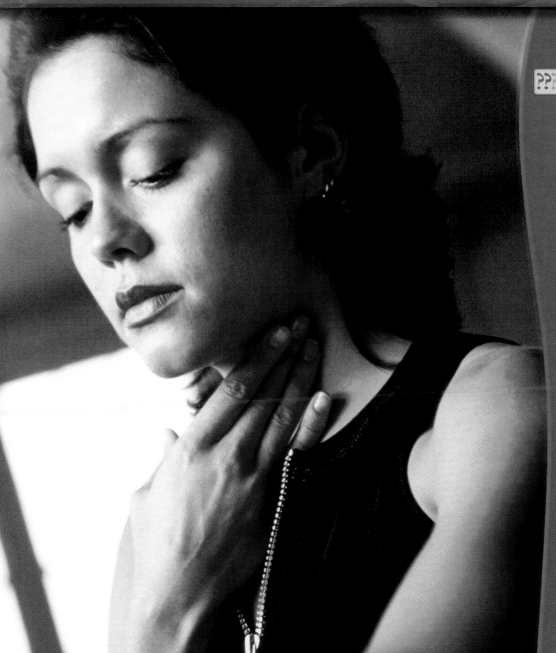

After studying the material in this chapter, you should be able to:

- **Explain** how the heart functions.
- **Identify** the risk factors for cardiovascular disease that you can control and those that you cannot control.
- **Describe** the types of cholesterol that compose your lipoprotein profile and the effects of each on heart health.
- **Define** hypertension, and **discuss** why it is dangerous and ways to prevent it.

- **Explain** how coronary artery disease occurs, and **list** effective treatments for it.
- **Explain** what happens during a myocardial infarction (MI) (heart attack) and what can be done to prevent and treat such attacks.
- **Define** stroke and transient ischemic attacks (TIAs), and **explain** their cause, prevention, and treatment.

How the Heart Works

The heart is a hollow, muscular organ with four chambers that serve as two pumps (see Figure 12-1). It is about the size of a clenched fist. Each pump consists of a pair of chambers formed of muscles. The upper two—each called an **atrium**—receive blood, which then flows through valves into the lower two chambers, the **ventricles,** which contract to pump blood out into the arteries through a second set of valves. A thick wall divides the right side of the heart from the left side; but even though the two sides are separated, they contract at almost the same time. Contraction of the ventricles is called **systole;** the period of relaxation between contractions is called **diastole.** The heart valves, located at the entrance and exit of the ventricular chambers, have flaps that open and close to allow blood to flow through the chambers of the heart.

The myocardium (heart muscle) consists of branching fibers that enable the heart to contract or beat between 60 and 80 times per minute, or about 100,000 times a day. With each beat, it pumps about 2 ounces of blood. This may not sound like much, but it adds up to nearly 5 quarts of blood pumped by the heart in one minute, or about 75 gallons per hour.

The heart is surrounded by the pericardium, which consists of two layers of a tough membrane. The space between the two contains a lubricating fluid that allows the heart muscle to move freely. The endocardium is a smooth membrane lining the inside of the heart and its valves.

Blood circulates through the body by means of the pumping action of the heart, as shown in Figure 12-2. The right ventricle (on your own right side) pumps blood, via the *pulmonary arteries,* to the lungs, where it picks up oxygen (a gas essential to the body's cells) and gives off carbon dioxide (a waste product of metabolism). The blood returns from the lungs via the *pulmonary veins* to the left side of the heart, which pumps it, via the **aorta,** to the arteries in the rest of the body.

The arteries divide into smaller and smaller branches, and finally into **capillaries,** the smallest blood vessels of all (only slightly larger in diameter than a single red blood cell). The blood within the capillaries supplies oxygen and nutrients to the cells of the tissues, and takes up vari-ous waste products. Blood returns to the heart via the veins: The blood from the upper body (except the lungs) drains into the heart through the *superior vena cava,* while blood from the lower body returns via the *inferior vena cava.*

The workings of this remarkable pump affect your entire body. If the flow of blood to or through the heart or to the rest of the body is reduced, or if a disturbance occurs in the small bundle of highly specialized cells in the heart that generate electrical impulses to control heartbeats, the result may at first be too subtle to notice. However, without diagnosis and treatment, these changes could develop into a life-threatening problem.

Perhaps the biggest breakthrough in the field of cardiology has been not a test or a treatment, but a realization: Heart disease is not inevitable. We can keep our hearts healthy for as long as we live, but the process of doing so must start early and continue throughout life.

Preventing Heart Problems

Risk factors related to lifestyle—smoking, physical inactivity, a high-fat diet, raised blood pressure—account for at least three in every four new cases of cardiovascular disease.[3] The best way to protect your heart is by making positive changes in your lifestyle, such as not smoking, exercising, controlling your weight, and limiting fat in your diet.[4]

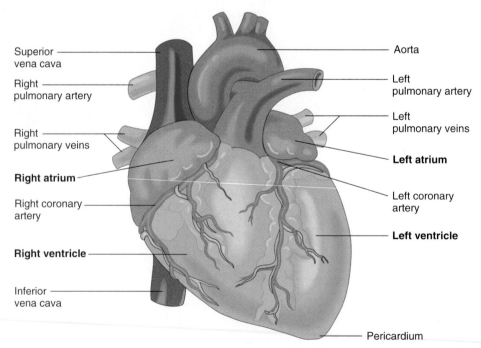

Superior vena cava
Right pulmonary artery
Right pulmonary veins
Right atrium
Right coronary artery
Right ventricle
Inferior vena cava

Aorta
Left pulmonary artery
Left pulmonary veins
Left atrium
Left coronary artery
Left ventricle
Pericardium

▲ **Figure 12-1** The healthy heart.
The heart muscle is nourished by blood from the coronary arteries, which arise from the aorta. The pericardium is the outer covering of the heart.

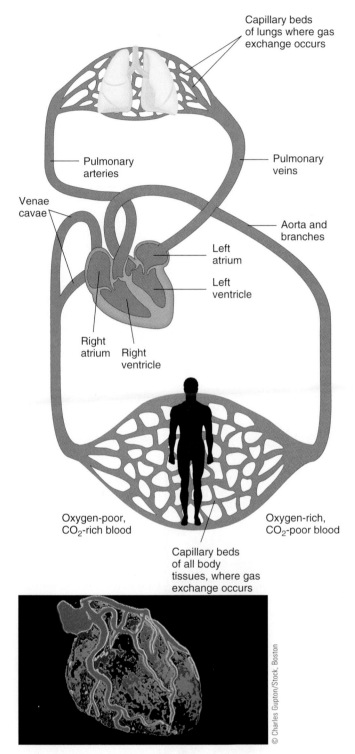

▲ **Figure 12-2** The path of blood flow.
Blood is pumped from the right ventricle into the pulmonary arteries, which lead to the lungs, where gas exchange (oxygen for carbon dioxide) occurs. Oxygenated blood returning from the lungs drains into the left atrium and is then pumped into the left ventricle, which sends the blood into the aorta and its branches. The oxygenated blood flows through the arteries, which extend to all parts of the body. Again, gas exchange occurs in the body tissues; this time oxygen is "dropped off" and carbon dioxide "picked up." The photo depicts a computer-enhanced image of a healthy heart.

Physical Activity

For years we've known that regular exercise reduces the risk of heart attack, helps maintain a healthy body weight, lowers blood pressure, and improves metabolism. If rigorous and frequent enough, it also may increase longevity. But you don't have to head to a gym or hit the bike path to keep your heart healthy. As recent studies have confirmed, "lifestyle" activities, such as walking, housecleaning, and gardening, are as effective as a structured exercise program in improving heart function, lowering blood pressure, and maintaining or losing weight.[5] (See Chapter 4 for a complete discussion of physical activity.)

The federal government and the American Heart Association recommend that adults try to get at least 30 minutes of moderate-intensity physical activity, such as brisk walking, or 45 minutes of recreational games like tennis, on most and preferably all days of the week.[6] While moderate exercise is beneficial, vigorous exercise is more clearly associated with longer life. In a study that followed Harvard alumni for several decades, those who participated in activities such as jogging and swimming lived, on average, a year and a half longer than those who engaged in less intense activities.[7]

What Kind of Diet Is Best for a Healthy Heart?

A balanced, low-fat diet is the best recipe for a healthy heart. In particular, foods rich in cell-protecting antioxidants have been linked with a lower risk of heart disease.

Free radicals—rogue molecules of oxygen—in the cardiovascular system combine with cholesterol and dangerous low-density lipoprotein to damage the inner lining of blood vessels. Vitamin E, a fat-soluble vitamin found in wheat germ, vegetable oils and nuts, short-circuits this process.[8] Americans spend more than $1 billion per year on vitamin E supplements. However, despite initial enthusiasm about its potential in reducing the risk of heart disease, several rigorous studies have shown that supplements of this nutrient do not protect either healthy individuals or those with heart disease or risk factors for it from heart attack, stroke, or death.[9]

Other antioxidants, particularly vitamin C and beta-carotene, also have not proved helpful in protecting the heart. In one study of 22,000 male physicians, 20 milligrams of beta-carotene, either alone or combined with vitamin E, did not reduce the risk of heart attacks. However, in epidemiological studies, individuals eating lots of dark green, yellow, and orange fruits and vegetables (good sources of vitamin C and beta-carotene) consistently have lower rates of coronary disease.

Increased intake of the B vitamins, particularly folate, can lower elevated levels of *homocysteine*, a naturally occurring amino acid and a recently identified risk factor for heart disease. The recommended daily dietary intake is 400 micrograms a day.[10]

Risk Factors for Cardiovascular Disease

Many people don't realize that they're at risk of heart disease; one-quarter of heart attack victims have no prior symptoms.[11] The best way of identifying individuals in potential danger is by looking for risk factors. About 35 percent of adults over age 25 have no elevated risk factors and can be categorized as "low risk." Roughly 40 percent with one or more elevated risk factors are at "intermediate risk." They should undergo regular testing by a physician. Approximately 25 percent of adults have multiple risk factors, some form of heart disease, or type 2 diabetes. They are considered at "high risk" and should work with their physicians on specific strategies to protect their hearts.

Why Should I Worry About Heart Disease?

Contrary to what many assume, heart disease is not a problem only for middle-aged and older individuals. Young hearts also can be in peril. Although the death rate from heart disease has declined overall in the United States, it has increased among individuals ages 15 to 34. (See Student Snapshot: "Young Hearts at Risk.") The underlying conditions that lead to heart disease, such as obesity and high blood pressure, often begin early in life.

The same risk factors endanger hearts at every age. A prime culprit is obesity, which is a growing problem among young people.[12] In a study that followed 11,016 men ages 18 to 39, younger men with the major risk factors for cardiovascular disease—high cholesterol level, high blood pressure, and cigarette smoking—were more likely to develop heart disease.[13] While heart attacks are rare in women under age 40, they are much more likely to occur in women who smoke.[14]

Student Snapshot Young Hearts at Risk

Age group with the greatest increase in sudden cardiac death rate		15- to 34-year-olds
Percentage of deaths occurring before age 24		21%
Percentage of deaths involving young men		71%
Increase in sudden cardiac death rate in young white men		14%
Increase in sudden cardiac death rate in young black men		18%

Source: Study by the Centers for Disease Control and Prevention and the American Heart Association, released in 2001.

When researchers have studied the hearts of young people—again aged 15 to 34—who died as a result of accidents, murder, or suicide, they found that those with cardiovascular risk factors were significantly more likely to show signs of atherosclerosis, such as fatty streaks.[15] According to another report, the teenagers with the highest blood pressure and weights had thicker arteries at age 30 and a greater risk of heart disease.[16]

Young athletes face special risks. Each year seemingly healthy youngsters die suddenly on playing fields and courts. The culprit in one of every three cases of sudden cardiac death in young athletes is a silent condition called hypertrophic cardiomyopathy (HCM), an excessive thickness of the heart muscle. Because of HCM, the heart is more prone to dangerous heart irregularities.

Risk Factors You Can Control

The choices individuals make and the habits they follow can have a significant impact on whether or not their hearts remain healthy. You can choose to avoid the following potential risks for the sake of your heart's health.

Physical Inactivity

Most Americans get too little physical activity. About one-quarter of U.S. adults are sedentary and another third are not active enough to reach a healthy level of fitness. People who are not even somewhat physically active face a much greater risk of fatal heart attack than those who engage in some form of exercise or activity. Individuals who work out rigorously and regularly have the healthiest hearts and the lowest risks of heart disease.

Tobacco Smoke

Each year smoking causes more than 250,000 deaths from cardiovascular disease—far more than it causes from cancer and lung disease. Smokers who have heart attacks are more likely to die from them than are nonsmokers. Smoking is the major risk factor for *peripheral vascular disease*, in which the blood vessels that carry blood to the leg and arm muscles get hardened and clogged. Cigar smoking causes a moderate, but significant increase in an individual's risk for coronary artery disease, as well as for cancers of the upper digestive tract and chronic obstructive pulmonary disease. Men who smoke five or more cigars per day have the highest risk, compared with those who do not smoke cigars at all.[17] Both active and passive smoking accelerate the process by which arteries become clogged and increase the risk of heart attacks and strokes.

The American Heart Association estimates that 37,000 to 40,000 nonsmokers die each year from cardiovascular diseases as a result of exposure to environmental tobacco smoke. Overall, nonsmokers exposed to environmental tobacco smoke are at a 25 percent higher relative risk of developing coronary heart disease than nonsmokers not exposed to environmental tobacco smoke. Cigarette smoking and second-hand smoke can damage the heart in several ways:

- The nicotine may repeatedly overstimulate the heart.
- Carbon monoxide may take the place of some of the oxygen in the blood, which reduces the oxygen supply to the heart muscle.
- The tars and other smoke residues may damage the lining of the coronary arteries, making it easier for cholesterol to build up and narrow the passageways.
- Smoking also increases blood clotting, leading to a higher incidence of clotting in the coronary arteries and subsequent heart attack. Clotting in the peripheral arteries is also increased, which can cause leg pain with walking and, ultimately, stroke.
- Even ex-smokers may have irreversible damage to their arteries.

High Blood Pressure (Hypertension)

Blood pressure is a result of the contractions of the heart muscle, which pumps blood through your body, and the resistance of the walls of the vessels through which the blood flows. Each time your heart beats, your blood pressure goes up and down within a certain range. It's highest when the heart contracts; this is called *systolic blood pressure.* It's lowest between contractions; this is called *diastolic blood pressure.* A blood pressure reading consists of the systolic measurement "over" the diastolic measurement, recorded in millimeters of mercury (mmHg) by a sphygmomanometer (see Figure 12-3).

High blood pressure, or **hypertension,** occurs when the artery walls become constricted so that the force exerted as the blood flows through them is greater than it should be. Physicians see blood pressure as a continuum: the higher the reading, the greater the risk of stroke and heart disease. (See the discussion of high blood pressure later in this chapter.)

As a result of the increased work in pumping blood, the heart muscle of a person with hypertension can become stronger and also stiffer. This stiffness increases resistance to filling up with blood between beats, which can cause shortness of breath with exertion. Hypertension can also act on the kidney arteries, which can lead to kidney failure in some cases. In addition, hypertension accelerates the development of plaque buildup within the arteries. Especially when combined with obesity, smoking, high cholesterol levels, or diabetes, hypertension increases the risks of cardiovascular problems several times. However, you can control high blood pressure through diet, exercise, and medication (if necessary).

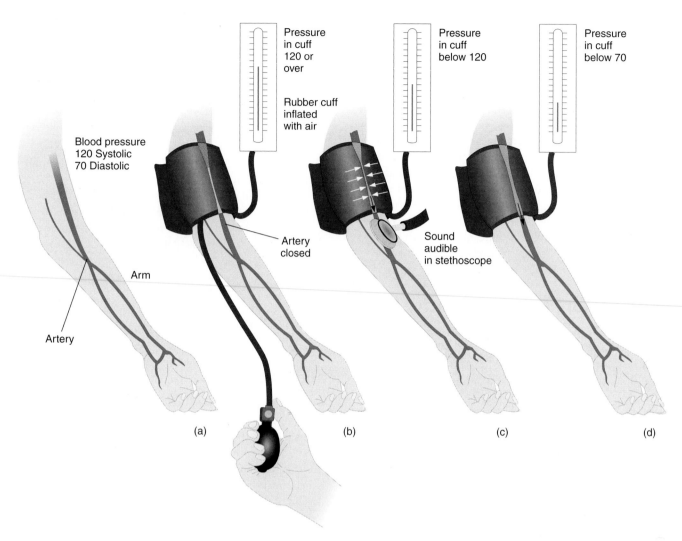

Pressure in cuff 120 or over

Rubber cuff inflated with air

Blood pressure 120 Systolic 70 Diastolic

Arm

Artery

Artery closed

Pressure in cuff below 120

Sound audible in stethoscope

Pressure in cuff below 70

(a)   (b)   (c)   (d)

▲ **Figure 12-3** Measurement of blood pressure.
Assume a blood pressure of 120/70 in a young, healthy individual. (a) The brachial artery of the arm is used to measure blood pressure. (b) The cuff of the sphygmomanometer (blood pressure cuff) is wrapped snugly around the arm just above the elbow and inflated until the blood flow into the brachial artery is stopped. This stoppage is detected with a stethoscope. (c) The cuff is gradually loosened, while the examiner listens carefully for pulse sounds with the stethoscope. The pressure reading as the first soft tapping sounds are heard (as a small amount of blood spurts through the constricted artery) is the systolic pressure. (d) As the cuff is loosened still further, the sounds become louder and more distinct. When the artery is no longer constricted and blood flows freely, however, the pulse sounds can no longer be heard. The reading at which the sounds disappear is recorded as the diastolic pressure.

Blood Fats

Cholesterol is a fatty substance found in certain foods and also manufactured by the body (see Chapter 5). The measurement of cholesterol in the blood is one of the most reliable indicators of the formation of plaque, the sludgelike substance that builds up on the inner walls of arteries. You can lower blood cholesterol levels by cutting back on high-fat foods and exercising more, thereby reducing the risk of a heart attack. According to the National Heart, Lung, and Blood Institute (NHLBI), for every 1 percent drop in blood cholesterol, studies show a 2 percent decrease in the likelihood of a heart attack.

Lipoproteins are compounds in the blood that are made up of proteins and fat. The different types are classified by their size or density. The heaviest are *high-density lipoproteins,* or HDLs, which have the highest portion of protein. These "good guys," as some cardiologists refer to them, pick up excess cholesterol in the blood and carry it back to the liver for removal from the body. An HDL Level of 40 mg/dL or lower substantially increases the risk of heart disease. The averagte HDL for men is about 45 mg/dL; for women, it is about 55 mg/dL. *Low-density lipoproteins,* or LDLs, and very-low-density lipoproteins (VLDLs) carry more cholesterol than HDLs and deposit it on the walls of arteries—they're the bad guys. The higher your LDL cholesterol, the greater your risk for heart disease. If you are at high risk of heart disease, any level of LDL higher than 100 mg/dL may increase your danger.

Triglycerides are fats that flow through the blood after meals and have been linked to increased risk of coronary artery disease, especially in women. Triglyceride levels tend to be highest in those whose diets are high in calories, sugar, alcohol, and refined starches. High levels of these fats may increase the risk of obesity, and cutting back on these foods can reduce high triglyceride levels.

Metabolic Syndrome

A cluster of risk factors, all linked to insulin resistance, make up what researchers call the *metabolic syndrome* and pose a threat to the heart as perilous as cigarette smoking. These factors include excessive abdominal fat (as indicated by a waist measurement of 40 inches or more in men and 35 or more inches in a women), elevated blood pressure, elevated triglycerides, and low HDL cholesterol.

Diabetes Mellitus

Diabetes mellitus, a disorder of the endocrine system, increases the likelihood of hypertension and atherosclerosis, thereby increasing the risk of heart attack and stroke.[18] A physician can detect diabetes and prescribe a diet, exercise program, and, if necessary, medication to keep it in check. Even before developing diabetes, individuals at high risk for this disease—those who are overweight, have a family history of the disease, have mildly elevated blood pressure and blood sugar levels, and above-ideal levels of harmful blood fats—may already be at increased risk of heart disease. Up to one-half of diabetics also have hypertension, another risk factor. Diabetics who develop heart disease are more likely to die if they suffer a heart attack or develop heart failure.[19] Two-thirds of people with diabetes die from cardiovascular disease.[20]

Weight

According to the NHLBI, losing weight at any age can help reduce the risk of heart problems. For women, obesity is as great a cause of excess death and disability from heart disease as smoking and heavy drinking. Even mild to moderately obese women are more likely to suffer chest pain or a heart attack than thinner women. Weight loss significantly reduces high blood pressure, another risk factor for heart disease. (See Chapter 6 for a discussion of weight control.)

Psychosocial Factors

How we respond to everyday sources of stress can affect our hearts as well as our overall health. While we may not be able to control the sources of stress, we can change how we habitually respond to it. Various psychological and social influences may affect vulnerability to heart disease. The most widely studied are Type A traits, particularly anger and hostility; depression and anxiety; work characteristics; and social supports. These factors may act alone or combine and may exert different effects at different ages and stages of life. They may influence behaviors such as smoking, diet, alcohol consumption, and physical activity, and they also may directly cause changes in physiology.

Although Type A behavior—especially anger—has long been linked with heart disease, a recent review of all prospective studies of its effects found no increased risk for Type A patients with coronary heart disease. However, women who bottle up their anger may be more likely to have a heart attack by age 60 than other women. According to a ten-year study of 200 women, those who conceal their anger or are concerned about their public appearance may have rising heart rates, elevated stress hormones, and high blood pressure—all associated with thickening of the carotid arteries.

Depression itself can be a risk factor for heart disease. Individuals who become depressed after a heart attack are significantly more likely to die or suffer a subsequent heart attack. Regardless of whether it's mild or severe, depression decreases ability to function on a daily basis by amplifying heart disease symptoms and reducing patients' interest in daily activities. New research from the University of Michigan School of Public Health shows a link between feelings of hopelessness—a sense of futility and negative expectations for the future—and the development of hypertension.[21]

Some psychological factors take a long-term toll. In a 20-year study of more than 2,000 Californians, women who were depressed and felt socially alienated and men who felt inadequate in their jobs were more likely than their peers to develop high blood pressure decades later. In women, much of the association between psychosocial factors and high blood pressure was the result of unhealthy lifestyle habits, such as smoking, obesity, and a sedentary lifestyle.[22]

Job stress also can be hard on the heart, particularly for employees who have little control over their work. A lack of social supports also seems to increase risk, possibly because intimate, caring relationships may buffer the effect of other stressors in life.

Illegal Drug Use

Illegal drugs, which are discussed in depth in Chapter 14, pose many dangers. One of the most serious is their potentially deadly impact on the cardiovascular system. An estimated one in four heart attacks in individuals between the ages of 18 and 45 can be linked to cocaine use.[23]

Cocaine, ecstasy, and amphetamines have similar harmful effects on the heart. They can cause a sudden rise in blood pressure, heart rate, and contractions of the left ventricle (the pumping chamber) of the heart, which can increase the risk of a heart attack. These drugs also tightly squeeze, or constrict, the coronary arteries that feed blood to the heart. If the artery constricts, blood flow to the heart and brain can be obstructed, causing a heart attack or stroke.

The hallucinogens lysergic acid diethylamide (LSD) and psilocybin (magic mushrooms) also have the potential for triggering irregular heartbeats and heart attacks, although less serious cardiac complications, such as a temporary rise in blood pressure, are more common. Morphine and heroin, which account for almost half of drug-related deaths, can lower blood pressure and affect the heart rate. Inhalants can produce fatal heartbeat irregularities.[24] Marijuana, the most widely used illegal drug among young adults, can affect blood pressure and heart rate, but it is not known whether it can trigger a heart attack.[25]

Risks You Can't Control

Heredity

Anyone whose parents, siblings, or other close relatives suffered heart attacks before age 50 is at increased risk of developing heart disease. Certain risk factors, such as abnormally high blood levels of lipids, can be passed down from generation to generation. Although you can't rewrite your family history, individuals with an inherited vulnerability to cardiovascular disease can lower the danger by changing the risk factors within their control. Your heart's health depends to a great extent on your behavior, including the decisions you make about the foods you eat, or the decision not to smoke. As an added preventive step, cardiologists may prescribe a small daily dose of aspirin to individuals with a history of coronary artery disease who are at risk of forming clots that could block blood supplies to the heart, brain, and other organs. (Note: Daily aspirin is not advised for individuals who are not at risk because of their age or health history.)

Race and Ethnicity

 African Americans are twice as likely to develop high blood pressure as are whites. African Americans also suffer strokes at an earlier age and of greater severity. Poverty may be an unrecognized risk factor for members of this minority group, who are less likely to receive medical treatments or undergo corrective surgery. Family history, lifestyle, diet, and stress may also play a role, starting early in life. However, researchers have found no single explanation for why

African-American youngsters, like their parents, tend to have higher blood pressure than white children.

Age

Almost four out of five people who die of heart attacks are over age 65. Heart disease accounts for more than 40 percent of deaths among people between 65 and 74 and almost 60 percent at age 85 and above. However, the risk factors that are likely to cause heart disease later in life, including high blood pressure and cholesterol levels, may begin to develop in childhood. Nevertheless, although cardiovascular function declines with age, heart disease is not an inevitable consequence of aging. Many 80- and 90-year-olds have strong, healthy hearts.

Gender

Men have a higher incidence of cardiovascular problems than women, particularly before age 40. The incidence of coronary artery disease in women remains lower than in men until the sixth and seventh decades of life, but heart disease often takes a greater toll on women.[26] The major risk factors for heart disease in women are diabetes and menopause; hypertension, smoking, and abnormal blood fats (lipids) are intermediate risks; sedentary lifestyle, obesity, age, and family history are relatively minor risk factors.[27]

The female sex hormone estrogen may have a protective effect by increasing HDL levels and decreasing harmful LDL levels. After menopause or surgical removal of the ovaries, women's estrogen levels drop and their LDL levels tend to go up.

Researchers long believed that postmenopausal hormone replacement therapy (HRT) protected women from heart disease. However, recent studies have challenged this belief. In the first two years of the major longitudinal study called the Women's Health Initiative (WHI), women beginning HRT experienced a slight increase in heart attacks, strokes, and blood clots in the lungs, as compared to those taking a placebo. The risk for these cardiovascular complications declined in subsequent years.[28]

The Heart and Estrogen/Progestin Replacement Study (HERS), which is following postmenopausal women with heart disease, found no cardiovascular benefit from HRT. Yet another report, the three-year Estrogen Replacement and Atherosclerosis (ERA) study, also concluded that postmenopausal women with heart disease did no better on HRT than they did on placebo.

Another possible risk of HRT is stroke. The most recent follow-up of participants in the ongoing Nurses' Health Study showed a significant increase in stroke risk for women using combined HRT. Estrogen use also increases the risk of blood clots, particularly in women already at risk for such problems (for example, because of surgery, hospitalization, or a leg fracture).[29]

Because heart disease has been perceived as a man's problem, research on women's hearts has lagged behind. The current recommendations for blood pressure, cholesterol levels, and prevention are based almost entirely on research on men. However, heart disease is the fourth-leading cause of death among women aged 30 to 34, third among women aged 35 to 39, second among women aged 40 to 64, and first among women over age 65. Although heart disease causes greater disability in women, it is routinely treated less aggressively than in men.[30] (See X & Y Files: "The Hearts of Men and Women.")

Heart disease takes different forms in men and women. Middle-aged men are more likely to have a heart attack or sudden heart stoppage, while women in their middle years are more likely to suffer angina or chest pain. However, the rate of heart attacks increases in women in their sixties or older.[31]

Male Pattern Baldness

Male pattern baldness (the loss of hair at the vertex, or top, of the head) is associated with increased risk of heart attack in men under age 55. A study of 1,437 men showed a "modest" increased risk for those men who'd lost hair at

---

The X & Y Files   The Hearts of Men and Women

Many people still think of heart disease as a "guy problem." However, in every year since 1984, heart disease has claimed the lives of more females than males. Cardiovascular diseases are the number-one killer of women as well as men. Yet most women are far more afraid of breast cancer (the cause of 1 in 27 female deaths) than heart disease (which is responsible for almost 1 in 2 female deaths).

The same risk factors—high cholesterol, high blood pressure, and obesity—endanger both sexes, but they play out differently in women than in men. Women with an HDL under 45 mg/dl are at greater risk, while men don't seem to be at risk unless their HDL dips below 40. Chest pain, or angina, is much more likely to predict coronary artery disease in men than women. About 50 to 60 percent of women with chest pain go on to develop heart disease, compared to 80 to 99 percent of men.

High blood pressure is more common in older women, but treating it may not be as beneficial for women as it is for men. In men, reducing blood pressure by any means reduces the mortality risk by 15 percent. The use of blood pressure medications to lower mild to moderate hypertension actually increases women's overall risk of dying.

For women, extra pounds spell extra danger. Even those who are moderately overweight (10 to 20 percent above their ideal weight) may have twice the risk of leaner women—particularly if they put on weight after age eighteen. In both men and women, the risk of heart disease increases if their extra pounds lodge around the waist rather than in the hips and thighs. Mid-torso fat seems more likely to move to the bloodstream, where it can build up and clog arteries.

Standard diagnostic tests are less precise in detecting heart disease in women. The traditional treadmill or exercise stress test, the gold standard for evaluating men, produces a high rate of false positive results in women. A thallium stress test also is less accurate than in men. Cardiologists recommend evaluation of a the female heart with an "echo stress test," an echocardiogram that uses sound waves to create a 3-D image of the heart at work.

If tests indicate a problem, the next step is an "invasive" diagnostic procedure called angiography or cardiac catheterization. But as recently as a decade ago, ten times as many men as women (40 percent versus 4 percent) were referred for this definitive test. Women still remain much less likely to undergo angiography—a critical prerequisite for angioplasty (balloon surgery to unclog arteries) or coronary bypass surgery.

Women who have heart attacks are less likely than men to survive over both the short and the long term. A woman's risk of dying within a month of a heart attack is 75 percent higher than a man's, in part because women typically take an hour longer to get to the hospital than men. Women also have more complications than men during hospitalization and a higher death rate. Men are more likely to receive therapy with aspirin, beta-blockers, or angiotensin-converting enzyme inhibitors and to undergo angioplasty or bypass surgery.

However, both men and women benefit from cardiac rehabilitation—an option that cardiologists often didn't even suggest for women in the past. Given the same opportunity to strengthen their hearts, women continue to show improvements for three years after they start an exercise program; men reach a certain performance plateau within months.

Sources: Bedinghaus, Joan, et al. "Coronary Artery Disease Prevention: What's Different for Women?" *American Family Physician,* Vol. 63, No. 7, April 1, 2001, p. 1393. Lawlor, D. A., et al. "Sex Matters: Secular and Geographical Trends in Sex Differences in Coronary Heart Disease Mortality." *British Medical Journal,* Vol. 323, No. 7312, September 8, 2001, p. 541. "One for 2001: Take Lifestyle to Heart." *Harvard Women's Health Watch,* Vol. 8, No. 5, January 2001.

the top of their heads but not for those with receding hair-lines. The speed at which men lose their hair also may be an indicator of risk. Scientists speculate that men with male pattern baldness who lose their hair quickly may metabolize male sex hormones differently than others, thereby increasing the likelihood of heart disease.[32]

Although it's premature to say that baldness is definitely "bad news for the heart," health experts advise bald men to follow basic guidelines, such as not smoking and controlling their cholesterol levels, to lower any possible risk.

Bacterial Infection

Unlike the illnesses discussed in Chapter 11, heart disease was never viewed as an illness caused by an infectious agent. However, recent investigations suggest that certain bacteria may indeed put the heart at risk. *Streptococcus sanguis,* the bacterium found in dental plaque, has been implicated in the buildup of atherosclerotic plaque. Individuals with periodontal disease are at increased risk of heart disease and stroke. Regular brushing, flossing, and dental visits can reduce this danger.

The link between gum disease and heart disease has been disputed by researchers who found that toothless individuals do not have a lower risk of heart disease. The American Heart Association advises, "It is not reasonable at this time to look at people's mouth and aggressively treat their periodontal disease—which usually involves antibiotics and surgery and other risks—for the sole purpose of reducing coronary disease risk. . . . You should treat your teeth for your teeth, not for your heart."[33]

Another common bacterium, *Chlamydia pneumoniae,* long linked to respiratory infections, also may threaten the heart. Individuals with high levels of antibodies to this bacteria are more likely to suffer a heart-related problem. Researchers have reported that antibiotics, taken to treat common infections, may protect against first-time heart attacks. A national clinical trial to determine whether antibiotics can reduce the risk of heart attack and stroke is underway.

Your Lipoprotein Profile

Medical science has changed the way it views and targets the blood fats that endanger the healthy heart. In the past, the focus was primarily on total cholesterol in the blood. The higher this number was, the greater the risk of heart disease. In 2001, the NHLBI's National Cholesterol Education Program revised federal guidelines and recommended more comprehensive testing, called a *lipoprotein profile,* for all individuals age 20 or older.[34] (See Savvy Consumer: "What You Need to Know About Testing Lipoproteins.")

This blood test, which should be performed after a 9- to 12-hour fast and repeated at least once every five years, provides readings of:

▷ Total cholesterol.
▷ LDL (bad) cholesterol, the main culprit in the buildup of plaque within the arteries.
▷ HDL (good) cholesterol, which helps prevent cholesterol buildup.
▷ Triglycerides, which are blood fats released into the bloodstream after a meal.

(See Table 12-1 for an interpretation of the test results.)

???? What Is a Healthy Cholesterol Reading?

The answer to this question has become more complex. In general, a total cholesterol reading of less than 200 mg/dL is considered healthy. However, one single cholesterol count no longer applies to everyone.

The greatest threat to your heart's health is LDL cholesterol. The degree of danger of a higher reading depends, not just on the number itself, but on whether or not you have

▼ Table 12-1 What Do Your Cholesterol Numbers Mean?*	
Total Cholesterol Level	**Category**
Less than 200 mg/dL	Desirable
200–238 mg/dL	Borderline high
240 mg/dL and above	High
LDL Cholesterol Level	**LDL Cholesterol Category**
Less than 100 mg/dL	Optimal
100–129 mg/dL	Near optimal/above optimal
130–159 mg/dL	Borderline High
160–189 mg/dL	High
190 mg/dL and above	Very high

HDL (good) Cholesterol

For HDL, higher numbers are better. A level less than 40 mg/dL is low and is considered a major risk factor because it increases your risk for developing heart disease. HDL levels of 60 mg/dL or more help to lower your risk for heart disease.

Triglycerides

Triglycerides can also raise heart disease risk. Levels that are borderline high (150–199 mg/dL) or high (200 mg/dL or more) may need treatment in some people.

*Cholesterol levels are measured in milligrams (mg) of cholesterol per deciliter (dL) of blood.
Source: "High Blood Cholesterol: What You Need to Know." National Cholesterol Education Program, 2001.

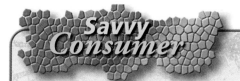

What You Need to Know About Testing Lipoproteins

- Go to your usual primary health-care provider to get a lipoprotein profile. Although cholesterol tests at shopping malls or health fairs can help identify people at risk, the analyzers are often not certified technicians, and the readings may occasionally be inaccurate. In addition, without a health expert to counsel them, some people may be unnecessarily frightened by a high reading—or falsely reassured by a low one.

- Ask about accuracy. Even at first-rate laboratories, cholesterol readings are often inaccurate. Find out if the lab is using the National Institutes of Health (NIH) standards, and ask about the lab's margin for error (which should be less than 5 percent).

- Fast beforehand. Lipoprotein tests are most accurate after a 9- to 14-hour fast. Schedule the test before breakfast if you can. Women may not want to get tested at the end of their menstrual cycles, when minor elevations in cholesterol levels occur because of lower estrogen levels. Cholesterol levels can also rise 5 to 10 percent during periods of stress. Reschedule the test if you come down with an intestinal flu, because the viral infection could interfere with the absorption of food and thus with cholesterol levels. Let your doctor know if you're taking any drugs. Common medications, including birth control pills and hypertension drugs, can affect cholesterol levels.

- Sit down before allowing blood to be drawn or your finger to be pricked, because fluids pool differently in the body when you're standing than when you're sitting. Don't let a technician squeeze blood from your finger, because that forces fluid from cells, diluting the blood sample and possibly leading to a falsely low reading.

- Get real numbers. Don't settle for "normal" or "high," because laboratories can label results inaccurately. Find out exactly what your reading is. Find out your HDL/LDL ratio and HDL and LDL levels.

- Some physicians advise getting two tests in the same month and averaging the result. A person's cholesterol levels vary so much from day to day that a single measurement may not be significant.

other risk factors for heart disease. These include age (over 45 in men, over 55 in women), smoking, high blood pressure, high blood sugar, diabetes, abdominal obesity ("belly" fat), and a family history of heart disease. Depending on your individual risk, your doctor may recommend lifestyle changes or medications that lower cholesterol.

An optimal LDL reading of less than 100 mg/dL should be the goal of those at highest risk of heart disease.

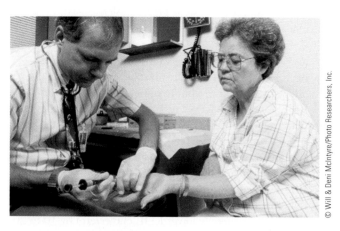

▲ Getting a cholesterol test is a quick, simple, and relatively painless procedure.

© Will & Deni McIntyre/Photo Researchers, Inc.

Those at moderate risk should keep their LDL level under 130 mg/dL; those at low risk should keep their LDL level at or below 160 mg/dL.[35]

HDL or good cholesterol also is important, particularly in women. The new federal guidelines define an HDL reading of less than 40 mg/dL as a major risk factor for developing heart disease. HDL levels of 60 mg/dL or more are protective and lower the risk of heart disease.

A lipoprotein profile also measures triglycerides, the free-floating molecules that transport fats in the bloodstream. Ideally these should be below 150 mg/dL. Individuals with readings of 150 to 199 mg/dL, considered borderline, as well as those with higher readings, may benefit from weight control, physical activity, and, if necessary, medication.

The NHLBI has developed an easy-to-use interactive website that weighs your risk factors, assesses your lipoprotein profile, and calculates how likely you are to have a heart attack in the next ten years. You can perform these calculations by clicking on www.nhlbi.nih.gov. Some doctors may recommend additional tests, such as measurements of homocysteine or hs-CRP or of the size and density of cholesterol particles. In general, small, dense particles of LDL cholesterol seem more dangerous.

Lowering Cholesterol

According to the new guidelines, about one in five Americans may require treatment to lower cholesterol level and the risk of dying from heart disease.[36] By the NCEP's estimates, some 36 million Americans should be watching their diet and exercising more. Another 65 million should be taking cholesterol-lowering drugs. Depending on your lipoprotein profile and assessment of other risk factors, your physician may recommend that you take steps to lower your LDL cholesterol. For some people, therapeutic life changes (TLC) can make a difference. Many require cholesterol-lowering medications.

Therapeutic Life Changes (TLC)

This approach involves several changes in the way of living of individuals with elevated cholesterol. These include:

▶ **The TLC Diet.** This eating plan is low in saturated fats (less than 7 percent of daily calories), total fat (no more than 35 percent of calories), and dietary cholesterol (less than 200 mg) a day. The TLC diet limits calories to the amount needed to maintain a desirable weight and avoid weight gain. Also recommended are foods rich in soluble fiber, such as oats, cereal grains, beans, peas, and legumes, which reduce saturated fat and cholesterol, and those containing plant stanols or plant sterols, such as cholesterol-lowering margarine and salad dressings, which help lower LDL.

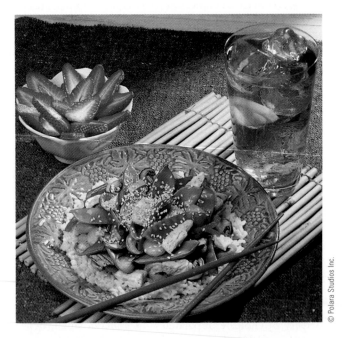

▲ A well-balanced, low-fat diet combined with physical activity is the best recipe for a healthy heart.

© Polara Studios Inc.

▶ **Weight management.** For individuals who are overweight, losing weight can help lower LDL. This is especially true for those with high triglyceride levels and/or low HDL levels and those who have a large waist measurement (more than 40 inches for a man and more than 35 inches for a woman).

▶ **Physical activity.** The recommended amount is 30 minutes on most, if not, all days. Regular activity can help lower LDL, lower blood pressure, reduce triglycerides, and, particularly importantly, raise HDL. Again, these benefits are especially important for those with high triglyceride levels or large waist measurements.

Cholesterol-Lowering Medication

The last decade has seen a revolution in treatment for high cholesterol, thanks to a new class of drugs called statins—better known by brand names such as Lipitor, Mevacor, Pravachol, and Zocor. These medications, which block cholesterol production in the liver, can cut the risk of dying of a heart attack by as much as 40 percent. Initially tested in men, statins have proven equally beneficial for women, including those whose cholesterol levels rise after menopause. Depending on your lipoprotein profile and other risk factors, your doctor may suggest one of the following or a combination of medications:

▶ **Statins.** These medications, among the most widely prescribed drugs in the United States, inhibit an enzyme called HMG-CoA reductase, which controls the rate of cholesterol production in the body. They thereby slow down cholesterol production and increase the liver's ability to remove the LDL cholesterol already in the blood. In several large studies, statins produced large reductions in total and LDL cholesterol—and in heart attacks and heart disease deaths. In some patients, statins can reduce LDL cholesterol by 20 to 60 percent. They also reduce elevated triglyceride levels and produce a modest increase in HDL cholesterol. In individuals with normal cholesterol levels but high levels of C-reactive protein, an indicator of inflammation, statins also have proven effective in lowering the risk of "coronary events," such as heart attacks.[37] Serious side effects, such as liver abnormalities and muscle problems, are rare. However, at least one statin, Baycol, was withdrawn from the U.S. market because of reports of a severe and sometimes fatal muscle adverse reaction. More common complaints include stomach upset, gas, constipation, and abdominal pain or cramps.

▶ **Bile acid sequestrants.** These drugs bind with bile acids that contain cholesterol and remove them in a person's stool. They generally lower LDL cholesterol by 10 to 20 percent. Often these agents are combined with statins to produce a greater reduction in LDL cholesterol. Side effects include constipation, bloating, nausea, and gas.

▶ **Nicotinic acid (niacin).** This B vitamin, taken in high doses and in various release forms, can lower LDL cholesterol, total cholesterol, and triglyceride levels. The niacin preparations used to lower cholesterol should be taken only under a doctor's supervision because of the danger of serious side effects. These include flushing, hot flashes, nausea, indigestion, gas, vomiting, diarrhea, peptic ulcers, gout, liver problems, and high blood pressure.

▶ **Fibrates.** These agents—Gemfibrozil is the most widely used—are most effective in lowering triglycerides and, to a lesser extent, increasing HDL cholesterol. Digestive complaints are the most common side effect. Fibrates also may increase the likelihood of gallstones and may increase the effects of blood-thinning medications.

In the past hormone replacement therapy (HRT) was standard therapy for postmenopausal women with high cholesterol. However, as discussed earlier, large-scale studies have not shown that HRT clearly offers women protection against heart disease. The National Cholesterol Education Project recommends statins or other cholesterol-lowering drugs rather than HRT to reduce a woman's heart attack risk.

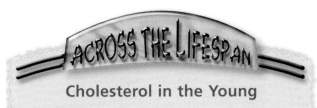

Cholesterol in the Young

Watching cholesterol levels isn't just for grown-ups anymore. In its guidelines for children, the National Cholesterol Education Program recommends cholesterol testing for youngsters at possible risk of heart disease, including those who have any of the following risk factors:

- A parent or grandparent who developed atherosclerosis (narrowing of the arteries due to plaque buildup) at or before age 55.
- A parent or grandparent who suffered a heart attack at or before age 55.
- A parent whose blood cholesterol level is over 240 mg/dL.

Federal health officials aren't advising cholesterol screening for all youngsters, in part because children with high cholesterol levels don't necessarily end up with high blood cholesterol as adults. For those with moderately elevated cholesterol levels, the suggested treatment is a low-fat, high-fiber diet, identical to the one most beneficial for adults' hearts.

Novel Risk Factors

"Half of the people who will have a heart attack or stroke do not have elevated cholesterol levels," says Paul Ridker, director of the Center for Cardiovascular Disease Prevention at Boston's Brigham and Women's Hospital.[38] To identify more individuals in danger, researchers have been investigating other potential cardiovascular villains. Most cardiologists do not test these "novel" risk factors, but some think they can provide an additional warning in patients with other abnormal test results.[39]

Homocysteine

Elevated levels of the amino acid **homocysteine** has been associated with greater risk of heart disease and stroke. A diet rich in fruits, vegetables, whole grains, poultry, fish, and low-fat dairy products can significantly reduce homocysteine. B-vitamin supplements, particularly folate, B_7, and B_{12}, also help, but no one yet knows whether lowering homocysteine will in itself lower the rate of heart attacks or strokes.

C-Reactive Protein (CRP)

C-reactive protein is a marker of inflammation in the blood vessels, which may make atherosclerotic plaque more likely to rupture. In a recent analysis of data on more than 28,000 individuals, a test called hs-CRP (for high-sensitivity CRP) or cardio-CRP proved a better predictor of future heart attacks than any other assessment, including cholesterol. A low-fat diet, exercise, losing weight, and stopping smoking all lower CRP, as do both aspirin and statins. There is no evidence that lowering CRP itself reduces heart attack risk. However, treatment with cholesterol-lowering statins both reduces CRP and does seem to lower the danger of dying as a result of heart disease.[40]

Lipoprotein-a

About 10 percent of the population have elevated levels of the fat-carrying particle called lipoprotein (a), or Lp (a). They are at two to three times greater risk of heart attack, coronary heart disease, and stroke. Unlike cholesterol, Lp (a) levels, primarily genetically determined, are not easily lowered with diet or lifestyle changes. There is no specific therapy for a high Lp (a), but lowering LDL levels is crucial because high LDL multiplies the danger. Niacin also can help bring down Lp (a) levels.

Lipoprotein Particle Size and Density

For some individuals, the size and density of their lipoprotein particles may be as important as their number. About 30 percent of Americans tend to have higher-than-normal concentrations of small LDL particles, which may multiply the risk of heart attack in some people. A tendency to small particle size is inherited, but diet and weight loss can make a difference. Niacin, or nicotinic acid, also can help increase particle size. However, there is no evidence that doing so lowers the risk of heart disease.[41]

The Silent Killers

The two most common forms of cardiovascular disease in this country are high blood pressure (hypertension) and coronary artery disease, the gradual narrowing of the blood vessels of the heart. Often these two problems go together.

▼ **Table 12-2 Heart Disease Deaths per 100,000 People**

	Men	Women
African American	841	553
White	666	388
Native American	465	259
Hispanic	432	265
Asian	372	221

Source: Centers for Disease Control and Prevention.

prevalent among southerners than among people of other regions of the same age and gender.[42] The absolute risk of heart disease related to elevated blood pressure varies in different geographic locations.[43] Physicians urge all adults to have their blood pressure checked at least once a year.

High Blood Pressure

Hypertension forces the heart to pump harder than is healthy. Because the heart must force blood into arteries that are offering increased resistance to blood flow, the left side of the heart often becomes enlarged. The term *essential hypertension* indicates that the cause is unknown, as is usually the case. Occasionally, abnormalities of the kidneys or the blood vessels feeding them, or certain substances in the bloodstream, are identified as the culprits. Whatever its cause, hypertension is dangerous because excessive pressure can wear out arteries, leading to serious cardiovascular diseases, vision problems, and kidney disease. See Figure 12-4.

About 50 million Americans—one in four adults—have high blood pressure that requires monitoring or treatment. (See Table 12-2.) Hypertension has become increasingly common among people in their twenties and thirties. High blood pressure is more

Eye damage
Prolonged high blood pressure can damage delicate blood vessels on the retina, the layer of cells at the back of the eye. If the damage, known as retinopathy, remains untreated, it can lead to blindness.

Heart attack
High blood pressure makes the heart work harder to pump sufficient blood through narrowed arterioles (small blood vessels). This extra effort can enlarge and weaken the heart, leading to heart failure. High blood pressure also damages the coronary arteries that supply blood to the heart, sometimes leading to blockages that can cause a heart attack.

Stroke
High blood pressure can damage vessels that supply blood to the brain, eventually causing them to rupture or clog. The interruption in blood flow to the brain is known as a stroke.

Damage to artery walls
Artery walls are normally smooth, allowing blood to flow easily. Over time, high blood pressure can wear rough spots in artery walls. Fatty deposits can collect in the rough spots, clogging arteries and raising the risk of a heart attack or stroke.

Rough artery walls

Clogged artery

Kidney failure
Prolonged high blood pressure can damage blood vessels in the kidney, where wastes are filtered from the bloodstream. In severe cases, this damage can lead to kidney failure and even death.

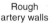

▲ **Figure 12-4** The consequences of high blood pressure.
If left untreated, elevated blood pressure can damage blood vessels in several areas of the body and lead to serious health problems.

A blood pressure reading that's slightly above normal isn't necessarily proof of a blood pressure problem. Due to nervousness, blood pressure may shoot up when anxious individuals enter a medical office, causing what's known as *white coat hypertension*. Other factors, such as warm weather or variations in how health-care practitioners do the test, also can cause elevated readings. It can help to take blood pressure readings at home and compare them with your physician's readings. (Equipment for measuring blood pressure is sold at most pharmacies.)

???? What Is a Healthy Blood Pressure?

Ideal blood pressure is 120/80 mmHg (120 systolic pressure, 80 diastolic pressure). Hypertension is diagnosed when blood pressure rises above 140/90 mmHg. (See Table 12-3). In the past, physicians relied mainly on the diastolic reading—the second and lower of the two blood pressure numbers—in diagnosing hypertension. In young people, diastolic pressure, a reflection of the constriction of the small blood vessels, continues to be a good indicator of cardiovascular risk. However, a rise in systolic blood pressure—the first and higher of the numbers in a blood pressure reading also can be dangerous. Systolic hypertension—a reading of 140 mmHg or higher—reflects stiffening or hardening of the large arteries and is the most common blood pressure problem in the United States (see Figure 12-5 on p. 424).[44]

"The traditional belief was that a systolic blood pressure of 100 plus your age is okay, but this is simply not true," says Joseph Izzo, M.D., an adviser to the NHLBI. "Research data have convinced us that it's time to blow the whistle about the danger of systolic hypertension."[45]

Systolic blood pressure typically rises with age and poses the greatest risk for those middle-aged and older.[46] However, the ideal time to start caring about blood pressure is in your twenties and thirties. In a young person, even mild hypertension can cause organs such as the heart, brain, and kidneys to start to deteriorate. By age 50 or 60, the damage may be irreversible.

Know Your Numbers

"Every one, regardless of age, should know his or her blood pressure—the actual numbers, not just that it's 'fine' or 'normal,' " says Claude Lenfant, M.D., director of the NHLBI. "If your reading is higher than 140 over 80 mmHg, ask your doctor why and find out what you can do about it."[47]

Although anyone can develop high blood pressure, some groups are at greater risk. In any decade of life, African Americans have higher blood pressure levels and suffer more consequences of high blood pressure. An African American with the same elevated blood pressure reading as a Caucasian faces a greater risk of stroke, heart disease, and kidney problems. No one knows why African Americans are more vulnerable, although some speculate that overweight or dietary factors may contribute.

Family history also plays a role. "If you study healthy college students with normal blood pressures, those who have one parent with hypertension will have blood pressure that's a little higher than average," notes Rose Marie Robertson, M.D., of the American Heart Association. "If two parents have high blood pressure, their levels will be a little higher, and they're destined to go higher still. If your parents have high blood pressure, have yours checked regularly."[48]

In a study that followed more than 10,000 healthy men for 25 years, those with high blood pressure in young adulthood were at higher risk for eventually dying from heart disease.[49]

▼ Table 12-3 **Classification of High Blood Pressure**

Category	Systolic Reading	Diastolic Reading	Follow-up Recommended
Normal	Less than 130	Less than 85	Check again in two years.
High normal	130–139	85–89	Check in one year. Many physicians recommend lifestyle modifications at this stage.
Hypertension			
Stage 1	140–159	90–99	Modify lifestyle. Begin drug treatment if lifestyle modifications are not effective within six months.
Stage 2	160–179	100–109	Begin drug treatment and modify lifestyle.
Stage 3	180–209	110–119	Begin drug treatment and modify lifestyle.
Stage 4	More than 210	More than 120	Immediate medical evaluation and treatment with drugs. Modify lifestyle.

Source: Joint National Committee on Detection, Evaluation, Treatment of High Blood Pressure.

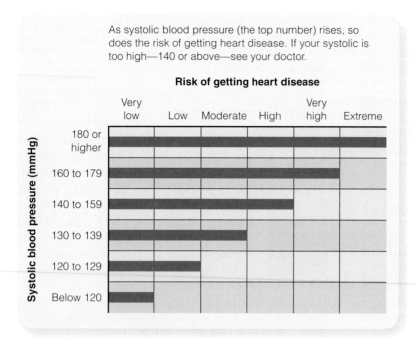

As systolic blood pressure (the top number) rises, so does the risk of getting heart disease. If your systolic is too high—140 or above—see your doctor.

Risk of getting heart disease

▲ **Figure 12-5** The dangers of systolic hypertension.

Source: Framingham Heart Study, National Heart, Lung, and Blood Institute, National Institutes of Health.

Men and women are equally likely to develop hypertension, but in women, blood pressure tends to rise around the time of menopause. Half of all women over age 45 have hypertension. For individuals who smoke, are overweight, don't exercise, or have high cholesterol levels, hypertension multiplies the risk of heart disease and stroke. At ultrahigh risk are people with diabetes or kidney disease.[50]

Preventing Hypertension

Prevention pays off when it comes to high blood pressure. The most effective preventive measures involve lifestyle changes. Losing weight is the best approach for individuals with high normal values. Exercise may be effective in lowering mildly elevated blood pressure. Among the approaches that have not proved effective are dietary supplements, such as calcium, magnesium, potassium, and fish oil.

The National Heart, Lung, and Blood Institute has developed what is known as the DASH diet. Following DASH, which stands for Dietary Approaches to Stop Hypertension, has proven as effective as drug therapy in lowering blood pressure.[51] An additional benefit: the DASH also lowers harmful blood fats, including cholesterol and low-density lipoprotein, and the amino acid homocysteine, (one of the new suspects in heart disease risk mentioned earlier).[52]

Restriction of sodium intake also helps. Most Americans consume more salt than they need. The current federal recommendation is to limit sodium to less than 2.4 grams (2,400 mg) a day. That equals 6 grams (about a teaspoon) of table salt a day. This total includes all sodium, including salt used in cooking and at the table. Doctors may advise those with high blood pressure to eat less salt. According to recent research, diets of less than 1,500 mg of sodium produce even greater benefits and help blood pressure medicines work better.

The lower the amount of sodium in the diet, the lower the blood pressure for both those with and without hypertension and for both genders and all racial and ethnic groups. However, reducing dietary sodium has an even greater effect on blood pressure in blacks than whites, in women than men, and in individuals with hypertension.[53]

The current recommendations for controlling blood pressure are:

▶ Achieve and maintain appropriate body weight.
▶ Limit alcohol to 1 ounce a day.
▶ Get some exercise daily.
▶ Keep sodium intake below 2.4 grams a day.
▶ Consume adequate dietary amounts of calcium and potassium.
▶ Don't smoke.
▶ Cut down on saturated fats, cholesterol, and trans fats.

If exercise, dietary changes, and restriction of salt intake fail to bring down blood pressure, some health experts argue that even those with mild hypertension should take drugs to prevent damage to the heart and blood vessels. There is controversy about the best medications for treating hypertension, however.

STRATEGIES FOR PREVENTION

Reducing Sodium in Your Diet

✔ Buy fresh, plain frozen, or canned "with no salt added" vegetables.

✔ Use fresh poultry, fish, and lean meat, rather than canned or processed types.

✔ Use herbs, spices, and salt-free seasoning blends in cooking.

✔ Check labels and choose "convenience" foods that are lower in sodium.

✔ Avoid frozen dinners, pizza, packaged mixes, canned soups or broths, and salad dressings, which often have large amounts of sodium.

Treating Hypertension

For some people, particularly those with mild hypertension, lifestyle changes alone can bring blood pressure down. "The most important thing is to be active—not just sit in front of the TV," says Dr. Lenfant. "Control your weight, watch what you eat, limit alcohol. Some people are more sensitive to salt than others and have to be especially careful, but everyone should monitor their salt intake."[54]

For other people, diet and exercise are not enough. "The good news is that today we can treat high blood pressure with medications that don't make people feel bad," says Dr. Robertson. "In the past, blood pressure medicines often caused so many side effects that people didn't take them. Now there are multiple classes of drugs, and many drugs in every class. With good communication between patient and doctor, virtually every case can be successfully treated with medications that are effective and don't cause side effects."[55]

Medications called beta-blockers and diuretics are recommended as the first-line treatment for hypertension, but newer drugs such as angiotensin-converting enzyme (ACE) inhibitors and calcium channel blockers are becoming increasingly popular. They account for 55 percent of prescriptions of antihypertensives in the United States. Nevertheless, there is no conclusive evidence that they are more effective and better tolerated. No single drug works well in everyone, so physicians have to rely on clinical judgment and trial-and-error to find the best possible medication for an individual patient.

Any form of high blood pressure is dangerous if not properly treated. The higher the diastolic pressure, the greater the risk for heart attacks, strokes, and kidney failure. As people become older, diastolic pressure typically begins to decrease, and systolic blood pressure starts to rise. Systolic hypertension also increases the danger of heart attacks, strokes, and kidney failure, as well as kidney damage, blindness, and other conditions. (See Pulse Points: "Ten Keys to a Healthy Heart.")

Coronary Artery Disease

The general term for any impairment of blood flow through the blood vessels, often referred to as "hardening of the arteries," is **arteriosclerosis.** The most common form is **atherosclerosis,** a disease of the lining of the arteries in which plaque—deposits of fat, fibrin (a clotting material), cholesterol, other cell parts, and calcium—narrows the artery channels.

Clogging the Arteries

Atherosclerosis, which may begin in childhood, worsens with the continued buildup of plaque on the arterial lining (see photos on this page). The arteries lose their ability to expand and contract. Blood moves with increasing difficulty through the narrowed channels, making it easier for a clot (thrombus) to form, perhaps blocking the channel and depriving vital organs of blood. When such a blockage is in a coronary artery, the result is coronary thrombosis, one form of heart attack. When the clot occurs in the brain, the result is cerebral thrombosis, one form of stroke (discussed later in this chapter).

ACROSS THE LIFESPAN

Treating Hypertension in the Elderly

Traditionally physicians viewed a rise in blood pressure as a normal age-related change and usually did not prescribe medications for hypertension in older men and women, particularly if only their systolic blood pressure (the first and higher blood pressure reading) was elevated. However, clinical trials have clearly shown that treating hypertension in the elderly can significantly reduce their risk of heart disease.

"We've found that treating high systolic pressure with diuretics (water pills), a simple, inexpensive treatment, dramatically reduces the risk of heart attack, stroke and congestive heart failure," says Richard Hodes, M.D., director of the National Institute on Aging. But even though we have a well-demonstrated therapy that can prevent terrible long-term consequences, a lot of people don't have their blood pressures checked or their doctors don't realize the importance of keeping systolic pressures low."[56]

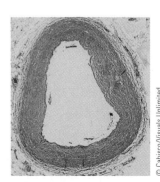 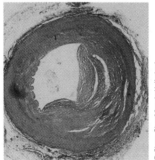

© Cabisco/Visuals Unlimited

© Sloop-Ober/Visuals Unlimited

▲ (A) A healthy coronary artery. (B) An artery partially blocked by the buildup of atherosclerotic plaque.

PULSE POINTS

Ten Keys to a Healthy Heart

1. **Don't smoke.** There's no bigger favor you can do your heart—and lungs!

2. **Watch your weight.** Even relatively modest gains can have a big effect on your risk of heart disease.

3. **Cut down on saturated fats and cholesterol.** This can help prevent high blood cholesterol levels, obesity, and heart disease.

4. **Get moving.** Engage in regular physical activity. A little is better than none; more is even better.

5. **Lower your stress levels.** If too much stress is a problem in your life, try the relaxation techniques described in Chapter 2.

6. **Know your family history.** Inheriting a predispositon to high blood pressure or heart disease means that your heart needs extra preventive care.

7. **Get your blood pressure checked regularly.** Knowing your numbers can alert you to a potential problem long before you develop any symptoms.

8. **Tame your temper.** Hostility can be hazardous to the heart. Look for other ways of releasing anger and frustration.

9. **Get a lipoprotein profile.** You can't know if your heart is in danger unless you know your cholesterol and lipoprotein levels. Get a blood test at your next physical, and discuss the results with your physician.

10. **Take appropriate medications.** Those with high cholesterol or high blood pressure should seek their physicians' advice.

Unstable Plaque

Extra cholesterol deposited on an artery wall creates a "bump" covered by a hard scar. This is called **plaque.** As plaque narrows the space in the arteries, the heart may not receive an adequate supply of oxygen-carrying blood, which may lead to chest pain (angina) or a heart attack.

Cardiologists long believed that the most dangerous plaques were the largest ones, which were most likely to cause total blockage of the coronary arteries. They are, in fact, the primary culprits in angina. However, small plaques are now thought to be very unstable and more likely to burst or rupture, spewing cholesterol into the bloodstream. This triggers blood clotting, which blocks the artery, stops blood flow, and leads to a heart attack.

Lowering cholesterol can make plaque more stable and less prone to rupture. (See Self-Survey: "Check Your Cholesterol and Heart Disease IQ.") A possible early warning of unstable plaque is an elevated level of C-reactive protein (see page 421). A variety of treatments, including a low-fat diet, exercise, weight loss, stopping smoking, aspirin, and statins, can all lower CRP.

Unclogging the Arteries

For years, heart specialists said that, once clogged, arteries couldn't be unclogged. However, research has now shown that it is possible to reverse the buildup of plaque inside the arteries by means of cholesterol-lowering drugs and a low-fat diet. A strict program of dietary and lifestyle change without any medication, developed by Dean Ornish, M.D., of the University of California, San Francisco, also has proven effective in reversing coronary artery disease. The following are the key elements of this approach:

▶ A very low-fat, vegetarian diet, including nonfat dairy products and egg whites, keeping fat intake to below 8 percent of total calories consumed. Ornish's recommended diet allows no meat, poultry, fish, butter, cheese, ice cream, or any form of oil.

▶ Moderate exercise, consisting of an hour of aerobic activity three times a week. Walking is recommended because more rigorous exercise might be dangerous for heart patients, who may develop increased risk of blood clots, irregular heartbeats, or coronary artery spasms during exertion.

▶ Stress counseling. Ornish's patients learn how the body's stress response can cause a rapid heartbeat and narrowing of the arteries, and how stress reduction can reduce cholesterol levels.

▶ An hour a day of yoga, meditation, breathing, and progressive relaxation. Some patients use visualization, for instance, imagining their arteries being cleared by a tunneling machine.[57]

Crises of the Heart

For many people, the first sign of heart disease is pain, ranging from mild to excruciating. They may be experiencing angina pectoris, spasms of the coronary artery, or myocardial infarction (heart attack). According to the American Heart Association (AHA), as many as 1.5 million men and women have heart attacks each year; almost

SELF SURVEY

Check Your Cholesterol and Heart Disease IQ

Instructions

Test your knowledge about high blood cholesterol. Mark each statement true or false.

1. High blood cholesterol is one of the risk factors for heart disease that you can do something about. _____
2. To lower your blood cholesterol level, you must stop eating meat altogether. _____
3. Any blood cholesterol level below 240 mg/dL is desirable for adults. _____
4. Fish oil supplements are recommended to lower blood cholesterol. _____
5. To lower your blood cholesterol level, you should eat less saturated fat, total fat, and cholesterol, and lose weight if you are overweight. _____
6. Saturated fats raise your blood cholesterol levels more than anything else in your diet. _____
7. All vegetable oils help lower blood cholesterol levels. _____
8. Lowering blood cholesterol levels can help people who have already had a heart attack. _____
9. All children need to have their blood cholesterol levels checked. _____
10. Women don't need to worry about high blood cholesterol and heart disease. _____
11. Reading food labels can help you eat the heart healthy way. _____

Answers

1. True. High blood cholesterol is one of the risk factors for heart disease that a person can do something about. High blood pressure, cigarette smoking, diabetes, being overweight, and physical inactivity are the others.
2. False. Although some red meat is high in saturated fat and cholesterol, which can raise your blood cholesterol, you do not need to stop eating it or any other single food. Red meat is an important source of protein, iron, and other vitamins and minerals. You should, however, cut back on the amount of saturated fat and cholesterol that you eat. One way to do this is by choosing lean cuts of meat with the fat trimmed. Another way is to watch your portion sizes and eat no more than 6 ounces of meat a day. Six ounces is about the size of two decks of playing cards.
3. False. A total blood cholesterol level under 200 mg/dL is desirable and usually puts you at a lower risk for heart disease. A blood cholesterol level of 240 mg/dL is high and increases your risk of heart disease. If your cholesterol level is high, your doctor will want to check your level of LDL-cholesterol ("bad" cholesterol). A *high* level of LDL-cholesterol increases your risk of heart disease, as does a *low* level of HDL-

cholesterol ("good" cholesterol). An HDL-cholesterol level below 35 mg/dL is considered a risk factor for heart disease. A total cholesterol level of 200–239 mg/dL is considered borderline-high and usually increases your risk for heart disease. All adults 20 years of age or older should have their blood cholesterol level checked at least once every five years.
4. False. Fish oils are a source of omega-3 fatty acids, which are a type of polyunsaturated fat. Fish oil supplements generally do not reduce blood cholesterol levels. Also, the effect of the long-term use of fish oil supplements is not known. However, fish is a good food choice because it is low in saturated fat.
5. True. Eating less fat, especially saturated fat, and cholesterol can lower your blood cholesterol level. Generally your blood cholesterol level should begin to drop a few weeks after you start on a cholesterol-lowering diet. How much your level drops depends on the amounts of saturated fat and cholesterol you used to eat, how high your blood cholesterol is, how much weight you lose if you are overweight, and how your body responds to the changes you make. Over time, you may reduce your blood cholesterol level by 10–50 mg/dL or even more.
6. True. Saturated fats raise your blood cholesterol level more than anything else. So, the best way to reduce your cholesterol level is to cut back on the amount of saturated fats that you eat. These fats are found in largest amounts in animal products such as butter, cheese, whole milk, ice cream, cream, and fatty meats. They are also found in some vegetable oils—coconut, palm, and palm kernel oils.
7. False. Most vegetable oils—canola, corn, olive, safflower, soybean, and sunflower oils—contain mostly monounsaturated and polyunsaturated fats, which help lower blood cholesterol when used in place of saturated fats. However a few vegetable oils—coconut, palm, and palm kernel oils—contain more saturated fat than unsaturated fat. Limit the total amount of any fats or oils, since even those that are unsaturated are rich sources of calories.
8. True. People who have had one heart attack are at much higher risk for a second attack. Reducing blood cholesterol levels can greatly slow down (and, in some people, even reverse) the buildup of cholesterol and fat in the wall of the coronary arteries and significantly reduce the chances of a second heart attack. If you have had a heart attack or have coronary heart disease, your LDL level should be around 100 mg/dL

(continued)

which is even lower than the recommended level of less than 130 mg/dL for the general population.

9. False. Children from high-risk families, in which a parent has high blood cholesterol (240 mg/dL or above) or in which a parent or grandparent has had heart disease at an early age (at 55 years or younger), should have their cholesterol levels tested. If a child from such a family has a cholesterol level that is high, it should be lowered under medical supervision, primarily with diet, to reduce the risk of developing heart disease as an adult. For most children, who are not from high-risk families, the best way to reduce the risk of adult heart disease is to follow a low saturated fat, low cholesterol eating pattern.

10. False. Blood cholesterol levels in both men and women begin to go up around age 20. Women before menopause have levels that are lower than men of the same age. After menopause, a woman's LDL-cholesterol level goes up—and so her risk for heart disease increases. For both men and women, heart disease is the number one cause of death.

11. True. Food labels have been changed. Look on the nutrition label for the amount of saturated fat, total fat, cholesterol, and total calories in a serving of the product. Use this information to compare similar products. Also, look for the list of ingredients. Here, the ingredient in the greatest amount is first and the ingredient in the least amount is last. So to choose food low in saturated fat or total fat, go easy on products that list fats or oil first, or that list many fat and oil ingredients.

Source: National Institutes of Health. http://www.nhlbi.nih.gov/health/public/heart.

5 million Americans alive today have had a heart attack, chest pain, or both.

Angina Pectoris

A temporary drop in the supply of oxygen to the heart tissue causes feelings of pain or discomfort in the chest known as **angina pectoris.** Some people suffer angina only when the demands on their hearts increase, such as during exercise or when under stress. Many people have angina for years and yet never suffer a heart attack; in some, the angina even disappears. However, angina should be considered a warning of danger if it becomes more severe or more frequent, occurs with less activity or exertion, begins to waken a person from a sound sleep at night, persists for more than ten to fifteen minutes, or causes unusual perspiration.

Angina is most commonly treated with beta-blockers, calcium channel blockers, or nitrates. The American College of Cardiology, the American Heart Association and the American College of Physicians have issued guidelines that call for daily aspirin, sublingual (under the tongue) nitroglycerine, and appropriate medications for lowering of cholesterol and control of diabetes.

Coronary Artery Spasms

Sometimes the arteries tighten suddenly or go into a spasm, cutting off or reducing blood flow. Spasms can pro-duce heart attacks, as well as angina, and can be fatal. Several factors may trigger spasms in the heart, including the following:

- **Clumping of platelets.** When *platelets* (a type of blood cell) clump together, they produce a substance called thromboxane A-2, which causes the narrowing of a blood vessel.
- **Smoking.** When some angina victims stop smoking, their chest pain declines or disappears.
- **Stress.** No one knows exactly how stress may lead to spasms, but many heart specialists believe that it's a culprit.
- **Increased calcium flow.** Calcium regularly flows into smooth muscle cells; too much calcium, however, may lead to a spasm. (This calcium flow is not regulated by the amount of calcium in your diet.)

What Happens During a Heart Attack?

According to the AHA, one person in the United States has a heart attack every 20 seconds, while one person dies of a heart attack every 60 seconds. The medical name for a heart attack, or coronary, is **myocardial infarction (MI).** The *myocardium* is the cardiac muscle layer of the wall of the heart. It receives its blood supply, and thus its oxygen and other nutrients, from the coronary arteries. If an artery is blocked by a clot or plaque, or by a spasm, the myocardial cells do not get sufficient oxygen, and the portion of the myocardium deprived of its blood supply begins to die (see Figure 12-6). Although such an attack may seem sudden, usually it has been building up for years, particularly if the person has ignored risk factors and early warning signs.

Individuals should seek immediate medical care if they experience the following symptoms:

- A tight ache, heavy, squeezing pain or discomfort in the center of the chest, which may last for 30 minutes or more and is not relieved by rest.
- The chest pain radiates to the shoulder, arm, neck, back, or jaw.
- Anxiety.
- Sweating or cold, clammy skin.
- Nausea and vomiting.
- Shortness of breath.
- Dizziness, fainting, or loss of consciousness.

The two hours immediately following the onset of such symptoms are the most crucial. About 40 percent of those who suffer an MI die within this time. According to the American Heart Association, most patients wait three hours after the initial symptoms begin before seeking help. By that time, half of the affected heart muscle may already be lost.

Heart attacks in the United States may be becoming less severe, as measured by the average size of myocardial infarcts. Prompt treatment may be one reason. However, this is not true for women.

Women's heart attacks are more likely to be fatal than men's. Heart attacks are twice as likely to kill women under age 50 than men in the same age range. A review of the records of 384,878 heart attack victims found that 17 percent of female heart attack victims die while still in the hospital, compared with 12 percent of males. The difference results entirely from a much higher death rate among the younger victims.[58]

Women wait hours longer after a heart attack before going to the hospital, then are treated less aggressively than men. This delay, which allows further damage to the oxygen-starved heart, results partly because women tend to experience less painful heart attack symptoms. Sometimes they feel only pressure or a burning feeling, not crushing pain. Younger female victims are more likely than men to have other health problems, such as diabetes, high blood pressure, and heart failure.[59]

In another study of 12,142 men and women who had bad heart attacks, milder ones, or severe chest pain, women were up to twice as likely to suffer serious complications. Among those who had heart attacks, the women were 50 percent more likely to die within 30 days.

More doctors' offices, airlines, and public meeting places, such as casinos, are purchasing heart defibrillators. This life-saving equipment may seem expensive, at an estimated $3,500, but the cost of defibrillators and training teams of nurses in their use comes to only about a nickel per paying patient. State-of the-art treatments for heart

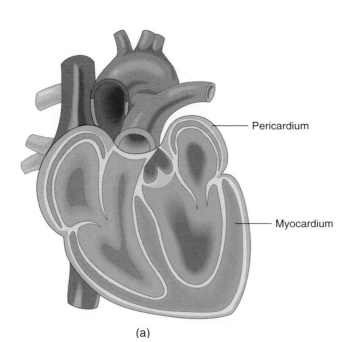

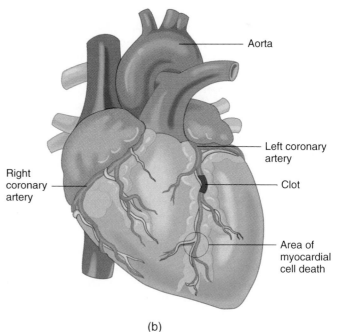

(a)   (b)

▲ **Figure 12-6** The making of a heart attack.
(a) The bulk of the heart is composed mainly of the myocardium, the muscle layer that contracts. (b) A clot in one of the arteries that feeds into the myocardium can cut off the blood supply to part of the myocardium, causing cells in that area to die. This is called a myocardial infarction, or heart attack.

STRATEGIES FOR PREVENTION

What to Do If a Heart Attack Strikes

✔ If you develop chest discomfort that lasts for two minutes or more, call the local emergency rescue service immediately.

✔ If you're with someone who's exhibiting the classic signs of heart attack, and if they last for two minutes or more, act at once. Expect the person to deny the possibility of anything as serious as a heart attack, but insist on taking prompt action.

✔ Call for help. Bystanders should call the emergency medical system (dial 911 in most places) immediately. The odds of survival are greatest if emergency teams get to a heart attack victim quickly and administer advanced cardiac life support. Individuals trained in **cardiopulmonary resuscitation (CPR),** a combination of mouth-to-mouth breathing and chest compression for victims of cardiac arrest, should use this technique only after calling or having someone else call for emergency help.

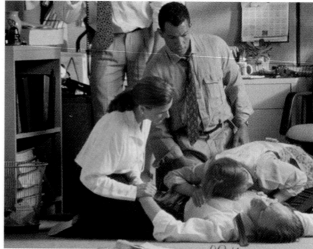

▲ If you witness someone who appears to be experiencing a heart attack, the best thing you can do is call for emergency help immediately. Only after medical emergency personnel are called should you begin any CPR efforts.

attacks include clot-dissolving drugs, early administration of medications to thin the blood, intravenous nitroglycerin, and, in some cases, a beta-blocker (which blocks many of the effects of adrenaline in the body, particularly its stimulating impact on the heart).

Clot-dissolving drugs called thrombolytic agents are the treatment of choice for acute myocardial infarction in most clinical settings. Administered through a *catheter* (flexible tube) threaded through the arteries to the site of the blockage (the more effective method of delivery) or injected intravenously (the faster, cheaper method of delivery), these agents can save lives and dissolve clots, but don't remove the underlying atherosclerotic plaque.

Two clot-thinning drugs may be better than one for treating heart attacks. One drug, called a thrombolytic, dissolves blood clots. The second drug, a platelet receptor blocker, keeps platelets from clumping and forming the blood clots that can obstruct blood flow and thereby trigger a heart attack or stroke. The platelet blockers, sometimes called "super aspirin," are more potent than aspirin. They are also administered through an intravenous drip or infusion. Patients receiving such therapy may require further procedures, such as bypass surgery or **angioplasty,** which can reduce their risk of another heart attack or death.

Emergency balloon angioplasty has shown greater effectiveness than clot-dissolving medication in restoring blood flow in arteries immediately after an attack. With this approach, arteries are less likely to close down again and patients have shorter hospital stays and fewer hospital readmissions. Angioplasty patients also are less likely to die of the heart attack or to experience repeat attacks. However, most American hospitals do not perform angioplasty, and not all can do it on an emergency basis.

Arrhythmias (Heart Rate Abnormalities)

The heart has its own electrical system, which produces an evenly timed, regular beat. When relaxed, most adults have a heart rate of between 60 and 80 beats per minute—slower if they're in good physical condition. During strenuous activity or stress, the heart beats faster. Sometimes the heart seems to skip a beat or experience premature (or early) heartbeats. In many cases, these irregularities or **arrythmias,** are no cause for alarm; but they can be dangerous in an MI victim. Caffeine, long suspected of triggering irregular heartbeats, doesn't seem to be a culprit.

A very fast heart rate (over 100 beats per minute) is known as **tachycardia;** a very slow one (under 60 beats per minute) is **bradycardia.** Resting heart rates of under 60 beats per minute aren't necessarily signs of illness, even though they meet the definition of bradycardia; in fact, they may reflect excellent physical condition. Portable monitors that patients wear around the clock are most likely to catch the heart in an irregular pattern. One, the Holter monitor,

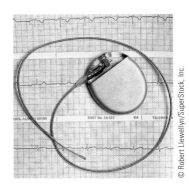

▲ The pacemaker can be surgically implanted in the chest to deliver electrical impulses that normalize a weak or irregular heartbeat.

provides a continuous 24-hour record of the heart rate. Another is a "loop" recorder or event monitor that "lies in ambush" for an attack.

Treatment options include medications, an artificial pacemaker about the size of a small beeper (to ensure that the heart keeps beating regularly), and radiofrequency ablation, a nonsurgical procedure that has revolutionized arrhythmia therapy. In this treatment, cardiologists thread a catheter with an electrode at its tip into the blood vessels of the heart. Using drugs to trigger an irregular heartbeat, they pinpoint its source and administer pulses of radiofrequency energy (similar to microwave heat) that destroy the cells sending errant signals. The risks are low, and more than 90 percent of patients report a complete cure.

As both sexes age, other arrhythmias, often linked with coronary artery disease, increase—and become increasingly perilous. Half of all deaths associated with coronary artery disease are due to arrhythmias. The most common such arrhythmia, affecting two million middle-aged and elderly Americans, is **atrial fibrillation** (AF), in which the upper chambers of the heart quiver rather than working together so blood pools in the heart rather than flowing through it. This greatly increases the risk of clotting, strokes, and death.

Mitral-Valve Prolapse

Mitral-valve prolapse (MVP) is a condition in which a valve in the heart is abnormally long and floppy. Normally, after blood rushes from the left atrium to the left ventricle, the valve between the two chambers slaps shut. But in some people, the closed valve bulges or prolapses back into the atrium. This often occurs because the valve doesn't close completely and blood leaks back into the atrium. This leakage, also called regurgitation, is what doctors may hear as a murmur when listening to your heart.

In the past doctors calculated that up to 30 percent of otherwise healthy young people had MVP. However, this problem is substantially less common and less serious than previously believed. According to recent estimates, MVP affects about 2 percent of the population rather than the 5 to 35 percent of the population previously believed. MVP, once thought to be more common in women, affects men and women equally.

In addition to being thought to have a high prevalence rate, MVP was seen as a disease with frequent and serious complications, including stroke and heart failure. New data show that these complications do not occur at higher rates among patients with mitral-valve prolapse compared to those patients without prolapse.

Congestive Heart Failure

When the heart's pumping power is well below normal capacity, fluid begins to collect in the lungs, hands, and feet. The heart is then said to be in failure. As blood fluids accumulate in the lungs, pulmonary congestion occurs, causing shortness of breath. In other parts of the body, fluid seeps through the thin capillary walls and causes swelling (edema), especially in the ankles and legs. **Congestive heart failure** usually results from myocardial infarction but can also be the result of rheumatic fever, birth defects, hypertension, or atherosclerosis. As many as 4.7 million Americans develop congestive heart failure, which causes 250,000 deaths a year. It is treated by reducing the workload on the heart, modifying salt intake, administering drugs that rid the body of excess fluid, and using medications (such as digitalis) to improve the heart's pumping efficiency. Adding the medication spironolactone, a standard diuretic, can reduce heart failure deaths by 30 percent.

Rheumatic Fever

Rheumatic fever, which strikes most often between the ages of 5 and 15, is a disease that causes painful, swollen joints; skin rashes; and heart damage in half its victims. It is always preceded by a streptococcal infection (see Chapter 11 on infectious diseases). A new strain of streptococcal bacteria has caused a resurfacing of rheumatic fever, which had been considered a disease of the past. The first step to prevention is early identification of the streptococcal infection; the second is treatment with antibiotics to avoid permanent scarring of the heart valves.

Congenital Defects

Approximately 8 out of every 1,000 children born in the United States have congenital heart disease. The most common defects are holes in the ventricular septum, the wall dividing the lower chambers of the heart. Holes may also occur in the atrial septum, the wall between the upper chambers. Sometimes the arteries delivering blood to the body and lungs are transposed and thus attached to the wrong ventricles. Such babies have a bluish color because their blood isn't carrying sufficient oxygen.

Heart Savers

A generation ago physicians had no way of detecting problems before the symptoms of heart disease began and could offer little more than bed rest as a therapy after they struck. Tremendous progress has been made in the diagnosis and treatment of heart problems. Today men and women with heart problems can learn of possible dangers much earlier than in the past and undergo treatments that may add years to their lives.

Diagnostic Tests

The **electrocardiogram (ECG, EKG),** a recording of the electrical activity of the heart, is the traditional method of evaluating the heart's health (see Figure 12-7). An exercise ECG—or *stress test*—is one method of finding out whether an area of the heart begins to run out of blood during the stress of an athletic workout. The subject walks or jogs on a treadmill while the ECG monitors the heart's response. This test is less accurate in women because of a high rate of false positives.

Thallium scintigraphy uses radioactive isotopes that are injected into the bloodstream. A special imaging device called a *scintillation,* or gamma camera, picks up the rays emitted by the isotopes; a computer translates these signals into images of the heart as it pumps. The test can be performed while the patient is either resting or exercising on a treadmill or bicycle. Adding a thallium scan to an exercise ECG increases the probability of detecting existing heart disease by 70 to 90 percent. A stress echocardiogram uses ultrasound to study the heart.

In **coronary angiography,** the most complete and accurate diagnostic test for heart problems, a thin tube is threaded through the blood vessels of the heart, a radiopaque dye is injected, and X rays are taken to detect any blockage of the arteries. Angiography is extremely precise, but it's also costly and risky: About one of every 1,500 patients dies as a result of the test. New methods of diagnosing the heart include ultrafast scans that can capture the heart as it beats.

Treatments

Most people with heart disease can be treated successfully with medications. Other alternatives are bypass surgery, balloon angioplasty, heart transplants, and external and implanted mechanical devices. Patients who respond positively, remain optimistic, and are conscientious in taking prescribed medications significantly reduce their risk of death, a subsequent heart attack, or another coronary event.

Aspirin Therapy

Daily aspirin is recommended as a preventive step for people at high risk of cardiovascular disease because it reduces the stickiness of platelets (cells that cause blood clotting). This lowers the risk of blood clots, which can block a blood vessel and trigger a heart attack or stroke. Several research studies, such as the Hypertension Optimal Treatment study, have demonstrated an association between aspirin use and reductions in heart attacks and strokes.[60] Aspirin lowers the risk of death from any cause, not just heart disease. Its protective effects are strongest in the elderly and those with heart disease.[61]

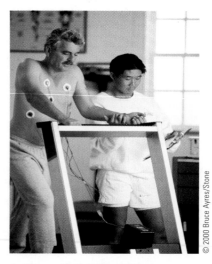
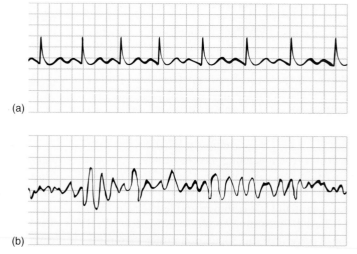

© 2000 Bruce Ayres/Stone

(a)

(b)

▲ **Figure 12-7** ECG readings.
(a) A recording of normal electrical activity in the heart. (b) Grossly irregular activity seen in an acute heart attack.

Only 26 percent of patients who could have benefited from aspirin therapy have ever used it. Aspirin can produce side effects, including gastrointestinal bleeding, allergic reactions, and peptic ulcers. However, the very low doses recommended for heart disease prevention generally do not cause serious problems. They are not advised for people taking anticlotting medication, who have stomach ulcers, or who have kidney or liver disease.

Medications

The main types of drugs used to treat high blood pressure and heart disease include diuretics; beta-blockers; calcium channel blockers; and angiotensin-converting enzyme (ACE) inhibitors, which block the hormone angiotensin that strongly influences blood pressure. Side effects range from lethargy and fatigue to an increased risk of chest pain and heart attack if certain drugs are discontinued abruptly. Calcium channel blockers and ACE inhibitors have become more popular, even though they have not proved more effective than older medications such as diuretics and beta-blockers. Unlike the older drugs, the new ones are less likely to cause side effects such as impotence, insomnia, lethargy, and depression. The newer drugs can be taken in lower doses with negligible side effects.

However, reports have found dangers associated with several widely used heart medications, including a modestly increased risk of heart attack in patients taking some calcium channel blockers, which are used to lower blood pressure, raise cardiac output in heart failure, relieve various forms of angina, and control arrhythmias. They work by countering the flow of calcium ions into the heart muscle cells; calcium is believed to stimulate and contract heart muscle, occasionally causing a sudden spasm that can completely close an artery.

Beta-blockers lower the heart's demand for blood by producing changes in the autonomic (involuntary) nervous system. A variety of beta-blockers are widely used for medical problems, including migraine headaches and glaucoma (a serious eye disease), as well as heart disease. Other cardiac medications include thrombolytic drugs and antiarrythmics. These drugs are not risk-free, and there have been recent reports that some may actually increase the likelihood of a heart attack.

Surgical Procedures and Mechanical Aids

A **coronary bypass** is a procedure in which an artery from the patient's leg or chest wall is grafted onto a coronary artery to detour blood around the blocked area. Each year hundreds of thousands of coronary bypasses are performed in the United States; about 1 to 5 percent of these patients die as a result of surgical complications.

For many patients, the results of bypass surgery are positive. But about one out of five patients suffers subtle, long-lasting impairment of mental performance, including problems concentrating and learning, remembering new information, and performing mental tasks as quickly as before the surgery. About 20 percent remain depressed a year after their operations; their mood changes may stem from damage sustained in the surgery.

Coronary bypasses do not extend life for individuals with mild to moderate angina unless the left main coronary artery was the one that was blocked. If drugs fail to control angina, a coronary bypass can eliminate pain. But surgery is not a cure for the atherosclerotic process that caused the blockage; indeed, in as many as 80 percent of bypass patients, the grafts themselves develop blockages within ten years.

Percutaneous transluminal coronary angioplasty (PTCA), also called balloon angioplasty, is the most often performed heart operation. Less costly and less risky than bypass surgery, PTCA opens blood vessels in the heart that are narrowed but not completely blocked. PTCA involves a precise, time-consuming technique called *cardiac catheterization*—the threading of a narrow tube or catheter through an artery to the heart. An X ray taken with a special dye injected into the arteries reveals the location and extent of a blockage. By inflating a tiny balloon at the tip of the catheter, physicians can break up the clog and widen the narrowed artery. When they deflate the balloon, circulation is restored. Balloon angioplasties are not without risks, however; and balloon-opened arteries can clog up again.

For a variety of heart disorders in which the heart muscle has become so damaged that it can no longer effectively pump blood throughout the body, the only hope is a heart transplant. In recent years the survival rates for transplant recipients have improved dramatically. *Left-ventricular-assist devices (LVADs)* enhance the pumping action of the heart. Used as external, temporary measures until a donor heart becomes available, fully implantable models may someday serve as permanent blood-pumping devices.

New Therapies

A variety of novel approaches are offering new promise for individuals with heart disease. In recent years researchers

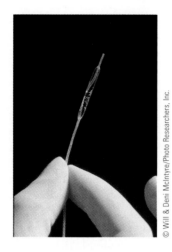

▲ A catheter with a tiny balloon is used in balloon angioplasty to widen a clogged artery.

© Will & Deni McIntyre/Photo Researchers, Inc.

have injected genes directly into the heart muscle to restore the flow of oxygen-rich blood and have used human stem cells to replace dead muscle in a failing heart.[62] Several models of artificial heart implant are currently undergoing clinical trials. In 2001 several patients suffering from chronic heart failure received a self-contained mechanical heart made by Abiomed, Inc. With no external wires, it runs by a short-term 30-minute battery implanted in the abdomen and an outside power source that transmits power through the skin. An implanted control device adjusts the heartbeat.[63]

In the near future, heart specialists may be able to sand plaque off artery walls with a tiny rotating sander, although this method has risks similar to those of balloon angioplasty. The most promising and commonly used nonballoon method is coronary stents, which can reduce complications and the risk of later renarrowing.

Stroke

When the blood supply to a portion of the brain is blocked, a cerebrovascular accident, or **stroke,** occurs. Someone in the United States suffers a stroke every 53 seconds; more than a quarter are under age 65. An estimated 20 percent of stroke victims die within three months; 50 to 60 percent are disabled. About half of those who have a stroke are partially paralyzed on one side of their bodies; between a quarter and a half are partially or completely dependent on others for daily living; a third become depressed; a fifth cannot walk.[64]

Strokes rank third, after heart disease and cancer, as a cause of death in this country.[65] After decades of steady decline, the number of strokes per year has begun to rise.[66] The main reasons seem to be that more people in the United States are living longer, advanced medical care is allowing more people to survive heart disease, and doctors are better able to diagnose and detect strokes. Yet 80 percent of strokes are preventable, and key risk factors can be modified through either lifestyle changes or drugs. The most important steps are treating hypertension, not smoking, managing diabetes, lowering cholesterol, and taking aspirin.

Strokes continue to occur 40 percent more often in the Southeast (the so-called Stroke Belt) than in other regions of the United States. However, stroke rates have fallen in Mississippi and Alabama while they've increased in Oregon, Washington, and Arkansas. The decline in deaths among stroke victims has been greatest in white men and smallest among black men.[67]

???? What Causes a Stroke?

There are two types of stroke: ischemic stroke, which is the result of a blockage that disrupts blood flow to the brain, and hemorrhagic stroke, which occurs when blood vessels rupture. One of the most common causes of ischemic stroke is the blockage of a brain artery by a thrombus, or blood clot—a *cerebral thrombosis.* Clots generally form around deposits sticking out from the arterial wall. Sometimes a wandering blood clot (embolus), carried in the bloodstream, becomes wedged in one of the cerebral arteries. This is called a *cerebral embolism,* and it can completely plug up a cerebral artery (see Figure 12-8a).

In hemorrhagic stroke, a diseased artery in the brain floods the surrounding tissue with blood. The cells nour-

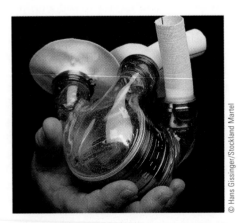

▲ Like a human heart, the AbioCor mechanical heart has two ventricles and its pumping device speeds up and slows down depending on activity level. Unlike a human heart, the AbioCor requires several external components including external batteries, backup batteries, and a power driver.

STRATEGIES FOR PREVENTION

How to Prevent a Stroke

✔ Quit smoking. Smokers have twice the risk of stroke that nonsmokers have. When they quit, their risk drops 50 percent in two years. Within five years after quitting, their risk is nearly the same as nonsmokers.

✔ Keep blood pressure under control. Treating hypertension with medication can lead to a 40 percent reduction in fatal and nonfatal strokes.

✔ Eat a low-fat, low-cholesterol diet, which reduces your risk of fatty buildup in blood vessels.

✔ Avoid obesity, which burdens the blood vessels as well as the heart.

✔ Exercise. Moderate amounts of exercise improve circulation and may help dissolve deposits in the blood vessels that can lead to stroke.

ished by the artery are deprived of blood and can't function, and the blood from the artery forms a clot that may interfere with brain function. This is most likely to occur if the patient suffers from a combination of hypertension and atherosclerosis. Hemorrhage (bleeding) may also be caused by a head injury or by the bursting of an aneurysm, a blood-filled pouch that balloons out from a weak spot in the wall of an artery (see Figure 12-8b).

Brain tissue, like heart muscle, begins to die if deprived of oxygen, which may then cause difficulty speaking and walking, and loss of memory. These effects may be slight or severe, temporary or permanent, depending on how widespread the damage is and whether other areas of the brain can take over the function of the damaged area. About 30 percent of stroke survivors develop dementia, a disorder that robs a person of memory and other intellectual abilities.

The following symptoms should alert you to the possibility that you or someone with you has suffered a stroke:

- Sudden weakness, loss of strength, or numbness of face, arm, or leg.
- Loss of speech, or difficulty speaking or understanding speech.
- Dimness or loss of vision, particularly double vision in one eye.
- Unexplained dizziness.
- Change in personality.
- Change in pattern of headaches.

Transient Ischemic Attacks (TIAs)

Sometimes a person will suffer **transient ischemic attacks (TIAs)**, "little strokes" that cause minimal damage but serve as warning signs of a potentially more severe stroke. One of three people who suffer TIAs will have a stroke during the following five years if they don't get treatment. The two major types of TIAs are:

- **Transient monocular blindness.** Blurring, a blackout or whiteout of vision, a sense of a shade coming down, or another visual disturbance in one eye.
- **Transient hemispheral attack.** Diminished blood flow to one side of the brain, causing numbness or weakness of one arm, leg, or side of the face, or problems speaking or thinking.

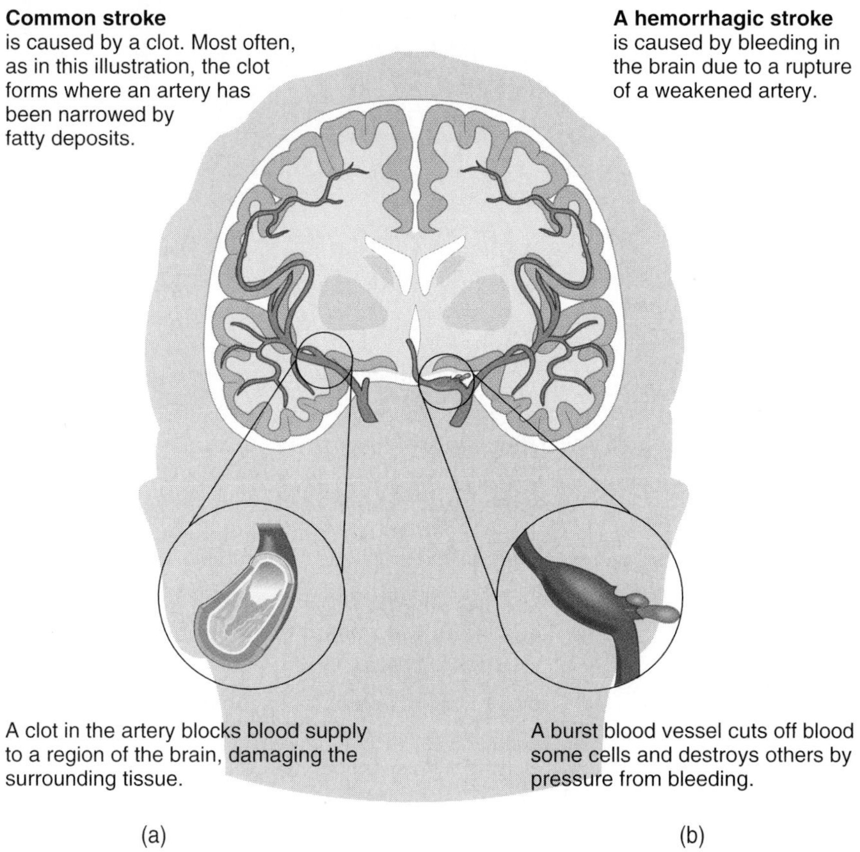

Many TIAs are caused by a narrowing of blood vessels in the neck (carotid arteries) because of a buildup of plaque. Specialists can diagnose this problem by feeling and listening to the arteries, by ultrasound, by measuring the pressure or circulation rate from the carotid arteries to the eyes, or by arterial angiography (injection of a dye into the arteries as X rays are taken), a procedure that can be dangerous, even deadly, or lifesaving.

Surgery to widen the carotid arteries may be recommended for individuals under age 60 with significant narrowing (50 to 80 percent or more). For other patients, aspirin and other drugs that make platelets less sticky and interfere with clotting may be effective.

Common stroke is caused by a clot. Most often, as in this illustration, the clot forms where an artery has been narrowed by fatty deposits.

A hemorrhagic stroke is caused by bleeding in the brain due to a rupture of a weakened artery.

A clot in the artery blocks blood supply to a region of the brain, damaging the surrounding tissue.

A burst blood vessel cuts off blood some cells and destroys others by pressure from bleeding.

(a)   (b)

▲ **Figure 12-8** Two types of strokes.
(a) Blockage of an artery by a blood clot can cause what is termed a common stroke. (b) The bursting of an artery in the brain is called a hemorrhagic stroke, or cerebral hemorrhage.

Risk Factors for Strokes

People who've experienced TIAs are at the highest risk for stroke. Other risk factors, like those for heart disease, include some that can't be changed (such as gender and race) and some that can be controlled:[68]

❱ **Gender.** Men have a greater risk of stroke than women do. However, women are at increased risk at times of marked hormonal changes, particularly pregnancy and childbirth. Past studies have shown an association between oral contraceptive use and stroke, particularly in women over age 35 who smoke. The newer low-dose oral contraceptives have not shown an increased stroke risk among women ages 18 to 44. A woman's stroke risk may increase markedly at menopause.

❱ **Race.** African Americans have a much greater risk of stroke than whites do. Hispanics also are more likely to develop hemorrhagic strokes than whites.

❱ **Age.** A person's risk of stroke more than doubles every decade after age 55.

❱ **Hypertension.** Detection and treatment of high blood pressure are the best means of stroke prevention.

❱ **High red blood cell count.** A moderate to marked increase in the number of a person's red blood cells increases the risk of stroke.

❱ **Heart disease.** Heart problems can interfere with the flow of blood to the brain; clots that form in the heart can travel to the brain, where they may clog an artery.

❱ **Blood fats.** Although the standard advice from cardiologists is to lower harmful LDL levels, what may be more important for stroke risk is a drop in the levels of protective HDL.

❱ **Diabetes mellitus.** Diabetics have a higher incidence of stroke than nondiabetics.

Treatments for Strokes

A small ("baby") aspirin a day cuts in half the risk of strokes caused by abnormal heartbeats, which strike 75,000 Americans each year. Extremely rapid beating of the heart's upper chambers causes blood clots to form; they may enter the bloodstream and travel to the brain, where they can get stuck and choke off the blood supply. In the past, the only way to prevent such strokes was regular use of a medication called warfarin, which inhibits blood clotting and therefore increases the risk of severe bleeding. However, aspirin proved as effective as warfarin—without that dangerous side effect.

Increasingly, surgeons are operating on carotid arteries that may have been narrowed by a buildup of atherosclerotic plaque—a condition that contributes to 20 to 30 percent of strokes, some in individuals with no symptoms—by cleaning them out in a procedure called *carotid endartectomy*. This procedure has been shown to be effective in preventing stroke in patients with and without early symptoms of stroke. An alternative is brain angioplasty, in which surgeons thread a catheter tipped with a tiny inflatable balloon into an artery and gently inflate it to restore blood flow.

It now seems possible to save brain cells for a brief time after a thrombotic stroke occurs. Thrombolytic drugs, used for heart attack victims, can restore brain blood flow after a thrombotic stroke; other medications called heparinoids can reduce the blood's tendency to clot. In order for thrombolytic drugs to be effective, they must be administered within three hours after the stroke; heparinoids must be given within 24 hours.[69] However, the average person does not seek help for 22 hours or longer.[70] The median time between onset of symptoms and calling for help ranges from two to six-and-a-half hours.[71]

In addition, drugs such as nimodipine and other agents undergoing clinical testing at major medical centers, are being used to protect brain cells from damage. Clinicians also are experimenting with ways to tie off tiny, bleeding, cranial arteries with tiny clothespins or to suction off blood that is exerting pressure on the brain. Using stereotactic radioimagery, which relies on a three-dimensional imaging system, surgeons can focus an X-ray beam on a clot or hemorrhage and destroy it.

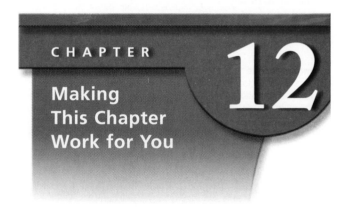

CHAPTER

Making This Chapter Work for You

12

1. The heart
   a. has four chambers, which are responsible for pumping blood into the veins for circulation through the body.
   b. pumps blood first to the lungs where it picks up oxygen and discards carbon dioxide.
   c. beats about 10,000 times and pumps about 75 gallons of blood per day.
   d. has specialized cells that generate electrical signals to control the amount of blood that circulates through the body.

2. You can help maintain a healthy heart by doing all the following except
   a. getting regular moderate levels of exercise every day.
   b. stopping smoking and avoiding regular exposure to secondhand smoke.
   c. eating a diet high in levels of free radicals.
   d. controlling your blood pressure.

3. Which of the following statements about blood pressure is true?
   a. blood pressure increases when the heart relaxes.

b. systolic blood pressure is the pressure of the blood entering the atrium of the heart.

c. high blood pressure is usually the cause of sudden cardiac death in young athletes.

d. blood pressure decreases during diastole.

4. Risk factors for heart disease that cannot be controlled include
   a. male pattern baldness
   b. diabetes mellitus
   c. sedentary lifestyle
   d. blood fat cells

5. Your lipoprotein profile
   a. provides a breakdown of the different types and levels of blood fats circulating in your body.
   b. is best obtained at a health fair where the results are uniformly accurate.
   c. will give a total cholesterol level, which is the amount of triglycerides and LDL cholesterol levels added together.
   d. should be evaluated after eating a full meal.

6. Hypertension
   a. is diagnosed when blood pressure is consistently less than 130/85 mmHg.
   b. may be treated with dietary changes, which include eating low-fat foods and avoiding sodium.
   c. can cause fatty deposits to collect on the artery walls.
   d. usually does not respond to medication, especially in severe cases.

7. Which of the following statements about coronary artery disease is false?
   a. In atherosclerosis, arteries are narrowed by deposits of plaques on the arterial walls.
   b. One successful approach to treatment combines a very low-fat diet, moderate exercise, and stress reduction.
   c. Once plaque appears in the arteries, it is impossible to reverse the effects of coronary artery disease.
   d. A coronary thrombosis may occur if a coronary artery is blocked by a blood clot.

8. A heart attack
   a. occurs when the myocardium receives an excessive amount of blood from the coronary arteries.
   b. is typically suffered by individuals who have irregular episodes of angina.
   c. can be treated successfully up to four hours after the event.
   d. occurs when the myocardial cells are deprived of oxygen-carrying blood, causing them to die.

9. Treatments for heart disease include all the following except
   a. daily aspirin to reduce the risk of blood clots.
   b. coronary bypass surgery to detour blood around a blocked artery.
   c. electrocardiogram to normalize the electrical activity of the heart.
   d. balloon angioplasty to open narrowed blood vessels.

10. Which of the following statements about stroke is true?
    a. A stroke occurs when the blood supply to the aorta is blocked.
    b. Ischemic stroke is usually caused by a blood clot in the brain.
    c. Little strokes, also called transient ischemic attacks, can cause permanent blindness and paralysis of one side of the body.
    d. Risk factors for stroke include gender and occupation.

Answers to these questions can be found on page 640.

 What are the greatest risk factors for heart disease?

Critical Thinking

1. Have you had your blood pressure checked lately? If your reading was high, what steps are you now taking to help reduce your blood pressure?

2. Have you had a lipoprotein profile lately? Do you think it's necessary for you to obtain one? If your reading was/is borderline or high, what lifestyle changes can you make to help control your cholesterol level?

3. The costs for a heart transplant are over $100,000. The annual price tag for a year's worth of cyclosporine, the drug that prevents rejection and must be taken for the rest of a transplant recipient's life, is about $5,000. The total medical bill can come to hundreds of thousands of dollars—enough to fund programs to improve the nutrition of poor pregnant women, to treat alcoholism, or to provide regular preventive care. Does treatment of any single individual justify such huge costs? Should our society try to balance the costs versus the benefits of such heroic measures as heart transplants? How would you go about making such decisions?

SITES & BYTES

American Heart Association Health Risk Awareness
http://www.americanheart.org
This site, sponsored by the American Heart Association, features nine simple questions about your personal characteristics and habits designed to determine your personal risk of having a heart attack or stroke. Risk factors are your personal characteristics, genetic makeup, and lifestyle behaviors that may increase your chances of having a heart attack or stroke. Some you can't change or control (age, gender, genetics); some you can, by making a few changes in your daily habits. Are you at risk? Find out by taking this short interactive quiz. The questions assess your risk based on age, family history, smoking habits, blood cholesterol level, blood pressure, physical activity, weight, diabetes, and past medical history of heart conditions. At the site, log on and follow the prompts to the quiz.

National Heart, Lung, and Blood Institute—National Cholesterol Education Program
http://rover.nhlbi.nih.gov/chd/
This interactive site describes the new 2001 cholesterol guidelines and has sites that allow you to create a heart healthy diet or take a heart disease quiz, print tipsheets, or find other heart resources.

HeartSite.com
http://www.heartsite.com
This site, developed by two prominent cardiologists at the Medical College of Georgia, features many color diagrams to illustrate cardiac disease, including diagnostic tests, procedures, and treatment. The site also features a multimedia lecture on heart disease and heart failure with slides and accompanying audio lecture.

Please note that links are subject to change. If you find a broken link, use a search engine such as **http://www.yahoo.com** and search for the website by typing in key words.

InfoTrac Activity "Major New Cholesterol Guidelines Issued by the National Cholesterol Education Program." *Medical Letter on the CDC & FDA*, June 10, 2001.

(1) List the major changes of the new cholesterol guidelines.

(2) What risk factors does the risk assessment tool described by the new cholesterol guidelines use to obtain a single easy-to-understand category of heart disease risk?

(3) What tests are measured by a lipoprotein profile? How often should this blood test be done in healthy adults?

You can find additional readings related to heart disease with InfoTrac College Edition, an online library of more than 900 journals and publications. Follow the instructions for accessing InfoTrac that were packaged with your textbook; then search for articles using a key word search.

For additional links, resources, and suggested readings on InfoTrac, visit our Health & Wellness Resource Center at **http://health.wadsworth.com**.

Key Terms

The terms listed here are used within the chapter on the page indicated. Definitions of the terms are in the Glossary at the end of the book.

References

1. "Analysts' Alert: There May Not Be as Many Heart Attack Patients as You Think." *Heart Care Strategic Management*, Vol. 19, No. 6, June 2001, p. 6.

2. Beaglehole, Robert. "Global Cardiovascular Disease Prevention: Time to Get Serious." *Lancet*, Vol. 358, No. 9282, August 25, 2001, p. 661.

3. Ibid.

4. Edwards, Thomas. "Lifestyle Influences and Coronary Artery Disease Prevention." *Physician Assistant*, Vol. 25, No. 8, August 2001, p. 19.

5. Lenfant, Claude. "Benefits of Exercise and Lifestyle Modification." National Heart, Lung, and Blood Institute, August 23, 2000.

6. "Exercise Standards Testing and Training." *Circulation*, October 2001.

7. Leiter, Lorene. "Study Finds Vigorous Exercise May Be Best." *Focus: News from Harvard Medical, Dental and Public Health Schools*, March 10, 2000.

8. Young I. S., and J. V. Woodside. "Antioxidants in Health and Disease." *Journal of Clinical Pathology*, Vol. 54, No. 3, March 2001, p. 176.

9. "Vitamin E Supplements: The Pendulum Swings Away." *Tufts University Health & Nutrition Letter*, Vol. 19, April 2001.

10. Tice, Jeffrey, et al. "Cost-effectiveness of Vitamin Therapy to Lower Plasma Homocysteine Levels for the Prevention of Coronary Heart Disease." *Journal of the American Medical Association*, Vol. 286, No. 8, August 22, 2001, p. 936.

11. "A Few Minutes of Risk Assessment Could Mean More of Life." News Release, *American Heart Association*, October 8, 2001.

12. "Heart Disease Prevention Should Start with the Young." *Lancet*, Vol. 357, No. 9260, March 24, 2001, p. 939.

13. Navas-Nacher, Elena. "Risk Factors for Coronary Heart Disease in Men 18 to 39 Years of Age." *Journal of the American Medical Association*, Vol. 285, No. 22, June 13, 2001, p. 2836.

14. Zajarias, Alejandro, et al. "Myocardial Infarction in Women Under 40 Years of Age." *Chest*, Vol. 118, No. 4, October 2000, p. 216S.

15. McCarthy, Michael. "Heart Disease Prevention Should Start with the Young, Studies Suggest." *Lancet*, Vol. 357, No. 9260, March 24, 2001, p. 939.

16. "Higher Blood Pressure in Youth Means Thicker Arteries at a Young Age." New Release, American Heart Association, September 24, 2001.

17. Iribarren, Carlos. "The Effect of Cigar Smoking on the Risk of Cardiovascular Disease, Chronic Obstructive Pulmonary Disease, and Cancer in Men." *New England Journal of Medicine*, Vol. 342, No. 12, March 23, 2000.

18. "Diabetes and Heart Disease: More Closely Linked than Most Think." *Tufts University Health & Nutrition Letter*, Vol. 19, No. 5, July 2001, p. 2.

19. American Diabetic Association. www.diabetes.org

20. "One for 2001: Take Lifestyle to Heart." *Harvard Women's Health Watch*, Vol. 8, No. 5, January 2001.

21. Reyes, Amy. "Link Between Hopelessness and Hypertension." University of Michigan News Service, February 18, 2000.

22. Levenstein, Susan, et al. "Psychosocial Predictors of Hypertension in Men and Women." *Archives of Internal Medicine*, Vol. 161, No. 10, May 28, 2001.

23. Lange, Richard, and David Hillis. "Cardiovascular Complications of Cocaine Use." *New England Journal of Medicine*, Vol. 345, No. 5, August 2, 2001, p. 351.

24. Ghuran, A., et al. "Cardiovascular Complications of Recreational Drugs." *British Medical Journal*, Vol. 323, No. 7311, September 1, 2001, p. 844.

25. Mittleman, Murray. "Triggering Myocardial Infarction by Marijuana." *Journal of the American Medical Association*, Vol. 286, No. 6, August 8, 2001, p. 655.

26. Anderson, Judith, and Cathy Kessenich. "Women and Coronary Heart Disease." *Nurse Practitioner*, Vol. 26, No. 8, August 2001, p. 12.

27. Hu, Frank, et al. "The Impact of Diabetes Mellitus on Mortality from All Causes and Coronary Heart Disease in Women: 20 Years of Follow-up." *Archives of Internal Medicine*, Vol. 161, No. 14, July 23, 2001, p. 1717.

28. Heckbert, Susan, et al. "Risk of Recurrent Coronary Events in Relation to Use and Recent Initiation of Postmenopausal Hormone Therapy." *Archives of Internal Medicine*, Vol. 161, No. 14, July 23, 2001, p. 1709.

29. "Hormone Replacement Therapy—Another Chapter in the Heart and Estrogen Story." *Harvard Women's Health Watch*, Vol. 8, No. 8, April 2001.

30. Roger, Veronique, et al. "Sex Differences in Evaluation and Outcome of Unstable Angina." *Journal of the American Medical Association*, Vol. 263, No. 5, February 2, 2000.

31. Mark, Daniel. "Sex Bias in Cardiovascular Care: Should Women Be Treated More Like Men?" *Journal of the American Medical Association*, Vol. 263, No. 5, February 2, 2000.

32. Lotufo, Paolo, et al. "Male Pattern Baldness and Coronary Heart Disease." *Journal of the American Medical Association*, Vol. 160, No. 2, January 24, 2000.

33. Larkin, Marilynn. "Link Between Gum Disease and Heart Disease." *Lancet*, Vol. 358, No. 9278, July 28, 2001, p. 303.

34. Expert Panel on Detection, Evaluation, and Treatment of High Blood Cholesterol in Adults. "Executive Summary of the Third Report of the National Cholesterol Education Program (NCEP) Expert Panel on Detection, Evaluation, and Treatment of High Blood Cholesterol in Adults." *Journal of the American Medical Association*, Vol. 285, No. 19, May 16, 2001, p. 2486.

35. "Cholesterol: Highlight of the New Guidelines." *Harvard Health Letter*, Vol. 26, No. 9, July 2001.

36. Expert Panel on Detection, Evaluation, and Treatment of High Blood Cholesterol in Adults. "Executive Summary of the Third Report."

37. "In Brief: C-Reactive Protein, Coronary Risk, and Statins." *Harvard Women's Health Watch*, Vol. 9, No. 1, September 2001.

38. Ridker, Paul. Personal interview.

39. Ridker, Paul. "Role of Inflammatory Biomarkers in Prediction of Coronary Heart Disease." *Lancet*, Vol. 357, No. 9260, March 24, 2001, p. 939.

40. Albert, Michelle, et al. "Effect of Statin Therapy on C-Reactive Protein Levels: A Randomized Trial and Cohort Study." *Journal of the American Medical Association*, Vol. 286, No. 1, July 4, 2001, p. 64.

41. "Getting a Handle on Heart Disease." *Tufts University Health & Nutrition Letter*, Vol. 19, No. 7, September 2001, p. 1.

42. Bullock, Carole. "Southerners at Risk for High Blood Pressure." *American Heart Association*, January 7, 2000.

43. Van den Hoogen, Peggy, et al. "The Relation Between Blood Pressure and Mortality Due to Coronary Heart Disease Among Men in Different Parts of the World." *New England Journal of Medicine*, Vol. 342, No. 1, January 6, 2000.

44. National Heart, Lung, and Blood Institute. "Clinical Advisory on Systolic Blood Pressure." May 4, 2000 available at www.nhlbi.nih.gov.

45. Izzo, Joseph. Personal interview.

46. Baker, C., et al. "Hypertension." *Heart*, Vol. 86, No. 3, September 2001, p. 251.

47. Lenfant, Claude. Personal interview.

48. Robertson, Rose Marie. Personal interview.

49. Miura, Katsuyuki, and Martha Daviglus. "Relationship of Blood Pressure to 25-Year Mortality Due to Coronary Heart Disease, Cardiovascular Diseases, and All Causes in Young Adult Men." *Archives of Internal Medicine*, Vol. 161, No. 12, June 2001, p. 1501.

50. Hales, Dianne. "The Stealth Killer." *Parade*, June 25, 2000.

51. Greenland, Philip. "Beating High Blood Pressure with Low-Sodium Dash." *New England Journal of Medicine*, Vol. 344, No. 1, January 4, 2001.

52. "DASH Hypertension Diet Also Lowers Cholesterol." NIH News Release, June 21, 2001.

53. Greenland, "Beating High Blood Pressure with Low-Sodium Dash."

54. Lenfant, Claude. Personal interview.

55. Hales, "The Stealth Killer."

56. Hodes, Richard. Personal interview.

57. Ornish, Dean, et al. "Intensive Lifestyle Changes for Reversal of Coronary Heart Disease." *Journal of the American Medical Association*, Vol. 280, No. 23, December 16, 1998.

58. Legato, Marianne. "Gender and the Heart: Sex-specific Differences in Normal Anatomy and Physiology." *Journal of Gender-Specific Medicine*, Vol. 3, No. 7, October 2000.

59. Mark, "Sex Bias in Cardiovascular Care."

60. Bedinghaus, Joan, et al. "Coronary Artery Disease Prevention: What's Different for Women?" *American Family Physician*, Vol. 63, No. 7, April 1, 2001, p. 1393.

61. Gum, Patricia, et al. "Aspirin Use and All-Cause Mortality Among Patients Being Evaluated for Known or Suspected Coronary Artery Disease: A Propensity Analysis." *Journal of the American Medical Association*, Vol. 286, No. 10, September 10, 2001, p. 1187.

62. "Stem Cell Transplantation Against Heart Attack." *British Medical Journal*, Vol. 323, No. 7306, July 28, 2001, p. 186.

63. "Artificial Heart Patients Faring Well, Doctors Say." *NHLBI Medline Plus*, September 26, 2001.

64. Liebman, Bonnie. "Brain Attack." *Nutrition Action Newsletter*, Vol. 28, No. 7, September 2001, p. 1.

65. "More People Are Hospitalized for Stroke, but Fewer Strokes Are Fatal. News release, American Heart Association, October 4, 2001.

66. "Strokes and Mini-Strokes on the Rise: Total May Exceed 1.2 Million." AHA News Media Relations, February 10, 2000.

67. "Stroke Mortality Varies by Race and Region." News release, American Heart Association, October 4, 2001.

68. Chatfield, Joanne. "American Heart Association Scientific Statement on the Primary Prevention of Ischemic Stroke." *American Family Physician*, Vol. 64, No. 3, August 1, 2001, p. 513.

69. Hankey, Graeme. "New Drugs, or New Trials of Current Drugs, for the Treatment of Acute Ischaemic Stroke?" *Lancet*, Vol. 358, No. 9283, September 1, 2001, p. 683.

70. Liebman, "Brain Attack."

71. "Patient Delay in Calling for Help: The Weakest Link in the Chain of Survival?" *Heart*, Vol. 85, No. 2, February 2001, p. 121.

13

Lowering Your Risk of Cancer and other Major Diseases

Celine knows that she inherited her mother's brown eyes and buoyant sense of humor. She wonders whether she's also inherited "the bad gene"—the cancer-causing one that killed her grandmother and great-grandmother. Celine's mother was 42 years old when she learned that she, too, had cancer. She died two years later, leaving behind eight sisters. Within the next decade, six had developed breast or ovarian cancer.

Unlike most college students, Celine never thinks of cancer as something that affects only people much older than she. Three of her five sisters have tested positive for what is called "the breast cancer gene." Celine is struggling to decide whether she too will undergo testing.

An estimated 10 percent of cancers are hereditary, but no one is immune from the threat of cancer or other serious diseases. Yet you do have some control over your risk of disease. Even if a major illness may be inevitable, you can often prevent or delay it for years or decades.

Prevention and health promotion hold great promise for cancer and for the other non-infectious illnesses discussed in this chapter: diabetes mellitus; epilepsy; respiratory diseases; anemias; liver disorders; kidney problems; digestive diseases; disorders of the muscles, joints, and bones; and skin disorders. This chapter also explains the causes, risk factors, development, diagnosis, and treatment of these disorders and discusses special needs related to differences in physical and mental abilities.

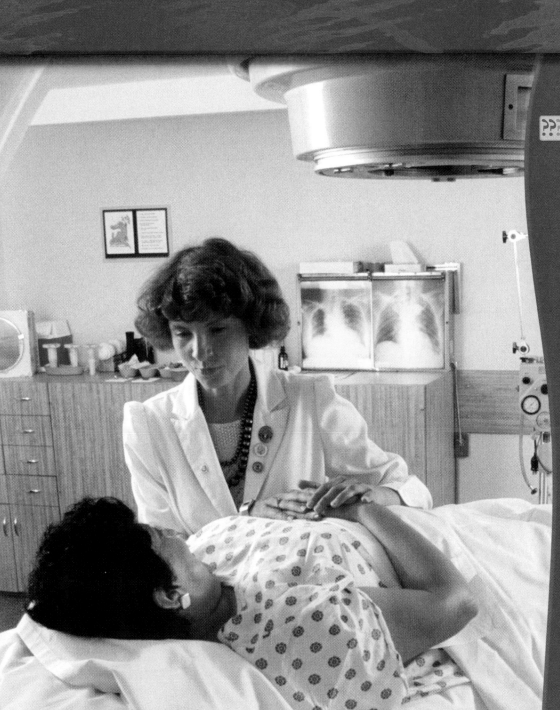

FREQUENTLY ASKED QUESTIONS

FAQ: Who is at risk for developing cancer? p. 444

FAQ: How can I reduce my cancer risk? p. 448

FAQ: Who is at risk for diabetes? p. 462

FAQ: What is asthma: p. 464

After studying the material in this chapter, you should be able to:

- **Explain** how cancer develops and how cancers are classified.
- **List** the risk factors for cancer, and **describe** ways you can reduce your risk of cancer.
- **Discuss** the most common types of cancer, and **describe** the treatments for each.
- **Explain** the disease process of diabetes mellitus, and **describe** the early symptoms and treatment for this disease.
- **Describe** the common major respiratory, liver, kidney, digestive, skeletal-muscular, and skin diseases.

Understanding Cancer

The uncontrolled growth and spread of abnormal cells causes cancer. Normal cells follow the code of instructions embedded in DNA (the body's genetic material); cancer cells do not. Think of the DNA within the nucleus of a cell as a computer program that controls the cell's functioning, including its ability to grow and reproduce itself. If this program or its operation is altered, the cell goes out of control. The nucleus no longer regulates growth. The abnormal cell divides to create other abnormal cells, which again divide, eventually forming **neoplasms** (new formations), or tumors.

Tumors can be either *benign* (slightly abnormal, not considered life-threatening) or *malignant* (cancerous). The only way to determine whether a tumor is benign is by microscopic examination of its cells. Cancer cells have larger nuclei than the cells in benign tumors, they vary more in shape and size, and they divide more often.

At one time cancer was thought to be a single disease that attacked different parts of the body. Now scientists believe that cancer comes in countless forms, each with a genetically determined molecular "fingerprint" that indicates how deadly it is. With this understanding, doctors can identify how aggressively a tumor should be treated.

Without treatment, cancer cells continue to grow, crowding out and replacing healthy cells. This process is called **infiltration,** or invasion. They may also **metastasize,** or spread to other parts of the body via the bloodstream or lymphatic system (see Figure 13-1). For many cancers, as many as 60 percent of patients may have metastases (which may be too small to be felt or seen without a microscope) at the time of diagnosis.

Although all cancers have similar characteristics, each is distinct. Some cancers are relatively simple to cure, whereas others are more threatening and mysterious. The earlier any cancer is found, the easier it is to treat and the better the patient's chances of survival.

Cancers are classified according to the type of cell and the organ in which they originate, such as the following:

▶ *Carcinoma,* the most common kind, which starts in the epithelium, the layers of cells that cover the body's surface or line internal organs and glands.
▶ *Sarcomas,* which form in the supporting, or connective, tissues of the body: bones, muscles, blood vessels.
▶ *Leukemias,* which begin in the blood-forming tissues (bone marrow, lymph nodes, and the spleen).
▶ *Lymphomas,* which arise in the cells of the lymph system, the network that filters out impurities.

???? Who Is at Risk for Developing Cancer?

Everyone and anyone can develop cancer. However, since the occurrence of cancer increases over time, most cases affect adults who are middle-aged or older (see Table 13-1). In the United States, men have a one in two lifetime risk of developing cancer; for women, the risk is one in three.[1] (See X & Y Files: "Gender Differences in Disease.")

The term **relative risk** compares the risk of developing cancer in persons with a certain exposure or trait to the risk in persons who do not have this exposure or trait. Smokers, for instance, have a ten-times-greater relative risk of developing lung cancer than nonsmokers. This means that smokers have a 900 percent increased risk of lung cancer. Most relative risks are smaller. For example, women who have a first-degree (mother, sister, or daughter) family history of breast cancer have about a twofold increased risk of developing breast cancer compared with women who do not have a family history of the disease. This means that they are about twice as likely to develop breast cancer.

Heredity

An estimated 13 to 14 million Americans may be at risk of a hereditary cancer. In hereditary cancers, such as retinoblastoma (an eye cancer that strikes young children) or certain colon cancers, a specific cancer-

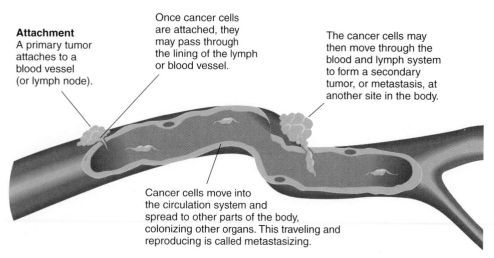

Attachment
A primary tumor attaches to a blood vessel (or lymph node).

Once cancer cells are attached, they may pass through the lining of the lymph or blood vessel.

The cancer cells may then move through the blood and lymph system to form a secondary tumor, or metastasis, at another site in the body.

Cancer cells move into the circulation system and spread to other parts of the body, colonizing other organs. This traveling and reproducing is called metastasizing.

▲ **Figure 13-1** Metastasis, or spread of cancer.
Cancer cells can travel through the blood vessels to spread to other organs, or through the lymphatic system to form secondary tumors.

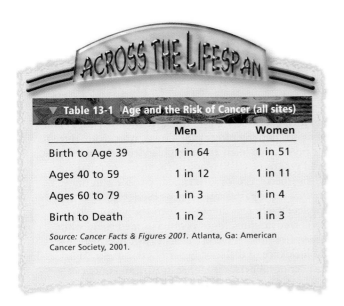

ACROSS THE LIFESPAN

▼ Table 13-1 Age and the Risk of Cancer (all sites)		
	Men	**Women**
Birth to Age 39	1 in 64	1 in 51
Ages 40 to 59	1 in 12	1 in 11
Ages 60 to 79	1 in 3	1 in 4
Birth to Death	1 in 2	1 in 3

Source: Cancer Facts & Figures 2001. Atlanta, Ga: American Cancer Society, 2001.

causing gene is passed down from generation to generation. The odds of any child with one affected parent inheriting this gene and developing the cancer are fifty-fifty. In familial cancers, close relatives develop the same types of cancer, but no one knows exactly how the disease is transmitted. Genetic tests can identify some individuals who are born with an increased susceptibility. Tracing cancers through a family tree is one simple way of checking your own risk.

The most likely sites for inherited cancers to develop are the breast, brain, blood, muscles, bones, and adrenal glands. The telltale signs of inherited cancers include:

▶ **Early development.** Genetic forms of certain diseases strike earlier than noninherited cancers. For example, the average age of women diagnosed with breast cancer is 62. But if breast cancer is inherited, the average age at diagnosis is 44, an 18-year difference.

▶ **Family history.** Anyone with a close relative (mother, father, sibling, child) with cancer has about three times the usual chance of getting the same type of cancer.

▶ **Multiple targets.** The same type of hereditary cancer often strikes more than once—in both breasts or both

GENES IN FOCUS

Cancer Genes

For decades researchers have tried to figure out exactly how a normal cell turns into a cancer cell. They've made dramatic progress in unraveling this mystery by studying **oncogenes,** normal genes that control growth but have gone awry. For reasons that scientists don't yet understand, the DNA in these genes changes and cells proliferate at a very rapid rate. In addition, other genes, called **tumor suppressor genes,** which normally control cell growth, fail to stop cells from dividing before they become cancerous. More than half of all known types of cancer, including those of the colon, brain, lung, breast, bone, and blood, have been linked to defects in one particular tumor suppressor gene: *p53.* Mismatch/repair genes correct mistakes in a cell's DNA when it is copied. If they do not function properly, mutations can occur in other genes, including oncogenes and tumor suppressor genes. (See Figure 13-2.)

In this sense, all cancers are genetic. Scientists have linked several cancers—including cancers of the ovaries, prostate, pancreas, gallbladder, bile duct, colon, and stomach, as well as malignant melanoma, the deadliest skin cancer—to two tumor suppressor genes, BRCA-1 and BRCA-2, initially linked only with breast cancer. Mutations in these genes, which are carried by 1 in 400 Americans, can be passed from a mother or father and can put both sons and daughters at increased risk of several cancers. Genetic tests can identify carriers of BRCA-1 and BRCA-2 mutations, but the results are often difficult to interpret.

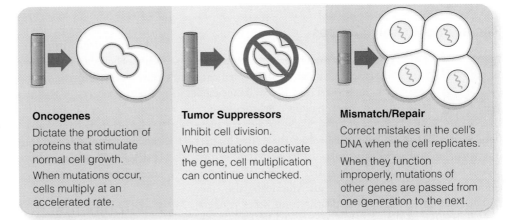

Oncogenes
Dictate the production of proteins that stimulate normal cell growth.
When mutations occur, cells multiply at an accelerated rate.

Tumor Suppressors
Inhibit cell division.
When mutations deactivate the gene, cell multiplication can continue unchecked.

Mismatch/Repair
Correct mistakes in the cell's DNA when the cell replicates.
When they function improperly, mutations of other genes are passed from one generation to the next.

▲ **Figure 13-2** Looking at cancer on the genetic level.
Three different gene types are linked to the development of cancer cells.

Source: New York Times, September 10, 1999. Reprinted by permission.

The X&Y Files — Gender Differences in Cancer

Disease doesn't discriminate. In general, men and women are vulnerable to the same illnesses, but there are differences in the diseases that strike each gender. Women are more prone to arthritis, osteoporosis, and joint problems, while more men are felled by heart attacks and cancer. Of the top ten causes of death in the United States—including heart disease, lung cancer, cirrhosis of the liver, and homicide—every single one kills roughly twice as many men as women.

Half of all men—compared to a third of women—develop cancer. Smoking, which for many years was much more prevalent among men, accounts for some of this difference. As more women became smokers in the last thirty years, lung cancer rates in women have doubled.

In some cancers, estrogen may somehow protect against distant metastases. This protection may be why women have a 12 percent lower death rate from cancer of the stomach and lung than do men and a 33 percent greater chance of surviving malignant melanoma. Men account for two of every three melanoma deaths. (See Figure 13-3 on gender differences in cancer sites and deaths in men and women.)

Some diseases, such as diabetes, afflict more women than men and pose a graver threat to their health. While more men develop ulcers and hernias, women are three to four times more likely to get gallbladder disease. Irritable bowel syndrome (IBS)—one of the most common digestive disorders—causes such varied symptoms in the genders that some gastroenterologists think of it as a completely different disease in men and women. IBS affects women three times as often as men—and white women five times more often than African Americans. The incidence of diabetes, hypertension, stroke, lupus, and other serious illnesses is higher in African American women than in other racial groups.

Sources: Wizeman, Theresa, and Mary-Lou Pardue. *Exploring the Biological Contributions to Human Health: Does Sex Matter?* Washington, DC: National Academy Press, 2001. Hales, Dianne. *Just Like a Woman.* New York: Bantam Books, 2000. Courtenay, Will. "Behavioral Factors Associated with Disease, Injury, and Death Among Men: Evidence and Implications for Prevention." *The Journal of Men's Studies,* Vol. 9, No. 1, Fall 2000, p. 81.

(continued)

kidneys, for instance, or in two separate parts of the same organ.

- **Unusual gender pattern.** Genes may be responsible for cancers that generally don't strike a certain gender—for example, breast cancer in a man.
- **Cancer family syndrome.** Some families, with unusually large numbers of relatives affected by cancer, seem clearly cancer-prone. For instance, in Lynch syndrome (a form of colon cancer), more than 20 percent of the family members in at least two generations develop cancer of both the colon and endometrium.

Racial and Ethnic Groups

 The American Cancer Society estimates 1,268,000 cases of cancer are diagnosed each year, with more cases in black Americans than in any other racial or ethnic group.[2] Blacks are about 33 percent more likely to die of cancer than whites. African-American women have the highest incidence of colorectal and lung cancers of any ethnic group, while black men have the highest rates of prostate, colorectal, and lung cancer. African Americans also have higher rates of incidence and deaths from other cancers, including those of the mouth, throat, esophagus, stomach, pancreas, and larynx. The National Cancer Institute (NCI) has launched the Southern Community Cohort Study to

determine why African Americans are more likely to develop and die from cancer.[3]

Cancer rates also vary in other racial and ethnic groups. Hispanics have six times lower risk of developing melanoma than Caucasians, yet tend to have a worse prognosis than Caucasians when they do develop this skin cancer.[4] The incidence of female breast cancer is highest among white women and lowest among Native American women.

Viruses

Researchers have long known that viruses can cause tumors in animals, but only recently have they shown a connection between several different viruses and cancer in humans. Viruses have been implicated in certain leukemias (cancers of the blood system) and lymphomas (cancers of the lymphatic system), cancers of the nose and pharynx, liver cancer, and cervical cancer. Human immunodeficiency virus (HIV) can lead to certain lymphomas and leukemias and to a type of cancer called Kaposi's sarcoma. Human papilloma virus (HPV) has been linked to an increased risk of cervical cancer and cancer of the penis.[5]

Environmental Risks

At any time during a person's lifetime, a genetic mutation that allows uncontrolled cell growth may be trig-

The X&Y Files — Gender Differences in Cancer—continued

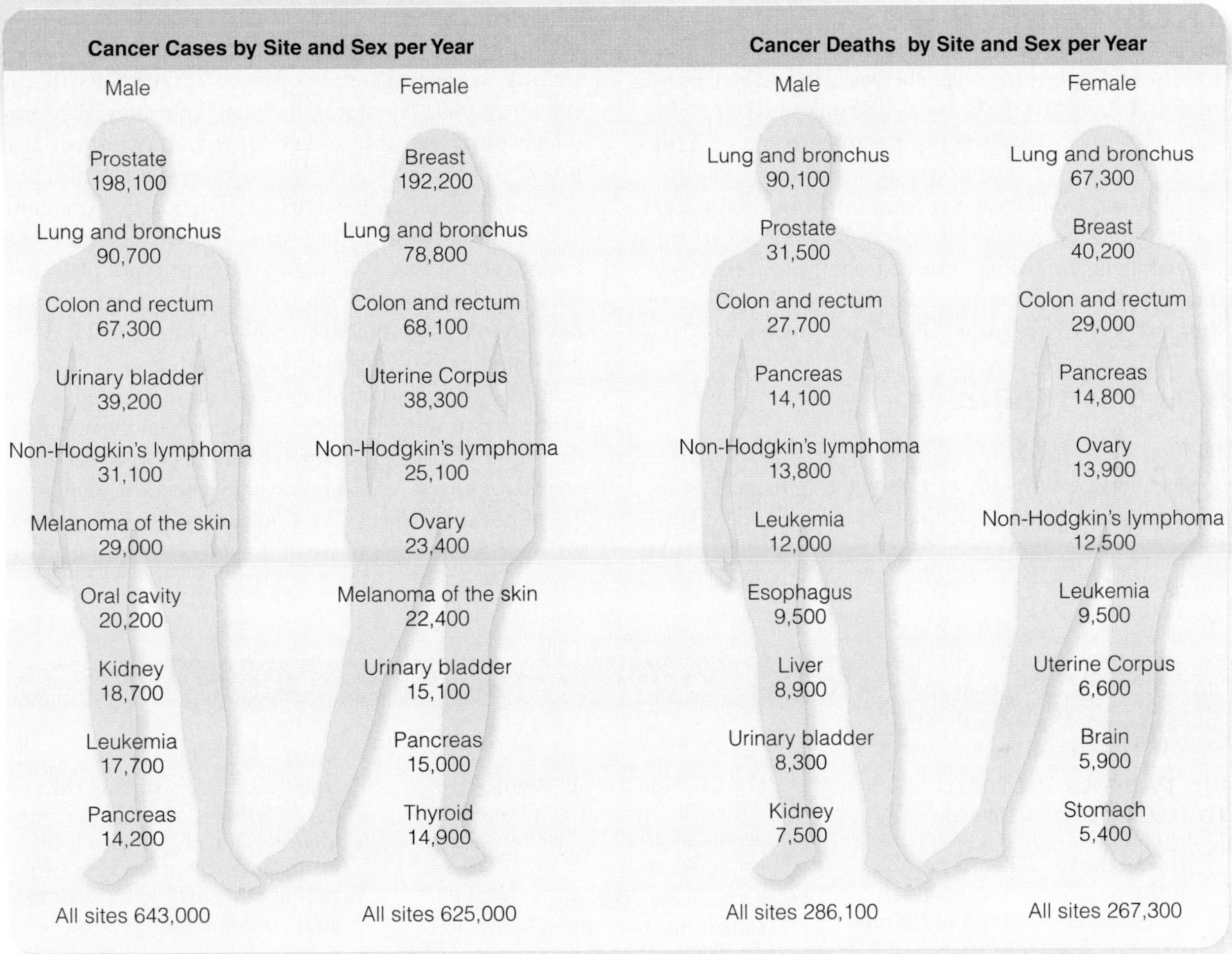

Cancer Cases by Site and Sex per Year		Cancer Deaths by Site and Sex per Year	
Male	Female	Male	Female
Prostate 198,100	Breast 192,200	Lung and bronchus 90,100	Lung and bronchus 67,300
Lung and bronchus 90,700	Lung and bronchus 78,800	Prostate 31,500	Breast 40,200
Colon and rectum 67,300	Colon and rectum 68,100	Colon and rectum 27,700	Colon and rectum 29,000
Urinary bladder 39,200	Uterine Corpus 38,300	Pancreas 14,100	Pancreas 14,800
Non-Hodgkin's lymphoma 31,100	Non-Hodgkin's lymphoma 25,100	Non-Hodgkin's lymphoma 13,800	Ovary 13,900
Melanoma of the skin 29,000	Ovary 23,400	Leukemia 12,000	Non-Hodgkin's lymphoma 12,500
Oral cavity 20,200	Melanoma of the skin 22,400	Esophagus 9,500	Leukemia 9,500
Kidney 18,700	Urinary bladder 15,100	Liver 8,900	Uterine Corpus 6,600
Leukemia 17,700	Pancreas 15,000	Urinary bladder 8,300	Brain 5,900
Pancreas 14,200	Thyroid 14,900	Kidney 7,500	Stomach 5,400
All sites 643,000	All sites 625,000	All sites 286,100	All sites 267,300

▲ **Figure 13-3** Gender differences in cancer sites and deaths.

Source: American Cancer Society, Inc., Surveillance Research, 2001.

gered, directly or indirectly, by environmental risk factors, such as tobacco smoke or toxic chemicals.[6] Mutations also can occur spontaneously when the body's self-monitoring systems do not detect an error made during cell division.

Often genetic and environmental risk factors interact. In colon cancer, for instance, an individual may inherit a gene that has been linked to colon cancer and develop hundreds to thousands of benign adenomatous polyps, which can progress to cancer if not treated. However, the trigger for polyp growth may be in a gene involved in fat metabolism; therefore, eating a high-fat diet increases any inherited vulnerability.

Many chemicals used in industry today are carcinogens, and employees as well as people living near a factory that creates smoke, dust, or gases are at risk. Among the known dangers are nickel, chromate, asbestos, and vinyl chloride. (See Chapter 19 for more information on environmental risks.)

Three to 5 percent of all cancers might be caused by radiation, including medical, occupational, and environmental exposures. Large doses clearly cause cancer; the effects of lower doses are not as clear. Among those at greater risk are workers at and residents near nuclear facilities, pregnant women and their fetuses, and children exposed to nuclear fallout. Clinical studies have revealed a long latent period before a radiation-induced cancer appears (usually a minimum of five years).

How Can I Reduce My Cancer Risk?

Environmental factors may cause between 80 and 90 percent of cancers and, at least in theory, can be prevented by avoiding cancer-causing substances (such as tobacco and sunlight) or using substances that protect against cancer-causing factors (such as antioxidants and vitamin D). How do you start protecting yourself? Simple changes in lifestyle—smart eating, not smoking, protecting yourself from the sun, exercising regularly—are essential. (See Pulse Points: "Ten Ways to Protect Yourself from Cancer" for practical guidelines.)

Cancer-Smart Nutrition

Diets high in antioxidant-rich fruits and vegetables have long been linked with lower rates of esophageal, lung, colon, and stomach cancer. At least in theory, antioxidants can block genetic damage induced by free radicals that could lead to some cancers. However, scientific studies have not proven conclusively that any specific antioxidant, particularly in supplement form, can prevent cancer.

In studies of beta-carotene, this carotenoid did not reduce overall cancer rates or mortality. In two studies of smokers, beta-carotene actually was associated with increased mortality from lung cancer. Researchers are continuing to investigate a variety of antioxidants that have shown promise as cancer-fighters. The mineral selenium, which promotes antioxidant activity, may protect against prostate cancer and possibly also lower the risk of cancer of the lung, colon, and esophagus. Diets rich in vitamin C and folate also may have some specific benefits against breast cancer. Eating as many different types of fruits and vegetables as possible—for a total of five to nine servings a day—remains a standard recommendation. However, a low-fat diet rich in fruit, vegetables, and fiber did not influence the risk of recurrence of colorectal polyps.[7] Some studies have found a correlation between very high consumption of fruits and vegetables and lower risk of breast cancer, but the overall findings have been inconclusive.[8]

Another way to lower your cancer risk is to reduce the fat in your diet. There is solid evidence that cutting back

PULSE POINTS

Ten Ways to Protect Yourself from Cancer

1. **Don't smoke.** Cigarette smoke is the number-one carcinogen in this country, responsible for one in every three cancers.

2. **Stay out of the sun.** Wearing sunscreen (with a Sun Protection Factor of at least 15) is better than not using any, but protective clothing is better— and staying in the shade is best.

3. **Limit your intake of alcohol.** Heavy drinkers are more likely to develop oral cancer and cancers of the larynx, throat, esophagus, liver, and breast.

4. **Watch your weight.** Obesity increases the risks of several cancers, including endometrial cancer and, particularly among postmenopausal women, breast cancer.

5. **Get moving.** Exercise—the heart strengthener and stamina builder—also can reduce the

risk of colon cancer. Women who exercised early in life are less likely to develop breast cancer as adults.

6. **Be sexually cautious.** Cervical cancer has been linked with intercourse at an early age, multiple sex partners, and infection with the human papilloma virus (HPV), the virus that causes genital warts. The incidence of prostate cancer in men increases with multiple sexual partners and a history of frequent sexually transmitted diseases.

7. **Check yourself out.** Scan your skin for suspicious moles every month. If you're a woman, examine your breasts. If you're a man, check your testicles. Follow ACS recommendations for other cancer checkups.

8. **Protect yourself from possible environmental carcinogens.** Many chemicals used in industry can increase the risk to employees and people living near a fac-

tory that creates smoke, dust, or gases. Follow safety precautions at work, and check with local environmental protection officials about possible hazards in your community.

9. **Watch what you eat.** Cut down on fat; eat more fruits, vegetables and whole grains. High-fat foods have been linked to several cancers, including breast, prostate, colon. Fruits, vegetables, and grains are rich in potentially protective antioxidants.

10. **Inform yourself.** Know the warning signs of cancer (see page 452), and see a physician if you develop any of them. Find out about any history of cancer in your family. Even though heredity accounts for a relatively small percentage of cancer cases, the more you know about potential risks, the more you can do to protect yours.

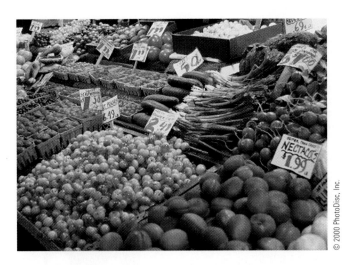

▲ Eating at least five servings of fruits and vegetables a day can help reduce your cancer risk.

on fat can lower the risks of colon, ovarian, and pancreatic cancer.

It's also important to pay attention to food processing and preparation. Whenever possible, select foods close to their natural state, grown locally and without pesticides. Avoid cured, pickled, or smoked meats. When cooking, try not to fry or barbecue often; these cooking methods can produce mutagens that induce cancer in animals. The process of smoking or charcoal-grilling releases carcinogenic tar that may increase the risk of cancer of the stomach and esophagus.

Tobacco Smoke

Cigarette smoking is the single most devastating and preventable cause of cancer deaths in the United States. People who smoke two or more packs of cigarettes a day are 15 to 25 times more likely to die of cancer than are nonsmokers. Cigarettes cause most cases of lung cancer and increase the risk of cancer of the mouth, pharynx, larynx, esophagus, pancreas, and bladder. Pipes, cigars, and smokeless tobacco also increase the danger of cancers of the mouth and throat.

Environmental tobacco smoke can increase the risk of cancer even among those who've never smoked. For example, researchers have found that exposure to others' tobacco smoke for as little as three hours a day can increase the risk of developing cancer threefold. (See the discussion of environmental tobacco smoke in Chapter 16.)

Possible Carcinogens

Although it may not be possible to avoid all possible **carcinogens** (cancer-causing chemicals), you can take

steps to minimize your danger. Many chemicals used in industry, including nickel, chromate, asbestos, and vinyl chloride, are carcinogens, and employees as well as people living near a factory that creates smoke, dust, or gases are at risk. If your job involves their use, follow safety precautions at work. If you are concerned about possible hazards in your community, check with local environmental protection officials.

Women and men who dye their hair frequently, particularly with very dark shades of permanent coloring, may be at increased risk for leukemia (cancer of blood-forming cells), non-Hodgkin's lymphoma (cancer of the lymph system), multiple myeloma (cancer of the bone marrow) and, in women, ovarian cancer. Lighter shades and less permanent tints do not seem to be a danger.

Early Detection

Cancers that can be detected by screening account for approximately half of all new cancer cases. Screening examinations, conducted regularly by a health-care professional, can lead to early diagnosis of cancers of the breast, colon, rectum, cervix, prostate, testicles, and oral cavity and can improve the odds of successful treatment. (See Table 13-2.) Self-examinations for cancers of the breast, testicles, and skin may also result in detection of tumors at earlier stages. The five-year relative survival rate for all these cancers is about 81 percent. If all Americans participated in regular cancer screenings, this rate could increase to more than 95 percent.[9] (See Self-Survey: "Are You at Risk of Cancer?")

Genetic Screening

Millions of Americans may be able to undergo tests to find out if they have genes that increase their risk of cancer, heart disease, alcoholism, and other common problems. But how many will want to know their possible fate? "That may depend on the type of problem," says geneticist Helga Toriello, M.D. "Knowledge can be frightening when little, if anything, can be done to alter the course of a disease. But in most cases, forewarned is forearmed."[10]

Yet genetic testing may never be able to tell individuals all that they want to know. "A test can tell you only whether you have a gene, a marker, or a predisposition for a disorder," says geneticist Reed Pyritz, M.D., of Johns Hopkins University. "It doesn't tell you when you might develop the disease, how it might affect you, whether your symptoms will be mild or severe, or what the course of the illness will be." In addition, he notes, "testing is a double-edged sword. Consumers aren't the only ones eager to find out about inherited risks. Insurance companies and employers also want to know who may be vulnerable. Testing could lead to genetic discrimination."[11]

▼ Table 13-2	American Cancer Society Recommendations for the Early Detection of Cancer in Asymptomatic People
Cancer Type	**Recommended Screening**
General cancer prevention	A cancer-related checkup is recommended every 3 years for people aged 20–40 and every year for people age 40 and older. The exam should include health counseling and depending on a person's age might include examinations for cancers of the thyroid, oral cavity, skin, lymph nodes, testes, and ovaries, as well as some nonmalignant diseases.
Breast	Women 40 and older should have an annual mammogram, an annual clinical breast examination (CBE) by a health-care professional, and should perform monthly breast self-exam (BSE). The CBE should be conducted close to and preferably before the scheduled mammogram. Women aged 20–39 should have a CBE by a health-care professional every 3 years and should perform monthly BSE.
Colon and Rectum	Beginning at age 50 men and women at average risk should follow one of the examination schedules below: • Fecal occult blood test (FOBT) every year • Flexible sigmoidoscopy every 5 years* • FOBT every year and flexible sigmoidoscopy every 5 years* (This is the option preferred by the American Cancer Society.) • Double-contrast barium enema every 5 years* • Colonoscopy every 10 years*
Prostate	Beginning at age 50, the prostate-specific antigen (PSA) test and the digital rectal exam should be offered annually to men who have a life expectancy of at least 10 years. Men at high risk (African-American men and men who have a first-degree relative who was diagnosed with prostate cancer at a young age) should begin testing at age 45. Patients should be given information about the benefits and limitations of tests so they can make an informed decision.
Uterus	**Cervix:** All women who are or have been sexually active or who are 18 and older should have an annual Pap test and pelvic examination. After three or more consecutive satisfactory examinations with normal findings, the Pap test may be performed less frequently. Discuss the matter with your physician. **Endometrium:** Beginning at age 35, women with or at risk for hereditary nonpolyposis colon cancer should be offered endometrial biopsy annually to screen for endometrial cancer.

*A digital rectal exam should be done at the same time. People at increased or high risk for colorectal cancer should talk with a doctor about a different testing schedule.
Source: © American Cancer Society, Inc., 2001. *Cancer Facts and Figures—2001.*

Chemoprevention

In recent years scientists have focused on what has long seemed revolutionary: **chemoprevention,** the use of natural or laboratory-made substances to reduce the risk of developing cancer. They are believed to work by halting or reversing the process by which a cell becomes cancerous.

The first medication that proved effective in preventing a major cancer is **tamoxifen,** a modified or "designer" estrogen that belongs to a group of medications called selective estrogen receptor modulators (SERMs), which have different effects in various parts of the body. In the breast, they block estrogen's harmful effects and lower cancer risk; in the skeleton, they mimic estrogen's beneficial impact and maintain bone density. Tamoxifen's primary disadvantage is an

increased risk of three rare but potentially life-threatening problems: endometrial cancer, deep vein thrombosis (a blood clot in a large vein), and pulmonary embolism (a clot in the lung) in women over age 50.

A second SERM—raloxifene (Evista), FDA-approved to prevent osteoporosis—also may lower breast cancer risk without such serious side effects. NCI's ongoing STAR (Study of Tamoxifen and Raloxifene) trial aims to find the answer. However, there is considerable debate over giving any drug that can cause significant side effects to healthy women.

NCI also is investigating the possible chemopreventive benefits of finasteride (Proscar), a drug used to treat benign swelling of the prostate, a common problem in older men. Unlike tamoxifen, it does not increase the risk

SELF-SURVEY

Are You at Risk of Cancer?

Answer the following questions:

1. Do you protect your skin from overexposure to the sun? _____
2. Do you abstain from smoking or using tobacco in any form? _____
3. If you're over 40 or if family members have had colon cancer, do you get routine digital rectal exams? _____
4. Do you eat a balanced diet that includes the RDA for vitamins A, B, and C? _____
5. If you're a woman, do you have regular Pap tests and pelvic exams? _____
6. If you're a man over 40, do you get regular prostate exams? _____
7. If you have burn scars or a history of chronic skin infections, do you get regular checkups? _____
8. Do you avoid smoked, salted, pickled, and high-nitrite foods? _____
9. If your job exposes you to asbestos, radiation, cadmium, or other environmental hazards, do you get regular checkups? _____
10. Do you limit your consumption of alcohol? _____
11. Do you avoid using tanning salons or home sunlamps? _____
12. If you're a woman, do you examine your breasts every month for lumps? _____
13. Do you eat plenty of vegetables and other sources of fiber? _____
14. If you're a man, do you perform regular testicular self-exams? _____
15. Do you wear protective sunglasses in sunlight? _____
16. Do you follow a low-fat diet? _____
17. Do you know the cancer warning signs? _____

Scoring:

If you answered no to any of the questions, your risk for developing various kinds of cancer may be increased.

Making Changes

Cutting Your Cancer Risk

You may not be able to control every risk factor in your life or environment, but you can protect yourself from the obvious ones.

▶ *Avoid excessive exposure to ultraviolet light.* If you spend a lot of time outside, you can protect your skin by using sunscreen and wearing long-sleeve shirts and a hat. Also, wear sunglasses to protect your eyes. Don't purposely put yourself at risk by binge-sunbathing or by using sunlamps.

▶ *Avoid obvious cancer risks.* Besides ultraviolet light, other environmental factors that have been linked with cancer include tobacco, asbestos, and radiation.

▶ *Keep yourself as healthy as possible.* The healthier you are, the better able your body is to ward off diseases that can predispose you to cancer. Get regular exercise; eat a balanced, high-fiber, low-fat diet; and avoid excessive alcohol use.

▶ *Be alert to changes in your body.* You know your body's rhythms and appearance better than anyone else, and only you will know if certain things aren't right. Changes in bowel habits, skin changes, unusual lumps or discharges—anything out of the ordinary—may be clues that require further medical investigation.

▶ *Don't put off seeing your doctor if you detect any changes.* Procrastination can't hurt anyone but you.

---

of other cancers, but it does have side effects, including sexual dysfunction.[12]

Cancer Staging

Once they diagnose a cancer, oncologists (specialists in cancer care) calculate the extent of the disease or the spread of cancer from the site of origin. This process, called staging, is essential in determining therapy and assessing prognosis. A cancer's stage is based on the primary tumor's size and location and whether it has spread to other areas of the body. According to one staging system, if cancer cells have not spread to other parts of the affected organ or elsewhere in the body, the stage is "in situ." If cancer cells have spread beyond the original layer of tissue, then the

cancer is considered invasive. If it has traveled to distant parts of the body, it has metastasized.

Common Types of Cancer

Cancer refers to a group of more than a hundred diseases characterized by abnormal cell growth. The most common are discussed in the following sections.

Skin Cancer

Sunlight is the primary culprit in the 1 million new cases of skin cancer that develop every year. Once scientists thought exposure to the B range of ultraviolet light (UVB),

STRATEGIES FOR PREVENTION

The Seven Warning Signs of Cancer

If you note any of the following seven warning signs, immediately schedule an appointment with your doctor:

✔ Change in bowel or bladder habits.

✔ A sore that doesn't heal.

✔ Unusual bleeding or discharge.

✔ Thickening or lump in the breast, testis, or elsewhere.

✔ Indigestion or difficulty swallowing.

✔ Obvious change in a wart or mole.

✔ Nagging cough or hoarseness.

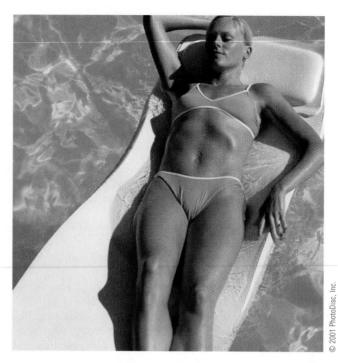

▲ The "healthy" glow of tanned skin may be the precursor to a severe, even fatal, case of skin cancer.

the wavelength of light responsible for sunburn, posed the greatest danger. However, longer-wavelength UVA, which penetrates deeper into the skin, also plays a major role in skin cancers.[13] An estimated 80 percent of total lifetime sun exposure occurs during childhood, so sun protection is especially important in youngsters. Tanning salons or sunlamps also increase the risk of skin cancer because they produce ultraviolet radiation. A half-hour dose of radiation from a sunlamp can be equivalent to the amount you'd get from an entire day in the sun.

The most common skin cancers are basal-cell (involving the base of the epidermis, the top level of the skin) and squamous-cell (involving cells in the epidermis). (See Figure 13-4.) Every year more than 5 million Americans develop skin lesions known as actinic keratoses (AKs), rough red or brown scaly patches that develop in the upper layer of the skin, usually on the face, lower lip, bald scalp, neck, and back of the hands and forearms. Forty percent of squamous cell carcinomas, the second leading cause of skin cancer deaths, begin as AKs. Treatments include surgical removal, cryosurgery (freezing the skin), electrodesiccation (heat generated by an electric current), topical chemotherapy, and removal with lasers, chemical peels, or dermabrasion.

Smoking and exposure to certain hydrocarbons in asphalt, coal tar, and pitch may increase the risk of squamous-cell skin cancer. Other risk factors include occupational exposure to carcinogens and inherited skin disorders, such as xeroderma pigmentosum and familial atypical multiple-mole melanoma.

Malignant melanoma, the deadliest type of skin cancer, causes 1 to 2 percent of all cancer deaths.[14] During the 1930s, the lifetime risk of melanoma was about 1 in 1,500. Today it is 1 in 75. This increase in risk is due mostly to overexposure to UV radiation. The use of a tanning bed ten times or more a year doubles the risk for individuals over age 30. For those younger than 30, this type of exposure increases the risk by a factor of 7.7.[15]

Melanoma occurs more often among people over 40 but is increasing in younger people, particularly those who had severe sunburns in childhood.[16] The rate of increase in melanoma also has risen more in men (4.6 percent a year) than for women (3.2 percent). Men are more likely than women to be diagnosed with melanoma after age 40.[17]

Individuals with any of the following characteristics are at increased risk:

▶ Fair skin, light eyes, or fair hair.
▶ A tendency to develop freckles and to burn instead of tan.
▶ A history of childhood sunburn or intermittent, intense sun exposure.
▶ A personal or family history of melanoma.
▶ A large number of *nevi*, or moles (200 or more, or 50 or more if under age 20), or dysplastic (atypical) moles.[18]

Detection

The most common predictor for melanoma is a change in an existing mole or development of a new and changing

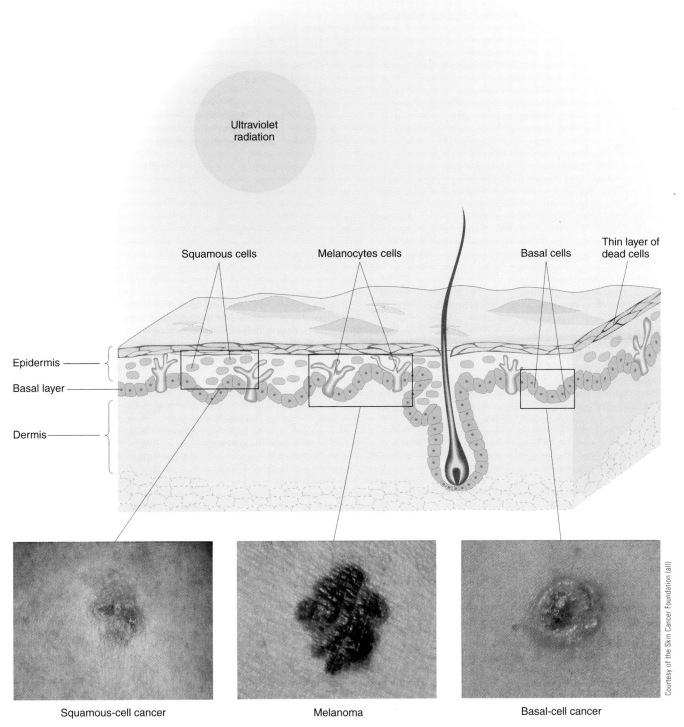

Ultraviolet
radiation

Squamous cells

Melanocytes cells

Basal cells

Thin layer of
dead cells

Epidermis

Basal layer

Dermis

Squamous-cell cancer

Melanoma

Basal-cell cancer

Courtesy of the Skin Cancer Foundation (all)

▲ **Figure 13-4** Three types of skin cancer.
Squamous-cell cancer arises from the squamous cells in the epidermis. Malignant melanoma, the deadliest form of skin cancer, arises from melanocyte cells. Basal-cell cancer arises from the basal cells.

pigmented mole. The most important early indicators are change in color, an increase in diameter, and changes in the borders of a mole. (See Figure 13-5.) An increase in height signals a corresponding growth in depth under the skin. Itching in a new or long-standing mole also should not be ignored.[19]

STRATEGIES FOR PREVENTION

Scanning Your Skin

Here's how to screen yourself for possible changes that may indicate skin cancer:

✔ Once a month, stand in front of a full-length mirror to examine your front and back, and your left and right sides with your arms raised. Check the backs of your legs, the tops and soles of your feet, and the surfaces between your toes. Use a hand mirror to check the back of your neck, behind your ears, and your scalp.

✔ Watch for changes in the size, color, number, and thickness of moles. Suspicious moles are likely to be asymmetrical (one half doesn't match the other), with ragged, notched, or blurred edges. Also look for any signs of darkly pigmented growth, oozing, scaliness, bleeding, or a change in sensation, itchiness, tenderness, or pain.

✔ Don't put too much faith in sunscreens. Wearing sunscreen (with a Sun Protection Factor, or SPF, of at least 15) is good, but protective clothing is better—and staying in the shade is best. Check your shadow. One simple guideline for reducing the risk of skin cancer risk is avoiding the sun anytime your shadow is shorter than you are. According to NCI, this shadow method—based on the principle that the closer the sun comes to being directly overhead, the stronger its ultraviolet rays—works for any location and at any time of year.

✔ Check for photosensitivity. If you are taking any drugs, ask your doctor or pharmacist to see if the medication could make you more sensitive to sun damage. Be especially cautious about sun exposure if you have been using a synthetic preparation derived from vitamin A (Retin A) as an acne or anti-wrinkle treatment; it can increase your susceptibility.

The most common types of melanoma are:

▷ Superficial spreading melanoma, which accounts for about 70 percent of cases, grows outward for a long time (one to seven years) before burrowing deeper into the skin.
▷ Nodular melanoma, which affects about 15 percent of cases, grows downward with no obvious changes in the skin. This type often remains undetected until it reaches an advanced stage.

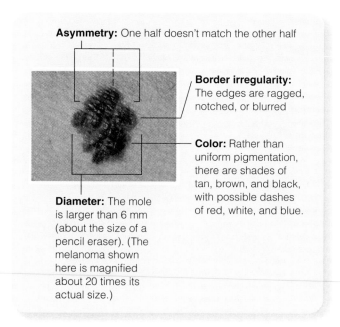

Asymmetry: One half doesn't match the other half

Border irregularity: The edges are ragged, notched, or blurred

Color: Rather than uniform pigmentation, there are shades of tan, brown, and black, with possible dashes of red, white, and blue.

Diameter: The mole is larger than 6 mm (about the size of a pencil eraser). (The melanoma shown here is magnified about 20 times its actual size.)

▲ **Figure 13-5** ABCD: The warning signs of melanoma. An estimated 95 percent of cases of melanoma arise from an existing mole. A normal mole is usually round or oval, less than 6 millimeters (about ¼ inch) in diameter and evenly colored (black, brown, or tan). Seek prompt evaluation of any moles that change in ways shown in the photo.

Source: American Academy of Dermatology. All rights reserved.

▷ Acral lentiginous melanoma, which accounts for 5 to 10 percent of melanomas, most commonly affects African Americans. It usually appears on the soles of the feet, the palms of the hands, or beneath the fingernails.
▷ Lentigo maligna melanoma, which represents about 5 percent of cases, affects mostly elderly people.

Treatment

If caught early, melanoma is highly curable, usually with surgery alone. Once it has spread, chemotherapy with a single drug or a combination can temporarily shrink tumors in some people. However, the five-year survival rate for metastatic melanoma is less than 10 percent.

Promising new therapies include immunotherapy (also called biological therapy), which uses agents such as interferon-alpha and interleukin-2 (IL-2) to marshal the body's own immune system to help attack cancer cells. Some patients in clinical trials have received a vaccine made up of entire melanoma cells or parts of cells to stimulate an immune response against tumors.

Breast Cancer

Every 3 minutes a woman in the United States learns that she has breast cancer. Every 12 minutes a woman dies of

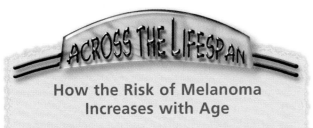

How the Risk of Melanoma Increases with Age

The incidence of melanoma is increasing faster than any other cancer in the United States, with more than 41,000 new cases diagnosed each year. While dermatology textbooks often report that crude rates of melanoma increase into middle age and then level off, cumulative damage to the immune system from exposure to ultraviolet light is expected to increase melanoma rates throughout the lifespan among aging baby boomers, as indicated by the adjusted rates depicted in Figure 13-6. Individuals who've had melanoma may be at high risk for developing this cancer again.

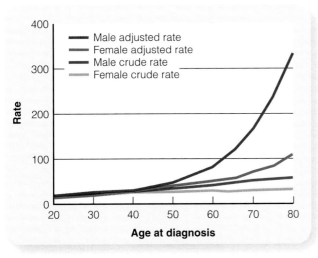

▲ **Figure 13-6** How the risk of melanoma increases with age.

breast cancer. But a new word has entered medical discussions about breast cancer: hope. "Death and incidence rates for breast cancer are heading down," says Harmon Eyre, M.D., chief medical officer of the American Cancer Society. "In 30 years in the field, this is the most optimistic time I have seen."[20]

Despite these encouraging trends, breast cancer remains the illness women worry about most—even though they are ten times more likely to die of heart disease. Many women misjudge their own likelihood of developing breast cancer, either overestimating or underestimating their susceptibility. In a recent national poll, one in every ten surveyed considered herself at no risk at all.

This is never the case. "Every woman is at risk for breast cancer simply because she's female," says Leslie Ford, M.D., associate director for early detection at NCI.[21]

However, not all women's risks are equal. NCI has developed a computerized Breast Cancer Risk Assessment Tool, based on data from more than 280,000 women, that allows a woman to sit down with her doctor and discuss her own odds of developing breast cancer within the next five years and over her entire lifetime. These calculations include a variety of risk factors, including the following:

▸ **Age.** As shown in Figure 13-7, at 25, a woman's chance of developing breast cancer is 1 in 19,608; at 45, 1 in 93; at 65, 1 in 17; at 85, 1 in 9. By age 90 to 95, 1 in 8 women will have developed breast cancer. The mean age at which women are diagnosed is 63.

▸ **Family history.** The overwhelming majority of breast cancers—90 to 95 percent—are not due to strong genetic factors. However, having a first-degree relative—mother, sister or daughter—with breast cancer does increase risk, and if the relative developed breast cancer before menopause, the cancer is more likely to be hereditary. Genetic testing, controversial but sometimes recommended for women in cancer-prone families, can identify these defects. However, it's not yet clear how many women with a defective gene actually will develop breast cancer; estimates range from 50 to 80 percent — or higher in families with many affected members.[22]

▸ **Age at menarche.** Women who had their first period before age 12 are at greater risk than women who began menstruating later. The reason is that the more menstrual cycles a woman has, the longer her exposure to estrogen, a hormone known to increase breast cancer danger. For similar reasons, childless women, who menstruate continuously for several decades, are also at greater risk.

▸ **Age at birth of first child.** An early pregnancy—in a woman's teens or twenties—changes the actual maturation of breast cells and decreases risk. But if a woman has her first child in her forties, precancerous cells may actually flourish with the high hormone levels of the pregnancy.

▸ **Breast biopsies.** Even if laboratory analysis finds no precancerous abnormalities, women who require such tests are more likely to develop breast cancer.

By age 25	1 in 19,608	By age 60	1 in 24
By age 30	1 in 2,525	By age 65	1 in 17
By age 35	1 in 622	By age 70	1 in 14
By age 40	1 in 217	By age 75	1 in 11
By age 45	1 in 93	By age 80	1 in 10
By age 50	1 in 50	By age 85	1 in 9
By age 55	1 in 33	Ever	1 in 8

▲ **Figure 13-7** A woman's risk of developing breast cancer.

Source: NCI Surveillance Program.

Fibrocystic breast disease, a term often used for "lumpy" breasts, is not a risk factor.

▶ **Race.** Breast cancer rates are lower in Hispanic and Asian populations than in whites, but higher in African-American women up to age 50. In post-menopausal African-American women, rates are lower. Nonetheless, African-American women are still more likely to die of breast cancer than whites. Scientists don't know if that's because they don't have equal access to care, if they don't get optimal care, or if the disease itself is more aggressive in black women.

▶ **Occupation.** Based on two decades of following more than a million women, Swedish researchers have developed a list of jobs linked with a high risk of breast cancer. These include pharmacists, certain types of teachers, schoolmasters, systems analysts and program-mers, telephone operators, telegraph and radio operators, metal platers and coaters, and beauticians.

▶ **Estrogen.** The role of estrogen replacement as a cancer risk factor remains controversial. Some studies have documented an increase in certain types of breast cancer in women who have used hormone replacement therapy (HRT) for more than five years. Some experts believe that the failure of well-designed epidemiological studies conducted over the last 25 years to confirm a risk indicates that the dangers, if they exist, are not great.

Detection

To detect lumps or changes that could signal breast cancer, all women should perform monthly breast self-exams seven to ten days after their periods (see Figure 13-8) and

Looking
Stand in front of a mirror with your upper body unclothed. Look for changes in the shape and size of the breast, and for dimpling of the skin or "pulling in" of the nipples. Any changes in the breast may be made more noticeable by a change in position of the body or arms. Look for any of the above signs or for changes in shape from one breast to the other.

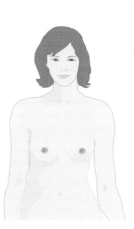
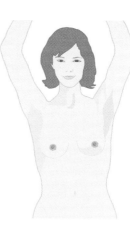
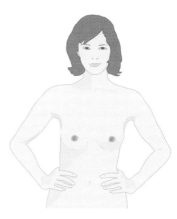

1. Stand with your arms down.

2. Raise your arms overhead.

3. Place your hands on your hips and tighten your chest and arm muscles by pressing firmly.

Feeling

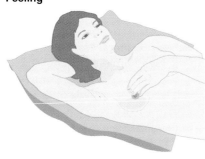
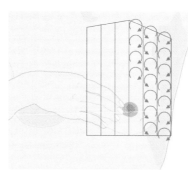
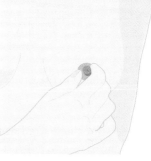

1. Lie flat on your back. Place a pillow or towel under one shoulder, and raise that arm over your head. With the opposite hand, you'll feel with the pads, not the fingertips, of the three middle fingers, for lumps or any change in the texture of the breast or skin.

2. The area you'll examine is from your collarbone to your bra line and from your breastbone to the center of your armpit. Imagine the area divided into vertical strips. Using small circular motions (the size of a dime), move your fingers up and down the strips. Apply light, medium, and deep pressure to examine each spot. Repeat this same process for your other breast.

3. Gently squeeze the nipple of each breast between your thumb and index finger. Any discharge, clear or bloody, should be reported to your doctor immediately.

▲ **Figure 13-8** Breast self-exam.
The best time to examine your breasts is after your menstrual period every month.

have a professional breast exam yearly if over 40 and every three years if between ages 20 and 40.

The best tool for early detection is the diagnostic X-ray exam called **mammography.** Overall, screening mammograms could reduce breast cancer deaths by 25 percent. Mammograms can detect a tumor two to three years before it can be detected by manual exam (see Figure 13-9). According to a recent report, annual mammography for women in their forties is more cost-effective than Pap smear tests for cervical cancer and installation of airbags and seat belts in vehicles. The ACS, AMA, and the National Cancer Society recommend that all women begin routine mammographic screening by age 40, although controversy continues over the effectiveness of screening mammograms in saving women's lives.[23] However, screening has been shown to lead to more aggressive treatment, increasing the number of mastectomies and lumpectomies by about 30 percent. About three percent of screening mam-

mograms yield suspicious results that require a biopsy; less than one-fifth of these cases turn out to be cancer.

 There are racial differences in mammography. Hispanic women undergo these potentially live-saving tests less often than white and African-American women and appear less likely than other women to seek follow-up memmograms in the recommended time frame.[24]

Hormone replacement therapy can increase breast density, decreasing the sensitivity of mammography.[25] Other new diagnostic methods, including digital ultrasound (computerized enhancement of images created with high-frequency sound waves), magnetic resonance imaging, and minimally invasive biopsy technique, are improving the odds of early detection.

Treatments

Breast cancer can be treated with surgery, radiation, and drugs (chemotherapy and hormonal therapy). Doctors may use one of these options or a combination, depending on the type and location of the cancer and whether the disease has spread.

Most women undergo some type of surgery. **Lumpectomy** or breast-conserving surgery removes only the cancerous tissue and a surrounding margin of normal tissue. A modified radical **mastectomy** includes the entire breast and some of the underarm lymph nodes. Radical mastectomy, in which the breast, lymph nodes, and chest wall muscles under the breast are removed, is rarely performed today because modified radical mastectomy has proven just as effective. Removing underarm lymph nodes is important to determine if the cancer has spread, but a new method, sentinel node biopsy, allows physicians to pinpoint the first lymph node into which a tumor drains (the sentinel node), and remove only the nodes most likely to contain cancer cells.

Radiation therapy is treatment with high-energy rays or particles given to destroy cancer. In almost all cases, lumpectomy is followed by six to seven weeks of radiation. Chemotherapy is used to reach cancer cells that may have spread beyond the breast—in many cases even if no cancer is detected in the lymph nodes after surgery.

The use of the drugs paclitaxe (Taxol) or docetaxel (Taxotere), which inhibit cell division, in addition to standard chemotherapy, can significantly lower the risk of recurrence.[26] A new "biotherapy"—a monoclonal antibody that zeros in on cancer cells like a miniature guided missile—also has shown promise against some aggressive breast tumors. The drug Herceptin targets a defective growth-promoting gene known as HER-2/neu, found in about 30 percent of women with breast cancer. The combination of Herceptin and standard chemotherapy has significantly improved survival rates in women with this gene.

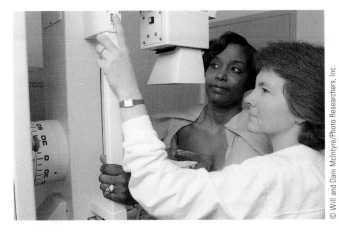

Cancer calcifications of this size and smaller can be seen on mammograms.

Average-size lump found by mammogram.

Average-size lump found by women practicing frequent breast self-exam.

Smallest-size cancer that can be felt by physician's palpation exam.

Average-size lump found by women practicing occasional breast self-exam.

▲ **Figure 13-9** Cancer sizes found by breast-cancer detection methods.
Mammography is able to detect a lump much smaller than a woman can find with regular breast self-exams.

Cervical Cancer

An estimated 12,900 cases of invasive cervical cancer are diagnosed in the United States every year, with about 4,400 annual deaths from this disease. The highest incidence rate occurs among Vietnamese women; Alaska Native, Korean, and Hispanic women also have higher rates than the national average. The mortality rate for African-American women is more than twice that of whites, largely because of a high number of deaths among older black women.

The primary risk factor for cervical cancer is infection with certain types of the human papillomavirus (HPV), discussed in Chapter 11. However, not every HPV infection becomes cervical cancer, and while HPV infection is very common, cervical cancer is not.

Other risk factors for cervical cancer include early age of first intercourse, multiple sex partners, genital herpes, and significant exposure to passive smoking. The standard screening test for cervical cancer is the Pap smear (described in Chapter 10). Each year this test detects about 1.2 million cases of abnormal cell growth. Since Pap tests were introduced, the death rate from cervical cancer has decreased by 70 percent. However, they can fail to detect cancerous cells in as many as 20 to 40 percent of the women tested. An estimated 5 to 10 percent of Pap smears require some follow-up.

Warning signs for cervical cancer include irregular bleeding or unusual vaginal discharge. In precancerous stages, cervical cells can be destroyed by laser surgery or freezing in a doctor's office.

The National Cancer Institute recommends a combination of chemotherapy and radiation rather than the standard use of radiation alone for invasive tumors. For women whose cervical cancer is detected early, cryotherapy (use of extreme cold), electrocoagulation (intense heat), or surgery are standard treatments.

Ovarian Cancer

Ovarian cancer is the leading cause of death from gynecological cancers, with 23,400 new cases diagnosed and 13,900 deaths each year. Risk factors include a family history of ovarian cancer; personal history of breast cancer; obesity; infertility (because the abnormality that interferes with conception may also play a role in cancer development); and low levels of transferase, an enzyme involved in the metabolism of dairy foods. Often women develop no obvious symptoms until the advanced stages, although they may experience painless swelling of the abdomen; irregular bleeding; lower abdominal pain; digestive and urinary abnormalities; fatigue; backache; bloating; and weight gain.

The lifetime risk of ovarian cancer in a woman with no affected relatives is 1 in 70. The risk for a woman with one first-degree relative with ovarian cancer is 1 in 20, and the risk increases with additional affected relatives. For women who may have a hereditary ovarian cancer syndrome and have mutations in BRCA-1 or BRCA-2, the lifetime risk may be as high as 1 in 2. Routine screening is not recommended for women who are not at known risk. For those at increased risk, an NIH consensus panel has recommended annual pelvic and rectal exams, and ultrasound imaging of the pelvic region and a blood test for a substance called CA125 every six months. In cases of very high risk, some oncologists (cancer specialists) recommend prophylactic removal of the ovaries when childbearing is completed or by no later than age 35. Treatment involves surgery, radiation therapy, and chemotherapy. The five-year survival rate is 50 percent.

Colon and Rectal Cancer

Colon and rectal or colorectal, cancer accounts for 10 percent of cancer deaths. Most cases occur after age 50. Both age and gender influence the risk of colon cancer. Older individuals and men are more likely to develop polyps (nonmalignant growths that may turn cancerous at some point) and tumors in the colon than young people and women. Men are 52 percent more likely to have polyps and 43 percent more likely to have cancer of the colon than women. When women do develop tumors, they are more likely to occur in the right side of the colon and are more responsive to chemotherapy.[27]

Risk factors include a personal or family history of colon and rectal cancer, polyps (growths) in the colon or rectum, and ulcerative colitis. Early signs of colorectal cancer are bleeding from the rectum, blood in the stool, or a change in bowel habits.

Sixty percent of eligible people in the United States have never been screened for colorectal cancer.[28] The simplest test for this common cancer—the Fecal Occult Blood Test—detects blood in a person's stool. According to the Congressional Office of Technology Assessment, such tests, which cost only about $4, could prevent 23,000 cancers a year among those aged 65 or older. The other standard screening tests for colon cancer are a digital rectal exam, which should be performed annually after age 40, a stool blood slide test that detects blood in feces (recommended every year after age 50), proctosigmoidoscopy, which involves inserting a fiber-optic tube for visual inspection of the colon and rectum (recommended every three to five years after age 50) and colonoscopy, a similar test that uses a longer tube to visualize the entire colon. In federal research, colonoscopy has proved far superior to other colon cancer tests, which missed one-quarter of the tumors and precancerous growths detected by colonoscopy.

Treatment may involve surgery, radiation therapy, or chemotherapy. Regular exercise can lower the risk of colon and rectal cancer in both men and women. Hormone replacement after menopause may significantly reduce women's risk of colon cancer.

Prostate Cancer

Prostate cancer is the most frequently diagnosed nonskin cancer among American men, with an estimated 179,000 new cases each year. A man's lifetime risk of prostate cancer is one in six.[29] African-American men have the highest rate of prostate cancer in the world; their death rate from this cancer is twice that of white men.

The risk of prostate cancer increases with age, family history, exposure to the heavy metal cadmium, high number of sexual partners, and history of frequent sexually transmitted diseases. An inherited predisposition may account for 5 to 10 percent of cases.

Several studies exploring a link between vasectomy and prostate cancer have produced conflicting results. In a recent investigation, men over age 55 who had had a vasectomy were at no greater risk for prostate cancer than men who had not had one. Men under age 55 who had prostate cancer were nearly twice as likely to have had a vasectomy as men under 55 who did not have cancer. However, researchers speculate that this finding may have been a statistical fluke, since it seems unlikely that vasectomy, a surgical procedure with permanent effects, would increase the risk only in younger men.

The development of a simple screening test that measures levels of a protein called prostate-specific antigen (PSA) in the blood has revolutionized the diagnosis of prostate cancer. Although PSA testing has proven more accurate than previous methods in detecting prostate cancers at early stages, it has created an ethical dilemma for physicians. Because PSA also can be elevated in men with a benign condition called prostatic hyperplasia, the test can indicate cancer where none exists.

In addition, there seem to be different forms of the cancer—some aggressive and deadly, some "low grade" and slow moving. Among men older than age 70, life expectancy without treatment is nearly identical to survival following definitive treatments. Many older men with low-grade prostate cancer may expect a normal lifespan without undergoing potentially debilitating surgery or radiation.

Men whose brothers or fathers had the disease and African Americans should begin getting tested at age 40. All men over age 50 should also undergo an annual rectal examination, in which a doctor inserts a gloved finger into the rectum and feels the prostate for abnormal growths that may indicate cancer.

Early warning signs of prostate cancer are frequent or difficult urination, blood in the urine, painful ejaculation, or constant lower-back pain. Treatments include surgical removal of the prostate, conventional radiation, implanting "seeds" of radioactive iodine in the prostate, and hormone therapy to suppress testosterone. Recent studies have shown that, in most men, prostate cancer does not progress after surgery. Another treatment, cryosurgery, has been used for men with prostate cancer who are not helped by radiation therapy. Its long-term effects are unclear. Short-term postoperative complications include incontinence, impotence, and obstructive urinary symptoms.

Testicular Cancer

In the last 20 years the incidence of testicular cancer has risen 51 percent in the United States—from 3.61 to 5.44 per 100,000. It is not clear why testicular cancer is on the rise, although researchers speculate that changing environmental or socioeconomic risk factors could have a role. Testicular cancer occurs mostly among young men between the ages of 18 and 35, who are not normally at risk of cancer. At highest risk are men with an undescended testicle (a condition that is almost always corrected in childhood to prevent this danger). To detect possibly cancerous growths, men should perform monthly testicular self-exams, as shown in Figure 13-10.

 Although college-age men are among those at highest risk of testicular cancer, three in four do not know how to perform a testicular self-examination. Only 8 to 14 percent examine their testicles regularly.[30]

Often the first sign of this cancer is a slight enlargement of one testicle. There also may be a change in the way it feels when touched. Sometimes men with testicular cancer report a dull ache in the lower abdomen or groin, along with a sense of heaviness or sluggishness. Lumps on the testicles also may indicate cancer.

A man who notices any abnormality should consult a physician. If a lump is indeed present, a surgical biopsy is

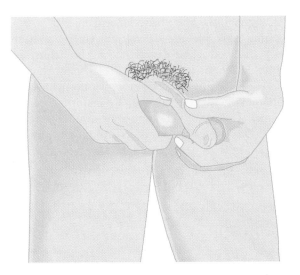

▲ **Figure 13-10** Testicular self-exam.
The best time to examine your testicles is after a hot bath or shower, when the scrotum is most relaxed. Place your index and middle fingers under each testicle and the thumb on top, and roll the testicle between the thumb and fingers. If you feel a small, hard, usually painless lump or swelling, or anything unusual, consult a urologist.

necessary to find out if it is cancerous. If the biopsy is positive, a series of tests generally is needed to determine whether the disease has spread. Treatment for testicular cancer generally involves surgical removal of the diseased testis, sometimes along with radiation therapy, chemotherapy, and the removal of nearby lymph nodes. The remaining testicle is capable of maintaining a man's sexual potency and fertility. Only in rare cases is removal of both testicles necessary. Testosterone injections following such surgery can maintain potency. The chance for a cure is very high if testicular cancer is spotted early.

Leukemia

Risk factors for this cancer of the blood include Down syndrome and other inherited abnormalities and excessive exposure to radiation or certain chemicals, such as benzene. Leukemia can be difficult to detect early because its symptoms are often similar to those of less serious conditions, such as influenza. Diagnosis is based on blood tests and a bone-marrow biopsy. Treatment may involve chemotherapy, drugs, blood transfusions, and bone-marrow transplants.

Lung Cancer

Cigarettes cause most cases of lung cancer, which is the leading cause of cancer deaths in women and in men. Risk factors include cigarette smoking; exposure to certain industrial substances, particularly asbestos; radiation or radon exposure; and environmental tobacco smoke. A smoker's risk of developing lung cancer drops almost to that of a nonsmoker within ten years after his or her last cigarette, although the lungs may still be damaged.

Warning signs include a persistent cough, sputum streaked with blood, chest pain, recurring bronchitis, or pneumonia. Diagnosis is based on a chest X ray, sputum cytology (cell) testing, and fiber-optic bronchoscopy (direct examination of the lungs by means of a specially lighted tube). The use of CT scans, which can detect tiny tumors, can lead to earlier diagnosis and might improve survival rates. Treatment generally involves surgery, chemotherapy, and/or radiation. The five-year survival rate for all stages combined is just 14 percent.

Oral Cancer

Heavy smoking of cigarettes, cigars, or pipes; excessive drinking; and the use of chewing tobacco increase the risk of oral cancer. Those who drink as well as smoke are particularly vulnerable. More young Americans are being diagnosed with oral and tongue cancer. Although the reasons remain unknown, suspected causes include smokeless tobacco and various forms of drug abuse.[31]

Early signs include a mouth sore that bleeds easily and doesn't heal; a lump or thickening; a reddish or whitish patch; and difficulty chewing, swallowing, or moving the tongue or jaws. Regular exams by your dentist or primary care physician can detect oral cancers. Surgery and radiation are the standard treatments.

New Hope Against Cancer

A variety of treatments, described below, have had a dramatic effect on improving the prognosis and decreasing mortality rates for most major cancers.[32] However, cancer therapy remains a challenging experience for patients and their families, and many turn to unproven alternative therapies. (See Savvy Consumer: "Alternative Cancer Treatments.") Conventional cancer therapies now include:

▸ *Surgery* to remove a tumor and surrounding cells. The oldest and most widely used approach, surgery is most effective for small, localized cancers.
▸ *Radiation therapy,* which exposes the involved area of the body to powerful radiation, which destroys cancer cells. Radiation therapy is sometimes used as an adjuvant, or supplementary, treatment along with surgery or chemotherapy.
▸ *Chemotherapy,* which uses powerful drugs or hormones, taken orally or through injection, to interfere with the reproduction of fast-multiplying cancer cells.
▸ *Targeted Therapies.* New drugs that target specific molecular abnormalities in cancer cells hold promise as extremely potent weapons against various cancers. Some researchers have described these medications as having the potential to change the way doctors treat cancer in much the same way the discovery of antibiotics changed the way doctors treated infections.[33] Some of these agents block signals that instruct a cancer cell to grow out of control. Others drive cancer cells to self-destruct or keep tumors from building new blood vessels to supply themselves with food and oxygen.

One compound that blocks an enzyme known as tyrosine kinase, the pill marketed as Gleevec, has produced dramatic results in patients with certain types of leukemia and a rare form of stomach cancer.[34] It is still not known whether Gleevec can actually extend life.[35] Other promising new cancer agents include Herceptin, which checks the growth of certain types of breast cancers, and Rituxan, a monoclonal antibody (a combination of a cancer cell and an antibody-forming cell) that targets proteins on cancer cells and is used for non-Hodgkin's lymphoma.

Bone-marrow transplantation involves extremely high doses of radiation or, increasingly, chemotherapy to kill cancer cells; however, the marrow in the patient's body is also destroyed. The patient then receives healthy bone-

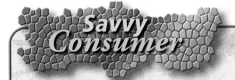

Alternative Cancer Treatments

About one-third of cancer patients use alternative medicine, such as meditation, reflexology, herbal medicine, food supplements, or homeopathy. None of these can cure cancer, but some may help ease patient suffering when used to complement mainstream treatments. Nonetheless, alternative therapies that are overused or used in lieu of mainstream treatments can be dangerous to a patient's health. Keep these points in mind when evaluating unconventional treatments for cancer:

- Special diets, especially those rich in high-antioxidant foods, may help prevent cancer. No diet can cure cancer.

- Vitamins, even in very high doses, cannot cure cancer. Excessive amounts of vitamins and minerals can be harmful and may even speed tumor growth.

- Over-the-counter herbal remedies for cancer can be contaminated or diluted with useless leaves.

- Detoxification regimens, such as high colonic irrigation to remove toxins thought to cause cancer, can be dangerous and have resulted in infection and death.

- Among the alternative therapies that can decrease pain and improve the quality of a cancer patient's life are relaxation techniques, massage, and aromatherapy.

- Patients should never put their trust in an alternative practitioner who encourages them to avoid or stop conventional cancer therapy.

- Many websites offering cancer information, particularly about unproven or alternative therapies, are unreliable. Always check that the website creators are clearly identified, that their credentials are reputable, and that the posting date is recent.

---

marrow cells, either his or her own (which may have undergone treatment in a laboratory) or a carefully matched donor's. *Autologous* transplants (those using the person's own blood) have produced long-term survival rates of more than 50 percent for certain leukemias and lymphomas (cancer of the immune system). Most patients with leukemia and other life-threatening cancers who survive the initial recovery period following bone marrow transplants have survival rates that approach that of the general population.

Cancer treatments affect normal, healthy cells as well as cancerous ones. Most vulnerable to radiation and chemotherapy are the fastest-growing body cells: hair cells, cells of the gastrointestinal tract, cells in the reproductive organs, and cells of the blood-producing tissue, the bone marrow.

Promising advances in cancer treatment that may save lives in the future include **gene therapy**, the insertion of genes into a patient, as a possible cancer treatment, and the development of cancer vaccines.[36] Immunotherapy, also called biological therapy, uses substances such as interferons (proteins produced by cells to resist viruses) and interleukins (proteins released by certain white blood cells to support the growth of others) to attack cancer cells.

Using the Mind to Help the Body

The powers of the mind also can be a powerful resource for cancer patients. In fact, knowledge itself can be powerful. Cancer patients who participate in educational programs that explain their disease and treatment have significantly higher survival rates. Support groups also affect both the quality and quantity of life. Patients with melanoma who attended support groups did much better both on psychological tests and on measures of tumor-fighting immune cells. Melanoma patients with strong religious and spiritual beliefs also were able to cope with their illness better and to view it in a positive, meaningful way.

Cancer Survivorship

Cancer survivors make up one of the fastest growing groups in the American population. Many have had no evidence of cancer for years; others are in remission, a state in which the spread of cancerous cells is presumed to be temporarily stopped. But for millions of men, women, and children who "win" their battle against cancer, survival, even when they live past the milestone five-year mark, does not mark the end of their cancer experience.

Many cancer survivors encounter difficulties that persist for years after initial diagnosis and treatment. These include physical problems, such as pain and fatigue, that can stem from the cancer itself or from cancer treatments. Sexual problems are a common consequence, affecting as many as 50 percent of women surviving breast and gynecologic cancers and as many as 70 percent of men surviving prostate cancer. Coping with cancer also causes psychological and emotional difficulties that can lead to depression, posttraumatic stress disorder, and profound fear of recurrence. Another source of anxiety is the cost of medical treatments, which, along with the loss of wages or a job, can be financially devastating.

Cancer survivors also are at risk of another bout with cancer. Of the 1.3 million new cancer cases diagnosed each year, almost 100,000 are second cancers. Patients surviving one cancer have almost twice the risk of developing a second cancer as the general population has of developing an initial cancer. Children under age 15 who have survived cancer have eight times the risk.[37]

Diabetes Mellitus

About 100 million people around the world—including nearly 16 million people in the United States—have **diabetes mellitus,** a disease in which the body doesn't produce or respond properly to insulin, a hormone essential for daily life.[38] In those who have diabetes, the pancreas, which produces insulin (the hormone that regulates carbohydrate and fat metabolism) doesn't function as it should. When the pancreas either stops producing insulin or doesn't produce sufficient insulin to meet the body's needs, almost every body system can be damaged.

Understanding Diabetes

Glucose is the primary form of sugar that the body cells use for energy. When a healthy person eats a meal, the level of glucose in the blood rises, triggering the production and release of insulin by special cell clusters in the pancreas called the islets of Langerhans. Insulin enhances the movement of glucose into various body cells, bringing down the level of glucose in the blood. In those who have diabetes, however, insulin secretion is either nonexistent (referred to as type 1 or *insulin-dependent diabetes*) or deficient (referred to as type 2 or *non–insulin-dependent diabetes*). Without sufficient insulin, the glucose in the blood is unable to enter most body cells, so the cells' energy needs aren't met. The levels of glucose in the blood rise higher and higher after each meal. This unused glucose eventually passes through the kidneys, which are unable to process the excessive glucose, and out of the body in urine.

Deprived of the fuel it needs, the body begins to break down stored fat as a source of energy. This process produces weak acids, called ketones. A buildup of ketones leads to ketoacidosis, an upheaval in the body's chemical balance that brings on nausea, vomiting, abdominal pain, lethargy, and drowsiness. Severe ketoacidosis can lead to coma and eventual death.

???? Who Is at Risk for Diabetes?

One in three Americans with diabetes is not aware of having an illness that increases the risk of blindness, kidney failure, cardiovascular disease, and premature death.[39] The incidence of this potential killer, which jumped about a third in the last decade, is growing so fast that Dr. Allen Spiegel, director of the National Institute of Diabetes and Digestive and Kidney Diseases (NIDDK), describes it as "a definite epidemic."[40] There has been a particularly dramatic rise in type 2 diabetes in children and adolescents, especially among minority populations.[41]

"The fact that kids just past puberty are getting type 2 diabetes blows us out of the water compared to what we were taught in medical school, which was that type 2 diabetes was a disease of aging," says Dr. Spiegel. Uncontrolled glucose levels slowly damage blood vessels throughout the body, thus individuals who become diabetic early in life may face devastating complications even before they reach middle age.

"Diabetes is already the number one cause of blindness, nontraumatic amputations, and kidney failure and increases by two or three times the risk of heart attack or stroke," says Dr. Robert Sherwin of Yale University, President of the American Diabetes Association, who estimates that the disease may affect 22 million Americans within the next two decades.[42]

Lifestyle factors, especially a lack of physical activity, greatly increase the risk for type 2 diabetes. Television watching, more so than other sedentary activities such as sewing, reading, writing, and driving, is strongly associated with weight and obesity, a risk factor for diabetes in both children and adults. In a ten-year study of 1,058 individu-

STRATEGIES FOR PREVENTION

Lowering the Risk of Diabetes

✔ Eat a diet rich in complex carbohydrates (bread and other starches) and high-fiber foods, and low in sodium and fat.

✔ Eat fruits and vegetables that are rich in antioxidants, substances that prevent oxygen damage to cells.

✔ Avoid alcohol.

✔ Keep your weight down. Weight loss for those who are overweight can sometimes decrease or eliminate the need for insulin or oral drugs. For individuals at high risk of developing type 2 diabetes, losing just half the pounds needed to reach their ideal weight can prevent the onset of the disease.

✔ Exercise regularly. Regular, vigorous aerobic activity reduces the risk of type 2 diabetes in men and women.

als with type 2 diabetes, watching television for 2 to 10 hours a week increased the risk of diabetes 66 percent; 21 to 40 hours per week more than doubled the risk; more than 40 hours a week nearly tripled the risk.[43]

To identify individuals with this disease as early as possible, the American Diabetes Association now recommends screening every three years for all men and women beginning at age 45. Those at highest risk include relatives of diabetics (whose risk is two and a half times that of others); obese persons (85 percent of diabetics are or were obese); older persons (four out of five diabetics are over age 45); and mothers of large babies, because this is an indication of maternal prediabetes. A child of two parents with type 2 diabetes faces an 80 percent likelihood of also becoming diabetic.

The early signs of diabetes are frequent urination, excessive thirst, a craving for sweets and starches, and weakness. Diagnosis is based on tests of the sugar level in the blood. Researchers are working to develop a test that would help identify telltale antibodies in the blood; this could indicate that pancreas cells are being destroyed years before the first signs of diabetes.

The Dangers of Diabetes

Before the development of insulin injections, diabetes was a fatal illness. Today diabetics can have normal life spans. However, both types of diabetes can lead to devastating complications, including increased risk of heart attack or stroke, kidney failure, blindness, and loss of circulation to the extremities. Although few people realize it, diabetes claims more than 100,000 women's lives a year—more than the number who succumb to breast cancer.

Diabetic women who become pregnant face higher risks of miscarriage and serious birth defects; however, precise control of blood sugar levels before conception and in early pregnancy can lower the likelihood of these problems. The development of diabetes during pregnancy—called gestational diabetes—may pose potentially serious health threats to mother and child years later. Women who develop gestational diabetes are more than three times as likely to develop type 2 diabetes if they have a second pregnancy; their infants may be at increased risk of cardiovascular disease later in life.

Diabetes and Ethnic Minorities

Several minority groups, especially African Americans, Native Americans, and Latinos, are at high risk of developing diabetes. One in every ten African Americans and Latinos has this disease. The members of some Native American tribes are 300 percent more likely to develop diabetes than the general population. For many, obesity and unhealthy food choices increase the risk. Researchers now believe that the interaction of environmental factors and genes varies among different racial and ethnic groups.

Treatments for Diabetes

There's no cure for diabetes at this time. The best treatment option is to keep blood sugar levels as stable as possible to prevent complications, such as kidney damage. Home glucose monitoring allows diabetics to check their blood sugar levels as many times a day as necessary and to adjust their diet or insulin doses as appropriate.

Those with type 1 diabetes require daily doses of insulin via injections, an insulin infusion pump, or oral medication. Those with type 2 diabetes can control their disease through a well-balanced diet, exercise, and weight management. However, insulin therapy may be needed to keep blood glucose levels near normal or normal, thereby reducing the risk of damage to the eyes, nerves, and kidneys.

Medical advances hold out bright hopes for diabetics. Laser surgery, for instance, is saving eyesight. Bypass operations are helping restore blood flow to the heart and feet. Dialysis machines and kidney and pancreas transplants save many lives. Researchers are exploring various approaches to prevention, including early low-dose insulin therapy, oral insulin to correct immune intolerance, and immunosuppressive drugs. Still on the horizon is the promise of a true cure through transplanting insulin-producing cells from healthy pancreases. In preliminary trials, this procedure has helped patients become insulin-independent.[44]

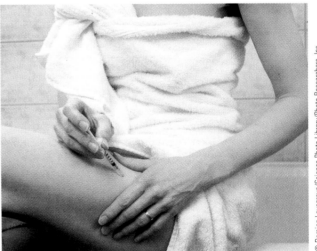

▲ Individuals with type 1 or insulin-dependent diabetes control their disease by injecting themselves with insulin.

Other Major Illnesses

Other noninfectious diseases besides cancer and diabetes have a debilitating effect on many people. But most of the diseases discussed in this section can be controlled, if not cured.

Epilepsy and Seizure Disorders

About 10 percent of all Americans will have at least one seizure at some time. Between 0.5 and 1 percent of all Americans have recurrent seizures. Derived from the Greek word for seizure, **epilepsy** is the term used to refer to a variety of neurological disorders characterized by sudden attacks (seizures) of violent muscle contractions and unconsciousness. Epilepsy is rarely fatal; the primary danger to life is to suffer an attack while driving or swimming.

Seizures can be major, referred to as *grand mal;* minor, referred to as *petit mal;* or psychomotor. In a grand-mal seizure, the person loses consciousness, falls to the ground, and experiences convulsive body movements. Petit-mal seizures are brief, characterized by a loss of consciousness for 10 to 30 seconds, by eye or muscle flutterings, and occasionally by a loss of muscle tone. About 90 percent of all epileptics have grand-mal seizures; 40 percent suffer both petit-mal and grand-mal seizures. The frequency of attacks defines the severity of the epilepsy. Diagnosis is based on a history of recurring attacks and a study of the brain's electrical activity, called an electroencephalogram (EEG).

About half of all cases of epilepsy have no known cause and are therefore classified as *idiopathic.* All others stem from conditions that affect the brain, such as trauma, tumors, congenital malformations, or inflammation of the membranes covering the brain. Idiopathic epilepsy usually begins between the ages of 2 and 14. Seizures before age 2 are usually related to developmental defects, birth injuries, or a metabolic disease affecting the brain. (Fever-induced convulsions are not related to epilepsy.) Seizures after age 14 are generally symptoms of brain disease or injury.

Seizure disorders don't reflect or affect intellectual or psychological soundness; people who suffer from them have normal intelligence. Therapy with anticonvulsant drugs can control seizures in most people, and once seizures are under control, epileptics can live full, normal lives by continuing to take their medications. However, about 10 to 20 percent of the 120,000 people who develop epilepsy every year continue to have seizures despite medical therapy. Early treatment of seizures by paramedics with benzodiazepines can prevent serious neurologic damage.[45]

Technological advances have allowed doctors to identify more accurately where seizures originate in the brain; and surgery, though risky and expensive, is offering new hope to many epileptics.

If you're with a person who suffers a grand-mal seizure, make sure he or she isn't injured during the attack. Don't try to restrain the person or interfere with his or her movements, and don't try to force anything into the person's mouth.

Respiratory Diseases

See Chapter 11 for the major infectious respiratory diseases and Chapter 16 for smoking-induced problems. In addition to the diseases treated below, chronic bronchitis and emphysema can also be causes of disability and death.

???? What Is Asthma?

Asthma is a disease characterized by constriction of the breathing passages. As with allergy, asthma rates have skyrocketed in the last two decades. Since 1980 U.S. mortality rates have doubled, with asthma claiming the lives of 5,000 Americans every year. The problem is especially severe in inner cities, where emergency room visits and asthma mortality rates run as high as eight times the national average.

The Centers for Disease Control and Prevention (CDC) estimates that approximately 17 million people in the United States, or 6.4 percent of the population, say they have asthma. Asthma is more common among blacks and other inner-city residents. The disease disproportionately affects African Americans. A black man in New York City is 11 times more likely to die from asthma than other men in the city.[46]

While asthma is not always linked to allergy, the two are related. Among people with asthma, 90 percent of the children, 70 percent of young adults, and 50 percent of older adults also have allergies. According to epidemiologic research, 23 percent of youngsters diagnosed with allergies by age 1 develop asthma by age 6. Of those diagnosed after age 1, 13 percent eventually become asthmatic. Symptoms include wheezing, coughing, shortness of breath, and chest tightness. If the symptoms are untreated or undertreated, they can worsen and damage the lungs.

The number of people with asthma continues to increase into adulthood. However, as shown by a study that followed college students for 23 years, most report that their symptoms improve or disappear.[47] See Student Snapshot: "Asthma in College—and Beyond.")

The two main approaches to asthma treatment are control of the underlying inflammation by means of anti-inflammatory drugs, such as corticosteroids, cromolyn sodium, and nedocromil, and short-term relief of symptoms with bronchodilators, such as albuterol, which expand the breathing passages. In its most recent official guidelines, the National Heart, Lung, and Blood Institute encouraged more frequent use of inhaled steroids and less reliance on bronchodilators, which have little effect on the underlying inflammation.

Other asthma medications directly target leukotriene, one of the chemicals involved in an inflammatory response. These drugs seem useful in cases of mild to moderate asthma, but specialists are still uncertain of exactly how they'll fit into long-term asthma management.

Chronic Obstructive Lung Disease (COLD)

Chronic obstructive lung disease (COLD), also called chronic obstructive pulmonary disease (COPD), is characterized by progressively more limited flow of air into, and out of, the lungs. COLD consists of two separate but closely related conditions: chronic bronchitis and emphysema. Most COLD patients develop both forms. The major cause is cigarette smoking, although air pollution may also play a role.

In chronic bronchitis, the bronchial passageways are constantly inflamed, and individuals develop a persistent, sputum-producing cough; shortness of breath; and wheezing. They must stop smoking, lose excess weight, exercise, and avoid or reduce contact with air pollutants.

Chronic bronchitis can lead to emphysema, a deterioration of the lungs that may begin in adolescence. Eventually, the alveoli, tiny air sacs in the lungs, tear, reducing the lungs' ability to exhale. This condition can lead to heart failure.

Anemias

The **anemias** are diseases affecting the oxygen-carrying capacity of the blood. Usually there's a reduced number of red blood cells or a reduced amount of hemoglobin, the oxygen-carrying component of red blood cells. Anemia can be caused by nutritional inadequacies; loss of blood, including heavy menstrual bleeding; deficiencies in red-cell production; or genetic disorders. Iron-deficiency anemia is a form of anemia caused by a lack of dietary iron, an essential component of the hemoglobin molecule that carries oxygen. It's the most common form of anemia and often goes undiagnosed in women.

Student Snapshot Asthma in College—and Beyond

In their initial study, researchers evaluated 1,837 freshman at Brown University for medical conditions, including asthma and allergy. Some 23 years later, 1,601 alumni completed a detailed questionnaire about asthma and allergies. The prevalence of asthma continues to increase until age 40 or 42. However, of the alumni with active asthma at follow-up, asthma symptoms had either improved or disappeared in three-fourths. Of the remaining fourth, most said their symptoms were unchanged; only a small number reported worsening of their symptoms.

Number of alumni with a history of asthma	84
Number who had asthma as freshmen	48
Number who had developed asthma after college	36
Number who had active asthma at time of follow-up	44
Number who were symptom free	40

Source: Skolnick, Helen, and Robert Wood. "Natural History of Asthma: A 23-Year Follow-Up of College Students. *Pediatrics,* Vol. 198, No. 2, August 2001, p. 547.

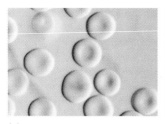 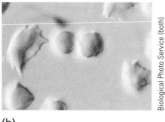

(a)   (b)

Biological Photo Service (both)

▲ Sickle-cell anemia. (a) Normal mature red blood cells are disk-shaped and concave. (b) In sickle-cell anemia, the red blood cells are crescent-shaped and jagged, causing them to pile up and obstruct small blood vessels. Areas of the body are thus deprived of oxygen and nutrients.

▷ *Sickle-cell anemia* is a genetic blood disorder that occurs when the hemoglobin contained in the red blood cells is abnormal. The red blood cells become crescent or sickle-shaped and unable to supply oxygen to body tissues (see photos above). This disease causes crippling, severe pain, and premature death. About 8 to 10 percent of African Americans carry the gene for sickle-cell anemia.

▷ *Pernicious anemia* results from a lack of vitamin B_{12} (cobalamine), which causes a deficiency in the formation of red blood cells. Although B_{12} is usually present in the diet, some people lack a substance needed to absorb it into their blood. Injections of B_{12} can control this condition.

▷ *Aplastic anemia*, most common in young adults and adolescents, interferes with the bone marrow's ability to form blood. Usually it results from ingesting a toxic agent, often a medication; symptoms include multiple internal hemorrhages. Whole-blood transfusions are the primary therapy, but the condition is usually fatal.

Liver Disorders

Cirrhosis is characterized by significant loss of liver cells and the formation of scar tissue that can interfere with circulation in the liver. The major cause of one of the most common forms of cirrhosis, Laennec's cirrhosis, is chronic alcoholism. Each year, about 30,000 Americans die of alcohol-related liver disorders. (See also Chapter 15.)

Early signs of liver damage include an enlarged liver (which your doctor can feel during a physical exam) and tiny, spiderlike blood vessels on the surface of the skin. Blood tests may show abnormal levels of certain enzymes or enlarged red blood cells. Even people with advanced liver disease feel better and live longer once they've stopped drinking alcohol. Cirrhosis symptoms, which occur only in the advanced stages of the disease, include yellow discoloration of the skin and eyes (jaun-

dice), accumulation of fluid in the abdomen, and mental confusion.

Liver transplants are the only hope for those with advanced liver disease. With improvements in surgical techniques and the use of antirejection drugs (including cyclosporin, a combination of cyclosporin and an antifungal medication, and a drug called FK-506), 70 percent or more of liver-transplant recipients—including some in their sixties and seventies—now live for at least a year. Some liver transplant recipients have lived longer than 20 years.

Kidney Diseases

A wide range of diseases can affect the kidneys and their ability to process fluids and waste. Some are acute, temporary problems; others are chronic, progressive illnesses that permanently impair kidney function.

Nephrosis refers to a cluster of symptoms indicating chronic damage to the kidneys, including chronic proteinuria (the loss of more than 1 gram of protein a day in the urine), hypercholesteremia (high levels of fats in the blood), and edema (fluid retention). The kidney damage can be the result of diabetes, heavy metal poisoning, allergic reactions to insect stings, or other disorders.

Kidney stones can form either from calcium salts or from minerals (the causes are unknown). Most stones eventually pass out of the body in urine, which can be extremely painful. They don't usually obstruct the flow of urine or interfere with kidney function. However, infection can develop behind a stone. Larger stones can be surgically removed or painlessly shattered into harmless fragments by high-frequency sound waves.

The various chronic and inflammatory diseases of the kidney can all lead to kidney failure. A mechanical process of clearing waste fluids from the body, called *dialysis*, can do the kidneys' job temporarily. Another alternative is a kidney transplant, either from a living, related donor or from a cadaver whose kidney has been carefully tissue-matched to the recipient to minimize the risk of rejection. On average, a transplanted kidney continues to function for only nine years. Kidneys that came from cadaver donors are especially likely to deteriorate slowly but steadily. The antirejection drugs that transplant recipients must take may themselves cause side effects and impair the functioning of the new kidney over time. High blood pressure and high glucose and cholesterol levels also can be harmful. A lack of organ donors remains a critical obstacle to performing more of these lifesaving operations.

Digestive Diseases

Most disorders of the digestive tract affect only one section: either the esophagus, the stomach and duodenum, the small intestine, the large intestine, the liver, the pancreas, the gallbladder, or the rectum. The most dangerous are Crohn's disease and ulcerative colitis. According to the National Digestive Diseases Advisory Board, almost half of the U.S. population will suffer a digestive problem at some time in their lives.

Ulcers

Open sores, often more than an inch wide, that develop in the lining of the stomach or the duodenum (the first part of the small intestine) are called **ulcers.** They are caused by excessive acidic digestive juices. The major symptom is a burning pain felt throughout the upper abdomen. The pain may come and go, lasting up to three hours. It may begin either right after eating or several hours later.

One in five men and one in ten women get ulcers of the stomach or duodenum, but the number of ulcers is declining. Risk factors include heavy use of cigarettes, alcohol, or caffeine; the ingestion of large amounts of painkillers that contain aspirin or ibuprofen; and advanced age. Bleeding is not common but may be dangerous, even life-threatening. An untreated stomach ulcer can lead to serious weight loss and anemia.

Researchers have identified a bacterium, *Helicobacter pylori* (formerly named *Campylobacter*) that may infect the digestive system and set the stage for ulcers. According to various studies, most ulcer patients carry this organism. One theory is that infection leads to an inflammation of the stomach lining called gastritis, which increases vulnerability to other stressors, such as smoking, alcohol, or anxiety.

H. pylori can be detected in several ways. A blood test can reveal the presence of infection by detecting antibodies against *H. pylori.* However, a blood test can be positive even if someone has long been free of the bacteria. The most definitive test requires endoscopy, a procedure in which a physician examines the lining of the stomach or duodenum by passing a thin flexible tube (an endoscope) down the patient's throat and snips a small bit of tissue for laboratory analysis to detect bacteria. Researchers are experimenting with a simpler diagnostic breath test in which patients drink a special liquid that triggers a response by *H. pylori* bacteria in the stomach. Treatment with antibiotics leads to improvement in most patients.

Conventional therapy for ulcers includes self-help measures, such as avoiding aspirin; eating small, frequent meals; taking antacids; and not smoking or drinking alcohol or caffeine. Drugs such as cimetidine, ranitidine, and sucralfate can reduce the amount of acid produced by the stomach and relieve ulcer symptoms. If a stomach ulcer doesn't heal after six to eight weeks of drug treatment, physicians may recommend surgery to remove the ulcer.

Inflammatory Bowel Disease (IBD)

As many as 2 million Americans—many in the prime of life—suffer from one of the two forms of **inflammatory bowel disease (IBD):** *Crohn's disease,* which causes inflammation anywhere in the digestive tract, and *ulcerative colitis,* which creates severe ulcers in the inner lining of the colon and rectum. Both illnesses can trigger frequent and intense diarrhea, abdominal pain, gas, fever, and rectal bleeding.

The specific causes of IBD remain unknown, but scientists speculate that some irritating substance—perhaps a bacterium, virus, or chemical or environmental agent—somehow leaks through the intestine's thin lining into the bowel's deep inner wall. Inflammation develops, setting into motion a chain of harmful reactions by the body's protective immune system and causing swelling, pain, and damage to the intestinal wall. Ulcers (small perforations or holes) may form, exposing cells and tissues to destructive intestinal bacteria and enzymes. Blood and fluid from body tissues may leak into the intestines, showing up as diarrhea or blood in the stool. Twenty percent of cases involve a genetic or familial predisposition.

Treatment for IBD consists primarily of drugs, including powerful steroids, antibiotics, and medications that fight inflammation. Dietary changes can also help. Crohn's patients who don't improve on medication or who develop life-threatening complications, such as a severe intestinal blockage, may undergo surgery to remove or bypass the diseased part of the intestine and reconnect two healthy segments. However, the disease very often recurs in another part of the intestinal tract. For those with ulcerative colitis, removal of the entire colon brings an end to troubling symptoms—and to the increased risk of colon cancer that these individuals face. Most gastroenterologists advise patients with ulcerative colitis to undergo annual examinations of the colon (colonoscopies) to detect precancerous changes in cells.

Irritable Bowel Syndrome

Irritable bowel syndrome (also called irritable colon or spastic colon) is a common problem caused by intestinal spasms. The muscular contractions that move waste material through the intestines become irregular and uncoordinated, causing frequent feelings of a need to defecate, nausea, cramping, pain, gas, and a sensation that the rectum is never emptied.

Diagnostic tests, including X rays, stool samples, and examination of the colon with a sigmoidoscope, can rule out colon cancer and other problems. Travel, stress, changes in diet, and smoking often worsen these symptoms. Many people respond well to a high-fiber diet; others prefer a bland diet. There's no standard medical treatment for irritable bowel syndrome; some physicians prescribe stool softeners, laxatives, or drugs to reduce intestinal spasms.

Gallstones

An estimated 25 million Americans—about 10 percent of the population—have **gallstones:** clumps of solid material, usually cholesterol, that form in bile stored in the gallbladder. One-third to one-half of all gallstones produce no symptoms. However, some gallstones, carried out of the liver with bile, get stuck in the bile duct and cause intense pain that lasts for several hours. Ultrasound and special X rays called cholecystograms can detect gallstones.

During an attack of gallstone pain, a physician may recommend a painkiller. Some gallstones can be dissolved by long-term drug treatment. Another alternative to traditional gallbladder surgery is laparoscopic surgery, in which gallstones are removed without having to cut through the major abdominal muscles.

Disorders of the Muscles, Joints, and Bones

Because they're constantly being used, muscles, joints, and bones are more susceptible to damage from injury than are most other parts of the body.

Arthritis

More than 22 million people suffer from some form of **arthritis,** an inflammatory disease of the joints that takes over a hundred forms. Rheumatoid arthritis is an autoimmune disease in which the body attacks its own connective tissue; it's fairly common among younger people. Degenerative arthritis, or osteoarthritis, characterized by changes in bone tissue and cartilage, primarily at the joints, seems to be the result of normal wear and tear.

Women are generally affected by arthritis three times more often than are men, until the seventh or eighth decade of life. Race and occupation don't seem to be factors; climate affects symptoms but not causes.

Aggressive treatment of arthritis pays off, but to be successful, early diagnosis before cartilage destruction occurs is critical. The most effective therapies include methotrexate and anti-inflammatory agents, which prevent or delay joint destruction. An educational arthritis self-help course can reduce physician visits by 40 percent and pain perception by about 20 percent. Relaxation training and cognitive-behavioral techniques also have proven highly effective in controlling arthritis pain.

The goal of all treatments for arthritis is to maintain the patient's ability to function. Drugs can relieve pain and reduce inflammation; surgical treatments, including total

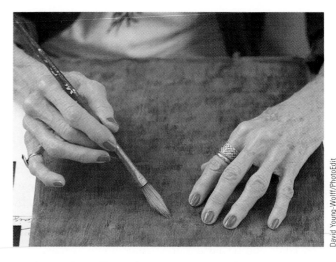

David Young-Wolff/PhotoEdit

▲ Those who suffer arthritis pain may tend to minimize movement in their joints, but moderate activity can help keep muscles functioning that stabilize the joints.

joint replacement, and physical therapy are also used to maintain motion and strength, and to correct deformities.

Hernias

A **hernia** is a bulge of soft tissue that forces its way through or between strained or weakened muscles. Hernias can occur in many parts of the body, but they're most common in the abdominal wall. A surgeon can push the protruding tissue back into place and tighten or sew together the loose muscles.

Backaches

Back woes, which rank second only to headaches among modern miseries, eventually afflict seven of every ten adults. Anyone from a college athlete to a retired grandparent can suffer a back injury, but the risks increase with time as the deeper muscles and tendons surrounding the spine become less resilient. Yet age itself is rarely the only factor in a disabling back attack; almost always tense, injured, or weak muscles are to blame. Other risk factors include extra pounds, particularly if stuffed into a pot belly; lack of exercise; poor posture; and bending from the waist to hoist a heavy load.

Strain from use or abuse accounts for 80 percent of back ailments. Most vulnerable is the lower, or lumbar, part of the spine, which bears the greatest pressure when bending and lifting. Five to 10 percent of back problems involve the discs between the vertebrae. Most common is the protrusion (or herniation) of the soft center of a disc through the casing so that it presses on spinal nerves. Another 10 percent of back problems involve structural defects, which may be the result of injuries, tumors, arthritis, congenital malformations, osteoporosis (the

STRATEGIES FOR PREVENTION

Preventing Back Problems

✔ When standing, shift your weight from one foot to the other. If possible, place one foot on a stool, step, or railing 4 to 6 inches off the ground. Hold in your stomach, tilt your pelvis toward your back, and tuck in your buttocks to provide crucial support for the lower back.

✔ Because sitting places more stress on the lower back than standing, try to get up from your seat at least once an hour to stretch or walk around. Whenever possible, sit in a straight chair with a firm back. Avoid slouching in overstuffed chairs or dangling your legs in midair. When driving, keep the seat forward so that your knees are raised to hip level; your right leg should not be fully extended. A small pillow or towel can help support your lower back.

✔ Sleep on a flat, firm mattress. The best sleep position is on your side, with one or both knees bent at right angles to your torso. The pillow should keep your head in line with your body so that your neck isn't bent forward or to the side.

✔ When lifting, bend at the knees, not from the waist. Get close to the load. Tighten your stomach muscles, but don't hold your breath. Let your leg muscles do the work.

✔ Don't smoke. Smoking may interfere with circulation to the lower back; and a chronic smoker's cough can be so irritating that it provokes a back spasm.

weakening of the bones), or scoliosis (side-to-side curving of the spine). Sometimes a sore back is a symptom of diseases of other organs, such as the kidneys, gallbladder, or stomach. A physical exam and various tests, including electrodiagnostic studies, X rays, CT scans, and MRIs (magnetic resonance imaging), may be necessary to pinpoint the problem.

Bed rest, supplemented by moist heat or other muscle relaxants and anti-inflammatory drugs, eases most backaches. However, the days when doctors advised two weeks of bed rest for a bad back are gone. After two or three days, most back patients are urged to get up, start walking, and resume light activity.

Back specialists tailor treatment programs to an individual's needs. Different forms of physical therapy—including specific exercises, massage, heat, ultrasound, and electrical stimulation—often relieve pain and speed recovery. Some people successfully use chiropractic, acupuncture, hypnosis, biofeedback, or relaxation techniques to cope with back pain. Regardless of treatment, more than 85 percent of back-injury patients get well within two weeks. Fewer than 2 percent eventually require surgery to repair a herniated disc.

Skin Disorders

Your skin is the largest organ of your body. Because of its visibility, none of its problems may seem trivial. Two serious skin diseases are discussed below.

Eczema and Dermatitis

Dermatitis is any inflammation of the skin. *Eczema,* a specific type of dermatitis usually caused by allergies, is a skin inflammation that results from internal processes. Symptoms of eczema include redness, flaking, blistering, and thickening of the skin. Self-help treatments include avoiding irritants, such as dishwater, and using steroid creams containing 0.5 percent hydrocortisone.

Psoriasis

In **psoriasis,** the rate of skin cell production is speeded up. As skin cells pile up faster than they can be shed, they produce scaly, deep pink, raised patches on the skin. Triggers of psoriasis are stress, skin damage, and illness. Self-help measures include sunbathing or using ultraviolet light to clear up the psoriasis. Physicians usually prescribe ointments, creams, or pastes, including some steroid preparations, or ultraviolet treatment.

Special Needs for Different Abilities

About 49 million Americans have physical or mental impairments, including blindness, deafness, disorders of the muscles or nerves, paralysis, loss of limbs, or mental retardation, that substantially limit one or more major life activities. Most are the result of illnesses, such as strokes, arthritis, or heart disease, and affect the ability to walk, speak, or live independently. Some congenital disorders, such as cerebral palsy, cause speech problems, muscular weakness, and mental retardation. Accidents are responsible for other disabilities, including paralysis.

Individuals with special needs and abilities can live full, happy, and productive lives. Famous people who've made major contributions to the world despite disabilities include the composer Ludwig van Beethoven, who wrote some of his most famous music after becoming deaf; the inventor Thomas A. Edison, who was deaf throughout much of his life; and President Franklin D. Roosevelt, who became paralyzed in both legs at the age of 39.

Few such problems can be cured, but a great deal can be done to overcome them. **Rehabilitation medicine,** the specialty dedicated to improving the condition of the disabled, can provide treatments such as surgery for certain types of blindness or deafness, medications to ease the crippling pain of arthritis, and physical therapy, including special exercises to build up endurance and muscle strength. Mechanical devices, such as electric wheelchairs, artificial limbs, and hearing aids, can open up wider worlds to people with disabilities. Occupational therapy teaches skills to help them gain confidence, and vocational training prepares them to find employment.

Individuals with special needs face special challenges in their daily lives. Some are primarily physical, such as difficulty bathing, lifting groceries, opening cans and bottles, or going someplace. They also face many social and economic challenges. Because some people feel uncomfortable about disabilities, they may not treat individuals with special needs with the same acceptance and respect that they show to others. This can lead to discrimination from employers.

The Americans with Disabilities Act protects people with disabilities from discrimination by private employers, requires wheelchair access to public buildings and mass transportation, and orders telephone companies to provide telephone relay services that allow people with impaired speech or hearing to make and receive calls. Many states require insurers to provide coverage for high-risk individuals such as cancer survivors. The names of many of the organizations that help the disabled, such as the National Coalition for Cancer Survivorship and the National Library Service for the Blind and Physically Handicapped, are in "Your Health Almanac" at the back of the book.

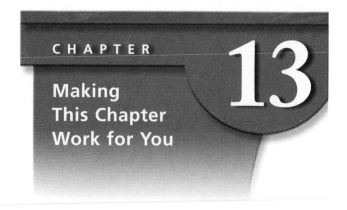

CHAPTER

Making This Chapter Work for You

13

1. Which of the following statements about cancer is true?
    a. The different types of cancers are classified according to the body system they affect.
    b. Cancer occurs when abnormal cells grow and spread uncontrollably until they form an ectoplasm.
    c. Those cancers that have been shown to be triggered by viruses are contagious.
    d. In some sense, all cancers are caused by genetic abnormalities.

2. Signs that a cancer might be inherited include all of the following except
    a. family history
    b. late development of the disease
    c. a diagnosis of retinoblastoma
    d. unusual gender pattern in the incidence of the disease

3. You can protect yourself from certain types of cancer by
    a. eating a diet rich in antioxidants.
    b. avoiding people who have had cancer.
    c. wearing sunscreen with an SPF of less than 15.
    d. using condoms during sexual intercourse.

4. Which of the following statements about skin cancer is true?
    a. Individuals with a large number of moles are at decreased risk for melanoma.
    b. The most serious type of skin cancer is squamous-cell carcinoma.
    c. The safest way to get a tan and avoid skin cancer is to use tanning salons and sunlamps instead of sunbathing in direct sunlight.
    d. Individuals with a history of childhood sunburn are at increased risk for melanoma.

5. A woman's risk of developing breast cancer increases if
    a. she is African American under the age of 50.
    b. she had her first child when in her teens or twenties.
    c. her husband's mother had breast cancer.
    d. she began menstruating when she was 15 or 16.

6. Prostate cancer
    a. occurs mostly among men between the ages of 18 and 35.
    b. is usually more aggressive in men older than 70.
    c. may be treated by implanting radioactive iodine in the prostate.
    d. can be detected through a screening test that measures the levels of prostate-serum antibody in the blood.

7. Which of the following statements about diabetes mellitus is false?
    a. The two types of diabetes are insulin-dependent and non–insulin-dependent.
    b. The incidence of diabetes has decreased in the last decade, especially among African Americans, Native Americans, and Latinos.

c. Individuals with diabetes must measure the levels of glucose in their blood to ensure that it does not rise to unsafe levels.

d. Untreated or uncontrolled diabetes can lead to coma and eventual death.

8. With asthma,
   a. the most common symptom is a persistent, sputum-producing cough.
   b. the recommended treatments include antibiotics to eliminate the underlying infection and bronchodilators to expand the breathing passages.
   c. an individual experiences wheezing and shortness of breath because of constricted breathing passages.
   d. if the disease is untreated, it may lead to emphysema.

9. Major disorders of the digestive system include all of the following except
   a. irritable bowel disease

b. Crohn's disease
c. gallstones
d. abdominal hernia

10. Which of the following statements is false?
    a. Psoriasis is the most severe form of dermatitis.
    b. In rheumatoid arthritis, the body attacks its own connective tissue.
    c. Sickle-cell anemia is a fatal genetic blood disorder of African Americans.
    d. Cirrhosis of the liver is commonly caused by chronic alcoholism.

Answers to these questions can be found on page 640.

 Can phytochemicals found in fruit, vegetables and whole grain stop the growth of cancer cells?

Critical Thinking

1. Do you have family members who have had cancer? Were these individuals at risk for cancer because of specific environmental factors, such as long-term exposure to tobacco smoke? If no particular cause was identified, what other factors could have triggered their diseases? Are you concerned that you might have inherited a genetic predisposition to any particular type of cancer because of your family history?

2. A friend of yours, Karen, discovered a small lump in her breast during a routine self-examination. When she mentions it, you ask if she has seen a doctor. She tells you that she hasn't had time to schedule an appointment; besides, she says she's not sure it's really the kind of lump one has to worry about. It's clear to you that Karen is in denial and procrastinating about seeing a doctor. What advice would you give her?

3. Because of advances in antirejection treatment, organ transplants have proven highly successful in helping many people who otherwise might have died. Even elderly patients have clearly benefited from donated kidneys and livers. However, because the demand for organs to transplant greatly exceeds the supply, health experts have debated setting priorities. Should a 30-year-old be placed higher on the waiting list for a particular organ than a 70-year-old? Should a nurse who needs a liver because she contracted hepatitis on the job get priority over an alcoholic whose liver has been destroyed by cirrhosis? Who, if anyone, should make such decisions? Would a lottery be a fair way to determine who receives an available organ?

SITES & BYTES

American Cancer Society
http://www.cancer.org
This comprehensive site features factual information on various types of cancers, as well as current cancer news events and information for professionals, patients, families, and friends of cancer patients. There is also information for cancer survivors.

Breast Cancer Interactive
http://www.tricaresw.af.mil/breastcd/index.html
Health Net: TriCare Southwest sponsors this site, which features an excellent personal breast cancer risk analysis, as well as several multimedia links, including a layperson site, self-exam video, clinical exam video, and a mammogram video. The site also contains teaching aids and resources.

American Diabetes Association
http://www.diabetes.org
This site features information on type 1 and type 2 diabetes, diet and exercise (healthy living), and community resources, as well as information for health professionals.

Please note that links are subject to change. If you find a broken link, use a search engine such as http://www.yahoo.com and search for the website by typing in key words.

 InfoTrac Activity "Cancer Treatment—New Drugs, New Hope." *Harvard Health Letter*, Vol. 26, No. 9, July 2001.

(1) What three types of new anticancer drugs are mentioned in the article?

(2) Name a specific type of cancer that illustrates how monoclonal antibodies work. Describe the mechanism of action.

(3) Why do tyrosine kinase inhibitors have a relatively low number of side effects?

You can find additional readings related to cancer with InfoTrac College Edition, an online library of more than 900 journals and publications. Follow the instructions for accessing InfoTrac that were packaged with your textbook; then search for articles using a key word search.

For additional links, resources, and suggested readings on InfoTrac, visit our Health & Wellness Resource Center at http://health.wadsworth.com.

Key Terms

The terms listed here are used within the chapter on the page indicated. Definitions of terms are in the Glossary at the end of the book.

anemia 465
arthritis 468
asthma 464
bone-marrow transplantation 460
carcinogen 449
chemoprevention 450
chronic obstructive lung disease (COLD) 465
cirrhosis 466
dermatitis 469
diabetes mellitus 462

epilepsy 464
gallstones 468
gene therapy 461
hernia 468
infiltration 444
inflammatory bowel disease (IBD) 467
irritable bowel syndrome 467
kidney stones 466
lumpectomy 457
mammography 457

mastectomy 457
metastasize 444
neoplasm 444
nephrosis 466
oncogene 445
psoriasis 469
rehabilitation medicine 470
relative risk 444
tamoxifen 450
tumor suppressor gene 445
ulcer 467

References

1. Wizeman, Theresa, and Mary-Lou Pardue. *Exploring the Biological Contributions to Human Health: Does Sex Matter?* Washington, DC: National Academy Press, 2001.

2. "Cancer in Minorities." *Cancer Facts and Figures—2001.* American Cancer Society, 2001.

3. "Why Blacks Get, Die from Cancer More." Press release, National Cancer Institute, October 18, 2001.

4. Franz, Rachel. "Hispanics: Watch Out for Hidden Melanomas." *Dermatology Nursing,* Vol. 13, No. 3, June 2001, p. 236.

5. Zenilman, Jonathan. "Chlamydia and Cervical Cancer." *Journal of the American Medical Association,* Vol. 285, No. 1, January 3, 2001.

6. Landua, Misia. "Environmentally Induced Cancers Target Genetic Achilles Heel." *Focus: News from Harvard Medical, Dental & Public Health Schools,* September 28, 2001, p. 1.

7. Velie, E.M., et al. "A Prospective Study of Dietary Patterns and Colorectal Cancer." *American Journal of Epidemiology,* Vol. 153, No. 11, June 1, 2001, p. S194.

8. Slattery, Martha. "Can an Apple a Day Keep Breast Cancer Away?" *Journal of the American Medical Association,* Vol. 285, No. 6, February 14, 2001.

9. Zoorob, Roger, et al. "Cancer Screening Guidelines." *American Family Physician,* Vol. 63, No. 6, March 15, 2001, p. 1101.

10. Toriello, Helga. Personal interview.

11. Pyritz, Reed. Personal interview.

12. Liebman, Bonnie. "Preventing Prostate Cancer: So Far, No Clear Answers." *Nutrition Action Newsletter,* Vol. 28, No. 6, July 2001, p. 1.

13. Goldstein, Beth, and Adam Goldstein. "Diagnosis and Management of Malignant Melanoma." *American Family Physician,* Vol. 63, No. 7, April 1, 2001, p. 1101.

14. Ibid.

15. Ibid.

16. "Skin Cancer—Shedding Light on Melanoma." *Harvard Women's Health Watch,* Vol. 9, No. 1, September 2001.

17. Beddingfield, Frederick. "Melanoma Strikes Men and Women Differently." Presentation, Society for Investigative Dermatory, Annual Meeting, Washington, DC, May 12, 2001.

18. "Skin Cancer—Shedding Light on Melanoma."

19. Goldstein and Goldstein, "Diagnosis and Management of Malignant Melanoma."

20. Eyre, Harmon. Personal interview.

21. Ford, Leslie. Personal interview.

22. Iversen, Edwin, Jr., et al. "Genetic Susceptibility and Survival: Application to Breast Cancer." *Journal of the American Statistical Association,* Vol. 95, No. 449, March 2000.

23. Gotzsche, Peter, and Ole Olsen. "Continuing Doubts About Screening for Breast Cancer." *Lancet,* Vol. 358, 2001, p. 1340.

24. Stidley, Christine, et al. "Mammography Utilization After a Benign Breast Biopsy Among Hispanic and Non-Hispanic Women." *Cancer,* Vol. 91, No. 9, May 1, 2001, p. 1716.

25. Rutter, Carolyn. "Changes in Breast Density Associated with Initiation, Discontinuation, and Continuing Use of Hormone Replacement Therapy." *Journal of the American Medical Association,* Vol. 285, No. 2, January 10, 2001.

26. Hellekson, Karen. "NIH Statement on Adjuvant Therapy for Breast Cancer." *American Family Physician,* May 1, 2001.

27. McCashland, Timothy, et al. "Age and Gender Influence Colon Cancer Risk." *American Journal of Gastroenterology,* Vol. 96, April 2001, p. 882.

28. Woolf, Steven. "The Best Screening Test for Colorectal Cancer—A Personal Choice." *New England Journal of Medicine,* Vol. 343, No. 22, November 30, 2000.

29. *Cancer Facts & Figures—2001.* Atlanta, GA; American Cancer Society, 2001.

30. Courtenay, Will. "Behavioral Factors Associated with Disease, Injury, and Death Among Men: Evidence and Implications for Prevention." *Journal of Men's Studies,* Vol. 9, No. 1, Fall 2000, p. 81.

31. Satterfield, Kenneth. "Oral and Tongue Cancer Rates Rise Among Young Americans." Press release, American Head and Neck Society, May 8, 2001.

32. Altman, Larry. "Cancer Doctors See New Era of Optimism." *New York Times,* May 22, 2001.

33. McCarthy, Michael. "Targeted Drugs Take Center Stage at US Cancer Meeting." *Lancet,* Vol. 357, No. 9268, May 19, 2001, p. 1593.

34. Druker, Brian, et al. "Activity of a Specific Inhibitor of the BCR-ABL Tyrosine Kinase in the Blast Crisis of Chronic Myeloid Leukemia and Acute Lymphoblastic Leukemia with the Philadelphia Chromosome." *New England Journal of Medicine,* Vol. 344, No. 14, April 5, 2001, p. 1038.

35. Charatan, Fred. "US Approves New Anti-leukaemia Drug." *British Medical Journal,* Vol. 322, No. 7296, May 19, 2001, p. 1201.

36. Jacobs, A., et al. "Positron-Emission Tomography of Vector-Mediated Gene Expression in Gene Therapy for Gliomas." *Lancet,* Vol. 358, No. 9283, September 1, 2001, p. 727.

37. *Cancer Facts & Figures—2001.*

38. CDC. "Facts About Diabetes." October 2000.

39. Hales, Dianne. "Should You Be Tested for Diabetes?" *Parade,* February 4, 2001.

40. Spiegel, Allen. Personal interview.

41. Levetan, Claresa. "Into the Mouth of Babes: The Diabetes Epidemic in Children." *Clinical Diabetes,* Vol. 19, No. 3, Summer 2001, p. 102.

42. Sherwin, Robert. Personal interview.

43. Hu, Frank, et al. "Diet, Lifestyle, and the Risk of Type 2 Diabetes Mellitus in Women." *New England Journal of Medicine,* Vol. 345, No. 11, September 13, 2001, p. 790.

44. Hales, "Should You be Tested for Diabetes?"

45. Reynolds, Tom. "Early Treatment of Seizure Patients May Limit Harm." *Focus: News from Harvard Medical, Dental & Public Health Schools,* September 14, 2001, p. 2.

46. Hopkins, Janice. "Asthma 'Crisis' for Black Americans." *British Medical Journal,* Vol. 323, No. 7308, August 11, 2001, p. 302.

47. Skolnick, Helen, and Robert Wood. "Natural History of Asthma: A 23-Year Follow-up of College Students." *Pediatrics,* Vol. 108, No. 2, August 2001, p. 547.

We constantly hear messages encouraging us to take risks with our health, to try drugs, to have a drink, to smoke cigarettes. We also live with the consequences of others' drug abuse, alcoholism, and smoking. That's why it's important to know about potentially harmful habits—even if you never rely on drugs to pick you up or bring you down, never smoke, and never drink to excess. This section provides information you can use to avoid or overcome habits that could destroy your health, happiness, and life.

14

Drug Use, Misuse, and Abuse

Amelia doesn't do drugs. That's what she says to anyone who asks. Sure, she and her friends occasionally pass a joint around while listening to music. She's tried a tab of ecstasy at a couple of raves. And when she was stressed out after finals, she took some of her roommate's Vicodin. But she thinks of drug users as desperate addicts craving a fix. She's not like that. That's what she tells herself.

Although she doesn't realize it, Amelia is at risk of drug-related problems—physical, psychological, and legal—and of developing a substance abuse disorder. Like Amelia, the people who try illegal drugs don't think they'll ever lose control. Even regular drug users are convinced that they are smart enough, strong enough, lucky enough not to get caught and not to get hooked. But with continued use, drugs produce changes in an individual's body, mind, and behavior. In time, a person's need for a drug can outweigh everything else, including the values, people, and relationships he or she once held dearest.

Drug use has declined in the last two decades—an estimated 14.8 million people in the United States currently use an illegal drug, nearly half the 25 million users in the peak year of 1979.[1] About half of American adults surveyed report having used an illicit drug at some time in their lives.

This chapter provides information on the nature and effects of drugs, the impact of drugs on individuals and society, and the drugs Americans most commonly use, misuse, and abuse.

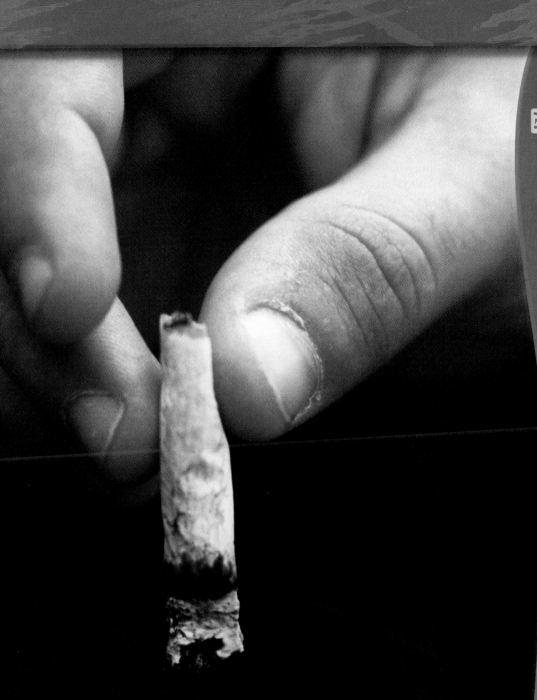

After studying the material in this chapter, you should be able to:

- **Describe** the different types of drug actions and factors affecting individuals' response to drugs.
- **Give examples** of appropriate and inappropriate use of over-the-counter and prescription medications.
- **Define** substance abuse disorders and **identify** the types of drug dependence.
- **Discuss** the factors affecting drug dependence.

- **Describe** the methods of use and effects of common drugs of abuse.
- **Describe** the treatment methods available for individuals seeking help for drug dependence.
- **Explain** codependency and some ways that a codependent person can enable another to continue an addictive behavior.

Understanding Drugs and Their Effects

A **drug** is a chemical substance that affects the way you feel and function. In some circumstances, taking a drug can help the body heal or relieve physical and mental distress. In other circumstances, taking a drug can distort reality, undermine well-being, and threaten survival. No drug is completely safe; all drugs have multiple effects that vary greatly in different people at different times. Knowing how drugs affect the brain, body, and behavior is crucial to understanding their impact and making responsible decisions about their use.

Drug misuse is the taking of a drug for a purpose or by a person other than that for which it was medically intended. Borrowing a friend's prescription for penicillin when your throat feels scratchy is an example of drug misuse. The World Health Organization defines **drug abuse** as excessive drug use that's inconsistent with accepted medical practice. Taking prescription painkillers to get high is an example of drug abuse.

There are risks involved with all forms of drug use. Even medications that help cure illnesses or soothe symptoms have side effects and can be misused. Some substances that millions of people use every day, such as caffeine, pose some health risks. Others—like the most commonly used drugs in our society, alcohol and tobacco—can lead to potentially life-threatening problems. With some illicit drugs, any form of use can be dangerous.

Many factors determine the effects a drug has on an individual. These include how the drug enters the body, the dosage, drug action, and presence of other drugs in the body—as well as the physical and psychological make-up of the person taking the drug and the setting in which the drug is used.

Routes of Administration

Drugs can enter the body in a number of ways (see Figure 14-1). The most common way of taking a drug is by swallowing a tablet, capsule, or liquid. However, drugs taken orally don't reach the bloodstream as quickly as drugs introduced into the body by other means. A drug taken orally may not have any effect for 30 minutes or more.

Drugs can enter the body through the lungs either by inhaling smoke, for example, from marijuana, or by inhaling gases, aerosol sprays, or fumes from solvents or other compounds that evaporate quickly. Young users of such **inhalants,** discussed later in this chapter, often soak a rag with fluid and press it over their noses. Or they may place

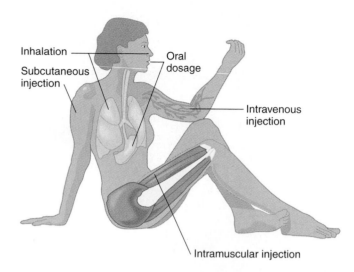

▲ **Figure 14-1** Routes of administration of drugs.

inhalants in a plastic bag, put the bag over their noses and mouths, and take deep breaths—a practice called *huffing* and one that can produce serious, even fatal consequences.

Drugs can also be injected with a syringe subcutaneously (beneath the skin), intramuscularly (into muscle tissue, which is richly supplied with blood vessels), or intravenously (directly into a vein). **Intravenous** (IV) injection gets the drug into the bloodstream immediately (within seconds in most cases); **intramuscular** injection, moderately fast (within a few minutes); and **subcutaneous** injection, more slowly (within ten minutes).

Approximately 1.5 million Americans use illegal IV drugs. This practice is extremely dangerous because many diseases, including hepatitis and infection with human immunodeficiency virus (HIV), can be transmitted by sharing contaminated needles. Injection-drug users who are HIV-positive are the chief source of transmission of HIV among heterosexuals. (See Chapter 11 for more on HIV infection and AIDS.)

Dosage and Toxicity

The effects of any drug depend on the amount an individual takes. Increasing the dose usually intensifies the effects produced by smaller doses. Also, the kind of effect may change at different dose levels. For example, low doses of barbiturates may relieve anxiety, while higher doses can induce sleep, loss of sensation, even coma and death.

The dosage level at which a drug becomes poisonous to the body, causing either temporary or permanent damage, is called its **toxicity.** In most cases, drugs are eventually broken down in the liver by special body chemicals called *detoxification enzymes.*

Individual Differences

Each person responds differently to different drugs, depending on circumstances or setting. The enzymes in our bodies reduce the levels of drugs in our bloodstream; because there can be 80 variants of each enzyme, every person's body may react differently.

Often drugs intensify the emotional state a person is in. If you're feeling depressed, a drug may make you feel more depressed. A generalized physical problem, such as having the flu, may make your body more vulnerable to the effects of a drug. Genetic differences among individuals also may account for varying reactions.

Personality and psychological attitude also play a role in drug effects, so that one person may have a frighteningly bad trip on the same LSD dosage on which another person has a positive experience. To a certain extent, this depends on each user's **set** (or mind-set)—his or her expectations or preconceptions about using the drug. Someone who snorts cocaine to enhance sexual pleasure may feel more stimulated simply because that's what he or she expects.

Setting

The setting for drug use also influences its effects. Passing around a joint of marijuana at a friend's is not a healthy or safe behavior, but the experience of going to a crack house is very different—and entails greater dangers.

Types of Action

A drug can act *locally*, as novocaine does to deaden pain in a tooth; *generally*, throughout a body system, as barbiturates do on the central nervous system; or *selectively*, as a drug does when it has a greater effect on one specific organ or system than on others, such as a spinal anesthetic. A drug that accumulates in the body because it's taken in faster than it can be metabolized and excreted is called *cumulative*; alcohol is such a drug.

Interaction with Other Drugs or Alcohol

A drug can interact with other drugs in four different ways:

- An **additive** interaction is one in which the resulting effect is equal to the sum of the effects of the different drugs used.
- A **synergistic** interaction is one in which the total effect of the two drugs taken together is greater than the sum of the effects the two drugs would have had if taken by themselves on separate occasions. Mixing barbiturates and alcohol, for example, has up to four times the depressant effect than either drug has alone.
- A drug can be **potentiating**—that is, one drug can increase the effect of another. Alcohol, for instance, can increase the drowsiness caused by antihistamines (antiallergy medications).
- Drugs can interact in an **antagonistic** fashion—that is, one drug can neutralize or block another drug with opposite effects. Tranquilizers, for example, may counter some of the nervousness and anxiety produced by cocaine.

The danger of mixing alcohol with other drugs cannot be emphasized too strongly. Alcohol and marijuana intensify each other's effects, making driving and many other activities extremely dangerous. Some people have mixed sedatives or tranquilizers with alcohol and never regained consciousness.

Medications

Many of the medications and pharmaceutical products available in this country do indeed relieve symptoms and help cure various illnesses. However, improper use of medications leads to more than 170,000 hospitalizations and costs of about $750 million every year. Because drugs are powerful, it's important to know how to use them appropriately.

What Should I Know About Buying Over-the-Counter Drugs?

More than half a million health products—remedies for everything from bad breath to bunions—are readily available without a doctor's prescription. This doesn't mean that they're necessarily safe or effective. Indeed, many widely used **over-the-counter (OTC) drugs** pose unsuspected hazards.

Among the most potentially dangerous is aspirin, the "wonder drug" in practically everyone's home pharmacy. When taken by someone who's been drinking (often to prevent or relieve hangover symptoms), for instance, aspirin increases blood-alcohol concentrations (see Chapter 15). Along with other nonsteroidal anti-inflammatory drugs, such as ibuprofen (brand names include Advil and Nuprin), aspirin can damage the lining of the stomach and lead to ulcers in those who take large daily doses for arthritis or other problems. Kidney problems have also been traced to some pain relievers including acetaminophen (Tylenol). Some health products that aren't even considered true drugs can also cause problems. Many Americans take food supplements, even though the FDA has never approved their use for any medical disorder. (See Chapter 4.)

A growing number of drugs that once were available only with a doctor's prescription can now be bought over the counter. These include Gyne-Lotrimin and Monistat, which combat vaginal yeast infections, and famotidine (sold as Pepcid AC) and cimetidine (sold as Tagamet), which offer an alternative to antacids for people suffering from heartburn and acid indigestion. For consumers, the advantages of this greater availability include lower prices and fewer visits to the doctor. The disadvantages, however, are the risks of misdiagnosing a problem and misusing or overusing medications.

Like other drugs, OTC medications can be used improperly, often simply because of lack of education about proper use. Among those most often misused are the following:

▶ **Nasal sprays.** Nasal sprays relieve congestion by shrinking blood vessels in the nose. If they are used too often or for too many days in a row, however, the blood vessels widen instead of contracting, and the surrounding tissues become swollen, causing more congestion. To make the vessels shrink again, many people use more spray more often. The result can be permanent damage to nasal membranes, bleeding, infection, and partial or complete loss of smell.

▶ **Laxatives.** Believing that they must have one bowel movement a day (a common misconception), many people rely on laxatives. Brands that contain phenol-phthalein irritate the lining of the intestines and cause muscles to contract or tighten, often making constipation worse rather than better. Bulk laxatives are less

dangerous, but regular use is not advised. A high-fiber diet and more exercise are safer and more effective remedies for constipation.

▶ **Eye drops.** Eye drops make the blood vessels of the eye contract. However, as in the case of nasal sprays, with overuse (several times a day for several weeks), the blood vessels expand, making the eye look redder than before.

▶ **Sleep aids.** Although over-the-counter sleeping pills are widely used, there has been little research on their use and possible risks.

▶ **Cough syrup.** Chugging cough syrup—or "roboing" as it is called, after the over-the-counter medication Robitussin—is a growing problem, in part because young people think of dextromethorphan (DXM), a common ingredient in cough medicine, as a "poor man's version" of the popular drug ecstasy.[2]

Prescription Drugs

Medications are a big business in this country. However, the latest, most expensive drugs aren't necessarily the best. Each year the Food and Drug Administration (FDA) approves about 20 new drugs, yet no more than 4 are rated as truly meaningful advances. The others often are no better or worse than what's already on the market. (For tips on using prescription drugs, see Savvy Consumer: "Getting the Most Out of Medications.")

College students, like other consumers, often take medicines, particularly nonprescription pain pills, without

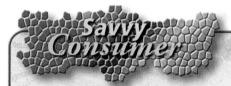

Getting the Most Out of Medications

Before you leave with a prescription, be sure to ask the following:

• What is the name of the drug? What's it supposed to do? How and when do I take it? For how long? What foods, drinks, other medications, or activities should I avoid while taking this drug? Are there any side effects? What do I do if they occur? What written information is available on this drug? Are there other, possibly cheaper alternatives? Why do you recommend this particular drug? Are there nondrug alternatives, such as using a vaporizer, gargling with salt water, and drinking plenty of liquids for a viral infection; or losing weight and exercising to lower blood pressure?

• If you're taking a medication, tell your doctor if you plan to change your diet significantly—cutting calories or fat, stopping or starting vitamin supplements, or changing the amount of fiber you consume.

• Don't keep old medications around, and don't take drugs prescribed for someone else unless your doctor tells you to. Keep medications out of reach of small children.

• Ask your pharmacist how best to store your prescriptions. (A hot, damp bathroom medicine chest is often the worst place.) Have all prescriptions filled at the same pharmacy, and ask your pharmacist to keep a record of your medications to avoid hazardous interactions.

discussing them with their physicians.[3] (See Table 14-1.) Both doctors and patients make mistakes when it comes to prescription drugs. The most frequent mistakes doctors make are over- or underdosing, omitting information from prescriptions, ordering the wrong dosage form (a pill instead of a liquid, for example), and not recognizing a patient's allergy to a drug.

Nonadherence

Many prescribed medications aren't taken the way they should be; millions simply aren't taken at all. As many as 70 percent of adults have trouble understanding dosage information and 30 percent of people can't read standard labels, according to the FDA, which has called for larger, clearer drug labeling. The dangers of nonadherence (not taking prescription drugs properly) include recurrent infections, serious medical complications, and emergency hospital treatment. The drugs most likely to be taken incorrectly are those that treat problems with no obvious symptoms (such as high blood pressure), that require complex dosage schedules, that treat psychiatric disorders, or that have unpleasant side effects.

Some people skip or stop taking medications because they fear that any drug can cause tolerance and eventual dependence. Others fail to let doctors know about side effects. For instance, patients may stop taking anti-inflammatory drugs because they irritate their stomachs. However, taking the drugs with food can eliminate this problem. The side effects of other drugs may disappear as the person's body becomes accustomed to the drug.

Physical Side Effects

Most medications, taken correctly, cause only minor complications. However, no drug is entirely without side effects for all individuals taking it. Serious complications that may occur include heart failure, heart attack, seizures, kidney and liver failure, severe blood disorders, birth defects, blindness, memory problems, and allergic reactions.

Allergic reactions to drugs are common. The drugs that most often provoke allergic responses are penicillin and other antibiotics (drugs used to treat infection). Aspirin, sulfa drugs, barbiturates, anticonvulsants, insulin, and local anesthetics can also provoke allergic responses. Allergic reactions range from mild rashes to hives to anaphylaxis—a life-threatening constriction of the airways and sudden drop of blood pressure that causes rapid pulse, weakness, paleness, confusion, nausea, vomiting, unconsciousness, and collapse. This extreme response, which is rare, requires immediate treatment with an injection of epinephrine (adrenaline) to open the airways and blood vessels.

Psychological Side Effects

Dozens of drugs—both over-the-counter and prescription—can cause changes in the way people think, feel, and behave. Unfortunately, neither patients nor their physicians usually connect such symptoms with medications. Doctors may not even mention potential mental and emotional problems because they don't want to scare patients away from what otherwise may be a very effective treatment. But what you don't know about a drug's effects on your mind can hurt you.

Among the medications most likely to cause psychiatric side effects are drugs for high blood pressure, heart disease, asthma, epilepsy, arthritis, Parkinson's disease, anxiety, insomnia, and depression. Some drugs—such as the powerful hormones called corticosteroids, used for asthma, autoimmune diseases, and cancer—can cause different psychiatric symptoms, depending on dosage and other factors. Other drugs, such as ulcer medications, can cause delirium and disorientation, especially when given in high doses or to elderly patients. More subtle problems, such as forgetfulness or irritability, are common reactions to many

▼ **Table 14-1**   **The Medicines Students Use Most**

Product	Percent Taking It	Percent Who Discussed It With Doctor
Advil	83.9	13.2
Midol	32.9	4.7
Excedrin	32.5	3.8
Ortho-Tricyclen	16.3	15.1
Monistat-3	13.4	4.2

Source: Based on a study of 471 undergraduates at a state college, a state university, and a private college. Burak, Lydia, and Amy Damico. "College Students' Use of Widely Advertised Medications." *Journal of American College Health,* Vol. 49, No. 3, November 2000, p. 118.

drugs—but also are more likely to be ignored or dismissed. The older you are, the sicker you are, and the more medications you're taking, the greater your risk of developing some psychiatric side effects. Even medications that don't usually cause problems, such as antibiotics, can cause psychiatric side effects in some individuals.[4]

Any medication that slows down bodily systems—as many high blood pressure and cardiac drugs do—can cause depressive symptoms. Estrogen in birth control pills can cause mood changes. As many as 15 percent of women using oral contraceptives have reported feeling depressed or moody. For many people, switching to another medication quickly lifts a drug-induced depression.

All drugs that stimulate or speed up the central nervous system can cause agitation and anxiety—including the almost 200 allergy, cold, and congestion remedies containing pseudoephedrine hydrochloride (Sudafed). Other common culprits in inducing anxiety are caffeine and theophylline, a chemical relative of caffeine found in many medications for asthma and other respiratory problems. These drugs act like mild amphetamines in the body, making people feel hyper and restless.

Drug Interactions

OTC and prescription drugs can interact in a variety of ways. For example, mixing some cold medications with tranquilizers can cause drowsiness and coordination problems, thus making driving dangerous. Moreover, what you eat or drink can impair or completely wipe out the effectiveness of drugs or lead to unexpected effects on the body. For instance, aspirin takes five to ten times as long to be absorbed when taken with food or shortly after a meal than when taken on an empty stomach. Or if tetracyclines encounter calcium in the stomach, they bind together and cancel each other out.

To avoid potentially dangerous interactions, check the label(s) for any instructions on how or when to take a medication, such as "with a meal." (See Figure 14-2.) If the directions say that you should take a drug on an empty stomach, do it at least one hour before eating or two or three hours after eating. Don't drink a hot beverage with a medication, because the temperature may interfere with the effectiveness of the drug. Don't open, crush, or dissolve tablets or capsules without checking first with your physician or pharmacist.

Whenever you take a drug, be especially careful of your intake of alcohol, which can change the rate of metabolism and the effects of many different drugs. Because it dilates the blood vessels, alcohol can add to the dizziness sometimes caused by drugs for high blood pressure, angina, or depression. Also, its irritating effects on the stomach can worsen stomach upset from aspirin, ibuprofen, and other anti-inflammatory drugs.

Generic Drugs

The **generic** name is the chemical name for a drug. A specific drug may appear on the pharmacist's shelf under a variety of brand names, which may cost more than twice the generic equivalent. About 75 percent of all prescriptions specify a brand name, but pharmacists may—and in some states must—switch to a generic drug unless the doctor specifically tells them not to. Prescriptions filled with generic drugs cost 20 to 85 percent less than their brand-name counterparts.

Generic drugs have the same active ingredients as brand-name prescriptions, but their fillers and binders, which can affect the absorption of a drug, may be different. For some serious illnesses, the generics may not be as effective; some experts recommend sticking with brand names for heart medications, psychiatric drugs, and anticonvulsant drugs (for epilepsy and other seizure disorders).

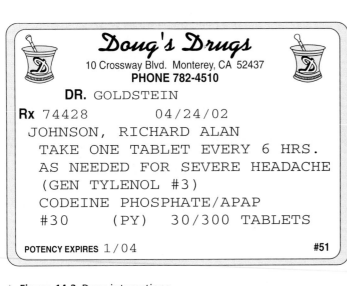
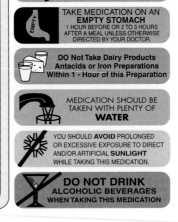

▲ **Figure 14-2 Drug interactions.**
When you take a prescription medication, be sure to read warning labels about interactions, possible side effects, and whether the medication interacts with certain foods.

To determine whether you should buy the generic version of a drug, ask your physician whether it matters if you get a brand-name or generic drug. If it does, ask which brand name is best. Also, find out if switching to a generic or from one generic to another might harm your condition in any way.

What Should I Know About Buying Drugs Online?

Millions of people in the United States purchase prescription medications online. Although some websites fill only faxed prescriptions from medical doctors, others ignore or sidestep traditional regulations and safeguards. Cyberspace distributors often ship pills across state lines without requiring a physical examination by a medical doctor. Instead, a "cyberdoc," who may or may not be qualified or up-to-date in a given specialty, reviews information submitted by a "patient." International pharmacies sometimes sell drugs that are not available or approved in the United States. And patients themselves use bulletin boards and other web areas to sell unused or unwanted medications to each other.

Many individuals turn to the Internet for "lifestyle" drugs such as Viagra for erectile dysfunction and Propecia, a baldness treatment. Other medications commonly bought online include Xenical, a diet pill; Zyban, an anti-smoking treatment; Celebrex, for arthritis; and Claritin, for allergies. Many customers turn to cyberspace because of the convenience and anonymity. Although many assume drugs cost less on the Internet, shipping costs tend to drive prices up to the same amount or more than the price at a pharmacy.

The dangers of unregulated distribution of medications have alarmed government agencies and medical groups. The American Medical Association has declared it unethical for physicians to write prescriptions for people they've never met. The National Association of Boards of Pharmacy has developed a seal of approval to help customers determine which sites are legitimate. The FDA and other federal agencies, such as the Federal Trade Commission, which regulates advertising, are trying to find ways to impose some controls.

Consumers have to be wary. Ordering a drug like Accutane, an acne treatment, online may seem harmless. However, without close monitoring by a physician, you could develop complications, such as a bad reaction that aggravates hepatitis or inflames the pancreas. Quality control is another concern. Cyberspace pharmacies provide no information on how the drug was stored or whether its expiration date has passed. In addition, since importing medications without a prescription is against the law, you could find yourself in legal trouble.

Abuse of Prescription Painkillers

Abuse of prescription painkillers such as Vicodin and Oxycontin has been increasing. According to a Department of Health and Human Services survey, some 1.5 million people take prescription painkillers for "nonmedical" purposes. Some pain medications, such as Percocet, Percodan, and Vicodin, are highly addictive. Oxycontin is particularly deadly. According to the Drug Enforcement Administration, since January 2000, 30 states have reported a total of more than 1,000 overdose deaths involving oxycodone, the active ingredient in the drug.[5] Most of those who died swallowed the pills whole or crushed them into powder, which had been considered less dangerous forms of administration than injecting or snorting crushed pills.

Many prescription painkillers work by blocking the pathway that pain signals travel to the brain and by triggering production of the chemical dopamine in the brain. Users can become accustomed to the changes dopamine causes in the brain. When they stop taking the medications, they develop a craving for the dopamine-induced feelings. Individuals who've had prior problems with drug dependence may be especially prone to addiction to prescription painkillers.

Caffeine Use and Misuse

Caffeine, which has been drunk, chewed, or swallowed since the Stone Age, is the most widely used **psychotropic** (mind-affecting) drug in the world. Eighty percent of Americans drink coffee, our principal caffeine source—an average of 3.5 cups a day. Coffee contains 100 to 150 milligrams of caffeine per cup; tea, 40 to 100 milligrams; cola, about 45 milligrams. Most medications that contain caffeine are one-third to one-half the strength of a cup of coffee. However, some, such as Excedrin, are very high in caffeine (Table 14-2).

The effects of caffeine vary. Because it is a **stimulant**, it relieves drowsiness, helps in the performance of repetitive tasks, and improves capacity for work. Some athletes feel that caffeine gives them an extra boost that allows them to go farther and longer in endurance events. Consumption of high doses of caffeine can lead to dependence, anxiety, insomnia, faster breathing, upset stomach and bowels, and dizziness.

Although there is no conclusive proof that caffeine causes birth defects, it does cross the placenta into the tissues of a growing fetus. Because of an increased risk of miscarriage, the U. S. surgeon general has recommended that pregnant women avoid or restrict their caffeine intake. Some fertility specialists also have urged couples trying to

▼ Table 14-2 Caffeine Counts

Substance (typical serving)	Caffeine (milligrams)
No Doz (one pill)	200
Coffee (drip), one 5-ounce cup	130
Excedrin (two pills)	130
Espresso (2-ounce cup)	100
Instant coffee (5-ounce cup)	74
Coca-Cola (12 ounces)	46
Tea (5-ounce cup)	40
Dark chocolate (1 ounce)	20
Milk chocolate	6
Cocoa (5 ounces)	4
Decaffeinated coffee	3

conceive to reduce caffeine to increase their chance of success. Women who are heavy caffeine users tend to have shorter menstrual cycles than nonusers.

Is It Possible to Overdose on Caffeine?

Yes, you can overdose on caffeine. The characteristic symptoms of caffeine intoxication are restlessness, nervousness, excitement, insomnia, flushed face, increased urination, digestive complaints, muscle twitching, rambling thoughts and speech, rapid heart rate or ar-

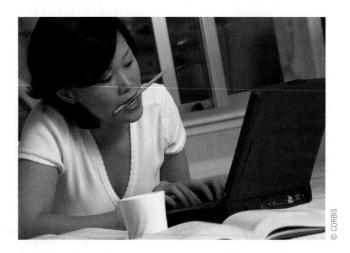

© CORBIS

▲ Coffee and work often go hand in hand, but too much caffeine can lead to dependence, anxiety, and other problems.

rhythmias, periods of inexhaustibility, and physical restlessness. Some people develop these symptoms after as little as 250 milligrams of caffeine a day; others, only with much larger doses. Higher doses may produce ringing in the ears or flashes of light, grand mal seizures, and potentially fatal respiratory failure.

Caffeine withdrawal for those dependent on this substance can cause headaches and other neurological symptoms. Those who must cut back should taper off gradually. One approach is to mix regular and decaffeinated coffee, gradually decreasing the quantity of the former.

Substance Use Disorders

People have been using mind-altering, or **psychoactive,** chemicals for centuries. Citizens of ancient Mesopotamia and Egypt used opium. More than 3,000 years ago Hindus included cannabis products in religious ceremonies. For centuries the Inca in South America have chewed the leaves of the coca bush. Yet while drugs existed in most societies, their use was usually limited to small groups. Today millions of people regularly turn to drugs to pick them up, bring them down, alter perceptions, or ease psychological pain.

Both men and women are vulnerable to substance use disorders, although they tend to have different patterns of drug use. (See X & Y Files: "Men, Women, and Drugs.") The 1960s ushered in an explosive increase in drug use and in the number of drug users in our society. Marijuana use soared in the 1960s and 1970s; cocaine, in the 1980s. In 1986, crack—a cheap, smokeable form of cocaine—hit the streets and cities of the United States, and the number of regular cocaine users zoomed. By the twenty-first century, overall drug use was down, but "club drugs," such as ecstasy (MDMA), were growing in popularity.[6]

Understanding Substance Use Disorders

In early Roman law, *addictus* referred to someone who, because he could not pay his debts, was sentenced into slavery. Indeed, one of the meanings of addiction given by the *Oxford Latin Dictionary* is "enslavement." For much of the twentieth century, addiction to drugs was viewed as a social or criminal problem, and the only people called addicts were "drug-crazed junkies" desperate for a fix. In the 1960s, however, when scientists switched to the *medical model* for understanding addictions, they began to view addictions to chemicals—such as alcohol and psychoactive drugs—as lifelong chronic diseases that affect a person's mind and body.

The X & Y Files

Men, Women, and Drugs

Beginning at a very early age, males and females show different patterns in drug use. Among 12-year-olds who have been offered drugs, boys are more likely to have received those offers from other males or their parents. Girls are most likely to have been offered drugs by a female friend or family member. The social settings and nature of drug offers also differ by gender. Boys are more likely to receive offers in a public setting, such as on the street or in a park, and the offers typically emphasize "benefits," such as improved status or self-image. Girls are more likely to receive a straightforward "do you want some?" offer or one that minimizes the risks of drug use. For girls, these offers are usually made in a private setting such as a friend's home.

Later in life men generally encounter more opportunities to use drugs than women, but given an opportunity to use drugs for the first time, both genders are equally likely to do so and to progress from initial use to addiction. Vulnerability to some drugs varies with gender. Both are equally likely to become addicted to or dependent on cocaine, heroin, hallucinogens, tobacco, and inhalants. Women are more likely than men to become addicted to or dependent on sedatives and drugs designed to treat anxiety or sleeplessness, and less likely than men to abuse alcohol and marijuana.

Males and females may differ in their biological responses to drugs. In studies of animals given the opportunity to self-administer intravenous doses of cocaine or heroin, females began self-administration sooner than males and administered larger amounts of the drugs. Women may be more sensitive than men to the cardiovascular effects of cocaine. In human studies, women and men given equal doses of cocaine experienced the same cardiovascular response despite the fact that blood concentrations of cocaine did not rise as high in women as in men. Male and female long-term cocaine users showed similar impairment in tests of concentration, memory, and academic achievement following sustained abstinence, even though women in the study had substantially greater exposure to cocaine. Women cocaine users also were less likely than men to exhibit abnormalities of blood flow in the brain's frontal lobes. These findings suggest a gender-related mechanism that may protect women from some of the damage cocaine inflicts on the brain. However, women are more vulnerable to poor nutrition and below-average weight, depression, physical abuse, and if pregnant, preterm labor or early delivery.

Substance abuse compounds the risk of AIDS for women, who may acquire it by sharing needles with other injection-drug users and by engaging in unprotected sex. In all, drug abuse is nearly twice as likely to be directly or indirectly associated with AIDS in women (66 percent) as in men (34 percent).

There are also differences between men and women who seek treatment for drug abuse. Women in treatment programs are less likely than men to have graduated from high school and to be employed, are more likely than men to have other health problems, to have sought previous drug treatment, to have attempted suicide, and to have suffered sexual abuse or other physical abuse. Traditional drug treatment programs, created for men, have proven to be less effective for women than programs that provide more comprehensive services, including child care, assertiveness training, and parenting training.

Sources: "Overview of NIDA Research on Women's Health and Gender Differences." http://www.nida.nih.gov. "Males and Females Respond to Amphetamines Differently Pre-Puberty." Press release, American Physiological Society, October 16, 2001. "Gender-specific Substance Abuse Treatment Promising." *Brown University Digest of Addiction Theory and Application*, Vol. 20, No. 7, July 2001, p. 4.

Today the word **addiction** has moved out of the realm of scientific terminology and into the cultural mainstream. Among laypeople, addiction refers to the habitual use of substances, such as alcohol, psychoactive drugs, and nicotine, and also to compulsive behaviors, such as overeating (discussed in Chapter 6). Like drugs, these activities can be used repeatedly to numb pain or enhance pleasure; some may alter a person's brain chemistry or create cravings; all can lead to a loss of internal control.

Chemical addiction is now viewed as a lifelong, chronic illness that affects mind, body, and spirit. Its key characteristics are repeated drug use, loss of control over how much or how often a person takes a drug, and continued use despite harmful consequences.[7] Because addiction is considered too broad and judgmental a term for scientific use, mental health professionals describe drug-related problems in terms of dependence and abuse. However, they agree that addiction has four characteristic symptoms: compulsion to use the substance, loss of control, negative consequences, and denial. (See Self-Survey: "Is It a Substance Use Disorder?")

Dependence

Individuals may develop **psychological dependence** and feel a strong craving for a drug because it produces pleasurable feelings or relieves stress or anxiety. **Physical**

SELF SURVEY

Individuals with a substance dependence or abuse disorder may

- Use more of an illegal drug or a prescription medication or use a drug for a longer period of time than they desire or intend. _____
- Try, repeatedly and unsuccessfully, to cut down or control their drug use. _____
- Spend a great deal of time doing whatever is necessary in order to get drugs, taking them, or recovering from their use. _____
- Be so high or feel so bad after drug use that they often cannot do their job or fulfill other responsibilities. _____
- Give up or cut back on important social, work, or recreational activities because of drug use. _____
- Continue to use drugs even though they realize that they are causing or worsening physical or mental problems. _____
- Use a lot more of a drug in order to achieve a "high" or desired effect or feel fewer such effects than in the past. _____
- Use drugs in dangerous ways or situations. _____
- Have repeated drug-related legal problems, such as arrests for possession. _____
- Continue to use drugs, even though the drug causes or worsens social or personal problems, such as arguments with a spouse. _____
- Develop hand tremors or other withdrawal symptoms if they cut down or stop drug use. _____
- Take drugs to relieve or avoid withdrawal symptoms. _____

The more blanks that you or someone close to you checks, the more reason you have to be concerned about drug use. The most difficult step for anyone with a substance use disorder is to admit that he or she has a problem. Sometimes a drug-related crisis, such as being arrested or fired, forces individuals to acknowledge the impact of drugs. If not, those who care—family, friends, boss, physician—may have to confront them and insist that they do something about it. This confrontation,

planned beforehand, is called an intervention and can be the turning point for drug users and their families.

Making Changes
Alternatives to Drugs

If you are an addict, you must first admit that you have a problem before you can begin the process of recovery. Then you should seek help from health-care professionals. If your answers raised doubts about your drug use, try to stop using them. Consider these alternatives instead of drugs:

- If you need physical relaxation, try athletics, exercise, or outdoor hobbies. For adventure, sign up for a wilderness survival outing, or take up windsurfing or rock climbing.
- If you want to stimulate your senses, train yourself to be more sensitive to nature and beauty. Take time to appreciate the sensations you experience when you're walking in the woods or embracing a person you love.
- If you're anxious, depressed, or uptight and want relief from emotional pain, turn to people—either friends or professional counselors or support groups. If you want to find meaning in life or expand your personal awareness, explore various philosophical theories through classes, seminars, and discussion groups. Study yoga or meditation.
- If you want to enhance your creativity or appreciation of the arts, challenge your mind through reading, classes, creative games, discussion groups, memory training, or travel. Pursue training in music, art, singing, or writing. Attend more concerts, ballets, or museum shows.
- If you want to be accepted, volunteer in programs in which you can assist others and not focus solely on yourself. If you want to promote political or social change, volunteer in political campaigns, or join lobbying and political-action groups.

dependence occurs when a person develops *tolerance* to the effects of a drug and needs larger and larger doses to achieve intoxication or another desired effect. Individuals who are physically dependent and have a high tolerance to a drug may take amounts many times those that would produce intoxication or an overdose in someone who was not a regular user.

Men and women with a substance dependence disorder may use a drug to avoid or relieve withdrawal symp-

toms or consume larger amounts of a drug or use it over a longer period than they'd originally intended. They may try repeatedly to cut down or control drug use without success; spend a great deal of time obtaining or using drugs or recovering from their effects; give up or reduce important social, occupational, or recreational activities because of their drug use; or continue to use a drug despite knowledge that the drug is likely to cause or worsen a persistent or recurring physical or psychological problem.

Specific symptoms of dependence vary with particular drugs. For instance, certain drugs, such as marijuana, hallucinogens, or phencyclidine, do not cause withdrawal symptoms. The degree of dependence also varies. In mild cases, a person may function normally most of the time. In severe cases, the person's entire life may revolve around obtaining, using, and recuperating from the effects of a drug.

Individuals with drug dependence become intoxicated or high on a regular basis—whether every day, every weekend, or several binges a year. They may try repeatedly to stop using a drug and yet fail—even though they realize that their drug use is interfering with their health, family life, relationships, and work.

Abuse

Some drug users do not develop the symptoms of tolerance and withdrawal that characterize dependence, yet they use drugs in ways that clearly have a harmful effect on them. These individuals are diagnosed as having a *psychoactive substance abuse disorder*. They continue to use drugs despite their awareness of persistent or repeated social, occupational, psychological, or physical problems related to drug use, or they use drugs in dangerous ways or situations (before driving, for instance). (See Pulsepoints: "Ten Ways to Tell If Someone Is Abusing Drugs.")

Intoxication and Withdrawal

Intoxication refers to maladaptive behavioral, psychological, and physiologic changes that occur as a result of substance use. **Withdrawal** is the development of symptoms that cause significant psychological and physical distress when an individual reduces or stops drug use. (Intoxication and withdrawal from specific drugs are discussed later in this chapter.)

Polyabuse

Most users prefer a certain type of drug but also use several others; this behavior is called **polyabuse.** The average user who enters treatment is on five different drugs. The more drugs anyone uses, the greater the chance of side effects, complications, and possibly life-threatening interactions.

Comorbidity

Mental disorders and substance abuse disorders have a great deal of overlap. "A little more than a third of those with a psychiatric disorder also have a chemical dependency problem, and a little more than a third of those with a chemical dependency problem have a psychiatric disorder," notes psychiatrist Richard Frances, M.D., the founding president of the American Association of Addiction

Psychiatry.[8] Individuals with such "dual diagnoses" require careful evaluation and appropriate treatment for the complete range of complex and chronic difficulties that they face.

What Causes Drug Dependence and Abuse?

No one fully understands why some people develop drug dependence or abuse disorders, while others, who may experiment briefly with drugs, do not. Inherited body chemistry, genetic factors, and sensitivity to drugs may make some individuals more susceptible. These disorders may stem from many complex causes.

The Biology of Addiction

Scientists now view addiction as a brain disease triggered by frequent use of drugs that change the biochemistry and anatomy of neurons and alter the way they work.[9] A major breakthrough in understanding the roots of addiction has been the discovery that certain mood-altering substances and experiences—a puff of marijuana, a slug of whiskey, a snort of cocaine, a big win at black jack—trigger a rise in a brain chemical called dopamine, which is associated with feelings of satisfaction and euphoria. This neurotransmitter, one of the crucial messengers that link neurons, or nerve cells, in the brain, rises during any pleasurable experience, whether it be a loving hug or a taste of chocolate.

STRATEGIES FOR PREVENTION

Saying No to Drugs

If people offer you a drug, here are some ways to say no:

✔ Let them know you're not interested. Change the subject. If the pressure seems threatening, just walk away.

✔ Have something else to do: "No, I'm going for a walk now."

✔ Be prepared for different types of pressure. If your friends tease you, tease them back.

✔ Keep it simple. "No, thanks," "No," or "No way" all get the point across.

✔ Hang out with people who won't ask you questions you have to say no to.

PULSE POINTS

Ten Ways to Tell If Someone Is Abusing Drugs

1. **An abrupt change in attitude.** Individuals may lose interest in activities they once enjoyed or in being with friends they once valued.

2. **Mood swings.** Drug users may often seem withdrawn or "out of it," or they may display unusual temper flareups.

3. **A decline in performance.** Students may start skipping classes, stop studying, or not complete assignments; their grades may plummet.

4. **Increased sensitivity.** Individuals may react intensely to any criti-

cism or become easily frustrated or angered.

5. **Secrecy.** Drug users may make furtive telephone calls or demand greater privacy concerning their personal possessions or their whereabouts.

6. **Physical changes.** Individuals using drugs may change their pattern of sleep, spending more time in bed or sleeping at odd hours. They also may change their eating habits and lose weight.

7. **Money problems.** Drug users may constantly borrow money, seem short of cash, or begin stealing.

8. **Changes in appearance.** As they become more involved with drugs, users often lose regard for their personal appearance and look disheveled.

9. **Defiance of restrictions.** Individuals may ignore or deliberately refuse to comply with deadlines, curfews, or other regulations.

10. **Changes in relationships.** Drug users may quarrel more frequently with family members or old friends and develop new, strong allegiances with new acquaintances, including other drug users.

Addictive drugs have such a powerful impact on dopamine and its receptors (its connecting cells) that they change the pathways within the brain's pleasure centers (Figure 14-3). Different substances create a craving for more of the same. According to this hypothesis, addicts do not specifically yearn for heroin, cocaine, or nicotine but for the rush of dopamine that these drugs produce. Other brain chemicals, including glutamate, GABA (gamma-amino-butyric-acid) and possibly norepinephrine, may also be involved. Some individuals, born with low levels of dopamine, may be particularly susceptible to addiction.

Other Routes of Addiction

Although scientists do not believe there is an "addictive" personality, certain individuals are at greater risk of drug dependence because of psychological risk factors, including difficulty controlling impulses, a lack of values that might constrain drug use (whether based in religion, family, or society), low self-esteem, feelings of powerlessness, and depression. The one psychological trait most often linked with drug use is denial. Young people in particular are absolutely convinced that they will never lose control or suffer in any way as a result of drug use.

Many diagnosed drug users have at least one mental disorder, particularly depression or anxiety. Disorders that emerge in adolescence, such as bipolar disorder, may increase the risk of substance abuse. Many people with psychiatric disorders abuse drugs. Individuals may self-

administer drugs to treat psychiatric symptoms; for example, they may take sedating drugs to suppress a panic attack.

Individuals who are isolated from friends and family, or who live in communities, such as poor inner-city areas where drugs are widely used, have higher rates of drug abuse. Young people from lower socioeconomic backgrounds are more likely to use drugs than their more affluent peers, possibly because of economic disadvantage; family instability; a lack of realistic, rewarding alternatives and role models; and increased hopelessness.

Those whose companions are substance abusers are far more likely to use drugs. Peer pressure to use drugs can be a powerful factor for adolescents and young adults. The likelihood of drug abuse is also related to family instability, parental rejection, and divorce.

When researchers followed families for a decade and a half and interviewed both children and their mothers, they found that youngsters who felt attached to their parents and showed greater responsibility and less rebelliousness were less likely to use drugs. Their attitudes and behaviors insulated them from socializing with drug-using peers, resulting in less drug use in their early and late twenties.[10] Clear rules and expectations from parents also can go a long way toward preventing or delaying alcohol and marijuana use in children, even if there is tension in the parent-child relationship.[11]

Parents' own attitudes and drug use history affect their children's likelihood of using marijuana, according to the Substance Abuse and Mental Health Services

NORMAL STATE

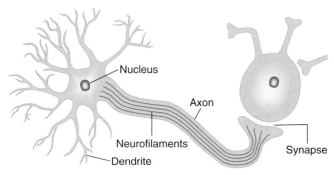

DRUG-ADDICTED STATE

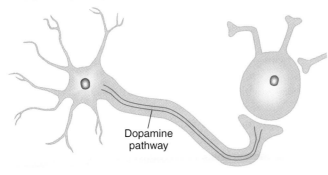

AFFECTED AREAS OF THE BRAIN

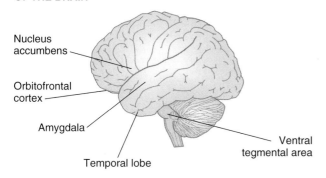

▲ **Figure 14-3** The normal vs. drug-addicted nervous system. Repeated drug doses overload normal neurotransmitter systems, and cells compensate by making dopamine less effective and becoming smaller. When doses stop, craving ensues.

Source: The Neuroscientist.

Administration. Parents who perceived little risk associated with marijuana use had children with similar attitudes, and the children of parents who had used marijuana were about three times more likely to try the drug than children whose parents had never used the drug.[12]

Drugs that produce an intense, brief high—like crack cocaine—lead to dependence more quickly than slower-acting agents, like cocaine powder. Drugs that cause uncomfortable withdrawal symptoms, such as barbiturates, may lead to continued use to avoid such discomfort.

Drug use involves certain behaviors, situations, and settings that users may, in time, associate with getting high. Even after long periods of abstinence, some former drug users find that they crave drugs when they return to a site of drug use or meet people with whom they used drugs. Former cocaine users report that the sight of white powder alone can serve as a cue that triggers a craving.

Most individuals who use drugs first try them as adolescents. Teens are likely to begin experimenting with tobacco, beer, wine, or hard liquor, then smoke marijuana or sniff inhalants. Teens who smoke cigarettes are more likely to use drugs and to drink heavily than non-smoking youths. Some then go on to try sedative-hypnotics, stimulants (including cocaine), and hallucinogens such as LSD. A much smaller percentage of teens try the opioids. Over time some individuals give up certain drugs, such as hallucinogens, and return to old favorites, such as alcohol and marijuana. A smaller number continue using several drugs.

The Toll of Drugs

Drugs affect a person's physical, psychological, and social health; their effects can be *acute* (resulting from a single dose or series of doses) or *chronic* (resulting from long-term use). Acute effects vary with different drugs. Stimulants may trigger unpredictable rage; an overdose of heroin may lead to respiratory depression, a breathing impairment that can be fatal.

Over time, chronic drug users may feel fatigued, cough constantly, lose weight, become malnourished, and ache from head to toe. They may suffer blackouts, flashbacks, and episodes of increasingly bizarre behavior, often triggered by escalating paranoia. Their risk of overdose rises steadily, and they must live with constant stress: the fear of getting busted for possession or of losing a job if they test positive for drugs, the worry of getting enough money for their next fix, the dangers of associating with dealers and other users.

The toll of drug use can be especially great on teenagers. Teenage drug use disrupts many critical developmental tasks of adolescence and young adulthood. Use of drugs during the teen years can lead to drug-related crime (including stealing), poor achievement in high school or college, and job instability.

Drugs in Society

Drug abuse remains a major problem even though drug use among teenagers has declined in recent years. The estimated medical and social costs of drug abuse are believed to exceed $276 billion. Addiction to drugs, alcohol, or tobacco accounts for a third of all hospital admissions and a quarter of all deaths. The number of emergency cases related to the use of the drug ecstasy has soared in recent years.[13]

An estimated 14 million Americans use illicit drugs, down from almost twice that number twenty years ago. According to the most recent figures from the Department of Health and Human Services, overall rates of illicit drug use have shown little change in the last few years. However, drug use has declined among young teenagers, with 9.7 percent of youths between ages 12 and 27 currently using drugs—down slightly from 9.8 percent in 1999. Among the very youngest of those surveyed—12- and 13-year-olds—3 percent reported that they had used drugs in the previous month, a drop from 3.9 percent in 1999. Rates of drug use increase through adolescence, peaking in those between ages 18 and 20; about one in five (19.6 percent) of these young adults report using illegal drugs.[14]

How Common Is Drug Use on Campus?

Alcohol is the number-one drug of abuse on college campuses. Marijuana remains the most commonly used illegal drug.[15] (See Student Snapshot: "Illegal Drug Use by Undergraduates.") However, there is a large gap between actual drug use on campus and how prevalent students believe drug use to be. When researchers have compared students' self-reports of frequency of drug use with what students perceived to be the frequency of drug use by "the average student," they greatly overestimate the use of a variety of drugs.[16]

Various factors influence which students use drugs, including the following:

 Race/ethnicity. In general, white students have higher levels of alcohol and drug use than do African-American students. In a comparison of African-American students at predominantly white and predominantly black colleges, those at historically black colleges had lower rates of alcohol and drug use than did either white or African-American students at white schools. The reason, according to the researchers, may be that these colleges provide a greater sense of self-esteem, which helps prevent alcohol and drug use.

Perception of risk. Students seem most likely to try substances they perceive as being "safe," or low risk. Of these, the top three are caffeine, alcohol, and tobacco; marijuana is listed fourth in terms of perceived safety. Other agents—barbiturates, heroin, cocaine, PCP,

Student Snapshot Illegal Drug Use by Undergraduates

Drug	Undergraduates reporting current use	Undergraduates reporting lifetime use
Marijuana	17%	43%
Cocaine	1%	7%
Other illegal drugs (ecstasy, LSD, PCP, etc.)	3%	16%

Source: Jones, Sherry, et al. "Binge Drinking Among Undergraduate College Students in the United States: Implications for Other Substance Use." *Journal of American College Health,* Vol. 50, No. 1, July 2001, p. 33.

speed, LSD, crack, and inhalants—are viewed as about equally risky and are used much less often.

- **Alcohol Use.** Often individuals engage in more than one "risk behavior," and researchers have documented correlations among smoking, drinking, and drug use. Among college students, researchers have found that those who report binge drinking (discussed in depth in Chapter 15) are much more likely than other students to report current or past use of marijuana, cocaine, or other illegal drugs.[17]
- **Environment.** As with alcohol use, students are influenced by their friends, their residence, the general public's attitude toward drug use, and even the Internet. Increasingly, college health officials are realizing that, rather than simply trying to change students' substance abuse, they also must change the environment to promote healthier lifestyle choices. One successful innovation are substance-free dorms.[18]

Drugs and Driving

One important impact of drugs is their effect on driving ability (see Chapter 17). Alcohol and drug use are equally common in drivers injured in traffic accidents. Often drivers using alcohol also test positive for other drugs. Different drugs affect driving ability in different ways. Here are the facts from the National Institute on Drug Abuse:

- Alcohol affects perception, coordination, and judgment, and increases the sedative effects of tranquilizers and barbiturates.
- Marijuana affects a wide range of driving skills—including the ability to track (stay in the lane) through curves, brake quickly, and maintain speed and a safe distance between cars—and slows thinking and reflexes. Normal driving skills remain impaired for four to six hours after smoking a single joint.
- Sedatives, hypnotics, and antianxiety agents slow reaction time, and interfere with hand–eye coordination and judgment; the greatest impairment is in the first hour after taking the drug. The effects depend on the particular drug: some build up in the body and can impair driving skills the morning after use; others make drivers very sleepy and, therefore, incapable of driving safely.
- Amphetamines, after repeated use, impair coordination. They can also make a driver more edgy and less coordinated, and thus more likely to be involved in an accident.
- Hallucinogens distort judgment and reality, and cause confusion and panic, thus making driving extremely dangerous.

Drugs on the Job

According to the National Household Survey on Drug Abuse, seven in ten illegal drug users have full-time jobs.

Workers of every variety—from truck drivers to stockbrokers—use drugs. However, young adults, men, whites, and those with less than a high school education are more likely to use drugs than other workers. At the very least, drug-abusing employees may affect their workplace by being unproductive, making poor decisions, and having strained relationships with coworkers. Even more frightening, however, is the threat to themselves and others from accidents due to their drug use.

Along with alcohol and nicotine, cocaine and marijuana are the primary drugs of abuse on or off the job. As a result of widespread drug use, the military and a growing number of companies are requiring drug tests of job applicants and employees. However, drug testing is not 100 percent precise. For example, individuals who have recently eaten poppy seeds (as in a muffin or bagel) can test positive for opiates. Increasingly, employers are shifting from policing employees to setting up programs to help those with drug problems overcome their drug dependence.

Drug use is also common among the unemployed. In particular, unemployed young adults are much more likely to use cocaine and marijuana than those who are working full-time.

Common Drugs of Abuse

The psychoactive substances most often associated with both abuse and dependence include alcohol (discussed in Chapter 15); amphetamines; cannabis (marijuana); cocaine; club drugs, hallucinogens; inhalants; opioids; phencyclidine (PCP); and sedative-hypnotic or anxiolytic (antianxiety) drugs. (See Table 14-3 on p. 492.)

Amphetamines

Amphetamines, stimulants that were once widely prescribed for weight control because they suppress appetite, have emerged as a global danger. They trigger the release of epinephrine (adrenalin), which stimulates the central nervous system. Amphetamines are sold under a variety of names: amphetamine (brand name Benzedrine, street-name "bennies"), dextroamphetamine (Dexedrine, or "dex"), methamphetamine (Methedrine, or "meth" or "speed"), and Desoxyn ("copilots"). Related *uppers* include the prescription drugs methylphenidate (Ritalin), pemoline (Cylert), and phenmetrazine (Preludin).

Amphetamines are available in tablet or capsule form. Abusers may grind and sniff the capsules, or make a solution and inject the drug. "Ice" is a smokeable form of methamphetamine that is highly addictive and produces an intense physical and psychological high that can last

▼ Table 14-3　Common Drugs of Abuse

Type of Drug	Drug Name	Street Name	Description	How It's Used	Related Paraphernalia	Signs and Symptoms of Use
Cannabis	Marijuana	Pot, grass, reefer, weed, Colombian hash, sinsemilla, joint, blunts, Acapulco Gold, Thai Sticks	Like dried oregano leaves, dark green or brown	Usually smoked in hand-rolled cigarettes, pipes, thin cigars or eaten	Rolling papers, pipes, bongs, baggies, roach clips	Sweet burnt odor, neglect of appearance, loss of motivation, slow reactions, red eyes, memory lapses
Depressants (Depress the nervous system)	Alcohol	Booze, hooch, juice, brew, Alcopops—hard lemonade or fruit juices	Clear or amber-colored liquid; sweet, fruit-flavored malt-based drinks	Swallowed in liquid form	Flask, bottles, cans, use of food color to disguise it. Colorful and innocent looking labels	Impaired judgment, poor muscle coordination, lowered inhibitions
	Barbiturates Amyl, Seconal, Nembutal, Butisol, Tuinal	Barbs, downers, yellow jackets, red devils, blue devils	Variety of tablets, capsules, powder	Swallowed in pill form or injected into the veins	Syringe, needles	Drowsiness, confusion, impaired judgment, slurred speech, needle marks, staggering gait
	Tranquilizers Valium, Librium, Miltown, Xanax	V's, blues, downers, candy	Variety of tablets	Swallowed in pill form or injected	Syringe, pill bottles, needles	Drowsiness, faulty judgment, disorientation
	Narcotics Heroin, Morphine	Dreamer, junk, smack, horse	White or brown powders, tablets, capsules, liquid	Injected, smoked, may be blended with marijuana	Syringes, spoon, lighter, needles, medicine dropper	Lethargy, loss of skin color, needle marks, constricted pupils, decreased coordination
Stimulants (Stimulate the nervous system)	Amphetamines Amphetamine, Dextroamphetamine Methamphetamine	Speed, uppers, pep pill, bennies, dexies, meth, crank, crystal, black beauties, white crosses	Variety of tablets, capsules, and crystal-like rock salt	Swallowed in pill or capsule form, or injected	Syringe, needles	Excess activity, irritability, nervousness, mood swings, needle marks, dilated pupils, talkativeness then depression
	Methylphenidate	Ritalin, MDMA Ecstasy	Tablets, imprinted logos	Crushed and sniffed	Razor blade, straws, glass surfaces	Increased alertness, excitation, insomnia, loss of appetite
	Cocaine	Coke, snow, toot, white lady	White odorless powder	Usually inhaled, can be injected, swallowed, or smoked	Razor blade, straws, glassy surfaces	Restlessness, dilated pupils, talkativeness, euphoric short-term high, followed by depression, oily skin
	Tobacco/ Nicotine	Smokes, butts, cigs, cancer sticks, snuff, dip, chew, plug	Dried brown organic material, "bidis" flavored with mint or chocolate; smokeless—moist	Tobacco is burned and inhaled as cigarettes, pipes, cigars, cigarillos; or is chewed or taken as snuff	Rolling papers, pipes, spit cups, cigar cutters, lighters, matches	Shortness of breath, respiratory illnesses, oral, lung, and other cancers

from four to fourteen hours. *Crank* is the street term for another central nervous system stimulant, propylexedrine, which is less potent than amphetamine. Abusers often extract the drug from the cotton plug of decongestant inhalants and inject it intravenously.

How Users Feel

Amphetamines produce a state of hyper-alertness and energy. Users feel confident in their ability to think clearly and to perform any task exceptionally well—although

▼ Table 14-3   Common Drugs of Abuse—continued

Type of Drug	Drug Name	Street Name	Description	How It's Used	Related Paraphernalia	Signs and Symptoms of Use
Hallucinogen (Alters perceptions of reality)	**PCP** (Phencyclidine)	Angel dust, killer weed, supergrass, hog, peace pill	White powder or tablet	Usually smoked, can be inhaled ("snorted"), injected, or swallowed in tablets	Tin foil	Slurred speech, blurred vision, lack of coordination, confusion, agitation, violence, unpredictability, "bad trips"
	LSD (Lysergic Acid Diethylamide)	Acid, cubes, purple haze, white lightning	Odorless, colorless, tasteless powder	Injected, or swallowed in tablets or capsules	Blotter papers, window panes, tin foil	Dilated pupils, illusions, hallucinations, disorientation, mood swings, nausea, flashbacks
	Mescaline caps, psilocybin, psilocin, mushrooms	Mesc, cactus, caps, magic mushroom, shrooms	Capsules, tablets, mushrooms	Ingested in their natural form or smoked, brewed as tea	Dried mushrooms	Same as LSD above
Inhalants (Substances abused by sniffing)	**Solvents, aerosols** airplane glue, gasoline, dry cleaning solution, correction fluid		Chemicals that produce mind-altering vapors	Inhaled or sniffed often with the use of paper or plastic bags	Cleaning rags, empty spray cans, tubes of glue, baggies	Poor motor coordination, bad breath, impaired vision, memory and thoughts, violent behavior
	Nitrates Amyl & Butyl	Poppers, locker room, rush, snappers	Clear yellowish liquid	Inhaled or sniffed from gauze or single dose glass vials	Cloth covered bulb that "pops" when broken, small bottles	Slowed thought, headache
	Nitrous oxide	Laughing gas, whippets	Colorless gas with sweet taste & smell	Inhaled or sniffed by mask or cone	Aerosol cans such as whipped cream, small canisters	Light-headed, loss of motor control
Club Drugs/ Designer Drugs (Stimulants, Depressants and/or Hallucinogens)	**MDMA, MDA, MDEA**	Ecstasy, XTC, X, Adam, Clarity	Tablet or capsule, colorless, tasteless and odorless	Swallowed, can be added to beverages by individuals who want to intoxicate others	Pacifiers, Glow Sticks (used at all night dance parties—"raves" or "trances")	Agitated state, confusion, sleep problems, paranoia
	Date rape drugs Rohypnol	Roofies, roche, love drug, forget-me pill	Tasteless, odorless, dissolves easily in all beverages	Swallowed, can be added to beverages by individuals who want to sedate others	Drinks, soda cans	1 mg can impair a victim for 8 to 12 hr, can cause amnesia, decreased blood pressure, urinary retention
	GHB	Liquid Ecstasy, Grievous Bodily Harm, G	Clear liquid, tablet, capsule	Swallowed, dissolved in drinks	Drinks, soda cans	Can relax or sedate

Source: "A Parent's Guide for the Prevention of Alcohol, Tobacco and Other Drug Use." © Copyright 2000 Lowe Family Foundation, Inc., Revised 2001. (Lowe Family Foundation, 3339 Stuyvesant Pl. NW, Washington DC, 20015, 202-362-4883.) Used with permission.

amphetamines do not, in fact, significantly boost performance or thinking. Higher doses make them feel "wired": talkative, excited, restless, irritable, anxious, moody.

If taken intravenously, amphetamines produce a characteristic "rush" of elation and confidence, as well as adverse effects, including confusion, rambling or incoherent speech, anxiety, headache, and palpitations. Individuals may become paranoid; be convinced they are having "profound" thoughts; feel increased sexual interest; and experience unusual perceptions, such as ringing in the ears, a sensation of insects crawling on their skin, or hearing their name called. Crank users may feel high and sleepy or may hallucinate and lose contact with reality. Methamphetamine, which produces a rapid high when inhaled, produces exceptionally long-lasting toxic effects, including psychosis, violence, seizures, and cardiovascular abnormalities. Brain-imaging studies show changes in heavy users' brains that may affect learning and memory for as long as a year.[19]

Risks

Dependence on amphetamines can develop with episodic or daily use. Users typically take amphetamines in large doses to prevent crashing. "Bingeing"—taking high doses over a period of several days—can lead to an extremely intense and unpleasant crash—characterized by a craving for the drug, shakiness, irritability, anxiety, and depression—that requires two or more days for recuperation.

Amphetamine intoxication may cause the following symptoms:

▶ Feelings of grandiosity, anxiety, tension, hypervigilance, anger, social hypersensitivity, fighting, jitteriness or agitation, paranoia, and impaired judgment in social or occupational functioning.

▶ Increased heart rate, dilated pupils, elevated blood pressure, perspiration or chills, and nausea or vomiting.

▶ Less frequent effects such as speeding up or slowing down of physical movement; muscular weakness, impaired breathing, chest pain, heart arrhythmia; confusion, seizures, impaired movements or muscle tone, or even coma.

▶ In high doses, a rapid or irregular heartbeat, tremors, loss of coordination, and collapse.

Smokeable methamphetamine, or "ice," also increases heart rate and blood pressure; high doses can cause permanent damage to blood vessels in the brain. Other physical effects of methamphetamine include dilated pupils, blurred vision, dry mouth, and increased breathing rate. Prolonged use can cause fatal lung and kidney disorders. Injecting propylexedrine can lead to convulsions, strokes, and respiratory and kidney failure. Abusers also may develop infected veins, and if they share needles, they risk HIV infection.

The long-term effects of amphetamine abuse include malnutrition; skin disorders; ulcers; insomnia; depression; vitamin deficiencies; and, in some cases, brain damage that results in speech and thought disturbances. Sexual dysfunction and impaired concentration or memory also may occur.

Withdrawal

When the immediate effects of amphetamines wear off, users experience a "crash"—they crave the drug and become shaky, irritable, anxious, and depressed. Amphetamine withdrawal usually persists for more than 24 hours after cessation of prolonged, heavy use. Its characteristic features include fatigue, disturbing dreams, much more or less than usual sleep, increased appetite, and speeding up or slowing down of physical movements. Those who are unable to sleep despite their exhaustion often take sedative-hypnotics (discussed later in this chapter) to help them rest and may become dependent on them as well as amphetamines. Symptoms usually reach a peak in two to four days, although depression and irritability may persist for months. Suicide is a major risk.

Cannabis Products

Marijuana ("pot") and **hashish**—the most widely used illegal drugs—are derived from the cannabis plant. The major psychoactive ingredient in both is *THC (delta-9-tetrahydrocannabinol)*. Nearly one of every three people in the United States over age 12 has tried marijuana at least once. Some 12 million Americans use it; more than 1 million cannot control this use.

THC triggers a series of reactions in the brain that ultimately lead to the high that users experience when they smoke marijuana. Heredity influences an individual's response to marijuana. Identical male twins, who share all their genes, are more likely than fraternal male twins, who share only about half their genes, to report similar responses to marijuana use, indicating a genetic basis for their sensations. Twins' shared or family environment before age 18 has no detectable influence on their response to marijuana.[20]

Different types of marijuana have different percentages of THC. Because of careful cultivation, the strength of today's marijuana is much greater than that used in the 1970s; the physical and mental effects are therefore greater. Usually, marijuana is smoked in a cigarette ("joint") or pipe; it may also be eaten as an ingredient in other foods (as when baked in brownies), though with a less predictable effect. The drug high is enhanced by holding the marijuana smoke in the lungs, and experienced smokers learn to hold the smoke for longer periods to increase the amount of drug diffused into the bloodstream. The circumstances in which marijuana is smoked, the communal aspects of its use, and the user's experience all can affect the way a marijuana-induced high feels.

Marijuana has been used therapeutically, primarily to ease the nausea of chemotherapy. A report from the Institute of Medicine (IOM) found "strong scientific evidence" that the active ingredients in marijuana (cannabinoids) are potentially effective in treating pain, nausea, and the severe weight loss associated with AIDS. Other studies have found that cannabinoids are more effective than conventional drugs in treating chemotherapy-related sickness, but there is no substantial proof of its effectiveness in easing pain.[21] In 2001, the American Medical Association rejected a proposal to endorse the medical use of marijuana under controlled circumstances.[22]

How Users Feel

In low to moderate doses, marijuana typically creates a mild sense of euphoria, a sense of slowed time (five minutes may feel like an hour), a dreamy sort of self-absorption, and some impairment in thinking and communicating. Users report heightened sensations of color, sound, and other stimuli, relaxation, and increased confidence. The sense of being "stoned" peaks within half an hour and usually lasts about three hours. Even when alterations in perception seem slight, as noted earlier, it is not safe to drive a car for as long as four to six hours after smoking a single joint. Some users—particularly those smoking marijuana for the first time or taking a high dose in an unpleasant or unfamiliar setting—experience acute anxiety, which may be accompanied by a panicky fear of losing control. They may believe that their companions are ridiculing or threatening them and experience a panic attack, a state of intense terror.

The immediate physical effects of marijuana include increased pulse rate, bloodshot eyes, dry mouth and throat, slowed reaction times, impaired motor skills, increased appetite, and diminished short-term memory (see Figure 14-4). High doses reduce the ability to perceive and to react; all the reactions experienced with low doses are intensified, leading to sensory distortion and—in the case of hashish—vivid hallucinations and LSD-like psychedelic reactions. The drug remains in the body's fat cells 50 hours or more after use, so people may experience psychoactive effects for several days after use. Drug tests may produce positive results for days or weeks after last use.

Risks

Marijuana produces a range of effects in different bodily systems, such as diminished immune responses and impaired fertility in men. Others include effects on the brain, lungs, and heart and on babies born to mothers who use marijuana.

Brain. THC produces changes in the brain that affect learning, memory, and the way in which the brain integrates sensory experiences with emotions and motivations. Short-term effects include problems with memory and learning; distorted perceptions; difficulty in thinking and problem-solving; loss of coordination; increased anxiety; and panic attacks. Long-term use produces changes in the brain similar to those seen with other major drugs of abuse.[23]

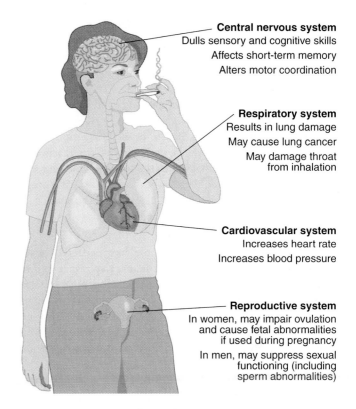

Central nervous system
Dulls sensory and cognitive skills
Affects short-term memory
Alters motor coordination

Respiratory system
Results in lung damage
May cause lung cancer
May damage throat
from inhalation

Cardiovascular system
Increases heart rate
Increases blood pressure

Reproductive system
In women, may impair ovulation
and cause fetal abnormalities
if used during pregnancy
In men, may suppress sexual
functioning (including
sperm abnormalities)

▲ **Figure 14-4** Some effects of long-term marijuana use on the body.

According to a study of college students, heavy marijuana use impairs critical skills related to attention, memory, and learning, even 24 hours after its use. "Heavy" users who smoked marijuana almost every day showed significant difficulty in sustaining attention, shifting attention to meet the demands of changes in the environment, and registering, processing, and using information.[24]

Teenagers below college age who use marijuana have lower achievement than nonusers, more acceptance of illegal or socially deviant behavior, more aggression, greater rebelliousness, poorer relationships with parents, and more delinquent and drug-using friends. Those who smoke marijuana regularly often lose interest in school and do not remember what they learned when they were high. Some long-term regular users may experience *burnout,* a dulling of their senses and responses termed *amotivational syndrome.*

Over time, continued heavy marijuana use can interfere with students' ability to learn and perform well in school and in challenging careers. Marijuana contributes significantly to accidental death and injury among adolescents, especially through motor vehicle crashes.

Lungs. Regular marijuana smokers have many of the same respiratory problems as tobacco smokers, including daily cough and phlegm, chronic bronchitis, and more frequent chest colds. The amount of tar inhaled by marijuana smokers and the level of carbon monoxide absorbed are three to five times greater than among tobacco smokers. The reason may be that marijuana users inhale more deeply and hold the smoke in the lungs and because marijuana smoke is unfiltered.

Chronic use can also lead to bronchitis, emphysema, and lung cancer. Smoking a single "joint," or marijuana cigarette, can be as damaging to the lungs as smoking five tobacco cigarettes. Frequent use of marijuana during pregnancy can lower birthweight and cause abnormalities in the fetus similar to those of fetal alcohol syndrome.

Heart. Otherwise healthy people have suffered heart attacks shortly after smoking marijuana. Experiments have also linked marijuana use to elevated blood pressure and decreased oxygen supply to the heart muscle. According to recent estimates, the risk of heart attack triples within an hour of smoking pot.[25] Smoking marijuana while shooting cocaine can potentially cause deadly increases in heart rate and blood pressure.[26]

Pregnancy. Babies born to mothers who use marijuana during pregnancy are smaller than those born to mothers who did not use the drug, and the babies are more likely to develop health problems.[27] A nursing mother who uses marijuana passes some of the THC to the baby in her breast milk. This may impair the infant's motor development (control of muscle movement).

Withdrawal

Marijuana users can develop a compulsive, often uncontrollable craving for the drug. More than 120,000 people enter treatment every year for marijuana addiction. In addition, animal studies suggest that marijuana causes physical dependence. Stopping after long-term marijuana use can produce "marijuana withdrawal syndrome," which is characterized by insomnia, restlessness, loss of appetite, and irritability. People who smoked marijuana daily for many years also may become aggressive after they stop using it and may relapse to prevent aggression and other symptoms.

Cocaine

Cocaine ("coke," "snow," "lady") is a white crystalline powder extracted from the leaves of the South American coca plant. Usually mixed with various sugars and local anesthetics like lidocaine and procaine, cocaine powder is generally inhaled. When sniffed or snorted, cocaine anesthetizes the nerve endings in the nose and relaxes the lung's bronchial muscles.

Cocaine can be dissolved in water and injected intravenously. The drug is rapidly metabolized by the liver, so the high is relatively brief, typically lasting only about 20 minutes. This means that users will commonly inject the drug repeatedly, increasing the risk of infection and damage to their veins. Many intravenous cocaine users prefer the practice of *speedballing*, the intravenous administration of a combination of cocaine and heroin.

Cocaine alkaloid—or *freebase*—is obtained by removing the hydrochloride salt from cocaine powder. "Freebasing" is smoking the fumes of the alkaloid form of cocaine. *Crack*, pharmacologically identical to freebase, is a cheap, easy-to-use, widely available, smokeable, and potent form of cocaine named for the popping sound it makes when burned. Because it is absorbed rapidly into the bloodstream and large doses reach the brain very quickly, it is particularly dangerous. However, its low price and easy availability have made it a common drug of abuse in poor urban areas.

How Users Feel

A powerful stimulant to the central nervous system, cocaine produces feelings of soaring well-being and boundless energy. This may be because cocaine targets, not one, but several chemical sites in the brain. Users feel that they have enormous physical and mental ability, yet are also restless and anxious. After a brief period of euphoria, users slump into a depression. They often go on cocaine binges, lasting from a few hours to several days, and consume large quantities of cocaine.

With crack, dependence develops quickly. As soon as crack users come down from one high, they want more crack. Whereas heroin addicts may shoot up several times a day, crack addicts need another hit within minutes. Thus, a crack habit can quickly become more expensive than heroin addiction. Some "crackheads" have $1,000-a-day habits. Police in big cities have traced many brutal crimes and murders to young crack addicts, who often are extremely paranoid and dangerous. Smoking crack doused with liquid PCP, a practice known as *space-basing*, has especially frightening effects on behavior.

With continuing use, cocaine users experience less pleasure and more unpleasant effects. Eventually they may reach a point at which they no longer experience euphoric effects and crave the drug simply to alleviate their persistent hunger for it. They think about it constantly, dream about it, spend all their money on it, and borrow, steal, or deal to pay for it. They cannot concentrate on work; they become increasingly irritable and confused. They may also become dependent on alcohol, sedatives, or opioids, which they use to calm down from cocaine's aftereffects.

Risks

Cocaine dependence is an easy habit to acquire. With repeated use, the brain becomes tolerant of the drug's stimulant effects, and users must take more of it to get high. Its grip is strong. Those who smoke or inject cocaine can develop dependence within weeks. Those who sniff cocaine may not become dependent on the drug for months or years. It is thought that 5 to 20 percent of all coke users—a group as large as the estimated total number of heroin addicts—are dependent on the drug.

The physical effects of acute cocaine intoxication include dilated pupils, elevated or lowered blood pressure, perspiration or chills, nausea or vomiting, speeding up or slowing down of physical activity, muscular weakness, impaired breathing, chest pain, and impaired movements or muscle tone. Prolonged cocaine snorting can result in ulceration of the mucous membrane of the nose and can damage the nasal septum (the membrane between the nostrils) enough to cause it to collapse.

Although some users initially try cocaine as a sexual stimulant, it does not enhance sexual performance. At low doses, it may delay ejaculation and orgasm and cause heightened sensory awareness, but men who use cocaine regularly have problems maintaining erections and ejaculating. They also tend to have low sperm counts, less active sperm, and more abnormal sperm than nonusers. Both male and female chronic cocaine users tend to lose interest in sex and have difficulty in reaching orgasm.

Cocaine use can cause blood vessels in the brain to clamp shut and can trigger a stroke, bleeding in the brain, and potentially fatal brain seizures. Cocaine users can also develop psychiatric or neurological complications (Figure 14-5). Repeated or high doses of cocaine can lead to impaired judgment, hyperactivity, nonstop babbling, feelings of suspicion and paranoia, and violent behavior. The brain never learns to tolerate cocaine's negative effects; users may become incoherent and paranoid and may experience unusual sensations, such as ringing in their ears, feeling insects crawling on the skin, or hearing their name called.

Cocaine can damage the liver and cause lung damage in freebasers. Smoking crack causes bronchitis as well as lung damage and may promote the transmission of HIV through burned and bleeding lips. Some smokers have died of respiratory complications, such as pulmonary edema (the buildup of fluid in the lungs).

Cocaine causes the heart rate to speed up and blood pressure to rise suddenly. Its use is associated with many cardiac complications, including arrhythmia (disruption of heart rhythm), angina (chest pain), and acute myocardial infarction (heart attack). These cardiac complications can lead to sudden death.[28] Cocaine-induced elevations in blood pressure can lead to kidney failure.

Cocaine users who inject the drug and share needles put themselves at risk for another potentially lethal problem: HIV infection. Other complications of injecting cocaine include skin infections, hepatitis, inflammation of the arteries, and infection of the lining of the heart.

The most common ways of dying from cocaine use are persistent seizures that result in respiratory collapse, cardiac arrest from arrhythmias, myocardial infarction, and intracranial hemorrhage or stroke. The combination of alcohol and cocaine is particularly lethal. Alcohol and cocaine together are second only to the combination of heroin and alcohol in causing deaths related to substance abuse. When people mix cocaine and alcohol, they compound the danger each drug poses. The human liver combines the two agents and manufactures a third substance, cocaethylene, which intensifies cocaine's euphoric effects, while possibly increasing the risk of sudden death.[29]

Cocaine is dangerous for pregnant women and their babies, causing miscarriages, developmental disorders, and life-threatening complications during birth. Women who use the drug while pregnant are more likely to miscarry in the first three months of pregnancy than women who do not use drugs or who use heroin and other opioids. When used early in pregnancy, cocaine can reduce the fetal oxygen supply, possibly interfering with the development of the fetus's nervous system. Infants born to cocaine and crack users can suffer withdrawal and may have major complications, or permanent disabilities. Cocaine babies have higher-than-normal rates of respiratory and kidney troubles, visual problems, and developmental retardation and may be at greater risk of sudden infant death syndrome.

Central nervous system
Repeated use or high dosages may cause severe psychological problems
Suppresses desire for food, sex, and sleep
Can cause strokes, seizures, and neurological damage

Cardiovascular system
Increases blood pressure by constricting blood vessels
Causes irregular heartbeat
Damages heart tissue

Respiratory system
Freebasing causes lung damage
Overdose can lead to respiratory arrest

Reproductive system
In men, affects ability to maintain erections and ejaculate; also causes sperm abnormalities
In women, may affect ability to carry pregnancy to term

Nose
Damages mucous membrane

▲ **Figure 14-5** Some effects of cocaine on the body.

Withdrawal

When addicted individuals stop using cocaine, they often become depressed. This may lead to further cocaine use to alleviate depression. Other symptoms of cocaine withdrawal include fatigue, vivid and disturbing dreams, excessive or too little sleep, irritability, increased appetite, and physical slowing down or speeding up. This initial crash may last one to three days after cutting down or stopping the heavy use of cocaine. Some individuals become violent, paranoid, and suicidal.

Symptoms usually reach a peak in two to four days, although depression, anxiety, irritability, lack of pleasure in usual activities, and low-level cravings may continue for weeks. As memories of the crash fade, the desire for cocaine intensifies. For many weeks after stopping, individuals may feel an intense craving for the drug. Experimental medical approaches for treating cocaine dependence include antidepressant drugs, anticonvulsant drugs, and the naturally occurring amino acids tryptophan and tyrosine. However, these have only limited benefit, and much more research into medical treatments is needed. Recent research has found that, depending on personal characteristics such as abstract reasoning ability and religious motivation, some cocaine abusers fare better with cognitive-behavioral therapy (discussed in Chapter 3); others, with 12-step programs.[30]

Club Drugs

Club drugs include MDMA (ecstasy), GHB, GBL, ketamine (Special-K), fentanyl, Rohypnol, amphetamines, methamphetamine, and LSD. (See Table 14-3.) Their primary users are teens and young adults at nightclubs, bars, and rave or trance events, night-long dances often held in warehouses. They try these low-cost drugs to increase their stamina and experience a high that supposedly deepens the rave or trance experience.

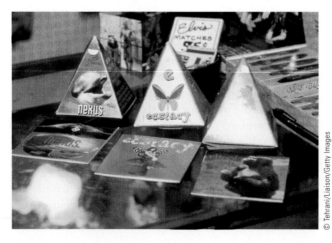

▲ Club drugs, made in the laboratory and sold on the street, aren't subject to quality controls and don't always contain what the buyer expects.

© Tehrani/Liaison/Getty Images

Some club drugs are legal and have legitimate medical uses. They include gamma hydroxybutyrate, or GHB, a depressant with potential benefits for people with narcolepsy, and Rohypnol, a tranquilizer used overseas that also can be slipped into women's drinks to knock them out and cause short-term amnesia (see Chapter 17 for a discussion of "date rape" drugs). Since the drugs are odorless and tasteless, a woman has no way of knowing whether her drink has been tampered with; the subsequent loss of memory leaves her with no explanation for where she's been or what's happened in the hours before she regains consciousness.

Although users may think of ecstasy and other club drugs as harmless and "fun," they can produce a range of unwanted effects, including hallucinations, paranoia, amnesia, and, in some cases, death. When used with alcohol, these drugs can be even more harmful because they involve the same brain mechanism. Also, there are great differences among individuals in how they react to club drugs. Some people have been known to have extreme, even fatal, reactions the first time they use club drugs. Club drugs found in party settings are often adulterated or impure and thus even more dangerous.[31]

Ecstasy

Ecstasy is a street name for methylenedioxymethamphetamine or MDMA, a synthetic compound with both stimulant and mildly hallucinogenic properties. Ecstasy is the only illicit drug whose use has been increasing substantially, particularly among young people. Use of ecstasy by teenagers has risen to what pediatricians describe as "epidemic" levels.[32] According to the federal government's National Household Survey, 8 percent of high school seniors took ecstasy at least once in the previous year. More college-age young adults are also trying ecstasy.[33]

Once used mostly by affluent white Americans, ecstasy is spreading into different racial, ethnic, and economic groups. More young people are using ecstasy, not just in clubs or at raves, but on a regular basis. In many big cities, ecstasy has become one of the most common causes of drug emergencies.

How It Feels. Although it can be smoked, inhaled (snorted), or injected, ecstasy is almost always taken as a pill or tablet. Its effects begin in 45 minutes and last for two to four hours.

MDMA belongs to a family of drugs called *enactogens*, which literally means "touching within." As a mood elevator, it produces a relaxed, euphoric state but does not produce hallucinations. Users of ecstasy often say they feel at peace with themselves and at ease and empathic with others. In some settings, they reveal intimate details of their lives (which they may later regret); in other settings, they join in collective rejoicing. Like hallucinogenic drugs, MDMA can enhance sensory experience, but it rarely causes visual distortions, sudden mood changes, or psychotic reactions. Regular users may experience depression and anxiety during the week after taking MDMA.

Psychologists have experimented with MDMA as a way to enhance self-revelation, self-criticism, and self-exploration and boost trust between a patient and a therapist. Most clinicians are highly skeptical of its benefits, and there has been no officially sanctioned research on its therapeutic benefits.[34]

Risks. Ecstasy poses risks similar to those of cocaine and amphetamines. These include psychological difficulties (confusion, depression, sleep problems, drug craving, severe anxiety, and paranoia) and physical symptoms (muscle tension, involuntary teeth clenching, nausea, blurred vision, rapid eye movement, faintness, chills, sweating, and increases in heart rate and blood pressure that pose a special risk for people with circulatory or heart disease).[35]

Like amphetamine, ecstasy affects brain receptors for the neurotransmitter dopamine; like LSD, mescaline, and other hallucinogens, it affects receptors for the neurotransmitter serotonin.[36] Repeated use may result in lasting neurological changes in the brain. According to brain-imaging studies, users, although as mentally alert as nonusers, fared far worse on measures of memory, learning, and general intelligence. The more frequently they took ecstasy, the worse they did. This is likely because ecstasy alters neuronal function in a brain structure called the hippocampus, which helps create short-term memory.[37] (See Figure 14-6). Other experiments have shown increased impulsiveness and attention deficits in MDMA users.

MDMA can produce nausea, vomiting, and dizziness. When combined with extended physical exertion like dancing, club drugs can lead to hyperthermia (severe overheating), severe dehydration, serious increases in blood pressure, stroke, and heart attack. Without sufficient water, dancers at raves may suffer dehydration and heat stroke, which can be fatal. Individuals with high blood pressure, heart trouble, or liver or kidney disease are in the greatest danger.[38]

MDMA has been implicated in some cases of acute hepatitis, which can lead to liver failure. Even after liver transplantation, the mortality rate for individuals with this condition is 50 percent.[39] Another danger comes from the practice of taking Prozac, a drug that modulates the mood-altering brain chemical serotonin, before ecstasy. This can cause jaw clenching, nausea, tremors, and in extreme cases, potentially fatal elevations in body temperature. Several deaths have occurred in teens who suffered brain damage by drinking too much water (MDMA users typically drink large amounts of water to counteract the raised body temperature induced by the drug).

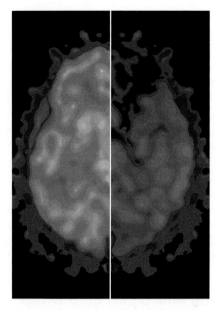

▲ **Figure 14-6** Effects of ecstasy on the brain. These brain scans show the sharp difference in human brain function for an individual who has never used drugs and one who used the club drug ecstasy many times but had not used any drugs for at least three weeks before the scan. In the left scan, the bright reddish color shows active serotonin sites in the brain. Serotonin is a critical neurochemical that regulates mood, emotion, learning, memory, sleep, and pain. In the right scan, the dark sections indicate areas where serotonin is not present even after three weeks without any drugs.

Source: www.clubdrugs.org.

Ecstasy also can pose risks to a developing fetus, including a greater likelihood of heart and skeletal abnormalities and long-term learning and memory impairments in children born to women who used MDMA during pregnancy.[40]

Although not a sexual stimulant (if anything, MDMA has the opposite effect), ecstasy fosters strong feelings of intimacy that may lead to risky sexual behavior. The psychological effects of ecstasy become less intriguing with repeated use, and the physical side effects become more uncomfortable.

GHB and GBL

The brain messenger chemical called **GHB (gammahydroxybutyrate)** stimulates the release of human growth hormone but has no known effects on muscle growth. Although this substance is banned by the FDA, users obtain it illegally either for its high, which is similar to that caused by alcohol or marijuana, or for its alleged ability to trim fat and build muscles.[41]

The main ingredient is **GBL (gamma butyrolactone),** an industrial solvent often used to strip floors. Once ingested,

GBL converts into GHB, an odorless, colorless sedative that can be slipped into a beverage to knock an individual out.

In small doses, GHB and GBL are believed to induce euphoria and enhance sex by increasing dopamine in the brain. However, a larger dose can cause someone to pass out in 15 minutes and fall into a coma within half an hour. Other side effects include nausea, amnesia, hallucinations, decreased heart rate, convulsions, and sometimes blackouts. Long-term use at high doses can lead to a withdrawal reaction: rapid heartbeat, tremor, insomnia, anxiety, and occasionally hallucinations that last a few days to a week.[42] According to the Drug Enforcement Administration, the use of GHB has been associated with more than 5,700 reported overdoses and at least 66 deaths, mainly from respiratory depression. The danger is greatest when mixed with alcohol or opiates.[43]

Ketamine and Other Club Drugs

"K," or ketamine, is an anesthetic used by veterinarians. When cooked, dried, and ground into a powder for snorting, K blocks chemical messengers in the brain that carry sensory input. As a result, the brain fills the void with hallucinations. Too much K can cause such massive sensory deprivation that researchers compare the impact to a near-death experience.

Another synthetic, developed by college students in Pennsylvania in the early 1990s, is *methcathinone*, or "cat," a powerful synthetic stimulant that can produce a high that lasts up to six days. Cat usually contains a mix of chemicals along with small doses of Drano or battery acid, which act as a catalyst.

College and street chemists have also produced synthetic opiates that are particularly dangerous because they're far more potent than those derived from natural substances. Derivatives of *fentanyl*, an anesthetic widely used for surgery in the United States, are 20 to 2,000 times as powerful as heroin, and the risk of a fatal overdose or brain damage is much greater.

"Herbal" drugs also are being marketed as substitutes for standard street drugs. With names such as "herbal ecstasy," "nexus," and "ritual spirit," these tablets and capsules are advertised as safe and potent agents that can lead to "sacred visions," "tingly happy-happy buzz," and better sex. However, critics warn that the herbal pills have dangerous and unpleasant side effects, including stroke, heart attack, and a disfiguring skin condition. They are sold at head shops, night clubs, and raves. The FDA has been investigating these agents, after receiving hundreds of complaints of strokes, seizures, and possibly even some deaths.

Hallucinogens

The drugs known as **hallucinogens** produce vivid and unusual changes in thought, feeling, and perception. The most widely used in the United States is *LSD (lysergic acid diethylamide,* or "acid"), which was initially developed as a tool to explore mental illness. It became popular in the 1960s and resurfaced among teenagers in the 1990s. LSD is taken orally, either blotted onto pieces of paper that are held in the mouth or chewed along with another substance, such as a sugar cube. Much less commonly used in this country is *peyote* (whose active ingredient is *mescaline*).

How Users Feel

LSD produces hallucinations, including bright colors and altered perceptions of reality. Effects from a single dose begin within 30 to 60 minutes and last 10 to 12 hours. During this time, there are slight increases in body temperature, heart rate, and blood pressure; sweating, chills, and goose pimples appear. Some users develop headache and nausea. Mescaline produces vivid hallucinations—including brightly colored lights, animals, and geometric designs—within 30 to 90 minutes of consumption. These effects may persist for 12 hours.

The effects of hallucinogens depend greatly on the dose, the individual's expectations and personality, and the setting for drug use. Many users report religious or mystical imagery and thoughts; some feel they are experiencing profound insights. Usually the user realizes that perceptual changes are caused by the hallucinogen, but some become convinced that they have lost their minds. Drugs sold as hallucinogens are frequently mixed with other drugs, such as PCP and amphetamines, which can produce unexpected and frightening effects.

Hallucinogens do not produce dependence in the same way as cocaine or heroin. Individuals who have an unpleasant experience after trying a hallucinogen may stop using the drugs completely without suffering withdrawal symptoms. Others continue regular or occasional use because they enjoy the effects.

Risks

Physical symptoms include dilated pupils, rapid heart rate, sweating, heart palpitations, blurring of vision, tremors, and poor coordination. These effects may last 8 to 12 hours. Hallucinogen intoxication also produces changes in emotions and mood, such as anxiety, depression, fear of losing one's mind, and impaired judgment.

LSD can trigger irrational acts. LSD users have injured or killed themselves by jumping out of windows, swimming out to sea, or throwing themselves in front of cars. Some individuals develop a delusional disorder, in which they become convinced that their distorted perceptions and thoughts are real. They may experience flashbacks (re-experiencing symptoms felt while intoxicated), which include geometric hallucinations, flashes of color, halos around objects, and other perceptual changes.

Individuals having a "bad trip" may blame themselves and feel excessively guilty, tense, and so agitated that they cannot stop talking and have trouble sleeping. They may fear that they have destroyed their brains and will never return to normal. Someone who already is depressed may take a hallucinogen to lift his or her spirits, only to become more depressed. Suicide is a real danger.

Inhalants

Inhalants or **deleriants** are chemicals that produce vapors with psychoactive effects. The most commonly abused inhalants are solvents, aerosols, model-airplane glue, cleaning fluids, and petroleum products like kerosene and butane. Some anesthetics and nitrous oxide (laughing gas) are also abused. Almost 21 percent of eighth graders surveyed have used household products, such as glue, solvents, and aerosols, to get high.[44]

To inhale intoxicating vapors, individuals soak a rag in the substance, place it against the mouth and nose, and inhale; or inhale fumes from a substance placed in a paper or plastic bag; or inhale vapors directly from their containers. Young people, especially those who may not have money for or access to other drugs, are those most likely to try inhalants. Children between the ages of 9 to 13 tend to use inhalants with a group of peers who are likely to use alcohol and marijuana as well. Users are in all racial, socioeconomic, and gender groups, but the incidence of use is higher among poor minority youth than among others. Many users come from families that have separated or been affected by alcohol or drug problems; they often have school difficulties, such as truancy and poor grades, or problems adjusting to work.

How Users Feel

Inhalants reach the lungs, bloodstream, and other parts of the body very rapidly. At low doses, users may feel slightly stimulated; at higher doses, they may feel less inhibited. Intoxication often occurs within five minutes and can last more than an hour. Inhalant users do not report the intense rush associated with other drugs, nor do they experience the perceptual changes associated with LSD. However, inhalants interfere with thinking and impulse control, so users may act in dangerous or destructive ways.

Often there are visible external signs of use: a rash around the nose and mouth; breath odors; residue on face, hands, and clothing; redness, swelling, and tearing of the eyes; and irritation of throat, lungs and nose that leads to coughing and gagging. Nausea and headache also may occur.

Risks

Regular use of inhalants leads to tolerance, so that the sniffer needs more and more to attain the desired effects.

Younger children who use inhalants several times a week may develop dependence. Older users who become dependent may use the drugs many times a day. Those who become dependent on inhalants are likely to have used many different substances as adolescents, and to have gradually turned to inhalants as their preferred substance.

Although some young people believe inhalants are safe to use, this is far from true. Inhalation of butane from cigarette lighters displaces oxygen in the lungs, causing suffocation. Users also can suffocate while covering their heads with a plastic bag to inhale the substance, or from inhaling vomit into their lungs while high. According to the International Institute on Inhalant Abuse, the effects of inhalants are unpredictable, and even a single episode could trigger asphyxiation or cardiac arrhythmia, leading to disability or death. Abusers also can develop difficulties with memory, with abstract reasoning, problems with coordination, and with uncontrollable movements of the extremities.[45]

Opioids

The **opioids** include *opium* and its derivatives (that is, *morphine, codeine,* and *heroin*) and nonopioid synthetic drugs that have similar sleep-inducing and pain-relieving properties. The opioids come from a resin taken from the seed pod of the Asian poppy. **Nonopioids,** such as *meperidine* (Demerol), *methadone,* and *propoxyphene* (Darvon), are chemically synthesized. These drugs are powerful narcotics, or painkillers.

Heroin, the most widely abused opioid, is illegal in this country. In other nations it is used as a potent painkiller for conditions such as terminal cancer. There are an estimated 600,000 heroin addicts in the United States, with men outnumbering women addicts by three to one.

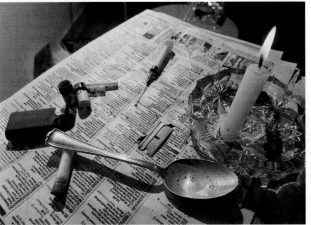

▲ Opioid drugs, made from the Asian poppy, come in both legal and illegal forms. In any form, these substances can readily become addictive.

© Roy Morsch/Corbis Stock Market

The number of young adults who use heroin is growing in suburban and rural areas, according to the CDC. Among people aged 18 to 25, the percentage of heroin users who inject the drug has doubled in the last decade. While the number of young heroin users in major cities has dropped by 50 percent, their numbers almost tripled in suburban and rural areas.[46]

Morphine, used as a painkiller and anesthetic, acts primarily on the central nervous system, eyes, and digestive tract and masks pain by producing mental clouding, drowsiness, and euphoria. It does not decrease the physical sensation of pain as much as it alters a person's awareness of the pain; in effect, he or she no longer cares about it.

Two semisynthetic derivatives of morphine are *hydromorphone* (trade name Dilaudid, or "little D"), with two to eight times the painkilling effect of morphine, and *oxycodone* (Oxycontin, Percocet, Percodan, or "perkies"), similar to codeine but more potent. The synthetic narcotic *meperidine* (Demerol, or "demies") is now probably second only to morphine for use in relieving pain. It is also used by addicts as a substitute for morphine or heroin.

Codeine is a weaker painkiller and sedative than morphine. It is an ingredient in liquid products prescribed for relieving coughs and in tablet and injectable form for relieving pain. The synthetic narcotic *propoxyphene* (Darvon) is a somewhat less potent painkiller than codeine—no more effective than aspirin in usual doses. It has been one of the most widely prescribed drugs for headaches, dental pain, and menstrual cramps. At higher doses, Darvon produces a euphoric high, which may lead to misuse.

Prescription opioids are taken orally in pill form but can also be injected intravenously. Heroin users typically inject the drug into their veins. However, individuals who experiment with recreational drugs often prefer *skin-popping* (subcutaneous injection) rather than *mainlining* (intravenous injection); they also may snort heroin as a powder, or dissolve it and inhale the vapors. To try to avoid addiction, some users begin by *chipping*, taking small or intermittent doses. Regardless of the method of administration, tolerance can develop rapidly.

Some individuals first take a medically prescribed opioid for pain relief or cough suppression, then gradually increase the dose and frequency of use on their own, often justifying this because of their symptoms rather than for the sensations the drug induces. They expend increasing efforts to obtain the drug, frequently seeking out several doctors to write prescriptions.

How Users Feel

All the opioids relax the user. When injected, they can produce an immediate "rush," or high, that lasts 10 to 30 minutes. For two to six hours thereafter, users may feel indifferent, lethargic, and drowsy; they may slur their speech and have problems paying attention, remembering, and going about their normal routine. The primary attractions of heroin ("horse," "junk," "smack," or "downtown") are the euphoria and pain relief it produces. However, some people experience very unpleasant feelings, such as anxiety and fear. Other effects include a sensation of warmth or heaviness, dry mouth, facial flushing, and nausea and vomiting (particularly in first-time users).

Some addicts report a rush when heroin is injected directly into their veins. Since the effects of heroin do not last long—usually only two to four hours—addicts have to "shoot up" two to five times a day. With large doses, the pupils become smaller; and the skin becomes cold, moist, and bluish. Breathing slows down; the user cannot be awakened and may stop breathing completely.

Risks

Addiction is common. Almost all regular users of opioids rapidly develop drug dependence, which can lead to lethargy, weight loss, loss of sex drive, and the continual effort to avoid withdrawal symptoms through repeated drug administration. In addition, they experience anxiety, insomnia, restlessness, and craving for the drug. Users continue taking opioids as much to avoid the discomfort of withdrawal—a classic sign of addiction—as to experience pleasure.

Opioid intoxication is characterized by changes in mood and behavior, such as initial euphoria followed by apathy or discontent and impaired judgment. Physical symptoms include constricted pupils (although pupils may dilate from a severe overdose), drowsiness, slurred speech, and impaired attention or memory. Morphine affects blood pressure, heart rate, and blood circulation in the brain. Both morphine and heroin slow down—depress—the respiratory system; overdoses can cause fatal respiratory arrest.

Opioid poisoning or overdose causes shock, coma, and depressed respiration and can be fatal. Emergency medical treatment is critical, often with drugs called narcotic antagonists that rapidly reverse the effects of opioids when administered intravenously.

Over time, users who inject opioids may develop infections of the heart lining and valves, skin abscesses, and lung congestion. Infections from unsterile solutions, syringes, and shared needles can lead to hepatitis, tetanus, liver disease, and HIV transmission. Depression is common and may be both an antecedent and risk factor for needle-sharing. The annual death rate among those dependent on opioids is 20 times higher than among other young people, primarily because of physical complications, overdose, suicide, and the violent lifestyle of many users. A long-term study that followed 581 heroin addicts for more than 33 years found that nearly half died in that time period, most in their forties and fifties. About 40 percent of the survivors had used heroin in the last year, while many used other illicit drugs.[47]

Withdrawal

If a regular user stops taking an opioid, withdrawal begins within 6 to 12 hours. The intensity of the symptoms depends on the degree of the addiction; they may grow stronger for 24 to 72 hours and gradually subside over a period of 7 to 14 days, though some symptoms, such as insomnia, may persist for several months. Individuals may develop craving for an opioid, irritability, nausea or vomiting, muscle aches, runny nose or eyes, dilated pupils, sweating, diarrhea, yawning, fever, and insomnia. Desperately craving the drug, users may plead, demand, or manipulate others to obtain more. Opioid withdrawal usually is not life-threatening.

Methadone Maintenance

Opioid dependence is a very difficult addiction to overcome. Studies demonstrate that only 10 to 30 percent of heroin users are able to maintain abstinence. This fact contributed to the development of a unique, yet still controversial, treatment for opioid dependence: the use of methadone, a long-acting opioid that users can substitute for heroin or other opioids.[48]

Methadone is used in two basic ways to treat opioid dependence: as an opioid substitute for detoxification, usually with a gradual tapering of methadone over a period of

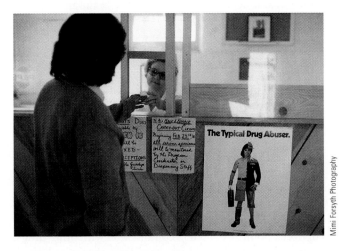

Mimi Forsyth Photography

▲ Methadone treatment has been criticized as a treatment for opioid addiction, but research clearly demonstrates positive benefits. Those who participate in long-term methadone maintenance programs usually move out of the drug culture and are candidates for eventually leaving methadone dependence behind them.

21 to 180 days, and as a maintenance treatment. Methadone maintenance has been criticized by some as nothing more than the substitution of a legal opioid, methadone, for an illegal opioid, heroin. Critics charge that since methadone maintenance does not have abstinence as its goal, it contributes to continued use of other drugs, such as cocaine or alcohol. There also is concern, especially by those in law enforcement, that methadone recipients will engage in "diversion," the sale of take-home doses of methadone for profit. Despite these charges, methadone maintenance remains the mainstay of opioid dependence treatment and is the most successful treatment currently available, whether offered by government programs or physicians in their offices.[49]

Methadone maintenance may be the most thoroughly studied drug treatment. Research has clearly documented several important positive benefits, including decreased use of illicit opioids; decreased criminal behavior; decreased risk of contracting HIV infection (through sharing of infected needles); and improvements in physical health, employment, and other lifestyle factors. Individuals who have been on methadone maintenance for a long time (often years), have stable relationships and employment, have assimilated themselves into the nondrug culture, and are highly motivated to get off methadone have the best chance for successful detoxification from methadone.

Phencyclidine (PCP)

PCP (phencyclidine—brand name Sernyl; street names "angel dust," "peace pill," "lovely," and "green")—is an illicit drug manufactured as a tablet, capsule, liquid, flake, spray, or crystal-like white powder that can be swallowed, smoked, sniffed, or injected. Sometimes it is sprinkled on crack, marijuana, tobacco, or parsley, and smoked. A fine-powdered form of PCP can be snorted or injected. Once PCP was thought to have medicinal value as an anesthetic, but its side effects, including delirium and hallucinations, made it unacceptable for medical use.

PCP use peaked in the 1970s, but it remains a popular drug of abuse in both inner-city ghettos and suburban high schools. Often users think that it is the PCP that they take together with another illegal psychoactive substance, such as amphetamines, coke, or hallucinogens, that is responsible for the highs they feel, so they seek it out specifically.

How Users Feel

The effects of PCP are utterly unpredictable. It may trigger violent behavior or irreversible psychosis the first time it is used, or the twentieth time, or never. In low doses, PCP produces changes—from hallucinations to euphoria to feelings of emptiness or numbness—similar to those produced by other psychoactive drugs. Higher doses may produce a stupor that lasts several days, increased heart rate and blood pressure, flushing, sweating, dizziness, and numbness.

Risks

Some first-time users feel PCP is too unpredictable and do not try it again. Others quickly become heavy users. Many go on PCP binges or runs that can last several days. Some people use it daily, often along with alcohol and marijuana. It takes only a short period of occasional use for dependence or abuse to develop.

The behavioral changes associated with PCP intoxication, which can develop within minutes, include belligerence, aggressiveness, impulsiveness, unpredictability, agitation, poor judgment, and impaired functioning at work or in social situations. The physical symptoms of PCP intoxication include involuntary eye movements, increased blood pressure or heart rate, numbness or diminished responsiveness to pain, impaired coordination and speech, muscle rigidity, seizures, and a painful sensitivity to sound. Some people experience repetitive motor movements, such as facial grimacing, hallucinations, and paranoia. Suicide is a definite risk. Intoxication typically lasts four to six hours, but some effects can linger for several days. Delirium may occur within 24 hours of taking PCP or after recovery from an overdose and can last as much as a week.

PCP can trigger an episode of depression or anxiety that may persist for months. Some users reproach themselves constantly in the fear that they have destroyed their brains and will never return to normal. Some feel so restless that they cannot stop talking; some think they have superhuman strength. Large amounts can lead to convulsions, coma, heart and lung failure, ruptured blood vessels in the brain, and death.

Sedative-Hypnotics or Anxiolytic (Antianxiety) Drugs

These drugs depress the central nervous system, reduce activity, and induce relaxation, drowsiness, or sleep. They include the benzodiazepines and the barbiturates.

The **benzodiazepines**—the most widely used drugs in this category—are commonly prescribed for tension, muscular strain, sleep problems, anxiety, panic attacks, anesthesia, and in the treatment of alcohol withdrawal. They include such drugs as *chlordiazepoxide* (Librium), *diazepam* (Valium), *oxazepam* (Serax), *lorazepam* (Ativan), *flurazepam* (Dalmane), and *alprazolam* (Xanax). They differ widely in their mechanism of action, absorption rate,

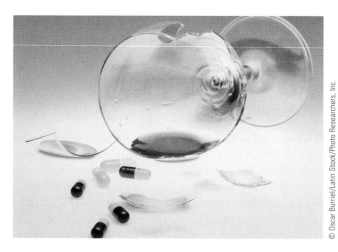

▲ Antianxiety drugs react dangerously with alcohol.

and metabolism, but all produce similar intoxication and withdrawal symptoms.

Benzodiazepine sleeping pills have largely replaced the **barbiturates,** which were used medically in the past for inducing relaxation and sleep, relieving tension, and treating epileptic seizures. These drugs are usually taken by mouth in tablet, capsule, or liquid form. When used as a general anesthetic, they are administered intravenously. Barbiturates such as *pentobarbital* (brand name Nembutal, or "yellow jackets"), *secobarbital* (Seconal, or "reds"), and *thiopental* (Pentothal) are short-acting and rapidly absorbed into the brain. The longer-acting barbiturates, such as *amobarbital* (brand name Amytal, or "blues" or "downers") and *phenobarbital* (Luminal, or "phennies"), which usually are taken orally and absorbed slowly into the bloodstream, take a while to reach the brain and have an effect for several days.

How Users Feel

The lower doses of these drugs may reduce or relieve tension, but increasing doses can cause a loosening of sexual or aggressive inhibitions. Individuals using this class of drugs may experience rapid mood changes, impaired judgment, and impaired social or occupational functioning. High doses produce slurred speech, drowsiness, and stupor.

Young people in their teens or early twenties who have used many illegal substances typically take sedative-hypnotic or anxiolytic drugs to obtain a high or a state of euphoria. Some use them in combination with other drugs. Less commonly, individuals may first obtain sedatives, hypnotics, or antianxiety medications by prescription from a physician for insomnia or anxiety and then gradually increase the dose or frequency of use on their own, often by seeking prescriptions from several physicians. While they justify this continued use because of their symptoms, the fact is that they reach a state in which they cannot function normally without the drug.

Risks

All the sedative-hypnotic and anxiolytic drugs can produce physical and psychological dependence within two to four weeks. A complication specific to sedatives is *cross-tolerance*—or cross-addiction—which occurs when users develop tolerance for one sedative or become dependent on it and develop tolerance for other sedatives as well. Individuals with a prior history of substance abuse are at greatly increased risk of abusing this class of drugs if they are prescribed by a physician. However, those who have not abused drugs or alcohol in the past rarely develop a substance-abuse problem from these medications when they are prescribed for legitimate psychiatric disorders, such as panic disorder or generalized anxiety disorder.

Intoxication with these drugs can produce changes in mood or behavior, such as inappropriate sexual or aggressive acts, mood swings, and impaired judgment. Physical signs include slurred speech, poor coordination, unsteady gait, involuntary eye movements, impaired attention or memory, and stupor or coma.

Taken in combination with alcohol, these drugs have a synergistic effect that can be dangerous or even lethal. For example, an individual's driving ability, already impaired by alcohol, will be made even worse, increasing the risk of an accident. Alcohol in combination with sedative-hypnotics leads to respiratory depression and may result in respiratory arrest and death. Regular users of any of these drugs who become physically dependent should not try to cut down or quit on their own. If they try to quit suddenly, they run the risk of seizures, coma, and death.

Sedative-hypnotic and anxiolytic drugs can easily cross through the placenta and cause birth defects and behavioral problems. Babies born to women who used these drugs during pregnancy may be physically dependent on the drugs and may develop breathing problems, feeding difficulties, disturbed sleep, sweating, irritability, and fever.

Withdrawal

Withdrawal from sedative-hypnotic and anxiolytic drugs may range from relatively mild discomfort to a severe syndrome with grand mal seizures, depending on the degree of dependence. Withdrawal symptoms include malaise or weakness, sweating, rapid pulse, coarse tremor of the hands, tongue, and eyelids, insomnia, nausea or vomiting, temporary hallucinations or illusions, physical restlessness, anxiety or irritability, and grand mal seizures. Withdrawal may begin within two to three days after stopping drug use, and symptoms may persist for many weeks.

Treating Drug Dependence and Abuse

The most difficult step for a drug user is to admit that he or she *is* in fact an addict. If drug abusers are not forced to deal with their problem through some unexpected trauma, such as being fired or going bankrupt, those who care—family, friends, coworkers, doctors—may have to confront them and insist that they do something about their addiction. Often this intervention can be the turning point for addicts and their families. Treatment has proven equally successful for young people and for older adults.[50]

Treatment may take place in an outpatient setting, a residential facility, or a hospital. Increasingly, treatment thereafter is tailored to address coexisting or dual diagnoses. A personal treatment plan may consist of individual psychotherapy, marital and family therapy, medication, and behavior therapy. Once an individual has made the decision to seek help for substance abuse, the first step usually is detoxification, which involves clearing the drug from the body. An exception is methadone maintenance, discussed earlier in this chapter, which does not rely on complete detoxification.

Controlled and supervised withdrawal within a medical or psychiatric hospital may be recommended if an individual has not been able to stop using drugs as an outpatient or in a residential treatment program. Detoxification is most likely to be complicated when a person is a polysubstance abuser and may require close monitoring and treatment of potentially fatal withdrawal symptoms. Other reasons for inpatient treatment include lack of psychosocial support for maintaining abstinence; the absence of a drug-free living environment; or a complicated drug history with addiction to multiple substances. However, restrictions on insurance coverage may limit the number of days of inpatient care. Increasingly, once individuals complete detoxification, they continue treatment in residential programs or as outpatients.

Medications are used in detoxification to alleviate withdrawal symptoms and prevent medical and psychiatric complications.[51] Once withdrawal is complete, adjunctive medications are discontinued, so the individual is in a drug-free state. However, those with mental disorders may require appropriate psychiatric medication to manage their symptoms and reduce the risk of relapse. For example, a person suffering from major depression or panic disorder may require ongoing treatment with antidepressant medication.

The aim of chemical dependence treatment is to help individuals establish and maintain their recovery from alcohol and drugs of abuse. Recovery is a dynamic process of personal growth and healing that takes place as one makes the transition from a lifestyle of active substance use to drug-free recovery.

Whatever their setting, chemical dependence treatment programs initially involve some period of intensive treatment followed by one or two years of continuing aftercare. Most freestanding programs—those not affiliated with a hospital—follow what is known as the *Minnesota model*, a treatment approach developed at Hazelden Recovery Center in Center City, Minnesota, more than 30 years ago. Its key principles include a focus on drug use as the primary problem, not as a symptom of underlying emotional problems; a multidisciplinary approach that addresses the physical, emotional, spiritual, family, and social aspects of the individual; a supportive community; and a goal of abstinence and health.

Outpatient programs for substance abuse, offered by freestanding centers, hospitals, and community mental health centers, often run four or five nights a week for four to eight weeks, or in daily eight-hour sessions for seven to eight days, followed by weekly group therapy. These outpatient programs allow recovering drug users to go on with their daily lives and learn to deal with day-to-day work and family stresses. Mental health professionals in private practice also offer individually structured outpatient treatment.

Therapy groups provide an opportunity for individuals who have often been isolated by their drug use to participate in normal social settings. Small groups with other drug users can be especially valuable because they all share the experience of drug use; the members can confront one another with frankness and cut through lies and rationalizations. A professional therapist keeps members of the group from ganging up on one person. After their discharge from inpatient treatment, individuals who became involved in self-help groups were less likely to use drugs, coped better with stress, and developed richer friendship networks.

In the 2000 elections, California voters passed a controversial initiative that would divert most nonviolent drug offenders in the state to treatment rather than incarceration. This landmark program will provide drug treatment services as an alternative to incarceration for all first- and second-time nonviolent drug possession offenders in the state, excluding those involved in the distribution or sale of drugs.[52]

12-Step Programs

Since its founding in 1935, Alcoholics Anonymous (AA)—the oldest, largest, and most successful self-help program in the world—has spawned a movement (see Chapter 15). As many as 200 different recovery programs are based on the spiritual **12-step program** of AA. Participation in 12-step programs for drug abusers, such as Substance Anonymous, Narcotics Anonymous, and Cocaine Anonymous, is of fundamental importance in promoting and maintaining long-term abstinence.

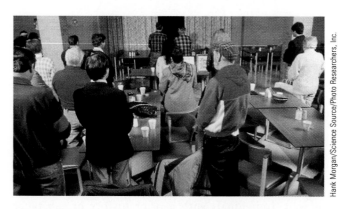

▲ Twelve-step programs, based on the Alcoholics Anonymous model, have helped many people overcome addictions. The one requirement for membership is a desire to stop following a pattern of addictive behavior.

The basic precept of 12-step programs is that members have been powerless when it comes to controlling their addictive behavior on their own. These programs don't recruit members. The desire to stop must come from the individual, who can call the number of a 12-step program, listed in the telephone book, and find out when and where the next nearby meeting will be held. A representative may offer to send someone to the caller's house to talk about the problem and to escort him or her to the next meeting.

Meetings of various 12-step programs are held daily in almost every city in the country. (Some chapters, whose members often include the disabled or those in remote areas, "meet" via electronic bulletin boards.) There are no dues or fees for membership. Many individuals belong to several programs because they have several problems, such as alcoholism, substance abuse, and pathological gambling. All have only one requirement for membership: a desire to stop an addictive behavior.

To get the most out of a 12-step program:

▶ Try out different groups until you find one you like and in which you feel comfortable.
▶ Once you find a group in which you feel comfortable, go back several times (some recommend a minimum of six meetings) before making a final decision on whether to continue.
▶ Keep an open mind. Listen to other people's stories and ask yourself if you've had similar feelings or experiences.
▶ Accept whatever feels right to you, and ignore the rest. One common saying in 12-step programs is, "Take what you like and leave the rest."

Relapse Prevention

The most common clinical course for substance abuse disorders involves a pattern of multiple relapses over the course of a lifespan. It is important for individuals with these problems and their families to recognize this fact. When relapses do occur, they should be viewed as neither a mark of defeat nor evidence of moral weakness. While painful, they do not erase the progress that has been achieved and ultimately may strengthen self-understanding. They can serve as reminders of potential pitfalls to avoid in the future.

One key to preventing relapse is learning to avoid obvious cues and associations that can set off intense cravings. This means staying away from the people and places linked with past drug use. Some therapists use conditioning techniques to give former users some sense of control over their urge to use the drug. The theory behind this approach, which is called *extinction* of conditioned behavior, is that with repeated exposure—for example, to videotapes of dealers selling crack cocaine—the arousal and craving will diminish. While this technique by itself cannot ward off relapses, it does seem to enhance the overall effectiveness of other therapies.

Another important lesson that therapists emphasize is that every "lapse" does not have to lead to a full-blown relapse. Users can turn to the skills acquired in treatment—calling people for support or going to meetings—to avoid a major relapse. Ultimately, users must learn much more than how to avoid temptation; they must examine their entire view of the world and learn new ways to live in it without turning to drugs. This is the underlying goal of the recovery process.

Outlook

Whatever the drug, recovery from dependence and abuse is a process of immense inner change that involves every aspect of a person's life. It does not follow a straight, even course, but moves back and forth between denial—of dependence, of loss of control, or of the severity of the problem—and awareness, ignorance and knowledge, craving and commitment. It often starts with a feeling of great relief, followed by a deep sense of emptiness. Individuals who have abused or become dependent on drugs must form a new identity, stop living in the past or future, give up their search for a quick fix, change the way they relate to family and old friends, find new things to do with the time they previously spent on their drug habit, learn new behaviors, and adopt new attitudes. Through treatment, education, and a reevaluation of what is meaningful in life, drug users can find a better way of living.

STRATEGIES FOR PREVENTION

Relapse-Prevention Planning

The following steps, from Terence Gorski and Merlene Miller's *Staying Sober* can lower the likelihood of relapses:

✔ *Stabilization and self-assessment.* Get control of yourself. Find out what's going on in your head, heart, and life.

✔ *Education.* Learn about relapse and what to do to prevent it.

✔ *Warning-sign identification and management.* Make a list of your personal relapse warning signs. Learn how to interrupt them before you lose control.

✔ *Inventory training.* Learn how to become consciously aware of warning signs as they develop.

✔ *Review of the recovery program.* Make sure your recovery program is able to help you manage your warning signs of relapse.

✔ *Involvement of significant others.* Teach them how to help you avoid relapses.

Codependence

Codependence refers to the tendency of the spouses, partners, parents, and friends of individuals who use drugs or alcohol to allow, or *enable,* their loved ones to continue their drug use and self-destructive behavior. (Codependence is also discussed in Chapter 15.)

Codependents Anonymous, founded in 1986 for "men and women whose common problem is an inability to maintain functional relationships," sponsors support programs throughout the country. Nar-Anon provides groups for people affected by drug abuse. Local chapters are in the white pages of the telephone directory.

If someone you love has a drug problem, get as much information as you can so that you understand what you—and your loved one—are up against. Also get some intervention training. Specially trained counselors work at most chemical-dependency units; some offer advice by phone. Here are some specific recommendations:

▶ Confront the user. Along with other loved ones and, if possible, a professional counselor, detail incident after incident in which the drug abuse affected or hurt you, other members of your family, or the user.

▶ Don't expect a drug abuser to quit without help. Chemical dependence is a medical and psychological disorder that requires professional treatment. Offer your support, but make it clear that you expect your loved one to undergo therapy.

▶ If your loved one agrees to treatment, make sure that the program is based on a complete evaluation, checking for medical and emotional problems, as well as chemical dependency.

▶ Don't believe abusers who say they've learned to control their drug use. Abstinence is a cornerstone of any good rehabilitation program.

▶ Encourage a user to attend support groups, such as Cocaine Anonymous or Narcotics Anonymous, for at least one year after rehabilitation. Get help for yourself. Most hospitals and chemical-dependency programs offer educational programs for codependents.

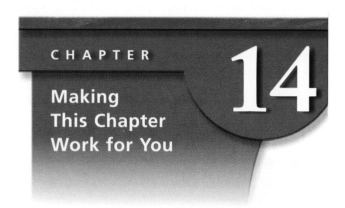

CHAPTER

14

Making This Chapter Work for You

1. Which of the following statements about drugs is false?
   a. A potentiating drug interaction is one in which one drug neutralizes or blocks the effects of another drug.
   b. Drugs can be injected into the body intravenously, intramuscularly, or subcutaneously.
   c. Drug misuse is the taking of a drug for a purpose other than that for which it was medically intended.
   d. An individual's response to a drug can be affected by the setting in which the drug is used.

2. To help ensure that an over-the-counter or prescription drug is safe and effective,
   a. take smaller dosages than indicated in the instructions.
   b. test your response to the drug by borrowing a similar medication from a friend.
   c. ask your doctor or pharmacist about possible interactions with other medications.
   d. buy all of your medications online.

3. Which of the following drugs does not cause withdrawal symptoms?
   a. caffeine

b. marijuana
   c. heroin
   d. aspirin

4. Individuals with substance use disorders
   a. are usually not physically dependent on their drug of choice.
   b. have a compulsion to use one or more addictive substances.
   c. require less and less of the preferred drug to achieve the desired effect.
   d. suffer withdrawal symptoms when they use the drug regularly.

5. Amphetamine is very similar to which of the following in its effects on the central nervous system?
   a. marijuana
   b. heroin
   c. cocaine
   d. Valium

6. Which of the following statements about marijuana is false?
   a. People who have used marijuana may experience psychoactive effects for several days after use.
   b. Marijuana has shown some effectiveness in treating chemotherapy-related nausea.
   c. Unlike long-term use of alcohol, regular use of marijuana does not have any long-lasting health consequences.
   d. Depending on the amount of marijuana used, its effects can range from a mild sense of euphoria to extreme panic.

7. Cocaine dependence can result in all of the following except
   a. stroke.
   b. paranoia and violent behavior.
   c. heart failure.
   d. enhanced sexual performance.

8. Which of the following statements about club drugs is true?
   a. The main ingredient of GHB is an industrial solvent used to strip floors.
   b. Most club drugs do not pose the same health dangers as "hard" drugs such as heroin.
   c. MDMA is the street name for ecstasy.
   d. When combined with extended physical exertion, club drugs can lead to hypothermia (lowered body temperature).

9. The opioids
   a. are not addictive if used in a prescription form such as codeine or Demerol.
   b. produce an immediate but short-lasting high and feeling of euphoria.
   c. include morphine, which is typically used for cough suppression.

d. are illegal in the United States, although they are allowed in other countries to help control severe pain.

10. Which of the following statements about drug dependence treatment is false?
    a. Chemical dependence treatment programs usually involve medications to alleviate withdrawal symptoms.
    b. Detoxification is usually the first step in a drug treatment program.
    c. Relapses are not uncommon for a person who has undergone drug treatment.

d. The 12-step recovery program associated with Alcoholics Anonymous has been shown to be ineffective with individuals with drug dependence disorders.

Answers to these questions can be found on p. 640.

 Drug Use, Misuse, and Abuse—Ritalin. Why is there a growing trend in ritalin abuse among college students?

Critical Thinking

1. Some argue that marijuana should be a legal drug like alcohol and tobacco. What is your opinion on this issue? Defend your position.

2. Some Web enthusiasts oppose any kind of government regulations on the Internet. Do you agree or disagree? How would you address the problems associated with distributing drugs online?

3. Suppose that a close friend is using amphetamines to keep her energy levels high so that she can continue to attend school full-time and hold down a job to pay her school expenses. You fear that she is developing a substance abuse disorder. What can you do to help her realize the dangers of her behavior? What resources are available at your school or in your community to help her deal with both her drug problem and her financial needs?

SITES & BYTES

National Institute on Drug Abuse
http://www.nida.nih.gov
This comprehensive site features information on a variety of drugs specifically written for students, current news topics, a list of publications, and information for researchers and professionals. The site also describes the current trends in drug use among college students.

Addiction Alternatives
http://www.addictionalternatives.com
This site features information on a variety of addictions, including alcohol, drugs, food, gambling, and personal interactive quizzes on alcohol, drugs, sex, sleep, attention/concentration, personality, and emotional quotient. The site also features tools to change behavior as well as consultations and information on self-help and professional therapy.

Center for Substance Abuse Prevention
http://www.samhsa.gov/centers/csap/csap.html
This site features information on model substance abuse prevention programs, youth substance abuse prevention initiative, a workplace program, resource links, and a clearinghouse of relevant topics including the National Mental Health Services Knowledge Exchange Network and Prevline (Prevention Online).

Please note that links are subject to change. If you find a broken link, use a search engine such as **http://www.yahoo.com** and search for the website by typing in key words.

InfoTrac Activity "New Ways to Stay Clean: Treatment—Beating an Addiction Is Tough, but Scientists Are Creating an Arsenal of Weapons, from Pills and Vaccines to Innovative Counseling." *Newsweek* (Special Report), February 12, 2001, p. 44.

(1) What percent of patients relapse within one year of rehabilitation? Why?

(2) Describe the physiological mechanisms of addiction on the brain chemistry.

(3) Describe several treatment approaches to addiction.

You can find additional readings related to drug abuse with InfoTrac College Edition, an online library of more than 900 journals and publications. Follow the instructions for accessing InfoTrac that were packaged with your textbook; then search for articles using a key word search.

For additional links, resources, and suggested readings on InfoTrac, visit our Health & Wellness Resource Center at **http://health.wadsworth.com.**

Key Terms

The terms listed here are used within the chapter on the page indicated. Definitions of terms are in the Glossary at the end of the book.

addiction 485
additive 479
amphetamine 491
antagonistic 479
barbiturates 504
benzodiazepines 504
club drugs 498
cocaine 496
codependence 507
delerians 501
drug 478
drug abuse 478
drug misuse 478
ecstasy (MDMA) 498

generic 482
GBL (gamma butyrolactone) 499
GHB (gamma hydroxybutyrate) 499
hallucinogen 500
hashish 494
inhalants 478
intoxication 487
intramuscular 478
intravenous 478
marijuana 494
nonopioids 501
opioids 501
over-the-counter (OTC) drugs 479
PCP (phencyclidine) 503

physical dependence 485
polyabuse 487
potentiating 479
psychoactive 484
psychological dependence 485
psychotropic 483
set 479
stimulant 483
subcutaneous 478
synergistic 479
toxicity 478
12-step program 506
withdrawal 487

References

1. "Fact Sheet: Substance Abuse—A National Challenge." Department of Health and Human Services Press Office, December 14, 2000.
2. "A Cough Syrup Ingredient Is a Popular Drug." *Pediatrics,* Vol. 106, No. 5, November 2000.
3. Burak, Lydia, and Amy Damico. "College Students' Use of Widely Advertised Medications." *Journal of American College Health,* Vol. 49, No. 3, November 2000, p. 118.
4. Hales, Robert, and Dianne Hales. *The Mind-Mood Pill Book.* New York: Bantam Books, 2001.
5. Meier, Barry. "Overdoses of Painkiller Are Linked to 282 Deaths." *New York Times,* October 28, 2001.
6. "Ecstasy Use Up Sharply; Use of Other Illegal Drugs Steady, or Declining." *Medical Letter on the CDC & FDA,* January 14, 2001.
7. "Why Addiction Is a Chronic Disease." *Brown University Digest of Addiction Theory and Application,* Vol. 20, No. 7, July 2001, p. S1.
8. Frances, Richard. Personal interview.
9. "Report Makes Case for Addiction as Chronic Disease." *Alcoholism & Drug Abuse Weekly,* Vol. 12, No. 43, November 6, 2000.

10. Brook, Judith, et al. "Longitudinally Foretelling Drug Use in the Late Twenties: Adolescent Personality and Social-Environment Antecedents." *Journal of Genetic Psychology,* Vol. 161, March 2000.
11. "Parental Ground Rules Work in Prevention." *Alcoholism & Drug Abuse Weekly,* Vol. 12, No. 30, July 31, 2000.
12. "Parental Attitudes, History Affect Children's Drug Use." *Alcoholism & Drug Abuse Weekly,* Vol. 13, No. 32, August 20, 2001, p. 7.
13. "Drug-related Emergency Room Visits Are on the Rise in Many Cities." *Behavioral Health Business News,* Vol. 7, No. 15, August 9, 2001, p. 6.
14. "HHS Report Shows Drug Use Rates Stable, Youth Tobacco Use Declines." *Medical Letter on the CDC & FDA,* October 21, 2001, p. 2.
15. Jones, Sherry, et al. "Binge Drinking Among Undergraduate College Students in the United States: Implications for Other Substance Use." *Journal of American College Health,* Vol. 50, No. 1, July 2001, p. 33.
16. Bon, Rebecca, et al. "Normative Perceptions in Relation to Substance Use and HIV-Risky Sexual Behaviors of College Students." *Journal of Psychology,* Vol. 135, No. 2, March 2001, p. 165.

17. Jones et al., "Binge Drinking Among Undergraduate College Students in the United States."

18. Wechsler, Henry, et al. "Drinking Levels, Alcohol Problems and Secondhand Effects in Substance-Free College Residences: Results of a National Study." *Journal of Studies on Alcohol,* Vol. 62, No. 1, January 2001, p. 23.

19. Volkow, Nora, et al. "Higher Cortical and Lower Subcortical Metabolism in Detoxified Methamphetamine Abusers." *American Journal of Psychiatry,* Vol. 158, March 2001, p. 383.

20. National Institute on Drug Abuse. http://www.nida.nih.gov.

21. "Research Casts Doubt on Marijuana for Pain." *Alcoholism & Drug Abuse Weekly,* Vol. 13, No. 27, July 16, 2001, p. 8.

22. "Doctors Reject Proposal Backing Medical Marijuana." *Alcoholism & Drug Abuse Weekly,* Vol. 13, No. 26, July 2, 2001, p. 8.

23. National Institute on Drug Abuse. http://www.nida.nih.gov.

24. Ibid.

25. Mittleman, Murray. "Triggering Myocardial Infarction by Marijuana." *Journal of the American Medical Association,* Vol. 286, No. 6, August 8, 2001, p. 655.

26. "Marijuana May Boost Heart Attack Risk." *Alcoholism & Drug Abuse Weekly,* Vol. 13, No. 37, October 1, 2001, p. 7.

27. Walling, Anne. "Marijuana Use During Pregnancy." *American Family Physician,* Vol. 63, No. 12, June 15, 2001, p. 2463.

28. Swift, Pauline, and Donald Singer. "Cocaine Use and Acute Left Ventricular Dysfunction." *Lancet,* Vol. 357, No. 9268, May 19, 2001, p. 1586.

29. National Institute on Drug Abuse. http://www.nida.nih.gov.

30. Shine, Barbara. "Some Cocaine Abusers Fare Better with Cognitive-Behavioral Therapy, Others with 12-Step Programs." *National Institute on Drug Abuse—NIDA Notes,* Vol. 15, No. 1, 2000.

31. "Officials Should Monitor Drugs Collected at Clubs." *Alcoholism & Drug Abuse Weekly,* Vol. 13, No. 36, September 24, 2001, p. 8.

32. "Ecstasy Epidemic Among Teens." Presentation, Academy of Pediatrics, Annual Meeting, San Francisco, October 2001.

33. "Report Finds Dramatic Increase in Ecstasy Use Nationwide." *Alcoholism & Drug Abuse Weekly,* Vol. 13, No. 14, April 2, 2001, p. 1.

34. "MDMA." *Harvard Mental Health Letter,* Vol. 18, No. 1, July 2001.

35. National Institute on Drug Abuse. http://www.nida.nih.gov.

36. "What Is MDMA Neurotoxicity?" *Brown University Child and Adolescent Behavior Letter,* Vol. 17, No. 8, August 2001, p. 4.

37. "Long-term Ecstasy Use Impairs Memory." *Science News,* Vol. 159, No. 18, May 5, 2001, p. 280.

38. "From MDMA to Ecstasy." *Brown University Digest of Addiction Theory and Application,* Vol. 20, No. 6, June 2001, p. 4.

39. Hilliard, Malaika. "Ecstasy, Liver Failure, and Death in a Young Adult." Press release, American College of Gastroenterology, October 22, 2001.

40. "Can Ecstasy's Effects Be Passed on to Offspring?" *Brown University Child and Adolescent Behavior Letter,* Vol. 17, No. 8, August 2001, p. 1.

41. "GHB: Its Use and Misuse." *Harvard Mental Health Letter,* Vol. 17, No. 9, March 2001.

42. Sadovsky, Richard. "Gamma-Hydroxybutyrate and Withdrawal Syndrome." *American Family Physician,* Vol. 64, No. 6, September 15, 2001, p. 1059.

43. Dyer, J. E., and C. A. Haller. "GHB-Related Fatalities." *Journal of Toxicology: Clinical Toxicology,* Vol. 39, No. 5, August 2001, p. 518.

44. "Inhalants." National Institute on Drug Abuse. http://www.nida.nih.gov.

45. "Getting High with Inhalants." *State Legislatures,* Vol. 27, No. 7, July 2001, p. 14.

46. "Heroin." National Institute on Drug Abuse. http://www.nida.nih.gov.

47. "33-year Study Shows Severe Long-term Effects of Heroin." *Brown University Digest of Addiction Theory and Application,* Vol. 20, No. 6, June 2001, p. 4.

48. Stancliff, Sharon, et al. "Methadone Maintenance." *American Family Physician,* Vol. 63, No. 12, June 15, 2001, p. 2335.

49. Fiellin, David, et al. "Methadone Maintenance in Primary Care: A Randomized Controlled Trial." *Journal of the American Medical Association,* Vol. 286, No. 14, October 10, 2001.

40. "Youth Treatment Study Shows Good Results, Parallels Findings for Adult Outcomes." *Alcoholism & Drug Abuse Weekly,* Vol. 13, No. 27, July 16, 2001, p. 1.

51. Sloves, Harold. "Drug Treatment for Drug Addiction." *Behavioral Health Management,* Vol. 20, No. 4, July 2000.

52. "California Voters Pass Controversial Treatment Initiative." *Alcoholism & Drug Abuse Weekly,* Vol. 12, No. 44, November 13, 2000.

15

Alcohol Use, Misuse, and Abuse

It was just another Friday night at the frat house. The drinking started early and usually didn't stop until dawn. One of the brothers, a popular easy-going guy named Ryan—not usually much of a drinker—was celebrating a big birthday: his twenty-first. Egged on by the hooting crowd, Ryan bolted down one drink after another, after another, after another.

By the time Ryan reached twelve, he was slurring his words. As he kept chugging drinks, his face looked flushed; he started sweating heavily. When Ryan lurched to his feet, he swayed unsteadily for a few moments and then collapsed. At first everyone laughed. Then two of his buddies tried to revive him. They couldn't.

"He's not breathing!" one of them shouted. Someone called 911, and paramedics rushed Ryan to the nearest hospital. His blood alcohol concentration was several times above the legal limit. Despite intensive efforts by the medical team, nothing helped. Ryan's twenty-first birthday was his last.

Ryan's death was a tragedy that didn't have to happen. Episodes of heavy drinking have increased on college campuses. When not used responsibly, alcohol can take an enormous toll. No medical conditions, other than heart disease, cause more disability and premature death than alcohol-related problems. No mental or medical disorders touch the lives of more families. No other form of disability costs individuals, employers, and the government more for treatment, injuries, reduced worker productivity, and property damage. The costs in emotional pain and in lost and shattered lives because of irresponsible drinking are beyond measure.

This chapter provides information about alcohol, its impact on the body, brain, behavior, and society, patterns of drinking, and the recognition, understanding, and treatment of drinking problems and of alcoholism.

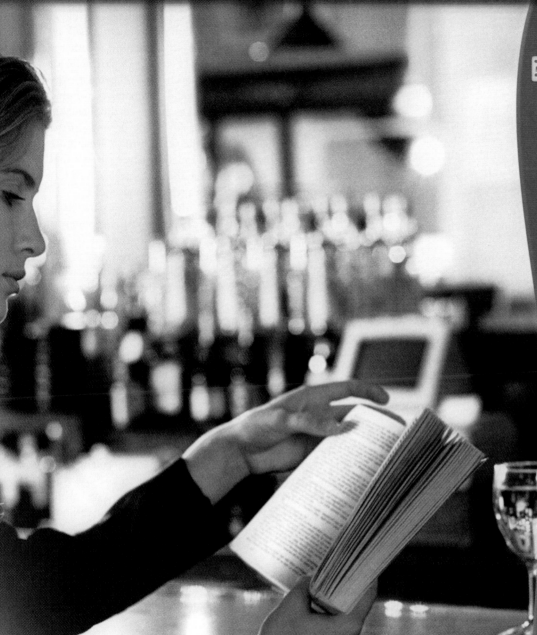

After studying the material in this chapter, you should be able to:

- **Describe** the factors affecting a drinker's response to alcohol consumption.
- **List** the effects of alcohol on the body systems.
- **Describe** the impact of alcohol misuse among college students, women, and different ethnic groups.
- **Define** alcoholism, and **list** common symptoms of this disease.
- **List** the negative consequences to individuals, and to our society, from alcohol abuse.
- **Explain** the common treatment methods for alcoholism.

Alcohol and Its Effects

Pure alcohol is a colorless liquid obtained through the fermentation of a liquid containing sugar. **Ethyl alcohol,** or *ethanol*, is the type of alcohol in alcoholic beverages. Another type—methyl, or wood, alcohol—is a poison that should never be drunk. Any liquid containing 0.5 to 80 percent ethyl alcohol by volume is an alcoholic beverage. However, different drinks contain different amounts of alcohol (see Figure 15-1).

One drink can be any of the following:

▶ One bottle or can (12 ounces) of beer, which is 5 percent alcohol.

▶ One glass (4 ounces) of table wine, such as burgundy, which is 12 percent alcohol.

▶ One small glass (2½ ounces) of fortified wine, which is 20 percent alcohol.

▶ One shot (1 ounce) of distilled spirits (such as whiskey, vodka, or rum), which is 50 percent alcohol.

All of these drinks contain close to the same amount of alcohol—that is, if the number of ounces in each drink is multiplied by the percentage of alcohol, each drink contains the equivalent of approximately ½ ounce of 100 percent ethyl alcohol. With distilled spirits (such as bourbon, scotch, vodka, gin, and rum), alcohol content is expressed in terms of **proof,** a number that is *twice* the percentage of alcohol: 100-proof bourbon is 50 percent alcohol; 80-proof gin is 40 percent alcohol.

But the words *bottle* and *glass* can be deceiving in this context. Drinking a 16-ounce bottle of malt liquor, which is 6.4 percent alcohol, is not the same as drinking a 12-ounce glass of 3.2 percent beer. Two bottles of high-alcohol wines (such as Cisco), packaged to resemble much less powerful wine coolers, can lead to alcohol poisoning, especially in those who weigh less than 150 pounds. This is one reason alcoholic drinks are a serious danger for young people.

expressed in terms of the percentage of alcohol in the blood and is often measured from breath or urine samples. Law enforcement officers use BAC to determine whether a driver is legally drunk. The Federal Department of Transportation has called on states to set 0.08 percent—the BAC that a 150-pound man would have after consuming about three mixed drinks within an hour—as the threshold at which a person can be cited for drunk driving. In the past, 0.1 percent was often the legal limit. (See Figure 15-2.) According to the National Institute on Alcohol Abuse and Alcoholism, lowering the BAC can lead to a significant drop in fatal car crashes related to alcohol.[1]

A BAC of 0.05 percent indicates approximately 5 parts alcohol to 10,000 parts other blood components. Most people reach this level after consuming one or two drinks and experience all the positive sensations of drinking—relaxation, euphoria, and well-being—without feeling intoxicated. If they continue to drink past the 0.05 percent BAC level, they start feeling worse rather than better, gradually losing control of speech, balance, and emotions (see Table 15-1). At a BAC of 0.2 percent, they may pass out. At a BAC of 0.3 percent, they could lapse into a coma; at 0.4 percent, they could die.

For some people, even very low blood alcohol concentrations can cause a headache, upset stomach, or dizziness. These reactions often are inborn. People who have suffered brain damage—often as a result of head trauma or encephalitis—may lose all tolerance for alcohol, either temporarily or permanently, and behave abnormally after drinking small amounts. The elderly, as well as those who are unusually fatigued or have a debilitating physical illness, may also have a low tolerance to alcohol and respond inappropriately to a small amount.

Your Body's Response to Alcohol

Many factors affect an individual's BAC and response to alcohol, including the following:

How Much Alcohol Can I Drink?

The best way to figure how much you can drink safely is to determine the amount of alcohol in your blood at any given time, or your **blood-alcohol concentration (BAC).** BAC is

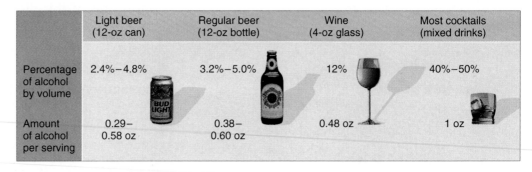

	Light beer (12-oz can)	Regular beer (12-oz bottle)	Wine (4-oz glass)	Most cocktails (mixed drinks)
Percentage of alcohol by volume	2.4%–4.8%	3.2%–5.0%	12%	40%–50%
Amount of alcohol per serving	0.29–0.58 oz	0.38–0.60 oz	0.48 oz	1 oz

▲ **Figure 15-1** The alcohol content of different drinks.

Men	Approximate blood alcohol percentage								
	Body weight in pounds								
Drinks	100	120	140	160	180	200	220	240	
0	.00	.00	.00	.00	.00	.00	.00	.00	Only safe driving limit
1	.04	.03	.03	.02	.02	.02	.02	.02	Impairment begins
2	.08	.06	.05	.05	.04	.04	.03	.03	
3	.11	.09	.08	.07	.06	.06	.05	.05	Driving skills significantly affected
4	.15	.12	.11	.09	.08	.08	.07	.06	
5	.19	.16	.13	.12	.11	.09	.09	.08	Possible criminal penalties
6	.23	.19	.16	.14	.13	.11	.10	.09	
7	.26	.22	.19	.16	.15	.13	.12	.11	
8	.30	.25	.21	.19	.17	.15	.14	.13	Legally intoxicated
9	.34	.28	.24	.21	.19	.17	.15	.14	Criminal penalties
10	.38	.31	.27	.23	.21	.19	.17	.16	

Subtract .01% for each 40 minutes of drinking.
One drink is 1.25 oz. of 80 proof liquor, 12 oz. of beer, or 5 oz. of table wine.

Women	Approximate blood alcohol percentage									
	Body weight in pounds									
Drinks	90	100	120	140	160	180	200	220	240	
0	.00	.00	.00	.00	.00	.00	.00	.00	.00	Only safe driving limit
1	.05	.05	.04	.03	.03	.03	.02	.02	.02	Impairment begins
2	.10	.09	.08	.07	.06	.05	.05	.04	.04	Driving skills significantly affected
3	.15	.14	.11	.10	.09	.08	.07	.06	.06	
4	.20	.18	.15	.13	.11	.10	.09	.08	.08	Possible criminal penalties
5	.25	.23	.19	.16	.14	.13	.11	.10	.09	
6	.30	.27	.23	.19	.17	.15	.14	.12	.11	
7	.35	.32	.27	.23	.20	.18	.16	.14	.13	Legally intoxicated
8	.40	.36	.30	.26	.23	.20	.18	.17	.15	Criminal penalties
9	.45	.41	.34	.29	.26	.23	.20	.19	.17	
10	.51	.45	.38	.32	.28	.25	.23	.21	.19	

Subtract .01% for each 40 minutes of drinking.
One drink is 1.25 oz. of 80 proof liquor, 12 oz. of beer, or 5 oz. of table wine.

▲ **Figure 15-2** Alcohol impairment charts.

Source: Data supplied by the Pennsylvania Liquor Control Board.

How much and how quickly you drink. The more alcohol you put into your body, the higher your BAC. If you chug drink after drink, your liver, which metabolizes about ½ ounce of alcohol an hour, won't be able to keep up—and your BAC will soar.

What you're drinking. The stronger the drink, the faster and harder the alcohol hits. Straight shots of liquor and cocktails such as martinis will get alcohol into your bloodstream faster than beer or table wine. Beer and wine not only contain lower concentrations of alcohol, but they also contain nonalcoholic substances that slow the rate of **absorption** (passage of the alcohol into your body tissues). If the drink contains water, juice, or milk, the rate of absorption will be slowed. However, carbon dioxide—whether in champagne, ginger ale, or a cola—whisks alcohol into your bloodstream. Also, the alcohol in warm drinks—such as a hot rum toddy or warmed sake—moves into your bloodstream more quickly than the alcohol in chilled wine or scotch on the rocks.

Your size. If you're a large person (whether due to fat or to muscle), you'll get drunk more slowly than someone smaller who's drinking the same amount of alcohol at the same rate. Heavier individuals have a larger water volume, which dilutes the alcohol they drink.

Your gender. Women have lower quantities of a stomach enzyme that neutralizes alcohol, so one drink for a woman has the impact that two drinks have for a man. Hormone levels also affect the impact of alcohol. Women are more sensitive to alcohol just before menstruation, and birth control pills and other forms of estrogen can intensify alcohol's impact. (See the section "Women and Alcohol" later in this chapter.)

Your age. The same amount of alcohol produces higher BACs in older drinkers, who have lower volumes of body water to dilute the alcohol than younger drinkers do.

Your race. Many members of certain ethnic groups, including Asians and Native Americans, are unable to break down alcohol as quickly as Caucasians. This can

▼ Table 15-1 Recognizing the Warning Signs of Alcoholism		
• Experiencing the following symptoms after drinking: frequent headaches, nausea, stomach pain, heartburn, gas, fatigue, weakness, muscle cramps, or irregular or rapid heartbeats. • Needing a drink in the morning to start the day.	• Denying any problem with alcohol. • Doing things while drinking that are regretted afterward. • Dramatic mood swings, from anger to laughter to anxiety. • Sleep problems.	• Depression and paranoia. • Forgetting what happened during a drinking episode. • Changing brands or going on the wagon to control drinking. • Having five or more drinks a day.

result in higher BACs, as well as uncomfortable reactions, such as flushing and nausea, when they drink.

▶ **Other drugs.** Some common medications—including aspirin, acetaminophen (Tylenol), and ulcer medications—can cause blood-alcohol levels to increase more rapidly. Individuals taking these drugs can be over the legal limit for blood-alcohol concentration after as little as a single drink.

▶ **Family history of alcoholism.** Some children of alcoholics don't develop any of the usual behavioral symptoms that indicate someone is drinking too much. It's not known whether this behavior is genetically caused or is a result of growing up with an alcoholic.

▶ **Eating.** Food slows the absorption of alcohol by diluting it, by covering some of the membranes through which alcohol would be absorbed, and by prolonging the time the stomach takes to empty.

▶ **Expectations.** In various experiments, volunteers who believed they were given alcoholic beverages but were actually given nonalcoholic drinks acted as if they were guzzling the real thing and became more talkative, relaxed, and sexually stimulated.

▶ **Physical tolerance.** If you drink regularly, your brain becomes accustomed to a certain level of alcohol. You may be able to look and behave in a seemingly normal fashion, even though you drink as much as would normally intoxicate someone your size. However, your driving ability and judgment will still be impaired.

Once you develop tolerance, you may drink more to get the desired effects from alcohol. In some people, this can lead to abuse and alcoholism. On the other hand, after years of drinking, some people become exquisitely sensitive to alcohol. Such reverse tolerance means that they can become intoxicated after drinking only a small amount of alcohol.

How Much Alcohol Is Too Much?

Federal health authorities at the National Institute of Alcohol Abuse and Alcoholism (NIAAA) recommend

that men have no more than two drinks a day and women, no more than one. The American Heart Association (AHA) advises that alcohol account for no more than 15 percent of the total calories consumed by an individual every day, up to an absolute maximum of 1.75 ounces of alcohol a day—the equivalent of three beers, two mixed drinks, or three and a half glasses of wine. Your own limit may well be less, depending on your gender, size, and weight. Some people—such as women who are pregnant or trying to conceive; individuals with problems, such as ulcers, that might be aggravated by alcohol; those taking medications such as sleeping pills or antidepressants; and those driving or operating any motorized equipment—shouldn't drink at all.

The dangers of alcohol increase along with the amount you drink. Heavy drinking destroys the liver, weakens the heart, elevates blood pressure, damages the brain, and increases the risk of cancer. Individuals who drink heavily have a higher mortality rate than those who have two or fewer drinks a day. However, the boundary between safe and dangerous drinking isn't the same for everyone. For some people, the upper limit of safety is zero: Once they start, they can't stop.

Intoxication

If you drink too much, the immediate consequence is that you get drunk—or, more precisely, intoxicated. According to the American Psychiatric Association's definition, **intoxication** consists of "clinically significant maladaptive behavioral or psychological changes," such as inappropriate sexual or aggressive behavior, mood changes, and impaired judgment and social and occupational functioning. Alcohol intoxication, which can range from mild inebriation to loss of consciousness, is characterized by at least one of the following signs: slurred speech, poor coordination, unsteady gait, abnormal eye movements, impaired attention or memory, stupor, or coma. Medical risks of intoxication include falls, hypothermia in cold climates, and increased risk of infections because of suppressed immune function.

Time and a protective environment are the recommended treatments for alcohol intoxication. Anyone who passes out after drinking heavily should be monitored regularly to ensure that vomiting (the result of excess alcohol irritating the stomach) doesn't block the breathing airway. Always make sure that an unconscious drinker is lying on his or her side, with the head lower than the body. Intoxicated drinkers can slip into shock, a potentially life-threatening condition characterized by a weak pulse, irregular breathing, and skin-color changes. This is an emergency, and professional medical care should be sought immediately.

The Impact of Alcohol

Unlike drugs in tablet form or food, alcohol is directly and quickly absorbed into the bloodstream through the stomach walls and upper intestine. The alcohol in a typical drink reaches the bloodstream in 15 minutes and rises to its peak concentration in about an hour. The bloodstream carries the alcohol to the liver, heart, and brain. (See Figure 15-3.)

Alcohol is a *diuretic,* a drug that speeds up the elimination of fluid from the body. Most of the alcohol you drink can leave your body only after metabolism by the liver, which converts about 95 percent of the alcohol to carbon dioxide and water. The other 5 percent is excreted unchanged, mainly through urination, respiration, and perspiration. Alcohol lowers body temperature, so you should never drink to get or stay warm.

Alcohol affects the major organ systems of the body, and its effects are cumulative. Light alcohol intake (no more than one drink a day for women and two for men) is associated with lower mortality than abstinence, but mortality rates increase with the amount of alcohol consumed. The mortality rate for alcoholics is two and a half times higher than for nonalcoholics of the same age. The leading alcohol-related cause of death is injury. Alcohol plays a role in at least half of all traffic fatalities, half of all homicides, and a quarter of all suicides. The second leading cause of alcohol-related deaths is cirrhosis of the liver, a chronic disease that causes extensive scarring and irreversible damage.

Digestive System

Alcohol reaches the stomach first, where it is partially broken down. The remaining alcohol is absorbed easily through the stomach tissue into the bloodstream. In the stomach, alcohol triggers the secretion of acids, which irritate the stomach lining. Excessive drinking at one sitting may result in nausea; chronic drinking may result in peptic ulcers (breaks in the stomach lining) and bleeding from the stomach lining.

The alcohol in the bloodstream eventually reaches the liver. The liver, which bears the major responsibility of fat metabolism in the body, converts this excess alcohol to fat. After a few weeks of four or five drinks a day, liver cells start to accumulate fat. Alcohol also stimulates liver cells to attract white blood cells, which normally travel throughout the bloodstream engulfing harmful substances and wastes. If white blood cells begin to invade body tissue, such as the liver, they can cause irreversible damage.

Cardiovascular System

Alcohol gets mixed reviews regarding its effects on the cardiovascular system. People who drink moderate amounts of alcohol have lower mortality rates after a heart attack, as well as a lower risk of heart attack compared to abstainers and heavy drinkers.[2] Moderate drinkers also have less buildup of cholesterol in their arteries, and are less likely to die of heart disease than heavy drinkers or teetotalers. French researchers have associated moderate drinking of only wine with lower mortality, although drinking both wine and beer reduced the risk of cardiovascular death.

However, heavier drinking triggers the release of harmful oxygen molecules called free radicals, which can increase the risk of heart disease, stroke, and cirrhosis of the liver. Alcohol use can weaken the heart muscle directly, causing a disorder called cardiomyopathy. The combined use of alcohol and other drugs, including tobacco and cocaine, greatly increases the likelihood of damage to the heart.

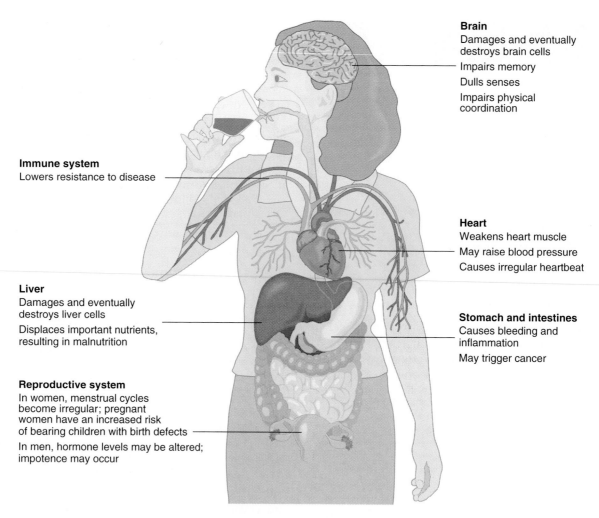

Brain
Damages and eventually destroys brain cells

Impairs memory

Dulls senses

Impairs physical coordination

Immune system
Lowers resistance to disease

Heart
Weakens heart muscle

May raise blood pressure

Causes irregular heartbeat

Liver
Damages and eventually destroys liver cells

Displaces important nutrients, resulting in malnutrition

Stomach and intestines
Causes bleeding and inflammation

May trigger cancer

Reproductive system
In women, menstrual cycles become irregular; pregnant women have an increased risk of bearing children with birth defects

In men, hormone levels may be altered; impotence may occur

▲ **Figure 15-3** The effects of alcohol abuse on the body.

Immune System

Chronic alcohol use can inhibit the production of both white blood cells, which fight off infections, and red blood cells, which carry oxygen to all the organs and tissues of the body. Alcohol may increase the risk of infection with human immunodeficiency virus (HIV), by altering the judgment of users so that they more readily engage in activities, such as unsafe sexual practices, that put them in danger. If you drink when you have a cold or the flu, alcohol interferes with the body's ability to recover. It also increases the chance of bacterial pneumonia in flu sufferers.

Brain and Behavior

At first, when you drink, you feel up. In low dosages, alcohol affects the regions of the brain that inhibit or control behavior, so you feel looser and act in ways you might not otherwise. However, you also experience losses of concen-

tration, memory, judgment, and fine motor control; and you have mood swings and emotional outbursts. Moderate and heavy drinkers show signs of impaired intelligence, slowed-down reflexes, and difficulty remembering. As recent research has shown, heavy drinking also depletes the brain's supplies of crucial chemicals, including dopamine, gamma aminobutyric acid, opioid peptides, and serotonin, that are responsible for our feelings of pleasure and well-being. At the same time, it promotes the release of stress chemicals, such as corticotropin releasing factor (CRF), that create tension and depression.

Heavy alcohol use may pose special dangers to the brains of drinkers at both ends of the age spectrum. Adolescents who drink regularly show impairments in their neurological and cognitive functioning.[3] Elderly people who drink heavily appear to have more brain shrinkage, or atrophy, than those who drink lightly or not at all. In general, moderate drinkers have healthier brains than those who don't drink and those who drink to excess.[4]

Because alcohol is a central nervous system depressant, it slows down the activity of the neurons in the brain, gradually dulling the responses of the brain and nervous system. One or two drinks act as a tranquilizer or relaxant. Additional drinks result in a progressive reduction in central nervous system activity, leading to sleep, general anesthesia, coma, and even death. Moderate amounts of alcohol can have disturbing effects on perception and judgment, including the following:

- **Impaired perceptions.** You're less able to adjust your eyes to bright lights because glare bothers you more. Although you can still hear sounds, you can't distinguish between them or judge their direction well.
- **Dulled smell and taste.** Alcohol itself may cause some vitamin deficiencies, and the poor eating habits of heavy drinkers result in further nutrition problems.
- **Diminished sensation.** You may walk outside without a coat on a freezing winter night and not feel the cold.
- **Altered sense of space.** You may not realize, for instance, that you have been in one place for several hours.
- **Impaired motor skills.** Writing, typing, driving, and other abilities involving your muscles are impaired. This is why law enforcement officers sometimes ask suspected drunk drivers to touch their nose with a finger or to walk a straight line. Drinking large amounts of alcohol impairs reaction time, speed, accuracy, and consistency, as well as judgment.
- **Impaired sexual performance.** While drinking may increase your interest in sex, it may also impair sexual response, especially a man's ability to achieve or maintain an erection. As Shakespeare wrote, "It provokes the desire, but it takes away the performance."

Interaction with Other Drugs

Alcohol can interact with other drugs—prescription and nonprescription, legal and illegal. Of the 100 most frequently prescribed drugs, more than half contain at least one ingredient that interacts adversely with alcohol. Because alcohol and other psychoactive drugs may work on the same areas of the brain, their combination can produce an effect much greater than that expected of either drug by itself. The consequences of this synergistic interaction can be fatal (see Savvy Consumer: "Alcohol and Drug Interactions"). Alcohol is particularly dangerous when combined with depressants and antianxiety medications.

Aspirin—long used to prevent or counter alcohol's effects—may actually enhance its impact by significantly lowering the body's ability to break down alcohol in the stomach. In a study of healthy men between the ages of 30 and 45, volunteers who took two extra-strength aspirin tablets an hour before drinking a glass and a half of wine had a 30 percent higher BAC than when they drank alcohol alone. This increase could make a difference in impairment for individuals driving cars or operating machinery.

If you want to drink while taking medication, be sure you read the warnings on nonprescription-drug labels or prescription-drug containers; ask your doctor about possible alcohol–drug interactions; and check with your pharmacist if you have any questions about your medications, especially over-the-counter (OTC) products.

Increased Risk of Dying

Alcohol kills. While light alcohol intake is associated with lower mortality than either abstinence or heavy drinking, mortality risks increase with the amount of alcohol consumed. Alcohol is responsible for 100,000 deaths each year and is the third leading cause of death after tobacco and improper diet and lack of exercise.[5]

The second leading cause of alcohol-related deaths is digestive disease, including cirrhosis of the liver, a chronic disease that causes extensive scarring and irreversible damage. In addition, as many as half of patients admitted to hospitals and 15 percent of those making office visits seek or need medical care because of the direct or indirect effects of alcohol.

Young drinkers—teens and those in their early twenties—are at highest risk of dying from injuries, mostly car accidents. Older drinkers over age 50 face the greatest danger of premature death from cirrhosis of the liver, hepatitis, and other alcohol-linked illnesses.

Drinking in America

According to the most recent statistics available from the National Institute on Alcohol Abuse and Alcoholism, about

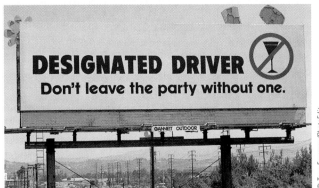

▲ Public awareness campaigns like this one for designated drivers can help prevent the high incidence of fatalities caused by drunk drivers.

Savvy Consumer

Alcohol and Drug Interactions

Drug	Possible effects of interaction
Analgesics (painkillers)	
Narcotic (Codeine, Demerol, Percodan)	Increase in central nervous system depression, possibly leading to respiratory failure and death.
Nonnarcotic (aspirin, acetaminophen)	Irritation of stomach, resulting in bleeding, and increased susceptibility to liver damage.
Antabuse	Nausea, vomiting, headache, high blood pressure, and erratic heartbeat.
Antianxiety drugs (Valium, Librium)	Increase in central nervous system depression; decreased alertness and impaired judgment.
Antidepressants	Increase in central nervous system depression; certain antidepressants in combination with red wine could cause a sudden increase in blood pressure.
Antihistamines (Actifed, Dimetap, and other cold medications)	Increase in drowsiness; driving more dangerous.
Antibiotics	Nausea, vomiting, headache; some medications rendered less effective.
Central nervous system stimulants (caffeine, Dexedrine, Ritalin)	Stimulant effects of these drugs may reverse depressant effect of alcohol but do not decrease intoxicating effects of alcohol.
Diuretics (Diuril, Lasix)	Reduction in blood pressure, resulting in dizziness upon rising.
Sedatives (Dalmane, Nembutal, Quaalude)	Increase in central nervous system depression, possibly leading to coma, respiratory failure, and death.

 60 percent of American adults use alcohol, although they vary in how much and how often they drink. Whites are more likely to be daily or near-daily drinkers than nonwhites. Men tend to drink more and more often than women. Young people between the ages of 21 and 34 are most likely to drink, and alcohol use typically declines with age.

Why People Drink

The most common reason why people drink alcohol is to relax. Because it depresses the central nervous system, alcohol can make people feel less tense. Other motivations for drinking include the following:

▸ **Celebration.** Unless alcohol use violates family, ethnic, or religious values, people raise their glasses together on life's important occasions—births, graduations, weddings, promotions.

▸ **Friendship.** When friends visit, you may have a drink, or you may meet them somewhere "for a drink." Young people are much more likely to experiment with alcohol if their friends drink.

▸ **Social ease.** When we use alcohol, we may seem bolder, wittier, sexier. At the same time, the people drinking with us become more relaxed and seem to enjoy our company more. Because alcohol lowers inhibitions, some people see it as a prelude to seduction.

▸ **Self-medication.** Like other drugs, alcohol may be the means some people use to treat—or escape from—painful feelings or bad moods.

▸ **Role models.** Athletes, some of the most admired celebrities in our country, have a long history of appearing in commercials for alcohol. Many advertisements feature glamorous women holding or sipping alcoholic beverages.

▸ **Advertising.** Brewers and beer distributors spend $15 to $20 million a year promoting the message: If you want to have fun, have a drink. Adolescents may be

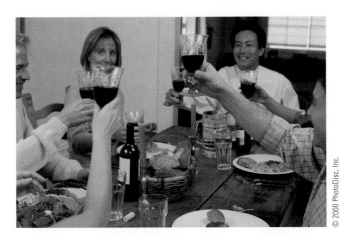

▲ Alcohol can be part of many enjoyable social situations, as long as individuals know when to say "no more." Increasingly, many people are substituting nonalcoholic drinks.

especially responsive to such sales pitches. Nearly two dozen national groups, including the American Medical Association, have petitioned the Federal Trade Commission to ban alcohol advertisements that link drinking to risky activities (such as driving, water skiing, and skydiving) and that target youth.

Patterns of Alcohol Use

Because of concern about alcohol's health effects, increasing numbers of Americans are choosing not to drink at all. (See Pulse Points: "Ten Steps to Responsible Drinking.") With alcohol consumption in the United States at its lowest level in 30 years, nonalcoholic beverages have grown in popularity. They appeal to drivers, boaters, pregnant women, individuals with health problems that could worsen with alcohol, those who are older and can't tolerate alcohol, anyone taking medicines that interact with alcohol (including antibiotics, antidepressants, and muscle relaxers), and everyone interested in limiting alcohol intake. Under federal law, these drinks can contain some alcohol, but a much smaller amount than regular beer or wine. Nonalcoholic beers and wines on the market also are lower in calories than alcoholic varieties.

Among adults who drink, fewer than 10 percent ever develop drinking problems. They also vary greatly in how much and how often they drink. Although there are no standard definitions for drinking patterns, the following are generally recognized as most common:

▶ **Light drinking.** This is defined as having fewer than three alcoholic drinks a week. (A drink equals 1 ounce of spirits, a 4-ounce glass of table wine, or a 12-ounce can of beer, each of which contains approximately 12 grams of absolute alcohol.)

▶ **Infrequent drinking.** This term refers to frequency, not quantity. Infrequent drinkers have less than one drink a month but drink at least once a year. Some "low maximum" infrequent drinkers drink one to three times a month but never have five or more drinks at a sitting. "High maximum" infrequent drinkers do not drink more often, but they occasionally have five or more drinks at a sitting.

PULSE POINTS

Ten Steps to Responsible Drinking

1. **Don't drink alone.** Cultivate friendships with nondrinkers and responsible moderate drinkers.

2. **Don't use alcohol as a medicine.** Rather than reaching for a drink to put you to sleep, help you relax, or relieve tension, develop alternative means of unwinding, such as exercise, meditation, or listening to music.

3. **Develop a party plan.** Set a limit on how many drinks you'll have before you go out—and stick to it.

4. **Alternate alcoholic and nonalcoholic drinks.** At a social occasion, have a nonalcoholic beverage to quench your thirst.

5. **Drink slowly.** Never have more than one drink an hour.

6. **Eat before and while drinking.** Choose foods high in protein (cheese, meat, eggs, or milk) rather than salty foods, like peanuts or chips, that increase thirst.

7. **Be wary of mixed drinks.** Fizzy mixers, like club soda and ginger ale, speed alcohol to the blood and brain.

8. **Don't make drinking the primary focus of any get-together.** Cultivate other interests and activities that you can enjoy on your own or with friends.

9. **Learn to say no.** A simple "Thank you, but I've had enough" will do.

10. **Stay safe.** During or after drinking, avoid any tasks, including driving, that could be affected by alcohol.

Underage Drinking

The age of first use of alcohol has declined since the 1960s.[6] According to the Substance Abuse and Mental Health Services Administration, the average age of first use is 16.1 years. The earlier young people start drinking, the more likely they are to develop alcohol dependence.[7] The rates of underage drinking declined significantly in the 1980s and have remained relatively constant. There also has been a decline in teen traffic deaths related to alcohol. The reasons for the drop include the increase in the legal drinking age to 21 and tougher legal penalties on alcohol use.[8]

Various psychosocial factors, such as low expectations for success, academic failure, and peer models for substance abuse, increase the risk of adolescent drinking.[9] In a national survey of 840 middle-school students, boys were more likely to drink than girls and more likely to increase their alcohol use over time. The factors that had the greatest influence on teens' drinking behavior were family support, religiosity, school performance, and peer influences.[10]

Adolescents who drink suffer both emotional and physical consequences, including sleep difficulties, chest discomfort, breathing symptoms, abdominal complaints, muscle and joint pain, headaches, and abnormalities in their liver function.[11] Researchers also have documented cognitive impairment and changes in brain structure in teens who drink heavily.

⬤ **Moderate drinking.** Moderate drinking generally is defined as having an upper limit of four standard drinks on any day, on no more than three days a week. For women, the upper limit is three drinks a day, on no more than three days a week.

⬤ **Social drinking.** This term—used by laypeople rather than health-care professionals or researchers—refers to drinking patterns that are accepted by friends and peers. If your friends drink only on special occasions, you may think that having one glass of wine at a party is social drinking. On the other hand, if the people you socialize with drink regularly and heavily, you may mistakenly think that having a six-pack of beer every night is social drinking.

⬤ **Problem drinking.** Any kind of drinking that interferes with a major aspect of life, such as sleep, energy, family relationships, health, or safety, qualifies as problem drinking. Some of the problems associated with drinking—getting into fights, unwanted sexual activity, car accidents—are obvious. Others, such as alcohol-related damage to the digestive system, heart, liver or brain, may remain invisible for years.

⬤ **Binge drinking.** When applied to alcohol, a binge consists of having five or more drinks at a single sitting for a man or four drinks at a single sitting for a woman. Binge drinking is most common among young men, especially those who are single, separated, or divorced, who drink beer, or who concentrate most of their drinking on weekends. Bingeing has been linked to a substantially increased risk of serious injury—especially from automobile accidents—as well as higher rates of unsafe sex, assault, and aggressive behavior. As discussed later in this chapter, binge drinking is common in college.

 ## How Common Is Drinking on College Campuses?

Most college students use alcohol, but they vary greatly in how often and how much they drink. The numbers of students abstaining from alcohol has increased over time (see Figure 15-4). About one in five students—20 percent of men and 18.7 percent of women—does not use alcohol.[12]

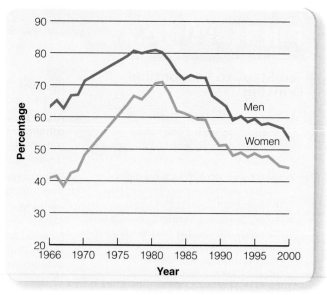

▲ **Figure 15-4** Percentage of freshmen who drink beer.

Source: Sax, Linda, et al. *The American Freshman: National Norms for Fall 2000.* Los Angeles: Higher Education Research Institute, UCLA, 2000.

Two in five students—44 percent—report at least occasional **binge drinking,** which generally means at least five drinks for men and four for women. Schools with large fraternity systems and rural colleges typically report more heavy drinking, while Christian and women's colleges have less drinking. However, heavy drinking has become more prevalent on most campuses.[13] An estimated 10 percent of college students drink more than 15 alcoholic beverages per week.[14]

Every year, students spend $5.5 billion on alcohol, mostly beer—more than they spend on books, soda pop, coffee, juice, and milk combined, for an average of $466 per student per year. The total amount of alcohol consumed by college students each year is 430 million gallons, enough for every college and university in the United States to fill an Olympic-size swimming pool.[15]

According to the Commission on Substance Abuse at Colleges and Universities, alcohol is involved in two-thirds of college student suicides, nine of ten rapes, and 95 percent of violent crimes on campus.[16]

According to a national survey released by the Higher Education Center for Alcohol and Other Drug Prevention, 75 to 90 percent of all violence on college campuses is alcohol-related. About 300,000 of today's college students will eventually die from alcohol-related causes, including drunk driving accidents, cirrhosis of the liver, various cancers, and heart disease, estimates the Core Institute, an organization that studies college drinking.

Drinking also increases sexual risks for college students. Heavy drinking has been correlated with increased casual sex without condoms, with increased numbers of sex partners, and with sexual attacks on women.

Why College Students Drink

Most college students drink for the same reasons undergraduates have always turned to alcohol. Away from home, often for the first time, many are both excited by and apprehensive about their newfound independence. When new pressures seem overwhelming, when they feel awkward or insecure, when they just want to let loose and have a good time, they reach for a drink.

Students may be especially vulnerable to dangerous drinking in their freshman year as they struggle to adapt to an often bewildering new world. In a study of freshmen at a medium-sized state university and at a small, predominantly African-American university who were nondrinkers as high school seniors, almost half (46.5 percent) started to drink in college. They were less likely to do so if they had friends who discouraged them from drinking.

Other studies have also linked alcohol consumption with where students live on campus and what they perceive as the norm for acceptable drinking.[17] Stress-related drinking is common. Students in competitive academic environments may turn to alcohol to reduce their anxiety and the pressure to perform. Athletes have higher drinking rates than nonathletes.[18] Members of sororities and fraternities rated all drinking norms as more extreme and perceived fraternity drinking as particularly heavy. Fraternity leaders are among the heaviest drinkers and most out-of-control partygoers, with the highest incidence of heavy drinking and bingeing.

The most dramatic increases in college drinking have been among women: Eight in ten female undergraduates say they drink; one in four get drunk three or more times in a month. (See X & Y Files: "Men, Women, and Drinking.")

Among both men and women, those with alcoholic parents and dysfunctional families are at greater risk of substance abuse. By some estimates, one of five college students comes from an alcoholic home and may be at increased risk of developing a drinking problem.

Binge Drinking

The Harvard School of Public Health College Alcohol Study, begun in 1993, has tracked how widespread and harmful binge drinking has become. It introduced the term *binge drinking,* defined as consumption of five or more alcoholic drinks by men or four or more alcoholic drinks by women in a row at least once in a two-week period. The proportion of students who binge drink (44 percent) has remained consistent over the last decade. However, the percentage of frequent binge drinkers has increased.[19] Frequent binge drinkers consume two-thirds of all the alcohol college students drink and account for more than three-fifths of the most serious alcohol-related problems on campus.

National surveys of college students at 119 colleges conducted since 1993 have shown a consistent rate of binge drinking. Two of five students reported occasional or frequent binge drinking at the time of the various surveys. However, student drinking patterns have become more extreme. More students in the most recent survey described themselves as frequent binge drinkers, reported being drunk three or more times in the previous month, drank on 10 or more occasions in the past month, usually binged when they drank, and drank for the sake of getting drunk. Those most likely to binge drink were fraternity or sorority house residents and students who were white, male, and binge drinkers in high school. In a recent survey, college athletes were 50 percent more likely to say they usually binged when they drank. Among men, 57 percent of athletes reported at least one drinking binge in the previous two weeks; among women, 48 percent reported a binge in the same period.[20] The students least likely to binge drink were African American or Asian, aged 24 years or older, married, and had not been binge drinkers in high school.[21]

The X&Y Files — Men, Women, and Drinking

According to conventional gender stereotypes, drinking is a symbol of manliness. In the past, far more men than women drank. In the United States today, both genders are likely to consume alcohol. However, there are well-documented differences in how often and how much men and women drink. In general, men drink more frequently, consume a larger quantity of alcohol per drinking occasion, and report more problems related to drinking.

The factors that create vulnerability to alcohol problems are the same in men and women. In both, genes are equally powerful influences. Sexual abuse in childhood also increases the likelihood of alcohol abuse in both men and women. Greater family support during adolescence protects both sexes from alcohol problems with alcohol use in adulthood.

Women are at greater risk of organ damage from heavy alcohol use and have higher rates of liver cirrhosis. One reason is that females do not respond to long-term heavy use of alcohol with the same protective physiological mechanisms as men. As a result, drinking the same amount of alcohol causes more damage to the female liver. As discussed later in the chapter, women drinkers also are at greater risk of heart disease, osteoporosis, and breast cancer. In recent years, researchers have been comparing and contrasting the reasons why men and women drink.

Undergraduate women and men are equally likely to drink for stress-related reasons; both perceive alcohol as a means of tension relaxation. In another study, psychologist Susan Nolen-Hoeksema of the University of Michigan interviewed approximately 1,300 adults (631 males, 697 females) about how they coped with sadness or distress. She asked about their tendency to ruminate or stew about how bad they felt, and about the extent to which they drank to cope with negative feelings, help themselves feel better, and deal with stress.

"The gender differences in both rumination and drinking to cope were quite pronounced," Nolen-Hoeksema reports. "In general, women think and men drink. But some men are ruminators and some women drink to cope, and for both men and women, rumination and drinking to cope are related." In other words, people who do one are at increased risk of doing the other.

In men, alcohol temporarily dampens rumination, says Nolen-Hoeksema, but in women, using alcohol just gives them one more thing to ruminate about—for reasons that are cultural as well as social and personal. For both men and women, she notes, the tendency to ruminate is linked not only to depression, but also to alcohol use. Therefore, both genders might benefit from learning more adaptive ways of coping with stress.

Other psychologists theorize that men engage in "confirmatory" drinking, that is, they drink to reinforce the image of masculinity associated with alcohol consumption. Both genders may engage in "compensatory" drinking and consume alcohol to heighten their sense of masculinity or femininity. Numerous studies in the past showed that men and women with low scores on various scales of masculinity and femininity are more vulnerable to problem drinking. High scores of masculinity have been associated with greater problem drinking by men, while high scores on femininity correlated with less problem drinking by women. However, the more men and women resemble each other on various measures of masculinity and femininity, the more similar their drinking patterns appear.

Sources: Eagon, P. K., et al. "Gender Differences in Hepatic Gene Expression in Response to Chronic Ethanol Exposure." Presentation, American Physiological Society, October 2001. Galaif, Elisha, et al. "Gender Differences in the Prediction of Problem Alcohol Use in Adulthood: Exploring the Influence of Family Factors and Childhood Maltreatment." *Journal of Studies on Alcohol,* Vol. 62, No. 4, July 2001, p. 486. Nolen-Hoeksema, Susan. Personal interview.

Binge-drinking rates have been decreasing among students living in dormitories and increasing among students living off campus. While two out of three students who live in fraternity or sorority houses are binge drinkers, one in three students in a campus residence hall or dormitory lives in an alcohol-free environment.

In a survey of 2,555 students at 52 campuses, residents of substance-free dormitories did not abstain entirely from alcohol. However, they drank less heavily and experienced fewer alcohol-related problems and secondhand effects of alcohol use than those in unrestricted housing. They also were less likely to engage in binge drinking.[22]

Beer drinkers and students under age 21 are much likelier to binge than other drinkers. (See Figure 15-5.) Binges tend to occur in the presence of friends, in drinking games, when other people are intoxicated, and when illegal drugs are available.[23]

Binge drinking is especially common in fraternities and sororities. By some estimates, more than 80 percent of "Greeks" who live in fraternity or sorority houses engage in binge drinking. The second highest rate occurs among athletes participating in intercollegiate sports. (See Student Snapshot: "Binge Drinking On Campus.")

Despite their heavy drinking as undergraduates, within three years of graduation, members of fraternities

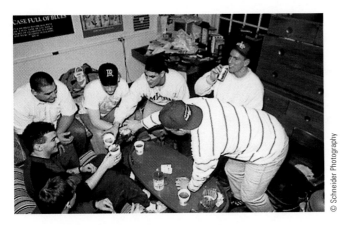

▲ Binge drinkers can get into—and cause—trouble. Dangerously large amounts of alcohol can cause death, and heavy party drinking often results in violence.

and sororities drink no more than students who did not join Greek houses. Heavy drinking may be the result of students' perceptions that excessive alcohol use is normal in Greek houses, along with the encouragement of peers.[24]

Surveys consistently show that students who engage in binge drinking, particularly those who do so more than once a week, experience a far higher rate of problems than other students. Frequent binge drinkers are likely to miss classes, vandalize property, and drive after drinking. Frequent binge drinkers are also more likely to experience five or more different alcohol-related problems and to use other substances, including nicotine, marijuana, cocaine, and LSD.[25]

Students on campuses with many binge drinkers report higher rates of secondhand problems caused by others' alcohol use, compared with students on campuses with lower rates of binge drinking. These problems include being assaulted, awakened, or kept from studying. The secondhand effects of binge drinking include interruption of studies, assaults, vandalization, and unwanted sexual advances. (See Table 15-2.) Students living on campuses with high rates of binge drinking are two or more times as likely to experience these effects as those living on campuses with low rates.[26]

Because of the danger it poses to drinkers and others, bingeing has become a major public health concern. In recent years, several students have died after consuming numerous drinks in a short period of time, sometimes as part of hazing rituals.

The American Medical Association has launched a campaign, "A Matter of Degree," to target binge drinking on campus by using strategies first tried with tobacco, such as limiting advertising for alcohol. Individual colleges also have taken steps, such as banning beer at sports events and curbing the opening of taverns near a campus.[27]

Virtually all colleges provide alcohol education programs. Many universities prohibit delivery of beer kegs to

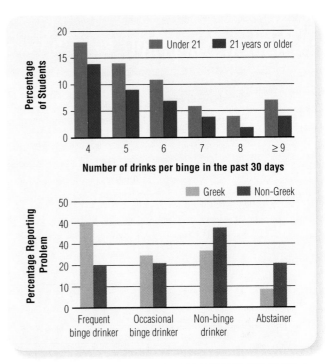

▲ **Figure 15-5** Binge drinking on college campuses in the United States.
Underage students binge drink at a higher frequency than students over 21 years of age. Two of five fraternity and sorority members are frequent binge drinkers compared to one of five non-Greek students.

Source: Henry Wechsler Harvard School of Public Health College Alcohol Study.

▼ Table 15-2	Secondhand Effects of Others' Drinking	
Type of Effect	**Percentage of students affected at schools with low and high frequency of bingeing**	
	Low	**High**
Insulted or humiliated	21	36
Unwanted sexual advance	15	23
Serious argument or quarrel	14	23
Pushed, hit, or assaulted	6	11
Had property damaged	7	16
Had studying/sleeping interrupted	43	71
Been a victim of sexual assault or date rape	6	1
Experienced at least one of the above problems	64	86

Source: Harvard School of Public Health Study. www.hsph.harvard.edu/cas.

Student Snapshot Binge Drinking on Campus

Student characteristics		Percentage who binge drink
Members of fraternities or sororities		80%
Athletes		29%
Nonathletes		22%
White		49%
African American		16%
Residents in substance-free housing		32%

Sources: Wechsler, Henry, et al. "Binge Drinking on American College Campuses." Harvard School of Public Health, 2001. Available at www.harvard.edu/cas. Wechsler, Henry, et al. "Drinking Levels, Alcohol Problems, and Secondhand Effects in Substance-Free College Residences: Results of a National Study." *Journal of Studies on Alcohol,* Vol. 62, No. 1, January 2001, p. 23.

dormitories or fraternity or sorority houses.[28] Some schools are studying whether they're scheduling too few classes on Fridays, which might spur Thursday-night partying. Other colleges are trying a "social norms" approach, spreading the message to students that their peers drink less than they think, in an attempt to make heavy drinking less socially acceptable.[29] Some have developed programs that extend beyond the campus to reach families or high school students.

The U.S. Department of Education has begun highlighting innovative antidrinking practices on campus; Mothers Against Drunk Driving (MADD) is planning to rank colleges based on how well they curb student drinking.[30] There has been an increase in on-campus chapters of national support groups such as AA, Al-Anon, Adult Children of Alcoholics, and a peer-education program called BACCHUS: Boost Alcohol Consciousness Concerning the Health of University Students.

Drinking and Race

Increasingly, experts in alcohol treatment are recognizing racial and ethnic differences in risk factors for drinking problems, patterns of drinking, and most effective types of treatment. Increases in drinking have been traced to stresses related to immigration, acculturation, poverty, racial discrimination, and powerlessness. Environmental factors, such as aggressive marketing and advertising of alcoholic beverages in minority neighborhoods, also play a role.

The African-American Community

Overall, African Americans consume less alcohol per person than whites, yet twice as many blacks die of cirrhosis of the liver each year. In some cities, the rate of cirrhosis is ten times higher among African-American than white

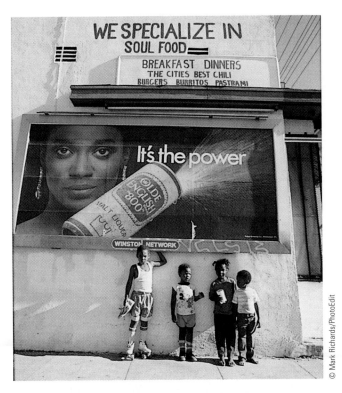

▲ The makers of alcoholic beverages market their products aggressively in poor urban neighborhoods, where liquor stores and bars are common.

men. Alcohol also contributes to high rates of hypertension, esophageal cancer, and homicide among African-American men.

The makers of alcoholic beverages market their products aggressively to African Americans, and there are many more liquor stores (per capita) in many African-American neighborhoods than in white communities. Peer pressure to drink, the easy accessibility of alcohol, and socioeconomic frustrations increase the likelihood of alcohol problems among African Americans. Moreover, recovery can be especially difficult because of the lack of treatment programs and role models in the African-American community and ongoing pressures to resume drinking.

The Latino Community

Latino societies discourage any drinking by women but encourage heavy drinking by men as part of machismo, or feelings of manhood. According to the Department of Health and Human Services, Latino men have higher rates of alcohol use and abuse than the general population and suffer a high rate of cirrhosis. Moreover, American-born Latino men drink more than those born in other countries.

Few Latinos enter treatment, partly because of a lack of information, language barriers, and poor community-based services. Latino families generally try to resolve problems themselves, and their cultural values discourage the sharing of intimate personal stories, which characterizes Alcoholics Anonymous and other support groups. Churches often provide the most effective forms of help.

The Native American Community

European settlers introduced alcohol to Native Americans. Because of the societal and physical problems resulting from excessive drinking, at the request of tribal leaders, the U.S. Congress in 1832 prohibited the use of alcohol by Native Americans. Many reservations still ban alcohol use, and thus Native Americans who want to drink may travel long distances to obtain alcohol, which may contribute to the high death rate from hypothermia and pedestrian and motor-vehicle accidents among Native Americans. (Injuries are the leading cause of death among this group.)

Certainly, not all Native Americans drink, and not all who drink do so to excess. However, they have three times the general population's rate of alcohol-related injury and illness. Cirrhosis of the liver is the fourth-leading cause of death among this cultural group. While many Native American women don't drink, those who do have high rates of alcohol-related problems, which affect both them and their children. Their rate of cirrhosis of the liver is 36 times that of white women. In some tribes, 10.5 out of every 1000 newborns have fetal alcohol syndrome, compared with 1 to 3 out of 1,000 in the general population. (See the discussion on fetal alcohol syndrome in the next section.)

Both a biological predisposition and socioeconomic conditions may contribute to alcohol abuse by Native Americans. In addition, according to their cultural beliefs, alcoholism is not a physical disease but a spiritual disorder—making it less likely that they'll seek appropriate treatment.

The Asian-American Community

Asian Americans tend to drink very little or not at all, in part because of an inborn physiological reaction to alcohol that causes facial flushing, rapid heart rate, lowered blood pressure, nausea, vomiting, and other symptoms. A very high percentage of women of all Asian-American nationalities abstain completely. Some sociologists have expressed concern, however, that as Asian Americans become more assimilated into American culture, they'll drink more—and possibly suffer very adverse effects from alcohol.

Women and Alcohol

More than half of women drink: Of these, 45 percent are light drinkers; 3 percent, moderate drinkers; 2 percent, heavy drinkers; and 21 percent, binge drinkers. According to the NIAAA, almost 4 million women suffer from alcohol abuse or dependence. But women who drink have different risk factors, potential dangers, and drinking patterns than men.[31]

Why Women Drink

In the past, most people, including physicians and therapists, assumed that women who drank heavily did so primarily for social and psychological reasons—because they were lonely, isolated, brokenhearted. Many of these assumptions have proven to be false. The following are more likely to lead to drinking problems in women.

▶ **Inherited susceptibility.** In women, as in men, genetics account for 50 to 60 percent of a person's vulnerability to a serious drinking problem. But while heredity increases the risk of alcoholism, life circumstances also play an important role in determining whether young women will have drinking problems. Female alcoholics are more likely than males to have a parent who abused drugs or alcohol, who had psychiatric problems, or who attempted suicide.

▶ **Childhood traumas.** Female alcoholics often report that they were physically or sexually abused as children or suffered great distress because of poverty or a parent's death.

▶ **Depression.** Women are more likely than men to be depressed prior to drinking and to suffer from both depression and a drinking problem at the same time. Even after women enter and complete treatment for their alcohol problems, depressive symptoms may persist.[32]

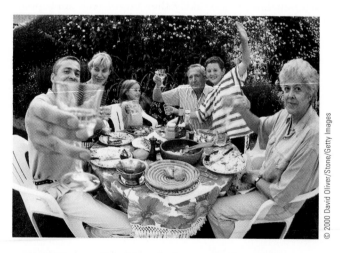

▲ Genetics as well as life experience contribute to a woman's vulnerability to heavy drinking and alcohol dependence. Risk factors and drinking patterns are different for women and men.

© 2000 David Oliver/Stone/Getty Images

▶ **Relationship issues.** Single, separated, or divorced women drink both more and more often than married women; women with live-in male partners have the highest rates of drinking problems. "Functioning women alcoholics may be very successful in other areas of their lives but have problems in their relationships," says Sharon Wilsnack, Ph.D., a professor at the University of North Dakota School of Medicine who studied the drinking habits of more than 1,100 women over ten years.[33]

▶ **Psychological factors.** Like men, women may drink to compensate for feelings of inadequacy. Women who tend to "ruminate" or mull over bad feelings may find that alcohol increases this tendency and makes them feel more distressed. Women involved with heavy drinkers are at risk of drinking heavily themselves, at least as long as the relationship continues.

▶ **Employment.** Women who work outside the home are less likely to become problem drinkers or alcoholics than those without paying jobs. The one exception: women in occupations still dominated by men, such as engineering, science, law enforcement and top corporate management. "Often women in these fields drink as a way of fitting in," observes Wilsnack. "Drinking takes on symbolic value. It's a way of signaling power, equality, status."

▶ **A lack or loss of roles.** Women of all ages, regardless of marital or employment status, tend to drink more and lean on alcohol when they lose a valued role, for example, when they're laid off from a job or their marriage ends in divorce.

▶ **Self-medication.** Some women feel it's permissible to use alcohol as if it were a medicine. As long as they're taking it for a reason, it seems acceptable to them, even if they're drifting into a drinking problem.

Alcohol's Effects on Women

Problems directly related to a woman's alcohol use range from the consequences of risky sexual behavior after alcohol consumption (such as unwanted pregnancy or STDs) to severe physiological problems related to fertility and pregnancy. Because they have far smaller quantities of a protective enzyme in the stomach to break down alcohol before it's absorbed into the bloodstream, women absorb about 30 percent more alcohol into their bloodstream than men do. The alcohol travels through the blood to the brain, so women become intoxicated much more quickly. And because there's more alcohol in the bloodstream to break down, the liver may also be adversely affected. In alcoholic women, the stomach seems to stop digesting alcohol completely, which may explain why women alcoholics are more likely to suffer liver damage than are men.

Among the other health dangers that alcohol holds for women are:

▶ **Gynecologic problems.** Moderate to heavy drinking may contribute to infertility, menstrual problems, sexual dysfunction, and premenstrual syndrome.

▶ **Pregnancy and fetal alcohol syndrome (FAS).** When a woman drinks during pregnancy, her unborn child drinks, too. According to CDC estimates, more than 8,000 alcohol-damaged babies are born every year. Women of all ages may be using alcohol and tobacco when they get pregnant; younger women are less likely to quit.[34] One of every 750 newborns has a cluster of physical and mental defects called **fetal alcohol syndrome (FAS):** small head, abnormal facial features (see photo), jitters, poor muscle tone, sleep disorders, sluggish motor development, failure to thrive, short stature, delayed speech, mental retardation, or hyperactivity. Many more babies suffer **fetal alcohol effects (FAE)**— low birthweight, irritability as newborns, and permanent mental impairment—as a result of their mothers' alcohol consumption.

Labels on alcoholic beverages have had a proven but modest effect on reducing drinking in pregnancy, while community-based education efforts have been much more effective. Drug and alcohol abuse also can affect the quality of a woman's mothering.

▶ **Breast cancer.** Numerous studies have suggested an increased risk of breast cancer among women who drink, and many physicians feel that those at high risk for breast cancer should stop, or at least reduce, their consumption of alcohol.

▶ **Osteoporosis.** As women age, their risk of osteoporosis, a condition characterized by calcium loss and bone thinning, increases. Alcohol can block the absorption of many nutrients, including calcium, and heavy drinking may worsen the deterioration of bone tissue.

▶ **Heart disease.** Women who are very heavy drinkers are more at risk of developing irreversible heart disease than are men who drink even more.

Alcohol Treatments for Women

Women who abuse alcohol also face a special burden: intense social disapproval. Many become cross-addicted to prescription medicines, or they develop eating disorders or sexual dysfunctions. Women often don't get the same care men do, frequently because of financial limitations and child-care responsibilities. Also, women are more likely to blame their symptoms on depression or anxiety, whereas men attribute them directly to alcohol. As a result, women often obtain treatment later in the course of their illness, at a point when their problems are more severe. Increasingly, prevention programs are targeting high-risk women to recognize alcohol problems early and to tackle underlying problems, such as depression and low self-esteem.

One of the most effective programs for women is Women for Sobriety, founded in 1975 by sociologist Jean Kirkpatrick, Ph.D. Its meetings focus on building self-esteem, self-confidence, and responsibility. "AA was started by men, and its message is very disempowering for women," says Kirkpatrick. "We view members as competent women who are struggling with issues that all women must face. Women don't need to recall the painful process of becoming alcoholics. They need to put the past behind them and move on, upward and onward."[35]

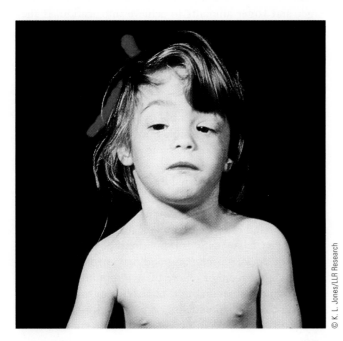

▲ A child with fetal alcohol syndrome (FAS) has distinctive facial characteristics that vary with the severity of the disease, including droopy eyelids, a thin upper lip, and a wide space between the nose and upper lip.

© K. L. Jones/LLR Research

Drinking and Driving

Drunk driving is the most frequently committed crime in the United States. In the last two decades, families of the victims of drunk drivers have organized to change the way the nation treats its drunk drivers. Because of the efforts of MADD (Mothers Against Drunk Driving), SADD (Students Against Destructive Decisions), and other lobbying groups, cities, counties, and states are cracking down on drivers who drink. Since courts have held bars liable for the consequences of allowing drunk customers to drive, many bars and restaurants have joined the campaign against drunk driving. Many communities also provide free rides home on holidays and weekends for people who've had too much to drink.

To keep drunk drivers off the road, many cities have set up checkpoints, where they stop automobiles and inspect the drivers for intoxication. The U.S. Supreme Court has ruled that a driver's refusal to submit to a blood-alcohol concentration test at such checkpoints or at any other time can be used as evidence to prosecute him or her for drunk driving. An increasing number of states have toughened their enforcement of drunk-driving penalties. Some suspend a driver's license for several months for a first offense; repeat offenders can lose their licenses for a year or more.

The National Highway Traffic Safety Administration estimates that setting the legal age limit for drinking at 21 has saved 16,500 lives in traffic crashes alone since 1975. The majority of states have made it illegal for people younger than 21 to drive with a measurable amount of alcohol in their blood. Research comparing states that adopted such zero tolerance laws to those that did not have found that zero tolerance states experienced 20 percent declines in the proportions of fatal single-vehicle, night crashes (the type most often alcohol-related) involving young drivers. Nationwide, alcohol-related traffic deaths among 15- to 20-year-olds have declined 57 percent. Raising the drinking age also has lowered the rate of pedestrian injuries.[36]

Alcohol-Related Problems

About 20 percent of Americans are "at risk" drinkers whose alcohol consumption exceeds the limits recommended by government studies (two drinks a day for men; one for women). These individuals are at increased risk of high blood pressure, stroke, violence, motor vehicle accidents, injury, and certain types of cancer.[37]

By the simplest definition, problem drinking is the use of alcohol in any way that creates difficulties or potential difficulties or health risks for an individual. Like alcoholics, problem drinkers are individuals whose lives are in some way impaired by their drinking. The only difference is one of degree. Alcohol becomes a problem, and a person becomes an alcoholic, when the drinker can't "take it or leave it." He or she spends more and more time anticipating the next drink, planning when and where to get it, buying and hiding alcohol, and covering up secret drinking.

Alcohol abuse involves continued use of alcohol despite awareness of social, occupational, psychological, or physical problems related to drinking, or drinking in dangerous ways or situations (before driving, for instance). A diagnosis of alcohol abuse is based on one or more of the following occurring at any time during a 12-month period:

▷ Recurrent alcohol abuse resulting in a failure to fulfill major role obligations at work, school, or home (such as missing work or school).
▷ Recurrent alcohol abuse in situations in which it is physically hazardous (such as before driving).
▷ Recurrent alcohol-related legal problems (such as drunk-driving arrests).
▷ Continued alcohol use despite persistent or recurring social or interpersonal problems caused or exacerbated by alcohol (such as fighting while drunk).

Alcohol dependence is a separate disorder, in which individuals develop a strong craving for alcohol because it produces pleasurable feelings or relieves stress or anxiety. Over time they experience physiological changes that lead to *tolerance* of its effects; this means that they must consume larger and larger amounts to achieve intoxication. If they abruptly stop drinking, they suffer *withdrawal*, a state of acute physical and psychological discomfort. A diagnosis of alcohol dependence is based on three or more of the following symptoms occurring during any 12-month period:

▷ Tolerance, as defined by either a need for markedly increased amounts of alcohol to achieve intoxication or desired effect, or a markedly diminished effect with continued drinking of the same amount of alcohol as in the past.
▷ Withdrawal, as manifested by characteristic symptoms, including at least two of the following: sweating, rapid pulse, or other signs of autonomic hyperactivity; increased hand tremor; insomnia; nausea or vomiting; temporary hallucinations or illusions; physical agitation or restlessness; anxiety; or grand mal seizures; or
▷ Drinking to avoid or relieve these symptoms.
▷ Consuming larger amounts of alcohol, or over a longer period than was intended.
▷ Persistent desire or unsuccessful efforts to cut down or control drinking.
▷ A great deal of time spent in activities necessary to obtain alcohol, drink it, or recover from its effects.
▷ Important social, occupational, or recreational activities given up or reduced because of alcohol use.

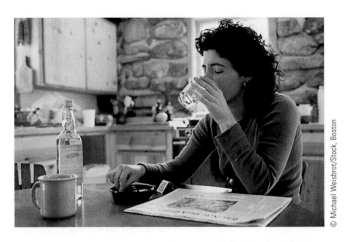

▲ Alcohol dependence may spring from the perception that alcohol relieves stress and anxiety, or creates a pleasant feeling. Chronic drinking—especially daytime drinking and drinking alone—can be a sign of serious problems, even though the drinker may otherwise appear to be in control.

▶ Continued alcohol use despite knowledge that alcohol is likely to cause or exacerbate a persistent or recurring physical or psychological problem.

Alcoholism, as defined by the National Council on Alcoholism and Drug Dependence and the American Society of Addiction, is a primary, chronic disease in which genetic, psychosocial, and environmental factors influence its development and manifestations. The disease is often progressive and fatal. Its characteristics include impaired control of drinking, a preoccupation with alcohol, continued use of alcohol despite adverse consequences, and distorted thinking, most notably denial. Like other diseases, alcoholism is not simply a matter of insufficient willpower, but a complex problem that causes many symptoms, can have serious consequences, yet can improve with treatment.

A lack of obvious signs of alcoholism can be deceiving. A person who doesn't drink in the morning but feels that he or she must always have a drink at a certain time of the day may have lost control over his or her drinking. A person who never drinks alone but always drinks socially with others may be camouflaging loss of control. If a person is holding a job or taking care of the family, he or she may still spend every waking hour thinking about that first drink at the end of the day (preoccupation).

Types of Alcoholism

Mental health professionals have developed different theoretical models to explain alcoholism. Although these models are used mainly by researchers and clinicians, they offer individuals with drinking problems and those close to them some insight into various personality and drinking patterns.

According to one long-established model, there are two primary types of alcoholics. *Type I*, or milieu-limited, alcoholics generally start heavy drinking, often in response to setbacks, losses, or other external circumstances, after age 25. They can abstain for long periods of time and frequently feel loss of control, guilt, and fear about their alcoholism. They also have characteristic personality traits: they tend to be anxious, shy, pessimistic, sentimental, emotionally dependent, rigid, reflective, and slow to anger. Because alcohol reduces their anxiety level, it serves as a positive reinforcer for continued use and contributes to the development of alcohol dependence.

Type II alcoholics are close relatives of an alcoholic male and become heavy drinkers before age 25. They drink regardless of what is going on in their lives; have frequent fights and arrests; and do not usually experience guilt, fear, or loss of control over their drinking. Unlike Type I alcoholics, they are impulsive and aggressive risk-takers, curious, excitable, quick-tempered, optimistic, and independent. Alcohol reinforces their feelings of euphoria and pleasant excitement. Often they abuse drugs as well as alcohol.

Newer research on male and female alcoholics classifies alcoholics as *Type A* or *Type B*. Type A alcoholism is a milder form, characterized by onset later in life, fewer childhood risk factors, less severe dependence, fewer alcohol-related physical and social consequences, fewer symptoms of other mental disorders, and less interference with work and family. Type B alcoholism is linked with childhood and familial risk factors, begins at an earlier age, involves more severe dependence and abuse of other substances, leads to more serious consequences, and often occurs along with other mental disorders. Type B alcoholics are younger, more inclined to experiment with other drugs and are more anxious, and of lower occupational status than Type A alcoholics.

How Common Are Alcohol-Related Problems?

According to the NIAAA, 9 percent of adults meet the criteria for alcohol abuse or dependence. White males 18 to 29 years old have 2.4 times greater prevalence of abuse and dependence than nonwhites. Among those over age 64, nonwhites have a prevalence rate of abuse and dependence 28.4 percent higher than whites.

Probably fewer than 5 percent of alcoholics and problem drinkers are "skid-row drunks." The other 95 percent are all around us, every day. (See Self-Survey: "Do You Have a Drinking Problem?") Alcoholism generally first appears between the ages of 20 and 40, although even children and young teenagers can become alcoholics. It takes 5 to 15 years of heavy drinking for an adult to become alcoholic, but just 6 to 18 months for an adolescent to develop the disease.

According to the National Comorbidity Survey, published in 1995, 23.5 percent of Americans may become dependent on or abuse alcohol in the course of a lifetime, while 9.7 percent experience these disorders in the course of a year. At all ages, men are two to five times more likely than women to abuse alcohol. In men, drinking usually starts in the late teens or twenties. Women tend to start drinking at a later age, are less likely to stop without help, and often have a history of depression.

SELF SURVEY

Do You Have a Drinking Problem?

This self-assessment, the Michigan Alcoholism Screening Test (MAST), is widely used to identify potential problems. This test screens for the major psychological, sociological, and physiological consequences of alcoholism.

To complete it, simply answer Yes or No to the following questions, and add up the points shown in the right column for your answers.

	Yes	No	Points
1. Do you enjoy a drink now and then?			(0 for either)
2. Do you think that you're a normal drinker? (By normal, we mean that you drink less than or as much as most other people.)			(2 for no)
3. Have you ever awakened the morning after some drinking the night before and found that you couldn't remember part of the evening?			(2 for yes)
4. Does your wife, husband, a parent, or other near relative ever worry or complain about your drinking?			(1 for yes)
5. Can you stop drinking without a struggle after one or two drinks?			(2 for no)
6. Do you ever feel guilty about your drinking?			(1 for yes)
7. Do friends or relatives think that you're a normal drinker?			(2 for no)
8. Do you ever try to limit your drinking to certain times of the day or to certain places?			(0 for either)
9. Have you ever attended a meeting of Alcoholics Anonymous?			(2 for yes)
10. Have you ever gotten into physical fights when drinking?			(1 for yes)
11. Has your drinking ever created problems for you and your wife, husband, a parent, or other relative?			(2 for yes)
12. Has your wife, husband, or other family members ever gone to anyone for help about your drinking?			(2 for yes)
13. Have you ever lost friends because of your drinking?			(2 for yes)
14. Have you ever gotten into trouble at work or school because of your drinking?			(2 for yes)
15. Have you ever lost a job because of your drinking?			(2 for yes)

	Yes	No	Points
16. Have you ever neglected your obligations, your family, or your work for two or more days in a row because of drinking?			(2 for yes)
17. Do you drink before noon fairly often?			(1 for yes)
18. Have you ever been told you have liver trouble? cirrhosis?			(2 for yes)
19. After heavy drinking, have you ever had delirium tremens (DTs) or severe shaking, or heard voices or seen things that weren't actually there?			(2 for yes*)
20. Have you ever gone to anyone for help about your drinking?			(5 for yes)
21. Have you ever been in a hospital because of your drinking?			(5 for yes)
22. Have you ever been a patient in a psychiatric hospital or on a psychiatric ward of a general hospital where drinking was part of the problem that resulted in hospitalization?			(2 for yes)
23. Have you ever been seen at a psychiatric or mental health clinic or gone to any doctor, social worker, or clergyman for help with any emotional problem where drinking was part of the problem?			(2 for yes)
24. Have you ever been arrested for drunk driving, driving while intoxicated, or driving under the influence of alcoholic beverages?			(2 for yes)
25. Have you ever been arrested, or taken into custody, even for a few hours, because of drunken behavior? (If Yes, How many times? ____ **)			(2 for yes)

*Five points for delirium tremens
**Two points for each arrest

Scoring:

In general, five or more points places you in an alcoholic category; four points suggests alcoholism; while three or fewer points indicates that you're *not* alcoholic.

???? What Causes Alcohol Dependence and Abuse?

Although the exact cause of alcohol dependence and abuse is not known, certain factors—including biochemical imbalances in the brain, heredity, cultural acceptability, and stress—all seem to play a role. They include the following:

▶ **Genetics.** Scientists who are working toward mapping the genes responsible for addictive disorders have not yet been able to identify conclusively a specific gene that puts people at risk for alcoholism. However, epidemiological studies have shown evidence of heredity's role. An identical twin of an alcoholic is twice as likely as a fraternal twin to have an alcohol-related disorder. The incidence of alcoholism is four times higher among the sons of Caucasian alcoholic fathers, regardless of whether they grow up with their biological or adoptive parents. The sons of alcoholic fathers have characteristic changes in brain wave activity. (See Genes in Focus: "The Genetics of Alcoholism.")

▶ **Stress and traumatic experiences.** Many people start drinking heavily as a way of coping with psychological problems. About half of all individuals who abuse or are dependent on alcohol also have another mental disorder. Alcohol often is linked with depressive and anxiety disorders. Men and women with these problems may start drinking in an attempt to alleviate their anxiety or depression.

▶ **Parental alcoholism.** According to researchers, alcoholism is four to five times more common among the children of alcoholics, who may be influenced by the behavior they see in their parents. The sons and daughters of alcoholics share certain characteristics, including early onset of problem drinking with severe social consequences, an unstable family, poor academic and social performance in school, and antisocial behavior.

▶ **Drug abuse.** Alcoholism is also associated with the abuse of other psychoactive drugs, including marijuana, cocaine, heroin, amphetamines, and various antianxiety medications. Adults under age 30 and adolescents are most likely to use alcohol plus several drugs of abuse, such as marijuana and cocaine. Middle-aged men and women are more likely to combine alcohol with benzodiazepines, such as antianxiety medications or sleeping pills, which may be prescribed for them by a physician. Whatever the reason they start, some people keep drinking out of habit. Once they develop physical tolerance and dependence—the two hallmarks of addiction—they may not be able to stop drinking on their own.

GENES IN FOCUS

The Genetics of Alcoholism

Alcoholism "runs" in families, and children of an alcoholic parent are more likely to become dependent on alcohol. Scientists long debated whether these youngsters inherit genes that increase their susceptibility to alcoholism or learn to abuse alcohol from the alcoholic parent or home environment. Increasingly, researchers have implicated the role of various genes as a major influence on vulnerability to alcoholism.

The Collaborative Study on the Genetics of Alcoholism (COGA) is a government-sponsored investigation of the genetic factors contributing to alcohol dependence and related disorders, including dependence on other drugs, such as nicotine. Its researchers have been studying several "candidate" genes on particular regions of certain chromosomes. Some affect dopamine, a brain chemical used by nerve cells in the brain's "reward center" and other regions to transmit signals. Others are involved with another neurotransmitter called GABA (gamma-aminobutyric acid).

Studies of twins—identical, who share the same genes, and fraternal, who like other siblings share about half their genes—suggest that heredity accounts for two-thirds of the risk of becoming alcoholic in both men and women. The same genes that confer a susceptibility for heavy drinking may also increase the risk of habitual smoking. These two dangerous behaviors are closely linked. COGA researchers also have found a genetic explanation for the increased prevalence of depression in alcoholics: The same genes may increase vulnerability to both conditions.

Because several genes undoubtedly influence alcohol and drug dependence, identifying them and unraveling the complex ways in which they interact with environmental factors will take some time. However, as science tells us more about genetic susceptibility to alcohol problems, individuals at risk will be able to do more to protect their health and their future.

Sources: Vanyukov, M. et al. "Dopamine System Genes, Sensation Seeking, and the Risk for Substance Use Disorders," *American Journal of Human Genetics,* Vol. 69, No. 4 (October 2001) p. 576. Nurnberger, John, et al. "Evidence for a Locus on Chromosome 1 That Influences Vulnerability to Alcoholism and Affective Disorder," *American Journal of Psychiatry,* Vol. 158, No. 5, May, 2001, p. 718.

Medical Complications of Alcohol Abuse and Dependence

Excessive alcohol use adversely affects virtually every organ system in the body, including the brain, the digestive tract, the heart, muscles, blood, and hormones. In addition, because alcohol interacts with many drugs, it can increase the risk of potentially lethal overdoses and harmful interactions. Among the major risks and complications are:

- **Liver disease.** Because the liver is the organ that breaks down and metabolizes alcohol, it is especially vulnerable to its effects. Chronic heavy drinking can lead to alcoholic hepatitis (inflammation and destruction of liver cells) and, in the 15 percent of people who continue drinking beyond this stage, cirrhosis (irreversible scarring and destruction of liver cells—see Figure 15-6). The liver eventually may fail completely, resulting in coma and death.
- **Cardiovascular system.** Heavy drinking can weaken the heart muscle (causing cardiac myopathy), elevate blood pressure, and increase the risk of stroke. The combined use of alcohol and tobacco greatly increases the likelihood of damage to the heart.
- **Cancer.** Heavy alcohol use may contribute to cancer of the liver, stomach, and colon, as well as malignant melanoma, a deadly form of skin cancer. Alcohol, in combination with tobacco use, also increases the risk of cancer of the mouth, tongue, larynx, and esophagus. Several major studies have implicated alcohol as a possible risk factor in breast cancer, particularly in young women, although the degree of danger remains unclear.
- **Brain damage.** Chronic brain damage resulting from alcohol consumption is second only to Alzheimer's disease as a cause of cognitive deterioration in adults. Long-term heavy drinkers may suffer memory losses, be unable to think abstractly or recall names of common objects, and not be able to follow simple instructions.
- **Vitamin deficiencies.** Alcoholics often tend to have very poor nutrition. Alcoholism is associated with vitamin deficiencies, especially of thiamin (B_1), which may be responsible for certain diseases of the neurological, digestive, muscular, and cardiovascular systems. Lack of thiamin, caused by alcoholism, may result in Wernicke-Korsakoff syndrome, characterized by disorientation, memory failure, hallucinations, and jerky eye movements, and it can be disabling enough to require life-long custodial care.
- **Digestive problems.** Alcohol triggers the secretion of acids in the stomach, which irritate the mucous lining and cause gastritis. Chronic drinking may result in peptic ulcers (breaks in the stomach lining) and bleeding from the stomach lining.

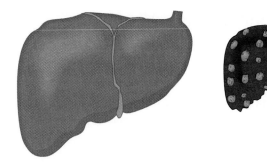

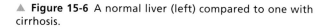
▲ **Figure 15-6** A normal liver (left) compared to one with cirrhosis.

- **Reproductive and sexual dysfunction.** Alcohol interferes with male sexual function and fertility through direct effects on testosterone and the testicles. In half of alcoholic men, increased levels of female hormones lead to breast enlargement and a feminine pubic hair pattern. Damage to the nerves in the penis by heavy drinking can lead to impotence. In women who drink heavily, a drop in female hormone production may cause menstrual irregularity and infertility.
- **Fetal alcohol syndrome.** The risk of this condition, discussed earlier in the chapter, is greatest if a mother-to-be drinks 3 ounces or more of pure alcohol (the equivalent of six or seven cocktails) a day. Consumption of lower quantities of alcohol can lead to fetal alcohol effects, including low birthweight, irritability in a newborn, and permanent mental impairment. Because no one knows how much—if any—alcohol is safe during pregnancy, the National Institute of Alcohol Abuse and Alcoholism recommends that pregnant women not drink at all.
- **Accidents and injuries.** Alcohol may contribute to almost half of the deaths caused by car accidents, burns, falls, and choking. Nearly half of those convicted and jailed for criminal acts committed these crimes while under the influence of alcohol.
- **Higher mortality.** The mortality rate for alcoholics is two to three times higher than that for nonalcoholics of the same age. The leading alcohol-related cause of death is injury, chiefly in auto accidents involving a drunk driver. The second leading cause of alcohol-related deaths is digestive disease, most notably cirrhosis of the liver. In addition, alcohol plays a role in about 30 percent of all suicides. Alcoholics who attempt suicide may have other risk factors, including major depression, poor social support, serious medical illness, and unemployment.
- **Withdrawal dangers.** Withdrawal can be life-threatening when accompanied by medical problems, such as grand mal seizures, pneumonia, liver failure, or gastrointestinal bleeding.

Alcoholism Treatments

Almost 600,000 Americans undergo treatment for alcohol-related problems every year. Until recent years, the only options for professional alcohol treatment were, as one expert puts it, "intensive, extensive and expensive," such as residential programs at hospitals or specialized treatment centers. Today individuals whose drinking could be hazardous to their health may choose from a variety of approaches. Treatment that works well for one person may not work for another. As research into the outcomes of alcohol treatments has grown, more attempts have been made to match individuals to approaches tailored to their needs and more likely to help them overcome their alcohol problems.

In a study of 222 men and women who had seriously abused alcohol, those who had remained sober for more than a decade credited a variety of approaches, including Alcoholics Anonymous (AA), individual psychotherapy, and other groups, such as Women for Sobriety. There is no one sure path to sobriety,—a wide variety of treatments may offer help and hope to those with alcohol-related problems.[38] In one of the few studies to follow adolescents for four years after alcohol treatment, about half either completely stopped drug and alcohol involvement or substantially reduced their use. Very few abstained entirely from any substances; over a third of youth treated showed fluctuations in their usage patterns over four years.[39]

Detoxification

The first phase of treatment for alcohol dependence focuses on **detoxification,** the gradual withdrawal of alcohol from the body. For 90 to 95 percent of alcoholics, withdrawal symptoms are mild to moderate. They include sweating; rapid pulse; elevated blood pressure; hand tremor; insomnia; nausea or vomiting; malaise or weakness; anxiety; depressed mood or irritability; headache; and temporary hallucinations or illusions.

Those who have drunk heavily for a prolonged period may develop more severe symptoms, including seizures or alcohol withdrawal delirium, commonly known as **delirium tremens,** or **DTs,** characterized by agitated behavior, delusions, rapid heart rate, sweating, vivid hallucinations, trembling hands, and fever. This problem is most likely to develop in chronic heavy drinkers who also suffer from a physical illness, fatigue, depression, or malnutrition. The symptoms usually appear over several days after heavy drinking stops. Individuals frequently report terrifying visual hallucinations, such as seeing insects all over their bodies. With treatment, most cases subside after several days, although delirium tremens has been known to last as long as four or five weeks. In some cases, complications such as infections or heart arrhythmias prove fatal.

 ## Are There Medications That Treat Alcoholism?

Antianxiety and antidepressive drugs are sometimes used in early treatment for alcoholism, especially for those with underlying mental disorders. Several medications, including certain antidepressant drugs that increase the neurotransmitter serotonin, are being studied as medical interventions to reduce cravings or prevent relapses. Two new medications, naltrexone and acamprosate, also have shown promise. Vitamin supplements, especially thiamin and folic acid, can help overcome some of the nutritional deficiencies linked with alcoholism.

The drug disulfiram (Antabuse), given to deter drinking, causes individuals to become nauseated and acutely ill when they consume alcohol. Antabuse interrupts the removal of acetaldehye by the liver, so this toxic substance accumulates and causes nausea or vomiting. If individuals taking Antabuse drink at all or consume foods with alcoholic content, they become extremely ill. They must avoid foods cooked or marinated in wine and cough syrup preparations containing alcohol. Some individuals have reactions to the alcohol in after-shave lotion. A large amount of alcohol can make them dangerously ill; fatalities have occurred. Side effects are usually mild and include drowsiness, bad breath, skin rash, and temporary impotence. Because Antabuse does not reduce cravings for alcohol, psychotherapy and support groups remain a necessary part of treatment.

The National Institute of Alcohol Abuse and Alcoholism is conducting a nationwide study evaluating the value of combining medication and behavioral inteventions.[40]

Inpatient or Residential Treatment

In the past, 28-day treatment programs in a medical or psychiatric hospital or a residential facility were the cornerstone of early recovery treatment. According to outcome studies, inpatient treatment was effective, with as many as 70 percent of "graduates" remaining abstinent or stable, nonproblem drinkers for five years after. However, because of cost pressures from the insurance industry, the length of stay has been reduced, and there's been increasing emphasis on outpatient care.

Outpatient Treatment

Outpatient treatment may involve group therapy, individual supportive therapy, marital or family therapy, regular attendance at Alcoholics Anonymous (AA) or another support group, brief interventions, and relapse prevention. According to outcome studies, intensive outpatient treatment at a day hospital (with individuals returning home every evening) are as effective as inpatient care. Outpatient therapy continues for at least a year, but many individuals continue to participate in outpatient programs for the rest of their lives.

Brief Interventions

These methods include individual counseling, group therapy, and training in specific skills—such as assertiveness—all packed into a six- to eight-week period. Offered at a growing number of centers, brief interventions may be most helpful for problem drinkers who are not physically dependent on alcohol. The University of Michigan's DrinkWise program offers clients the options of one-on-one therapy, group sessions, or telephone counseling. In its first year of operation, DrinkWise reported a success rate of 90 percent in helping clients quit or control their drinking.

Moderation Training

Highly controversial, this approach uses cognitive-behavioral techniques, such as keeping a diary to chart drinking patterns and learning "consumption management" techniques, such as never having more than one drink an hour.

Treatment programs in other countries, such as Great Britain and Canada, have long offered moderation training for problem drinkers who consume too much alcohol. However, most experts agree that the best—and perhaps only—hope for recovery for chronic alcoholics who are physically dependent on alcohol is complete abstinence. Because support is critical for maintaining moderation as well as abstinence, those trying to cut back on alcohol can turn to a new support network called Moderation Management. Aimed at problem drinkers rather than alcoholics, it teaches members how to use alcohol responsibly. After a period of abstinence, members follow drinking guidelines that restrict the number of drinks they have per day and the number of days per week that they drink.

Self-Help Programs

The best-known and most commonly used self-help program for alcohol problems is Alcoholics Anonymous (AA), which was founded more than 60 years ago and which has grown into an international organization that includes 2 million members and 185,000 groups worldwide. Acknowledging the power of alcohol, AA offers support from others struggling with the same illness, from a sponsor available at any time of the day or night, and from fellowship meetings that are held every day of the year. Because anonymity is a key part of AA, it has been difficult for researchers to study its success, but it is generally believed to be a highly effective means of overcoming alcoholism and maintaining abstinence. Its 12 steps, which

emphasize honesty, sobriety, and acknowledgment of a "higher power," have become the model for self-help groups for other addictive behaviors, including drug abuse (discussed in Chapter 14) and compulsive eating.

The average age of entry into AA is 30; about 60 percent of the members are men. Members encompass a wide range of ages, occupations, nationalities, and socioeconomic classes. People generally attend 12-step meetings every day when they first begin recovery; most programs recommend 90 meetings in 90 days. Many people taper off to one or two meetings a week as their recovery progresses. No one knows exactly how 12-step programs help people break out of addictions. Some individuals stop their drinking, or other destructive behavior, simply on the basis of the information they get at meetings. Others bond to the group and use it as a social support and refuge while they explore and release their inner feelings—a process similar to what happens in psychotherapy.

Alternatives to AA

Secular Organizations for Sobriety (SOS) was founded in 1986 as an alternative for people who couldn't accept the spirituality of AA. Like AA, SOS holds confidential meetings, celebrates sobriety anniversaries, and views recovery as a one-day-at-a-time process.

Rational Recovery, which also emphasizes anonymity and total abstinence, focuses on the self rather than spiri-

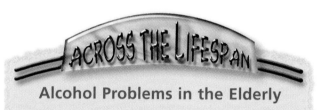

Alcohol Problems in the Elderly

Community surveys suggest that persons older than 65 years consume less alcohol and have fewer alcohol-related problems than younger drinkers. In contrast, surveys conducted in healthcare settings have found increasing prevalence of alcoholism among older adults. In acute care hospitals, rates of alcohol-related admissions are similar to rates for heart attacks, and some surveys have found the prevalence of problem drinking in nursing homes to be as high as 49 percent. In addition to the direct risks of alcohol, older individuals face additional dangers when they drink, including falls, fractures, traffic crashes, medication interactions, depression, and cognitive changes.[41]

Brief treatment can be effective in helping the elderly overcome alcohol problems.

tuality. Members use reason instead of prayer and learn to control the impulse to drink by learning how to control the emotions that lead them to drink. Women for Sobriety (WFS), discussed earlier in the chapter, addresses the unique needs of women with drinking problems.

Recovery

Recovery from alcoholism is a lifelong process of personal growth and healing. The first two years are the most difficult, and relapses are extremely common. By some estimates, more than 90 percent of those recovering from substance use will use alcohol or drugs in any one 12-month period after treatment. However, approximately 70 percent of those who get formal treatment stop drinking for prolonged periods. Even without treatment, 30 percent of alcoholics are able to stop drinking for long periods. Those most likely to remain sober after treatment have the most to lose by continuing to drink: they tend to be employed, married, and upper-middle class.

Most recovering alcoholics experience urges to drink, especially during early recovery when they are likely to feel considerable stress. These urges are a natural consequence of years of drinking and diminish with time. Mood swings are common during recovery, and individuals typically describe themselves as alternately feeling relieved or elated and then discouraged or tearful. Such disconcerting ups and downs also decrease over time. Patience—learning to take "one day at a time"—is crucial.

Increasingly, treatment programs focus on **relapse prevention,** which includes the development of coping strategies and learning techniques that make it easier to live with alcohol cravings and rehearsal of various ways of saying "no" to offers of a drink. According to outcomes research, social skills training—a combination of stress management therapy, assertiveness and communication skills training, behavioral self-control training, and behavioral marital therapy—has proven effective in decreasing the duration and severity of relapses after one year in a group of alcoholics.

A medication called nalmefene, an opioid antagonist, has proven effective in preventing relapse in alcohol-dependent individuals. In one trial, patients receiving nalmefene were 2.4 times less likely to relapse to heavy drinking than those who received a placebo.

Alcoholism's Impact on Relationships

Alcoholism shatters families and creates unhealthy patterns of communicating and relating. Separation and divorce rates are high among alcoholics. Another common occurrence is **codependence,** a term used to describe the behavior of close family members or friends who act in ways that enable their spouses, parents, or friends to continue their self-destructive behavior.

Codependence and Enabling

Codependent spouses of alcoholics follow a predictable pattern of behavior: While trying to control the drinkers, they act in ways that enable the drinkers to keep drinking. If an alcoholic finds it hard to get up in the morning, his wife wakes him up, pulls him out of bed and into the shower, and drops him off at work. If he is late, she makes excuses to his boss. By helping him evade his responsibilities, his wife is helping him continue drinking. Indeed, he might not be able to keep up his habit without her cooperation.

Such behavior is harmful for individuals who are dependent on alcohol because it reinforces their denial. They do not feel out of control or powerless over alcohol because the person or persons closest to them are constantly protecting them from the consequences of their actions. Every crisis—a missed deadline, a forgotten appointment, a child's disappointment when a parent doesn't come to an important event—should be seen as a chance for the individual to recognize what alcohol is doing to the lives of all those close to him or her. If family members let their loved one experience the consequences of drinking, the person may be able to come to the moment of truth concerning alcohol.

Codependents often need help in acknowledging their own feelings and needs. National self-help organizations, such as Al-Anon, help adult family members recognize dysfunctional behaviors in their relationships and start looking at their own problems. Similar self-help groups, such as Alateen, provide support for the teenaged children of alcoholics. These organizations also help family members cope with their loved one's alcoholism—whether or not codependence is a problem.

Growing Up with an Alcoholic Parent

According to recent estimates, 28 million children in the United States (or one of every four) are living in a household with an alcoholic adult.[42] Parental alcoholism increases the likelihood of childhood ADHD, conduct disorder, and anxiety disorders. The experience often leads youngsters to play certain roles: The adjuster or "lost child" does whatever the parent says. The responsible child, or "family hero," typically takes over many household tasks and responsibilities. The acting-out child, or "scapegoat," shows his or her anger early in life by causing problems at home or in school and taking on the role of troublemaker. The "mascot" disrupts tense situations by focusing attention on himself or herself, often by clowning. Regardless of which roles they assume, the children of alcoholics are prone to learning disabilities, eating disorders, and addictive behavior.

Numerous studies have linked child abuse and neglect to parental drinking. Children of women who are problem drinkers have twice the risk of serious injury as children of mothers who don't drink. Children with two parents who are problem drinkers are at even higher risk. As teenagers, children of alcoholics are more likely to report early sexual intercourse and face a greater risk of adolescent pregnancy.

Adult Children of Alcoholics

Growing up with an alcoholic parent can have a long-lasting effect. Adult children of alcoholics are at risk for many problems. Some try to fill the emptiness inside with alcohol, drugs, or addictive habits. Others find themselves caught up in destructive relationships that repeat the patterns of their childhood. They are likely to have difficulty solving problems, identifying and expressing their feelings, trusting others, and being intimate. In addition to their own increased risk of addictive behavior, they are likely to marry individuals with some form of addiction and keep on playing out the roles of their childhood. They may feel inadequate, not know how to set limits or recognize normal behavior, be perfectionistic, and want to control all aspects of their lives. However, not all adult children are alike or necessarily suffer from psychological problems or face an increased risk of substance abuse themselves.

Because the impact of alcoholism can be so enduring, support groups—such as Adult Children of Alcoholics, Children of Alcoholics, and Adult Children of Dysfunctional Families—have spread throughout the country in the last decade. These organizations provide adult children of alcoholics a mutually supportive group setting to discuss their childhood experiences with alcoholic parents and the emotional consequences they carry into adult life. Through such groups or other forms of therapy, individuals may learn to move beyond anger and blame, see the part they themselves play in their current state of unhappiness, and create a future that is healthier and happier than their past.

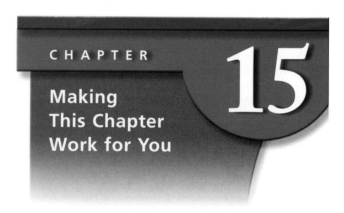

CHAPTER

Making This Chapter Work for You

15

STRATEGIES FOR CHANGE

If Someone Close to You Drinks Too Much

✔ Try to remain calm, unemotional, and factually honest in speaking about the drinker's behavior. Include the drinker in family life.

✔ Discuss the situation with someone you trust: a member of the clergy, social worker, friend, or someone who has experienced alcoholism directly.

✔ Never cover up or make excuses for the drinker, or shield him or her from the consequences of drinking. Assuming the drinker's responsibilities undermines his or her dignity and sense of importance.

✔ Refuse to ride with the drinker if he or she is driving while intoxicated.

✔ Encourage new interests and participate in leisure-time activities that the drinker enjoys.

✔ Try to accept setbacks and relapses calmly.

1. An individual's response to alcohol depends on all of the following except
   a. the rate at which the drink is absorbed into the body's tissues.
   b. the blood alcohol concentration.
   c. socioeconomic status.
   d. gender and race.

2. Which of the following statements about the effects of alcohol on the body systems is true?
   a. In most individuals, alcohol sharpens the responses of the brain and nervous system, enhancing sensation and perception.
   b. Moderate drinking may have a positive effect on the cardiovascular system.
   c. French researchers have found that drinking red wine with meals may have a positive effect on the digestive system.
   d. The leading alcohol-related cause of death is liver damage.

3. Responsible drinking includes which of the following behaviors?
   a. avoiding eating while drinking because eating speeds up absorption of alcohol

b. limiting alcohol intake to no more than four drinks in an hour

c. taking aspirin while drinking to lower your risk of a heart attack

d. socializing with individuals who limit their alcohol intake

4. Which of the following statements about drinking on college campuses is true?
   a. The percentage of students who frequently binge drink has increased.
   b. As a result of school crackdowns, the proportion of students who binge drink has decreased.
   c. Because of peer pressure, students in fraternities and sororities tend to drink less than students in dormitories.
   d. Students who live in substance-free dormitories tend to binge drink when alcohol is available.

5. Racial and ethnic patterns related to alcohol use include which of the following?
   a. Asian-American women tend to have higher rates of alcoholism than Asian-American men.
   b. Socioeconomic conditions increase the likelihood of alcohol problems in African Americans and Native Americans.
   c. White Americans tend to have higher rates of cirrhosis of the liver than African Americans or Native Americans.
   d. The Latino culture discourages men from drinking because heavy drinking indicates a lack of machismo.

6. Women who have drinking problems
   a. often have suffered from fetal alcohol syndrome as a result of their mothers' alcohol consumption.
   b. are less likely to have an alcoholic parent than men with drinking problems.
   c. are at higher risk for osteoporosis than women who are not heavy drinkers.
   d. are less likely to suffer liver damage than men.

7. Alcoholism
   a. is considered a chronic disease with genetic, psychosocial, and environment components.
   b. is characterized by a persistent lack of willpower.
   c. may be classified as either Type A, which affects people who are high-strung, or Type B, which affects people who are more mild mannered.
   d. is easily controlled by avoiding exposure to social situations where drinking is common.

8. Which of the following statements about alcohol abuse and dependence is false?
   a. Alcohol dependence involves a persistent craving for and an increased tolerance to alcohol.
   b. An individual may have a genetic predisposition for developing alcoholism.
   c. Alcoholics often abuse other psychoactive drugs.
   d. Alcohol abuse and alcohol dependence are different names for the same problem.

9. Health risks of alcoholism include all of the following except
   a. hypertension.
   b. lung cancer
   c. peptic ulcers.
   d. hepatitis.

10. Which of the following statements about alcoholism treatment is true?
    a. Inpatient treatment has been shown to be more effective than outpatient treatment.
    b. Alcoholism can be cured by detoxifying or ridding the body of all traces of alcohol.
    c. Antabuse is a medication given to alcoholics with underlying mental disorders.
    d. A combination of medical, behavioral, and self-help approaches may be necessary to treat alcohol abuse and dependence.

Answers to these questions can be found on page 640.

 Alcohol Addictions. What does research say about Ondansetion, a drug used to diminish alcohol cravings?

Critical Thinking

1. Driving home from his high school graduation party, 18-year-old Rick has had too much to drink. As he crosses the dividing line on the two-lane road, the driver of an oncoming car—a young mother with two young children in the backseat—swerves to avoid an accident. She hits a concrete wall and dies instantly, but her children survive. Rick has no record of drunk driving. Should he go to prison? Is he guilty of manslaughter? How would you feel if you were the victim's husband? If you were Rick's friend?

2. Some groups concerned about alcohol abuse advocate greater restrictions on availability, such as prohibiting the sale of alcoholic beverages in supermarkets, convenience stores, and gas stations. They would like to see a ban on advertisements, especially those aimed at young people. Opponents argue that laws have never

been effective in controlling alcohol abuse. Do you think our society is too permissive in the way we allow alcohol to be promoted or sold? Would you support anti-alcohol laws? Why or why not?

3. Have you ever been around people who have been intoxicated when you have been sober? What did you think of their behavior? Were they fun to be around? Was the experience not particularly enjoyable, boring, or difficult in some way? Have you ever been intoxicated? How do you behave when you are drunk? Do you find the experience enjoyable? What do the peo-

ple around you think of your actions when you are drunk?

4. What effects has alcohol use had in your life? Try making a list of the positive and negative effects your own alcohol use has had. Be specific. If you continue to drink at your current rate, what positive and negative effects do you think it will have on your future? What effects has other people's drinking had on your life? List family members and friends who drink regularly, and how their drinking has affected you.

SITES & BYTES

Facts On Tap: Alcohol and Your College Experience
http://www.factsontap.org

The Children of Alcoholics Foundation and the American Council for Drug Education, two of the nation's leaders in substance abuse prevention education, sponsor this excellent website written specifically for college students. The interactive site features activities and straightforward information, including alcohol and the college experience, the effects of alcohol on the nondrinker, alcohol and the family, and a true/false quiz to test your knowledge about alcohol and its effects.

Students Against Destructive Decisions (SADD)
http://www.saddonline.com

This site features resources and relevant information to empower students to help their peers understand the consequences of destructive decisions related to alcohol use and abuse, and to live safe and happy lives.

BACCHUS & GAMMA Peer Education Network for Colleges
http://www.bacchusgamma.org

This site designed for college students and health services professionals features information on college and university peer health education programs focusing on alcohol abuse prevention and other student health and safety issues.

Please note that links are subject to change. If you find a broken link, use a search engine such as **http://www.yahoo.com** and search for the website by typing in key words.

InfoTrac Activity Henry Wechsler and Meichun Kuo. "College Students Define Binge Drinking and Estimate Its Prevalence: Results of a National Survey." *Journal of American College Health,* Vol. 49, No. 2, September 2000, p. 57.

(1) At the median, what are college students' predictions of peer binge-drinking rates? What do you think accounts for this?

(2) Why are social norms programs effective in college health education programs designed to promote responsible alcohol consumption?

You can find additional readings related to alcohol use with Infotrac College Edition, an online library of more than 900 journals and publications. Follow the instructions for accessing InfoTrac that were packaged with your textbook; then search for articles using a key word search.

For additional links, resources, and suggested readings on InfoTrac, visit our Health & Wellness Resource Center at **http://health.wadsworth.com**.

Key Terms

The terms listed here are used within the chapter on the page indicated. Definitions of terms are in the Glossary at the end of the book.

absorption 515	**alcohol abuse** 530	**alcohol dependence** 530

References

1. NIAAA. http://www.niaaa.nih.gov.
2. Mukamal, Kenneth, et al. "Prior Alcohol Consumption and Mortality Following Acute Myocardial Infarction." *Journal of the American Medical Association*, Vol. 285, No. 15, April 18, 2001, p. 1965.
3. "New Study Shows Alcohol May Affect Cognition in Young People." *The Dana Brain Daybook*, Vol. 4, No. 2, March–April 2000.
4. Mukamal et al., "Prior Alcohol Consumption and Mortality Following Acute Myocardial Infarction."
5. "Targeting the At-Risk Drinker with Screening and Advice." *Facts of Life: Issue Briefing for Health Reporter*, Vol. 6, No. 1, January 2001.
6. "Alcohol Use and Abuse: A Pediatric Concern." *Pediatrics*, Vol. 108, No. 1, July 2001, p. 185.
7. "SAMHSA Guide Focuses on Underage Drinking." *Alcoholism & Drug Abuse Weekly*, Vol. 13, No. 30, August 6, 2001, p. 6.
8. "Findings About Teen Drinking." *American Psychological Association*, July 5, 2001.
9. Olds, R. Scott, et al. "The Relationship of Adolescent Perceptions of Peer Norms and Parent Involvement to Cigarette and Alcohol Use." *Journal of School Health*, Vol. 71, No. 6, August 2001, p. 223.
10. "Family Support Tops List of Protective Factors for Alcohol Misuse." *Brown University Digest of Addiction Theory and Application*, Vol. 20, No. 8, August 2001, p. 3.
11. "Researchers Find Health Problems Among Teen Drinkers." *Alcoholism & Drug Abuse Weekly*, Vol. 13, No. 36, September 24, 2001, p. 6.
12. Wechsler, Henry, et al. "College Binge Drinking in the 1990s: A Continuing Problem." *Journal of American College Health*, Vol. 48, No. 5, March 2000.
13. Gose, Ben. "Harvard Researchers Note a Rise in College Students Who Drink Heavily and Often." *Chronicle of Higher Education*, Vol. 46, No. 20, March 24, 2000.
14. Anding, Jenna, et al. "Dietary Intake, Body Mass Index, Exercise, and Alcohol." *Journal of American College Health*, Vol. 49, January 2001, p. 167.
15. Federal Office of Substance Abuse Prevention.
16. Jones, Sherry, et al. "Binge Drinking Among Undergraduate College Students in the United States: Implications for Other Substance Use." *Journal of American College Health*, Vol. 50, No. 1, July 2001, p. 33.
17. Wood, Mark, et al. "Social Influence Processes and College Student Drinking: The Mediational Role of Alcohol Outcome Expectancies." *Journal of Studies on Alcohol*, Vol. 62, No. 1, January 2001, p. 32.
18. Hildebran, Kathryn, and Dewaynef Johnson. "Comparison of Patterns of Alcohol Use Between High School and College Athletes and Nonathletes." *Research Quarterly for Exercise and Sport*, Vol. 72, March 2001.
19. Wechsler, Henry, et al. "Binge Drinking on America's College Campuses." Harvard School of Public Health, 2001. Available at www.hsph.harvard.edu/cas.
20. Dreyfuss, Ira. "Athletes Drink More Alcohol." *Associated Press*, January 21, 2001.
21. Wechsler et al., "Binge Drinking on America's College Campuses."
22. Wechsler, Henry, et al. "Drinking Levels, Alcohol Problems, and Secondhand Effects in Substance-Free College Residences: Results of a National Study." *Journal of Studies on Alcohol*, Vol. 62, No. 1, January 2001, p. 23.
23. Clapp, John, and Audrey Shilington. "Environmental Predictors of Heavy Episodic Drinking." *American Journal of Drug and Alcohol Abuse*, Vol. 27, No. 2, May 2001, p. 301.
24. Wilenz, Pam. "Greek Membership Does Not Predict Post-College Drinking Levels." *American Psychological Association*, March 1, 2001.
25. Jones et al., "Binge Drinking Among Undergraduate College Students in the United States." p. 33.
26. Wechsler et al., "Drinking Levels, Alcohol Problems and Secondhand Effects in Substance-Free College Residences."
27. "Curbing Binge Drinking on Campus." *Facts of Life Issue Briefing for Health Reporters*, Vol. 6, No. 1, January 2001, p. 1.
28. Carter, Colleen, and William Kahnweiler. "The Efficacy of the Social Norms Approach to Substance Abuse Prevention Applied to Fraternity Men." *Journal of American College Health*, Vol. 49, No. 20, September 2000.
29. Werch, Chudley, et al. "Results of a Social Norm Intervention to Prevent Binge Drinking Among First-Year Residential College Students." *Journal of American College Health*, Vol. 49, No. 20, September 2000.
30. McGinn, Daniel. "Scouting a Dry Campus." *Newsweek*, November 27, 2000.
31. NIAAA. http://www.niaaa.nih.gov.
32. Hales, Dianne. *Just Like a Woman*. New York: Bantam Books, 2000.
33. Wilsnack, Sharon. Personal interview.
34. "Younger Women Less Likely to Stop Using Alcohol and Tobacco During Pregnancy." *Medical Letter on the CDC & FDA*, November 26, 2000.
35. Kirkpatrick, Jean. Personal interview.
36. "10th Special Report to Congress on Alcohol and Health." National Institute on Alcohol and Alcohol Abuse, December 2000.
37. "Targeting the At-Risk Drinker with Screening and Advice."
38. Fletcher, Anne. *Sober for Good*. New York: Houghton Mifflin, 2001.
39. Brown, Sandra, et al. "Four-Year Outcomes from Adolescent Alcohol and Drug Treatment." *Journal of Studies on Alcohol*, Vol. 62, No. 3, May 2001, p. 381.
40. NIAAA. http://www.niaaa.nih.gov.
41. Thomas, Vince, et al. "Alcohol Abuse, Cognitive Impairment, and Mortality Among Older People." *Journal of the American Geriatric Society*, Vol. 49l, No. 4, April 2001, p. 415.
42. "When Parents Have a Drinking Problem." *Contemporary Pediatrics*, Vol. 18, No. 1, January 2001, p. 67.

16

Tobacco Use, Misuse, and Abuse

Andrea didn't really want her first cigarette. Her tent mate at camp had snatched one from a counselor's pack, and the two of them had climbed to a remote rock to share it. Andrea hated everything about her first drag: the taste, the smell, the horrible burning in her throat and lungs. But she loved feeling more grown-up and sophisticated than other seventh graders. By the time she reached high school, Andrea would sneak off to smoke with friends at least once a week. By graduation, she was smoking daily.

As a college freshmen, Andrea discovered that she was part of an unpopular minority. Even though her dorm didn't ban smoking, her roommate declared their room a smoke-free zone. Her college didn't allow smoking in any classrooms or public areas. And many of her new friends reacted as if smoking was a sign of impaired intelligence. Andrea has decided to quit, but she's discovered that nicotine dependence is very difficult to overcome. "I just wish I'd never started smoking in the first place," she says.

More young people are indeed deciding not to smoke. According to the most recent federal data, cigarette smoking has declined among youths aged 12 to 17 and young adults between the ages of 18 and 25. The number of young people becoming daily smokers has dropped by a third.[1]

About one in three people in the United States—29.3 percent—currently smoke. Tobacco use remains the leading preventable cause of death in the United States, claiming more than 400,000 lives each year and costing more than $50 billion in direct medical costs every year. Each year, smoking kills more people than AIDS, alcohol, drug abuse, car crashes, murders, suicides, and fires combined. Nationally, smoking results in more than 5 million years of potential life lost each year.[2]

This chapter discusses the effects of tobacco on the body, smoking patterns, tobacco dependence, quitting smoking, smokeless tobacco, and environmental tobacco smoke. The information it provides may help you to breathe easier today—and may help ensure cleaner air for others to breathe tomorrow.

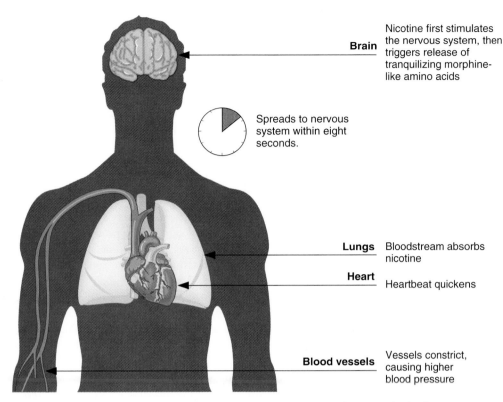

Brain Nicotine first stimulates the nervous system, then triggers release of tranquilizing morphine-like amino acids

Spreads to nervous system within eight seconds.

Lungs Bloodstream absorbs nicotine

Heart Heartbeat quickens

Blood vessels Vessels constrict, causing higher blood pressure

▲ **Figure 16-2** The effects of nicotine, a fast-acting and potent drug, on the body.

Sources: American Cancer Society, National Cancer Institute

ity of the hemoglobin in the blood to carry oxygen, impairs normal functioning of the nervous system, and is at least partly responsible for the increased risk of heart attack and strokes in smokers.

The Impact of Tobacco

About one in every five deaths in the United States and between $50 billion and $73 billion in medical expenses can be attributed to tobacco use.[3] Tobacco causes more than 400,000 deaths among smokers and another 50,000 deaths among nonsmokers exposed to environmental tobacco smoke.[4] Cigarette smoking is associated with elevated risk of mortality from all causes, several cardiovascular diseases, and cancer. Teenagers who smoke are more likely to engage in binge drinking.[5]

Health Effects of Cigarette Smoking

If you're a smoker who inhales deeply and started smoking before the age of 15, you're trading a minute of future life for every minute you now spend smoking. On average smokers die nearly seven years earlier than nonsmokers.[6] Smoking not only eventually kills, it also ages you: Smokers get more wrinkles than nonsmokers. But the effects of smoking are far more than skin-deep. A cigarette smoker is 10 times more likely to develop lung cancer than a nonsmoker and 20 times more likely to have a heart attack. Those who smoke two or more packs a day are 15 to 25 times more likely to die of lung cancer than are nonsmokers. Moreover, the danger of lung cancer skyrockets when smokers are also exposed to other carcinogens, such as asbestos. This double threat increases the risk of lung cancer to as much as 92 times that for nonsmokers not exposed to asbestos.

Heart Disease and Stroke

Although a great deal of publicity has been given to the link between cigarettes and lung cancer, heart attack is actually the leading cause of deaths for smokers. Smoking doubles the risk of heart disease, and smokers who suffer heart attacks have only a 50 percent chance of recovering. Smokers have a 70 percent higher death rate from heart disease than do nonsmokers, and those who smoke heavily have a 200 percent higher death rate.

The federal Office of the Surgeon General blames cigarettes for one of every ten deaths attributable to heart disease. Smoking is more dangerous than are the two most notorious risk factors for heart disease: high blood pressure and high cholesterol. If smoking is combined with one of these, the chances of heart attack are four times greater. Women who smoke and use oral contraceptives have a ten times higher risk of suffering heart attacks than women who do neither.

Smoking also causes a condition called *cardiomyopathy*, which weakens the heart's ability to pump blood and results in the death of about 10,000 people a year. Although researchers don't know precisely how smoking poisons the heart muscle, they speculate that either nicotine or carbon monoxide has a direct toxic effect. Other coronary diseases may be associated with smoking. *Aortic aneurysm* is a bulge in the aorta (the large artery attached to the heart) caused by a weakening of its walls. *Pulmonary heart disease* is a heart disorder caused by changes in blood vessels in the lungs.

Even people who have smoked for decades can reduce their risk of heart attack if they quit smoking. However, recent studies indicate some irreversible damage to blood vessels. Progression of atherosclerosis—hardening of the arteries—among past smokers continues at a faster pace than among those who never smoked.

In addition to contributing to heart attacks, cigarette smoking increases the risk of stroke two to three times in men and women, even after other risk factors are taken into account. According to one study of middle-aged men, giving up smoking leads to a considerable decrease in the risk of stroke within five years of quitting, particularly in smokers of fewer than 20 cigarettes a day. Those with hypertension show the greatest benefit. The risk for heavy smokers declines but never reverts back to that of men who never smoked.

Cancer

The American Cancer Society estimates that tobacco smoking is the cause of 28 percent of all deaths from cancer and the cause of more than 85 to 90 percent of all cases of lung cancer. The more people smoke, the longer they smoke, and the earlier they start smoking, the more likely they are to develop lung cancer.

Smokers of two or more packs a day have lung cancer mortality rates 15 to 25 times greater than nonsmokers. If smokers stop smoking before cancer has started, their lung tissue tends to repair itself, even if there were already precancerous changes. Former smokers who haven't smoked for 15 or more years have lung cancer mortality rates only somewhat above those for nonsmokers.

Chemicals in cigarette smoke and other environmental pollutants switch on a particular gene in the lung cells of some individuals. This gene produces an enzyme that helps manufacture powerful carcinogens, which set the stage for cancer. The gene seems more likely to be activated in some people than others, and people with this gene are at much higher risk of developing lung cancer. However, smokers without the gene still remain at risk, because other chemicals and genes also may be involved in the development of lung cancer.

Smokers who are depressed are more likely to get cancer than nondepressed smokers. Although researchers don't know exactly how smoking and depression may work together to increase the risk of cancer, one possibility is that stress and depression cause biological changes that

lower immunity, such as a decline in natural killer cells that fight off tumors.

Despite some advances in treating lung cancer, however, the prognosis for sufferers is not good. Even with vigorous therapy, fewer than 10 percent survive for five years after diagnosis. This is one of the lowest survival rates of any type of cancer. And if the cancer has spread from the lungs to other parts of the body, only 1 percent survive for five years after diagnosis.

Respiratory Diseases

Smoking quickly impairs the respiratory system. Even some teenaged smokers show signs of respiratory difficulty—breathlessness, chronic cough, excess phlegm production—when compared with nonsmokers of the same age. Cigarette smokers are up to 18 times more likely than are nonsmokers to die of noncancerous diseases of the lungs.

Cigarette smoking is the major cause of chronic obstructive lung disease (COLD), which includes emphysema and chronic bronchitis, in men and women. COLD is characterized by progressive limitation of the flow of air into and out of the lungs. In emphysema, the limitation of air flow is the result of disease changes in the lung tissue, affecting the bronchioles (the smallest air passages) and the walls of the alveoli (the tiny air sacs of the lung) (see Figure 16-3). Eventually, many of the air sacs are destroyed, and the lungs become much less able to bring in oxygen and remove carbon dioxide. As a result, the heart has to work harder to deliver oxygen to all organs of the body.

In chronic bronchitis, the bronchial tubes in the lungs become inflamed, thickening the walls of the bronchi, and the production of mucus increases. The result is a narrowing of the air passages. Smoking is more dangerous than any form of air pollution, at least for most Americans, but exposure to both air pollution and cigarettes is particularly harmful. Although each may cause bronchitis, together they have a synergistic effect—that is, their combined impact exceeds the sum of their separate effects.

Other Smoking-Related Problems

Smokers are more likely than nonsmokers to develop gum disease, and they lose significantly more teeth. Even those who quit have worse gum problems than people who never smoked at all. Smoking may also contribute to the loss of teeth and teeth supporting bone, even in individuals with good oral hygiene.

Cigarette smoking is associated with stomach and duodenal ulcers; mouth, throat, and other types of cancer; and cirrhosis of the liver. Smoking may worsen the symptoms or complications of allergies, diabetes, hypertension, peptic ulcers, and disorders of the lungs or blood vessels. Some men who smoke ten cigarettes or more a day may

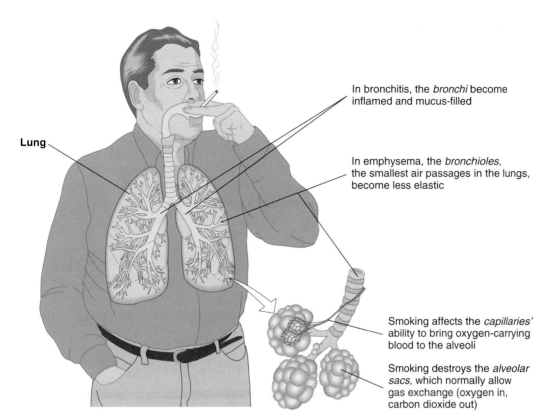

In bronchitis, the *bronchi* become inflamed and mucus-filled

In emphysema, the *bronchioles*, the smallest air passages in the lungs, become less elastic

Lung

Smoking affects the *capillaries'* ability to bring oxygen-carrying blood to the alveoli

Smoking destroys the *alveolar sacs*, which normally allow gas exchange (oxygen in, carbon dioxide out)

▲ **Figure 16-3** How smoking affects the lungs.

experience sexual impotence. Cigarette smokers also tend to miss work one-third more often than do nonsmokers, primarily because of respiratory illnesses. In addition, each year cigarette-ignited fires claim thousands of lives.

Cigarette smoking may increase the likelihood of anxiety, panic attacks, and social phobias, according to a study that followed 688 teenagers into adulthood. Those who smoked a pack a day or more were at 6.8 times greater risk of agoraphobia, 5.5 times greater risk of general anxiety disorder, and 15.6 times greater risk of panic disorder. The exact mechanism is unknown, but one theory is that nicotine may have anxiety-generating effects that act on the nervous system.[7]

Smoking and Medication

Smokers use more medications—aspirin, painkillers, sleeping pills, tranquilizers, antihistamines, cough medicines, stomach medicines, laxatives, diuretics, and antibiotics—than nonsmokers do. According to the American Pharmaceutical Association, nicotine and other tobacco ingredients speed up the process by which the body uses and eliminates drugs, so they may not be able to do what they're intended to do. As a result, smokers may have to take a medication more frequently than do nonsmokers. If you smoke, let your physician know so that he or she can adjust any prescriptions, if necessary.

The Financial Cost of Smoking

The total costs of cigarette smoking to American society include greater work absenteeism, higher insurance premiums, disability payments, and training costs to replace employees who die prematurely from smoking. In the course of a lifetime, the average smoker can expect to spend $10,000 to $20,000 on cigarettes—but that's only the beginning. The potential costs for medical services for a man between the ages of 35 and 39 who smokes heavily may be as high as $60,000. But the greatest toll—the pain and suffering of cancer victims and their loved ones—obviously cannot be measured in dollars and cents.

Why Do People Start Smoking?

Most people are aware that there is a health risk associated with smoking, but many don't know exactly what that risk is or how it might affect them.

The two main factors linked with the onset of a smoking habit are age and education. The vast majority of white men (93 percent) with less than a high school education are current or former daily cigarette smokers. White women with similar educational backgrounds are also very likely to smoke or to have smoked every day. Latino men and women without a high school education are less likely to be or become daily smokers. Other factors associated with the reasons for smoking are discussed in the following sections.

Genetics

Researchers speculate that genes may account for about 50 percent of smoking behavior, with environment playing an equally important role. Studies have shown that identical twins, who have the same genes, are more likely to have matching smoking profiles than fraternal twins. If one identical twin is a heavy smoker, the other is also likely to be; if one smokes only occasionally, so does the other.

According to Swedish research that has followed 25,000 pairs of same-sex twins since 1886, smoking patterns in men suggested both genetic and environmental influences. The smoking patterns in female twins, however, were quite different. Among those born before 1925, when smoking was socially unacceptable for women, the overall rate of smoking was low, and the genetic influence was absent. However, among those born after 1940, when smoking had become much more acceptable for women, rates of tobacco use increased, and the role of genetic influences rose as well—essentially to the same level as that among men. This suggests that some individuals do have a strong genetic predisposition toward tobacco use. However when smoking is strongly discouraged, they do not express that genetic tendency. On the other hand, if smoking is socially acceptable, the genetic tendency to smoke emerges.[8]

Parental Role Models

Children who start smoking are 50 percent more likely than youngsters who don't smoke to have at least one smoker in their families. A mother who smokes seems a particularly strong influence on making smoking seem acceptable. The majority of youngsters who smoke say that their parents also smoke and are aware of their own tobacco use.

Adolescent Experimentation and Rebellion

Young people who are trying out various behaviors may take up smoking because they're curious or because they want to defy adults. Others simply want to appear grown-up or cool. A comprehensive, youth-led prevention program in Florida that emphasizes the truth about tobacco has significantly reduced smoking among middle and high school students.[9] In studies conducted by the CDC, about seven out of ten high school students said they wanted to stop smoking, but only a small percentage were successful.

Teens often misjudge the addictive power of cigarettes. Many, sure that they'll be able to quit any time they want, figure that smoking for a year or two won't hurt them. But when they try to quit, they can't. Like older smokers, most young people who smoke have tried to quit at least once. The American Cancer Society has found that young smokers tend to become heavy smokers and that the longer anyone is exposed to smoke, the greater the health dangers.

Limited Education

People who have graduated from college are much less likely to smoke than are high school graduates; those with fewer than 12 years of education are most likely to smoke. An individual with 8 years or less of education is 11 times more likely to smoke than someone with postgraduate training.

Weight Control

Smokers burn up an extra 100 calories a day compared with nonsmokers—the equivalent of walking a mile—probably because nicotine increases metabolic rate. Once they start smoking, many individuals say they cannot quit because they fear they'll gain weight. The CDC estimates that women who stop smoking gain an average of 8 pounds, while men put on an average of 6 pounds. One in eight women and one in ten men who stop smoking put on 29 pounds or more. The reasons for this weight gain include nicotine's effects on metabolism as well as emotional and behavioral factors, such as the habit of frequently putting something into one's mouth. Yet as a health risk, smoking a pack and a half to two packs a day is a greater danger than carrying 60 pounds in extra weight.

Weight gain for smokers who quit is not inevitable, however. Aerobic exercise helps increase metabolic rate, and limiting alcohol and foods high in sugar and fat can help smokers control their weight as they give up cigarettes.

Aggressive Marketing

Cigarette companies spend billions each year on advertisements and promotional campaigns, with manufacturers targeting ads especially at women, teens, minorities, and the poor. Most controversial are cigarette advertisements in magazines and media aimed at teenagers and even younger children. As part of a nationwide antismoking campaign, health and government officials have called for restrictions on cigarette ads, and manufacturers have agreed not to aim their sales efforts at children and teens.

Stress

In studies that have analyzed the impact of life stressors, depression, emotional support, marital status, and income, researchers have concluded that an individual with a high stress level is approximately 15 times as likely to be a smoker than a person with low stress. About half of smokers identify workplace stress as a key factor in their smoking behavior.

Addiction

According to recent research, the first symptoms of nicotine addiction can start within a few days of starting to smoke and after just a few cigarettes, particularly in teenagers.[10] The findings, based on a study of almost 700 adolescents, challenges the conventional belief that nicotine dependence is a gradual process that takes hold after prolonged daily smoking.

Why People Keep Smoking

Whatever the reasons for lighting up that first cigarette, very different factors keep cigarettes burning pack after pack, year after year. In national polls, four out of five smokers say that they want to quit but can't. The reason isn't a lack of willpower. Medical scientists have recognized tobacco dependence as an addictive disorder that may be more powerful than heroin dependence and that may affect more than 90 percent of all smokers.

Pleasure

According to the American Cancer Society, 87.5 percent of regular smokers find smoking pleasurable. Nicotine—the addictive ingredient in tobacco—is the reason. Researchers have shown that nicotine reinforces and strengthens the desire to smoke by acting on brain chemicals that influence feelings of well-being. This drug also can improve memory, help in performing certain tasks, reduce anxiety, dampen hunger, and increase pain tolerance.

Mental Disorders

Individuals with mental disorders are twice as likely to smoke as others, and people with mental illness may account for nearly one-half of the tobacco market in the United States. Heavy smoking also is linked with an almost elevenfold risk of anxiety disorders in early adulthood.[11]

People with a history of depression are significantly more likely to be smokers and to be diagnosed as nicotine-dependent. Smokers are more likely than nonsmokers to report depressive symptoms—and these symptoms may interfere with quitting. According to researchers, the likelihood of quitting smoking is about 40 percent lower among depressed than nondepressed smokers.

Dependence

Nicotine has a much more powerful hold on smokers than alcohol does on drinkers. Whereas about 10 percent of alcohol users lose control of their intake of alcohol and become alcoholics, as many as 80 percent of all heavy smokers have tried to cut down on or quit smoking but cannot overcome their dependence.

Nicotine causes dependence by at least three means:

- It provides a strong sensation of pleasure.
- It leads to fairly severe discomfort during withdrawal.
- It stimulates cravings long after obvious withdrawal symptoms have passed.

Few drugs act as quickly on the brain as nicotine does. It travels through the bloodstream to the brain in seven seconds—half the time it takes for heroin injected into a blood vessel to reach the brain. And a pack-a-day smoker gets 200 hits of nicotine a day—73,000 a year.

After a few years of smoking, the most powerful incentive for continuing to smoke is to avoid the discomfort of withdrawal. Generally, ten cigarettes a day will prevent withdrawal effects. For many who smoke heavily, signs of withdrawal, including changes in mood and performance, occur within two hours after smoking their last cigarette. Smokeless tobacco users also get constant doses of nicotine. However, absorption of nicotine by the lungs is more likely to lead to dependence than absorption through the linings of the nose and mouth. As with other drugs of abuse, continued nicotine intake results in tolerance (the need for more of a drug to maintain the same effect), which is why only 2 percent of all smokers smoke just a few cigarettes a day, or smoke only occasionally. (See Self-Survey: "Are You Addicted to Nicotine?")

Use of Other Substances

Many smokers also drink or use drugs. According to the Addiction Research Foundation in Canada, tobacco smokers say cigarettes are harder to abandon than other drugs, even when they find them less pleasurable than their preferred drug of abuse. Individuals who drink excessively also find their cigarette habit a hard one to break.

Smoking in America

Tobacco use remains the most serious and widespread addictive behavior in the world and the major cause of preventable deaths in our society. About one in three Americans (29.3 percent) currently use tobacco products. Cigarettes are the most popular, with 24.9 percent of Americans over age 12 reporting current use, while 10.7 percent smoke cigars, 3.4 percent use smokeless tobacco, and 1 percent smoke pipes.[12] Half of those who continue to smoke will die from a smoking-related disease.

Tobacco Use on Campus

 College-age individuals make up the youngest age group that tobacco manufacturers can legally target with their marketing efforts. Smoking by college students rose dramatically during the 1990s and has remained high. The actual percentage of students who smoke varies in different

SELF SURVEY

Are You Addicted to Nicotine?

Answer the following questions as honestly as you can by placing a check mark in the appropriate column:

	Yes	No
1. Do you smoke every day?	—	—
2. Do you smoke because of shyness and to build up self-confidence?	—	—
3. Do you smoke to escape from boredom and worries or while under pressure?	—	—
4. Have you ever burned a hole in your clothes, carpet, furniture, or car with a cigarette?	—	—
5. Have you ever had to go to the store late at night or at another inconvenient time because you were out of cigarettes?	—	—
6. Do you feel defensive or angry when people tell you that your smoke is bothering them?	—	—
7. Has a doctor or dentist ever suggested that you stop smoking?	—	—
8. Have you ever promised someone that you would stop smoking, then broken your promise?	—	—
9. Have you ever felt physical or emotional discomfort when trying to quit?	—	—
10. Have you ever successfully stopped smoking for a period of time, only to start again?	—	—
11. Do you buy extra supplies of tobacco to make sure you won't run out?	—	—
12. Do you find it difficult to imagine life without smoking?	—	—
13. Do you choose only those activities and entertainments during which you can smoke?	—	—
14. Do you prefer, seek out, or feel more comfortable in the company of smokers?	—	—
15. Do you inwardly despise or feel ashamed of yourself because of your smoking?	—	—
16. Do you ever find yourself lighting up without having consciously decided to?	—	—
17. Has your smoking ever caused trouble at home or in a relationship?	—	—
18. Do you ever tell yourself that you can stop smoking whenever you want to?	—	—
19. Have you ever felt that your life would be better if you didn't smoke?	—	—
20. Do you continue to smoke even though you are aware of the health hazards posed by smoking?	—	—

If you answered Yes to one or two of these questions, there's a chance that you are addicted or are becoming addicted to nicotine. If you answered Yes to three or more of these questions, you are probably already addicted to nicotine.

Source: Nicotine Anonymous World Services, San Francisco.

Making Changes

Breaking the Habit

Here's a six-point program to help you or someone you love quit smoking. (*Caution:* Don't undertake the quit-smoking program until you have a two- to four-week period of relatively unstressful work and study schedules or social commitments.)

1. *Identify your smoking habits.* Keep a daily diary (a piece of paper wrapped around your cigarette pack with a rubber band will do) and record the time you smoke, the activity associated with smoking (after breakfast, in the car), and your urge for a cigarette (desperate, pleasant, or automatic). For the first week or two, don't bother trying to cut down; just use the diary to learn the conditions under which you smoke.

2. *Get support.* It can be tough to go it alone. Phone your local chapter of the American Cancer Society, or otherwise get the names of some ex-smokers who can give you support.

3. *Begin by tapering off.* For a period of one to four weeks, aim at cutting down to, say, 12 or 15 cigarettes a day; or change to a lower-nicotine brand, and concentrate on not increasing the number of cigarettes you smoke. As indicated by your diary, begin by cutting out those cigarettes you smoke automatically. In addition, restrict the times you allow yourself to smoke. Throughout this period, stay in touch, once a day or every few days, with your ex-smoker friend(s) to discuss your problems.

4. *Set a quit date.* At some point during the tapering-off period, announce to everyone—friends, family, and ex-smokers—when you're going to quit. Do it with flair. Announce it to coincide with a significant date, such as your birthday or anniversary.

5. *Stop.* A week before Q-day, smoke only five cigarettes a day. Begin late in the day, say after 4:00 P.M. Smoke the first two cigarettes in close succession. Then, in the evening, smoke the last three, also in close succession, about 15 minutes apart. Focus on the negative aspects of cigarettes, such as the rawness in your throat and lungs. After seven days, quit and give yourself a big reward on that day, such as a movie or a fantastic meal or new clothes.

6. *Follow up.* Stay in touch with your ex-smoker friend(s) during the following two weeks, particularly if anything stressful or tense occurs that might trigger a return to smoking. Think of the person you're becoming—the very person cigarette ads would have you believe smoking makes you. Now that you're quitting smoking, you're becoming healthier, sexier, more sophisticated, more mature, and better looking—and you've earned it!

Sources: American Cancer Society; National Cancer Institute.

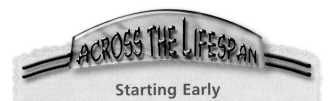

Starting Early

Every day nearly 3,000 young people under the age of 18 become regular smokers. More than 5 million children will die prematurely because they decide to start smoking. Eighty to 90 percent of adults who currently smoke began to do so before the age of 18, at an average age of 12.5 years, and most were regular smokers by the age of 14. Among high school smokers who thought they wouldn't be smoking in five years, 73 percent still are.[13]

The earlier that smokers light up, the greater the dangers they face. Recent studies suggest that smoking in adolescence may trigger changes in DNA that put young people at higher risk for cancer even if they later quit. In studies of lung cancer patients, those with the worst genetic damage were not those who'd smoked the longest but those who started the youngest. And the earlier they started, the more severe the damage.

An estimated 13.4 percent of teens report current use of cigarettes. More girls (14.1 percent) than boys (12.8 percent) are smokers. Among young adults, 38.3 percent smoke.

Many factors influence teens' decision to smoke, including aggressive marketing by tobacco companies, peer pressure, and psychological vulnerability. Studies of teens have found very high awareness of tobacco advertising, branding, and sponsorship of sports events. Thirty percent of teen smokers had received free gifts through coupons in cigarette packs.[14] Athletes, beginning in high school and continuing into college, use tobacco more frequently and in greater amounts than nonathletes.[15] Teenagers with aggressive tendencies or even low levels of depression also are more likely to smoke.[16]

Starting to smoke at an early age may lead to heavier smoking and other unhealthy behaviors, including binge drinking.[17] Researchers have documented a significantly higher proportion of anxiety disorders, including generalized anxiety and panic disorder, among adolescents who are heavy smokers (defined as smoking at least 20 cigarettes a day) than among teens who smoked less or not at all.[18]

Treatment for nicotine dependence has proven effective for adolescents as well as adults.[19] Teens who underwent treatment have consistently higher abstinence rates from six months to five years afterward than those who try to quit on their own.[20]

STRATEGIES FOR PREVENTION

Why Not to Light Up
Before you start smoking—before you ever face the challenge of quitting—think of what you have to gain by *not* smoking:

✔ A significantly reduced risk of cancer of the lungs, larynx, mouth, esophagus, pancreas, and bladder.

✔ Half the risk of heart disease that smokers face.

✔ A lower risk of stroke, chronic obstructive lung disease (COLD), influenza, ulcers, and pneumonia.

✔ A lower risk of having a low-birthweight baby.

✔ A longer lifespan.

✔ Potential savings of tens of thousands of dollars that you would otherwise spend on tobacco products and medical care.

surveys, ranging from 29 percent to as high as 50 percent.[21] Today's students also use a broader range of tobacco products: cigarettes, cigars, pipes, and smokeless tobacco. In one study, nearly half (46 percent) of college students reported having used tobacco products in the previous year.[22]

 Among African-American students, almost half (49 percent) have tried smoking (that is, smoked at least one cigarette but less than 100 during their lifetime); 9.3 percent were "lifetime smokers" (smoked more than 100 cigarettes during their lifetime). More black women than men have tried smoking.[23]

College men and women have nearly identical rates for cigarette smoking, but more men use cigars and smokeless tobacco. White students used more cigarettes and smokeless tobacco than Hispanics, African Americans, or Asians. Among tobacco users, 51.3 percent used more than one tobacco product in the past year; the most frequent combination was cigars and cigarettes. The median age of first cigarette use for students of both genders was 14 years; for first cigar use, it was 17 years for men and 18 years for women.

Students who use tobacco are more likely to smoke marijuana, binge drink, have more sexual partners, have lower grades, rate parties as important, and spend more time socializing with friends. They are less likely than nonusers to rate athletics or religion as important. Tobacco use is lower in western colleges. Unlike cigarette smokers, cigar users rate fraternities and sororities and attending

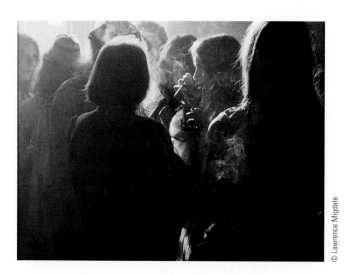

▲ Smoking often goes hand in hand with drinking.

encourages all schools to work toward a campus-wide tobacco/smoke-free environment. Among its recommendations to the nation's institutions of higher learning are the following:

▶ Prohibition of campus-controlled advertising, sales, or free sampling of tobacco products and of sponsorship of campus events by tobacco-promoting organizations.
▶ Prohibition of smoking in all public areas, including classrooms, auditoriums, laboratories, libraries, gymnasiums, meeting rooms, stadiums, buses, vans, meeting rooms, private offices, and dining facilities.
▶ Prohibition of smoking in all residence halls, dormitories, and campus housing, including lounges, stairwells, hallways, restrooms, and bedrooms.
▶ Prevention and education initiatives directed against tobacco use.
▶ Programs that include practical steps to quit tobacco use.[26]

sporting events as important. College students who use smokeless tobacco tend to be white men attending schools in rural areas.

In a survey of 393 colleges and universities, 85 percent of student health center directors considered student smoking a problem or a major problem. Those at public institutions were more likely to perceive smoking as a major problem, while those at religiously affiliated schools were less likely to do so. Most schools—97 percent—restricted smoking in some way, usually in public areas but not in offices or student residences. (See Student Snapshot: "Smoking on Campus.") Schools in the northeast and north-central regions of the country were significantly less likely to prohibit smoking than those in the west.

An estimated 44 percent of students live in smoke-free dorms, while another 29 percent who do not would like to move into one. Freshmen who did not smoke regularly in high school and who live in smoke-free dorms are 40 percent less likely to take up smoking than those in unrestricted housing, according to a study of the smoking behavior of 4,495 students at 101 schools.[24]

Despite concern about student smoking, more than 40 percent of schools do not offer smoking cessation programs to students who want to quit. Those that do primarily refer students to campus support groups or community-based programs like Nicotine Anonymous, they report little student demand for these options. Colleges are much less likely to offer individualized support, medical screening and assistance, or FDA-approved cessation products. Few provide smoking awareness programs, peer education, or quitting incentive programs.[25]

Researchers warn that experimentation with tobacco products in college could evolve into nicotine dependence and daily cigarette smoking. The American College Health Association has adopted a no-smoking policy that

Smoking and Minorities

Cigarette smoking is a major cause of disease and death in all population groups. However, tobacco use varies within and among racial/ethnic minority groups. Among adults, Native Americans and Alaska Natives have the highest rates of tobacco use—37.9 percent of the men smoke cigarettes, compared with 25 percent of adults in the overall U.S. population. African-American men (32.1 percent) and Southeast Asian men also have a high smoking rate. Asian-American and Hispanic women have the lowest rates of smoking. Tobacco use is significantly higher among white college students.[27]

However, tobacco has taken the greatest toll on the health of African Americans. Middle-aged and older African Americans are far more likely than their counterparts in other major racial/ethnic minority groups to die from coronary heart disease, stroke, or lung cancer. In the 1970s and 1980s, death rates from respiratory cancers (mainly lung cancer) increased among both African-American men and women. In the last decade, these rates declined substantially among African-American men and leveled off in African-American women.

As several studies have shown, many African-American adolescents experiment with smoking but then stop. Among black college students, the risk factors for smoking include friends who smoke, parents who smoked, and a view of religion as unimportant. For lifetime smoking, being single, having had no or few childhood friends who smoked and having no current friends who smoke decrease the likelihood that an African American would continue to smoke.[28]

African-American teens who smoke are at greater risk of developing long-term consequences than are other

Student Snapshot   Smoking on Campus

College students who smoke		29%
College health center directors who view student smoking as a problem or major problem		85%
Colleges that prohibit smoking in all public areas	NO SMOKING	81%
Colleges that prohibit smoking in student residents		27%
Colleges that allow smoking everywhere on campus		3%

Source: Wechsler, Henry, et al. "College Smoking Policies and Smoking Cessation Programs: Results of a Survey of College Health Center Directors." *Journal of American College Health,* Vol. 49, No. 5, March 2001, p. 205.

youths, even when they smoke less. The reason for their increased susceptibility to asthma, allergies and depression may be potential differences in the way that ethnic groups metabolize nicotine.[29]

Tobacco is the substance most abused by Hispanic youths, and their smoking rates have soared in the last ten years.[30] In general, smoking rates among Hispanic adults increase as they adopt the values, beliefs, and norms of American culture. Recent declines in the prevalence of smoking have been greater among Hispanic men with at least a high school education than among those with less education.

According to the U.S. Surgeon General, "adverse infant health outcomes," such as low-birthweight babies, sudden infant death syndrome (SIDS), and infant mortality, are especially high for African Americans, Native Americans, and Alaska Natives who smoke. Cigarette smoking also increases these risks, especially for SIDS, among Asian Americans, Pacific Islanders, and Hispanics.

Smoking and Women

Approximately one in five women (22 percent) smoke. Smoking rates are even higher among teenage girls: 30 percent of female high school seniors report having smoked within the past 30 days. Globally, smoking prevalence among women varies from as low as 7 percent in developing countries to 24 percent in developed countries.[31]

Women with less than a high school education are three times more likely to smoke than those with a college degree.[32] As discussed in The X & Y Files: "Men, Women, and Tobacco," women smoke for different reasons and in different ways than men. They also suffer unique consequences.

According to the U.S. Surgeon General, women account for 39 percent of smoking-related deaths each year, a proportion that has doubled since 1965. Since 1980 approximately three million women in the United States have died from smoking-related diseases. Each year,

The X & Y Files — Men, Women, and Tobacco

In the past, men were far more likely than women to smoke—and to suffer the health consequences. More women today, particularly young women, smoke. According to the Centers for Disease Control and Prevention, 28 percent of men and 22 percent of women are smokers. Among teens, more girls than boys smoke.

Male and female smokers share certain characteristics: Most start smoking as teenagers; the lower their educational level, the more likely they are to smoke. But there are gender differences in tobacco use. In the last decade, smoking rates among adult women stopped their previous decline and have risen sharply among teenage girls. Men of all ages are more likely than women to use other forms of tobacco, such as cigars and chewing tobacco.

The genders smoke for different reasons. Men smoke to decrease boredom and fatigue and to increase arousal and concentration. Women smoke to control their weight and to decrease stress, anger, and other negative feelings.

Men respond more intensely to the pleasurable and painkilling effects of nicotine on brain chemistry. While nicotine affects appetite and weight in both genders, its effects are more pronounced in women. Yet accumulating evidence shows that, for women, nicotine intake may be less important in smoking behavior than it is for men. Women take fewer and shorter puffs from cigarettes and are less sensitive to some of nicotine's effects, but they may be more sensitive to external stimuli, such as the presence of a lit cigarette or the smell of smoke.

Women tend to be less successful than men in quitting smoking. Possible reasons include gender differences in the effectiveness of therapies, a greater fear of weight gain among women, the inability to take certain anti-smoking drugs while pregnant, and the menstrual cycle's effect on withdrawal symptoms. Women drop out at higher rates from traditional stop-smoking programs and are less responsive to nicotine replacement therapies. The approaches that work best for them combine medication and behavioral treatments, including support groups.

Sources: http://www.nida.nih.gov. "Women Less Successful in Quitting Smoking." *Alcoholism & Drug Abuse Weekly,* Vol. 13, No. 21, May 28, 2001, p. 8. *Women and Smoking: A Report of the Surgeon General—2001.* Washington, DC: U.S. Department of Health and Human Services, 2001.

American women lose an estimated 2.1 million years of life due to premature deaths attributable to smoking.

If she smokes, a woman's annual risk of dying more than doubles after age 45 compared with a woman who has never smoked. Lung cancer now claims more women's lives than breast cancer. Smoking also is a major cause of cancer of the pharynx and bladder and may increase the risk of liver, colon, cervical, kidney, and pancreatic cancer.

Women who smoke face an increased risk of depression, stroke, bleeding in the brain, diseases of the blood vessels, and respiratory diseases such as chronic obstructive pulmonary disease (COPD). The risk of heart attack in women who smoke 25 or more cigarettes a day is more than 500 percent greater than the risk in women who don't smoke. Even smoking just one to four cigarettes a day doubles the risk. Women who smoke low-nicotine cigarettes are four times more likely to have a first heart attack than women who don't smoke—the same risk as for those who smoke high-nicotine cigarettes.

Women who smoke also are more likely to develop osteoporosis, a bone-weakening disease. They tend to be thin, which is a risk factor for osteoporosis, and they enter menopause earlier, thus extending the period of jeopardy from estrogen loss.

Smoking directly affects women's reproductive organs and processes. Women who smoke are less fertile and experience menopause one or two years earlier than women who don't smoke. Smoking also boosts a woman's likelihood of developing cervical cancer and greatly increases the possible risks associated with taking oral contraceptives. Older women who smoke are weaker, have poorer balance, and are at greater risk of physical disability than nonsmokers.

Women who smoke during pregnancy increase their risk of miscarriage and pregnancy complications, including bleeding, premature delivery, and birth defects such as cleft lip or palate. Women who smoke are twice as likely to have an ectopic pregnancy (in which a fertilized egg develops in the fallopian tube rather than in the uterus) and to have babies of low birthweight as those who have never smoked. However, women who stop smoking before pregnancy reduce their risk of having a low-birthweight baby to that of women who don't smoke. Even those who quit three or four months into the pregnancy have babies with higher birthweights than those who continue smoking throughout pregnancy. (See Chapter 9 for more information on the health risks associated with smoking during pregnancy.)

Other Forms of Tobacco

Some 10.7 million Americans smoke cigars; 7.6 million use smokeless tobacco, and 2.1 million smoke pipes.[33]

Ingesting tobacco may be less deadly than smoking cigarettes, but it is dangerous. Smoking cigars, clove cigarettes, and pipes, and chewing or sucking on smokeless tobacco all put the user at risk of cancer of the lip, tongue, mouth, and throat—as well as other diseases and ailments.

Cigars

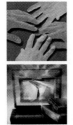

Cigar use has declined in the last few years. However, after cigarettes, cigars are the tobacco products most widely used by college students. According to the first national survey to report on undergraduate cigar use, more than a third reported ever smoking a cigar (including more than half of men and a quarter of women), while 23 percent had smoked a cigar within the past year and 8.5 percent had smoked one within the previous 30 days. About one in five students smoke both cigars and cigarettes. Most cigar use is occasional. Fewer than 1 percent of current cigar users on campus smoked daily. Cigar use is similar in white and black students but lower in Hispanics and Asians. In contrast to the ratio for men, more African-American than white women reported smoking cigars (6.8 versus 4 percent).[34]

Cigar smoking is as dangerous even though smokers do not inhale. Cigars are known causers of cancers of the lung and the digestive tract. The risk of death related to cigars approaches that of cigarettes, as the number of cigars smoked and the amount of cigar smoke inhaled increases (see Figure 16-4). Cigar smoking can lead to nicotine addiction, even if the smoke is not inhaled. The nicotine in the smoke from a single cigar can vary from an amount roughly equivalent to that in a single cigarette to that in a pack or more of cigarettes.

Clove Cigarettes

Sweeteners have long been mixed into tobacco, and clove, a spice, is the latest ingredient to be added to the recipe for cigarettes. Clove cigarettes typically contain two-thirds tobacco and one-third cloves. Consumers of these cigarettes are primarily teenagers and young adults.

Many users believe that clove cigarettes are safer than regular ones because they contain less tobacco, but this isn't necessarily the case. The CDC reports that people who smoke clove-containing cigarettes may be at risk of serious lung injury. Smoking clove cigarettes during a mild upper respiratory tract illness can lead to severe breathing difficulty. And clove cigarette smokers, like other cigarette smokers, can become addicted to the tobacco.

Clove cigarettes may be more harmful than conventional cigarettes. They deliver twice as much nicotine, tar, and carbon monoxide as moderate-tar American brands. Eugenol, the active ingredient in cloves (which dentists have used as an anesthetic for years), deadens sensation in the throat, allowing smokers to inhale more deeply and hold smoke in their lungs for a longer time. Chemical relatives of eugenol can produce the kind of damage to cells that may lead to cancer.

???? What Are Bidis?

Skinny, sweet-flavored cigarettes called **bidis** (pronounced "beedees") have become a smoking fad among teens and young adults. For centuries, bidis were popular in India, where they are known as the "poor man's cigarette" and sell for less than five cents a pack. Although they look strikingly like clove cigarettes or marijuana joints, bidis, available in flavors like grape, strawberry, and mandarin orange, are legal for adults and even minors in some states and are sold on the Internet as well as in stores.

Although bidis contain less tobacco than regular cigarettes, their unprocessed tobacco is more potent. Smoke from bidis has about three times as much nicotine and carbon monoxide and five times as much tar as smoke from regular filtered cigarettes.[35] Because bidis are wrapped in nonporous brownish leafs, they don't burn as easily as cigarettes, and smokers have to inhale harder and more often to keep them lit. In one study, smoking a single bidi required 28 puffs, compared to 9 puffs for cigarettes.

Health authorities view bidis as "cigarettes with training wheels"—products that could lead to a lifetime of nicotine addiction because they are easy to buy and lack the health-warning labels required of cigarettes. Unlike

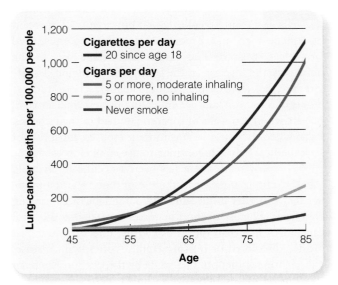

▲ **Figure 16-4** The dangers of cigarettes versus cigars.

Sources: American Cancer Society, National Cancer Institute.

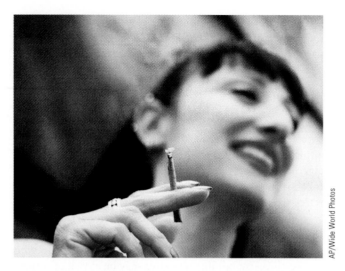

AP/Wide World Photos

▲ The smoke produced by bidis—skinny, flavored cigarettes—can contain higher concentrations of toxic chemicals than that in regular cigarettes.

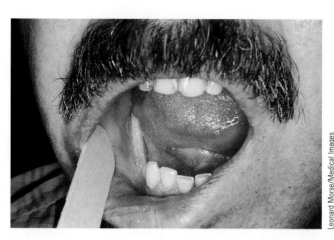

Leonard Morse/Medical Images

▲ Chewing smokeless tobacco can damage the tissues of the mouth. In addition to causing oral cancer, the use of smokeless tobacco can lead to cancer of the larynx, esophagus, kidney, pancreas, and bladder.

regular cigarettes, which are smoked mostly by white youths, bidis also are popular among young Hispanics and blacks.

Pipes

Many cigarette smokers switch to pipes to reduce their risk of health problems. But former cigarette smokers may continue to inhale, even though pipe smoke is more irritating to the respiratory system than cigarette smoke. People who have only smoked pipes and who do not inhale are much less likely to develop lung and heart disease than are cigarette smokers. However, they are as likely as cigarette smokers to develop—and die of—cancer of the mouth, larynx, throat, and esophagus.

Smokeless Tobacco

The sale and consumption of smokeless tobacco products are rising, particularly among young males. These substances include snuff, finely ground tobacco that can be sniffed or placed inside the cheek and sucked, and chewing tobacco, which consists of tobacco leaves mixed with flavoring agents such as molasses. With both, nicotine is absorbed through the mucous membranes of the nose or mouth.

Every day approximately 2,200 U.S. youths, ages 11 to 19, try smokeless tobacco for the first time. About 830 become regular users. Many of these users lack awareness of its dangers.[36] Smokeless tobacco can cause cancer and noncancerous oral conditions and lead to nicotine addiction and dependence. Smokeless tobacco users are more

likely than nonusers to become cigarette smokers. Powerful carcinogens in smokeless tobacco include nitrosamines, polycyclic aromatic hydrocarbons, and radiation-emitting polonium. Its use can lead to the development of white patches on the mucous membranes of the mouth, particularly on the site where the tobacco is placed. Most lesions of the mouth lining that result from the use of smokeless tobacco dissipate six weeks after the use of tobacco products is stopped, according to a U.S. Air Force study. However, when first found, about 5 percent of these lesions are cancerous or exhibit changes that progress to cancer within ten years if not properly treated. Cancers of the lip, pharynx, larynx, and esophagus have all been linked to smokeless tobacco.

More than 7 million people, many of them young, use snuff and chewing tobacco. In a national survey of 5,894 men and women from 72 colleges and universities, 22 percent of college men and 2 percent of college women used smokeless tobacco. The lowest percentage was in the northeast, the highest, in the south-central region. In different regions, 8 to 36 percent of male high school students are regular users. Many are emulating professional baseball players who keep wads of tobacco jammed in their cheeks. Even when they spot lesions in their mouths, most do not seek medical help but continue to use smokeless tobacco.

In recent years, there has been a decline in chewing tobacco, but an increase in the use of moist snuff, a product that is higher in nicotine and potential cancer-causing chemicals. The use of snuff increases the likelihood of oral cancer by more than four times. Other effects include bad breath, discolored or missing teeth, cavities, gum disease, and nicotine addiction. In a study by the Oregon Research Institute, dental patients were three times more likely to quit snuff and chewing tobacco after hygienists taught them that smokeless tobacco was responsible for their mouth sores, bleeding gums, and receding gums. Self-help approaches, such as using oral substitutes like nicotine gum or mint chew, also have proven effective.[37]

Environmental Tobacco Smoke

Maybe you don't smoke—never have, never will. That doesn't mean you don't have to worry about the dangers of smoking, especially if you live or work with people who smoke. **Environmental tobacco smoke,** or secondhand cigarette smoke, the most hazardous form of indoor air pollution, ranks behind cigarette smoking and alcohol as the third-leading preventable cause of death.

Mainstream and Sidestream Smoke

On average, a smoker inhales what is known as **mainstream smoke** eight or nine times with each cigarette, for a total of about 24 seconds. However, the cigarette burns for about 12 minutes, and everyone in the room (including the smoker) breathes in what is known as **sidestream smoke.**

According to the American Lung Association, incomplete combustion from the lower temperatures of a smoldering cigarette makes sidestream smoke dirtier and chemically different from mainstream smoke. It has twice as much tar and nicotine, five times as much carbon monoxide, and 50 times as much ammonia. And because the particles in sidestream smoke are small, this mixture of irritating gases and carcinogenic tar reaches deeper into the lungs. If you're a nonsmoker sitting next to someone smoking seven cigarettes an hour, even in a ventilated room, you'll take in almost twice the maximum amount of carbon monoxide set for air pollution in industry—and it will take hours for the carbon monoxide to leave your body.

What Are the Risks of Secondhand Smoke?

Even a little secondhand smoke is dangerous.[38] According to the Centers for Disease Control and Prevention (CDC), every year environmental tobacco smoke causes 3,000 deaths from lung cancer. In a Harvard University study that tracked 10,000 healthy women who never smoked over ten years, regular exposure to other people's smoke at home or work almost doubled the risk of heart

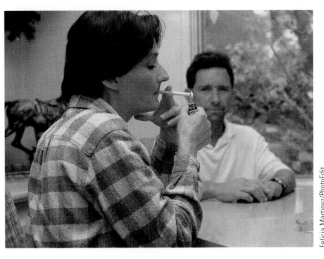

Felicia Martinez/PhotoEdit

▲ Secondhand (or environmental tobacco) smoke is the most hazardous form of indoor air pollution.

disease. On the basis of their findings, the researchers estimated that up to 50,000 Americans may die of heart attacks from environmental tobacco smoke every year, while 3,000 to 4,000 die of other forms of heart disease. As a cancer-causing agent, secondhand smoke may be twice as dangerous as radon gas and more than a hundred times more hazardous than outdoor pollutants regulated by federal law. Secondhand smoke also increases the sick leave rates among employees.[39]

Families of Smokers: Living Dangerously

Just thirty minutes of exposure to secondhand smoke at home may have a substantial impact on health.[40] The most vulnerable nonsmokers are the spouses and children of smokers. Numerous epidemiological and autopsy studies have linked environmental tobacco smoke with lung cancer and other disorders. The nonsmoking spouses of smokers, for instance, are 30 percent more likely to die of heart disease than other nonsmokers.

Prenatal exposure to tobacco can have significant effects that may extend from infancy into adulthood. Smoking during pregnancy affects a child's growth, cognitive development, and behavior both before and after birth. Birthweight decreases in direct proportion to the number of cigarettes smoked. The babies of teenage mothers who smoke have lower birthweight, length, head circumference, and chest circumference.[41] As they grow, children of smokers tend to be shorter and weigh less than children of nonsmokers.[42]

A mother's smoking during pregnancy may have cognitive and behavioral effects as well. These include abnormal neurological responses, such as more tremors and startles. Among older children, researchers have found deficits in language and reading abilities and poorer visual perception. Youngsters whose mothers smoked during pregnancy also tend to have problems with hyperactivity, inattention, and impulsivity. Some of these behavior problems persist through the teenage years and even into adulthood. At ages 16 to 18, children exposed to prenatal smoking have higher rates of conduct disorder, substance use, and depression than others.

Even if their mothers don't smoke, children exposed to secondhand smoke before birth also are likely to weigh less and to perform more poorly on tests of speech, language skills, intelligence, and visual-spatial abilities and to develop behavior problems. These youngsters perform at a level between that of children of active smokers and children of nonsmokers.

Exposure to smoke after birth increases the risk of sudden infant death syndrome (SIDS) and is associated with lower IQ scores and deficits in cognitive development.

Children who breathe environmental tobacco smoke suffer from more asthma, wheezing, and bronchitis than children in smoke-free homes.[43] They also face increased risk of lung cancer, heart disease, and stroke.

The negative effects of childhood exposure to environmental tobacco smoke persist even after youngsters leave home. In recent research at Ohio State University, college students who grew up in a smoking household had higher blood pressure and resting heart rates at rest and during psychological stress than those who grew up in smoke-free homes.

The Politics of Tobacco

More than three decades after government health authorities began to warn of the dangers of cigarette smoking, tobacco remains a politically hot topic. After many years of difficult negotiations, the tobacco industry and attorneys general from nearly 40 states reached a historic settlement. Major tobacco companies have agreed to pay more than $200 billion to settle smoking-related lawsuits filed by 46 states, to finance antismoking campaigns, to restrict marketing, to permit federal regulation of tobacco, and to pay fines if tobacco use by minors does not decline.

The federal government has launched a seven-year grassroots antismoking coalition called Americans Stop Smoking

Intervention Study (ASSIST) to combat cigarette smoking. Community leaders in some neighborhoods have whitewashed billboard ads for cigarettes. Some civic and consumer associations have proposed boycotting athletic events sponsored by tobacco companies. In some states, school-based tobacco prevention campaigns and tough antismoking campaigns, financed by taxes on cigarettes, have led to impressive declines in cigarette sales.[44]

The Fight for Clean Air

Nonsmokers, realizing that their health is being jeopardized by environmental tobacco smoke, have increasingly turned to legislative and administrative measures to clear the air and protect their rights. (See Figure 16-5.) Thousands of cities, towns, and counties now restrict smoking in public places and/or regulate the sale of tobacco to minors. Nationally, the airlines have banned smoking on domestic flights. Many institutions, including medical centers and some universities, no longer allow smoking on their premises. Some cities restrict smoking in bars, restaurants, and other public places.

Supporters of smoking restrictions argue that no one should be subjected involuntarily to the dangers of environmental tobacco smoke. (See Savvy Consumer: "How Nonsmokers Can Clear the Air.") Besides the health hazards, smokers jeopardize nonsmokers by increasing the danger of fire.

Opponents of smoking restrictions contend that banning smoking on the job might impair rather than enhance productivity, because employees would take more frequent breaks to go to lounges where smoking is permitted—or else would suffer the negative effects of nicotine withdrawal.

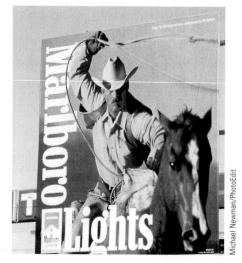
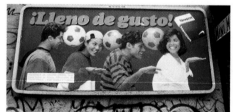
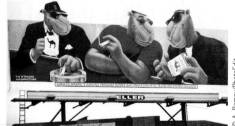

▲ Tobacco advertising is aggressive, but tough antismoking campaigns have led to declines in cigarette sales.

Nonsmoker's Bill of Rights

Nonsmokers Help Protect the Health, Comfort, and Safety
of Everyone by Insisting on the Following Rights:

The Right to Breathe Clean Air

*Nonsmokers have the right to breathe clean air, free from harmful and irritating
tobacco smoke. This right supersedes the right to smoke when the two conflict.*

The Right to Speak Out

*Nonsmokers have the right to express — firmly but politely — their discomfort
and adverse reactions to tobacco smoke. They have the right to voice their objections
when smokers light up without asking permission.*

The Right to Act

*Nonsmokers have the right to take action through legislative means — as
individuals or in groups — to prevent or discourage smokers from polluting the
atmosphere and to seek the restriction of smoking in public places.*

▲ **Figure 16-5** Nonsmoker's bill of rights.

Quitting

Tobacco dependence may be the toughest addiction to overcome. One-third of smokers try to quit annually, but fewer than 10 percent succeed. Current cigarette smokers who stop smoking, even as late as 60 years of age, can avoid most of the excess risk of lung cancer later in life. Quitting at an earlier age further reduces the risk of lung cancer.[45] Most people who eventually quit on their own have already tried other methods. Nicotine withdrawal symptoms can behave like characters in a bad horror flick: Just when you think you've killed them, they're back with a vengeance. In recent studies, some people who tried to quit smoking reported a small improvement in withdrawal symptoms over two weeks, but then their symptoms leveled off and persisted. Others found that their symptoms intensified rather than lessened over time. For reasons scientists cannot yet explain, former smokers who start smoking again put their lungs at even greater jeopardy than smokers who never quit.[46]

According to therapists, quitting usually isn't a one-time event but a "dynamic process" that may take several years and four to ten attempts. The good news is that half of all living Americans who ever smoked have managed to quit. And thanks to new products and programs, it may be easier now than ever before to become an ex-smoker.

Quitting on Your Own

More than 90 percent of former smokers quit on their own—by throwing away all their cigarettes, by gradually cutting down, or by first switching to a less potent brand. One characteristic of successful quitters is that they see themselves as active participants in health maintenance and take personal responsibility for their own health.

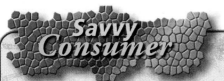

Savvy Consumer

How Nonsmokers Can Clear the Air

• Let people know your feelings in advance by putting up "No Smoking" signs in your office, home, or car. If you're in a car and someone pulls out a cigarette, ask politely if the smoker can hold off until you reach your destination or stop for a break.

• When giving a party, designate a smoking room. Suggest that friends do the same for parties at their houses.

• If you're about to participate in a long meeting or class, suggest regular smoking breaks to avoid a smoke-filled room.

• At restaurants, always ask for a table in the nonsmoking section or, if there is none, one in a well-ventilated part of the restaurant.

• If someone's smoke is bothering you, speak up. Be polite, not pushy. Say something like, "Excuse me, but smoke bothers me."

Often they experiment with a variety of strategies, such as learning relaxation techniques. In women, exercise has proven especially effective for quitting and avoiding weight gain. Making a home a "smoke-free" zone also increases a smoker's likelihood of successful quitting. (See Pulse Points: "Ten Ways to Kick the Habit.")

Stop-Smoking Groups

Joining a support group doubles your chances of quitting for good. The American Cancer Society's FreshStart Program runs about 1,500 stop-smoking clinics, each with about 8 to 18 members meeting for eight 2-hour sessions over four weeks. Instructors explain the risks of smoking, encourage individuals to think about why they smoke, and suggest ways of unlearning their smoking habit. A quitting day is set for the third or fourth session.

The American Lung Association's Freedom from Smoking Program consists of eight 1- to 2-hour sessions over seven weeks. The approach is similar to the American Cancer Society's, but smokers keep diaries and team up with buddies. Ex-smokers serve as advisers on quitting day. Both groups estimate that 27 or 28 percent of their participants successfully stop smoking.

Stop-smoking classes are also available through health-science departments and student-health services on many college campuses, as well as through community public health departments. The Seventh-Day Adventists sponsor a four-week Breathe Free Plan, in which smokers commit themselves to clean living (no smoking, alcohol, tea, or coffee, along with a balanced diet and regular exercise). Many businesses sponsor smoking-cessation programs for employees, which generally follow the approaches of professional groups. Motivation may be even higher in these programs than in programs outside the workplace, however, because some companies offer attractive incentives to participants, such as lower rates on their health insurance.

Some smoking-cessation programs rely primarily on **aversion therapy,** which provides a negative experience every time a smoker has a cigarette. This may involve taking drugs that make tobacco smoke taste unpleasant, undergoing electric shocks, having smoke blown at you, or rapid smoking (the inhaling of smoke every six seconds until you're dizzy or nauseated).

Nicotine Replacement Therapy

This approach uses a variety of products that supply low doses of nicotine in a way that allows smokers to taper off gradually over a period of months. They include nicotine gum (available in two doses) and slow-release skin patches. Although still experimental, a nasal spray also has shown promise.

In research studies, nicotine replacement is the only treatment for nicotine addiction that has proven clearly ben-

PULSE POINTS

Ten Ways to Kick the Habit

1. **Use delaying tactics.** Have your first cigarette of the day 15 minutes later than usual, then 15 minutes later than that the next day, and so on.
2. **Distract yourself.** When you feel a craving for a cigarette, talk to someone, drink a glass of water, or get up and move around.
3. **Establish nonsmoking hours.** Instead of lighting up at the end of a meal, for instance, get up immediately, brush your teeth, wash your hands, or take a walk.
4. **Never smoke two packs of the same brand in a row.** Buy cigarettes only by the pack, not by the carton.
5. **Make it harder to get to your cigarettes.** Lock them in a drawer, wrap them in paper, or leave them in your coat or car.
6. **Change the way you smoke.** Smoke with the hand you don't usually use. Smoke only half of each cigarette.
7. **Keep daily records.** Chart your daily cigarette tally to see what progress you're making.
8. **Stop completely for just one day at a time.** Promise yourself 24 hours of freedom from cigarettes; when the day's over, make the same commitment for one more day. At the end of any 24-hour period, you can go back to smoking and not feel guilty.
9. **Spend more time in places where you can't smoke.** Take up bike-riding or swimming. Shower often. Go to movies or other places where smoking isn't allowed.
10. **Go cold turkey.** If you're a heavily addicted smoker, try a decisive and complete break. Smokers who quit completely are less likely to light up again than those who gradually decrease their daily cigarette consumption, switch to low-tar and low-nicotine brands, or use special filters and holders.

eficial. When measured against a look-alike placebo treatment, nicotine gum and patches have doubled the initial quitting rate and the numbers of smokers who remain abstinent six months to one year later. However, even with these approaches, only about one smoker in four quits completely; about half of these remain abstinent over the long term.

Nicotine Gum

Nicotine gum, sold as Nicorette, contains a nicotine resin that's gradually released as the gum is chewed. Absorbed through the mucous membrane of the mouth, the nicotine doesn't produce the same rush as a deeply inhaled drag on a cigarette. However, the gum maintains enough nicotine in the blood to diminish withdrawal symptoms. A month's supply of Nicorette costs roughly $45.

Although this gum is lightly spiced to mask nicotine's bitterness, many users say that it takes several days to become accustomed to its unusual taste. Its side effects include mild indigestion, sore jaws, nausea, heartburn, and stomachache. Also, because Nicorette is heavier than regular chewing gum, it may loosen fillings or cause problems with dentures. Drinking coffee or other beverages may block absorption of the nicotine in the gum; individuals trying to quit smoking shouldn't ingest any substance immediately before or while chewing nicotine gum.

Nicotine in any form is harmful, and nicotine gum should not be used during pregnancy or by people with heart disease. Most people use nicotine gum as a temporary crutch and gradually taper off until they can stop chewing it relatively painlessly. However, 5 to 10 percent of users transfer their dependence from cigarettes to the gum. When they stop using Nicorette, they experience withdrawal symptoms, although the symptoms tend to be milder than those prompted by quitting cigarettes.

Intensive counseling to teach smokers coping methods can greatly increase the success rates.

Nicotine Patches

Nicotine transdermal delivery system products, or patches, provide nicotine, their only active ingredient, via a patch attached to the skin by an adhesive. Like nicotine gum, the nicotine patch minimizes withdrawal symptoms, such as intense craving for cigarettes. Some insurance programs pay for patch therapy. Nicotine patches, which cost between $3.25 and $4 each, are replaced daily during therapy programs that run between 6 and 16 weeks. However, there is no evidence that continuing their use for more than 8 weeks provides added benefit.

Some patches deliver nicotine around the clock and others for just 16 hours (during waking hours). Those most likely to benefit from nicotine patch therapy are people who smoke more than a pack a day, are highly motivated to quit, and participate in counseling programs. However, the nicotine patch is not a cure for a smoking habit. While using the patch, 37 to 77 percent of people are able to abstain from

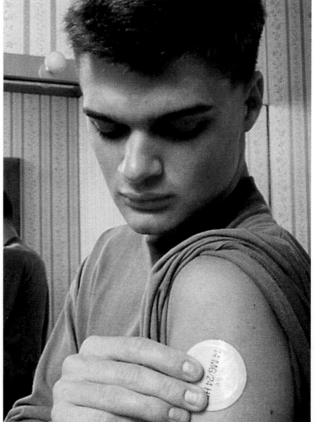

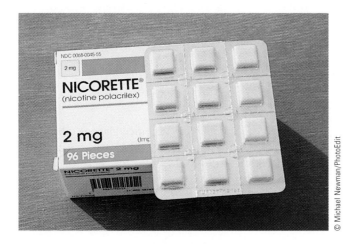

▲ Nicorette gum, when chewed, gradually releases a nicotine resin and helps some smokers break their habit. Nicorette is now available without a prescription.

▲ A nicotine patch releases nicotine transdermally (through the skin) in measured amounts, which are gradually decreased over time.

smoking. But the patch doesn't affect the psychological dependence that makes quitting smoking so hard. That's why the key to long-term success in quitting smoking is getting support. When combined with counseling, the patch can be about twice as effective as a placebo, enabling 26 percent of smokers to abstain for six months.

Because nicotine is a powerful, addictive substance, the use of nicotine patches for a prolonged period is not advised. Pregnant women and individuals with heart disease shouldn't use them. Patch wearers who smoke or use more than one patch at a time can experience a nicotine overdose; some users have even suffered heart attacks. Occasional side effects include redness, itching, or swelling at the site of the patch application; insomnia; dry mouth; and nervousness.

Bupropion (Zyban)

An alternative to the patch is **bupropion,** a drug initially developed to treat depression that is marketed in a slow-release form for nicotine addiction as Zyban. In studies that have combined Zyban with nicotine replacement and counseling, 40 to 60 percent of those treated have remained smoke-free for at least a year after completing the program. This success rate is much higher than the 10 to 26 percent reported among smokers who try to quit using nicotine replacement alone. The combination of Zyban and nicotine replacement also prevented the initial weight gain that often accompanies quitting.[47] Other

medications used to treat nicotine addiction are clonidine, mecamylamine, and buspirone.

Smoke-Free Days

Since 1976, a November day has been set aside in the United States for the annual Great American Smoke-Out, an idea promoted by the American Cancer Society to encourage smokers to give up cigarettes for 24 hours. As many as 36 percent of American smokers have given up cigarettes on Smoke-Out Day; about 5 to 6 percent have quit permanently; 15 percent reduced smoking for extended periods. In addition, the World Health Organization has established World No-Tobacco Days in May to call on nations to urge tobacco users to abstain for at least one day and perhaps quit for good.

Other Ways to Quit

Hypnosis may help some people quit smoking. Hypnotherapists use their techniques to create an atmosphere of strict attention and give smokers in a mild trance positive suggestions for breaking their cigarette habit.

Acupuncture, in which a circular needle or staple is inserted in the flap in front of the opening to the ear, has also had some success. When smokers feel withdrawal symptoms, they gently move the needle or staple, which may increase the production of calming chemicals in the brain.

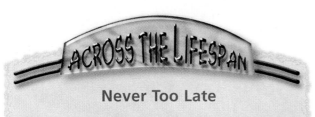

Never Too Late

The sooner a smoker stops using tobacco, the greater the health benefits. However, it is never too late to quit. Quitting at any age, even after age 65, can improve health and extend life—even after thirty or more years of regular smoking. A person who smokes more than 20 cigarettes a day and quits at age 65 increases life expectancy by two or three years.

Despite the well-documented benefits of quitting, an estimated 13 percent of seniors over age 65 smoke. They account for about 70 percent of the smoking-related deaths in the country. When older people stop tobacco use, their circulation and lung function increase; they suffer less cardiovascular illness; and their quality of life improves.[48]

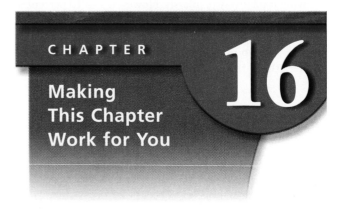

CHAPTER

Making This Chapter Work for You

16

1. Which of the following statements about tobacco and its components is true?
    a. Nicotine settles in the lungs, eventually causing precancerous changes.
    b. Tobacco stimulates the kidneys to form urine.
    c. Carbon monoxide contained in tobacco smoke impairs oxygen transport in the body.
    d. Tar is the addictive substance in tobacco.

2. Cigarette smokers
    a. are more likely to die of lung cancer than heart disease.

b. usually develop lung problems after years of tobacco use.

c. have two to three times the risk of suffering a stroke than nonsmokers.

d. may completely reverse the damage to their blood vessels if they quit smoking.

3. Which of the following statements about smoking is false?

a. Smoking behavior may have a genetic component.

b. People who graduate college are less likely to smoke than those who complete only high school.

c. Most regular smokers enjoy smoking.

d. Smoking two packs of cigarettes daily is as dangerous as carrying 40 pounds of extra weight.

4. Tobacco use on college campuses

a. is most often in the form of smokeless tobacco products used by students to avoid detection.

b. is more prevalent among those students who also use marijuana, binge drink, and spend more time socializing with friends.

c. has decreased in the past 10 years because almost all schools have adopted a no-smoking policy on their premises.

d. is considered a minor problem by most student health center directors, since less than a third of students smoke.

5. Which of the following statements about smoking and minorities is true?

a. Hispanic men are less likely to smoke than Hispanic women.

b. Native American women who smoke are at low risk of having babies with health problems.

c. African Americans are at greater risk for dying from heart disease, lung cancer, and stroke than those of other population groups.

d. Smoking is culturally unacceptable among Southeast Asian men.

6. Women smokers

a. tend to be less successful than men in quitting smoking.

b. are more likely to die from breast cancer than lung cancer.

c. experience menstruation earlier than women who don't smoke.

d. who smoke low-nicotine cigarettes lower their risk of having a heart attack to the same level as women who don't smoke.

7. Cigarette smokers may switch to which of the following products to reduce their risk of health problems?

a. cigars

b. snuff

c. clove cigarettes

d. pipes

8. Secondhand tobacco smoke is

a. the smoke inhaled by a smoker.

b. more hazardous than outdoor pollution as a cancer-causing agent.

c. less hazardous than mainstream smoke.

d. less likely to cause serious health problems in children than in adults.

9. Quitting smoking

a. usually results in minor withdrawal symptoms.

b. will do little to reverse the damage to the lungs and other parts of the body.

c. can be aided by using nicotine replacement products.

d. is best done by cutting down on the number of cigarettes you smoke over a period of months.

10. Ways to help yourself quit include all of the following except

a. join a support group.

b. make your home a smoke-free zone.

c. try acupuncture.

d. switch to bidis.

Answers to these questions can be found on page 640.

 Kids and Tobacco Addictions. Why are teen smokers at a greater risk for cancer and other diseases?

Critical Thinking

1. Has smoking become unpopular among your friends or family? What social activities continue to be associated with smoking? Can you think of any situation in which smoking might be frowned upon?

2. How would you motivate someone you care about to stop smoking? What reasons would you give for them to stop? Describe your strategy.

3. According to the chapter, environmental tobacco smoke is even more dangerous than mainstream smoke. If you're a nonsmoker, how would you react to someone who's smoking in the same room as you? Define the rights of smokers and nonsmokers.

SITES & BYTES

Centers for Disease Control and Prevention on Smoking and Tobacco Control
http://www.cdc.gov/health/smoking.htm
This site features comprehensive educational materials on smoking, quitting tips, surgeon general reports, research data on tobacco use among specific populations and minority groups, and helpful information for educators and youth.

Joe Chemo Antismoking Site
http://www.joechemo.org
Based on the character Joe Chemo, an antismoking parody of Joe Camel, this site is highly interactive and allows visitors to test their "Tobacco IQ," get a personalized "Smoke-o-Scope," and send free Joe Chemo E-Cards. There is also extensive information for teachers, antismoking activists, health-care providers, journalists, and smokers who wish to quit.

American Lung Association Tobacco Control
http://www.lungusa.org/tobacco/index.html
This site features information on smoking cessation, including seven steps to a smoke-free life, as well as information on tobacco control, smoking and special populations, and several fact sheets on secondhand smoke, data and statistics, and current news events.

Please note that links are subject to change. If you find a broken link, use a search engine such as http://www.yahoo.com and search for the website by typing in key words.

InfoTrac Activity Sharon Scott Morey. "PHS Updates Smoking Cessation Guideline." *American Family Physician*, Vol. 63, No. 8, April 15, 2001, p. 1635.

(1) What are the five first-line pharmacologic agents that can be used, either alone or in combination, to help smokers break nicotine dependency?

(2) Besides pharmacologic therapy, what other interventions are proven to increase the likelihood of cessation from smoking?

You can find additional readings related to tobacco use with InfoTrac College Edition, an online library of more than 900 journals and publications. Follow the instructions for accessing InfoTrac that were packaged with your textbook; then search for articles using a key word search.

For additional links, resources, and suggested readings on InfoTrac, visit our Health & Wellness Resource Center at http://health.wadsworth.com.

Key Terms

The terms listed here are used within the chapter on the page indicated. Definitions of terms are in the Glossary at the end of the book.

aversion therapy 560	**carbon monoxide** 544	**nicotine** 544
bidis 555	**environmental tobacco smoke** 557	**sidestream smoke** 557
bupropion 562	**mainstream smoke** 557	**tar** 544

References

1. "HHS Report Shows Drug Use Rates Stable, Youth Tobacco Use Declines." *Medical Letter on the CDC & FDA*, October 21, 2001, p. 2.
2. http://www.cdc.gov/tobacco.
3. "Reducing Tobacco Use: The Quest to Quit." *Facts of Life: Issue Briefing for Health Reporters*, Vol. 6, No. 3, March–April 2001.
4. Malarcher, Ann, et al. "Methodological Issues in Estimating Smoking-Attributable Mortality in the United States." *American Journal of Epidemiology*, Vol. 152, No. 5, September 15, 2000.
5. Johnson, Patrick, et al. "The Co-occurrence of Smoking and Binge Drinking in Adolescence." *Addictive Behaviors*, Vol. 25, No. 5, September–October 2000.
6. "Reducing Tobacco Use: The Quest to Quit."
7. Johnson, Jeffrey, et al. "Association Between Cigarette Smoking and Anxiety Disorders During Adolescence and Early Adulthood." *Journal of the American Medical Association*, Vol. 284, No. 18, November 8, 2000.

8. "Genes That Cause Smoking?" *Harvard Heart Letter,* Vol. 11, No. 7, March 2001.

9. Bauer, Ursula, et al. "Changes in Youth Cigarette Use and Intentions Following Implementation of a Tobacco Control Program." *Journal of the American Medical Association,* Vol. 284, No. 6, August 9, 2000.

10. DiFranza, Joseph. "Initial Symptoms of Nicotine Dependence in Adolescents." *Tobacco Control,* Vol. 9, 2000.

11. Charatan, Fred. "Mental Illness and Smoking Show Strong Links." *Bulletin of the World Health Organization,* Vol. 79, No. 1, January 2001, p. 79.

12. "HHS Report Shows Drug Use Rates Stable, Youth Tobacco Use Declines."

13. http://www.cdc.gov/tobacco.

14. "Teenagers Susceptible to Tobacco Marketing." *Brown University Child and Adolescent Behavior Letter,* Vol. 17, No. 4, April 2001, p. 3.

15. Bogle, Kimberly, et al. "Comparisons of Patterns of Tobacco Use between High School and College Athletes and Nonathletes." *Research Quarterly for Exercise and Sport,* Vol. 72, No. 1, March 2001, p. A-24.

16. "Youth Smoking Linked to Disposition Factors." *Alcoholism & Drug Abuse Weekly,* Vol. 13, No. 18, May 7, 2001, p. 8.

17. "Early Smoking May Predict Dependence in Adulthood." *Alcoholism & Drug Abuse Weekly,* Vol. 13, No. 6, February 5, 2001, p. 7.

18. Charatan, "Mental Illness and Smoking Show Strong Links."

19. Patten, Christi. "Tobacco Use Outcomes of Adolescents Treated Clinically for Nicotine Dependence." *Journal of the American Medical Association,* Vol. 286, No. 15, October 17, 2001, p. 1819.

20. "Nicotine Dependence Treatment Shows Success in Adolescents." *Alcoholism & Drug Abuse Weekly,* Vol. 13, No. 28, July 23, 2001, p. 8.

21. Wechsler, Henry, et al. "College Smoking Policies and Smoking Cessation Programs: Results of a Survey of College Health Center Directors." *Journal of American College Health,* Vol. 49, No. 5, March 2001, p. 205.

22. http://substanceabuse.rwjf.org.

23. Hestick, Henrietta, et al. "Trial and Lifetime Smoking Risks Among African-American College Students." *Journal of American College Health,* Vol. 49, No. 5, March 2001, p. 205.

24. Wechsler et al., "College Smoking Policies and Smoking Cessation Programs."

25. Wechsler, Henry, et al. "Cigarette Use by College Students in Smoke-Free Housing: Results of a National Study." *American Journal of Preventive Medicine,* Vol. 20, No. 3, March 2001.

26. "Position Statement on Tobacco on College and University Campuses." American College Health Association. http://www.acha.org.

27. Rigotti, Nancy, et al. "US College Students' Use of Tobacco Products: Results of a National Survey." *Journal of the American Medical Association,* Vol. 284, No. 6, August 9, 2000.

28. Hestick et al., "Trial and Lifetime Smoking Risks among African-American College Students."

29. "African-American Teens at High Risk from Smoking." *Alcoholism & Drug Abuse Weekly,* Vol. 13, No. 10, March 5, 2001, p. 8.

30. Guinn, Bobby, et al. "Association of Tobacco Use with Acculturative Status, Knowledge and Attitudes Among Early Adolescent Mexican Americans." *Research Quarterly for Exercise and Sport,* Vol. 72, No. 1, March 2001, p. A-29.

31. "Report: Tobacco-related Deaths Increase Among Women." *Alcoholism & Drug Abuse Weekly,* Vol. 13, No. 14, April 2, 2001, p. 5.

32. *Women and Smoking: A Report of the Surgeon General—2001.* Washington, DC: U.S. Department of Health and Human Services, 2001.

33. "HHS Report Shows Drug Use Rates Stable, Youth Tobacco Use Declines."

34. Rigotti et al., "US College Students' Use of Tobacco Products."

35. Malson, Jennifer, et al. "Comparison of the Nicotine Content of Tobacco Used in Bidis and Conventional Cigarettes." *Tobacco Control,* Vol. 10, No. 2, June 2001, p. 181.

36. Goebal, Lynne, et al. "Young Users of Smokeless Tobacco Lack Awareness of Its Dangers." *Nicotine & Tobacco Research,* December 2000.

37. Severson, Herbert. "Self-Help Programs Help Smokeless Tobacco Users Quit." *Nicotine & Tobacco Research,* December 2000.

38. Glantz, Stanton, and William Parmley. "Even a Little Secondhand Smoke Is Dangerous." *Journal of the American Medical Association,* Vol. 286, No. 4, July 25, 2001, p. 436.

39. Heloma, Antero et al. "The Short-Term Impact of National Smoke-Free Workplace Legislation on Passive Smoking and Tobacco Use." *American Journal of Public Health,* Vol. 91, No. 9, September 2001, p. 1416.

40. Otsuka, Ryo, et al. "Acute Effects of Passive Smoking on the Coronary Circulation in Healthy Young Adults." *Journal of the American Medical Association,* Vol. 286, No. 4, July 25, 2001, p. 436.

41. England, Lucinda, et al. "Effects of Smoking Reduction During Pregnancy on the Birth Weight of Term Infants." *American Journal of Epidemiology,* Vol. 154, No. 8, October 15, 2001, p. 694.

42. "Tobacco Exposure Linked with Long-term Adverse Effects." *Brown University Digest of Addiction Theory and Application,* Vol. 20, No. 10, October 2001, p. 3.

43. Larsson, Matz, et al. "Environmental Tobacco Smoke Exposure During Childhood Is Associated with Increased Prevalence of Asthma in Adults." *Chest,* Vol. 120, No. 3, September, 2001, p. 1711.

44. Wang, Li Yan, et al. "Cost-effectiveness of a School-Based Tobacco-Use Prevention Program." *Archives of Pediatrics & Adolescent Medicine,* Vol. 155, No. 9, September 2001.

45. *Cancer Prevention & Early Detection: Facts & Figures 2001.* Atlanta, GA: American Cancer Society, 2001.

46. "Study Shows Dangers of Resuming Smoking." *Alcoholism & Drug Abuse Weekly,* Vol. 13, No. 40, October 22, 2001, p. 8.

47. Hales, Robert, and Dianne Hales. *The Mind-Mood Pill Book.* New York: Bantam Books, 2001.

48. "Even for Older Adults, It's Not Too Late to Quit." *Facts of Life: Issue Briefing for Health Reporters,* Vol. 6, No. 3, March–April 2001, p. 5.

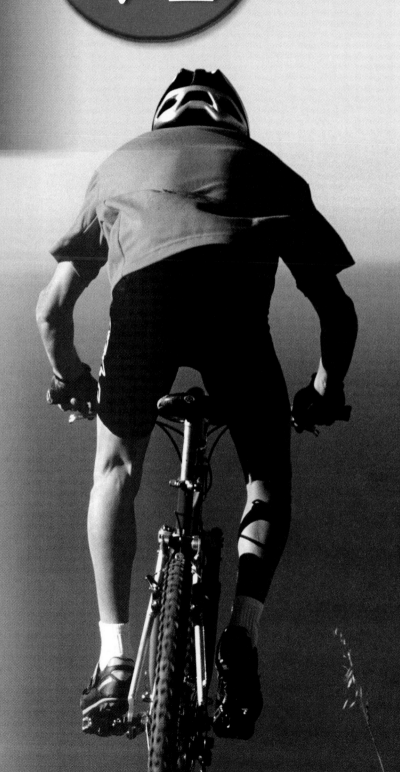

SECTION VI

HEALTH IN CONTEXT

Personal health involves more than a single individual. We are social beings, and we live our lives as part of a network of family, friends, acquaintances, colleagues, neighbors. Our actions affect others; others' behaviors have a significant impact on our well-being.

This social context is particularly pertinent in issues such as injury, violence, and sexual victimization. For college students, staying safe is an essential part of staying healthy. Injury claims more lives of young Americans than illness. Threats such as violence and terrorism are too serious and wide-spread to ignore.

Ultimately, all lives end in the same way. Death is as much as part of the real world as life itself. The quest to find meaning in dying is one of the challenges of living. All of us share something else: our planet. The problems of creating a healthy environment are many and complex. They too demand our attention and commitment.

17

Staying Safe: Preventing Injury, Violence, and Victimization

"This can't be happening to me!" This was the phrase that first ran through Parker's mind when the car swerved out of control. He kept repeating it to himself as he heard the sickening sound of metal hitting metal and felt a terrible crushing pain shoot up through his legs. Later at the hospital, when he woke up after surgery, it was his first thought. And all through the long months of rehabilitation, on the days when he thought life would never go back to normal, he'd try to tell himself that this too couldn't be happening to him.

Most young people think the same way. Accidents, injuries, assaults, crimes—all seem like things that happen only to other people, only in other places. But no one, regardless of how young, healthy, or strong, is immune from danger.

Recognizing the threat of intentional and unintentional injury is the first step to ensuring your personal safety. You may think that the risk of something bad happening is simply a matter of chance, of being in the wrong place at the wrong time. That's not the case. Certain behaviors, such as using alcohol or drugs or not buckling your seat belt, greatly increase the risk of harm. Ultimately, you have more control over your safety than anyone or anything else in your life.

This chapter is a primer in self-protection that could help safeguard—perhaps even save—your life. Included are recommendations for common sense safety on the road, at home, and outdoors. This chapter also explores other serious threats to personal safety in our society—violence, both public and domestic, and sexual victimization.

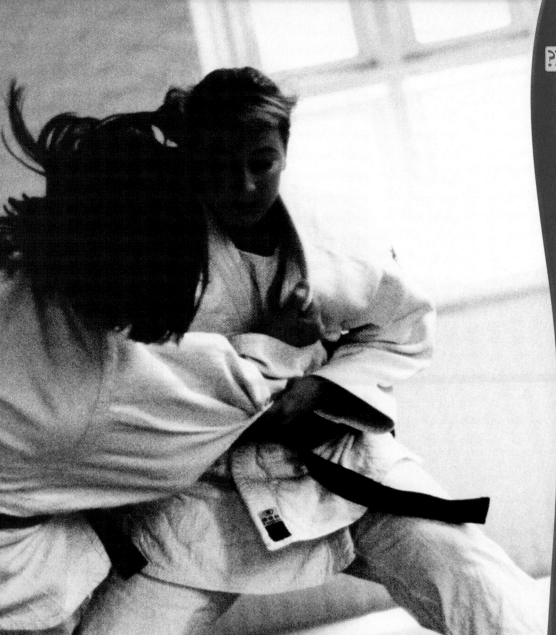

FREQUENTLY ASKED QUESTIONS

FAQ: What should I do in an emergency situation? p. 572

FAQ: Is it safe to use a car phone while driving? p. 575

FAQ: Can my computer be a health hazard? p. 578

FAQ: What is sexual harassment? p. 585

FAQ: How can I prevent date rape? p. 590

After studying the material in this chapter, you should be able to:

- **List** and **explain** factors that increase the likelihood of an accident.
- **Describe** safety procedures for road, residential, worksite, and outdoor safety.
- **Discuss** the factors contributing to aggression and violence.
- **Define** sexual victimization, sexual harassment, and sexual coercion.
- **List** the different types of rape, and describe recommended actions for preventing rape.
- **Explain** the consequences of sexual violence.

Unintentional Injury: Why Accidents Happen

The major threats to the lives of college students aren't illnesses but injuries. Almost 75 percent of deaths among Americans aged 15 to 24 years are caused by unintentional injuries (a term public health officials prefer), suicides, and homicides.[1] The odds of dying from an injury in any given year are about one in 765; over a lifetime they rise to one in 23.[2] In all, injuries—intentional and unintentional—claim almost 150,000 lives a year. Accidents, especially motor vehicle crashes, kill more college-age men and women than all other causes combined; the greatest number of lives lost to accidents is among those 25 years of age.

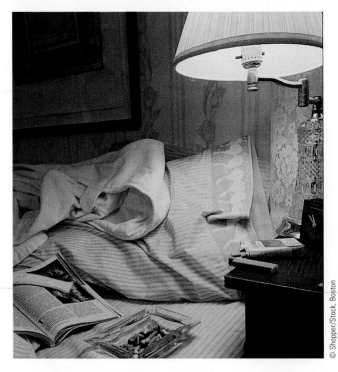

© Shopper/Stock, Boston

▲ Home is a dangerous place. Many accidents happen at home—perhaps because we let down our guard there.

Unsafe Attitudes

Where do you feel safest? Chances are you'll answer by naming the places that are most familiar to you: your room, your home, your car. Yet that's where you're most likely to have an accident—often because you let your guard down. While listening to the morning news, you may forget to shut off a burner on the stove. Since there usually isn't much traffic on your street, you may back out of your driveway without looking both ways. Most of the time you, or someone with you, is able to correct such dangerous situations before a fire or collision occurs. But you can't count on always being so lucky.

Keep in mind that *feeling* safe is not the same as *being* safe. Away from home, unsafe attitudes can set the stage for unsafe behaviors. If you're overly confident in your driving skills, you may speed on a winding or wet road. If you're daydreaming, you may trip and fall as you hike. Keeping your wits about you is essential to keeping yourself safe. (See Self-Survey: "Are You Doing Enough to Prevent Accidents?")

Individual Risk Factors

Many factors influence an individual's risk of accident or injury, including those discussed in the following sections.

Age

The very young and the very old are the most susceptible to serious injury. Children may not recognize the danger of running into the street or jumping into a pool. In older people, a combination of factors—poor health, vision and hearing impairments, a faltering sense of balance, decreased agility, slower reflexes, and reduced resilience—make accidents a greater threat. Most victims of fatal accidents are males, often in their teens and twenties. Feeling full of life and energy, they may take dangerous risks because they think they're invulnerable.

Alcohol and Drugs

An estimated 40 percent of Americans are involved in an alcohol-related accident sometime during their lives. In nearly half of motor-vehicle deaths, either the driver or a pedestrian was intoxicated at the time of the crash. Other drugs also affect driving ability by impairing judgment and perceptions.

Stress

In times of tension and anxiety, we all pay less attention to what we're doing. We rush about; we don't take time to relax or rest. One common result is an increase in accidents during busy or stressful periods. If you find yourself having a series of small mishaps or "near-misses," it's important to do something to lower your stress level, rather than wait for something more harmful to happen. (See Chapter 2 on stress.)

Situational Factors

Some situations—such as driving on a curvy, wet road in a car with worn tires—are so inherently dangerous that they greatly increase the odds of an accident. But even when there's greater risk, you can lower the danger—for instance,

SELF SURVEY

Are You Doing Enough to Prevent Accidents?

These questions are designed to test how well you protect yourself and your family from accidental injury—answer Yes or No to each. The first group of questions concentrates on guarding against possible hazards in and around your house or apartment. The second group deals with safety measures against accidents on the road, whether in a vehicle or as pedestrians. The third group is concerned mainly with safety on vacations, when unfamiliar surroundings and activities present special hazards.

Group 1: Safety at Home

1. Do you make it a point never to smoke in bed?
2. If you have fireplaces, do you keep screens around them?
3. When cooking, do you guard against accidental hot spills by positioning pan handles so that they don't extend outward?
4. Do you keep electrical cords out of the reach of children and avoid overloading electrical outlets?
5. Are you careful never to leave small children unsupervised in the kitchen or bathroom?
6. Are nightclothes and soft toys labeled to show that they're made of nonflammable materials?
7. Are medicines in your house kept in a secure place, out of children's reach and away from beds?
8. Are you careful never to store drugs or dangerous chemicals (bleach, paint-stripper, and so on) within children's reach or in incorrectly labeled containers?
9. If you own a gun, do you keep it unloaded, separate from the ammunition, and locked away?
10. Do you make a point of preventing your children from playing with objects small enough to be swallowed or inhaled?
11. Do you keep plastic bags away from your children?
12. When working around the house, do you wear safety glasses, earplugs, and protective clothing such as sturdy shoes?
13. Are your carpets firmly fixed, with no ragged spots or edges, and are loose rugs placed to minimize the risk of sliding or tripping?
14. Are your stairs, halls, and other passages lit brightly enough to read a newspaper?
15. Is it a rule in your house that nothing gets left on the stairs?
16. If you spill or drop something on the floor that might be slippery, do you always clean it up right away?
17. Do you keep nonslip mats both in and alongside the bath or shower?

Group 2: Safety on the Road

18. Have you taught your children exactly how, when, and where to cross streets safely?
19. Have your children been taught the basic rules of the road to use when bicycling?
20. When walking in streets or open roads at twilight or in the dark, do all members of your family carry a flashlight or wear a markedly visible outer garment, such as a white or luminous jacket?
21. Do you always drive within the speed limit and defensively?
22. Are you always careful not to drink if you're going to drive a car soon afterward?
23. Do you avoid driving when you feel unusually tired or ill, or if you're taking drugs (such as antihistamines) known to impair alertness?
24. Do you have your car fully serviced, including checking the lights, tires, windshield washer and wipers, brakes, and steering, either every 6,000 miles (10,000 km) or at least every six months?
25. Do you check at least once a week to make sure that your car windows, lights, mirrors, and reflectors are clean?
26. When driving, do you always try to keep a gap between your car and the one in front of you of at least a yard (or meter) for each mile-per-hour you're traveling?
27. Do you always make sure that you and all passengers in your car use available seat belts?
28. Are any infants or toddlers riding in your car securely strapped into infant car seats?

Group 3: Safety on Vacations

29. Are all members of your family able to swim or in the process of learning how to swim?
30. Do you test the depth of the water and go in feet first?
31. In a boat, does everyone always wear a life jacket?
32. If you do any skiing, hiking, or climbing, do you always go properly prepared with the right clothing and equipment?
33. When going on an excursion for a day or longer, do you tell someone what your route is and when you expect to return?
34. Do you and your family take full safety precautions and have the proper equipment when you engage in contact and other possibly dangerous sports?
35. Before taking up a new and potentially dangerous activity, such as hang gliding, do you make sure you get proper instruction?
36. During a vacation, do you make sure you get adequate rest and relaxation?

(continued)

Evaluation

A No answer to any of the above questions indicates that you're not doing all you can to minimize your risk of accidents. You can and should take all the protective steps suggested by the questions.

Source: Kunz, Jeffrey, and Asher Finkel, eds. *The AMA Family Medical Guide.* New York: Random House, 1987. Reprinted by permission of the publisher.

you can't make the road dry, but you can make sure your tires and brakes are in good condition.

Thrill-Seeking

Some people crave the sensation of danger. To them, activities that others might find terrifying—such as sky-diving or parachute-jumping—are stimulating. The reason may be that they have lower than normal levels of the brain chemicals that regulate excitement. Because the stress of potentially hazardous sports may increase the levels of these chemicals, they feel pleasantly aroused rather than scared. However, their desire for this sensation could lead them to ignore safety precautions and jeopardize their safety.

What Should I Do in an Emergency Situation?

Life-threatening situations rarely happen more than once or twice in any person's life. When they do, you must think and act quickly to prevent disastrous consequences.

▶ **Don't panic.** Your immediate response to an emergency may be overwhelming fear and anxiety. Take several deep breaths. Start by assessing the circumstances. Shout for help if you're in a public place. Look for any possible dangers to you or the victim, such as a live electrical wire or a fire. Seek medical assistance as quickly as possible. Don't attempt rescue techniques, such as cardiopulmonary resuscitation (CPR), unless you're trained. (For advice on what to do in case of a heart attack, see the "Emergency!" section at the back of this book.)

▶ **Don't wait for symptoms to go away or get worse.** If you suspect that someone is having a heart attack or stroke, or has ingested something poisonous, *phone for help immediately.* A delay could jeopardize the person's life. Stay on the line long enough to give your name, address, and a brief description of the emergency.

▶ **Don't move a victim.** The person may have a broken neck or back, and attempting to move him or her could cause extensive damage or even death.

▶ **Don't drive.** Even if the hospital is just ten minutes away, you're better off waiting for a well-equipped ambulance with trained paramedics who can deliver emergency care on the spot. People rushing to emergency rooms are more likely to get into accidents themselves.

▶ **At home, keep a supply of basic first-aid items in a convenient place.** Make sure that emergency telephone numbers (ambulance service, police and fire departments, poison control center, your doctor and neighbors) are handy. If you can't find a number quickly, call the operator.

▶ **Don't do too much.** Often well-intentioned Good Samaritans make injuries worse by trying to tie tourniquets, wash cuts, or splint broken limbs. Also, don't give an injured person anything to eat or drink. (See "Emergency!" in the Hales Health Almanac at the back of this book for more on first-aid and emergency care.)

Safety on the Road

After a five-year decline, the number of people killed on American highways appears to be rising, particularly for motorcycle riders and teenagers between ages 16 and 20.[3] Every 14 seconds someone in America is injured in a traffic crash; every 12 minutes someone is killed. Motor vehicle accidents in the United States claim about 42,000 lives annually, more than any other form of unintentional injury. They are the leading cause of all deaths for people ages 1 to 24; only cancer and heart attacks claim more American lives.[4] Far more people—more than 3.5 million annually—are injured in motor vehicle accidents. The proper use of automatic shoulder belts could reduce this number.[5] (See Table 17-1.) The use of child safety and booster seats also could prevent many injuries. Placing children in the back seat in itself reduces the risk of fatal injury by 30 percent or more.[6] The economic toll of motor vehicle accidents also is high: an estimated total of $150 billion a year, including $17 billion in medical and emergency expenses, lost productivity, and property loss.

▼ Table 17-1 Staying Alive	
Strategy	Reduction in risk of death
Motor vehicle passengers	
Wear three-point restraints properly	47%
Always use lap belt if your car has automatic seat belts	58%
Choose a car with an air bag	20%
Do not ride with an intoxicated driver	Greater than 90%
Drivers	
Avoid driving at night for first year after getting license	Greater than 50%
Cyclists	
Wear a helmet	85% (bicycle) 55% (motorcycle)
Boaters	
Do not drink alcohol while boating	Greater than 90%

Source: Grossman, David. "Adolescent Injury Prevention and Clinicians: Time for Instant Messaging." *Western Journal of Medicine*, Vol. 172, No. 3, March 2000.

In various studies, posttraumatic stress disorder (PTSD), discussed in Chapter 3, has developed in 8 to 39 percent of individuals injured in motor vehicle crashes or other accidents. It is more likely to develop after a motor vehicle accident when other distressing events occur at the same time, when the victim feared death, when the accident was extremely serious, or when the victim was socially isolated afterward.[7]

Safe Driving

Car crashes aren't accidents that just happen. Most are the result of unsafe vehicles, unsafe drivers, or unsafe driving techniques. Basic precautions can greatly increase your odds of reaching a destination alive. Vehicles equipped with seat belts, air bags, padded dashboards, safety glass windows, a steel frame, and side-impact beams all help protect against injury or death.

The size and weight of a vehicle also matter. According to the National Highway Traffic Safety Administration (NHTSA), sport-utility vehicles (SUVs) are two-and-a-half times as likely as other vehicles to kill the occupants of another vehicle in a collision. Many of the larger models either ram their heavily reinforced bumpers straight into the passenger cabin of the other car or climb up and over the other car.[8]

Seat Belts and Air Bags

Seat belts have proven to be the most effective means of reducing fatalities and serious injuries when traffic crashes

STRATEGIES FOR PREVENTION

How to Drive Safely

✔ Don't drive while under the influence of alcohol or other drugs, including medications that may impair your reflexes, cause drowsiness, or affect your judgment. Never get into a car if you suspect the driver may be intoxicated or affected by a drug.

✔ Remain calm when dealing with drivers who are reckless or rude. Be alert and anticipate possible hazards. Don't let yourself be distracted by conversations, children's questions, arguments, food or drink, or scenic views. If you become exhausted, pull over and rest.

✔ Don't get too comfortable. Alertness matters. Use the rearview mirror often. Don't let passengers or packages obstruct your view. Use the turn signals when changing lanes or making a turn. If someone cuts you off, back off to a safe distance. When you can, drive so that you have enough space around you.

✔ Make sure small children are in safety seats. Unless pets are trained to ride quietly in a car, keep them in carrying cases.

✔ Drive more slowly if weather conditions are bad. Avoid driving at all during heavy rain, snow, or other conditions that affect visibility and road conditions. If you must drive in hazardous conditions, make sure that your car has the proper equipment, such as chains or snow tires, and that you know how to respond in case of a skid.

✔ Maintain your car properly, replacing windshield wipers, tires, and brakes when necessary. Keep flares and a fire extinguisher in your car for use in emergencies.

✔ To avoid a head-on collision, generally veer to the right—onto a shoulder, lawn, or open space. Steer your way to safety; avoid hitting the brakes hard once you leave the pavement. If you have to hit something stationary, look for a "soft" target—bushes, parked cars, woodframe buildings—as opposed to "hard" boulders, brick walls, trees, concrete abutments, and so on.

occur. They save an estimated 9,500 lives in the United States each year. When lap/shoulder belts are used properly, they reduce the risk of fatal injury to front seat

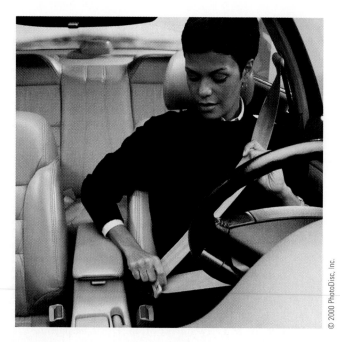

▲ Buckling up is one of the simplest and most effective ways of protecting yourself from injury.

passengers by 45 percent and the risk of moderate-to-critical injury by 50 percent. For light truck occupants, seat belts reduce the risk of fatal injury by 60 percent and moderate-to-critical injury by 65 percent.

Seat belts save lives in several ways. When a crash occurs, occupants continue to travel at the vehicle's original speed at the moment of impact. After the vehicle comes to a complete stop, unbelted occupants slam into the steering wheel, windshield, or into another part of the car. Seat belts reduce injuries from this second collision and also prevent ejection from the car.

More Americans are buckling up—an estimated 71 percent, up from 58 percent in 1994.[9] State laws that require motorists to "click it or ticket" make a difference, usually boosting seat belt use about 15 percentage points. However, even so, a significant percentage of drivers do not use seat belts regularly.

Typically, nonusers of seat belts also are high-risk drivers. They are more likely than others to drive after drinking and to be involved in a serious crash, yet they're the least likely to take responsibility for the social and economic consequences of their behavior. Although nonusers come from all segments of society, they are frequently male, younger than 30 years of age, unmarried, have little or no postsecondary education, and often drive pickup trucks or sport-utility vehicles. In NHTSA surveys, the female seat belt use rate is generally 10 percentage points higher than the male use rate. Overall seat belt use rates are highest in the suburbs, followed by cities, then rural areas.

Air bags also can save adult lives. Federal law requires all cars manufactured since 1998 to be equipped with air bags, but there is controversy over the potential hazard

they pose to children. NHTSA has given automobile owners permission to deactivate air bags if a small child might be a front seat passenger. However, the American Academy of Pediatrics has argued that deactivation might pose an even greater risk by jeopardizing the safety of older children, teens, and adult passengers. It recommends that children be placed in the back seat, whether or not the car is equipped with a passenger air bag.

Unsafe Driving Behaviors

Drunk driving is the number one cause of serious motor vehicle accidents. In recent years, there has been a decline in the number of fatalities caused by drunk driving, particularly among young people. The NHTSA attributes this decline to increases in the drinking age, to educational programs aimed at reducing nighttime driving by teens, to the formation of Students Against Destructive Decisions (SADD) and similar groups, and to changes in state laws that penalize drivers younger than age 21 for driving with even lower blood-alcohol concentration levels than were previously acceptable (from 0.01 to 0.05 percent). (See Chapter 15 for more information on blood-alcohol concentrations and drunk driving.)

Falling asleep at the wheel is second only to alcohol as a cause of serious motor-vehicle accidents. According to the National Commission on Sleep Disorders Research, each year 200,000 sleep-related motor vehicle accidents claim more than 5,000 lives, cause hundreds of thousands of injuries, and lead to billions of dollars in indirect costs. Too little sleep, recent research suggests, may be as detrimental to driving skills as drinking too much. Employees who work night shifts, long hours, or more than one job run an increased risk of falling asleep at the wheel and being in a sleep-induced crash.[10]

Certain driving behaviors, such as speeding, tailgating, or running yellow lights, also increase the risk of an accident. Self-described aggressive drivers are not only more aggressive and angry on the road, but in other circumstances. Their bodies seem more "reactive," with greater facial muscle tension and blood pressure when under stress.[11]

Teenage drivers are more likely to be in a car crash than any other age group. The risk is highest among 16- and 17-year-old drivers, particularly during the first few months and first 500 miles of driving.[12]

More than 30 states have enacted graduated driver licensing (GDL) systems to reduce crash rates among young novice drivers.[13] They require teenage drivers to gain experience and maturity under relatively low-risk conditions before gaining full driving privileges. Researchers are working to determine which aspects of the new approach, such as limits on teenage passengers and night driving, are most effective.[14]

Road Rage

The emotional outbursts known as road rage are a factor in as many as two-thirds of all fatal car crashes and one-third of nonfatal accidents, according to the NHTSA.[15] Psychologist Arnold Nerenberg of Whittier, California, a specialist in motorway mayhem, estimates 1.78 billion episodes of road rage a year, resulting in more than 28,000 deaths and 1 million injuries.[16]

Some strategies for reducing road rage include the following:

▷ **Lower the stress in your life.** Take a few moments to breathe deeply and relax your shoulders before putting the key in the ignition.

▷ **Consciously decide not to let other drivers get to you.** Decide that whatever happens, it's not going to make your blood pressure go up.

▷ **Slow down.** If you're going five or ten miles over the speed limit, you won't have the time you need to react to anything that happens.

▷ **Modify bad driving habits one at a time.** If you tend to tailgate slow drivers, spend a week driving at twice your usual following distance. If you're a habitual horn honker, silence yourself.

▷ **Be courteous—even if other drivers aren't.** Don't dawdle in the passing lane. Never tailgate or switch lanes without signaling. Don't use your horn or high beams unless absolutely necessary.

▷ **Never retaliate.** Whatever another driver does, keep your cool. Count to ten. Take a deep breath. If you yell or gesture at someone who's upset with you, the conflict may well escalate.

▷ **If you do something stupid, show that you're sorry.** On its website, the AAA Foundation for Traffic Safety solicited suggestions for automotive apologies. The most popular: slapping yourself on your forehead or the top of your head to indicate that you know you goofed. Such gestures can soothe a miffed motorist—and make the roads a slightly safer place for all of us.

Is It Safe to Use a Car Phone While Driving?

Any activity that takes a driver's hands off the wheel and mind off the road is dangerous. Driver distraction contributes to as many as 25 percent of all vehicle crashes, according to the NHTSA.[17] And talking on the phone seems to be the greatest distraction of all. Drivers using a cellular phone are four times more likely to have a collision than those listening to the radio or talking to passengers.[18] According to actual accident reports, drivers using cell phones have crashed into trees, struck stopped vehicles, and caused other cars to swerve out of control. Some communities have banned the use of cellular phones while driving.

On the other hand, car phones are helpful in alerting authorities to road hazards, congestion, or problem drivers and in summoning help in case of a breakdown or another emergency. For safety's sake, it's best to restrict calls to such circumstances or to pull over to the side of the road to make an important call.

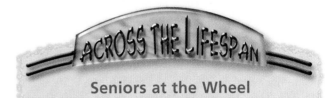

Seniors at the Wheel

About a third of all drivers are over age 55; their number will increase as the baby boom generation ages. Driving is very important to seniors, and most want to stay on the road as long as possible. While age alone is not an indicator of impairment, age-related changes can affect driving ability.

The rate of drivers involved in car accidents, including fatal ones, rises after age 70. Drivers aged 70 to 74 are twice as likely to die in an accident than those between ages 30 to 59. The risk for drivers over 80 is five times higher. The most common contributing factors in accidents involving older drivers include pulling out from the side of the road or changing lanes, careless backing, inaccurate turning, and difficulty giving right of way and reading traffic signs. Unlike younger drivers, older drivers' accidents seldom involve high speeds or alcohol use. Rather, problem driving in older adults involves visual, cognitive, and motor skills, which may decline with aging.[19] Older drivers who have heart disease, arthritis, or a history of stroke are at an increased risk for car crashes.[20]

Although half the people over age 85 meet motor vehicle bureau vision standards, many suffer weaknesses in other critical aspects of vision, such as recovery from glare and depth perception. The ability of those over 85 to operate a vehicle when they have to divide their attention is half that of people under age 65.

As various regulatory agencies struggle with ways to evaluate the safety of older drivers, seniors can lower their risks by taking simple steps such as limiting night driving, avoiding freeways, driving during less crowded periods of the day, making practice runs of new or difficult routes, and identifying and using alternate means of transportation. The insurance industry has recommended changes that could reduce accidents in senior drivers, such as road signs with bigger letters and air bags that inflate with less force.[21]

Safe Cycling

Mile for mile, motorcycling is far more risky than automobile driving. The most common motorcycle injury is head trauma, which can lead to physical disability, including paralysis and general weakness, as well as problems reading and thinking. It can also cause personality changes and psychiatric problems, such as depression, anxiety, and uncontrollable mood swings and anger. Some improvement may occur naturally as swelling diminishes and the brain heals. However, complete recovery from head trauma can take four to six years, and the costs can be staggering. Head injury can also result in permanent disability, coma, and death. To prevent head trauma, motorcycle helmets are required in most states. Federal law dictates that a certain percentage of highway construction funds be reallocated for safety programs in states that don't require motorcycle helmets.

Approximately 80.6 million people ride bicycles. Each year, bicycle crashes kill about 900 of these individuals; about 200 of those killed are children under age 15. Men are more likely to suffer cycling injuries. The risk increases with high speed; collisions with motor vehicles are most likely to be fatal.[22] About 567,000 people go to hospital emergency departments annually with bicycle-related injuries; 350,000 of the injured are children under age 15.

According to a national survey, 50 percent of all bicycle riders in the United States regularly wear bike helmets—43 percent every time they ride and 7 percent more than half the time. Safety is the primary reason that 98 percent of those surveyed gave for wearing a helmet, followed by the insistence of a parent or spouse. The reasons for not wearing a bike helmet included riding only a short distance, forgetting to put it on, or feeling that the helmet was uncomfortable. (See Savvy Consumer: "Buying a Bike Helmet.")

Safety at Home

Every year home accidents cause nearly 25 million injuries. Poison poses the greatest threat, causing more than 17,000 deaths every year. Half a million children swallow poisonous materials each year; 90 percent are under age 5. Adults may also be poisoned by mistakenly taking someone else's prescription drugs or taking medicines in the dark and swallowing the wrong one. In most cities, you can call a poison control center for advice.

Falls

Falls of all kinds are the second leading cause of death from unintentional injury in the United States.[23] High heels or worn footgear, poor lighting, slippery or uneven walkways, broken stairs and handrails, loose or worn rugs, or objects left where people walk all increase the likelihood of a slip.

Falls are an especially serious health risk for the elderly. Each year about one-third of all people 65 years of age or older who live at home fall; 6 to 10 percent of these falls result in injury, including fractures, muscle injuries, sprains, lacerations, and dislocations. Falls are the number-one cause of injury-related death in older men and women. Muscle weakness and impaired balance are risk factors that increase the risk of falls in older people.[24]

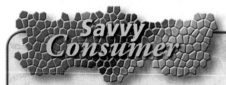

Buying a Bike Helmet

What should you look for in buying a helmet? Here are some basic guidelines:

- A government regulation requires all helmets produced after 1999 to meet the Consumer Product Safety Commission standard; look for a CPSC sticker inside the helmet. The Snell Memorial Foundation's B-90 standard and the ASTM standard are comparable to CPSC. The Snell B-95 standard is even better.

- Check the fit. The helmet should sit level on your head, touching all around, comfortably snug but not tight. The helmet should not move more than about an inch in any direction, regardless of how hard you tug at it.

- Pick a bright color for visibility. Avoid dark colors, thin straps, or a rigid visor that could snag in a fall.

- Look for a smooth plastic outer shell, not one with alternating strips of plastic and foam. Watch out for excessive vents, which put less protective foam in contact with your head in a crash. Mirrors should have a breakaway mount; the wire type mounted on eyeglasses can gouge an eye in a fall.

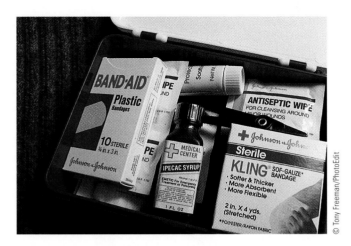

▲ Your home first-aid kit should include (at minimum) bandages, sterile gauze pads, adhesive tape, scissors, cotton, antibiotic ointment, a needle, safety pins, calamine lotion, syrup of ipecac to induce vomiting, and a thermometer.

Fires

You can prevent fires by making sure that the three ingredients of fire—fuel, a heat source, and oxygen—don't get a chance to mix. Almost anything can act as fuel for fire, including paper, wood, and, of course, flammable liquids such as oils, gasoline, and some paints. A heat source can be a spark from a lighted match, pilot light, or an electrical wire. Oxygen is necessary for the chemical reaction between the fuel and heat source that causes combustion.

If a fire starts and it's small, you may be able to put it out with a portable fire extinguisher before it spreads. However, if the fire does get out of control, you might have only two to five minutes to get out of the house or building alive. A fire-escape plan can save time and lives. Sketch a plan of your house, apartment building, dormitory, or fraternity or sorority house. Identify two ways out of each room or apartment. Make sure everyone is familiar with these escape routes. Designate an area outside where all family members or dorm residents should meet after escaping from a fire.

If a fire breaks out in your dorm room, get out as quickly as possible, but don't run. Before opening a room door, place your hand on it. If it's hot, don't open it. If the door feels cool, open it slightly to check for smoke. If there's none, leave by your planned escape route. If you're on an upper floor and your escape routes are blocked, open a window (top and bottom, if possible) and wait or signal from the window for help. Never try to use an elevator in a fire.

If you can't leave your room safely during a fire, call for help and turn off the air-conditioning or heating systems. To block smoke, press sheets and towels (wet, if possible) around and under the door. Keep as close to the floor as

STRATEGIES FOR PREVENTION

Staying Safe at Home

✔ Wear gloves when using household cleaning products. Read labels carefully, and use the products only in well-ventilated rooms. Never combine cleaning products; doing so could produce a dangerous chemical reaction.

✔ Light stairways well. Remove clutter, cords, wires, and furniture from walking paths in living areas. Make sure carpets are attached firmly and area rugs are secure. Install nonskid mats in bathtubs and showers.

✔ Carry only loads you can see over. Clean up spills immediately, or mark the spill with a paper towel or wastebasket until you get a chance to clean it up. If you must walk over wet or slippery surfaces, take short steps to keep your center of balance beneath you. Slow down.

✔ To avoid shocks, be careful about anything involving electricity and water. Avoid using power tools in the rain; be careful with electrical heaters and other appliances, such as radios and hair dryers, in the bathroom; and use tools with nonconducting handles.

possible (where there's likely to be more oxygen), and place a wet washcloth over your face to filter out smoke particles.

On-the-Job Safety

The workplace is second only to the home as the most frequent site of accidents. More than 5,500 injury deaths occur on the job every year.[25] The industries with the highest fatality rates are mining; transportation, communication, and public utilities; construction; and agriculture, forestry, and fishing. Whatever your job, find out about potential hazards and learn the proper safety regulations. (Chapter 19 discusses some potential environmental hazards at work, including noise, toxic substances, and video display terminals.)

According to a report by the National Research Council and Institute of Medicine, about one million workers annually suffer musculoskeletal disorders of the lower back and upper extremities as a result of their "particular jobs and working conditions—including heavy lifting, repetitive and forceful motions, and stressful working conditions." Many can be prevented.[26]

?⁇? Can My Computer Be a Health Hazard?

As computers have become part of daily life for everyone from preschoolers to seniors, health professionals have learned a great deal about potential health problems, including repetitive motion injuries and vision-related difficulties.

Repetitive Motion Injuries

Repetitive motion injuries (RMI) have surpassed back and neck injuries as the number one claim for workers compensation injuries. Repeated motions—such as the hand and arm movements made while using a computer keyboard—all day, every day, can result in muscle and tendon strain and inflammation. About 20 percent of people with pain, tingling, or numbness in the hands may have carpal tunnel syndrome, an overuse injury caused by repetitive motions in the hands and wrists. Symptoms include pain, swelling, and numbness and weakness in the hands or the arms. If these problems are identified early, permanent damage can generally be avoided by altering the work environment and allowing for more breaks during the day.

The slope and height of a computer keyboard can affect the likelihood of repetitive motion injuries.[27] If you work at a computer, good posture and correct positioning of the computer screen and keyboard can help prevent repetitive motion injuries, eyestrain, and back strain (see Figure 17-1). Here are some additional tips:

▶ Place the keyboard so that your elbows are bent at a 90° angle and you don't have to bend your wrists to type.
▶ Use a chair that provides ample back support. Keep your thighs parallel to the floor and your feet on the floor. If your feet don't reach the floor, use a footrest.
▶ If you experience neck strain, place a document holder next to your screen so that you can view the materials more easily.
▶ Every 15 minutes take a 30-second break, stretch your arms, and walk around the office. Take a 15-minute break at least once every two hours.

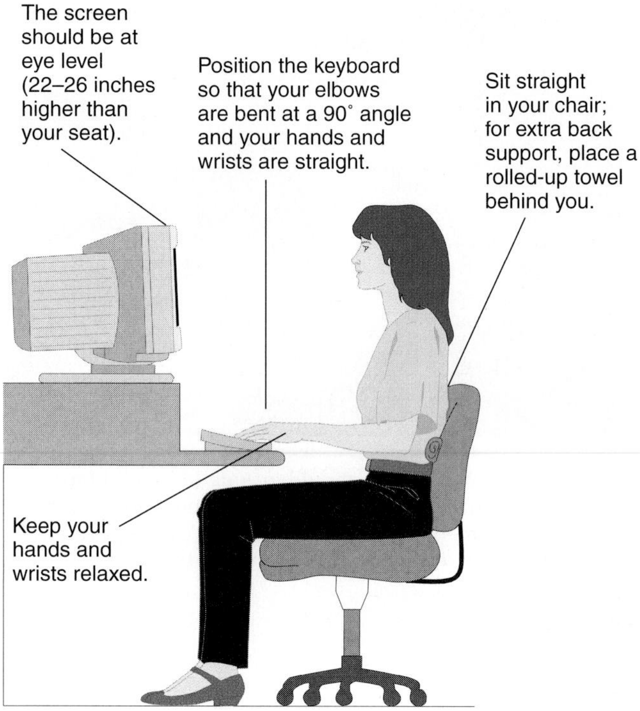

Vision Problems

Computer vision syndrome is a condition marked by tired and sore eyes, blurred vision, headaches and neck, shoulder, and back pain. The American Optometric Association estimates that it afflicts nearly 90 percent of workers who use computers and also is common among children and students of all ages. The symptoms result from repeatedly

The screen should be at eye level (22–26 inches higher than your seat).

Position the keyboard so that your elbows are bent at a 90° angle and your hands and wrists are straight.

Sit straight in your chair; for extra back support, place a rolled-up towel behind you.

Keep your hands and wrists relaxed.

▲ **Figure 17-1** Safe computing.
By paying attention to your posture and your computer's position, you can help protect yourself from repetitive motion injury, back strain, and eyestrain.

stressing some aspect of the visual system, but they often disappear as soon as the person stops working at the computer.

The eye focuses on a computer image differently from the way it focuses on a printed one. The pixels that appear on a computer screen, unlike printed characters, are bright in the center and gradually fade away into the background color. This makes it difficult for the eye to sustain focus. Optometrists have developed a specific method, called a PRIO examination, that simulates how the eye responds to pixels on a computer screen. It can determine the need and proper prescription for computer-only eyeglasses.

Working with Chemicals

Many different workers, from laboratory technicians to professional artists, must use dangerous chemicals to perform their jobs. Employers and manufacturers of these chemicals are required by federal law to inform workers about any potential hazards, as well as first-aid measures in case they're accidentally exposed.

Here are some safety guidelines to follow if you work with dangerous substances:

▶ Make sure your work space is adequately ventilated. This doesn't mean a fan, which just blows dust and fumes around, but the equivalent of a filtered vacuum cleaner at the source of the toxic material.

▶ Be careful with the storage and handling of flammable solvents. Label all toxic materials clearly and carefully. Store them in nonbreakable containers. Discard them according to the manufacturer's instructions.

▶ Wash yourself thoroughly with soap and water before taking a break. Don't sweep up: vacuum or wet mop.

▶ Do not eat or smoke when using toxic materials. Wear appropriate protective gear: air respirators, goggles, gloves, earplugs, and so on.

▶ If you're pregnant or planning to conceive, check with your doctor about any potential risks to an unborn child.

Recreational Safety

When you want to take a break, exercise, or simply enjoy yourself, you probably go outside. But if you aren't careful, even a simple stroll or swim can turn into a hazardous event. According to a study by the Johns Hopkins School of Public Health, every year 750,000 Americans are injured during recreational activities such as horseback riding, skiing, sledding, skating, and playground activities; 82,000 suffer head injuries requiring emergency room or hospital treatment. Two dangers on the increase are snowboarding and riding electric scooters. Young men under age 30 have the highest incidence of snowboarding injuries; wrist fractures are the most common.[28] Public health experts urge helmet use for sports such as inline skating and skateboarding because such activities combine high speeds with exposure to traffic.

Handling Heat

Each year as many as 1,000 Americans die from heat-caused illnesses that are almost always preventable. Two common heat-related maladies are **heat cramps** and **heat stress.** Heat cramps are caused by hard work and heavy sweating in the heat. Heat stress may occur simultaneously or afterward, as the blood vessels try to keep body temperature down. **Heat exhaustion,** a third such malady, is the result of prolonged sweating with inadequate fluid replacement. (See Table 17-2.)

The first step in treating these conditions is to stop exercising, move to a cool place, and drink plenty of water. Don't resume work or activity until all the symptoms have disappeared; see a doctor if you're suffering from heat exhaustion. **Heat stroke** is a life-threatening medical emergency caused by the breakdown of the body's mechanism for cooling itself. The treatment is to cool the body down: Move to a cooler environment; sponge down with cool water, and apply ice to the back of the neck, armpits,

▼ **Table 17-2** **Heat Dangers**

Illness	Symptoms	Treatment
Heat cramps	Muscle twitching or cramping; muscle spasms in arms, legs, and abdomen	Stop exercising; cool off; drink water.
Heat stress	Fatigue, pale skin, blurred vision, dizziness, low blood pressure	Stop exercising; cool off; drink water.
Heat exhaustion	Excessive thirst, fatigue, lack of coordination, increased sweating, elevated body temperature	See a doctor.
Heat stroke	Lack of perspiration, high body temperature (over 105°F), dry skin, rapid breathing, coma, seizures, high pulse	Cool the body; sponge; get medical help.

and groin. Immersion in cold water could cause shock. Get medical help immediately.

Coping with Cold

The tips of the toes, fingers, ears, nose, chin, and cheeks are most vulnerable to exposure to high wind speeds and low temperatures, which can result in **frostnip.** Because frostnip is painless, you may not even be aware of it occurring. Watch for a sudden blanching or lightening of your skin. The best early treatment is warming the area by firm, steady pressure with a warm hand; blowing on it with hot breath; holding it against your body; or immersing it in warm (not hot) water. As the skin thaws, it becomes red and starts to tingle. Be careful to protect it from further damage. Don't rub the skin vigorously or with snow, as you could damage the tissue.

More severe is **frostbite,** which can be either *superficial* or *deep.* Superficial frostbite, the freezing of the skin and tissues just below the skin, is characterized by a waxy look and firmness of the skin, although the tissue below is soft. Initial treatment should be to slowly rewarm the area. As the area thaws, it will be numb and bluish or purple, and blisters may form. Cover the area with a dry, sterile dressing, and protect the skin from further exposure to cold. See a doctor for further treatment. Deep frostbite, the freezing of skin, muscle, and even bone, requires medical treatment. It usually involves the tissues of the hands and feet, which appear pale and feel frozen. Keep the victim

STRATEGIES FOR PREVENTION

Protecting Yourself from the Cold

✔ Dress appropriately. Choose several layers of loose clothing made of wool, cotton, down, or synthetic down. Make sure your head, feet, and hands are well protected. A pair of cotton socks inside a pair of wool socks will keep your feet warm.

✔ Don't go out in the cold after drinking. Alcohol can make you more susceptible to cold (see Chapter 15) and can impair your judgment and sense of time.

✔ When snowshoeing or cross-country skiing, always let a responsible person know where you're heading and when you expect to be back. Stick to marked trails. Don't eat snow; it could lower your body temperature.

✔ Carry an emergency kit that includes waterproof matches, a compass, a map, high-energy food, and water.

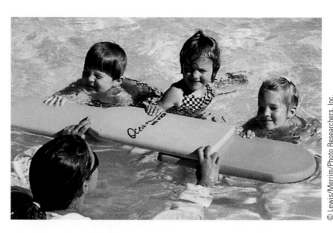

© Lewis/Merrim/Photo Researchers, Inc.

▲ Water safety training can begin in early childhood. Swimming, treading water, and engaging in safe water practices are all important to preventing drownings.

dry and as warm as possible on the way to a medical facility. Cover the frostbitten area with a dry, sterile dressing.

The gradual cooling of the center of the body may occur at temperatures above, as well as below, freezing—usually in wet, windy weather. When body temperature falls below 95°F, the body is incapable of rewarming itself because of the breakdown of the internal system that regulates its temperature. This state is known as **hypothermia.** The first sign of hypothermia is severe shivering. Then the victim becomes uncoordinated, drowsy, listless, confused, and is unable to speak properly. Symptoms become more severe as body temperature continues to drop, and coma or death can result.

Hypothermia requires emergency medical treatment. Try to prevent any further heat loss: Move the victim to a warm place, cover him or her with blankets, remove wet clothing, and replace it with dry garments. If the victim is conscious, administer warm liquids, not alcohol.

Drowning

Over the last few decades, deaths from drowning have declined. Possible reasons include less use of alcohol by swimmers and boaters, and an increase in body fat, which makes floating easier. Toddlers under age 4 and teenage boys between 15 and 19 remain at greatest risk. Among young children, 90 percent of drownings occur in residential swimming pools.

Drowning is the second leading cause of unintentional injury death among children ages 1 to 19 years. Young children are most likely to drown in swimming pools; teenagers, in natural bodies of freshwater.[29] The causes of drowning, in order of frequency, are becoming exhausted, being swept into deep water, losing support, becoming trapped or entangled, having a cramp or other attack, and striking an underwater object. Many drowning victims were strong swimmers. Most drownings occur at unorganized facilities, such as ponds or pools with no lifeguard present. Health officials believe that pool fencing alone, along with adequate gates and latches, could prevent as many as half of all drownings or near-drownings of children.

Intentional Injury: Living in a Dangerous World

Acts of violence are a significant threat to health and well-being, whether they are committed by terrorists, criminals, acquaintances, or family members.

Violence in the United States

Although the United States remains the most violent country in the Western world, violent crime has dropped to its lowest level in more than 25 years.[30] The rates for rape, robberies, and assaults dropped by more than one-third during the 1990s.[31]

Gun-related injuries and deaths have declined, but guns remain the second-leading cause of injury-related death in the United States after car accidents. About 260 Americans are injured by firearms every day; one-third die from their wounds.[32] Despite the decline in crime, gun violence annually takes the lives of nearly 30,000

STRATEGIES FOR CHANGE

Coping with the Threat of Violence and Terrorism

Uncertainty can be the most difficult aspect of living in a dangerous world. While you cannot eliminate risk, the following strategies can help you deal with it:

✔ Focus on the here-and-now. Make a daily to-do list. Check off each chore as you complete it. Break down large projects into a series of manageable steps.

✔ Act despite fear. Take that first step even if you are anxious, trusting that the second will be easier.

✔ Adjust your attitude. The way you appraise a situation—as a threat that endangers your life or as a challenge that can be overcome—has a tremendous impact on your psychological and physical responses.

✔ Draw on your spiritual beliefs. Faith and values provide a bridge over the unknown.

✔ Dare to hope. This may be the most life-affirming coping strategy of all.

Over half the increase in the prison population is due to an increase in convictions for violent crimes. The number of prisoners on death row also has increased.[34]

Violence touches many Americans' lives in ways that aren't always reported to the police. More than half of women (51.9 percent) and men (66.4 percent) say they have been physically assaulted at some point in their lives. Every year an estimated 1.9 million women and 3.2 million men experience a physical assault. The most frequent forms are slapping and hitting, followed by pushing, grabbing, shoving, and hitting with an object.[35]

 There are ethnic and racial differences in patterns of violence. African Americans are at greater risk of victimization by violent crime than white or persons of other racial groupings; Hispanics are at greater risk of violent victimization than non-Hispanics. There is little difference between white women and nonwhite women in rape, physical assault, or stalking. Native American/Alaska Native women are significantly more likely than white women or African-American women to report being raped. Mixed-race women also have a significantly higher incidence of rape than white women. Native American/Alaska Native men report significantly more physical assaults than Asian/Pacific Islander men do. (See Table 17-3.)

Alcohol availability increases the rates of total crime, violent crime, property crime, and homicides.[36] (See The X & Y Files: "Which Gender Is at Greater Risk?")

Americans, including 10 children every day. The proportion of youth involved in crime has actually risen. Almost half the victims of violent crime are under 25 years of age.[33] Although men commit more violent crimes than women, the rates are getting closer.

Many more criminals are behind bars. The incarceration rate nationwide has more than tripled since 1980.

Teen Violence

Today's adolescents, according to federal statistics, seem the least violent generation in decades. Fewer teens are being arrested for murder, robbery, and rape. Violent crime by teenagers fell by 30 percent from 1993 to 1998; murder,

▼ Table 17-3	Lifetime Victimization (Percentage of People)					
Type of Victimization	Total	White	African American	Asian/Pacific Islander	Native American/ Alaska Native	Mixed Race
Women	(n = 7,850)	(n = 6,452)	(n = 780)	(n = 133)	(n = 88)	(n = 397)
Rape	18.2	17.7	18.8	6.8	34.1	24.4
Physical assault	51.8	51.3	52.1	49.6	61.4	57.7
Stalking	8.2	8.2	6.5	4.5	17.0	10.6
Men	(n = 7,759)	(n = 6,424)	(n = 659)	(n = 165)	(n = 105)	(n = 406)
Rape	3.0	2.8	3.3	—	—	4.4
Physical assault	66.6	66.5	66.3	58.8	75.2	70.2
Stalking	2.3	2.1	2.4	—	—	3.9

Source: Tjaden, Patricia, and Nancy Thoennes. *Full Report of the Prevalence, Incidence and Consequences of Violence against Women.* Washington, DC: National Center for Justice, November 2000.

The X & Y Files — Which Gender Is at Greater Risk?

Just like illness, injury doesn't discriminate against either gender. Both men and women can find themselves in harm's way—but for different reasons. Here are some gender differences in vulnerability:

- Men are ten times more likely to die of an occupational injury than women.
- Males are most often the victims and the perpetrators in homicides in the United States. In about 68 percent of cases reported by the Bureau of Justice Statistics, both the offender and the victim were male. In 22 percent, the offender was male, and the victim female. In 7.8 percent of all cases, the offender was female and the victim male, while in 2.3 percent both the offender and victim were female.
- Overall, men are 3.6 times more likely than women to be murdered and 9 times more likely to commit murder. Both men and women are more likely to kill or attempt to kill male victims than female victims.
- Boys and men are more likely to be perpetrators of interpersonal violence, including homicide, physical assaults, sexual assaults, domestic abuse, and hate-related crimes. They are three to five times more likely than women and girls to carry weapons, thus increasing their risks for homicide and suicide. Men are 1.5 times more likely than women to be assaulted as an adult.

Each year 3.2 million men, compared with 1.9 million women, are physically attacked.

- Women are more often the targets of partner violence. Approximately 1.3 million women and 835,000 men are assaulted by an intimate partner annually. At some point in their lifetime, 22.1 percent of women—compared with 7.4 percent of men—report a physical attack by a spouse, partner, boyfriend or girlfriend, or date. About two-thirds (64 percent) of women who report being raped, physically assaulted, or stalked as adults were victimized by a current or former husband, cohabiting partner, boyfriend, or date.
- Physical assaults are more likely to injure women than men. Of female assault victims, 39 percent—compared with 24.8 percent of male assault victims—reported being injured during their most recent attack. Female rape victims also report more injuries than men who've been raped.

Sources: National Center for Health Statistics. Bureau of Justice statistics. Hong, Luoluo. "Toward a Transformed Approach to Prevention: Breaking the Link Between Masculinity and Violence." *Journal of American College Health,* Vol. 48, No. 6, May 2000. Tjaden, Patricia, and Nancy Thoennes. *Full Report of the Prevalence, Incidence and Consequences of Violence Against Women.* Washington, DC: National Center for Justice, November 2000.

by more than 56 percent. America's schools are reporting fewer serious crimes, both violent and nonviolent.[37]

Yet the reality behind the numbers is complex. Teen violence—though less prevalent than during the 1980s—remains "an ongoing, startlingly pervasive problem," according to the first-ever report on youth violence by the Office of the Surgeon General. Homicide is the second leading cause of death (after accidents) for young people between the ages of 15 and 20. Murder rates for young people in the United States remain the highest in the world—10 times higher than in Canada, 15 times higher than in Australia, 28 times higher than in France or Germany. American teenagers are more likely to die of gunshot wounds than of all natural causes combined. And despite the overall drop in teen crime, mass murders by teens on school grounds have risen sharply since 1996.[38]

Experts offer a host of explanations for the high rates of violence in American adolescents: the breakdown of families, violence-saturated media, easy access to guns, bullying and harassment in schools, undiagnosed mental disorders, abuse of alcohol and drugs. Teenagers involved in violent crime weren't necessarily victimized as children.

They often show no early signs of aggressive behavior, and they aren't more likely to belong to any one racial or ethnic group.[39]

Most of the teenagers who've committed high-profile mass murders are white, middle-class males raised in small towns or suburbs. In a study of 34 adolescent males who committed a total of 27 mass murders between 1958 and 1999, researchers found no common characteristics, other than suspicious comments or behavior prior to committing a violent act.[40]

The Roots of Aggression and Violence

While anger is considered a normal, sometimes inevitable emotion, aggression—behavior with the intent to control or dominate—is a threat to individuals and to society. Angry people may want to push or punch someone; aggressive people carry through on such impulses and become violent. Why? The reasons, discussed in the following sections, are complex.

Biological Causes

Traumatic brain injury, which can lead to violent outbursts of explosive anger, is one of many medical factors associated with violence. As many as 70 percent of those who suffer head injuries report some degree of irritability or explosive rage. The use of alcohol or drugs before or after a head injury may increase the likelihood of such problems. Illnesses that affect the brain—stroke and neurologic diseases, brain tumors, infectious illnesses, epilepsy, metabolic disorders (such as hyperthyroidism or hypothyroidism), multiple sclerosis, and systemic lupus erythematosus—can also lead to aggressive behavior.

Certain medications—painkillers, antianxiety agents, steroids, antidepressants, and over-the-counter sedatives (which may produce delirium)—can trigger aggression. Alcohol abuse, which lowers inhibitions against violent behavior and interferes with judgment, and many street drugs, including amphetamines, cocaine, and hallucinogens, are also associated with violence.

In searching for other biological abnormalities that may be linked with violence, neuroscientists have noted low levels of the neurotransmitter serotonin in men convicted of homicide. Serotonin is involved in the control of impulses, particularly toward violent or self-destructive acts. Other neurotransmitters also may play important roles in aggression, and the relations among these chemicals ultimately may prove more critical than the levels of any single one of them.

Sex chromosome abnormalities have been investigated but do not seem to lead to a greater tendency toward violence in, for example, men with an extra Y chromosome. The role of the male sex hormone testosterone also has been investigated. The highly competitive men most likely to dominate a situation or group—whether it's a seminar or a street gang—tend to have higher testosterone levels than other men. But testosterone in itself does not make men aggressive. Rather, scientists explain, it is only one of many contributing factors.

Individuals with serious mental disorders may be somewhat more violent than the general population, especially immediately after discharge from the hospital. Individuals with a serious mental illness (such as schizophrenia) report having been violent much more often than those with no mental disorder. However, alcohol and drug users are, as a group, more violent than individuals with serious mental illnesses.

Developmental Factors

For years, experts have debated whether some individuals are violent from a very young age or whether they "learn" violent behavior as they grow. According to current research, teen violence can develop in either way.

Most children who are highly aggressive or have behavioral disorders early in life do not become serious violent offenders. However, some offenders follow the "early onset" path and commit their first serious violent act before puberty. Early-onset offenders commit more and more serious crimes in adolescence and are more likely to remain violent throughout their lives.

Teens who develop "late-onset" violence—the majority of male adolescent offenders—do not become violent until puberty, at about age 13. As children, they show few or no signs of problem behavior, aggression, or behavioral disorders. As teenagers, their offenses tend to be less frequent and less serious. Most give up their violent behavior as they reach adulthood.

While some risk factors for violence, such as simply being born male, are biological, most come from a child's environment or ability to respond to his or her environment. Children of violent parents who become violent themselves are more likely to have learned this behavior than to have inherited a tendency to act this way.

The strongest risk factor during childhood are involvement in serious, but not necessarily violent, criminal behavior, substance use, physical aggression, poverty, and parents who are violent or criminal. During adolescence, when peers become more influential, the strongest

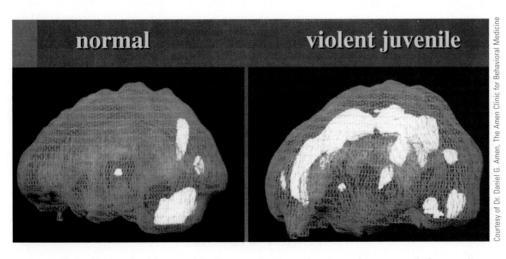

normal   violent juvenile

Courtesy of Dr. Daniel G. Amen, The Amen Clinic for Behavioral Medicine

▲ Scans of the brain of a 16-year-old who assaulted another teen show several abnormalities compared with a normal brain. They may reflect some combination of early head injuries, depression, and exposure to violence as a child.

risk factors are weak ties to conventional teens, relationships with antisocial or delinquent peers, gang membership, and involvement in other criminal acts.

Being "at risk" does not doom any child to become violent. Most children whose childhoods are shadowed by abuse or poverty do not turn to violence. And some children with no risk factors in their early lives become ensnared in dangerous lifestyles that include not only violence, but drugs, alcohol, and other risky behaviors. There is no one single underlying trigger for teen violence, but a combination of factors that may all play a role.

According to a federal survey of 15,686 public and private school students, nearly one of every three U.S. children in sixth through tenth grades is bullied. Verbal and physical harassment—which many contend is more demeaning than in the past—can create deep-seated humiliation and a desire for revenge.[41]

Exposure to violence in the media may have some effect on violent behavior. Early viewing of violent TV programs has been linked to later aggression, including violent crimes, spousal abuse, and child abuse. Sensationalized news reports that exaggerate or romanticize danger also can desensitize youngsters to the loss and horror violence cause—and can inspire "copycats," who imitate kids who receive intense attention after committing a crime.

Adding to this volatile mix are drugs and weapons. In numerous analyses, school violence has been linked with tobacco, alcohol, and marijuana use and with the availability of illegal drugs on school property. In one study of teen mass murders, the majority used a variety of legal and illegal drugs as well as alcohol.

Both fights and revenge fantasies are more likely to become deadly when guns are readily available. Firearms are the most commonly used weapons in mass murders by teens. In some cases, school shooters took guns from a parent's or relative's home. Some became fascinated with firearms at early ages.

Hate Crimes

Recent years have seen the emergence of violent crimes motivated by hatred of a particular person's or group of persons' race, religion, sexual orientation, or political values. They have included the dragging death of a young African-American man, the beating of a young gay man, the shooting of children and teachers at a Jewish community center in Los Angeles, and the vandalizing of Muslim-owned businesses after the terrorist attacks of September 11, 2001. Politicians and government leaders have called for an expansion of hate-crime laws that would inflict especially severe sentences on those who commit violence on the basis of racism, sexism, homophobia, anti-Semitism, or other forms of prejudice.

Hate may have been the motivation in some of the most baffling and disturbing of recent crimes: school shootings. The two young men who murdered classmates, teachers, and themselves at Columbine High School in 1999 felt hated by others and eventually released their hatred and anger in a horrible shooting spree. Some school districts and national advocacy groups are offering violence prevention programs to children as young as age 4, using techniques such as taking turns and dealing with angry feelings.

Crime on Campus

 Once considered havens from the meanness of America's streets, colleges and universities have seen a dramatic rise in crime in recent years. However, crime rates in these institutions are lower than in the general community.[42] According to the U.S. Department of Education, the criminal homicide rate on campus is 0.07 per 100,000 students—compared with a criminal homicide rate of 5.7 per 100,000 persons overall in the United States and of 14.1 per 100,000 for young people ages 17 to 29.[43]

Colleges must compile annual security reports with statistics on violent crime, as well as drug and alcohol violations.[44] The most recent crime statistics for the nation's 6,269 colleges, universities, and career schools are posted on the Internet at http://ope.ed.gov/security. Under the Federal Student Right to Know and Campus Security Act, all colleges and universities receiving federal funds must publish and make readily available the number of campus killings, assaults, sexual assaults, robberies, burglaries and other crimes, and their security policies.[45] (See discussions of sexual harassment and assault later in this chapter.)

Because of concerns about safety on campus, more schools are taking tougher stands on student behavior. Many have established codes of conduct barring the use of alcohol and drugs, fighting, and sexual harassment. Many also have instituted policies requiring suspension or expulsion for students who violate this code.

Many campuses have set up public safety programs, which include late-night shuttle buses and escorts, student bicycle patrols, outdoor emergency phones, and increased numbers of police and security guards. Sexual-assaults services provide counseling, crisis intervention, and educational programs. Students are urged to walk in groups, lock doors and windows, and limit alcohol consumption. Freshman orientation often includes mandatory sessions on campus safety and sexual assault.

Family Violence

Violence doesn't stop at the front doors of America's homes. According to the Federal Bureau of Investigation, the most common and least-reported violent crimes are attacks in which the victim and the perpetrator knew each other at the time of or before the incident. One-third of all murders occur within families. Physical violence may occur in 20 to 30 percent of all American households. As with other forms of violent crime, there has been a decline in assaults and murders by intimates.

Partner Abuse

During their lifetime, at least one of every five women will be assaulted by a partner or ex-partner. Domestic violence is the single most common cause of injury to women—more common than car accidents, muggings, and rapes combined—and accounts for 42 percent of female murders.

Battered women (who outnumber battered men ten to one) are victims of severe, deliberate, and repeated physical assaults, often accompanied by psychological abuse and threats on their lives. A significant proportion of women who visit emergency departments seek help for symptoms related to ongoing abuse, yet only 5 percent are identified as victims of domestic violence by the physicians who treat them.

The primary factors contributing to physical abuse are the degree of frustration and stress a man is under, his use of alcohol (involved in up to 60 percent of battering cases), and whether he was raised in an abusive home. Only one in twenty men who beat their partners is violent outside the home; nine in ten refuse to admit that they have a problem. In homes where a wife is beaten, children also may be abused. The primary risk factors for domestic murder are poverty and household crowding; the lower a family's socioeconomic status—regardless of its racial or ethnic background—the greater the risk of deadly violence.

Abused wives and children are often trapped in terror. Wives may stay with abusive husbands because of love, financial dependence, shame, guilt, fear of being pursued, harmed, or killed if they leave, or a sense of responsibility to their children. The incidence of alcoholism, substance abuse, depression, and suicide attempts is higher in battered women than others.

Emotional violence causes a variety of physical problems, including chronic neck and back pain, migraine, high blood pressure, and ulcers. In one study of more than 1,000 women, those who'd experienced only emotional battering were 70 percent more likely than the average woman to have poor physical as well as mental health.[46]

Sexual Victimization and Violence

Sexual victimization refers to any situation in which a person is deprived of free choice and forced to comply with sexual acts. It is not only a woman's issue; in fact, men are also victimized. In recent years, researchers have come to view acts of sexual victimization along a continuum, ranging from behaviors such as street hassling, stalking, and obscene telephone calls to rape, battering, and incest.

???? What Is Sexual Harassment?

All forms of sexual harassment or unwanted sexual attention—from the display of pornographic photos to the use of sexual obscenities to a demand for sex by anyone in a position of power or authority—are illegal.

Sexual Harassment on the Job

As defined by the Equal Employment Opportunity Commission, sexual harassment takes two basic forms: in **quid pro quo** harassment, a person in power or authority makes unwanted sexual advances as a condition for receiving a job, a promotion, or another type of favor; in harassment by means of a **hostile or offensive environment,** supervisors or coworkers engage in persistent inappropriate behaviors that make the workplace hostile, abusive, or otherwise unbearable.[47]

"There's a spectrum of verbal, nonverbal and physical acts, ranging from making off-color remarks to grabbing someone's breast or buttocks," says consultant Susan L. Webb of Seattle, author of *Step Forward: Sexual Harassment in the Workplace.* "But sexual harassment always involves behavior that is related to or based on sex, that is deliberate or repeated, and that is not welcome, not asked for, and not returned." Sexual comments, propositions, dirty jokes, suggestive looks or remarks, displays of pinups or pornography, "accidental" touches, pats, squeezes, pinches, fondling, and ogling are all potentially offensive.[48]

"There isn't always a clear line," says Webb. "Each sexual harassment case has to be considered in its own context." The standard the courts use is whether a reasonable person would consider the behavior or environment abusive or hostile. Since most targets of sexual harassment are women, that usually translates into what a reasonable *woman* would think—which may be quite different from a man's view.

Sexual harassment can affect employees in many ways—financially, psychologically, even physically. If they are fired because they refuse to endure sexual harassment, they may jeopardize their own and their family's economic security. Common psychological effects include crying spells, loss of self-esteem, anger, humiliation, shame, alienation, helplessness, and degradation. Many victims also suffer physical symptoms that stem directly from pressures associated with sexual harassment, including headache, stomach ailments, decreased appetite, weight loss, back and neck pain, decreased sleep, and other stress-related problems.

Workers who feel victimized by sexual harassment should document their complaints by writing down specific incidents (including dates, times, places, and what happened). It sometimes helps initially to confront the harasser, either in person or by writing a note, and state that you're not interested in his or her attention. Many companies have established grievance procedures for handling sexual harassment complaints. The courts have awarded substantial payments of both punitive and compensatory damage to victims of physical and verbal harassment and have held companies liable for failing to halt offensive actions.

Sexual Harassment on Campus

Sexual harassment starts early. In a survey conducted by the American Association of University Women, 81 percent of students in grades 9 through 11 said they had been harassed at least once. A recent study of third to fifth graders indicated that both girls and boys had experienced harassment by their peers.[49] Among 11- to 16-year-olds, half of the females and 37 percent of the males reported some form of sexual harassment, including sexual comments and advances, calls, letters, and pressure for dates.

As many as 30 to almost 50 percent of female undergraduates and 12 to 18 percent of male undergraduates have experienced some form of sexual harassment.[50] Professors or supervisors may pressure students into sexual involvement for the sake of a grade, recommendation, or special opportunity. If a student tries to end a sexual relationship, the professor or supervisor may threaten reprisals. Most harassment comes from male faculty members, but both men and women report having been harassed by either male or female faculty. In a University of Washington study, college men were almost as likely as women to report unwanted sexual contact and coercion.

Sexual harassment can undermine students' well-being and academic performance. Its effects include diminished ambition and self-confidence, reduced ability to concentrate, sleeplessness, depression, physical aches, and ailments. Some students avoid classes or work with certain faculty members because of the risk of sexual advances. However, few file official grievances.

Because college administrations can be held legally responsible for allowing a hostile or offensive sexual environment, many schools have set up committees to handle such student reports and to take action against faculty members. Universities also are discouraging and, in some cases, restricting consensual relationships between teachers and students, especially any dating of students by their academic professors or advisers. Although such relation-

ships may seem consensual, in reality they may not be because of the power faculty members have to determine students' grades and futures. In some cases, students have sued their universities for failing to protect them from professors who pressured them into sexual liaisons.

If you encounter sexual harassment as a student, report it to the department chair or dean. If you don't receive an adequate response to your complaint, talk with the campus representatives who handle matters involving affirmative action or civil rights. Federal guidelines prevent any discrimination against you in terms of grades or the loss of a job or scholarship if you report harassment. Schools that do not take measures to remedy harassment could lose federal funds.

Sexual Victimization of Students

As the nation has become more aware of issues such as sexual harassment and coercion, there has been growing recognition that college campuses are not ivory towers isolated from these dangers. Recent federal legislation requires colleges and universities to report crimes of all sorts, including sexual victimization.

In 2000 the National Institute for Justice and the Bureau of Justice Statistics published the findings of the National College Women Sexual Victimization Study, a survey of a randomly selected, national sample of 4,446 women attending two- or four-year colleges or universities. The survey represents the most thorough investigation to date of the nature, incidence, and impact of sexual victimization on campus. Included were twelve types of victimization, ranging from threat of contact without force to attempted and completed rape. As shown in the Student Snapshot: "Sexual Violence on Campus," 2.8 percent of the women surveyed—about one in 36—had experienced an attempted or completed rape. Because some women had been victimized more than once, the rate of incidents was higher than the rate of victims: 35.3 per 1,000 students. This means that there might be more than 350 rapes on a campus with 10,000 women.[51]

Based on these findings, the researchers estimate that nearly 5 percent of college women are victimized in a calendar year. Over the course of a college career, which now averages five years, as many as 20 to 25 percent of women may become victims of a sexual assault.

In the sample, 15.5 percent of the women who'd been victimized had encountered either physical or nonphysical force. Most knew their assailants, who had been boyfriends, ex-boyfriends, classmates, friends, acquaintances, or coworkers. More than a third of the attempted rapes (35 percent) took place on a date, as did 22.9 percent of the threatened rapes and 12.8 percent of completed rapes. More than half of the completed rapes (51.8 per-

Student Snapshot Sexual Violence on Campus

Type of violence	Victims			Incidents	
	Number of victims in sample	Percentage of sample	Rate per 1000 students	Number of incidents	Rate per 1000 students
Completed rape	74	1.7%	16.6	86	19.3
Attempted rape	49	1.1%	11.0	71	16.0
Total	123	2.8%	27.7	157	35.3

Source: Based on a survey of 4,446 women at two- or four-year colleges and universities. Fisher, Bonnie, et al. *The Sexual Victimization of College Women.* Washington, DC: U.S. Department of Justice, December 2000.

cent) took place after midnight, while 36.6 percent occurred between 6:00 P.M. and midnight, and 11.8 percent between 6:00 A.M. and 6:00 P.M.

The report identified certain college women as being at higher risk of sexual victimization. Among the risk factors were frequently drinking enough to get drunk, being unmarried, and having been a victim of a sexual assault prior to the start of the school year. Fewer than 5 percent of the rapes, either completed or attempted, were reported to law enforcement officials. However, in about two-thirds of the rape incidents, the victim did tell another person, most often a friend, about what had happened.

The survey also asked about stalking, which it defined as following, watching, phoning, writing, e-mailing, or communicating in other ways that seemed obsessive and made a woman afraid or concerned for her safety. Of the women in the sample, 13.1 percent said they had been stalked in the current school year. Four in five knew their stalkers, and the stalking lasted an average of 60 days. In nearly three-fourths of these incidents, the women took some action as a result of the stalking, most often avoiding the stalker or confronting him.

The most common forms of sexual victimization involved sexual or sexist remarks, catcalls, and whistles. One in five women reported obscene phone calls or being asked intrusive questions about her sex or romantic life. One in ten had false rumors spread about her sex life.

About 6 percent confronted pornographic pictures, while 5 percent encountered a man exposing his sexual organs.

Approximately one in five teenage girls—or about 20 percent—are victims of dating violence. Girls assaulted by a date are more likely to develop other problems, including substance abuse, unhealthy dieting, and risky sexual behaviors.[52]

Sexual Coercion and Rape

At a bar on a weekend night, a group of intoxicated young men grab a woman and squeeze her breasts as she struggles to get free. At a party, a man offers his date drugs and alcohol in the hope of lowering her resistance to sex. Although some people don't realize it, such actions are forms of sexual coercion (forced sexual activity), which is very common, on and off college campuses. In fact, about one in five college women report being forced to have sexual intercourse.

Sexual coercion can take many forms, including exerting peer pressure, taking advantage of one's desire for popularity, threatening an end to a relationship, getting someone intoxicated, stimulating a partner against his or her wishes, or insinuating an obligation based on the time or money one has expended. Men may feel that they need to live up to the sexual stereotype of taking advantage of every opportunity for sex. Women are far more likely than men to encounter physical force.

Rape refers to sexual intercourse with an unconsenting partner under actual or threatened force. Sexual intercourse between a male over the age of 16 and a female under the "age of consent" (which ranges from 12 to 21 in different states) is called *statutory* rape. In *acquaintance* rape, or *date* rape, discussed in depth later in this chapter, the victim knows the rapist; in stranger rape, the rapist is an unknown assailant. Both stranger and acquaintance rapes are serious crimes that can have a devastating impact on their victims.

At least one in every five women experiences rape or attempted rape during her lifetime. Worldwide, rates reported to authorities vary greatly.[53] One in six U.S. women and one in 33 U.S. men have been victims of completed or attempted rape. In the National Violence against Women Survey, 17.6 percent of the women surveyed and 3 percent of men surveyed reported experiencing a completed or attempted rape at some time in their life; 0.3 percent of the women and 0.1 percent of the men had been raped in the previous 12 months. These findings indicate that some 302,091 women and 92,748 men are forcibly raped in the United States every year.[54] (See Table 17-3.)

The motives of rapists vary. Those who attack strangers often have problems establishing intimate relationships, have poor self-esteem, feel inadequate, and may have been sexually abused as children. Some rapists report a long history of fantasizing about rape and violence, generally while masturbating. Others commit rape out of anger that they can't express toward a wife or girlfriend. The more sexually aggressive men have been, the more likely they are to see such aggression and violence as normal and to believe rape myths, such as that it's impossible to rape a woman who doesn't really want sex. Sexually violent and degrading photographs, films, books, magazines, and videos may contribute to some rapists' assaultive

behaviors. Hard-core pornography depicting violent rape has been strongly associated, not only with judging oneself capable of sexual coercion and aggression, but also with engaging in such acts.

Alcohol and drugs also play a major role. About 25 percent of both men and women report unwanted sexual experiences as a result of alcohol use. Many rapists drink prior to an assault, and alcohol may interfere with a victim's ability to avoid danger or resist attack.

STRATEGIES FOR PREVENTION

Reducing the Risk of Stranger Rape

Rape prevention consists primarily of making it as difficult as possible for a rapist to make you his victim:

✔ Don't advertise that you're a woman living alone. Use initials on your mailbox. Install and use secure locks on doors and windows, changing door locks after losing keys or moving into a new residence.

✔ Don't open your door to strangers. If a repairman or public official is at your door, ask him to identify himself and call his office to verify that he is a reputable person on legitimate business.

✔ Lock your car when it is parked, and drive with locked car doors. Should your car break down, attach a white cloth to the antenna and lock yourself in. If someone other than a uniformed officer stops to offer help, ask this person to call the police or a garage but do not open your locked car door.

✔ Avoid dark and deserted areas, and be aware of the surroundings where you're walking. Should a driver ask for directions when you're a pedestrian, avoid approaching his car. Instead, call out your reply from a safe distance.

✔ Have house or car keys in hand as you approach the door. Check the back seat before getting into your car.

✔ Carry a device for making a loud noise, like a whistle or, even better, a small pint-sized compressed air horn available in many sporting goods and boat supply stores. Sound the noise alarm at the first sign of danger.

✔ Take a self-defense class to learn techniques of physical resistance that can injure the attacker or distract him long enough for you to escape.

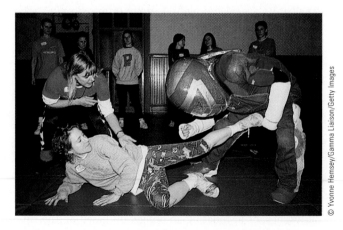

© Yvonne Hemsey/Gamma Liaison/Getty Images

▲ Model mugging courses train women to actively resist assault and rape.

For many years, the victims of rape were blamed for doing something to bring on the attack. Researchers have since shown that women are raped because they encounter sexually aggressive men, not because they look or act a certain way. However, while no woman is immune to attack, many rape victims are children or adolescents. Women who were sexually abused or raped as children are at greater risk than others. Scientists are exploring the reasons for this greater vulnerability.

Women who successfully escape rape attempts do so by resisting verbally and physically, usually by yelling and fleeing. Women who use forceful verbal or physical resistance (screaming, hitting, kicking, biting, running, and so on) are more likely to avoid rape than women who try pleading, crying, or offering no resistance.

Types of Rape

Although rape has long been viewed as an act of violence and domination, recent studies indicate that not all rapes fit into a single pattern. Within the broad category of rape are specific, but not mutually exclusive, subcategories of the crime, including anger rape, power rape, sadistic rape, gang rape, and sexual gratification rape.

Anger rape, usually on a total stranger, is motivated by hatred and a desire for revenge for the rejection the rapist feels he's suffered from women. Anger rapists often harbor long-standing hostility toward women, use far more physical violence than is needed for submission, and usually don't find the rape sexually gratifying.

Power rape is a generally premeditated attack motivated by a desire to dominate and control another person. Power rapists, unable to deal with stress and their sense of failure, may rape to regain a sense of power. They use only as much force as needed to make their victims submit and may find the rape sexually gratifying, even though that's not their primary motive.

Sadistic rape is a premeditated assault that often involves bondage, torture, or sexual abuse. Sadistic rapists find power and anger sexually arousing and may subject victims to rituals of humiliation or torture. They're often preoccupied with violent pornography; their motives are more complex and difficult to understand than those of other types of rapists.

Gang rape involves three or more rapists. Men in close groups that drink and party together—such as fraternities or athletic teams—are more likely to participate in such assaults. The reasons may go beyond aggression and sexual gratification to the excitement and camaraderie the men feel while sharing the experience.

Sexual gratification rape is usually an impulsive attack by someone willing to use physical coercion for the sake of sex. These rapists generally use no more force than needed to get a partner to submit and may stop the attack if it becomes clear they'll have to use extreme violence to overcome resistance. Many acquaintance rapes fit into this category.

Certain myths can contribute to rape and reactions to it. One is the myth of female precipitation, which blames the victim, often for dressing or behaving provocatively. Others are the myths of male pathology, which views the rapist as mentally ill, and of male's supposedly uncontrollable sexuality.[55] In research with college students, women were more likely to see male hostility and dominance in society as causes of rape while men believed more strongly in female provocation.

Acquaintance or Date Rape

Most rapes are committed by someone who is known to the victim. Both women and men report having been forced into sexual activity by someone they know. Many college students are in the age group most likely to face this threat: women aged 16 to 25 and men under 25. Women are most vulnerable and men are most likely to commit assaults during their senior year of high school and their first year of college.

Often women who describe incidents of sexual coercion that meet the legal definition of rape don't label it as such. Often they have a preconceived notion that true "rape" consists of a blitzlike attack by a stranger. Or they

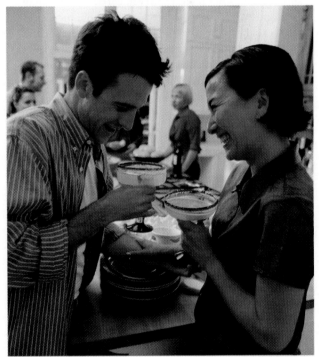

▲ Acquaintance rape and alcohol use are very closely linked. Both men and women may find their judgment impaired or their communications unclear as a result of drinking.

may blame themselves for getting into a situation in which they couldn't escape, or they may feel some genuine concern for others who would be devastated if they knew the truth (for example, if the rapist were the brother of a good friend or the son of a neighbor). In studies of university students, both men and women who held less traditional gender roles tended to view rape scenarios involving acquaintances or spouses as more serious and were less likely to blame the victim.

Men who admit to being sexually aggressive don't see themselves as would-be rapists. The reasons stem from our society's ambivalence about sexual violence and standards for "normal" interactions between potential sexual partners. According to various studies, 25 to 60 percent of college men have engaged in some form of sexual coercion. Most often these men simply ignored a woman when she said no or protested. In addition, many college men report engaging in sexual activity against their own wishes, most often because of male peer pressure or a desire to be popular.

The same factors that lead to other forms of sexual victimization can set the stage for date rape. Socialization into an aggressive role, acceptance of rape myths, and a view that force is justified in certain situations increase the likelihood of a man's committing date rape. Other factors can also play a role, including the following:

▶ **Personality and early sexual experiences.** Psychological studies haven't found that date rapists are more disturbed than other men. However, certain factors may predispose individuals to sexual aggression, including first sexual experience at a very young age, earlier and more frequent than usual childhood sexual experiences (both forced and voluntary), hostility toward women, irresponsibility, lack of social consciousness, and a need for dominance over sexual partners.

▶ **Situational variables (what happens during the date).** Men who initiate a date, pay all expenses, and provide transportation are more likely to be sexually aggressive, perhaps because they feel that they can call all the shots. For instance, a man may drive to an isolated area and park his car, setting the stage for a sexual assault.

▶ **Acceptance of sexual coercion.** Some social groups, such as fraternities or athletic teams, may encourage the use of alcohol; reinforce stereotypes about masculinity; and emphasize violence, force, and competition. The group's shared values, including an acceptance of sexual coercion, may keep individuals from questioning their behavior. In studies comparing self-admitted date rapists with college men who had not sexually victimized women, the rapists were more likely to have taken advantage of women—for example, by saying that they loved them—for the sake of sex. They also were much more likely to have friends who viewed rough sex and rape as justified—or even as something that would enhance their reputation among their peers.

▶ **Drinking.** Alcohol use is one of the strongest predictors of acquaintance rape. Men who've been drinking may not react to subtle signals, may misinterpret a woman's behavior as come-ons, and may feel more sexually aroused. At the same time, drinking may impair a woman's ability to communicate her wishes effectively and to cope with a man's aggressiveness. Alcohol also affects the way rape is perceived: Assailants suffer less blame when drunk than when sober, while victims may be considered more responsible for the rape if they were drunk.

▶ **Date rape drugs.** Drugs such as Rohypnol (roofie, La Rocha, rope, Mexican Valium, Rib Roche, R-2), a tranquilizer used overseas, and gammahydroxybutrate or GHB, a depressant with potential benefits for people with narcolepsy, have been implicated in cases of acquaintance or date rape. Since both are odorless and tasteless, a woman has no way of knowing whether her drink has been tampered with. The subsequent loss of memory leaves her with no explanation for where she's been or what's happened in the hours before she regains consciousness. Women have reported waking up naked in college fraternity houses or in the apartments of dates or casual acquaintances with no recall of what happened.[56]

Rohypnol can cause impaired motor skills and judgment, lack of inhibitions, dizziness, confusion, lethargy, very low blood pressure, coma, and death. Its use has been outlawed in this country; rapists found guilty of giving this drug to one of their victims can get 20 years added to their prison sentences. Deaths also have been attributed to GHB overdoses. Some drug makers have developed legal substitutes for GHB that are odorless and tasteless chemicals and easily mixed in drinks.[57]

▶ **Gender differences in interpreting sexual cues.** In research comparing college men and women, the men typically overestimated the woman's sexual availability and interest, seeing friendliness, revealing clothing, and attractiveness as deliberately seductive. In one study of date rapes, the men reported feeling "led on," in part because their female partners seemed to be dressed more suggestively than usual. They didn't define their behavior as rape, placed equal responsibility on their partners for what happened, and said that they'd behave similarly again. They also disagreed with their victims about the amount of force used and viewed the women's protests as token resistance.

???? How Can I Prevent Date Rape?

For men:

▶ Remember that it's okay not to "score" on a date. Don't assume that a sexy dress or casual flirting is an invitation to sex.

▶ Be aware of your partner's actions. If she pulls away or tries to get up, understand that she's sending you a message—one you should acknowledge and respect.

▶ Restrict drinking, drug use, or other behaviors (such as hanging out with a group known to be sexually aggressive in certain situations) that could affect your judgment and ability to act responsibly.

▶ Think of the way you'd want your sister or a close woman friend to be treated by her date. Behave in the same manner.

For women:

▶ Be wary if the man calls all the shots (ordering for you at restaurants, planning what to do on your date); he may do the same when it comes to sex. If he pays for all expenses, he may think he's justified in using force to get "what he paid for." If you cover some of the costs, he may be less aggressive.

▶ Back away from a man who pressures you into other activities you don't want to engage in on a date, such as chugging beer or drag racing with his friends.

▶ Avoid misleading messages and avoid behavior that may be interpreted as sexual teasing. Don't tell him to stop touching you, talk for a few minutes, and then resume petting. If you know or feel at the onset of a relationship that you don't want to have sex with this person, say so.

▶ If, despite your clearly stated intentions, your date behaves in a sexually coercive manner, use a strategy of escalating forcefulness—direct refusal, vehement verbal refusal, and, if necessary, physical force.

▶ Avoid using alcohol or other drugs when you definitely do not wish to be sexually intimate with your date.

Male Rape

No one knows how common male rape is because men are less likely to report such assaults than women. In a recent survey in England, nearly 3 percent of men reported nonconsensual sexual experiences as adults. Other researchers estimate that the victims in about 10 percent of acquaintance rape cases are men. These "hidden victims" often keep silent because of embarrassment, shame, or humiliation and their own feelings and fears about homosexuality and conforming to conventional sex roles.

Although many people think that men who rape other men are always homosexuals, most male rapists consider themselves to be heterosexual. Young boys aren't the only victims. The average age of male rape victims is 24. Rape is a serious problem in prison, where men may experience brutal assaults by men who usually resume sexual relations with women once they're released.

There have been reports of men forced by women to participate in sexual intercourse. Typically, these men feel very upset afterward because they functioned sexually in circumstances that they thought should have made it impossible to obtain an erection. They suffer a postassault syndrome comparable to the rape trauma syndrome women experience, including psychological and sexual difficulties. Men raped by other men also suffer extreme emotional distress after an attack.

The Impact of Rape

Only a small percentage of college women who are raped report their assaults to the police; many don't even tell a close friend or relative about the assault. However, women who survive a rape can benefit from the support of others. If you are raped, call a friend or rape crisis center. Before you take a bath or shower, go to a doctor—you may later decide to report the rape. If you must go to a hospital, remember that you don't necessarily have to talk to the police. Talk to a counselor or health-care workers at the hospital about testing and antibiotics for sexually transmitted diseases and postintercourse contraception.

Sexual violence has both a physical and a psychological impact. Rape-related injuries include unexplained vaginal discharge, bleeding, infections, multiple bruises, and fractured ribs. Victims of sexual violence often develop chronic symptoms, such as headaches, backaches, high blood pressure, sleep disorders, pelvic pain, and sexual fertility problems.

The psychological scars of a sexual assault take a long time to heal. Therapists have linked sexual victimization with hopelessness, low self-esteem, high levels of self-criticism, and self-defeating relationships. Some have described a "rape trauma syndrome," similar to posttraumatic stress disorder, in which women suffer both acute symptoms, such as crying, shortly after the rape and long-term symptoms, which can

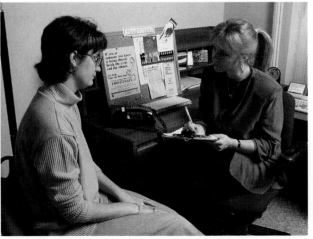

▲ Counseling from a trained professional can help ease the trauma suffered by a rape victim.

persist for years and often include deeply disturbing flashbacks in which they relive the rape.

Acquaintance rape may cause fewer physical injuries but greater psychological torment. The victims of date rape are less likely to notify the police, in part because they fear that no one will believe their stories. Often too ashamed to tell anyone what happened, they may suffer alone, without skilled therapists or sympathetic friends to reassure them. Women raped by acquaintances blame themselves more, see themselves less positively, question their judgment, have greater difficulty trusting others, and have higher levels of psychological distress. Nightmares, anxiety, and flashbacks are common. The women may avoid others, become less capable of protecting themselves, and come to accept victimization as part of being a woman.

According to some researchers, victims of acquaintance rape rate themselves as less recovered than women raped by strangers for up to three years after the assault. Years after a rape, victims of date rape may still be struggling with rage against men and having problems establishing trusting relationships. Women who remain haunted by the sexual violence should seek professional help. A therapist can help them begin the slow process of healing.

What to Do in Case of Rape

If a woman has been raped, she will have to decide whether to report the attack to the police. Even an unsuccessful rape attempt should be reported because the information a woman may provide about the attack—the assaulter's physical characteristics, voice, clothes, car, even an unusual smell—may prevent another woman from being raped. A woman shouldn't bathe or change her clothes before calling the police. Semen, hair, and material under her fingernails or on her apparel all may be useful in identifying the man who raped her. Many rape victims find it very helpful to contact a rape crisis center, where qualified staff members assist in dealing with the trauma. Many colleges, universities, and large urban communities in the United States have such programs. Friends and family members should remember that many women will mistakenly blame themselves for the rape. However, the victim hasn't committed a crime—the man who raped her has.

Halting Sexual Violence: Prevention Efforts

Sexual violence has its roots in social attitudes and beliefs that demean women and condone aggression. As colleges and universities have become more aware of the different forms of sexual danger, many have taken the lead in setting up primary prevention programs (including newspaper articles; seminars in dormitories, fraternities, and sorori-

ties; and lectures) to help students examine their attitudes and values, understand cultural influences, and develop skills for avoiding or escaping from dangerous situations. All men and women should understand the impact of socialization on their willingness to tolerate or participate in sexual victimization, recognize misleading rape myths, and develop effective ways of communicating to avoid misinterpretation of sexual cues. Students should also know where they can turn to learn more about and seek help for sexual victimization: counselors, campus police, deans of student affairs, fraternity or sorority representatives, campus ministers, and so on. (See Pulse Points: "Ten Ways to Prevent Sexual Victimization.")

While most campuses provide self-defense seminars for potential female victims of rape and general campus safety measures, some have tried innovative approaches, such as Men Against Violence, a peer education program that confronts male students' conceptions of manhood and appropriate gender roles to reduce their likelihood of sexually or physically violent behavior.[58] Such all-male, peer-guided approaches that challenge myths about rape and rape victims also have proven effective in targeting college fraternity men. Past research on sexual violence has documented an increased rate of gang rapes and sexual coercion among this group.[59]

In addition, practical institutional steps—such as providing adequate lighting, escort services, and clear policies

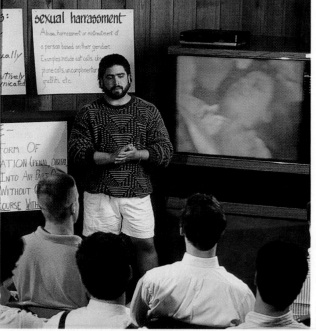

▲ All-male workshops can generate discussion about gender roles, violence, and other societal ideas. These discussions may also provide positive pressure against rape and other forms of aggression against women.

PULSE POINTS

Ten Ways to Prevent Sexual Victimization

1. **Challenge gender stereotypes.** Just because you're male doesn't mean you have to act in a macho, sexually aggressive way. Just because you're female doesn't mean you have to be passive and accepting of male behavior.

2. **Don't tolerate inappropriate language or behavior.** If you find someone's sexually crude language offensive, say so. If you don't like to be touched by casual acquaintances, back away, and keep your distance.

3. **Be careful of your sexual signals.** Men often assume that women who smile, make conversation, and flirt are signaling sexual availability. Women typically think they're just being friendly. Make sure you know the message you want to send—and don't assume you can tell what someone else is trying to signal.

4. **Choose safe settings.** If you're going out with someone you don't know well or have reservations about being alone with, suggest meeting in a public place or participating in a group activity.

5. **Think about your sexual expectations for a relationship.** What are you willing to do? How much sexual activity is enough? Where do you want to draw the line? Remember, your partner will be making decisions about the same things.

6. **Talk about sex.** Using the communication guidelines in Chapters 7 and 8, bring up the topic of sexual involvement. Let your date know from the beginning how you feel about sexual activity on first, second, third, or twentieth dates.

7. **Think ahead.** Rather than letting yourself get carried away by passion, anticipate what could happen if, for instance, you agree to go to your date's apartment for a drink or park in an isolated spot. State your feelings clearly.

8. **Say "no" clearly when you mean it, and accept "no" when you hear it.** If you're the one saying no, use a firm, even loud voice, and back up what you say with body language. If you're on the receiving end of a no, pay attention. A "no"—even if said quietly and shyly—still means no.

9. **Keep your wits about you.** Alcohol and other drugs can affect your judgment and inhibitions. You may become more sexually aggressive under their influence, or you may greatly increase your risk of being victimized.

10. **Call it like it is.** If you're the target of sexual taunts or unwanted propositions on campus or at work, say, "What you're doing is sexual harassment, and I'm going to report it." If a date or acquaintance won't respect your limits, one of the most effective defensive tactics is saying, "This is rape, and I'm calling the cops."

---

against both violence and drug and alcohol abuse—can help. Self-defense classes teach women how to avoid becoming victims either by escaping or protecting themselves. Individuals who advocate such training believe that it can strengthen women's physical capacities and encourage them to be less passive in encounters with potential victimizers. Others, however, view self-defense behaviors as violent actions in themselves, and are concerned that they may lead to an increased risk of injury or death. Followup studies of college women have found that self-defense training increased their feelings of self-improvement, a sense of control over their life, confidence, security, independence, and physical prowess.

Campuses are also providing "secondary prevention" by getting help to victims of sexual violence as soon as possible through rape crisis teams and emergency mental-health services, and "tertiary prevention" by working with victims to ameliorate the long-term effects of their experience through psychotherapy, educational services, and medical care.

Helping the Victims of Violence

As their numbers have grown and their anguish has been recognized, the victims of violence have received greater attention. In the last decade, hundreds of shelters for battered wives and their children have been set up across the country. They offer physical and psychological treatment, and a haven where women can begin to rebuild their shattered self-esteem, as well as their daily lives. Rape counseling and crisis centers on college campuses and in the community provide various forms of assistance to victims of rape. In many cities, the telephone directory lists hot lines and resources. More than 400 victims' advocacy groups have been set up across the country to advise those hurt by crime. Support organizations help many survivors deal with the emotional aftermath of their experiences.

(See "Your Health Almanac" at the back of this book for listings.)

Sometimes well-intentioned friends and relatives add to the stress felt by the victims of violence. Here's how to offer comfort without implying criticism:

▶ Don't blame the victim. Even when no one doubts that the victim is completely innocent, individuals may be plagued by regrets and self-accusation: Why didn't I lock the windows? Why did I park on that dark street? Any second-guessing or implied criticism adds to this burden of blame and shame.

▶ Don't try to deny that it happened. Although it may be hard to talk about—or even listen to—what happened, the reality of the event must not be ignored. Denial makes victims doubt their own experience and question themselves at a time when they crave reassurance.

▶ Don't pressure the victim to talk—or not to talk. Some individuals need to go over every detail of what happened, again and again, until they work out their feelings of outrage and become ready to get on with their lives. Others find going into details too humiliating. Let the victim set the tone and limits for disclosure. Don't pry or prod.

▶ Don't try to rush the victim to leave the past behind and get on with his or her life. Recovery from any traumatic event takes time, and only the victim knows the appropriate pace. If, however, months pass without any lessening of symptoms or improvement in day-to-day functioning, family members and friends shouldn't hesitate to recommend that their loved one see a mental health professional.

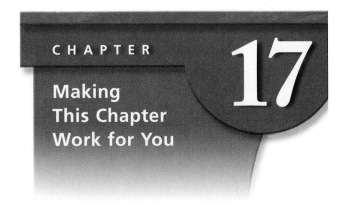

CHAPTER

Making
This Chapter
Work for You

17

1. You can keep yourself safe by doing all of the following except
   a. using seatbelts when driving or a passenger.
   b. wearing pajamas made of nonflammable materials.
   c. removing or fixing loose carpets.
   d. allowing a spilled liquid to dry on a slippery floor before cleaning it up.

2. Which of the following factors affects an individual's risk of accident or injury?
   a. hunger level
   b. stress level
   c. amount of automobile insurance coverage
   d. knowledge of CPR

3. Safe driving tips include all of the following except
   a. Avoid driving at night for the first year after getting a license.
   b. Make sure that your car has snow tires or chains before driving in hazardous snowy conditions.
   c. If riding with an intoxicated driver, keep talking to him so that he doesn't fall asleep at the wheel.
   d. Don't let packages or people obstruct the rear or side windows.

4. Which of the following statements about home safety is true?
   a. Falls pose the greatest threat of injury in the home, followed by poison.
   b. The three ingredients of fire are fuel, a heat source, and oxygen.
   c. The risk of falls is lowest in the elderly.
   d. When using cleaning products, make sure that windows are tightly closed.

5. Health hazards related to computer use include all of the following except
   a. exposure to toxic materials.
   b. computer vision syndrome.
   c. repetitive motion injuries.
   d. back strain.

6. Which of the following statements about recreational safety hazards is true?
   a. Hypothermia is a life-threatening medical emergency caused by the inability of the body to cool itself.
   b. The most common heat-related conditions are heat stroke and heat exhaustion.
   c. Most drownings occur at organized facilities.
   d. Frostbite usually affects the tissues of the hands and feet

7. Which of the following statements about violence in the United States is false?
   a. Almost half the victims of violent crime are under 25 years of age.
   b. More than 5 million people are physically assaulted annually.
   c. Homicide is the leading cause of death for teenagers, followed by automobile accidents.
   d. Boys and men are most likely to be the perpetrators of homicide, domestic abuse, and hate-related crimes.

8. Sexual victimization
   a. includes sexual harassment, sexual coercion, and rape.
   b. is gender-specific, affecting women who are violated emotionally or physically by men.
   c. is rare in academic environments such as college campuses.
   d. most commonly takes the form of physical assault and stalking.

9. Which of the following statements about rape is true?
   a. When a person is sexually attacked by a stranger, it is referred to as rape. When a person is sexually attacked by an acquaintance, it is referred to as sexual coercion.
   b. Statutory rape is defined as sexual intercourse initiated by a woman under the age of consent.
   c. Men who rape other men usually consider themselves heterosexuals.
   d. Women who flirt and dress provocatively are typically more willing to participate in aggressive sex than women who dress conservatively and do not flirt.

10. Ways to protect or prevent rape include:
    a. Use alcohol and drugs in familiar surroundings only.
    b. Take a self-defense class.
    c. To avoid angering him or her, become passive and quiet when around a sexually aggressive person.
    d. Do not discuss your sexual limits on a first or second date because just talking about sex will encourage your date to think that you are interested in a sexual relationship.

Answers to these questions can be found on page 640.

 Are courses in conflict management and peace studies a solution to preventing school violence?

Critical Thinking

1. Can you name two risk factors in your daily life that might increase the likelihood of accidental injury? What actions have you taken to keep yourself safe? Are there other risk factors you could minimize or eliminate? What might you do about them?

2. A friend of yours, Eric, frequently makes crude or derogatory comments about women. When you finally call him on it, his response is, "I didn't say anything wrong. I like women." What might you say to him?

3. At one college, women raped by acquaintances or dates scrawled the names of their assailants on the walls of women's restrooms on campus. Several young men whose names appeared on the list objected, protesting that they were innocent and were being unfairly accused. How do you feel about this method of fighting back against date rape? Do you think it violates the rights of men? How do you feel about naming women who've been raped in news reports? Are there circumstances in which a woman's identity should be revealed? Would fewer women report a rape if not assured of privacy?

SITES & BYTES

National Organization for Victim Assistance
http://www.try-nova.org
This site features current news events as well as information on victim rights, how to get help after victimization, and resources for victims/survivors.

American Psychological Association
http://helping.apa.org/daily/terrorism.html
At this site, the American Psychological Association offers practical advice on coping with terrorism and trauma.

First Aid Online
http://www.scivolutions.com/fistaid/index.html
This site features printable materials for managing a variety of conditions requiring first aid, including cuts and wounds, insect bites, burns, choking, hypothermia, allergies, and shock.

Please note that links are subject to change. If you find a broken link, use a search engine such as **http://www.yahoo.com** and search for the website by typing in key words.

 InfoTrac Activity "CDC Provides Strategies on How to Help Prevent Illness from Heat Exposure." *Medical Letter on the CDC & FDA,* August 19, 2001.

(1) List five risk factors for the development of heat-related illness.

(2) What are the warning signs of heat stroke? What are the warning signs of heat exhaustion?

(3) List four specific strategies that can help prevent heat-related illness.

You can find additional readings related to violence and injury with InfoTrac College Edition, an online library of more than 900 journals and publications. Follow the instructions for accessing InfoTrac that were packaged with your textbook; then search for articles using a key word search.

For additional links, resources, and suggested readings on InfoTrac, visit our Health & Wellness Resource Center at **http://health.wadsworth.com**.

Key Terms

The terms listed here are used within the chapter on the page indicated. Definitions of terms are in the Glossary at the end of the book.

computer vision syndrome 578	**heat stress** 579	**rape** 588
frostbite 579	**heat stroke** 579	**repetitive motion injury (RMI)** 578
frostnip 579	**hostile or offensive environment** 585	**sexual coercion** 587
heat cramps 579	**hypothermia** 580	
heat exhaustion 579	**quid pro quo** 585	

References

1. Grossman, David. "Adolescent Injury Prevention and Clinicians: Time for Instant Messaging." *Western Journal of Medicine,* Vol. 172, No. 3, March 2000.
2. National Safety Council. www.nsc.org.
3. Department of Transportation's National Highway Traffic Safety Administration.
4. Quinlan, Kyran, et al. "Characteristics of Child Passenger Deaths and Injuries Involving Drinking Drivers." *Journal of the American Medical Association,* Vol. 283, No. 17, May 3, 2000.
5. Rivara, Fredrick, et al. "Effectiveness of Automatic Shoulder Belt Systems in Motor Vehicle Crashes." *Journal of the American Medical Association,* Vol. 283, No. 21, June 7, 2000.
6. Burke, Michael. "Deaths in Car Accidents Neither Rise nor Fall." *Contemporary Pediatrics,* Vol. 17, No. 5, May 2000.
7. Schnyder, U., et al. "Incidence and Prediction of Posttraumatic Stress Disorder Symptoms in Severely Injured Accident Victims." *American Journal of Psychiatry,* Vol. 158, No. 4, April 2001, p. 594.
8. "Out of My Way!" *The Wilson Quarterly,* Vol. 25, No. 3, Summer 2001, p. 85.
9. National Safety Council. www.nsc.org.
10. Martin, Melissa. "Asleep at the Wheel." *Occupational Hazards,* Vol. 63, No. 7, July 2001, p. 39.
11. Malta, Loretta, et al. "Psychological Reactivity in Aggressive Drivers." *Applied Psychophysiology & Biofeedback,* June 2001.
12. McCarrt, Anne. "Graduated Driver Licensing Systems Reducing Crashes Among Teenage Drivers." *Journal of the American Medical Association,* Vol. 286, No. 13, October 3, 2001.
13. Foss, D. "Initial Effects of Graduated Driver Licensing on 16-Year-Old Driver Crashes in North Carolina." *Journal of the American Medical Association,* Vol. 286, No. 13, October 3, 2001.
14. Shope, Jean, et al. "Graduated Driver Licensing in Michigan: Early Impact on Motor Vehicle Crashes Among 16-Year-Old Drivers." *Journal of the American Medical Association,* Vol. 286, No. 13, October 3, 2001.
15. AAA Foundation for Traffic Safety.
16. Nerenberg, Arnold. Personal interview.
17. Moser, Phil. "The Mobile Communications Threat: Drivers in Danger." *Risk Management,* Vol. 48, No. 5, May 2001, p. 28.
18. "Cell Phone Use in Motor Vehicles 'Distinctly More Risky' Than Other Distractions." *Medical Letter on the CDC & FDA,* June 17, 2001.
19. Messinger-Rapport, Barbara, and Erin Rader. "High Risk on the Highway: How to Identify and Treat the Impaired Older Driver." *Geriatrics,* Vol. 55, No. 1, October 2000.

20. "Drivers with History of Heart Disease, Stroke at Risk for Car Crashes." *Geriatrics*, Vol. 55, No. 1, October 2000.

21. Institute for Highway Safety.

22. Thompson, Matthew, and Fredrick Rivara. "Bicycle-Related Injuries." *American Family Physician*, May 15, 2001.

23. Preboth, Monica. "AAP Statement on Falls in Children." *American Family Physician*, Vol. 64, No. 8, October 15, 2001, p. 1468.

24. Gardner, Melinda, et al. "Practical Implementation of an Exercise-Based Falls Prevention Programme." *Age and Ageing*, Vol. 30, No. 1, January 2001, p. 77.

25. National Center for Health Statistics (NCHS).

26. Reichard, John. "Report Cites One Million Annual Ergonomics Injuries." *Medicine & Health*, Vol. 55, No. 5, January 29, 2001, p. 3.

27. Simoneau, Guy, and Richard Marklin. "Effect of Computer Keyboard Slope and Height on Wrist Extension Angle." *Human Factors*, Vol. 43, No. 2, Summer 2001, p. 287.

28. Idzikowski, Jan, et al. "Upper Extremity Snowboarding Injuries: Ten-Year Results from the Colorado Snowboard Injury Survey." *American Journal of Sports Medicine*, Vol. 28, No. 6, November 2000.

29. Brenner, Ruth, et al. "Where Children Drown." *Pediatrics*, Vol. 108, No. 1, July 2001, p. 85.

30. Bureau of Justice Statistics.

31. Statement on the National Crime Victimization Survey. Weekly Compilation of Presidential Documents, Vol. 36, No. 35, September 4, 2000.

32. Centers for Disease Control and Prevention (CDC).

33. Purugganan, Ruth, et al. "Exposure to Violence Among Urban School-Aged Children: Is It Only on Television?" *Pediatrics*, Vol. 106, No. 4, October 2000.

34. Department of Justice. www.ojp.usdoj.gov/bjs.

35. Tjaden, Patricia, and Nancy Thoennes. *Full Report of the Prevalence, Incidence and Consequences of Violence Against Women.* Washington, DC: National Center for Justice, November 2000.

36. Gyimah-Brempong, Kwabena. "Alcohol Availability and Crime: Evidence from Census Tract Data." *Southern Economic Journal*, Vol. 68, No. 1, July 2001, p. 2.

37. Small, Margaret, and Kellie Tetrick. "School Violence: An Overview." *Juvenile Justice*, Vol. 8, No. 1, p. 3.

38. *Youth Violence: A Report of the Surgeon General.* Washington, DC: Department of Health and Human Services, 2001.

39. Hales, Dianne. "Teen Violence." *Worldbook Annual*, 2002.

40. Meloy, J. Reid, et al. "Offender and Offense Characteristics of a Nonrandom Sample of Adolescent Mass Murderers." *Journal of the American Academy of Child and Adolescent Psychiatry*, Vol. 40, No. 6, June 2001, p. 719.

41. Hales, "Teen Violence."

42. Carter, Daniel. "Covering Crime on College Campuses." *Quill*, Vol. 88, No. 8, September 2000.

43. Department of Education.

44. Dervarics, Charles. "College Groups Battle Safety Advocates over Reform Plan." *Community College Week*, Vol. 13, No. 26, August 6, 2001, p. 3.

45. "Database Will List Campus Crime Figures." *Black Issues in Higher Education*, Vol. 17, No. 11, July 20, 2000.

46. "Some Physical Effects of Emotional Violence." *Harvard Mental Health Letter*, Vol. 17, No. 10, April 2001.

47. "Prevention of Sexual Harassment in the Workplace and Educational Settings." *Pediatrics*, Vol. 106, No. 5, December 2000.

48. Webb, Susan. Personal interview.

49. Murnen, Sarah, and Linda Smolak. "The Experience of Sexual Harassment Among Grade-School Students: Early Socialization of Female Subordination?" *Sex Roles: A Journal of Research*, July 2000.

50. Ibid.

51. Fisher, Bonnie, et al. *The Sexual Victimization of College Women.* Washington, DC: U.S. Department of Justice, December 2000.

52. Wingood, Gina. "Dating Violence and the Sexual Health of Black Adolescent Females." *Pediatrics*, Vol. 107, No. 5, May 2001, p. 1169.

53. MacDonald, Rhona. "Time to Talk About Rape: If Men Remember That Women Are Their Mothers, Daughters, and Wives They May Change Their Laws." *British Medical Journal*, Vol. 321, No. 7268, October 28, 2000.

54. Tjaden and Thoennes, *Full Report of the Prevalence, Incidence and Consequences of Violence Against Women.*

55. Cowan, Gloria. "Beliefs About the Causes of Four Types of Rape." *Sex Roles: A Journal of Research*, May 2000.

56. Walling, Anne. "Helping Patients Recognize and Avoid 'Date Rape' Drugs." *American Family Physician*, Vol. 62, No. 11, December 1, 2000.

57. "Legal Chemicals Being Used for Date Rape." *State Legislatures*, Vol. 27, No. 2, February 2001, p. 9.

58. Hong, Luoluo. "Toward a Transformed Approach to Prevention: Breaking the Link Between Masculinity and Violence." *Journal of American College Health*, Vol. 48, No. 6, May 2000.

59. Fourbert, John. "The Longitudinal Effects of a Rape-Prevention Program on Fraternity Men's Attitudes, Behavioral Intent, and Behavior." *Journal of American College Health*, Vol. 48, No. 4, January 2000.

18

When Life Ends

On September 11, 2001, at colleges and universities across the United States, professors stopped lecturing. Students closed their notebooks and looked up from their computers. Silence fell over classrooms, auditoriums, dormitories, gymnasiums. Death—sudden, horrific, on an almost unimaginable scale—became the lesson of the day.

Many in what has been dubbed "Generation 9-11," growing up in times of peace and prosperity, had no prior experience of loss. They stared at television images that defied comprehension. In the days after the tragic hijackings and attacks, they, like others around the nation and the globe, cried, prayed, lit candles, sang songs, and held each other close. Large or small, urban or bucolic, college campuses became something they were never meant to be: places of sorrow and grief.

"College seems a life-or-death matter to students, professors, and staff scurrying about campus, but it isn't. It's a matter of life," a philosophy professor observed months before September 11. "Admissions offices are powerful, but not powerful enough to keep out death. It crashes in when it will."[1] When it does, we not only mourn for those who died but also have to confront the inescapable reality that every life ends in death.

In time we all lose people we cherish: grandparents, aunts and uncles, parents, siblings, friends, coworkers, teachers, and neighbors. With each loss, part of us may seem to die, yet each loss also reaffirms how precious life is.

This chapter explores the meaning of death, describes the process of dying, provides practical information on medical and legal arrangements, and offers advice on comforting the dying and helping their survivors.

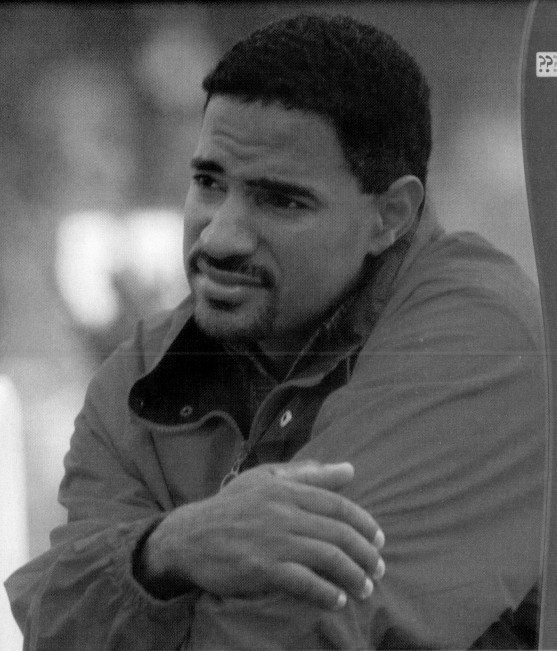

After studying the material in this chapter, you should be able to:

- **Define** death and **explain** the stages of emotional reaction experienced in facing death.
- **Explain** the purposes of advanced directives, a living will, and a holographic will.
- **Discuss** the factors that can affect an individual's death experience.
- **Explain** the controversy surrounding the right to die, including the influence of culture on life-and-death decisions.
- **List** and **explain** factors affecting the length and intensity of grief.

Living and Dying

The French writer Albert Camus once wrote that there could be no lasting peace in the hearts of individuals until death is outlawed. The human race has not been able to ban death, but scientific, technical, and public health advances have delayed it by decades. Life expectancy in the United States has risen to a record high of 76.9 years; age-adjusted death rates have fallen to record lows.[2]

How long can human beings live? Scientific evidence suggests that, for most people, maximum life expectancy is 85 years.[3] However, the number of centenarians is growing dramatically, and some individuals have survived for more than 110 years. While genes may play a role in longevity (see Genes in Focus: "Is There a Methuselah Gene?"), lifestyle and healthful behaviors can influence both how long and how well we live. In a landmark study that has tracked the mental and physical health of 724 men as they aged over a 60-year period, seven factors predicted long life and successful aging: moderate alcohol use, no smoking, a stable marriage, exercise, appropriate weight, positive coping mechanisms, and no depressive illness.[4]

More than two million people die in the United States each year. Although most are older, death occurs in all age groups. The causes of death vary both with age and gender. Among those under age 35, intentional and nonintentional injury is the primary cause of death. (See Student Snapshot: "Dying Young.") Among older Americans, cancer and heart disease are the top killers. Men typically die at younger ages than women. (See The X&Y Files: "Why Do Men Die Sooner than Women?")

Defining Death

In our society, death isn't a part of everyday life, as it once was. Because machines can now keep people alive who, in the past, would have died, the definition of death has become more complex. Death has been broken down into the following categories:

▶ **Functional death.** The end of all vital functions, such as heartbeat and respiration.
▶ **Cellular death.** The gradual death of body cells after the heart stops beating. If placed in a tissue culture or, as is the case with various organs, transplanted to another body, some cells can remain alive indefinitely.
▶ **Cardiac death.** The moment when the heart stops beating.
▶ **Brain death.** The end of all brain activity, indicated by an absence of electrical activity (confirmed by an electroencephalogram, or EEG) and a lack of reflexes. The

GENES IN FOCUS

Is There a Methuselah Gene?

Scientists have identified a genetic marker known as apolipoprotein E (ApoE) that, depending on the variation we inherit, can affect how our hearts, brains, and bodies age. Recent studies have linked the ApoE gene with diabetes, macular degeneration, Alzheimer's disease, coronary artery disease, multiple sclerosis, and longevity.

All of us inherit the ApoE gene, which comes in three varieties, each associated with low, intermediate, and high risk of cardiovascular and neurological disease. About 60 percent of people carry ApoE-3, which neither significantly increases nor decreases health risks. At least 10 percent are born with ApoE-4, a bad-news gene that has been linked to greater risk of Alzheimer's and other degenerative diseases. The so-called Methuselah gene, ApoE-2, shows up in the genetic profiles of healthy centenarians with no signs of dementia, cancer, or heart disease.

A simple blood test can identify which type of ApoE gene a person has. Most individuals who undergo testing learn that they have ApoE-3, which has a more or less neutral impact on their health and longevity. About 20 percent get good news: They carry the ApoE-2 variation, which boosts their odds of a long and healthy life. But even those who discover that they have the ominous ApoE-4 gene, shouldn't feel fated for illness or early death. By changes in lifestyle and nutrition, researchers estimate that even those with ApoE-4 can add years to their lifespans.

Sources: Corder, Elizabeth. "Apolipoprotein E Polymorphisms in Aging and Human Disease." *Gerontologist,* October 15, 2001, p. 152. Peila, R., et al. "Type 2 Diabetes, APOE Gene and the Risk of Dementia and Dementia-related Pathologies," *American Journal of Human Genetics,* Vol. 69, No. 4, October 2001, p. 385.

notion of brain death is bound up with what we consider to be the actual person, or self. The destruction of a person's brain means that his or her personality no longer exists; the lower brain centers controlling respiration and circulation no longer function.
▶ **Spiritual death.** The moment when the soul, as defined by many religions, leaves the body.

When does a person actually die? The traditional legal definition of death is failure of the lungs or heart to func-

Student Snapshot Dying Young

The Five Leading Causes of Death for College-Age Americans

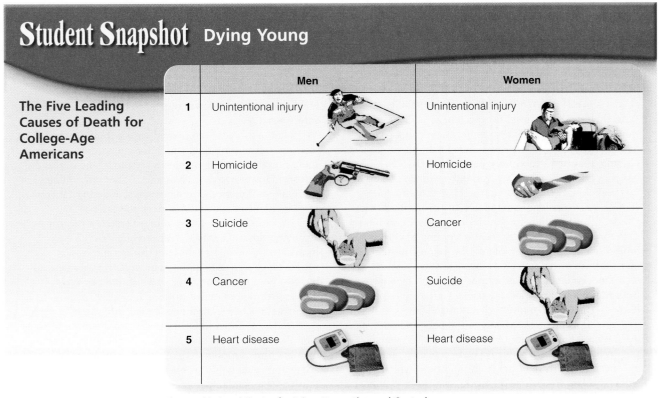

	Men	Women
1	Unintentional injury	Unintentional injury
2	Homicide	Homicide
3	Suicide	Cancer
4	Cancer	Suicide
5	Heart disease	Heart disease

Source: National Center for Injury Prevention and Control.

tion. However, because modern medicine is often able to maintain respiration and circulation by artificial means, most states have declared that an individual is considered dead only when the brain, including the brain stem, completely stops functioning. Brain-death laws prohibit a medical staff from "pulling the plug" if there is any hope of sustaining life.

The Meaning of Death

Death is not a mystery to those who have died. The living are the ones who struggle to find meaning in it. As far back as 60,000 years ago, prehistoric people observed special ceremonies when burying their dead. Many early cultures believed that people continued to exist after death and had the same needs that they did in life; hence they buried their loved ones with food, dishes, weapons, and jewels. Some religions, such as Christianity, believe that the dead will rise again; to them, the burial of the body is symbolic, like the planting of a seed in the earth to await rebirth. Many Eastern religions share the belief that death marks the end only of physical existence and of the limited view of reality that human beings can grasp.

Death itself is a remote experience in most lives today, something that takes place off-stage in a hospital or nursing home. In earlier times, dying was a much more visible part of daily living. Families, friends, and other loved ones in a community would share in caring for those at the end of life.[5] Most deaths occurred at home, often following a brief illness and unaffected by the limited medical care available. Today, the process of dying has become invisible.[6]

Our attitudes toward dying also have changed with the development of medical technology and the extension of the human lifespan. Some people will do anything to delay aging or defeat death itself through medical science or other means. Others see death as part of a natural biological process and work toward the goal of dying well, with dignity and without undue suffering.

Denial and Death

Most of us don't quite believe that we're going to die. A reasonable amount of denial helps us focus on the day-to-day realities of living. However, excessive denial can be life-threatening. Some drivers, for instance, refuse to buckle their seat belts, because they refuse to acknowledge

The X&Y Files — Why Do Men Die Sooner than Women?

The gender gap in longevity has been shrinking since 1990. According to the National Center for Health Statistics, life expectancy for American women now stands at 79.5 years; for men, it is a record high of 74.1 years. In other developed nations—Australia, Canada, France, Greece, Italy, Japan, Netherlands, Norway, Spain, Sweden, Switzerland—women live up to two years longer than those in the United States and about seven years longer than men. In the former Soviet Union, life expectancy for females is thirteen years longer than for males. By the year 2020, according to current projections for the United States, the average woman's life may increase by ten years—the average man's, by six.

The gender difference in mortality rates emerges from the moment of conception. Baby girls are less likely to die in the womb or after delivery than baby boys. Once past age 30 women consistently outnumber and outlive men. By age 85, there are three women for every man.

Why do men die sooner? The female edge may begin at conception with the extra X chromosome, which provides a backup for defects on the X gene and a double dose of the genetic factors that regulate the immune system. In addition, the female hormone estrogen bolsters immunity and protects heart, bone, brain, and blood vessels. In contrast, testosterone may dampen the immune response—possibly to prevent attacks on sperm cells, which might otherwise be mistaken as alien invaders. When the testes are removed from mice and guinea pigs,

their immune systems become more active. In men, lessened immunity may lower resistance to cancer as well as infectious disease.

Half of all men—compared with a third of women—develop cancer. Smoking, which for a long time was much more prevalent among men, accounts for some of this difference. However, this is changing. About one in four—23 percent—of American women smoke, and lung cancer rates in women have doubled since the early 1970s.

In some cancers, estrogen may somehow protect against distant metastases. Testosterone also has been implicated in men's risk of heart disease and stroke. Originally designed to equip men with an instantaneous burst of power—essential for survival in Stone Age times—this potent male hormone may surge so intensely that it wreaks havoc throughout the cardiovascular system.

Males, as noted in Chapter 17, also die more often as a result of intentional and nonintentional injury. Overall, men are three times more likely than women to die in accidents—mainly in cars and on the job. Men also are four times more likely to die violently. Nine in ten murderers—and eight in ten murder victims—are men.

Sources: Minino, Arialdi, and Betty Smith. "Deaths: Preliminary Data for 2000." *National Vital Statistics Reports,* Vol. 49, No. 12, October 9, 2001. Wizemann, Theresa, and Mary-Lou Pardue, *Exploring the Biological Contributions to Human Health: Does Sex Matter?* Washington, DC: National Academy Press, 2001. Hales, Dianne. *Just Like a Woman.* New York: Bantam Books, 2000.

that a drunk driver might collide with them. Similarly, cigarette smokers deny that lung cancer will ever strike them, and people who eat high-fat meals deny that they'll ever suffer a heart attack.

One important factor in denial is the nature of the threat. It's easy to believe that death is at hand when someone's pointing a gun at you; it's much harder to think that cigarette smoking might cause your death 20 or 30 years down the road. (See the Self-Survey: "How Do You Feel About Death?") Yet as Elisabeth Kübler-Ross, a psychiatrist who has extensively studied the process of dying, writes in *Death: The Final Stage of Growth:*

> It is the denial of death that is partially responsible for people living empty, purposeless lives; for when you live as if you'll live forever, it becomes too easy to postpone the things you know that you must do. You live your life in preparation for tomorrow or in the remembrance of yesterday,—and meanwhile, each today is lost. In contrast, when you fully understand that each day you awaken could be the last you have, you take the time that day to grow, to become more of who you really are, to reach out to other human beings.[7]

Emotional Responses to Death

Kübler-Ross has identified five typical stages of reaction that a person goes through when facing death (see Figure 18-1).

1. *Denial ("No, not me").* At first knowledge that death is coming, a terminally ill patient rejects the news. The denial overcomes the initial shock and allows the person to begin to gather together his or her resources. Denial, at this point, is a healthy defense mechanism. It can become distressful, however, if it's reinforced by the relatives and friends of the dying patient.
2. *Anger ("Why me?").* In the second stage, the dying person begins to feel resentment and rage regarding imminent death. The anger may be directed at God or at the patient's family and caregivers, who can do little but try to endure any expressions of anger, provide comfort, and help the patient on to the next stage.
3. *Bargaining ("Yes, me, but . . .").* In this stage, a patient may try to bargain, usually with God, for a way to

SELF SURVEY

How Do You Feel About Death?

This questionnaire isn't designed to test your knowledge. Instead, it should encourage you to think about your present attitudes toward death and how these attitudes may have developed. Answer the questions, to the best of your knowledge, by circling the appropriate letter.

1. Who died, in your first personal involvement with death?
   a. Grandparent or great-grandparent
   b. Parent
   c. Brother or sister
   d. Friend or acquaintance
   e. Stranger
   f. Public figure
   g. Animal

2. To the best of your memory, at what age were you first aware of death?
   a. Under 3 years
   b. 3–5 years
   c. 5–10 years
   d. 10 years or older

3. When you were a child, how was death talked about in your family?
   a. Openly
   b. With some sense of discomfort
   c. Only when necessary, and then with an attempt to exclude children
   d. As though it were a taboo subject
   e. Don't recall any discussion

4. Which of the following best describes your childhood conceptions of death?
   a. Heaven-and-hell concept
   b. Afterlife
   c. Death as sleep
   d. Cessation of all physical and mental activity
   e. Mysterious and unknowable
   f. Something other than the above
   g. No conception
   h. Can't remember

5. To what extent do you believe in a life after death?
   a. Strongly believe in it
   b. Tend to believe in it
   c. Uncertain
   d. Tend to doubt it
   e. Convinced it doesn't exist

6. Regardless of your belief about life after death, what is your wish about it?
   a. I strongly wish that there were a life after death.
   b. I am indifferent about life after death.
   c. I definitely prefer that there not be a life after death.

7. Has there been a time in your life when you wanted to die?
   a. Yes, mainly because of great physical pain
   b. Yes, mainly because of great emotional upset
   c. Yes, mainly to escape an intolerable social or interpersonal situation
   d. Yes, mainly because of great embarrassment
   e. Yes, for a reason other than one above
   f. No

8. What does death mean to you?
   a. The end, the final process of life
   b. The beginning of a life after death, a transition, a new beginning
   c. A joining of the spirit with a universal cosmic consciousness
   d. A kind of endless sleep, rest, and peace
   e. An interim period before being born again
   f. Termination of this life but survival of the spirit
   g. Don't know
   h. Other (specify)

9. What aspect of your own death is the most distasteful to you?
   a. I could no longer have any experiences.
   b. I'm afraid of what might happen to my body after death.
   c. I'm uncertain about what might happen to me if there is a life after death.
   d. I could no longer provide for my dependents.
   e. It would cause grief to my relatives and friends.
   f. All my plans and projects would come to an end.
   g. The process of dying might be painful.
   h. Other (specify)

10. How do you rate your present physical health?
    a. Excellent
    b. Very good
    c. Moderately good
    d. Moderately poor
    e. Extremely poor

11. How do you rate your present mental health?
    a. Excellent
    b. Very good
    c. Moderately good
    d. Moderately poor
    e. Extremely poor

12. Based on your present feelings, what is the probability of your taking your own life in the near future?
    a. Extremely high (feel very much like killing myself)
    b. Moderately high
    c. Between high and low
    d. Moderately low
    e. Extremely low (very improbable that I would kill myself)

(continued)

13. In your opinion, at what age are people most afraid of death?
    a. Up to 12 years
    b. 13–19 years
    c. 20–29 years
    d. 30–39 years
    e. 40–49 years
    f. 50–59 years
    g. 60–69 years
    h. 70 years and older
14. When you think of your own death (or when circumstances make you realize your own mortality), how do you feel?
    a. Fearful
    b. Discouraged
    c. Depressed
    d. Purposeless
    e. Resolved, in relation to life
    f. Pleasure, in being alive
    g. Other (specify)
15. What is your present orientation to your own death?
    a. Death-seeker
    b. Death-hastener
    c. Death-accepter
    d. Death-welcomer
    e. Death-postponer

f. Death-fearer
16. If you were told that you had a terminal disease and a limited time to live, how would you want to spend your time until you died?
    a. I would make a marked change in my lifestyle to satisfy hedonistic needs (travel, sex, drugs, or other experiences).
    b. I would become more withdrawn—reading, contemplating, or praying.
    c. I would shift from my own needs to a concern for others (family and friends).
    d. I would attempt to complete projects, to tie up loose ends.
    e. I would make little or no change in my lifestyle.
    f. I would try to do one very important thing.
    g. I might consider committing suicide.
    h. I would do none of the above.
17. How do you feel about having an autopsy done on your body?
    a. Approve
    b. Don't care one way or the other
    c. Disapprove
    d. Strongly disapprove

Source: Shneidman, Edwin. "You and Death Questionnaire." *Psychology Today,* August 1970. Reprinted by permission of Sussex Publishers, Inc.

reverse, or at least postpone, dying. The patient may promise, in exchange for recovery, to do good works or to see family members more often. Alternatively, the patient may say, "Let me live long enough to see my grandchild born" or "to see the spring again."

4. *Depression ("Yes, it's me").* In the fourth stage, the patient gradually realizes the full consequences of his or her condition. This may begin as grieving for health that has been lost and then become anticipatory grieving for the loss that is to come of friends, loved ones, and life itself. This stage is perhaps the most difficult time: The dying person should not be left alone during this period. Neither should one try to cheer the patient, however, who must be allowed to grieve.

5. *Acceptance ("Yes, me; and I'm ready").* In this last stage, the person has accepted the reality of death: The moment looms as neither frightening nor painful, neither sad nor happy—only inevitable. The person who waits for the end of life may ask to see fewer visitors, to separate from other people, or perhaps to turn to just one person for support.

Several stages may occur at the same time and some may happen out of sequence. Each stage may take days or only hours or minutes. Throughout, denial may come back to assert itself unexpectedly—and hope for a medical breakthrough or a miraculous recovery is forever present.

Some experts dispute Kübler-Ross's basic five-stage theory as too simplistic and argue that not all people go through such well-defined stages in the dying process. The way a person faces death is often a mirror of the way he or she has faced other major stresses in life: Those who have

1	2	3	4	5
Denial	**Anger**	**Bargaining**	**Depression**	**Acceptance**
"No, not me"	"Why me?"	"Yes, me, but..."	"Yes, it's me..."	"Yes, me; and I'm ready"

▲ **Figure 18-1** Kübler-Ross's five stages of adjustment to death.

had the most trouble adjusting to other crises will have the most trouble adjusting to the news of their impending death.

An individual's will to live can postpone death for a while. In a study of elderly Chinese women, researchers found that their death rate decreased before and during a holiday during which the senior women in a household play a central role; it increased after the celebration. A similar temporary drop occurs among Jews at the time of Passover. However, different events may have different effects. The prospect of an upcoming birthday postpones death in women but hastens it in men. The will to live typically fluctuates in terminal patients, varying along with depression, anxiety, shortness of breath, and sense of well-being.[8]

The family of a dying person experiences a spectrum of often wrenching emotions. Family members, too, may deny the verdict of death, rage at the doctors and nurses who can't do more to save their loved one, bargain with God to give up their own health if necessary, sink into helplessness and depression, and finally accept the reality of their anticipated loss.

One way of reducing the mystery and fear of death is to learn more about it. **Thanatology,** a term derived from the Greek god of death, Thanatos, refers to "the discipline of humanitarian caregiving for critically ill patients and their grieving family members and friends." Such care, which may be provided by physicians, nurses, social workers, psychologists, and others, helps ensure that terminally ill patients receive the compassionate, respectful care they deserve. The more we all learn about the process of dying and about what can be done to help more people die more peacefully, the better we can understand, and offer support to, the terminally ill.

Ethical Dilemmas

Modern medicine can do more to delay or defy death than was once thought possible. However, the ability to sustain life in patients with no hope of recovery has created wrenching medical and moral dilemmas. Increasingly, lawyers, ethicists, and consumer advocates are arguing that health-care providers must recognize a fundamental right of patients: the right to die.

Health economists, noting that more than half of U.S. health-care dollars are spent in the last year of life, have questioned "heroic" measures to prolong the life of chronically ill elderly patients or those with fatal diseases. Policies on such aggressive measures vary from hospital to hospital and state to state; often medical staffs are not aware of patients' wishes. In one study of HMOs, a third of seniors had filed advance directives stating their end-of-life preferences, but only 15 percent had discussed them with a health-care professional.

Some health-care facilities require that staff members try to resuscitate any patient whose heart stops unless a do-not-resuscitate (DNR) order has been written, usually with the family's permission. (DNR documents are discussed in the next section.) In other cases, physicians may decide against resuscitation despite the family's wishes if they think that treatment would be futile and that the family's objections are not based on the patient's values or best interests.

Another major ethical concern is the fate of an estimated 5,000 to 10,000 unconscious Americans who are being kept alive by artificial means. Some are in a **coma,** a state of total unconsciousness. They may have no sense of where they are, no memory, and no experience of pain. Others are in a **persistent vegetative state,** in which they're awake and yet unaware. They open their eyes; their brain waves show the characteristic patterns of waking and sleep. They can usually breathe on their own after a few weeks on artificial respiration; they can cough; the pupils of their eyes respond to light; but they do not respond to pain. The questions of when to use and when to discontinue artificial means of life support remain among the most challenging ethical dilemmas facing health-care workers and the families of critically ill patients.

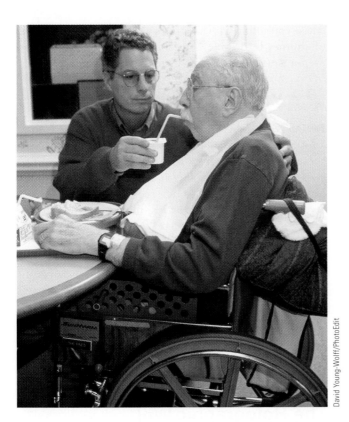

▲ Humanitarian caregiving for both critically ill patients and their loved ones can help to take some of the fear out of death.

Preparing for Death

Throughout this book we have stressed the ways in which you can determine how well and how long you live. You can also make decisions about the end of your life, particularly its impact on other people. To clarify your thinking on this difficult subject, ask yourself the following questions:

▶ Would I prefer to receive or not to receive any specific treatments if I were unconscious or incapable of voicing my opinion?

▶ Would I like my bodily systems to be kept functioning by extraordinary life-sustaining measures, even though my natural systems had failed? If I could not survive without mechanical assistance, would I want to be kept alive or resuscitated if my heart were to stop?

▶ Would I like the state to decide how to distribute my property or provide for my children (if any), or my family to decide how to handle my funeral arrangements?

▶ Would I care to give someone else, by donating my organs, the same possibilities for life that I have had?

You can assure that your wishes are heeded by several means, including advance directives, such as health-care proxies and living wills; a holographic will; and an organ donation card.

[????] What Are Advance Directives?

Every state and the District of Columbia have laws authorizing the use of **advance directives** to specify the kind of medical treatment individuals want in case of a medical crisis. However, few Americans have any type of advance directive. These documents are important because, without clear indications of a person's preferences, hospitals and other institutions often make decisions on an individual's behalf, particularly if family members are not available or disagree.

According to the Patient Self-Determination Act, health-care facilities that receive Medicare or Medicaid reimbursements must advise patients of their rights to sign advance directives for health-care decisions, such as whether they want to be kept alive by artificial means. (See Figure 18-2.) These statements allow medical professionals to know and follow an individual's wishes, or the wishes of a person to whom the patient has given authority to make decisions on his or her behalf. Although the idea of advance directives is popular among patients and physicians, they are rarely discussed. In one study of patients who were either seriously ill or over age 70, only 2 percent had discussed advance directives with their doctors.[9]

A *health-care proxy* is an advance directive that gives someone else the power to make decisions on your behalf. People typically name a relative or close friend as their

agent. Let family and friends know your thoughts about treatments and life support. You also should let your primary physician know about the type of care you would or wouldn't want to receive in various circumstances, such as an accident that results in an irreversible coma, but you should not designate your doctor as your agent. Many states prohibit this. Even when allowed, it is not a good idea because your doctor's primary responsibility is to administer care.

You can also sign an advance directive specifying that you do not want to be resuscitated in case your heart stops beating or that you want to be allowed to die naturally. **Do-not-resuscitate (DNR)** orders apply mainly to hospitalized, terminally ill patients. However, in some states, it is possible to complete a "nonhospital DNR" form that specifies an individual's wish not to be resuscitated at home. Patients in the final stages of advanced cancer or AIDS may choose to use such forms to protect their rights in case paramedics are called to their home.

Whereas a health-care proxy allows you to name someone to make health-care decisions for you, a power of attorney designates someone to make financial decisions on your behalf. An aging parent might give a son or daughter the power to file tax returns, pay bills, or handle other financial matters. One partner might give similar authorization to another. Power-of-attorney forms are sold at many large stationery or office supply stores. Some experts advise consulting with an attorney to make sure your power of attorney is "durable"—meaning that it remains in effect even if you should become mentally incapacitated.

[????] What Is a Living Will?

Living wills aren't just for people who don't want to be kept alive by artificial means. Individuals can also use these advance directives to indicate that they want all possible medical treatments and technology used to prolong their lives. Most states recognize living wills as legally binding, and a growing number of health-care professionals and facilities are offering patients help in drafting living wills. You can obtain state-specific forms for living wills and health-care proxies free from Partnership for Caring (www.partnershipforcaring.org, 1-800-989-WILL). Computer software for preparing such documents also is available. (See Figure 18-3.)

Once the forms are completed, make copies of your living will and other advance directives and give them to anyone who might have input in decisions on your behalf. Also give copies to your physician or health-care organization, and ask that they be made part of your medical record.

The Holographic Will

Perhaps you think that only wealthy or older people need to write wills. However, if you're married, have children, or

Except in California, where they must be renewed every five years, living wills are effective until they're revoked. Still, it's considered a good idea to initial and date your living will every few years to show that it still expresses your wishes.

"Imminent" is used on many living wills to express the inevitability and timing of death, but it's open to varying interpretations. A recent Virgina court decision found that it doesn't necessarily mean "immediately, at once, within a few days," and that a comatose person who's within a few months of death falls within the definition.

Except in California, Idaho, and Oregon, living wills have a space to specify treatment you do or don't want. Ask your physician what to include here. You can:

• Ask for or prohibit use of artificial feeding tubes, cardiopulmonary resuscitation, antibiotics, dialysis, and respirators.

• Ask for pain medication to keep you comfortable.

• State whether you would prefer to die in the hospital or at home.

• Designate a proxy—someone to make decisions about your treatment when you're unable.

• Donate organs or other body parts.

If your directions are contrary to state law, they'll be ignored, but the rest of the

DIRECTIVE TO PHYSICIANS

Directive made this _____ day of _____ (month, year). I, _____ being of sound mind, willfully and voluntarily make known my desire that my life shall not be artificially prolonged under the circumstances set forth below, and do hereby declare:

If at any time I should have an incurable condition caused by injury, disease, or illness certified to be a terminal condition by two physicians, and where the application of life-sustaining procedures would serve only to artificially prolong the moment of death and where my attending physician determines that my death is imminent whether or not life-sustaining procedures are utilized, I direct that such procedures be withheld or withdrawn, and that I be permitted to die naturally.

In the absence of my ability to give directions regarding the use of such life-sustaining procedures, it is my intention that this directive shall be honored by my family and physicians as the final expression of my legal right to refuse medical or surgical treatment and accept the consequences from such refusal.

If I have been diagnosed as pregnant and that diagnosis is known to my physician, this directive shall have no force or effect during the course of my pregnancy.

Other directions:
This directive shall be in effect until it is revoked. I understand the full import of this directive, and I am emotionally and mentally competent to make this directive. I understand that I may revoke this directive at any time.

Signed _____

City, County, and State of Residence _____

The declarant has been personally known to me and I believe him/her to be of sound mind. I am not related to the declarant by blood or marriage, nor would I be entitled to any portion of the declarant's estate on his/her decease, nor am I the attending physician of the declarant or an employee of the attending physician or a health facility in which the declarant is a patient, or a patient in the health care facility in which the declarant is a patient, or any person who has a claim against any portion of the estate of the declarant upon his/her decease.

Witness _____ Witness _____

"Life-sustaining procedures" are those that only prolong the process of dying. Most states include feeding and hydration tubes in this definition.

In some states a physician who will not carry out a patient's wishes must make a "good faith effort" to locate a doctor who will; other states require the physician to actually find someone and specify penalties—in some cases, jail terms—for failure to do so.

In some states the living will is valid for pregnant women. Others exclude women during all or part of their pregnancy, although that has been challenged on the grounds that a woman's right to privacy doesn't end when she becomes pregnant.

You can revoke or amend your living will at any time simply by making a statement to a physician, nurse, or other health-care worker.

Several states provide for the appointment of a proxy. In others decisions may be delegated through a document called a Durable Power of Attorney.

In some states, your signature must be notarized. Elsewhere, the signature of the witnesses is adequate although if you're in a hospital or nursing home in some states you may need as an additional witness the chief of staff or medical director.

▲ **Figure 18-2** Preparing a physician's directive.

Source: A Guide to the Living Will, Hippocrates (May/June, 1988).

A LIVING WILL

To My Family, Doctors, and All Those Concerned with My Care:

I, _____, being of sound mind, make this statement as a directive to be followed if I become unable to participate in decisions regarding my medical care.

If I should have an incurable or irreversible mental or physical condition with no reasonable expectation of recovery. I direct my attending physician to withhold or withdraw treatment that merely prolongs my dying. I further direct that treatment be limited to measures to keep me comfortable and to relieve pain.

> This declaration sets forth your directions regarding medical treatment.

These directions express my legal right to refuse treatment. Therefore, I expect my family, doctors, and everyone concerned with my care to regard themselves as legally and morally bound to act in accord with my wishes, and in so doing to be free of any legal liability for having followed my directions.

> You have the right to refuse treatment you do not want, and you may request the care you do want.

I especially do not want _____
_____
_____
_____
_____
_____

> You may list specific treatment you do not want (for example, cardiac resuscitation, mechanical respiration, artificial feeding/fluids by tube); otherwise, your general statement, top left, will stand for your wishes.

Other instructions/comments: _____
_____
_____
_____

> You may want to add instructions or care you do want— for example, pain medication, or that you prefer to die at home if possible.

Proxy Designation Clause: Should I become unable to communicate my instructions as stated above, I designate the following person to act on my behalf:

Name _____

Address _____

If the person I have named above is unable to act on my behalf, I authorize the following person to do so:

Name_____

Address_____

This living will declaration expresses my personal treatment preferences. The fact that I may have also executed a document in the form recommended by state law should not be construed to limit or contradict this living will declaration, which is an expression of my common-law and constitutional rights.

> If you want, you can name someone to see that your wishes are carried out, but you do not have to do this.

Signed: _____ Date: _____

Witness:_____ Witness:_____

Address:_____ Address:_____

Keep the assigned original with your personal papers at home. Give signed copies to doctors, family, and proxy. Review your declaration from time to time: initial and date it to show it still expresses your intent.

> Sign and date here in the presence of two adult witnesses, who should also sign.

▲ **Figure 18-3** A sample form for a living will. From American Health, April, 1991, 40. 1991, the Reader's Digest.

own property, you should either hire a lawyer to draw up a will, or write a **holographic will** yourself, specifying who you wish to raise your children or who should have your property. If you die *intestate* (without a will), the state will make these decisions for you. Even a modest estate can be tied up in court for a long period of time, depriving family members of money when they need it most.

Many states will recognize a handwritten (not typed) statement by you, through which you can accomplish the following:

▶ Name a family member or friend as the executor, the person who sees that your wishes are carried out.

▶ List the things you own and to whom you want them to go; include addresses and telephone numbers, if possible.

▶ Select a guardian for your children (if any), presumably someone whose ideas about raising children are similar to your own. Be sure that they are willing and able to accept this responsibility before writing them into your will.

▶ Specify any funeral arrangements.

▶ Be sure to keep the will in a safe place, where your executor, family members, or closest beneficiary can get to it quickly and easily; tell them where it is.

The Gift of Life

If you're at least 18 years old, you can fill out a donor card (see Figure 18-4), agreeing to designate, in the event of your death, any organs or tissues needed for transplantation. Corneas may help a blind person see, for example. Kidneys, or even a heart, may be transplanted. The donation takes effect upon your death and is a generous way of giving others the possibilities for life that you have had yourself. The card should be filled out and signed; some must be signed in the presence of two witnesses. Attach the

donor card to the back of your driver's license or I.D. card. (Whole-body donations may require other arrangements.)

The Process of Dying

Most people who have a fatal or **terminal illness** prefer to know the truth about their health and chances for recovery. (See Table 18-1.) Even when they're not officially informed by a doctor or relative, most fatally ill people know or strongly suspect that they're dying. Dying people usually make it clear whether they want to talk about death and to what extent. The most frequent concern is how much time is left. Usually physicians can give only a rough estimate, such as "several weeks or months."

Once death was a taboo topic even between doctors and patients. Filled with a zeal to heal, physicians viewed death as the enemy; it caused a sense of medical impotence and failure that often led them to pull away from dying patients. However, surveys of physicians show changes in the last decades. Today's doctors are much more open to communicating with dying patients and their families on issues concerning death. They, too, benefit from open, honest conversations with their patients.

A "Good" Death

As life expectancy has increased and high-technology interventions have multiplied, many health-care professionals as well as citizens and social organizations have begun to demand a better way of caring for those who are dying. Individuals have different perspectives on what is a "good death." In a survey in Japan, for instance, old people expressed a preference for heart disease as the cause of death rather than dementia, cancer, or stroke.[10] The Center to Improve Care of the Dying in Washington, DC, has set goals for reintegrating dying within living, thus enhancing the prospect for growth at the end of life. These experts talk of "dying well," "living while dying," and "physician-assisted living." They aim to change our way of thinking about dying so that we view the end of life as a time of love and reconciliation, and transcendence of suffering.[11]

As discussed later in this chapter, physicians who care for the dying are being urged to do all that they can to eliminate pain. They are encouraged not to withhold opioid drugs, such as morphine, simply out of fear of addiction. More efforts are being made for patients to be taken care of at home, with appropriate support and well-informed guidance.

Various psychological factors can affect those at risk of dying. In a study of nearly 800 elderly people, those who

UNIFORM DONOR CARD

OF _____
Print or type name of donor

In the hope that I may help others, I hereby make this anatomical gift, if medically acceptable, to take effect upon my death. The words and marks below indicate my desires.

I give (a) ____ any needed organs or parts
I give (b) ____ only the following organs or parts

_____
Specifiy the organ(s) or part(s)

for the purposes of transplantation, therapy, medical research, or education:

I give (c) ____ my body for anatomical study if needed

Limitations or
special wishes, if any _____

▲ **Figure 18-4** Example of a uniform donor card.

▼ **Table 18-1 Attitudes Toward the Dying**

Percent of Ethnic Group Who Believe:	Korean Americans	Mexican Americans	African Americans	European Americans
A patient should be told a diagnosis of metastatic cancer.	47%	65%	89%	87%
A patient should be told of terminal prognosis.	35	48	63	69
A patient should decide about the use of life support.	28	41	60	65

Source: The University of Southern California

lacked hope in the future were much more likely to die within the next few years. No one knows exactly how hopelessness affects mortality. Researchers speculate that hopelessness may lead to biochemical and nervous system abnormalities or that hopeless individuals may not eat well, take medications as prescribed, or follow a doctor's recommendations.[12]

Spirituality also plays a major role. In various surveys, 41 to 94 percent of patients say they want their doctors and nurses to address their spiritual concerns. In one survey, even 45 percent of nonreligious patients thought physicians should inquire politely about patients' spiritual needs. However, some worry that such queries may be inappropriate or detract from a doctor's primary mission.[13]

There are few data on the impact of spiritual approaches on the dying. In a survey of relatives of deceased patients, 63 percent thought that their loved one's faith was of help at the time of death. In a study of nursing home residents, traditional religious beliefs and values affected acceptance, endurance, coping, and security in the face of impending death.[14]

Relieving Pain

Pain remains a major problem for the terminally ill. At least 20 percent of terminally ill patients experience moderate to severe pain; among cancer patients, the percentage may be as high as 75 percent.[15] Individuals who suffer widespread pain have a higher risk of death, particularly from cancer that may not yet have been diagnosed.[16]

Various factors might get in the way of adequate pain relief for the dying, including medical care providers' hesitancy to prescribe opioid medications, family members who have concerns about these drugs, and patients who either don't report pain or fear medication.

However, a painful death is not inevitable, even for patients with advanced cancer. The World Health Organization has developed pain relief guidelines that would provide effective pain relief for most terminal cancer patients in their own homes. The guidelines include several med-

ications, including nonopioid pain relievers, anti-ulcer drugs, antinausea drugs, and, if needed, opioids. In addition to standard pain medication, researchers have also experimented with such restricted drugs as marijuana (for the relief of nausea in cancer patients undergoing chemotherapy) and heroin (as a painkiller for people who don't respond well to other narcotics).

Caregiving

When someone becomes terminally ill, a woman—usually the patient's wife, daughter, or sister—is most likely to provide day-to-day care, often for periods longer than a year.[17] Caregiving takes a different toll on men and women. In one study of adult daughters and husbands caring for terminally ill breast cancer patients, the daughters experienced more symptoms of anxiety and depression and greater family strain.[18]

The impact of caregiving continues even after the death of an ill spouse. In one study, the health of older caregivers who had experienced strain prior to a spouse's death did not deteriorate. They showed no increase in depressive symptoms or use of antidepressant drugs and did not lose weight. Those who had not been caregivers were more likely to experience depression and weight loss.[19]

Hospice: Caring When Curing Isn't Possible

A **hospice** is a homelike health-care facility or program that helps dying men and women who can afford such care to live their final days to the fullest, as free as possible from disabling pain and mental anguish. Hospice workers generally work in teams, usually consisting of a nurse, physician, social worker, chaplain, and trained volunteers. Other professionals, such as a physical therapist, may join the team when needed. These workers provide the comfort, support, and care dying patients need until they do die.

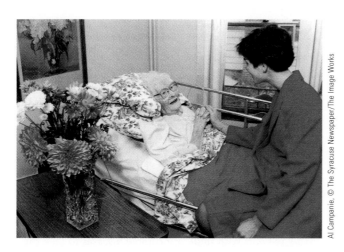

▲ A hospice provides care and support and helps people die with comfort and dignity.

Hospice programs offer a combination of medical and emotional care that involves not only the patient but also the family members or others concerned with caring for the patient. Most hospice patients have life expectancies of six months or less, and are no longer receiving treatments aimed at curing their diseases. When someone is available to provide care, patients remain in their own homes. Hospice nurses regularly visit all home patients and are available around the clock.

For patients requiring care that the family cannot provide, round-the-clock care is available at the hospice facility. Unlike a traditional hospital, where the focus is on diagnosis, cure, and treatment, a hospice works to make what is left of life pain-free and comfortable. Visiting hours for relatives and friends are flexible, with no restrictions on visits by children and grandchildren. Hospice services are covered, in full or in part, by most major insurance companies.

??? What Do We Know About Near-Death Experiences?

In recent years, the number of reports of **near-death experiences** has grown, thanks largely to advances in emergency medical care. Most such experiences are remarkably similar, whether they occur in children or adults, whether they're the result of accidents or illnesses, even whether the individuals actually are near death or only think they are. Some individuals who have survived a close brush with death report **autoscopy** (watching, from several feet in the air, resuscitation attempts on their own bodies) or **transcendence** (the sense of passing into a foreign region or dimension). Some see light, often at the end of a tunnel. Their vision seems clearer; their hearing, sharper. Some recall scenes from their lives or feel the presence of loved ones who have died. Many report profound

feelings of joy, calm, and peace. Fewer than 1 percent of those who've reported near-death experiences described them as frightening or distressing, although a larger number recall transitory feelings of fear or confusion.

Many near-death experiences occur in individuals who've been sedated or given other medications; however, many others do not. Several studies have shown that individuals who received medication or anesthesia were actually less likely to remember near-death experiences than those who hadn't had any drugs. Some scientists have speculated that lack of oxygen, changes in blood gases, altered brain functioning, or the release of neurotransmitters (messenger chemicals in the brain) may play a role in near-death experiences. However, there's little solid evidence that physiological events are responsible. There's also no proof that wishful thinking, cultural conditioning, posttraumatic stress, or other psychological mechanisms may be at work. For now, the most that scientists can say for sure about this medical mystery is that it needs further study.

Suicide

Suicide is among the ten leading causes of death in the United States; each year 25,000 to 55,000 people kill themselves. And for every completed suicide, there are 10 to 40 unsuccessful attempts. (Chapter 3 presents a detailed discussion of the risk factors and warning signs of suicide.)

One of the main factors leading to suicide is illness, especially terminal illness. A great deal of debate centers on quality of life, yet there is no reliable or consistent way to measure this. Patients who are dying may feel some quality of life, even when others do not recognize it, or their evaluations of the quality of their lives may fluctuate. Dying patients who say their lives are not worth living may be suffering from depression; hopelessness is one of its characteristic symptoms.[20]

Approximately three-fourths of those who commit suicide consult a physician, most with medical complaints, within the six-month period prior to their deaths. Disease, medication, and the fear of pain or of being a burden to one's family can breed depression; treatment can make a difference. Only 10 to 14 percent of those who survive a suicide attempt take their lives in the next ten years. Fatally ill individuals who talk about suicide should be taken seriously; family physicians can arrange for them to talk with psychotherapists. (Physician-assisted suicide is discussed below.)

"Rational" Suicide

An elderly widow suffering from advanced cancer takes a lethal overdose of sleeping pills. A young man with several

AIDS-related illnesses shoots himself. A woman in her fifties, diagnosed as having Alzheimer's disease, asks a doctor to help her end her life. Are these suicides "rational" because these individuals used logical reasoning in deciding to end their lives?

The question is intensely controversial. Advocates of the right to "self-deliverance" argue that individuals in great pain or faced with the prospect of a debilitating, hopeless battle against an incurable disease can and should be able to decide to end their lives. As legislatures and the legal system tackle the thorny questions of an individual's right to die, mental health professionals worry that, even in those with fatal diseases, suicidal wishes often stem from undiagnosed depression.

In one classic study of 44 terminally ill individuals, 34 had never been suicidal or wished for death. The remaining ten (seven who did desire early death and three who specifically considered suicide) all had severe depression. Their despair and preoccupation with dying may well have contributed to their willingness to consider suicide. Numerous studies have indicated that most patients with painful, progressive, or terminal illnesses do not want to kill themselves. The percentage of those who report thinking about suicide ranges from 5 to 20 percent; most of these have major depressions. Many mental health professionals argue that what makes patients with severe illnesses suicidal is depression, not their physical condition.

Because depression may indeed warp the ability to make a rational decision about suicide, mental health professionals urge physicians and family members to make sure individuals with chronic or fatal illnesses are evaluated for depression and given medication, psychotherapy, or both. It is also important for everyone to allow enough time—an average of three to eight weeks—to see if treatment for depression will make a difference in their desire to keep living.

Physician-Assisted Suicide

According to U.S. surveys, there is greater support for physician-assisted suicide and euthanasia among patients and the general public than among physicians.[21] More Caucasians support these practices than members of ethnic minority groups.[22]

If patients have a right to die, should doctors help them end their lives? Physicians have been willing to stop any extraordinary efforts to sustain life (for example, by withholding oxygen or ending intravenous feedings); such actions are referred to as passive **euthanasia,** or **dyathanasia.** Euthanasia, the active form of so-called mercy killing, has generally been viewed as illegal and unethical. Euthanasia has been tolerated for years in the Netherlands, but it is not technically legal there.[23]

Oregon has passed the "Death with Dignity" act and is the first state to legalize physician-assisted suicide for

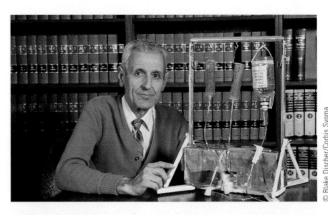

▲ Dr. Jack Kevorkian designed this suicide machine to enable patients with fatal or incurable diseases to take their own lives.

terminally ill patients. Legal challenges to it continue. This law bars suicide assistance for anyone whose judgment may be impaired by a mental disorder.

Jack Kevorkian, M.D., a Michigan pathologist, has stirred public debate by using a "suicide machine" to help end the life (at their request) of dozens of people suffering from chronic, but not necessarily fatal, illnesses. He has been found guilty of murder charges. The Michigan Supreme Court has since ruled physician-assisted suicide a "common law felony." Some medical groups, such as the American Medical Association, oppose as unethical any physician's involvement in euthanasia. Others argue that individuals have the right to end their own lives and that physicians who provide prescriptions for lethal doses of certain drugs are acting out of compassion.

A study that compared Kevorkian euthanasia cases with Oregon physician-assisted suicides found that only 25 percent of the patients euthanized by Kevorkian were terminally ill, compared with 100 percent of the Oregon cases. The individuals who sought physician-assisted suicide in Oregon were significantly more likely to have cancer than Kevorkian's patients.[24] Women and those who were divorced or never married were significantly more likely to seek euthanasia.

The Practicalities of Death

At a time of great emotional pain, grieving family members must cope with medical, legal, and practical concerns, including obtaining a medical certificate of the cause of death, registering the death, and making funeral arrangements. They may also want to arrange for organ donations and, in some circumstances, an autopsy.

Funeral Arrangements

A burial is typically the third most expensive purchase of a lifetime, behind the cost of a house and car. The average national costs range as high as $6,000, although they vary considerably. (See Savvy Consumer: "What You Should Know About Funeral Costs.") Memorial societies are voluntary groups that help people plan in advance for death. They obtain services at moderate cost, keep the arrangements simple and dignified, and—most importantly, perhaps—ease the emotional and financial burden on the rest of the family when death finally does come.

A body can be either buried or cremated. Burial requires the purchase of a cemetery plot, which many families do decades before death. If the body is to be cremated, you must comply with some additional formalities, with which the funeral director can help you. After a cremation (incineration of the remains), you can either collect the ashes to keep, bury, or scatter yourself, or ask the crematorium to dispose of them.

The tradition of a funeral may help survivors come to terms with the death, enabling them both to mourn their loss and to celebrate the dead person's life. Alternatively, the body may be disposed of immediately, through burial, cremation, or bequeathal to a medical school, and a memorial service held later.

Funerals are usually held two to four days after the death. Many have two parts: a religious ceremony at a church or funeral home, and a burial ceremony at the grave site. In a memorial service, the body is not present, which may change the focus of the service from the person's death to his or her life.

Autopsies

An autopsy is a detailed examination of a body after death, also called a post-mortem exam. There are two types:

▸ **Medicolegal.** This type of autopsy is performed to establish the cause of death and to gather information about the death for use as evidence in any legal proceedings. It is done to detect any crimes and to help identify the proper person for prosecution, to investigate possible industrial hazards or contagious diseases that

may endanger the public health, or to establish the cause of death for insurance purposes.

▸ **Medical/educational.** This type of autopsy is performed, usually in the hospital where the person died, to increase medical knowledge and to determine a more exact cause of death. It may be requested by the attending physician or the family, but it cannot be performed without the family's permission.

Autopsies can be extremely valuable in establishing an accurate cause of death, revealing a different diagnosis that might have led to a change in therapy and prolonged survival in about 10 percent of cases. Thirty years ago about 50 percent of patients who died in hospitals were autopsied. However, the autopsy rate in the United States has been steadily declining, and today about 10 to 20 percent of deaths in teaching hospitals are autopsied. Physicians are arguing for an increase in autopsies as the best method for establishing the cause of death, helping to spot infectious diseases, aiding medical education, and helping assure the high quality of medical practice.

Grief

An estimated 8 million Americans lose a member of their immediate families each year. The death of a loved one may be the single most upsetting and feared event in a person's life.

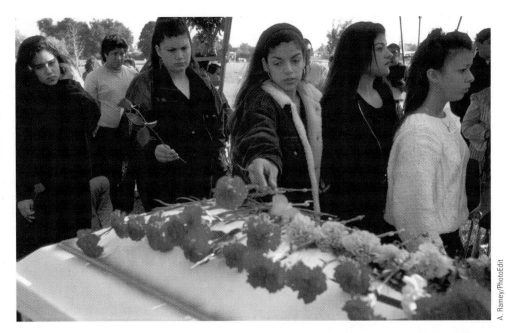

▲ Funerals and memorial services allow those in mourning to honor the deceased and to come to terms with their loss.

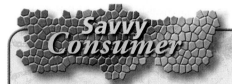

Savvy Consumer

What You Should Know About Funeral Costs

About half the people responsible for making or for overseeing final arrangements report that, before meeting with a funeral director, they had no idea of how much a funeral might cost. Survivors are usually not only grieving and emotionally distressed but also pressed for time when it comes to making final arrangements. One local cemeterian estimated that there are more than 70 tasks to be completed after a family death. It would be wise to review the following information before you need it:

- Have an idea of what your final costs are likely to be before meeting with the funeral director. This puts you and other family members in a better position to understand the options, to serve as your own advocate, and to make an informed purchase.

- Final costs may vary considerably depending on which funeral home you choose, and whether you choose burial or cremation.

- The Federal Trade Commission requires that all funeral homes provide a "General Price List" to anyone who requests it in person. Check with the local chapter of the Funeral and Memorial Society (if available) for additional information.

- The American Association of Retired Persons (AARP) is an excellent source of consumer-oriented information on final arrangements. Other community agencies may also sponsor talks and seminars on the subject.

Losing a parent in childhood, as thousands of children did on September 11, can have a lasting impact. A study that followed 100 orphans found that as young adults they suffered significantly higher depressive symptoms.[25] The death of a family member produces a wide range of reactions, including anxiety, guilt, anger, and financial concern. Many see the death of an old person as less tragic (usually) than the death of a child or young person. A sudden death is more of a shock than one following a long illness. A suicide can be particularly devastating, because family members may wonder whether they could have done anything to prevent it. The cause of death can also affect the reactions of friends and acquaintances. Some people express less sympathy and support when individuals are murdered or take their own lives.

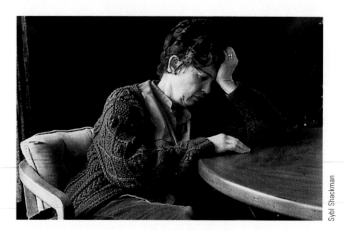

Sybil Shackman

▲ Grief can take an enormous physical and psychological toll on family members and loved ones.

Encountering death can make us feel alone and vulnerable. The most common and one of the most painful experiences is the death of a parent. When both parents die, individuals may feel like orphaned children. They mourn, not just for the father and mother who are gone, but for their lost role of being someone's child.

The death of a child can be even more devastating. Grieving may continue for many years. Eventually parents may be able to resolve their grief and accept the death as "God's will" or as "something that happens." Time erases their pain, and they feel a desire to get on with their lives, consciously putting the loss behind them. Others deal with their grief by keeping busy, or by substituting other problems or situations to take their minds off their loss. Yet many parents who lose a child continue to grieve for many years. Although the pain of their loss diminishes with time, they view it as part of themselves and describe an emptiness inside—even though most have rich, meaningful, and happy daily lives.

The loss of a mate can also have a profound impact, although men's and women's responses to the death—and their subsequent health risks—may depend on how their spouses died. Men whose wives die suddenly face a much greater risk of dying themselves than those whose wives die after a long illness. On the other hand, women whose husbands die after a long illness face greater risk than other widows. The reason may be that men whose wives were chronically ill learned how to cope with the loss of their nurturers, while women who spend a long time caring for an ill husband may be at greater risk because of the combined burdens of caregiving and loss of financial support.

All grieving people continue to need support for many months. The anniversary of a death or the first several holidays spent alone can be particularly difficult. (See Pulse Points: "Ten Ways to Cope with Grief.") For individuals who remain intensely distressed, or whose grief does not ease over time, therapy and medication can be enormously helpful—and potentially life-saving. Grieving parents, partners, or adult children are at increased risk of serious physical and mental illness, suicide, and premature death. The family members of a suicide victim are especially likely to need, and benefit from, professional help in sorting out their feelings of failure, anger, and sorrow.

Bereavement is not a rare occurrence on college campuses, but it is largely an ignored problem. Counselors have called upon universities to help students who have lost a loved one through initiatives such as training nonbereaved students to provide peer support and raising consciousness about bereavement.[26]

Grief's Affect on Health

Men and women who lose partners, parents, or children endure so much stress that they're at increased risk of serious physical and mental illness, and even of premature death. Studies of the health effects of grief have found the following:

▶ Grief produces changes in the respiratory, hormonal, and central nervous systems, and may affect functions of the heart, blood, and immune systems.

▶ Grieving adults may experience mood swings between sadness and anger, guilt and anxiety. They may feel physically sick, lose their appetites, sleep poorly, or fear that they're going crazy because they "see" the deceased person in different places.

▶ Friends and remarriage offer the greatest protection against health problems.

▶ Some widows may have increased rates of depression, suicide, and death from cirrhosis of the liver. The greatest risk factors are poor previous mental and physical health, and a lack of social support.

Methods of Mourning

Grief is a psychological necessity, not self-indulgence. Psychotherapists refer to grief as work, and it is—slow, tedious, and painful. Yet only by working through grief, by dealing with feelings of anger and despair, and adjusting emotionally and intellectually to the loss, can bereaved individuals make their way back to the living world of hope and love.

Some widows and widowers move through the grieving process without experiencing extreme distress. Others stop somewhere in the midst of normal grieving and become clinging and overreliant, continue to pine for the deceased, or show signs of denial, avoidance, or anxiety. Individuals who lose children or spouses in car accidents are particularly likely to remain depressed and anxious years later. One of the most devastating losses is the death of a child killed by a drunk driver. Many years afterward parents often cannot find any "meaning" in what happened.

PULSE POINTS

Ten Ways to Cope with Grief

1. **Accept your feelings**—sorrow, fear, emptiness, whatever—as normal.

2. **Don't try to deny emotions** such as anger, guilt, despair, or relief.

3. **Let others help you**—by bringing you food, by taking care of daily necessities, by providing companionship and comfort. (It will make them feel better, too.)

4. **Express your feelings**—through tears, recollections, and talking with others—so that you can accept the loss.

5. **Don't feel that you must be strong and brave and silent,** though you have every right to keep your grief private.

6. **Face each day as it comes.** Let yourself live in the here-and-now until you're ready to face the future.

7. **Give yourself time**—perhaps more than you ever imagined— for the pain to ebb, the scars to heal, and your life to move on.

8. **Commemorate.** A funeral or memorial service can help you come to terms with a loved one's death and provides an opportunity to celebrate the dead person's life.

9. **Don't think there's a right or wrong way to grieve.** Mourning takes many forms, and there's no set timetable for working through the various stages of grief.

10. **Seek professional counseling** if you remain intensely distressed for more than six months or your grief does not ease over time. Therapy can be enormously helpful—and can help prevent potentially serious physical and psychological problems.

???? How Can You Help Survivors of a Loss?

Although we grieve for the dead, the living are the ones who need our help. Bereavement is such an intense state that survivors may be too numb or too stunned to ask for help. Family and friends must take the initiative and spend time with them, even if that means sitting together silently. Offer empathy and support, and let the grieving person know with verbal and nonverbal expressions that you care and wish to help. Simply being there is enough to let your friend know you care.

You may also wish to write a simple note expressing your sympathy. A phrase, such as "I want to let you know I'm thinking of you and praying for you," can mean a great deal. A small gift, such as a book or plant, is also thoughtful. Or you can invite your friend to do something with you. Choose something you know your friend might enjoy—a walk in the country or a concert. And don't just give your help over the first few days or weeks and then withdraw. Grieving people continue to need support for many months. The first anniversary of a death or the first holiday spent alone can be particularly difficult.

Most bereaved people don't need professional psychological counseling. In most instances, sharing their feelings with friends is all that's needed. However, you should urge a friend or relative to seek help if he or she shows no sign of grieving, or exhibits as much distress a year after the loss as during the first months. The family members of a suicide victim are those most likely to need, and benefit from, professional help in sorting out their feelings of failure, anger, and sorrow.

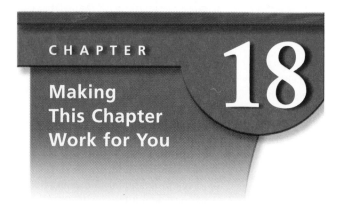

CHAPTER

Making This Chapter Work for You

18

1. Factors that contribute to a long life and successful aging include all of the following except
   a. healthy weight.
   b. moderate smoking.
   c. regular exercise.
   d. positive coping mechanisms.

2. The categories of death include
   a. functional death
   b. sexual death
   c. organ death
   d. respiratory death

3. According to Kübler-Ross, an individual facing death goes through all of the following emotional stages except
   a. bargaining.
   b. acceptance.
   c. denial.
   d. repression.

4. The gender gap related to longevity
   a. is related to deficiencies in the Y chromosome.
   b. results from the presence of the ApoE gene.
   c. may be due to hormonal influences on the immune system.
   d. is about 13 years in the United States.

5. An advance directive
   a. indicates who should have your property in the event you die.
   b. may authorize which individuals may not participate in your health care if you are unable to care for yourself.
   c. can specify your desires related to the use of medical treatments and technology to prolong your life.
   d. should specify which physician you designate to be your health-care proxy.

6. Which of the following statements about terminal illness is true?
   a. Most health-care professionals believe that it is harmful to tell patients that they are dying.
   b. Factors that may hasten a person's death include hopelessness and inadequate pain relief.
   c. Religious beliefs and values appear to have little affect on how an individual handles impending death.
   d. Opioid medications such as morphine should not be given to terminally ill patients because of the risk of addiction.

7. Passive euthanasia
   a. is legal in most states.
   b. occurs when a terminally ill patient has a near-death experience.
   c. is suicide by nonviolent means such as carbon monoxide poisoning.
   d. is the stopping of extraordinary efforts to sustain life.

8. An autopsy
   a. is also called a postmortem exam.
   b. is performed after a body has been cremated.
   c. can help establish the time of disease onset.

d. is used by teaching hospitals to help teach medical students anatomy and physiology.

9. Which of the following recommendations for coping with grief is probably most helpful?
   a. To avoid reminders of your loss, do not interact with others who are also grieving.
   b. Put a limit on the amount of time you will allow yourself to grieve so that you can get on with your life.
   c. If your grief does not subside over time, see a therapist who specializes in grief counseling.
   d. Look at how other people handle their grief to best determine the style that works for you.

10. You can best help a friend who is bereaved by
    a. encouraging him to have a few drinks to forget his pain.
    b. simply spending time with her.
    c. avoiding talking about his loss because it is awkward.
    d. reminding her about all she still has in her life.

Answers to these questions can be found on page 640.

 What are the stages of death?

Critical Thinking

1. Have your living parents and grandparents provided you or other family members with written advanced directives or a living will? Have you discussed with them their preferences regarding medical treatment in the event of a medical crisis? If you haven't had this discussion with your family yet, how can you help to begin the process of helping your parents or grandparents communicate their wishes?

2. Do you think that coming to terms with mortality allows an individual to live each day to its fullest, rather than putting off what he or she would like to do until tomorrow? How does this concept affect your own life? Explain. Do you believe in a next life or a greater reality? If so, how does this affect your view of life and death?

3. In 20 cases over the last 50 years, family members accused of mercy killings of fatally ill relatives have gone to trial. One was a father who held off hospital workers with a pistol while he unplugged his baby's respirator. Another was a man who suffocated his wife, who had Alzheimer's disease, with a pillow. Only three of the defendants were sentenced to jail. Do you think these individuals should have been put on trial? Should all have been punished? Are there circumstances that would make mercy killing a crime in some cases but not in others?

4. As many as 10,000 people in this country are chronically unconscious, kept alive by artificial respirators and feeding tubes. What if you were in an accident that left you in a vegetative state? Would you want doctors to do everything possible to fight for your life? Would you want to spend months or even years totally unaware of your surroundings? Should health-care professionals have the right to declare that anyone is too old, too ill, or too frail to try to save? Should they have the right to insist that someone live on even if that person isn't experiencing much of a "life"?

SITES & BYTES

Beyond Indigo—Death and Dying
http://www.death-dying.com
This site features information on caregiving and illness, support groups for grief, quizzes, and emotional and inspirational stories about coping with death.

Hospice Association of America
http://www.nahc.org/HAA
This site offers consumers general information about hospice, including consumer guides, fact sheets, historical perspectives, and other background information.

Defining Wellness Through the End of Life
http://www.dyingwell.org
This site features resources for people facing life-limiting illness, their families, and their professional caregivers. Dr. Ira Byock, an experienced palliative care physician and advocate for improved end-of-life care, provides written resources and referrals to organizations, websites, and books designed to empower persons with life-threatening illness and their families to live fully.

Please note that links are subject to change. If you find a broken link, use a search engine such as **http://www.yahoo.com** and search for the website by typing in key words.

InfoTrac Activity Mercedes Bern-Klug, Charles Gessert, and Sarah Forbes. "The Need to Revise Assumptions About the End of Life: Implications for Social Work Practice." *Health and Social Work,* Vol. 26, No. 1, February 2001, p. 38.

(1) What were the three leading causes of death in 1900? What are the three leading causes of death today?

(2) From 1900 to 2000, how much has life expectancy increased? Name four major reasons for this dramatic improvement.

(3) What is an advance directive? How should family members and the dying patient deal with impending death?

You can find additional readings related to death and dying with InfoTrac College Edition, an online library of more than 900 journals and publications. Follow the instructions for accessing InfoTrac that were packaged with your textbook; then search for articles using a key word search.

For additional links, resources, and suggested readings on InfoTrac, visit our Health & Wellness Resource Center at **http://health.wadsworth.com**.

Key Terms

The terms listed here are used within the chapter on the page indicated. Definitions of terms are in the Glossary at the end of the book.

advance directives 606	**euthanasia** 612	**persistent vegetative state** 605
autoscopy 611	**holographic will** 609	**terminal illness** 609
coma 605	**hospice** 610	**thanatology** 605
do-not-resuscitate (DNR) 606	**living will** 606	**transcendence** 611
dyathanasia 612	**near-death experiences** 611	

References

1. Romano, Carlin. "When Death Breaches the Campus Walls." *Chronicle of Higher Education,* Vol. 47, No. 24, February 23, 2001, p. B12.
2. Minino, Arialdi, and Betty Smith. "Deaths: Preliminary Data for 2000." *National Vital Statistics Reports,* Vol. 49, No. 12, October 9, 2001.
3. Indrayan, A. "Can I Choose the Cause of My Death?" *British Medical Journal,* Vol. 322, No. 7292, April 21, 2001, p. 1003.
4. Vaillant, George, and Kenneth Mukamal. "Successful Aging." *American Journal of Psychiatry,* June 2001, p. 839.
5. Schulz, Richard, et al. "Involvement in Caregiving and Adjustment to Death of a Spouse." *Journal of the American Medical Association,* Vol. 285, June 27, 2001, p. 3123.
6. Bern-Krug, Mercedes, et al. "The Need to Revise Assumptions About the End of Life." *Health and Social Work,* Vol. 26, No. 1, February 2001, p. 38.
7. Kübler-Ross, Elisabeth. *Death: The Final Stage of Growth.* Englewood Cliffs, NJ: Prentice Hall, 1975.
8. Carpenter, E. "The End of Life Odyssey." *Gerontologist,* October 15, 2001, p. 51.

9. Tierney, William, et al. "Discussion of Advance Care Directives." *Journal of General Interest Medicine,* January 2001.

10. Indrayan, "Can I Choose the Cause of My Death?"

11. Roman, Marlene. "Care for the Dying." *MedSurg Nursing,* Vol. 10, No. 1, February 2001, p. 5.

12. Stern, Stephen, et al. "Hopelessness and the Risk of Dying." *Psychosomatic Medicine,* May 2001.

13. Sulmasy, Daniel. "Addressing the Religious and Spiritual Needs of Dying Patients." *Western Journal of Medicine,* Vol. 175, No. 4, October 2001, p. 251.

14. Gibson, D., et al. "Impact of Spirituality on the Living-Dying of Terminally Ill Black and White Nursing Home Residents." *Gerontologist,* October 15, 2001, p. 338.

15. Ramsden, Elsa, and James Stephens. "Factors Considered Important at the End of Life by Patients, Family, Physicians, and Other Care Providers." *Physical Therapy,* Vol. 81, No. 7, July 2001, p. 1360.

16. Macfarlane, Gary, et al. "Widespread Body Pain and Mortality: Prospective Population-based Study." *British Medical Journal,* Vol. 323, No. 7314, September 22, 2001, p. 662.

17. Brazil, K., et al. "The Role of Families in Caring for the Terminally Ill." *Gerontologist,* October 15, 2001, p. 300.

18. Bernard, L., and C. Guarnaccia. "Husband's and Daughter's Role Strain During Breast Cancer Hospice Patient Caregiving." *Gerontologist,* October 15, 2001, p. 100.

19. Schulz et al., "Involvement in Caregiving and Adjustment to Death of a Spouse."

20. Farsides, Bobbie, and Robert Dunlop. "Is There Such a Thing as a Life Not Worth Living?" *British Medical Journal,* Vol. 322, No. 7300, June 16, 2001, p. 1481.

21. Kayashima, R., and K. L. Braun. "Examining the Variance in Support for Assisted Death Among Physicians, Patients, and the General Public." *Gerontologist,* October 15, 2001, p. 166.

22. Braun, Kathryn, et al. "Support for Physician-Assisted Suicide: Exploring the Impact of Ethnicity and Attitudes Toward Planning for Death." *Gerontologist,* Vol. 41, No. 1, February 2001, p. 51.

23. Alagra, Wybo. "A Release from Life." *UNESCO Courier,* July 2001, p. 54.

24. Roscoe, Lori, et al. "A Comparison of Characteristics of Kevorkian Euthanasia Cases and Physician-Assisted Suicides in Oregon." *Gerontologist,* Vol. 41, No. 4, August 2001, p. 439.

25. Ifeagwazi, Chuka, et al. "The Influence of Early Parents' Death on Manifestations of Depressive Symptoms Among Young Adults." *Omega—The Journal of Death and Dying,* Vol. 42, No. 2, March 2001, p. 151.

26. Balk, David. "College Student Bereavement, Scholarship, and the University." *Death Studies,* Vol. 25, No. 1, January 2001, p. 67.

19

Working Toward a Healthy Environment

As a teenager, Ocean Robbins wanted to change the world. At age 16, he founded Youth for Environmental Sanity (YES!) to mobilize his generation to save the planet. Now in his late twenties, Robbins has seen his California-based organization grow into what *Time* magazine describes as "a mini-movement that spans environmental consciousness raising, leadership training and community building." Over the last eleven years, more than 600,000 students in seven countries have taken part in YES! events in schools, summer camps, and workshops. "Part of my mandate is to help my generation see the power we have," says Robbins.[1]

No one has more stake in the future of the planet than the young. Environmental concerns may seem so enormous that nothing any individual can do will have an effect. This is not the case. Some individuals, like Ocean Robbins, become international advocates. But all of us, as citizens of the world, can help find solutions to the challenges confronting our planet. The first step is realizing that you have a personal responsibility for safeguarding the health of your environment and, thereby, your own well-being.

This chapter explores the complex interrelationships between your world and your well-being. It discusses major threats to the environment—including atmospheric changes; air, water, and noise pollution; chemical risks; and radiation—and provides specific guidance on what you can do about them.

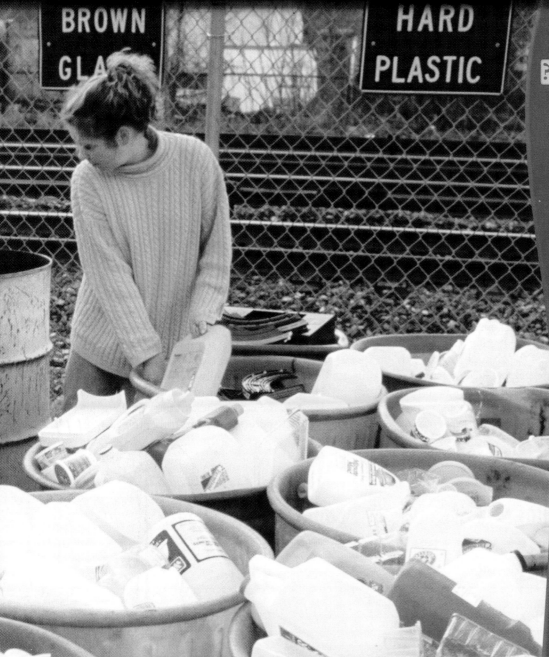

BROWN GLA...

HARD PLASTIC

???? FREQUENTLY ASKED QUESTIONS

FAQ: What is global warming? p. 624

FAQ: What can I do to protect the planet? p. 625

FAQ: What is acid rain? p. 628

FAQ: Is bottled water better? p. 632

FAQ: What health risks are caused by pesticides? p. 633

FAQ: Are cellular phones safe to use? p. 635

After studying the material in this chapter, you should be able to:

- **Discuss** the health effects of the major environmental hazards.
- **List** the major types of outdoor and indoor pollution.
- **List** and **describe** actions that individuals can take to protect the environment.
- **Describe** ways to protect your ears from noise-induced hearing loss.
- **Identify** the primary contaminants that can affect water quality.
- **List** the key sources and health risks of electromagnetic fields.
- **Discuss** ways that you can protect yourself from environmental dangers.

The State of the Environment

The planet Earth—once taken for granted as a ball of rock and water that existed for our use for all time—now is seen as a single, fragile **ecosystem** (a community of organisms that share a physical and chemical environment). Our environment is a closed ecosystem, powered by the sun. The materials needed for the survival of this planet must be recycled over and over again. Increasingly, we're realizing just how important the health of this ecosystem is to our own well-being and survival. However, as shown in Student Snapshot: "Do Students Care About the Environment?" the majority of undergraduates do not share this concern.

At the beginning of the twenty-first century, environmental experts predict new dangers to human life and health. These include acts of biological or chemical terrorism, natural disasters, contamination of water supplies, and hazardous waste disposal. One of the greatest challenges is the creation of a shared vision of a global society that is fair and equitable to all people today and for generations to come. Making this happen will require a different type of health decision-making—one that takes into account both individual and societal risks and that may lead to recommended action, such as bans on potential toxins, before definitive scientific knowledge is available.

Our Planet, Our Health

Our environment affects our well-being both directly and indirectly. Changes in temperature and rainfall patterns disturb ecological processes in ways that can be hazardous to health. The environment may account for 25 to 40 percent of diseases worldwide. Children are the most vulnerable because of their greater sensitivity to toxic threats.[2]

No individual is immune to environmental health threats. Depletion of the ozone layer has already been implicated in the increase in skin cancers and cataracts. Global warming, according to some theorists, might lead to change in one-third to one-half of the world's vegetation types and to the extinction of many plant and animal species. A warmer world is expected to produce more severe flooding in some places and more severe droughts in others, jeopardizing natural resources and the safety of our water supply. Warmer weather—a consequence of changes in atmospheric gases and climate discussed later in this chapter—worsens urban-industrial air pollution and, if the air also is moist, increases concentrations of allergenic pollens and fungal spores. These are truly problems without borders.

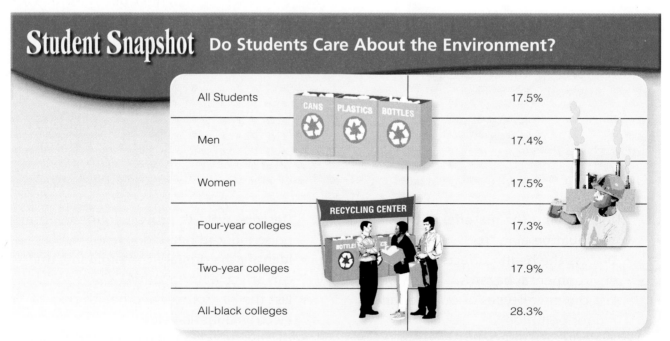

Student Snapshot Do Students Care About the Environment?

All Students	17.5%
Men	17.4%
Women	17.5%
Four-year colleges	17.3%
Two-year colleges	17.9%
All-black colleges	28.3%

Source: Sax, Linda et al. *The American Freshman: National Norms for Fall 2000.* Los Angeles: Higher Education Research Institute, UCLA, 2000.

For good or for ill, we cannot separate our individual health from that of the environment in which we live. The air we breathe, the water we drink, the chemicals we use all have an impact on the quality of our lives. At the same time, the lifestyle choices we make, the products we use, the efforts we undertake to clean up a beach or save wetlands affect the quality of our environment.

Multiple Chemical Sensitivity

The proliferation of chemicals in modern society has led to an entirely new disease, **multiple chemical sensitivity (MCS),** also called environmentally triggered illness, universal allergy, or chemical AIDS. MCS was first described almost a half century ago when a Chicago allergist treated a number of patients who reported becoming ill after being exposed to various petrochemicals. Since that time, many more cases of MCS have been reported, yet there is no agreed-upon definition for the condition, no medical test that can diagnose it, and no proven treatment.

According to medical theory, people become chemically sensitive in a two-step process: First, they experience a major exposure to a chemical, such as a pesticide, a solvent, or a combustion product. The sensitized person then begins to react to low-level chemical exposures from ordinary substances, such as perfumes and tobacco smoke. In other words, these low-level exposures trigger a physiological response. Over time, chemically unrelated substances may induce symptoms such as chest pain, depression, difficulty remembering, dizziness, fatigue, headache, inability to concentrate, nausea, and aches and pains in muscles and joints.

Individuals who may be at risk of MCS include Persian Gulf veterans, industrial workers, occupants of "sick buildings" with high levels of indoor pollutants, and people who live near contaminated sites. Because of the variety of racial, ethnic, and socioeconomic groups affected, medical professionals have become convinced that MCS is a real and serious health problem that requires investigation.[3]

Pollution

Any change in the air, water, or soil that could reduce its ability to support life is a form of **pollution.** Natural events, such as smoke from fires triggered by lightning, can cause pollution. The effects of pollution depend on the concentration (amount per unit of air, water, or soil) of the **pollutant,** how long it remains in the environment, and its chemical nature. An *acute effect* is a severe immediate reaction, usually after a single, large exposure. For example, pesticide poisoning can cause nausea and dizziness, even death. A *chronic effect* may take years to develop or may be a recurrent or continuous reaction, usually after repeated

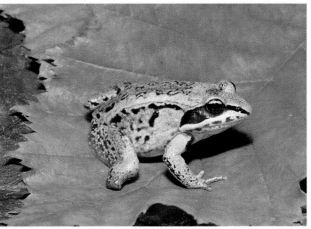

Glenn M. Oliver/Visuals Unlimited

▲ Environmental factors may be to blame for a rise in the number of deformed frogs, toads, and salamanders that have been discovered in recent years.

exposures. The development of cancer after repeated exposure to a pollutant such as asbestos is an example of a chronic effect.

Environmental agents that trigger changes, or **mutations,** in the genetic material, the DNA, of living cells are called **mutagens.** The changes that result can lead to the development of cancer. A substance or agent that causes cancer is a *carcinogen:* All carcinogens are mutagens; most mutagens are carcinogens. Furthermore, when a mutagen affects an egg or a sperm cell, its effects can be passed on to future generations. Agents that can cross the placenta of a pregnant woman and cause a spontaneous abortion or birth defects in the fetus are called **teratogens.**

Pollution is a hazard to all who breathe. Deaths caused by air pollution exceed those from motor vehicle injuries, according to research in Austria, France, and Switzerland.[4] Those with respiratory illnesses are at greatest risk during days when smog or allergen counts are high. However, even healthy joggers are affected; carbon monoxide has been shown to impair their exercise performance. The effects of carbon monoxide are much worse in smokers, who already have higher levels of the gas in their blood.

Toxic substances in polluted air can enter the human body in three ways: (1) through the skin, (2) through the digestive system, and (3) through the lungs. The combined interaction of two or more hazards can produce an effect greater than that of either one alone. Pollutants can affect an organ or organ system directly or indirectly.

Among the health problems that have been linked with pollution are the following:

◗ Headaches and dizziness.
◗ Eye irritation and impaired vision.
◗ Nasal discharge.
◗ Cough, shortness of breath, and sore throat.
◗ Constricted airways.

▸ Chest pains and aggravation of the symptoms of colds, pneumonia, bronchial asthma, emphysema, chronic bronchitis, lung cancer, and other respiratory problems.
▸ Birth defects and reproductive problems.
▸ Nausea, vomiting, and stomach cancer.

⁇⁇⁇ What Is Global Warming?

Earth's average surface temperature has risen by an estimated 0.6–1.2 degrees Fahrenheit in the last century (see Figure 19-1).[5] More of the warming has occurred over land than over water, more at night than during the day, and more in winter than in summer. No one can predict exactly what effects a continuing temperature rise may have, but some experts have predicted severe drought and a rise in ocean levels of 2 to 20 feet—conditions that will affect everyone on Earth. Ways to prevent these consequences include increasing the globe's tree cover (which accelerates carbon dioxide removal) and reducing fossil fuel combustion.[6]

Why is our planet getting warmer? Scientists and policy makers have been heatedly debating this question for years. Global warming may have many causes, including natural processes like volcanic activity and solar radiation and human activities that have resulted in atmospheric changes (See Figure 19-2). Some scientists argue that the mean surface temperatures of the last 100 years are not unusual, but the extremely rapid warming in the last 15 years cannot be explained by natural forces alone.[7]

The consequences of global warming are many and even include planetary motion. According to French scientists, higher temperatures may be slowing Earth's daily spin by around half a millisecond every century. A more visible consequence is the melting of the Antarctic ice shelves, flat expanses of ice up to 1,000 feet thick, which extend into the ocean from opposite sides of the Antarctic Peninsula. Satellite imagery shows that chunks of ice, some the size of aircraft carriers, are breaking off the shelves and drifting into the sea. The shelves themselves will probably disappear within a few years, but most scientists do not now think they will raise sea levels since they are already displacing ocean water in their frozen state. Within the next century, though, if global warming continues, the sea level will probably creep up more modestly, by about a foot or two, enough to endanger beachfront property and cost billions of dollars of damage.

Rising temperature during the summer on the arctic tundra may increase both snowfall and the emission of carbon dioxide. This may further contribute to atmospheric changes. However, farms, forests, and grasslands—if protected from development—may help counterbalance this trend. According to scientists' calculations, agricultural lands could remove from 40 to 80 billion metric tons of carbon from the atmosphere over the next 50 to 100 years and store it in the soil. In addition to significant climate changes, global warming is affecting both plants and animals, with some species dying off.[8]

For the last ten years, world leaders have been focusing on global warming and its potential consequences. Politicians and scientific experts continue to debate which measures—if any—should be taken to slow or stop global warming. Meanwhile, emissions of greenhouse gases are rising faster than expected, and it seems unlikely that any of the international goals for reducing emissions early in the twenty-first century will be met.[9]

In 2001, 165 countries—not including the United States—signed the first international treaty to fight global warming by implementing the rules known as the Kyoto Protocol. These call on about 40 industrialized nations to

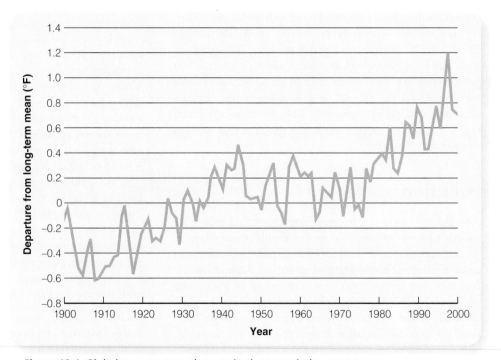

▲ **Figure 19-1** Global temperature changes in the twentieth century.

Source: National Climatic Data Center, 2000 (http://www.epa.gov/globalwarming/climate/index.html).

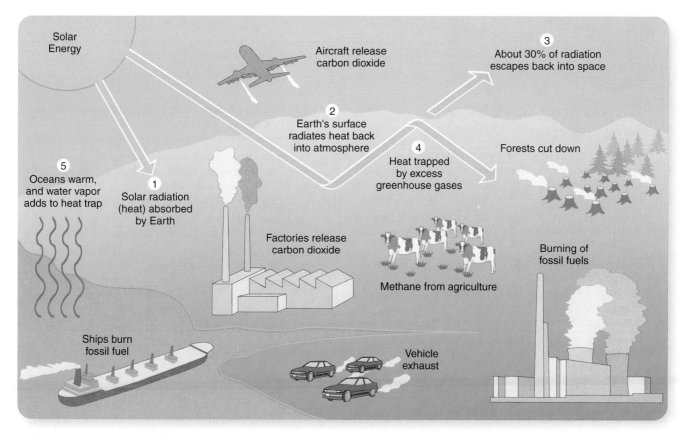

▲ **Figure 19-2** Why the world is heating up.
The buildup of carbon dioxide and other greenhouse gases in the atmosphere could result in the greatest climate change in human history. A combination of factors, including the burning of fossil fuels and deforestation, is causing the atmosphere to retain heat. Scientists estimate that the world will become hotter within a hundred years—the hottest it's been in two million years.

limit carbon emissions or reduce them to levels below those of 1990. The United States rejected the accord as harmful to the U.S. economy and unfair because it excused heavily polluting nations, such as India and China, from any obligation.[10]

???? What Can I Do to Protect the Planet?

By the choices you make and the actions you take, you can improve the state of the world. (See Savvy Consumer: "Save Energy, Save Money, Save the Planet.") No one expects you to sacrifice every comfort or spend great amounts of money. However, for almost everyone, there's plenty of room for improvement. If enough people make small individual changes, they can have an enormous impact. (See the Self-Survey: "Are You Doing Your Part for the Planet?")

A basic environmental action is **precycling:** buying products packaged in recycled materials. According to Earthworks, a consumer group, packaging makes up a third of what people in the United States throw away. When you precycle, you consider how you're going to dis-

pose of a product and the packaging materials before purchasing it. For example, you might choose eggs in recyclable cardboard packages rather than plastic ones and look for refillable bottles.

Recycling—collecting, reprocessing, marketing, and using materials once considered trash—has become a necessity for several reasons. We've run out of space for all the garbage we produce; waste sites are often health and safety hazards; recycling is cheaper than landfill storage or incineration (which is a major source of air pollution); and recycling helps save energy and natural resources. Different communities take different approaches to recycling. Many provide regular curbside pickup of recyclables, which is so convenient that a majority of those eligible for such services participate. Most programs pick up bottles, cans, and newspapers—either separated or mixed together. Other communities have drop-off centers where consumers can leave recyclables. Conveniently located and sponsored by community organizations (such as charities or schools), these centers accept beverage containers, newspapers, cardboard, metals, and other items.

Buy-back centers, usually run by private companies, pay for recyclables. Many centers specialize in aluminum

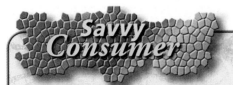

Savvy Consumer

Save Energy, Save Money, Save the Planet

Simple steps can help save energy, lower carbon dioxide emissions, and cut down on energy costs. Here are some recommendations from the Environmental Defense and World Wildlife Fund:

- Wash laundry in warm or cold water, not hot. *Average annual CO_2 reduction: up to 500 pounds for two loads of laundry a week.*

- Buy products sold in the simplest possible packaging. Carry a tote bag or recycle shopping bags. *Average annual CO_2 reduction: 1,000 pounds because garbage is reduced 25 percent.*

- Switch from standard light bulbs to energy-efficient fluorescent ones. *Average annual CO_2 reduction: about 500 pounds per bulb.*

- Set room thermostats lower in winter and higher in summer. *Average annual CO_2 reduction: about 500 pounds for each two-degree reduction.*

- Run dishwashers only when full, and choose the energy-saving mode rather than the regular setting. *Average annual CO_2 reduction: 200 pounds.*

- Bike, carpool, or take mass transit whenever possible. *Average annual CO_2 reduction: 20 pounds for each gallon of gasoline saved.*

---

cans, which offer the most profit. Some operate in supermarket parking lots; other centers have regular hours and staff members who carefully weigh and evaluate recyclables. In some places, reverse vending machines accept returned beverage containers and provide deposit refunds, in the form of either cash or vouchers. Enthusiasm and support for recycling has grown, and, thanks to these

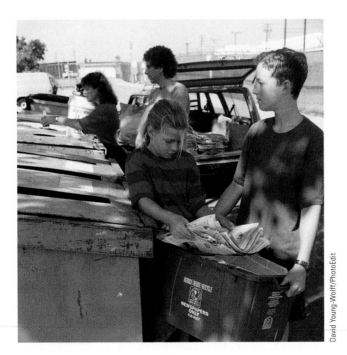

David Young-Wolff/PhotoEdit

▲ Recycling is an easy way to help save energy and conserve resources.

efforts along with new manufacturing techniques and other technological advances, people in the United States are consuming some natural materials, such as aluminum and steel, at lower rates.

With *composting*—which some people describe as nature's way of recycling—the benefits can be seen as close as your backyard. Organic products, such as leftover food and vegetable peels, are mixed with straw or other dry material and kept damp. Bacteria eat the organic material and turn it into a rich soil. Some people keep a compost pile (which should be stirred every few days) in their backyards; others take their organic garbage (including mowed grass and dead leaves) to community gardens or municipal composting sites. (See Pulse Points: "Ten Ways to Protect the Planet.")

Clearing the Air

In most places in the United States, you can breathe easier today than you would have a quarter century ago. Smog has declined by about a third, although there are now 85 percent more vehicles being driven 105 percent more miles a year. Current model automobiles emit an average of 80 percent less pollution per mile than was emitted by new cars in 1970. However, tailpipe emissions from cars and trucks still account for almost a third of the air pollution in the United States.[11]

According to the Harvard School of Public Health, living in a city with even moderately sooty air may shorten your lifespan by about a year. In fact, air pollution can be as

SELF SURVEY

Are You Doing Your Part for the Planet?

You may think that there is little you can do, as an individual, to save Earth. But everyday acts can add up and make a difference in helping or harming the planet on which we live.

	Almost Never	Sometimes	Always
1. Do you walk, cycle, carpool, or use public transportation as much as possible to get around?	_____	_____	_____
2. Do you recycle?	_____	_____	_____
3. Do you reuse plastic and paper bags?	_____	_____	_____
4. Do you try to conserve water by not running the tap as you shampoo or brush your teeth?	_____	_____	_____
5. Do you use products made of recycled materials?	_____	_____	_____
6. Do you drive a car that gets good fuel mileage and has up-to-date emission control equipment?	_____	_____	_____
7. Do you turn off lights, televisions, and appliances when you're not using them?	_____	_____	_____
8. Do you avoid buying products that are elaborately packaged?	_____	_____	_____
9. Do you use glass jars and waxed paper rather than plastic wrap for storing food?	_____	_____	_____
10. Do you take brief showers rather than baths?	_____	_____	_____
11. Do you use cloth towels and napkins rather than paper products?	_____	_____	_____
12. When listening to music, do you keep the volume low?	_____	_____	_____
13. Do you try to avoid any potential carcinogens, such as asbestos, mercury, or benzene?	_____	_____	_____
14. Are you careful to dispose of hazardous materials (such as automobile oil or antifreeze) at appropriate sites?	_____	_____	_____
15. Do you follow environmental issues in your community and write your state or federal representative to support "green" legislation?	_____	_____	_____

Making Changes

Count the number of items you've checked in each column. If you've circled 10 or more in the "always" column, you're definitely helping to make a difference. If you've circled 10 or more in the "never" column, read this chapter carefully, particularly the "Strategies for Change" to find out how and why you should make some changes. If you've mainly circled "sometimes," you're moving in the right direction, but you need to be more consistent and more conscientious.

---

harmful to breathing capacity as smoking. Residents of polluted cities are exposed to some of the same toxic gases, such as nitrogen oxide and carbon monoxide, found in cigarettes.

Air pollution of any sort can cause numerous ill effects. As pollutants destroy the hairlike cilia that remove irritants from the lungs, individuals may suffer chronic bronchitis, characterized by excessive mucus flow and continuous coughing. Emphysema may develop or worsen, as pollutants constrict the bronchial tubes and destroy the air sacs in the lungs, making breathing more difficult. In addition to respiratory diseases, air pollution also contributes to heart disease, cancer, and weakened immunity. For the elderly and people with asthma or heart disease, polluted air can be life-threatening. Even healthy individuals can be affected, particularly if they exercise outdoors during high-pollution periods.

Smog

A combination of smoke and fog, **smog** is made up of chemical vapors from auto exhaust and industrial and commercial pollutants that react with sunlight, including volatile organic compounds, carbon monoxide, nitrogen oxides, sulfur oxides, particulates, and ozone. The most obvious sources of these pollutants are motor vehicles, industrial factories, electric utility plants, and wood-burning stoves.

PULSE POINTS

Ten Ways to Protect the Planet

1. **Plant a tree.** Even a single tree helps absorb carbon dioxide and produces cooling that can reduce the need for air-conditioning.

2. **Look for simply packaged items.** Whenever possible, choose items packed in recycled materials or something recyclable.

3. **Bring your own bag.** Whenever possible, avoid using plastic or paper bags for items you could carry in a cloth or string carryall.

4. **Hit the switch.** Turn off all electrical appliances (TVs, CD players, radios, lights) when you're not in the room or paying attention to them.

5. **Avoid disposables.** Use a mug instead of a paper or Styrofoam cup, a sponge instead of a paper towel, a cloth napkin instead of a paper one.

6. **Be water wise.** Turn off the tap while you shave or brush your teeth. Install water-efficient faucets and shower heads. Wash clothes in cold water.

7. **Cancel junk mail.** It consumes 100 million trees a year. To get off mailing lists, write: Direct Mail Association, Mail Preference Service, P.O. Box 9008, Farmingdale, NY 11735-9008

8. **Spare the seas.** If you live near the coast or are picnicking or hiking near the ocean, don't use plastic bags (which are often blown into the water) or plastic six-pack holders (which can get caught around the necks of sea birds).

9. **Don't buy products made of endangered substances.** Examples include coral, ivory, tortoise shell, or wood from endangered forests (teak, mahogany, ebony, rosewood).

10. **Speak out.** Write to your senators and congressional representatives, who vote on pollution controls, budgets for the enforcement of safety regulations, and the preservation of forests and wildlife. Identify the particular bill or issue you're addressing. Be as specific, brief, and to the point as possible, and make sure you have the correct addresses: Hon. [Your District's Congressperson] United States House of Representatives, Washington, DC 20515

or

Senator [Your State's Senator], United States Senate, Washington, DC 20510

Gray-air, or *sulfur-dioxide,* smog, often seen in Europe and much of the eastern United States, is produced by burning oil of high sulfur content. Among the cities that must deal with gray-air smog are Chicago, Baltimore, Detroit, and Philadelphia. Like cigarette smoke, gray-air smog affects the cilia in the respiratory passages; the lungs are unable to expel particulates, such as soot, ash, and dust, which remain and irritate the tissues. This condition is hazardous to people with chronic respiratory problems.

Brown-air, or *photochemical,* smog is found in large traffic centers such as Los Angeles, Salt Lake City, Denver, Mexico City, and Tokyo. This type of smog results principally from nitric oxide in car exhaust reacting with oxygen in the air, forming nitrogen dioxide, which produces a brownish haze and, when exposed to sunlight, other pollutants.

One of these, *ozone,* the most widespread pollutant, can impair the body's immune system and cause long-term lung damage. (Ozone in the upper atmosphere protects us by repelling harmful ultraviolet radiation from the sun, but ozone in the lower atmosphere is a harmful component of air pollution.) Automobiles also produce carbon monoxide, a colorless and odorless gas that diminishes the ability of red blood cells to carry oxygen. The resulting oxygen deficiency can affect breathing, hearing, and vision.

STRATEGIES FOR CHANGE

Doing Your Part for Cleaner Air

✔ Drive a car that gets high gas mileage and produces low emissions. Keep your speed at or below the speed limit.

✔ Keep your tires inflated and your engine tuned. Recycle old batteries and tires. (Most stores that sell new ones will take back old ones.)

✔ Turn off your engine if you're going to be stopped for more than a minute.

✔ Collect all fluids that you drain from your car (motor oil, antifreeze) and recycle or dispose of them properly.

???? What Is Acid Rain?

The burning of fossil fuels, such as oil and gas, and the smelting of certain ores, such as copper and nickel, can produce **acid rain**—rain, sleet, snow, mist, fog, and clouds

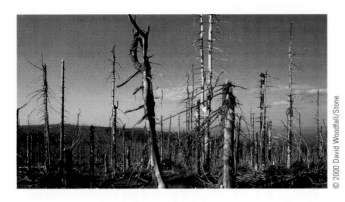

▲ The effects of acid rain on a forest.

containing sulfuric acid and nitric acid. These pollutants are carried through the atmosphere long distances from their sources and fan to Earth when it rains. Acid rain, which is believed to be declining in some regions, has damaged buildings, monuments, and other structures.

During the last 30 years, acid rain has contributed to the death of more than half of certain trees, including red spruce and sugar maples, in the Northeast.[12] More than a decade after the passage of the Clean Air Act in 1990, habitats in the northeastern states have not yet recovered from acid rain damage.[13]

Indoor Pollutants

Because people in industrialized nations spend more than 90 percent of their time in buildings, the quality of the air they breathe inside can have an even greater impact on their well-being than outdoor pollution. The most hazardous form of indoor air pollution is cigarette smoke. Passive smoking—inhaling others' cigarette smoke—may rank behind active smoking and alcohol use as the third-leading preventable cause of death. Each year secondhand cigarette smoke kills 53,000 nonsmokers.

Formaldehyde

Unlike outdoor contaminants from exhaust pipes or smokestacks, indoor pollutants come from the very materials the buildings are made of and from the appliances inside them. For instance, formaldehyde, commonly used in building materials, carpet backing, furniture, foam insulation, plywood, and particle board, can cause nausea, dizziness, headaches, heart palpitations, stinging eyes, and burning lungs. Formaldehyde has been shown to cause cancer in animals. Most manufacturers have voluntarily quit using it, but many homes already contain materials made with urea-formaldehyde, which can seep into the air. To avoid formaldehyde exposure, buy solid wood or non-wood products whenever possible, and ask about the formaldehyde content of building products, cabinets, and furniture before purchasing them.

Asbestos

Asbestos, a mineral widely used for building insulation, has been linked to lung and gastrointestinal cancer among asbestos workers and their families, although it may take 20 to 30 years for such cancer to develop. If fibers from asbestos home insulation or fireproofing become airborne, they can cause progressive and deadly lung diseases, including cancer. More than 200,000 lawsuits have been filed for asbestos-related injuries, and as many as 300,000 American workers may have died from asbestos-linked diseases, including lung cancer. The danger may be greatest for those who smoke and are also exposed to asbestos.

If you're concerned about asbestos in your home, don't waste money searching for asbestos in the air. The results of such tests are meaningless. To check a building material for asbestos, put three small pieces in a film canister and send it to an EPA-approved laboratory. The cost for testing is usually $25 to $75 per sample. If you find asbestos in your house, sealing it may be safer than removing it. Contact your state or city health department for advice. If asbestos must be removed, have it done by professionals.

Lead

A danger both inside and outside our homes is lead, which lurks in some 57 million American homes, most built before 1960, with walls, windows, doors, and banisters coated with more than 3 million metric tons of lead paint. The CDC estimates that one of every twenty U.S. children suffers from some sort of lead poisoning.[14] Millions more are at risk of poisoning from lead in the air they breathe or the water they drink. "In terms of the number of children

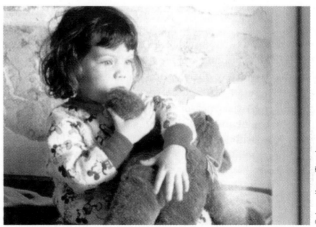

▲ Lead-based paint poses a hazard, especially to young children, who can be poisoned even by ingesting small amounts of paint chips.

affected, the number at risk and the dire effects of exposure, lead is the number-one environmental threat to our youngsters," says pediatrician John Rosen, M.D., chairman of the advisory committee on childhood lead poisoning for the CDC.

Fetuses and children under age 7 are particularly vulnerable to lead because their nervous systems are still developing and because their body mass is so small that they ingest and absorb more lead per pound than adults. Even 10 micrograms (millionths of a gram) of lead per deciliter of blood—the CDC standard for lead poisoning—can kill a child's brain cells and cause poor concentration, reduced short-term memory, slower reaction times, and learning disabilities.

Adults exposed to low levels of lead (which once were thought to be safe) may develop headaches, high blood pressure, irritability, tremors, and insomnia. Health effects increase with exposure to higher levels and include anemia, stomach pain, vomiting, diarrhea, and constipation. Long-term exposure can impair fertility and damage the kidneys. Workers exposed to lead may become sterile or suffer irreversible kidney disease, damage to their central nervous system, stillbirths, or miscarriages.

The CDC and the American Academy of Pediatrics recommend annual testing of blood levels of lead in all children from age 9 months to 6 years, regardless of where they live. High-risk youngsters—those who live or play in older housing (especially if a building is in poor condition or undergoing renovation), those who live with someone who uses lead for a job or hobby, and those who live near a lead smelter, a processing plant, or a heavily traveled road or highway—should be screened every two or three months until age 3 and every six months until age 6. High levels of ascorbic acid (vitamin C) have been associated with a lower rate of elevated blood lead levels.

Mercury

While free of lead, some popular, easy-to-use latex paints may contain potentially hazardous mercury, which manufacturers routinely added, until a 1990 ban, to prevent the growth of mold and mildew. The threat of mercury poisoning is greatest during painting and immediately after. Even mercury in medical devices, such as sphygmomanometers that measure blood pressure, can be a hazard. Symptoms of mercury poisoning include a racing heartbeat, sweating, aching limbs, kidney problems, hand tremors, peeling skin, and emotional problems.

Carbon Monoxide and Nitrogen Dioxide

Carbon monoxide (CO) gas, which is tasteless, odorless, colorless, and nonirritating, can be deadly. Produced by the incomplete combustion of fuel in space heaters, furnaces, water heaters, and engines, it reduces the delivery of oxygen in the blood. Every year an estimated 10,000 Americans seek treatment for CO inhalation; at least 250 die because of this silent killer. Those most at risk are the chronically ill, the elderly, pregnant women, and infants. Typical symptoms of CO poisoning are headache, nausea, vomiting, fatigue, and dizziness. A blood test can measure CO levels; inhaling pure oxygen speeds removal of the gas from the body. Most people who don't lose consciousness as a result of CO poisoning recover completely.

Another dangerous gas, nitrogen dioxide, can reach very high levels if you use a natural gas or propane stove in a poorly ventilated kitchen. This gas may lead to respiratory illnesses. Pilot lights are a steady source of nitrogen dioxide; to reduce exposure, switch to spark ignition.

Radon

Radioactive radon—which diffuses from rock, brick, and concrete building materials and natural soil deposits under some homes—produces charged decay products that cling to dust particles, which often lodge in the lungs. Once trapped inside, radon can reach levels that may increase the risk of lung cancer. EPA estimates that the inhalation of indoor radon is responsible for approximately 14,000 lung cancer deaths per year. Radon levels tend to be highest in areas with granite and black shale topped with porous soil. If you live in a high-radon area, don't panic. Your hypothetical risk of dying from radon-caused lung cancer is about equal to the known risk of dying in a home fire or fall. Check with the geology department at the nearest university or with your state health department to find out if they've performed radon tests in your area. If there may be danger, you can buy a radon detector. In most homes, the readings turn out to be low. If not, your state health department can provide guidelines for bringing them down.

Protecting Your Hearing

Loud noises cause hearing loss in an estimated 10 million Americans every year.[15] Loudness, or the intensity of a sound, is measured in **decibels (dB).** A whisper is 20 decibels; a conversation in a living room is about 50 decibels. On this scale, 50 isn't two and a half times louder than 20, but 1,000 times louder: Each 10-dB rise in the scale represents a tenfold increase in the intensity of the sound. Very loud but short bursts of sounds (such as gunshots and fireworks) and quieter but longer-lasting sounds (such as power tools) can induce hearing loss.

Sounds under 75 dB don't seem harmful. However, prolonged exposure to any sound over 85 dB (the equivalent of a power mower or food blender) or brief exposure to louder sounds can harm hearing. The noise level at rock concerts can reach 110–140 dB—about as loud as an air raid siren. Personal sound systems (boom boxes) can blast sounds of up to 115 dB. Cars with extremely loud music systems, known as boom cars, can produce an earsplitting 145 dB—louder than a jet engine or thunderclap. (See Figure 19-3.)

Most hearing loss occurs on the job. The people at highest risk are firefighters, police, military personnel, construction and factory workers, musicians, farmers, and truck drivers. Other sources of danger include live or recorded high-volume music, recreational vehicles, airplanes, lawn-care equipment, woodworking tools, some appliances, and chain saws.

Common "sound offenders" are clubs (with sustained levels of well over 100 decibels), restaurants (with levels of 80 to 96 decibels), and street traffic (90 decibels or more).[16] However, even low-level office noise can undermine well-being and increase health risks.[17]

The Effects of Noise

Noise-induced hearing loss is 100 percent preventable—and irreversible. Hearing aids are the only treatment, but they do not correct the problem, they just amplify sound to compensate for hearing loss.

The healthy human ear can hear sounds within a wide range of frequencies (measured in hertz), from the low-frequency rumble of thunder at 50 hertz to the high-frequency overtones of a piccolo at nearly 20,000 hertz. High-frequency noise damages the delicate hair cells that serve as sound receptors in the inner ear. Damage first begins as a diminished sensitivity to frequencies around 4,000 hertz—the highest notes of a piano. Early symptoms of hearing loss include difficulty understanding speech and tinnitus (ringing in the ears). Brief, very loud sounds, such as an explosion or gunfire, can produce immediate, severe, and permanent hearing loss. Longer exposure to less intense but still hazardous sounds, such as those common at work or in public places, can impair hearing gradually, often without the individual's awareness.

Conductive hearing loss, often caused by ear infections, cuts down on perception of low-pitched sounds. Sensorineural loss involves damage or destruction of the sensory cells in the inner ear that convert sound waves to nerve signals.

Noise can harm more than our ears: High-volume sound has been linked to high blood pressure and other stress-related problems that can lead to heart disease, insomnia, anxiety, headaches, colitis, and ulcers. Noise frays the nerves; people tend to be more anxious, irritable,

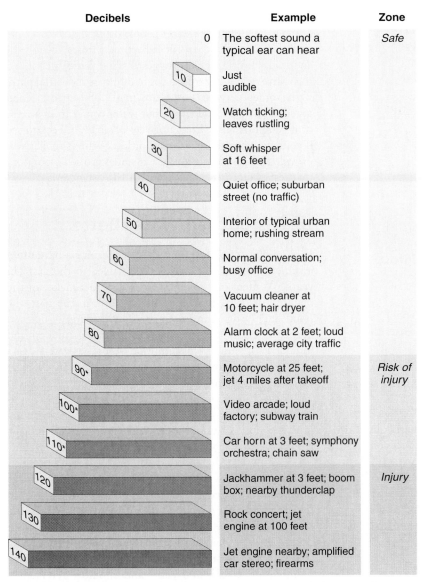

Decibels	Example	Zone
0	The softest sound a typical ear can hear	Safe
10	Just audible	
20	Watch ticking; leaves rustling	
30	Soft whisper at 16 feet	
40	Quiet office; suburban street (no traffic)	
50	Interior of typical urban home; rushing stream	
60	Normal conversation; busy office	
70	Vacuum cleaner at 10 feet; hair dryer	
80	Alarm clock at 2 feet; loud music; average city traffic	
90*	Motorcycle at 25 feet; jet 4 miles after takeoff	Risk of injury
100*	Video arcade; loud factory; subway train	
110*	Car horn at 3 feet; symphony orchestra; chain saw	
120	Jackhammer at 3 feet; boom box; nearby thunderclap	Injury
130	Rock concert; jet engine at 100 feet	
140	Jet engine nearby; amplified car stereo; firearms	

*Note: The maximum exposure allowed on the job by federal law, in hours per day, is as follows: 90 decibels—8 hours; 100 decibels—2 hours; 110 decibels—½ hour.

▲ **Figure 19-3** Loud and louder.
The human ear perceives a 10-decibel increase as a doubling of loudness. Thus, the 100 decibels of a subway train sounds much more than twice as loud as the 50 decibels of a rushing stream.

STRATEGIES FOR PREVENTION

Protecting Your Ears

✔ If you must live or work in a noisy area, wear hearing protectors to prevent exposure to blasts of very loud noise. Don't think cotton or facial tissue stuck in your ears can protect you; foam or soft plastic earplugs are more effective. Wear them when operating lawn mowers, weed trimmers, or power tools.

✔ Soundproof your home by using draperies, carpets, and bulky furniture. Put rubber mats under washing machines, blenders, and other noisy appliances. Seal cracks around windows and doors.

✔ When you hear a sudden loud noise, press your fingers against your ears. Limit your exposure to loud noise. Several brief periods of noise seem less damaging than one long exposure.

✔ Be careful if you wear Walkman-type stereos. The volume is too high if you can feel the vibrations.

✔ Beware of large doses of aspirin. Researchers have found that eight aspirins a day can aggravate the damage caused by loud noise; twelve aspirins daily can cause ringing in the ears (tinnitus).

✔ Don't drink in noisy environments. Alcohol intensifies the impact of noise and increases the risk of lifelong hearing damage.

and angry when their ears are constantly barraged with sound. Chronic airport noise can affect children's physical and mental health.[18] Even unborn babies respond to sounds; some researchers speculate that noise, particularly if it stresses the mother, may be hazardous to the fetus.

As a result of exposure to damaging noise levels, 12.5 percent of young Americans—an estimated 5.2 million—between ages 6 and 19 have incurred permanent damage to the hair cells within the ear.[19]

Is Your Water Safe to Drink?

According to a survey by the Water Quality Association, some 86 percent of the people in the United States are concerned about th quality of their tap water, while 32 percent think their water is not as safe as it should be. About two-thirds take steps to drink purer water, either by using filtration and distillation methods or by drinking bottled water.[20] Fears about the public water supply have led many Americans to turn off their taps. However, Consumer Union, a nonprofit advocacy group, maintains that the United States has the safest water supply in the world.[21] The U.S. Environmental Protection Agency (EPA) has set standards for some 80 contaminants. These include many toxic chemicals and heavy metals—including lead, mercury, cadmium, and chromium—that can cause kidney and nervous system damage and birth defects.

Each year the CDC reports an average of 7,400 cases of illness related to the water people drink. The most common culprits include parasites, bacteria, viruses, chemicals, and lead. Health officials suggest having your water tested if you live near a hazardous waste dump or industrial park, if the pipes in your house are made of lead or joined together with lead solder, if your water comes from a well, or if you purchase it from a private company. Check to see if your state health department or local water supplier will provide free testing. If not, use a state-certified laboratory that tests water in accordance with EPA standards.

???? Is Bottled Water Better?

Is bottled water better? That's what consumers have often assumed. Bottled water sales have tripled in the past ten years. Women and college-age Americans make up the majority of bottled-water drinkers.[22] Yet in the past, the Food and Drug Administration (FDA) simply defined bottled water as "sealed in bottles or other containers and intended for human consumption." Bottled water wasn't required to be "pure" or even to be tested for toxic chemicals. One survey found chemical contaminants associated with cancer in 22 of 100 brands tested.[23]

The FDA has called for federal monitoring of the purity of bottled water. Some states, including California and New York, have their own bottled-water safety standards to ensure that bottled water is at least as safe as drinking water. In cases where public drinking water has been contaminated (for instance, by a toxic spill) and health authorities advise using bottled waters, check the label to make sure that the brand you purchase has been tested or undergone purification treatment. Health experts also caution against bottled waters "fortified" with vitamins or minerals, which you can—and should—get from a healthful diet.[24]

Fluoride

About half (53 percent) of Americans drink water containing fluoride, an additive to water and toothpaste that helps teeth resist decay. According to the American Dental Association (ADA), the incidence of tooth decay is 50 to 70 percent lower in areas with fluoridated water. However, laboratory rats given fluoridated water have shown a high rate of bone cancer. The more fluoride they drank in their water, the more likely they were to develop this cancer. But this type of cancer is extremely rare in humans, and the estimated lifetime risk to any individual from drinking fluoridated water is less than one in 5,000.

Federal health officials have found no evidence that fluoride causes cancer in humans and have concluded that its benefits far outweigh any risks. However, excessive fluoride can increase bone loss and fractures in pre- and postmenopausal women. Health professionals advise consumers to use only small amounts of fluoridated toothpastes, rinse thoroughly after brushing, and use fluoride supplements only when the home water supply is known to be deficient.

Chlorine

Three-quarters of the population of the United States drinks water treated with chlorine to kill disease-causing bacteria. The Council on Environmental Quality has warned that people drinking chlorinated water have a 53 percent greater risk of getting colon and bladder cancer and a 13 to 93 percent greater risk of getting rectal cancer than those not drinking chlorinated water. There may even be a link between soft water and a higher rate of cardiovascular disease, perhaps because soft water in some areas tends to have more sodium in it.

Lead

Long recognized as a hazard in paint and dust, lead can also leach from pipes into the drinking supply. The highest risk exists in cities with older housing and lead pipes or water lines.

Chemical Risks

According to a 2001 report by the CDC, there have been declines of levels of potentially harmful chemicals, including pesticides and lead, in the country's blood.[25] No relationship has been found between fertility, as measured by time to pregnancy (that is, the time taken for a couple to conceive once they decide they want to), and male exposure to pesticides. Exposure to pesticides may, however, pose a risk to pregnant women and their unborn children. Exposure to toxic chemicals cause about 3 percent of developmental defects.[26]

An estimated 50,000–70,000 U.S. workers die each year of chronic diseases related to past exposure to toxic substances, including lung cancer, bladder cancer, leukemia, lymphoma, chronic bronchitis, and disorders of the nervous system. **Endocrine disruptors,** chemicals that act as or interfere with human hormones, particularly estrogen, may pose a different threat. Scientists are investigating their impact on fertility, falling sperm counts, and cancers of the reproductive organs.

What Health Risks Are Caused by Pesticides?

The FDA estimates that 33 to 39 percent of our food supply contains residues of pesticides, which may pose a long-term danger to our health.[27] Scientists have detected traces of pesticides in groundwater in both urban and rural areas.[28]

Various chemicals, including benzene, asbestos, and arsenic, have been shown to cause cancer in humans. Probable carcinogens include DDT and PCBs. Risks can be greatly increased with simultaneous exposures to more than one carcinogen, for example, tobacco smoke and asbestos.[29] Chronic exposure to pesticides also has been linked to Parkinson's disease.[30]

Chlorinated hydrocarbons include several high-risk substances—such as DDT, kepone, and chlordane—that have been restricted or banned because they may cause cancer, birth defects, neurological disorders, and damage to wildlife and the environment. They are extremely resistant to breakdown.

Organic phosphates, including chemicals such as malathion, break down more rapidly than do the chlorinated hydrocarbons. Most are highly toxic, causing cramps, confusion, diarrhea, vomiting, headaches, and

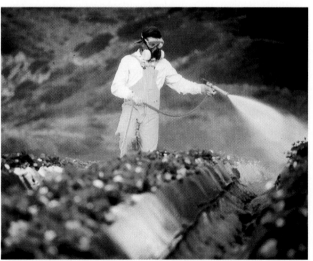

▲ Pesticides protect crops from harmful insects, plants, and fungi but may endanger human health.

breathing difficulties. Higher levels in the blood can lead to convulsions, paralysis, coma, and death.

Farm workers and those in the surrounding communities are at greatest risk for pesticide exposure. However, even city dwellers aren't out of range. About half (52 percent) of the nation uses insect repellents, including some made with potent insecticides.

Invisible Dangers

Among the unseen threats to health are various forms of radiation.

Electromagnetic Fields

Any electrically charged conductor generates two kinds of invisible fields: electric and magnetic. Together they're called **electromagnetic fields (EMFs).** For years, these fields, produced by household appliances, home wiring, lighting fixtures, electric blankets, and overhead power lines, were considered harmless. However, epidemiological studies revealed a link between exposure to high-voltage lines and cancer (especially leukemia, a blood cancer) in electrical workers and children.

Laboratory studies on animals have shown that alternating current, which changes strength and direction 60 times a second (and electrifies most of North America), emits fields that may interfere with the normal functioning of human cell membranes, which have their own electromagnetic fields. The result may be mood disorders, changes in circadian rhythms (our inner sense of time), miscarriage, developmental problems, or cancer. Researchers have documented an increase in breast cancer deaths in women who worked as electrical engineers, electricians, or in other high-exposure jobs and a link between EMF exposure and an increased risk of leukemia and possibly brain cancer.

After six years of congressionally mandated research, the National Institute of Environmental Health Sciences concluded that the evidence of a risk of cancer and other human disease from the electric and magnetic fields around power lines is "weak." This finding applies to the extremely low frequency electric and magnetic fields surrounding both the big power lines that distribute power and the smaller but closer electric lines in homes and appliances. However, the researchers also noted that EMF exposure "cannot be recognized as entirely safe."

The strongest evidence for health effects came from statistical associations of childhood leukemia and chronic lymphocytic leukemia in adults exposed to EMFs on the job, such as electric utility workers, machinists, and welders.

"While the support from individual studies is weak," according to the report, "these epidemiological studies demonstrate, for some methods of measuring exposure, a fairly consistent pattern of a small, increased risk." Laboratory studies and investigations of basic biological function do not support these epidemiological associations.

Appliances that are used only briefly, such as hair dryers, are probably less dangerous than electric blankets, which people sleep under for an entire night. Expectant mothers who often use electric blankets or heated water beds during winter have a higher miscarriage rate than nonusers; babies conceived in the winter by electric blanket-users grow more slowly in the womb and tend to have a lower birthweight than others. Federal officials urge "prudent avoidance" of electric blankets for women who are pregnant or hoping to conceive.

Video Display Terminals (VDTs)

Chances are there's a **video display terminal (VDT)** in your life—at the school library, at the office where you work, or maybe in your home. Is it a health hazard? The answer is a definite maybe. Although VDTs have been blamed for increases in reproductive problems, miscarriages, low birthweights, and cataracts, repeated measurements of radiation from VDTs have shown that leakage is well below present standards for safe occupational exposure. However, VDTs emit electromagnetic fields from all sides, not just the screen, and the strongest emissions are from the sides, backs, and tops of monitors. At least in theory, working next to someone using a computer may be more hazardous than using one yourself. Scientists are continuing to investigate possible links between VDT use and health hazards.

Microwaves

Microwaves (extremely high frequency electromagnetic waves) increase the rate at which molecules vibrate; this vibration generates heat. There's no evidence that existing levels of microwave radiation encountered in the environment pose a health risk to people, and all home microwave ovens must meet safety standards for leakage.

Another concern about the safety of microwave ovens stems from the chemicals in plastic wrapping and containers used for them, which may leak into food. Some, such as DEHA, a chemical that makes plastic more pliable, can cause cancer in mice in high concentrations. Consumers should be cautious about using clingy plastic wrap when reheating leftovers, and plastic-encased metal "heat susceptors" included in convenience foods such as popcorn and pizza. Although these materials seem safe when tested in conventional ovens at temperatures of 300°F–350°F, microwave ovens can boost temperatures to 500°F.

Are Cellular Phones Safe to Use?

Since cellular phone service was introduced in the United States in 1984, mobile and handheld phones have become ubiquitous. More than 86 million people use cell phones, and concern has grown about their possible health risks, particularly brain cancer. Because of the close proximity of the antenna to the brain, researchers hypothesized that radiofrequency signals might increase the danger. In experimental studies, researchers have documented changes in biological tissues exposed to radiofrequency waves.[31]

Researchers have found no link between cell phone use and brain cancer, but further studies are needed to determine whether exposure to radio waves from radio phones might cause slow-growing brain tumors.[32] One study compared 469 men and women between ages 18 and 80 with primary brain cancer with 422 individuals without brain cancer and found no correlation between short-term exposure to handheld cell phones and brain cancer.[33] Another compared about 800 adults with brain tumors with 800 people without brain tumors and found no evidence that cell phones cause brain tumors.[34] A large Danish study of 420,000 cell phone users concluded that callers are no more likely than anyone else to suffer cancer.[35] None of these studies have continued long enough to rule out any long-term risk of cancer, however.

Irradiated Foods

The use of radiation on food, from either radioactive substances or devices that produce X rays, is known as **irradiation.** It doesn't make the food radioactive—its primary benefit is to prolong the food's useful life. Like the heat in canning, irradiation can kill all the microorganisms that might grow in a food; the sterilized food can then be stored for years in sealed containers at room temperature without spoiling. In addition, low-dose irradiation can inhibit the sprouting of vegetables such as potatoes and onions, and delay the ripening of some fruits, such as bananas, mangoes, tomatoes, pears, and avocados—cost-saving benefits of great appeal to the food industry.

Irradiated foods are believed to be safe to eat, and the federal government has approved their distribution. Most research has focused on low-dose irradiation to delay ripening and destroy insects. Nutritional studies have shown no significant decreases in the quality of the foods, but high-dose treatments may cause vitamin losses similar to those that occur during canning. It's also possible that the ionizing effect of radiation creates new compounds in foods that may be mutagenic/carcinogenic.

Ionizing Radiation

Radiation that possesses enough energy to separate electrons from their atoms, leaving charged ions, is called **ionizing radiation.** Its effects on health depend on many factors, including the amount, length of exposure, type, part of the body exposed, and the health and age of the individual.

We're surrounded by low-level ionizing radiation every day. Most comes from cosmic rays and radioactive minerals, which vary according to geography. (Denver has more than Atlanta, for instance, because of its altitude.) Man-made sources, including medical and dental X rays, account for approximately 18 percent of the average person's lifetime exposure.

Radiation exposure in humans is measured in units called rads and rems. A *rad (radiation absorbed dose)* is a measure of the energy deposited by ionizing radiation when it's absorbed by an object. A *rem (roentgen equivalent man)* is a measure of the biological effect of ionizing radiation. Different types of radiation cause different amounts of damage. The rem measurement takes this into account. For X rays, rads and rems are equivalent. A quantity of 1 rad or 1 rem is a substantial dose of radiation. Smaller doses are measured in *millirads* (thousandths of a rad) or *millirems* (thousandths of a rem). The average annual radiation exposure for a person in the United States is about one-tenth of a rem.

Virtually any part of the body can be affected by ionizing radiation, although bone marrow and the thyroid are especially vulnerable. Radon exposures in homes can increase the risk of lung cancer.[36] Although high levels of radiation are most dangerous, even low-level radiation can be harmful to health. According to the National Research Council, the risk of getting cancer from small amounts of radiation is four times more than had been previously estimated, and there's much greater danger of mental retardation among babies exposed to radiation in the womb from eight to fifteen weeks after conception.

Diagnostic X Rays

The EPA estimates that 30 to 50 percent of the 700 million X rays taken every year in the United States are unnecessary. However, doctors sometimes prescribe X rays or newer imaging techniques involving radiation, such as CT scans, to protect themselves from malpractice suits, and hospitals benefit financially from the heavy use of X-ray equipment.

Dental X rays involve little radiation, but many people receive so many so often that they're second only to chest examinations in frequency. Dentists typically obtain radiographs of all the teeth at the beginning of a patient's care, and again every three to five years. However, you can cut down on total X rays by bringing previous films with you or having your dentist forward copies when you switch dentists.

Always ask why an X ray is being ordered. Don't give your consent unless there's a clear need. Keep a record of the date and location of every X-ray exam. Some of these X rays may someday provide information that would make more X rays unnecessary. Ask the radiologist to explain specifically how much radiation you'll be exposed to, and be sure to wear a protective leaded apron. There's no sense in refusing a needed medical X ray just because you're afraid of the radiation exposure. Under certain circumstances, the benefits far outweigh the risks.

Into the Future

Environmental problems can seem so complex that you may think there's little you an do about them. That's not the case. This world can be made better instead of worse. The job isn't easy, and all of us have to do our part. Just as many diseases of the previous century have been eradicated, so, in time, we may be able to remove or reduce many environmental threats. Your future—and our planet's future—may depend on it.

CHAPTER 19

Making This Chapter Work for You

1. Threats to the environment include
   a. an open ecosystem
   b. depletion of the oxygen layer
   c. ecological processes
   d. global warming

2. Mutagens
   a. are caused by birth defects.
   b. result in changes to the DNA of body cells.
   c. are agents that trigger changes in the DNA of body cells.
   d. are caused by repeated exposure to pollutants.

3. Which of the following statements about global warming is true?
   a. The primary cause of global warming is the melting of the Antarctic ice shelves.
   b. Global warming may result in severe drought and a rise in ocean levels.
   c. Increasing tree cover and agricultural lands will contribute to global warming.
   d. Increasing carbon dioxide production will slow the progress of global warming.

4. One of the most important things you can do to help protect the environment is
   a. recycle paper, bottles, cans, and unwanted food.
   b. use as much water as possible to help lower the ocean water levels.
   c. avoid energy-depleting fluorescent bulbs.
   d. use plastic storage containers and plastic wrap to save trees from being cut down.

5. Which of the following statements about air pollution is false?
   a. Acid rain is produced by the burning of fossil fuels and the smelting of ores such as copper and nickel.
   b. The three types of smog include sulfur-dioxide smog, produced by burning oil; photochemical smog, resulting from car exhaust; and carbon-monoxide smog, caused by fossil fuels.
   c. Ozone in the upper atmosphere protects us from harmful ultraviolet radiation from the sun, but in the lower atmosphere, it is a harmful air pollutant.
   d. Air pollution can cause the same types of respiratory health problems as smoking.

6. Indoor pollutants include
   a. lead, which is often found in paint and can result in nervous system damage in adults and impaired fertility and kidney damage in children.
   b. radon, which is found in building materials and can cause heart disease.
   c. asbestos, which may be found in building insulation and can cause lung diseases.
   d. carbon monoxide, which can be produced by furnaces and engines and can result in chronic illnesses such as emphysema.

7. You can protect your hearing by
   a. avoiding prolonged exposure to sounds under 75 decibels.
   b. using foam earplugs when operating noisy tools or attending rock concerts.

c. limiting noise exposure to short bursts of loud sounds such as fireworks.

d. drinking alcohol in noisy environments to mute the sounds.

8. Drinking water safety
   a. may be compromised if your water comes from a well.
   b. is high in the United States because of the use of sodium chloride to kill disease-causing bacteria.
   c. can be guaranteed by using bottled water, which is completely free of chemical contaminants.
   d. has been significantly decreased in those communities that add fluoride to the water.

9. Which of the following statements about electromagnetic fields is true?
   a. Overwhelming evidence indicates a strong link between electromagnetic fields around power lines and cancer and other diseases.
   b. The electromagnetic fields emitted by electric blankets are probably less dangerous than those from hair dryers.

c. The amount of radiation from video display terminals exceeds present standards for safe occupational exposure.

d. Electrical engineers and electricians who have high exposure to EMFs may be at greater risk for developing leukemia.

10. Radiation
    a. can be used to sterilize food and for medical imaging procedures.
    b. is measured in units called reds and rams.
    c. is always more dangerous in low levels than in high levels.
    d. from natural sources, such as the sun and radioactive minerals, is safer than the radiation from diagnostic X rays.

Answers to these questions can be found on page 640.

 Can the sights and smells of nature improve your health?

Critical Thinking

1. How do you personally contribute to environmental pollution? How might you change your practices to protect the environment instead?

2. An excerpt from a recent newspaper article stated, "Children living in a public housing project near a local refinery suffer from a high rate of asthma and allergies, and an environmental group says the plant may be to blame." The refinery has met all the local air quality standards, employs hundreds in the community, and pays substantial city taxes, which supports police, fire, and social services. If you were a city council member, how would you balance health and environmental concerns with the need for industry in your community? What actions would you recommend in this particular situation?

3. In one Harris poll, 84 percent of Americans said that, given a choice between a high standard of living (but with hazardous air and water pollution and the depletion of natural resources) and a lower standard of living (but with clean air and drinking water), they would prefer clean air and drinking water and a lower standard of living. What about you? What exactly would you be willing to give up: air conditioning, convenience packaging and products, driving your own car rather than using public transportation? Do you think that most people are willing to change their lifestyles to preserve the environment?

SITES & BYTES

Environmental Health
http://www.cdc.gov/health/environm.htm
This CDC site features excellent links including air pollution, carbon monoxide poisoning, temperature extremes, natural disasters, lead poisoning, and more.

U.S. Geological Society
http://water.usgs.gov/education.html
This site contains information on a variety of environmental topics, including water pollution, natural resources, pesticides, and acid rain, and is designed for the public, teachers, and students.

Environmental Protection Agency
http://www.epa.gov/globalwarming
This site contains a wealth of information on environmental hazards affecting climate and the impacts to the environment such as the greenhouse effect. The site also features information on the actions being taken to curb the effects of global warming.

Please note that links are subject to change. If you find a broken link, use a search engine such as **http://www.yahoo.com** and search for the website by typing in key words.

 InfoTrac Activity   Kirk R. Smith. "Environment and Health: Issues for the New U.S. Administration." *Environment*, Vol. 43, No. 4, May 2001, p. 34.

(1) What factors constitute environmental agents of disease?

(2) In terms of disease etiology, what is the relationship between nature and nurture?

(3) What constitutes the greatest environmental health risk to people in developing countries?

You can find additional readings related to environmental health with InfoTrac College Edition, an online library of more than 900 journals and publications. Follow the instructions for accessing InfoTrac that were packaged with your textbook; then search for articles using a key word search.

For additional links, resources, and suggested readings on InfoTrac, visit our Health & Wellness Resource Center at **http://health.wadsworth.com**.

Key Terms

The terms listed here are used within the chapter on the page indicated. Definitions of terms are in the Glossary at the end of the book.

acid rain 628
chlorinated hydrocarbons 633
decibel (dB) 630
ecosystem 622
electromagnetic fields (EMFs) 634
endocrine disruptors 633
ionizing radiation 635

irradiation 635
microwaves 634
multiple chemical sensitivity (MCS) 623
mutagen 623
mutation 623
organic phosphates 633

pollutant 623
pollution 623
precycling 625
recycling 625
smog 627
teratogen 623
video display terminal (VDT) 634

References

1. "Ocean Robbins: Youth for Environmental Sanity." *Time International*, Vol. 158, No. 16, October 22, 2001, p. 71.
2. Crain, Ellen. "Environmental Threats to Children's Health." *Pediatrics*, Vol. 106, No. 4, October 2000.
3. Sadovsky, Richard. "Assessing Patients with Medically Unknown Symptoms." *American Family Physician*, Vol. 61, No. 11, June 1, 2000.
4. Richter, Elihu, and Tamar Berman. "Speed, Air Pollution, and Health: A Neglected Issue." *Archives of Environmental Health*, Vol. 56, No. 4, July 2001, p. 296.
5. Environmental Protection Agency's website on global warming: http://www.epa.gov/globalwarming/.
6. Aber, John, et al. "Forest Processes and Global Environmental Change: Predicting the Effects of Individual and Multiple Stressors." *BioScience*, Vol. 51, No. 9, September 2001, p. 735.
7. Weaver, Andrew, et al. "The Causes of 20th Century Warming." *Science*, Vol. 290, No. 5499, December 15, 2000.

8. Stolzenburg, William. "Nature Feels the Heat: As Climate Goes Awry, Wildlife Goes Away." *Nature Conservancy*, Vol. 51, No. 5, September–October, 2001, p. 12.
9. Begley, Sharon. "The Mercury's Rising." *Newsweek*, December 4, 2000.
10. Staver, A. "The Collapse of the Kyoto Protocol and the Struggle to Slow Global Warming." *Choice*, Vol. 39, No. 2, October 2001, p. 347.
11. Environmental Protection Agency. http://www.epa.gov.
12. "Hard Rain Keeps Falling." *National Wildlife*, August–September 2001.
13. Ember, Lois. "Acid Rain Is Still a Menace." *Chemical & Engineering News*, Vol. 79, No. 14, April 2, 2001, p. 11.
14. Crain, "Environmental Threats to Children's Health."
15. "Noise-induced Hearing Loss: Common Condition Easily Prevented." *Facts of Life: Issue Briefing for Health Reporters*, Vol. 6, No. 5, July–August 2001.

16. "Recent Findings Suggest Urban Setting Means More Noise Exposure and More Hearing Loss." *Facts of Life: Issue Briefing for Health Reporters*, Vol. 6, No. 5, July–August 2001.

17. Lang, Susan. "Even Low-Level Office Noise Can Increase Health Risks." Cornell University News Office, January 22, 2001.

18. "Aircraft Noise and Public Health." *Journal of Environmental Health*, Vol. 63, No. 5, December 2000.

19. "Noise-induced Hearing Loss."

20. "Water, Water, Everywhere." *American Demographics*, October 1, 2001, p. 50.

21. Napoli, Maryann. "Consumer Reports Look at Bottled Water." *HealthFacts*, August 2000.

22. "Water, Water, Everywhere."

23. "Don't Bottle It Up." *The Ecologist*, Vol. 30, No. 5, July 2000, p. 12.

24. "Whatever Happened to Plain Old H_2O?" *Environmental Nutrition*, Vol. 23, No. 8, August 2000.

25. Revkin, Andrew. "Study of Chemicals in Americans Shows Encouraging Trends." *New York Times*, March 22, 2001.

26. "Advances in Biology Could Help in Assessing the Impact of Chemicals on Children." *Journal of Environmental Health*, Vol. 63, No. 3, October–September 2000.

27. Crain, "Environmental Threats to Children's Health."

28. Koplin, Dana, et al. "Pesticides in Ground Water of the United States." *Ground Water*, Vol. 38, No. 6, November 2000.

29. "Environmental Cancer Risks." *Cancer Facts & Figures 2001*, American Cancer Society, 2001.

30. Berger, Abi. "Parkinson's Disease Linked with Pesticide." *British Medical Journal*, Vol. 321, No. 7270, November 11, 2000.

31. Frey, Allan. "Cellular Phones: Are They Safe to Use?" *Scientists*, Vol. 14, No. 23, November 27, 2000.

32. Jones, David. "Phones and the Brain." *Nature*, Vol. 411, No. 6841, June 28, 2001, p. 1012.

33. Muscat, Joshua, et al. "Handheld Cellular Telephone Use and Risk of Brain Cancer." *Journal of the American Medical Association*, Vol. 284, No. 23, December 20, 2000.

34. Inskip, Peter, et al. "Cellular-Telephone Use and Brain Tumors." *New England Journal of Medicine*, Vol. 344, January 11, 2001.

35. Boice, John, et al. "Cell Phones and Brain Tumors." *Journal of the National Cancer Institute*, February 2001.

36. "Environmental Cancer Risks."

Making This Chapter Work for You

Answers to multiple choice questions

Chapter 1
1. b; 2. a; 3. d; 4. c; 5. a; 6. d; 7. b; 8. c; 9. a; 10. d

Chapter 2
1. b; 2. d; 3. a; 4. a; 5. c; 6. d; 7. b; 8. a; 9. c; 10. d

Chapter 3
1. b; 2. d; 3. a; 4. c; 5. c; 6. a; 7. b; 8. a; 9. d; 10. b

Chapter 4
1. c; 2. c; 3. b; 4. a; 5. d; 6. c; 7. b; 8. d; 9. a; 10. d

Chapter 5
1. c; 2. a; 3. d; 4. d; 5. b; 6. a; 7. c; 8. a; 9. d; 10. b

Chapter 6
1. d; 2. b; 3. b; 4. c; 5. a; 6. c; 7. d; 8. a; 9. c; 10. b

Chapter 7
1. c; 2. b; 3. a; 4. d; 5. a; 6. d; 7. c; 8. b; 9. c; 10. b

Chapter 8
1. b; 2. d; 3. a; 4. d; 5. c; 6. d; 7. b; 8. c; 9. a; 10. a

Chapter 9
1. c; 2. d; 3. a; 4. c; 5. b; 6. d; 7. a; 8. b; 9. c; 10. d

Chapter 10
1. c; 2. b; 3. d; 4. a; 5. b; 6. c; 7. a; 8. d; 9. d; 10. b

Chapter 11
1. a; 2. c; 3. d; 4. b; 5. c; 6. a; 7. a; 8. d; 9. b; 10. c

Chapter 12
1. b; 2. c; 3. d; 4. a; 5. a; 6. b; 7. c; 8. d; 9. c; 10. b

Chapter 13
1. d; 2. b; 3. a; 4. d; 5. a; 6. c; 7. b; 8. c; 9. d; 10. a

Chapter 14
1. a; 2. c; 3. d; 4. b; 5. c; 6. c; 7. d; 8. a; 9. b; 10. d

Chapter 15
1. c; 2. b; 3. d; 4. a; 5. b; 6. c; 7. a; 8. d; 9. b; 10. d

Chapter 16
1. a; 2. c; 3. d; 4. b; 5. c; 6. a; 7. d; 8. b; 9. c; 10. d

Chapter 17
1. d; 2. b; 3. c; 4. b; 5. a; 6. d; 7. c; 8. a; 9. c; 10. b

Chapter 18
1. b; 2. a; 3. d; 4. c; 5. c; 6. b; 7. d; 8. a; 9. c; 10. b

Chapter 19
1. d; 2. c; 3. b; 4. a; 5. b; 6. c; 7. b; 8. a; 9. d; 10. a

Almanac

Health Information on the Internet

Your Health Directory

Emergency!

A Consumer's Guide to Medical Tests

Counting Your Calories and Fat Grams

Health Information on the Internet

Using the Internet

The Internet: A Gateway to Health Information

What are the very latest statistics on the incidence of AIDS? Are any new drugs in the works for the treatment of diabetes? How can I get in touch with others who suffer from asthma? Is it possible to make a low-fat chocolate cake? You can answer these kinds of questions from your home or computer lab, with the help of the Internet. A gold mine of information for the student of health, the Internet can help you with research for your schoolwork and also with personal questions and concerns about your own health. But the Internet is not comprehensively catalogued, and finding information can be daunting. This guide will introduce you to health resources on the Internet and how to find them.

What are the practical uses of the Internet for the student of health and the health care consumer?

- **Educational resources.** Most colleges and universities now have Internet websites. Faculty often post course information and syllabi on line, and some courses are even offered entirely online. Some instructors require students to do tutorials, research, or other projects on the Internet. In addition, you may be able to get general information about policies, programs, graduation requirements, and faculty on your school's website.

- **Research.** The Internet is a repository for many health journals, government statistics, archives, and other sources of scholarly information. Subscribing to a mailing list or posting to a newsgroup in an area of interest can yield new sources of information that would be hard to get elsewhere.

- **Graduate school and career information.** The Internet is a great resource for those interested in a career in a health-related field. Most graduate schools have websites that list their programs, entrance requirements, faculty profiles, and other information of interest to prospective students. And once you get that degree you can consult online listings of jobs available in many areas of health care.

- **Self-help and support.** Dozens of newsgroups and mailing lists offer support and advice for people dealing with all kinds of health-related issues, from

Alzheimer's caregivers to people with eating disorders to athletes comparing training programs.

- **Goods and services.** Online shopping is easy. People with concerns about health can order books, software, or journals of interest, sign up for classes or conferences, or even get online professional consultations (though we're not recommending that).

The World Wide Web

The World Wide Web is an information retrieval system with a user-friendly graphic interface with the Internet. You can surf the Web using any one of a number of different programs called browsers, such as Netscape or Microsoft Explorer. Many websites offer audio, video, animation clips, and interactivity. Each website has its own unique address, or URL. To go to a website, type its URL into the box at the top of your browser or click on a hyperlink from another page that will take you to the new site. Hyperlinks often appear as color or underlined text and offer links to other websites.

Thousands of websites are related to health and wellness. As a starting point, go to any of the sources listed in the Sites & Bytes in this book or at this book's website at http://health.wadsworth.com. Or you can look for specific information by doing a web search.

Bookmarks

When you find a website you will want to return to again, "bookmark" it. To bookmark a site, go to that site and choose "bookmark" from your menu bar. Your browser will record the address of that site in your bookmark folder. Anytime you want to return to that site, you simply open the bookmark folder and click on the title of that website.

Tips for Using the World Wide Web

- **Be patient.** Accessing a website can take time depending on how elaborate the site is, how fast your modem can download the information, and what time of day you are surfing. You can speed things up a bit by turning off the "auto load image" option in your browser.

- **Keep in mind that glitches can occur in the transfer process.** Sometimes the server of the website you are trying to reach may be down, there may be a lot of activity on that site, or there may be line noise. Just try again to load the website, or try again later.

- **Sites and links change every day.** Some links on web pages go nowhere if the link has moved to a new server or address.

- **Remember that not everything on the web is true.** It is up to you to evaluate the information you get from the Web; see the section on Thinking Critically about Health Information on the Internet.

Searching the Web

One way to find websites of interest to you is to use a search engine. A search engine allows you to type in key words on the topic you are interested in, and it will retrieve sites that contain those words. Some of the larger and more popular search engines are:

- **Yahoo!**
  http://www.yahoo.com

- **AltaVista**
  http://www.altavista.com

- **Excite**
  http://www.excite.com

- **Lycos**
  http://www.lycos.go.com

- **WebCrawler**
  http://webcrawler.com

- **Google**
  http://www.google.com

To use a search engine, type in one of the URLs listed above. When the home page for the site comes up, type one or more key words or phrases into the "search" box. The engine will then search all the sites in its index and return a list to you, with hyperlinks and sometimes short descriptions, of those that contain your key words.

No single search engine contains all the contents of the Internet. After connecting to a search engine for the first time, it is a good idea to read the tool's description, search options, and rules and restrictions. Each engine offers a different "view" of the Web and you'll want to tailor your query to make the best use of that system. Some search engines contain indexes to huge amounts of online information, so it pays to make precise queries so you don't get thousands of sites returned to you. It is also possible to make queries that are too precise and retrieve no results.

The key to an effective search is picking the right key words. Commonly used words make poor search key words; try to find distinctive words or combinations of words. If you use several key words, separate them with one of these three operators: AND, OR, and NOT. Using the word AND actually narrows the results you obtain in a search. For example, if you search for "pregnancy AND teen," you will get back only sites that contain both these keywords. The word "OR" broadens the search results. You may try searching "pregnancy AND teen OR adolescent," to find sites that refer to teen or adolescent pregnancy. To limit your results, you can use the word NOT. Searching for "pregnancy AND teen NOT United States" might help you find sites that deal with teen pregnancy in other countries.

Your search may turn up hundreds or even thousands of results—or only a few. If you have more results than you can handle, try making the key words in your search more precise. See if you can think of words that uniquely identify what you are looking for, and use several relevant key words. If you have too few results, try another search engine, using synonyms or variations on your key words, or be less specific in your query.

News Groups/Discussion Forums

News groups and discussion forums are ways of discussing topics over the Internet with other people who share the same interests or concerns. They are a popular way to establish an online community, share information, and give and receive support. For example, a person suffering from a relatively rare disorder may not know anyone else with the same problems and concerns on campus or in town, but he or she can frequent a news group specifically for people with that disorder to learn about other peoples' experiences, the latest treatments, and just to commiserate. Or a person who is trying to quit smoking can participate in a news group to share frustrations, tips, and successes. But, as always, be aware that not everything posted to a news group is necessarily true; you must be a critical thinker.

Many commercial online services offer members-only news groups to their subscribers, but many other news groups are available to anyone. To find a news group on a topic of interest to you, try going to http://groups.google.com.

News group addresses are grouped into several broad categories called hierarchies. Listed below are some of the standard hierarchies that relate to health.

- **alt**
  groups generally alternative in nature (i.e., alt.sex)

- **bionet**
  groups discussing biology and biological sciences (i.e., bionet.immunology)

- **misc**
  groups that don't fit into other categories (i.e., misc.fitness)

- **rec**
  groups discussing hobbies, sports, music, and art (i.e., rec.food)

- **sci**
  groups discussing subjects related to the science and scientific research (i.e., sci.epidemiology)

- **soc**
  groups discussing social issues including politics, social programs, etc. (i.e., soc.college)

- **talk**
  public debating forums on controversial issues (i.e., talk.abortion)

Before you make a posting to a news group, you may want to "lurk" for awhile, that is, read the discussion without contributing your own posting. Lurking will give you a sense of the kinds of postings that are appropriate for that news group and what the news group culture is like. Read the news group's "FAQ," or list of answers to frequently asked questions before joining the discussion.

Postings to many news groups are updated frequently, so if an item is of interest to you, you should print it or save it to your computer since it may be gone the next day. After lurking for awhile, you can join in the discussion by posting a message to the news group. You may also want to reply only to the originator of a certain message. You may want to join in on the discussion of an already-existing topic, or start your own "thread."

Mailing Lists

Mailing lists (or listservs) are groups of people who "get together" via e-mail to discuss a specific topic. Mailing lists offer a way to participate in lively discussions, stay up on current research, or find out answers to burning questions. There are mailing lists on nearly every topic imaginable. Mailing lists are similar to news groups in that they are forums for discussion, but the messages are delivered to your e-mail account instead of to a public bulletin board. Here's how it works:

- First, find a mailing list dealing with a subject you are interested in discussing with others (i.e., attention deficit disorder).

- To get involved in a discussion group, you have to subscribe to it. To subscribe, send an e-mail to that mailing list's "subscribe" address with the word "subscribe" in the subject line and in the main body of the text. Also include your e-mail address.

- Usually, the listserv will then subscribe you to the list and send you instructions on how to "post" to the group. "Posting" means that you send out a comment to the entire mailing list that you have subscribed to.

- Every time any member posts to the listserv, all the subscribers get that posting as an e-mail message.

- Once you have subscribed you will begin to receive e-mail messages from the mailing list. Be careful though: Some discussion groups have a large following and you may find your mailbox filling up faster than you can read the messages.

- Again, evaluate carefully any information you get from a mailing list to make sure it is accurate.

Thinking Critically About Health Information on the Internet

Unlike information in most books and journals, anyone can post information or advice on the Internet. Some of this information can be misleading or downright harmful, so it is important to use your best critical thinking skills to evaluate health information you find on the Internet. Ask yourself the following questions:

- **Who is the author or sponsor of the information?** The author of the site is usually listed at the top or bottom of a site's home page. Be very wary of any anonymous site. Sites that are maintained by established schools or universities, government agencies, professional organizations, or other established organizations like the American Cancer Society are probably trustworthy. Sites created by individuals or other groups may or may not contain valid information; see if you can verify their information in other places. And keep in mind that many sites contain links to other pages which may be maintained by other less (or more) reliable sources.

- **Is it current?** Many sites post the date of their most recent modification. Look for sites where you can determine when the information was created or modified; many of the best sites are updated weekly or even daily.

- **What is the purpose of the site?** The hidden purpose of some health websites is to sell products or act as a vehicle for advertisements. Be wary of any site that tries to sell you things or get your money. Also beware of sites that seem to be trying to persuade you of things, promote "miracle cures" or anything that seems too good to be true. There are also people who use news groups and other chat forums to sell or persuade. Be skeptical and use your common sense.

- **Who is the intended audience?** Some Internet information is intended for doctors and other health-care professionals; although the information may be accurate, it may be too difficult for a layperson to interpret. Other websites or Internet forums are targeted toward people with specific problems or disorders, students, or the general public.

- **Is the information verifiable?** To get a better perspective on information from the Internet, see if you can verify it with other sources. Before you follow any health advice you get from the Net, check it out with your physician.

Health Resources on the Internet

"Your Health Directory" (next pages) contains web adresses for several health-related organizations. And hundreds of health-related Internet addresses can be found at http://health.wadsworth.com.

Your Health Directory

In *An Invitation to Health*, I emphasize that you shoulder a great deal of responsibility for your health and the quality of your life. Given the complexity of our minds and bodies and the many social and environmental factors that affect us, this responsibility can be a very heavy burden. But your load can be made lighter if you know where to turn for health information, services, and support.

In this directory, you will find more than 100 health-related topics and about 250 resources, including addresses, phone numbers, and websites for government agencies, community organizations, professional associations, recovery groups, and Internet sources. Many of these organizations and groups have toll-free 800 or 888 phone numbers, and most have websites (one caution: as you may have experienced, website addresses—like street addresses and phone numbers—change on occasion). Much of the material available from these groups is free.

Also included in Your Health Directory are clearinghouses and information centers that are especially rich sources of health knowledge. Their main purpose is to collect, help manage, and disseminate information. Clearinghouses often perform other services as well, such as creating original publications and providing tailored responses to individual requests. These organizations also may provide referrals to other groups that can help you.

Many of the groups listed here have local offices or chapters. You can call, write, or visit the websites of these organizations to find out if there is a branch in your vicinity, or you can check your local telephone directory.

The purpose of this directory is to help you be in control of your health. If you know where to turn for answers to your questions and if you know what choices you have, you may find that you have more control over your life.

Resources by Topic

▶ Abortion

National Abortion Federation
(provides information about abortion and referral for abortion services)
1755 Massachusetts Ave., N.W.
Suite #600
Washington, DC 20036
(202) 667-5881
(800) 772-9100
http://www.prochoice.org

▶ Accident Prevention

Centers for Disease Control and Prevention
1600 Clifton Rd. N.E.
Atlanta, GA 30333
(404) 639-3311
http://www.cdc.gov

National Safety Council
1121 Spring Lake Drive
Itasca, IL 60143-3201
(630) 285-1121
(800) 621-7619
http://www.nsc.org

▶ Adoption

AASK (Adopt a Special Kid)
(provides assistance to families who adopt older and handicapped children)
1025 N. Reynolds Rd.
Toledo, OH 43615
(419) 534-3350
http://www.adoptamerica.org

▶ Aging

Administration on Aging
U.S. Department of Health and Human Services
330 Independence Ave., S.W.
Washington, DC 20201
(800) 677-1116 (Eldercare Locator - to find services for an older person in his or her locality)
(202) 619-7501 (AoA's National Aging Information Center)
Fax: (202) 260-1012
E-mail: aoainfo@aoa.gov
http://www.aoa.gov

American Association of Retired Persons
601 E St., N.W.
Washington, DC 20049
(800) 424-3410
(202) 434-2277
http://aarp.org

Gray Panthers
733 15th St., N.W., Suite 437
Washington, DC 20005
(800) 280-5362
(202) 737-6637
http://graypanthers.org

▶ AIDS (Acquired Immunodeficiency Syndrome)

National Center for HIV, STD, and TB Prevention (NCHSTP)
Centers for Disease Control and Prevention
1600 Clifton Rd. N.E.
Atlanta, GA 30333
(800) 311-3435
(404) 639-3311
http://www.cdc.gov/hiv/dhap.htm

University of California at San Francisco AIDS Research Institute
74 New Montgomery, Suite 600
San Francisco, CA 94105
Campus Mail Box 0886
(415) 597-9203
Fax: (415) 597-9213
E-mail: ari@psg.ucsf.edu
http://hivinsite.ucsf.edu

Gay Men's Health Crisis
119 West 24th Street
New York, NY 10011
(212) 807-6664
http://www.gmhc.org

National AIDS Hotline
(800) 342-2437

San Francisco AIDS Foundation
995 Market Street
San Francisco, CA 94103
(415) 487-3000
http://www.sfaf.org

▌ Alcohol Abuse and Alcoholism

Al-Anon and Alateen
(support groups for friends and
    relatives of alcoholics)
281 Independence Blvd.
Virginia Beach, VA 23462
(757) 499-1443
http://www.al-anon-alateen.org
See also white pages of telephone
    directory for listing of local chapter

Alcohol Hotline
(800) ALCOHOL

Alcoholics Anonymous
307 Seventh Ave., 2nd Floor
New York, NY 10001
(212) 647-1680
http://alcoholics-anonymous.org
See also white pages or telephone
    directory for listing of local chapter

**National Association of Children
    of Alcoholics**
11426 Rockville Pike, Suite 100
Rockville, MD 20852
(888) 554-COAS (554-2627)
(301) 468-0985
http://health.org/nacoa

**National Clearinghouse for
    Alcohol and Drug Information**
P.O. Box 2345
Rockville, MD 20847-2345
(800) 729-6686
(301) 468-2600
http://www.health.org/index.htm

**National Institute on Alcohol
    Abuse and Alcoholism**
6000 Executive Blvd.
Willcom Building

Bethesda, MD 20892-7003
(301) 443-3860
http://www.niaaa.nih.gov
See also Drug Abuse; Drinking &
    Driving Groups

▌ Allopathic Medicine

American Medical Association
515 N. State Street
Chicago, Il 60610
(312) 464-5000
http://www.ama-assn.org

▌ Alternative Medicine

**National Center for
    Complementary and
    Alternative Medicine (NCCAM)**
P.O. Box 7923
Gaithersburg, Maryland 20898
(888) 644-6226
International: 301-519-3153
TTY: 1-866-464-3615 (toll-free)
http://nccam.nih.gov

▌ Alzheimer's Disease

**Alzheimer's Association
    National Office**
919 N. Michigan Ave., Suite 1000
Chicago IL 60611-1676
(800) 272-3900
(312) 335-8700
www.alz.org

▌ Arthritis

Arthritis Foundation
1330 West Peachtree St.
Atlanta, GA 30309
(800) 283-7800
(404) 872-7100
http://www.arthritis.org

**National Institute of Arthritis
    and Musculoskeletal
    and Skin Diseases**
National Institutes of Health
Bldg. 31, Rm. 4C05
Bethesda, MD 20892-2350
(301) 496-8188
(877) 22-NIAMS (226-4267)
E-mail: NIAMSInfo@mail.nih.gov
http://www.nih.gov/niams

▌ Asthma

**Asthma and Allergy Foundation
    of America**
1233 Twentieth St., N.W., Suite 402

Washington, DC 20036
(800) 7-ASTHMA (727-8462)
(202) 466-7643
Fax: (202) 466-8940
http://www.aafa.org

Lung Line
National Jewish Center for
    Immunology and Respiratory
    Medicine
(information and referral service)
1400 Jackson St.
Denver, CO 80206
(800) 222-5864
(303) 388-4461
http://www.njc.org

▌ Attention Deficit Disorder

**National Attention Deficit
    Disorder Association
    (National ADDA)**
1788 Second St., Suite 200
Highland Park, IL 60035
(847) 432-ADDA
http://www.add.org

**Children and Adults
    with Attention Deficit
    Disorder (CHADD)**
8181 Professional Place,
    Suite 201
Landover, MD 20785
(301) 306-7070
http://www.chadd.org/

▌ Automobile Safety

**American Automobile
    Association (AAA)**
1000 AAA Drive #28
Heathrow, FL 32746-5080
(407) 444-4240
http://www.aaa.com
See also white or yellow pages of
    telephone directory for listing of
    local chapter

**Insurance Institute
    for Highway Safety**
1005 North Glebe Rd., Suite 800
Arlington, VA 22201
(703) 247-1500
www.highwaysafety.org/

**National Highway Traffic Safety
    Administration**
Office of Publications

400 7th St., S.W.
Room 6123
Washington, DC 20590
(202) 366-02587
http://www.nhtsa.dot.gov

Auto Safety Hotline
(for consumer complaints about auto
    safety and child safety seats, and
    requests for information on recalls)
(800) 424-9393

▶ Birth Control and Family Planning

Advocates for Youth
(develops programs and material to
    educate youth on sex and sexual
    responsibility)
1025 Vermont Ave. N.W., Suite 200
Washington, DC 20005
(202) 347-5700
Fax: (202) 347-2263
E-mail: info@advocatesforyouth.org
www.advocatesforyouth.org

**American College of Obstetricians
    and Gynecologists**
(provides literature and
    contraceptive information)
409 12th Street, S.W.
P.O. Box 96920
Washington, DC 20090-6920
(202) 638-5577
http://www.acog.com

**Association for Voluntary
    Surgical Contraception (AVSC)**
(provides information and referrals
    to individuals considering tubal
    ligation or vasectomy)
440 Ninth Ave.
New York, NY 10001
(212) 561-8000

**Planned Parenthood Federation
    of America (PPFA)**
810 Seventh Ave.
New York, NY 10019
(212) 541-7800
http://www.plannedparenthood.org
See also white or yellow pages of
    telephone directory for listing of
    local chapter

▶ Birth Defects

Cystic Fibrosis Foundation (CFF)
6931 Arlington Rd.
Bethesda, MD 20814

(800) FIGHT-CF (344-4823)
(301) 951-4422
Fax: (301) 951-6378
http://www.cff.org

**March of Dimes Birth Defects
    Foundation**
1275 Mamaroneck Ave.
White Plains, NY 10605
(888) 663-4637
(914) 428-7100
http://www.modimes.org

▶ Blindness

American Foundation for the Blind
11 Penn Plaza, Suite 300
New York, NY 10001
(800) AFB-LINE (232-5463)
(212) 502-7661
http://www.afb.org

National Federation of the Blind
1800 Johnson St.
Baltimore, MD 21230
(800) 638-7518
(410) 659-9314
http://www.nfb.org

**National Library Service
    for the Blind and
    Physically Handicapped**
Library of Congress
1291 Taylor St., N.W.
Washington, DC 20011
(800) 424-8567
(202) 707-5100
http://www.loc.gov/nls

▶ Blood Banks

American Red Cross
11th Floor
1621 N. Kent St.
Arlington, VA 22209
(703) 248-4222
http://www.redcross.org
See also white or yellow pages of
    telephone directory for listing of
    local chapter

▶ Breast Cancer

Reach to Recovery
(support program for women who
    have undergone mastectomies as
    a result of breast cancer)
American Cancer Society
2200 Lake Blvd.
Atlanta, GA 30319

(800) ACS-2345 (227-2345)
(404) 816-7800
http://www2.cancer.org

▶ Cancer

American Cancer Society
American Cancer Society
2200 Lake Blvd.
Atlanta, GA 30319
(800) 227-2345
(404) 816-7800
http://www.cancer.org

Cancer Information Service
National Cancer Institute
31 Center Dr., MSC 2580
Building 31, Room 10A03
Bethesda, MD 20892-2580
(800) 4-CANCER (422-6237)
(301) 435-3848
http://www.nci.nih.gov/hpage/
    cis.htm

**Leukemia & Lymphoma Society
    of America**
1311 Mamaroneck Ave.
White Plains, NY 10605
(914) 949-5213
Fax: (914) 949-6691
http://www.leukemia.org

**National Coalition
    for Cancer Survivorship**
1010 Wayne Ave., Suite 770
Silver Spring, MD 20910-5600
(301) 650-9127
 (877) NCCS-YES (622-7937)
Fax: (301) 565-9670
http://www.cansearch.org

**R. A. Bloch Cancer Foundation
    (Cancer Connection)**
(support group that matches cancer
    patients with volunteers who are
    cured, in remission, or being
    treated for same type of cancer)
4400 Main St.
Kansas City, MO 64111
(800) 433-0464
(816) 932-8453
http://www.blochcancer.org

▶ Child Abuse

**National Child Assault
    Prevention**
(provides services to children,
    adolescents, mentally retarded
    adults, and elderly)

606 Delsea Drive
Sewell, NJ 08080
(800) 258-3189
(609) 582-7000
http://www.ncap.org

National Child Abuse Hotline
(800) 422-4453

**National Committee for the
Prevention of Child Abuse**
(provides literature on child abuse
prevention programs)
200 S. Michigan Ave., 17th Floor
Chicago, IL 60604-2404
(312) 663-3520
http://www.
preventchildabuse.org

Parents Anonymous
(self-help group for abusive
parents)
675 W. Foothill Blvd., Suite 220
Claremont, CA 91711-3475
(909) 621-6184
Fax: (909) 625-6304
http://www.
parentsanonymous-natl.org

▶ **Childbirth**

**American College
of Nurse-Midwives**
(R.N.s who provide services through
the maternity cycle)
818 Connecticut Ave., N.W.
Suite 900
Washington, DC 20006
(202) 728-9860
www.midwife.org

**American College of
Obstetricians and
Gynecologists**
409 12th St., S.W.
P.O. Box 96920
Washington, DC 20090-6920
(202) 638-5577
http://www.acog.com

Lamaze International
2025 M St., Suite 800
Washington DC 20036-3309
(202) 367-1128
(800) 368-4404
Fax: (202) 367-2128
http://www.lamaze-
childbirth.com

**International Childbirth
Education Association**
P.O. Box 20048
Minneapolis, MN 55420
(952) 854-8660
Fax: (952) 854-8772
http://www.icea.org

▶ **Child Health
and Development**

**National Center for Education in
Maternal and Child Health**
2000 15th St., N.
Suite 701
Arlington, VA 22201
(703) 524-7802

**National Institute of Child
Health & Human
Development**
Bldg. 31, Rm. 2A32, MSC 2425
31 Center Drive
Bethesda, MD 20892-2425
(800) 370-2943
http://www.nichd.nih.gov

▶ **Chiropractic**

**American Chiropractic
Association**
1701 Clarendon Blvd.
Arlington, VA 22209
(800) 986-4632
Fax: (703) 243-2593
http://www.amerchiro.org

▶ **Consumer Information**

**Federal Consumer Information
Center**
(catalog of publications developed by
federal agencies for consumers)
Department WWW
Pueblo, CO 81009
(888) 878-3256
http://www.pueblo.gsa.gov

**U.S. Consumer Product Safety
Commission**
Office of Information Services
4330 East-West Highway
Bethesda, MD 20814-4408
(800) 638-2772
(301) 504-0990
Fax: (301) 504-0124 and
(301) 504-0025
E-mail: info@cpsc.gov
http://www.cpsc.gov

**Consumers Union of Untied
States**
(tests quality and safety of
consumer products: publishes
Consumer Reports magazine)
101 Truman Ave.
Yonkers, NY 10703
(914) 378-2000
http://www.
consumerreports.org

**Council of Better Business
Bureaus**
4200 Wilson Blvd., Suite 800
Arlington, VA 22203-1804
(703) 276-0100
Fax: (703) 525-8277
http://www.bbb.org
See also white or yellow pages of
telephone directory for listing of
local chapter

**Food and Drug
Administration (FDA)**
Office of Consumer Affairs
Consumer Inquiries
5600 Fishers Lane (HFE-88)
Rockville, MD 20857
(888) INFO-FDA (463-6332)
http://www.fda.gov

▶ **Crime Victims**

**Crisis Prevention
Institute, Inc.**
(offers programs on nonviolent
physical crisis interventions)
3315-K North 124th St.
Brookfield, WI 53005
(800) 558-8976 (US and Canada)
(262) 783-5787
http://www.crisisprevention.com

**National Association for Crime
Victims Rights (NACVR)**
P.O. Box 16161
Portland, OR 97292
(503) 252-9012

▶ **Death and Grieving**

Share
(support group for parents who have
suffered loss of newborn baby)
c/o St. John's Hospital
800 E. Carpenter St.
Springfield, IL 62769
(217) 544-6464

Dental Health

American Dental Association (ADA)
211 E. Chicago Ave.
Chicago, IL 60611
(312) 440-2500
http://www.ada.org

National Institute of Dental Research
Office of Communication
9000 Rockville Pike
Bldg. 31, Rm. 2C35
Bethesda, MD 20892-2190
(301) 496-4251
http://www.nidr.nih.gov

Depressive Disorders

American Psychiatric Association
1400 K St., N.W.
Washington, DC 20005
(202) 682-6000
(888) 357-7924
Fax: (202) 682-6850
E-mail: apa@psych.org
http://www.psych.org

American Psychological Association
750 First St., N.E.
Washington, DC 20002-4242
(202) 336-5510
(800) 374-2721
TDD/TTY: (202) 336-6123
http://www.apa.org

National Depressive and Manic-Depressive Association (NDMA)
730 N. Franklin, Suite 501
Chicago, IL 60610-3526
(312) 642-0049
(800) 826-3632
Fax: (312) 642-7243
http://www.ndmda.org

DES (Diethylstibestrol)

DES Action, USA
(support group for persons exposed to DES)
1615 Broadway, Suite 510
Oakland, CA 94612
(510) 465-4011
Fax: (510) 465-4815
http://www.desaction.org

Diabetes

American Diabetes Association
National Center
1701 North Beauregard St.
Alexandria, VA 22311
(800) DIABETES (342-2383)
(703) 549-1500
http://www.diabetes.org

Juvenile Diabetes Research Foundation International (JDRFI)
120 Wall St.
New York, NY 10005-4001
(800) JDF-CURE (533-2873)
(212) 785-9500
Fax: (212) 785-9595
http://www.jdfcure.org

National Diabetes Information Clearinghouse
1 Information Way
Bethesda, MD 20892-3560
(301) 654-3327
(800) 860-8747
E-mail: ndic@info.niddk.nih.gov
http://www.niddk.nih.gov/health/diabetes/ndic.htm

Digestive Diseases

National Institute of Diabetes & Digestive & Kidney Diseases (NIDDK)
2 Information Way
Bethesda, MD 20892-3570
(301) 654-3810
www.niddk.nih.gov

Disabled Services

American Alliance for Health, Physical Education, Recreation & Dance (AAHPERD)
(provides information about recreation and fitness opportunities for the disabled)
1900 Association Drive
Reston, VA 20191
(800) 213-7193
Fax: (703) 476-9527
http://www.aahperd.org

National Library Service for the Blind and Physically Handicapped
Library of Congress
1291 Taylor St., N.W.

Washington, D.C. 20011
(800) 424-8567
(202) 707-5100
TDD: (202) 707-0744
Fax: (202) 707-0712
http://www.loc.gov/nls

Special Olympics International (SOI)
1325 G St., N.W.
Suite 500
Washington, DC 20005
(202) 628-3630
Fax: (202) 824-0200
http://www.specialolympics.org

Domestic Violence

National Coalition Against Domestic Violence (NCADV)
P.O. Box 18749
Denver, CO 80218
(303) 839-1852
Fax: (303) 831-9851
www.ncadv.org

National Domestic Violence Hotline
(800) 799-SAFE (799-7233)

National Network to End Domestic Violence
701 Pennsylvania, N.W., Suite 900
Washington, DC 20004
(202) 347-9520

Down Syndrome

National Association for Down Syndrome (NADS)
P.O. Box 4542
Oak Brook, IL 60522-4542
(630) 325-9112
http://www.nads.org

National Down Syndrome Society
666 Broadway, 8th Floor
New York, NY 10012-2317
(800) 221-4602
(212) 460-9330
http://www.ndss.org

Drug Abuse

Cocaine Anonymous World Services
P.O. Box 2000
Los Angeles, CA 90049-8000 or
3740 Overland Ave., Ste. C

Los Angeles, CA 90034
(800) 347-8998
(310) 559-5833
http://www.ca.org

Narcotics Anonymous (NA)
(support group for recovering
   narcotics addicts)
P.O. Box 9999
Van Nuys, CA 91409
(818) 773-9999
Fax: (818) 700-0700
http://www.wsoinc.com
See also white or yellow pages of
   telephone directory for local
   chapter

National Cocaine Hotline
(800) COCAINE (262-2463)

**National Institute
   on Drug Abuse**
6001 Executive Blvd.
Bethesda, MD 20892-9651
(301) 443-1124
Helpline: (800) 662-4357
http://www.nida.nih.gov

**National Parents Resource
   Institute for Drug Education
   (PRIDE)**
4684 S. Evergreen
Newaygo, MI 49337
(231) 652-4400
(800) 668-9277
Fax: (231) 652-2461
http://www.prideusa.org

Substance Abuse Prevention
Alcohol, Drug Abuse, and Mental
   Health Administration
5600 Fishers Lane
Rockwall 2 Building
Rockville, MD 20857
(301) 443-0365

▶ **Drinking
   and Driving Groups**

Mothers Against Drunk Driving
P.O. Box 541688
Dallas, TX 75354-1688
(800) GET-MADD (438-6233)
http://www.madd.org
See also white or yellow pages of
   telephone directory for local
   chapter

**Students Against Destructive
   Decisions (also Students
   Against Driving Drunk (SADD)**
P.O. Box 800
Marlboro, MA 01752
(508) 481-3568
Fax: (508) 481-5759
www.saddonline.com

▶ **Eating Disorders**

**National Eating Disorders
   Association**
(self-help groups that provide
   information and referrals to
   physicians and therapists)
165 West 46th St., #1108
New York, NY 10036
(212) 575-6200
www.NationalEatingDisorders.org

**Anorexia Nervosa and Related
   Eating Disorders (ANRED)**
(provides information and referrals
   for people with eating disorders)
P.O. Box 5102
Eugene, OR 97405
(800) 931-2237
(541) 344-1144
http://www.anred.com

▶ **Environment**

**U.S. Environmental Protection
   Agency (EPA)**
Ariel Rios Building
1200 Pennsylvania Ave., N.W.
Washington, DC 20460
(202) 260-2090
http://www.epa.gov

Greenpeace, USA
702 H St. N.W.
Washington, DC 20001
(800) 326-0959
(202) 462-1177
http://www.greenpeaceusa.org

**Natural Resources Defense
   Council**
40 West 20th St.
New York, NY 10011
(212) 727-2700
Fax: (212) 727-1773
http://www.nrdc.org

Sierra Club
85 2nd St., 2nd Floor
San Francisco, CA 94105-3441

(415) 977-5500
(415) 977-5799
http://www.sierraclub.org

World Wildlife Fund
1250 24th St., N.W.
P.O. Box 97180
Washington, DC 20077-7180
(800) CALL-WWF (225-5993)
(202) 293-4800
Fax: (202) 293-2911
http://www.wwfus.org

▶ **Epilepsy**

**Epilepsy Foundation
   of America**
4351 Garden City Drive
Landover, MD 20785-2267
(800) EFA-1000 (332-1000)
(301) 459-3700
http://www.efa.org

▶ **Gay and Lesbian
   Organizations
   and Services**

Human Rights Campaign
919 18th St.
Washington, DC 20006
(202) 628-4160
Fax: (202) 347-5323
http://www.hrc.org

**National Gay and Lesbian Task
   Force (NGLTF)**
1700 Kalorama Rd., N.W.
Washington, DC 20009-2624
(202) 332-6483
Fax: (202) 332-0207
http://www.ngltf.org

**Parents, Families, and Friends of
   Lesbians and Gays (PFLAG)**
1726 M St., N.W. Suite 400
Washington, DC 20036
(202) 467-8180
Fax: (202) 467-8194
http://www.pflag.org

▶ **Genetics**

**American College of Medical
   Genetics**
9650 Rockville Pike
Bethesda, MD 20814-3998
(301) 530-7127
Fax: (301) 571-0677
E-mail: acmg@faseb.org
http://www.acmg.net

The Human Genome Organization
HUGO Americas
Laboratory of Genetics
National Institute on Aging
NIH/NIA-IRP. GRC, Box 31
5600 Nathan Shock Drive
Baltimore, MD 21224-6825
(410) 558-8337
Fax: (410) 558-8331
E-mail: schlessingerd@grc.nia.
nih.gov

GeneTests—GeneClinics
(a database of information for
patients and families with
genetic disorders, providing
access to support groups)
University of Washington School
of Medicine
Seattle, WA
http://www.genetests.org

Hazardous Waste

Environmental Protection Agency (EPA)
Ariel Rios Building
1200 Pennsylvania Ave., N.W.
Washington, DC 20460
(202) 260-2090
http://www.epa.gov

Hazardous Waste Hotline Information
(800) 424-9346

Health Care

Association for Applied and Therapeutic Humor (AATH)
(publishes a newsletter and
sponsors seminars for people in
the helping professions)
1951 W. Camelback Rd., Suite 445
Phoenix, AZ 85015
http://www.aath.org

American Medical Association
515 N. State St.
Chicago, IL 60610
(312) 464-5000
http://www.ama-assn.org

American Nurses Association
600 Maryland Ave., S.W.
Suite 100 West
Washington, DC 20024-2571
(800) 274-4ANA (274-4262)

(202) 651-7000
http://www.ana.org

Health Education

National Center for Chronic Disease Prevention and Health Promotion
Centers for Disease Control and
Prevention
Mail Stop A34
1600 Clifton Rd., N.E.
Atlanta, GA 30333
(404) 639-3534
(800) 311-3435
http://www.cdc.gov/nccdphp

Hearing Impairment

American Society for Deaf Children
(resource group for parents of
hard of hearing and deaf
children)
P.O. Box 3355
Gettysburg, PA 17325
(717) 334-7922
Fax: (717) 334-8808
(800) 942-ASDC (Parent Hotline)
www.deafchildren.org

Better Hearing Institute (BHI)
(provides educational and resource
materials on deafness)
Better Hearing Institute
515 King St., Suite 420
Alexandria, VA 22314
Phone: (703) 684-3391
http://www.betterhearing.org

Heart Disease

American Heart Association (AHA)
7272 Greenville Ave.
Dallas, TX 75231
(800) 242-8721
(214) 373-6300
http://www.americanheart.org

National Heart, Lung, and Blood Institute
(provides information on
cardiovascular risk factors and
disease)
4733 Bethesda Ave., Suite 530
Bethesda, MD 20814
(800) 575-9355
http://www.nhlbi.nih.gov/index.htm

Helping Others

United Way of America
701 N. Fairfax St.
Alexandria, VA 22314-2045
(703) 836-7100
http://www.unitedway.org

Hospice

The National Hospice and Palliative Care Organization
1700 Diagonal Rd., Suite 300
Alexandria, VA 22314
(703) 837-1500
http://www.nhpco.org

Immunization

National Center for Prevention Services
Centers for Disease Control
1600 Clifton Rd., N.E.
Atlanta, GA 30333
(404) 639-3311
(800) 311-3435
http://www.cdc.gov/nip/diseases/
adult-vpd.htm

Immunization Action Coalition
(information for children,
adolescents, and adults)
1573 Selby Ave., Suite 234
St. Paul, MN 55104
(651) 647-9009
Fax: (651) 647-9131
http://www.immunize.org

Infant Care

American Red Cross
1621 N. Kent St., 11th Floor
Arlington, VA 22209
(703) 248-4222
E-mail: info@usa.redcross.org.
http://www.redcross.org/services/
youth/kids/

La Leche League International
(provides information and support
to women interested in breast-
feeding)
1400 N. Meacham Rd.
Schaumburg, IL 60168-4079
(800) LA-LECHE (525-3243)
(847) 519-7730
http://www.lalecheleague.org

Infectious Diseases

Centers for Disease Control and Prevention
1600 Clifton Rd., N.E.
Atlanta, GA 30333
(404) 639-3534
http://www.cdc.gov

Infertility

Resolve: The National Infertility Association
(offers counseling, information, and support to people with problems of infertility)
1310 Broadway
Somerville, MA 02144-1779
(617) 623-0744
http://www.resolve.org

Kidney Disease

American Kidney Fund (AKF)
(provides information on financial aid to patients, organ transplants, and kidney-related diseases)
6110 Executive Blvd., Suite 1010
Rockville, MD 20852
(800) 638-8299
(301) 881-3052
http://www.akfinc.org

American Association of Kidney Patients (AAKP)
100 S. Ashley Dr., Suite 280
Tampa, FL 33602-5346
(800) 749-2257
Fax: (813) 223-0001
http://www.aakp.org

National Kidney Foundation (NKF)
30 East 33rd St., Suite 1100
New York, NY 10016
(800) 622-9010
(212) 889-2210
Fax: (212) 689-9261
http://www.kidney.org

Liver Disease

American Liver Foundation (ALF)
75 Maiden, Suite 603
New York, NY 10038
(800) 465-4837
www.liverfoundation.org/

Lung Disease

American Lung Association
1740 Broadway
New York, NY 10019
(212) 315-8700
http://lungusa.org

National Heart, Lung, and Blood Institute
(provides information on cardiovascular risk factors and disease)
4733 Bethesda Ave., Suite 530
Bethesda, MD 20814
(800) 575-9355
http://www.nhlbi.nih.gov/index.htm

Lupus Erythematosus

Lupus Foundation of America (LPA)
1300 Piccard Drive, Suite 200
Rockville, MD 20850-4303
(301) 670-9292
(800) 558-0121
http://www.lupus.org/lupus/index.html

Marriage and Family

Women Work! The National Network for Women's Employment
(national advocacy group for women over 35 who have lost their primary means of support through death, divorce, or disabling of spouse)
1625 K St. N.W., Suite 300
Washington, DC 20006
(202) 467-6346

Alliance for Children & Families
11700 West Lake Park Drive
Milwaukee, WI 53224-3099
(414) 359-1040
Fax: (414) 359-1074
E-mail: info@alliance1.org
http://www.alliance1.org

Stepfamily Association of America
(provides information and publishes quarterly newsletter)
650 J St., Suite 205
Lincoln, NE 68508
(402) 477-7837
(800) 735-0329
Fax: (402) 477-8317
http://www.stepfam.org

Medications

(Prescriptions and Over-the-Counter)

Food and Drug Administration (FDA)
Office of Consumer Affairs Public Inquiries
5600 Fishers Lane (HFE-88)
Rockville, MD 20857-0001
(888) 463-6332 (INFO-FDA)
http://www.fda.gov

Mental Health

American Psychiatric Association
1400 K St., N.W.
Washington, DC 20005
(202) 682-6000
(888) 357-7924
Fax: (202) 682-6850
E-mail: apa@psych.org
http://www.psych.org

American Psychological Association
750 First St., N.E.
Washington, DC 20002-4242
(202) 336-5510
(800) 374-2721
TDD/TTY: (202) 336-6123
http://www.apa.org

American Psychoanalytic Foundation
1636 Connecticut Ave., N.W.
2nd Floor
Washington, DC 20009
(202) 667-6363
Fax: (202) 667-4477
E-mail: APF@cyberpsych.org
http://www.cyberpsych.org/apf

National Alliance for the Mentally Ill (NAMI)
(self-help advocacy organization for persons with schizophrenia and depressive disorders and their families)
Colonial Place Three
2107 Wilson Blvd., Suite 300
Arlington, VA 22201
(703) 524-7600
HelpLine: (800) 950-NAMI (950-6264)
www.nami.org/

National Institute of Mental Health
Information Resources and Inquiries Branch
6001 Executive Blvd., Rm. 8184
MSC 9663
Bethesda, MD 20892-9663
(301) 443-4513
Fax: (301) 443-4279
TTY: (301) 443-8431
E-mail: nimhinfo@nih.gov
http://www.nimh.nih.gov/

National Mental Health Association (NMHA)
1021 Prince St.
Alexandria, VA 22314-2971
(800) 969-NMHA (969-6642)
(703) 684-7722
Fax: (703) 684-5968
http://www.nmha.org

Mental Retardation

Association for Retarded Citizens (ARC)
1010 Wayne Ave., Suite 650
Silver Spring, MD 20910
(301) 565-3842
E-mail: info@thearc.org
http://www.thearc.org

Missing and Runaway Children

Child Find of America
(800) I-AM-LOST (426-5678)
Runaway Hotline
(800) 621-4000

National Center for Missing and Exploited Children (NCMEC)
699 Prince St., Suite 550
Alexandria, VA 22314
(703) 274-3900
Fax: (703) 274-2200
24-hour Hotline:
(800) THE-LOST (843-5678)
http://www.missingkids.org

Neurological Disorders

National Institute of Neurological Disorders and Stroke
National Institutes of Health
31 Center Drive, Rm. 8A18
Bethesda, MD 20892-2540
(301) 496-5751

(800) 352-9424
Fax: (301) 402-2186
E-mail: braininfo@ninds.nih.gov
http://www.ninds.nih.gov

Nutrition

American Dietetic Association
216 West Jackson Blvd.
Chicago, IL 60606-6995
(312) 899-0040
http://www.eatright.org

American Society for Nutritional Sciences
9650 Rockville Pike, Suite 4500
Bethesda, MD 20814-3990
(301) 530-7050
Fax: (301) 571-1892
http://www.faseb.org/ain

Food and Drug Administration (FDA)
Office of Consumer Affairs
Public Inquiries
5600 Fishers Lane (HFE-88)
Rockville, MD 20857
(888) 463-6332 (INFO-FDA)
http://www.fda.gov

Food and Nutrition Information Center
U.S. Dept. of Agriculture
National Agricultural Library
10301 Baltimore Ave.
Beltsville, MD 20705-2351
(301) 504-5719
Fax: (301) 504-6409
TTY: (301) 504-6856
E-mail:fnic@nal.usda.gov
http://www.nal.usda.gov/fnic

Center for Nutrition in Sport and Human Performance
206A Chenoweth Lab
University of Massachusetts
Amherst, MA 01002
(413) 545-1076
Fax: (413) 545-1074
E-mail: volpe@nutrition.umass.edu
http://www.umass.edu/cnshp/

National Dairy Council
10255 W. Higgins Rd., Suite 900
Rosemont, IL 60018-5616
(800) 426-8271
www.nationaldairycouncil.org

Occupational Safety and Health

Occupational Safety and Health Administration (OSHA)
U.S. Dept. of Labor
Office of Public Affairs, Rm. N3647
200 Constitution Ave.
Washington, DC 20210
(202) 693-1999
(800) 321-OSHA (6742)
TTY: (877) 889-5627
http://www.osha.gov

Organ Donations

The Living Bank (TLB)
(provides information and acts as registry and referral service for people wanting to donate organs for research or transplantation)
P.O. Box 6725
Houston, TX 77265
(800) 528-2971

Osteopathic Medicine

American Osteopathic Association (AOA)
142 East Ontario St.
Chicago, IL 60611
(800) 621-1773
Fax: (312) 202-8200
E-mail: info@aoa-net.org
http://www.aoa-net.org

Parent Support Groups

National Organization of Mothers of Twins Clubs (NOMOTC)
P.O. Box 438
Thompson Station, TN 37179-0438
(615) 595-0936
(877) 540-2200
www.nomotc.org

Parents Anonymous
(self-help group for abusive parents)
675 W. Foothill Blvd., Suite 220
Claremont, CA 91711-3475
(909) 621-6184
Fax: (909) 625-6304
E-mail: parentsanonymous@ parentsanonymous.org
http://www.parentsanonymous.org

Parents Without Partners, Inc.
1650 South Dixie Highway, Suite 510
Boca Raton, FL 33432

(561) 391-8833
Fax: (561) 395-8557
E-mail: pwp@jti.net
www.parentswithoutpartners.org

▶ Parenting

National Parent Information Network
National Library of Education
400 Maryland Ave., S.W.
Washington, DC 20202
(800) 424-1616
Fax: (202) 401-0552
http://www.npin.org

▶ Phobias

Anxiety Disorders Association of America (ADAA)
(provides information about phobias and referrals to therapists and support groups)
11900 Parklawn Drive, Suite 100
Rockville, MD 20852
(301) 231-9350
http://www.adaa.org

TERRAP Programs
(headquarters for national network of treatment clinics for agoraphobia)
932 Evelyn St.
Menlo Park, CA 94025
(415) 327-1312
(800) 2-PHOBIA (274-6242)
www.terrap.com

▶ Physical Fitness

See local yellow and white pages of telephone directory for listing of local health clubs and YMCAs, YWCAs, and Jewish Community Centers

Cooper Institutes for Aerobics Research
12330 Preston Rd.
Dallas, TX 75230
(972) 341-3200
Fax: (972) 341-3227
E-mail: courses@cooperinst.org
www.cooperinst.org

President's Council on Physical Fitness and Sports
200 Independence Ave., S.W.
H. H. Humphrey Bldg., Room 738 H

Washington, DC 20201
(202) 690-9000

American College of Sports Medicine
ACSM National Center
P.O. Box 1440
Indianapolis, IN 46206-1440
(317) 395-8557
http://www.acsm.org

Center for Nutrition in Sport and Human Performance
206A Chenoweth Lab
University of Massachusetts
Amherst, MA 01002
(413) 545-1076
Fax: (413) 545-1074
E-mail: volpe@nutrition.umass.edu
http://www.umass.edu/cnshp/

▶ Poisoning

See emergency numbers listed in the front of your local phone directory

National Poison Hotline
(800) 962-1253

▶ Pregnancy

National Institute of Child Health & Human Development
Bldg. 31, Rm. 2A32, MSC 2425
31 Center Drive
Bethesda, MD 20892-2425
(800) 370-2943
http://www.nichd.nih.gov

▶ Product Safety

U.S. Consumer Product Safety Commission
4330 East-West Highway
Bethesda, MD 20814-4408
(800) 638-CPSC (638-2772)
http://www.cpsc.gov

▶ Radiation Control and Safety

Center for Devices and Radiological Health
U.S. Food and Drug Administration
Office of Consumer Affairs
5600 Fishers Lane HFC-210
Rockville, MD 20850

(301) 443-6220
http://www.fda.gov/cdrh/index.html

National Institute of Environmental Health Sciences
National Institutes of Health
P.O. Box 12233
Research Triangle Park, NC 27709
(919) 541-3345
http://www.niehs.nih.gov

▶ Rape, Victimization

See white pages of telephone directory for listing of local rape crisis and counseling centers

National Center for Victims of Crime
2000 M St., N.W., Suite 480
Washington, DC 20036
(202) 467-8700
Fax: (202) 467-8701
http://www.ncvc.org

National Coalition Against Sexual Assault
912 N. 2nd St.
Harrisburg, PA 17102
(717) 232-6745

National Organization for Victim Assistance (NOVA)
1730 Park Rd. N.W.
Washington, DC 20010
(202) 232-6683
Fax: (202) 462-2255
http://www.try-nova.org

National Sexual Violence Resource Center
123 North Enola Drive
Enola, PA 17025
(877) 739-3895
(717) 909-0710
Fax: (717) 909-0714
TTY: (717) 909-0715
E-mail: resources@nsvrc.org
http://www.nsvrc.org

▶ Reye's Syndrome

National Reye's Syndrome Foundation
426 North Lewis
P.O. Box 829
Bryan, OH 43506-0829
(800) 233-7393 (U.S. only)
(419) 636-2679

Fax: (419) 636-9897
E-mail: nrsf@reyessyndrome.org
www.reyessyndrome.org

Self-Care/Self-Help

National Self-Help Clearinghouse (NSHC)
(provides information about self-help groups)
365 5th Ave., Suite 3300
New York, NY 10016
(212) 354-8525
http://selfhelpweb.org

Sex Education

American Association of Sex Educators, Counselors and Therapists (AASECT)
P.O. Box 5488
Richmond, VA 23220-0488
E-mail: AASECT@mediaone.net
http://www.aasect.org

Advocates for Youth
(develops programs and material to educate youth on sex and sexual responsibility)
1025 Vermont Ave. N.W., Suite 200
Washington, DC 20005
(202) 347-5700
Fax: (202) 347-2263
E-mail: info@advocatesforyouth.org
www.advocatesforyouth.org

Planned Parenthood Federation of America (PPFA)
810 Seventh Ave.
New York, NY 10019
(212) 541-7800
http://www.
plannedparenthood.org

Sexuality Information and Education Council of the U.S. (SIECUS)
(maintains an information clearinghouse on all aspects of human sexuality)
130 West 42nd St., Suite 350
New York, NY 10036-7802
(212) 819-9770
Fax: (212) 819-9776
E-mail: siecus@siecus.org
http://www.siecus.org

Sexual Abuse and Assault

National Center for Assault Prevention
(provides services to children, adolescents, mentally retarded adults, and elderly)
606 Delsea Drive
Sewell, NJ 08080
(856) 582-7000
(800) 258-3189

National Committee for Prevention of Child Abuse
200 S. Michigan Ave., Suite 1700
Chicago, IL 60604
(312) 663-3520

Sexually Transmitted Diseases

Centers for Disease Control and Prevention
1600 Clifton Rd. N.E.
Atlanta, GA 30333
(404) 639-3311
http://www.cdc.gov

American Social Health Association
P.O. Box 13827
Research Triangle Park, NC 27709
(919) 361-8400
Fax: (919) 361-8425
http://www.ashastd.org

Herpes Resource Center
American Social Health Association
P.O. Box 13827
Research Triangle Park, NC 27709-3827
(919) 361-8488
http://www.ashastd.org/hrc/index.html

National STD Hotline
(800) 227-8922

Sexuality Information and Education Council of the U.S. (SIECUS)
(maintains an information clearinghouse on all aspects of human sexuality)
130 West 42nd St., Suite 350
New York, NY 10036-7802
(212) 819-9770

Fax: (212) 819-9776
E-mail: siecus@siecus.org
http://www.siecus.org

Sickle-Cell Disease

Sickle Cell Disease Association of America
200 Corporate Pointe, Suite 495
Culver City, CA 90230-7633
(310) 216-6363
(800) 421-8453
http://sicklecelldisease.org

The Sickle Cell Information Center
The Georgia Comprehensive Sickle Cell Center—Emory School of Medicine
P.O. Box 109, Grady Memorial Hospital, 80 Butler St. S.E.
Atlanta, GA 30303
(404) 616-3572
Fax: (404) 616-5998
E-mail: aplatt@emory.edu
http://www.emory.edu/PEDS/SICKLE

Skin Diseases

American Academy of Dermatology
930 N. Meacham Rd.
P.O. Box 4014
Schaumburg, IL 60168-4014
(847) 330-0230
Fax: (847) 330-0050
http://www.aad.org

University of Iowa Hospitals and Clinics
Department of Dermatology
200 Hawkins Drive BT 2045-1
Iowa City, IA 52242-1090
(319) 356-7500 (appointments only)
(319) 356-2274 (business only)
Fax: (319) 356-8317 (business only)
http://tray.dermatology.uiowa.edu

National Psoriasis Foundation
6600 SW 92nd Ave., Suite 300
Portland, OR 97223-7195
(503) 244-7404
(800) 723-9166
Fax: (503) 245-0626
getinfo@npfusa.org
http://www.psoriasis.org

Sleep and Sleep Disorders

American Sleep Apnea Association
1424 K St. N.W., Suite 302
Washington, DC 20005
(202) 293-3650
Fax: (202) 293-3656
E-mail: asaa@sleepapnea.org
http://www.sleepapnea.org

American Academy of Sleep Medicine
6301 Bandel Rd., N.W., Suite 101
Rochester, MN 55901
(507) 287-6006
Fax: (507) 287-6008
http://www.asda.org

Better Sleep Council
501 Wythe St.
Alexandria, VA 22314
(703) 683-8371
www.bettersleep.org/

National Sleep Foundation
1522 K St., N.W., Suite 500
Washington, DC 20005
(202) 347-3471
Fax: (202) 347-3472
http://www.sleepfoundation.org

Smoking and Tobacco

Action on Smoking and Health (ASH)
(provides information on nonsmokers' rights and related subjects)
2013 H St., N.W.
Washington, DC 20006
(202) 659-4310
http://ash.org

American Cancer Society
(provides information about quitting smoking and smoking cessation programs)
2200 Lake Blvd.
Atlanta, GA 30319
(800) 227-2345
(404) 816-7800
http://www.cancer.org

American Heart Association
(provides information about quitting smoking and smoking cessation programs)

7272 Greenville Ave.
Dallas, TX 75231
(800) 242-8721
(214) 373-6300
http://www.americanheart.org

American Lung Association
(provides information about quitting smoking and smoking cessation programs)
432 Park Ave., South, 8th Floor
New York, NY 10016
(800) LUNG-USA (586-4872)
(212) 889-3370
http://www.lungusa.org

Americans for Nonsmokers' Rights
2530 San Pablo Ave., Suite J
Berkeley, CA 94702
(510) 841-3032
Fax: (510) 841-3060
E-mail: anr@no-smoke.org
http://www.no-smoke.org

Stress Reduction

American Institute of Stress
124 Park Ave.
Yonkers, NY 10703
(914) 963-1200
Fax: (914) 965-6267
E-mail: stress124@earthlink.net
http://www.stress.org

American Psychological Association
750 First St., N.E.
Washington, DC 20002-4242
(202) 336-5510
(800) 374-2721
TDD/TTY: 202-336-6123
http://www.apa.org

Association for Applied Psychophysiology and Biofeedback
10200 W. 44th Ave., Suite 304
Wheat Ridge, CO 80033
www.aapb.org

Stroke

Council on Stroke
American Heart Association
7272 Greenville Ave.
Dallas, TX 75231
(214) 373-6300
www.americanheart.org

National Institute of Neurological Disorders and Stroke
National Institutes of Health
P.O. Box 5801
Bethesda, MD 20824
(301) 496-4000
www.ninds.nih.gov/

Stuttering

National Center for Stuttering
200 East 33rd St.
New York, NY 10016
Hotline: (800) 221-2483
(212) 532-1460
http://www.stuttering.com

Sudden Infant Death Syndrome (SIDS)

SIDS Alliance
(provides information and referrals to families who have lost an infant because of SIDS)
1314 Bedford Ave., Suite 210
Baltimore, MD 21208
(800) 221-7437
(410) 653-8226
Fax: (410) 653-8709
E-mail: info@sidsalliance.org
www.sidsalliance.org

Suicide Prevention

American Association of Suicidology (AAS)
4201 Connecticut Ave., N.W., Suite 408
Washington, DC 20008
(202) 237-2280
National Hopeline: 1-800-SUICIDE
Fax: (202) 237-2282
E-mail: ajkulp@suicidology.org
http://www.suicidology.org

American Psychoanalytic Foundation
1636 Connecticut Ave., N.W., 2nd Floor
Washington, DC 20009
(202) 667-6363
Fax: (202) 667-4477
E-mail: APF@cyberpsych.org
http://www.cyberpsych.org/apf

Terminal Illness

Make-A-Wish Foundation of America (MAWFA)
(dedicated to granting the special wishes of terminally ill children)

3550 North Central Ave., Suite 300
Phoenix, AZ 85012-2127
(602) 279-WISH (279-9474)
(800) 722-WISH (722-9474)
Fax: (602) 279-0855
E-mail: mawfa@wish.org
http://www.wish.org

Make Today Count (MTC)
(self-help group for persons with
    terminal illness)
St. Johns Hospital
1235 E. Cherokee St.
Springfield, MO 65804
(800) 432-2273
(417) 885-3324

▶ **Victimization**

**National Center for Victims
    of Crime**
2000 M St., N.W., Suite 480
Washington, DC 20036
(202) 467-8700
Fax: (202) 467-8701
http://www.ncvc.org

**National Coalition Against
    Domestic Violence**
P.O. Box 18749
Denver, CO 80218
(303) 839-1852
Fax: (303) 831-9251
http://www.ncadv.org

**National Coalition Against
    Sexual Assault**
912 N. 2nd St.
Harrisburg, PA 17102
(717) 232-6745

**National Organization for Victim
    Assistance (NOVA)**
1730 Park Rd. N.W.
Washington, DC 20010
(202) 232-6683
Fax: (202) 462-2255
http://www.try-nova.org

▶ **Weight Control**

Overeaters Anonymous (OA)
P.O. Box 44020

Rio Rancho, NM 87174-4020
(505) 891-2664
Fax: (505) 891-2664
E-mail: info@overeatersanonymous.
    org
http://www.oa.org

**Weight-control Information
    Network (WIN)**
National Institute of Diabetes and
    Digestive and Kidney Diseases
1 WIN Way
Bethesda, MD 20892-3665
(202) 828-1025
(877) 946-4627
Fax: (202) 828-1028
E-mail: win@info.niddk.nih.gov
http://www.niddk.nih.gov/health/
    nutrit/win.htm

Take Off Pounds Sensibly (TOPS)
P.O. Box 07360
4575 S. Fifth St.
Milwaukee, WI 53207-0360
(800) 932-8677
(414) 482-4620
www.tops.org

Weight Watchers International
175 Crossways Park West
Woodbury, NY 11797
(516) 390-1657
http://www.weight-watchers.com

▶ **Wellness**

National Wellness Institute
University of Wisconsin—
    Stevens Point
P.O. Box 827
Stevens Point WI 54481-0827
(715) 342-2969
Fax: (715) 342-2979
E-mail: NWI@nationalwellness.org
http://www.nationalwellness.org

Wellness Associates
(publishes *The Wellness Inventory*)
706 West Junior Terrace
Chicago, IL 60613
(773) 935-6377
Fax: (773) 929-4446

E-mail: info@wellness-
    associates.com
www.wellness-associates.com

▶ **Women's Health**

**National Women's Health
    Network (NWHN)**
514 10th St. N.W., Suite 400
Washington, DC 20004
(202) 347-1140
Health Info: (202) 628-7814
Fax: (202) 347-1168
www.womenshealthnetwork.org

**National Women's Health
    Information Center**
**U.S. Public Health Service
    on Women's Health**
8550 Arlington Blvd., Suite 300
Fairfax, VA 22031
(800) 994-WOMAN (994-9662)
http://www.4women.gov

**GenneX Healthcare
    Technologies, Inc.**
**Estronaut: A Forum
    for Women's Health**
GenneX Healthcare
    Technologies, Inc.
207 E. Ohio, 186
Chicago, IL 60611
(312) 335-0095
E-mail: ask@gennexhealth.com
http://www.estronaut.com

Planned Parenthood
810 Seventh Ave.
New York, NY 10019
(212) 541-7800
http://www.plannedparenthood.org
See also white or yellow pages of
    telephone directory for listing of
    local chapter

Emergency!

By definition, an emergency is a situation in which you have to think and act fast. Start by assessing the circumstances. Shout for help if you're in a public place. Look for any possible dangers to you or the victim, such as a live electrical wire or a fire. Seek medical assistance as quickly as possible. Dial 911, the operator, or a local emergency phone number, and keep it near every phone in your house. Don't attempt rescue techniques, such as cardiopulmonary resuscitation (CPR), unless you are trained. If you have a car, be sure you know the shortest route from your home to the nearest 24-hour hospital emergency department.

Supplies

Every home should have a kit of basic first aid supplies kept in a convenient location out of the reach of children. Stock it with the following:

- Bandages and sterile gauze pads
- Adhesive tape
- Scissors
- Cotton balls or absorbent cotton
- Cotton swabs
- Thermometer
- Syrup of ipecac to induce vomiting
- Antibiotic ointment
- Sharp needle
- Safety pins
- Calamine lotion

Keep a similar kit in your car or boat. You might want to add some extra items from your home, such as a flashlight, soap, blanket, paper cups, and any special equipment that a family member with a chronic illness may need.

Bleeding

Blood loss is frightening and dangerous. Direct pressure stops external bleeding. Since internal bleeding can also be life-threatening, you must be aware of the warning signs.

For an Open Wound

1. Apply direct pressure over the site of the wound. Cover the entire wound.
2. Use sterile gauze, a sanitary napkin, a clean towel, sheet, or handkerchief or, if necessary, your washed bare hand. Ice or cold water in a pad will help stop bleeding and decrease swelling.
3. Apply firm, steady pressure for five to fifteen minutes. Most wounds stop bleeding within a few minutes.
4. If the wound is on a foot, hand, leg, or arm, use gravity to help slow the flow of blood. Elevate the limb so that it is higher than the victim's heart.
5. If the bleeding doesn't stop, press harder.
6. Seek medical attention if the bleeding was caused by a serious injury, if stitches will be needed to keep the wound closed, or if the victim has not had a tetanus booster within the last ten years.

For Internal Bleeding

1. Suspect internal bleeding if a person coughs up blood, vomits red or brown material that looks like coffee grounds, passes blood in urine or stool, or has black, tarlike bowel movements.
2. Do not let the victim take any medication or fluids by mouth until seen by a doctor, because surgery may be necessary.
3. Have the victim lie flat. Cover him or her lightly.
4. Seek immediate medical attention.

For a Bloody Nose

1. Have the victim sit down, leaning slightly forward so the blood does not run down his or her throat. The person should spit out any blood in his or her mouth.
2. Use the thumb and forefingers to pinch the nose. If the victim can do the pinching, apply a cold compress to the nose and surrounding area.
3. Apply pressure for ten minutes without interruption.
4. If pinching does not work, gently pack the nostril with gauze or a clean strip of cloth. Do not use

absorbent cotton, which will stick. Let the ends hang out so you can remove the packing easily later. Pinch the nose, with the packing in place, for five minutes.

5. If a foreign object is in the nose, do not attempt to remove it. Ask the person to blow gently. If that does not work, seek medical attention.

6. The nose should not be blown or irritated for several hours after a nosebleed stops.

Breathing Problems

If a person appears to be unconscious, approach carefully. The victim may be in contact with electrical current. If so, make sure the electricity is shut off before touching the victim. The first function you should check is respiration. Tap or shake the victim's shoulder gently, shouting, "Are you all right?" Look for any signs of breathing: Can you hear breath sounds? Can you feel breath on your cheek? If the person is breathing, do not perform mouth-to-mouth resuscitation.

If you aren't certain if the victim is breathing, or if there are no signs of breath, follow these steps:

1. Lay the person on his or her back on the floor or ground. Roll the victim over if necessary, being careful to turn the head with the remainder of the body as a unit to avoid possible neck injury. Loosen any tight clothing around the neck or chest.

2. Check for any foreign material in the mouth or throat and remove it quickly.

3. Open the airway by tilting the head back and lifting the chin up.

4. Pinch the nostrils shut with your thumb and index finger.

5. Take a deep breath, open your mouth wide and place it securely over the victim's, and give two slow breaths, each lasting 1 to 10 seconds. Remove your mouth, turn your head, and check to see if the victim's chest rises and falls. If you hear air escaping from the victim's mouth and see the chest fall, you know that you are getting air into the lungs.

6. Repeat once every five seconds (twelve breaths per minute) until professional help takes over, or the victim begins breathing on his or her own. It may take several hours to revive someone. If you stop, the victim may not be able to breathe on his or her own. Once the person does begin to breathe independently, always get professional help.

7. If air doesn't seem to be entering the chest, or the chest doesn't fall between breaths, tilt the head further back. If that doesn't work, follow the directions for choking emergencies later in this section.

8. If the victim is a child, do not pinch the nose shut. Cover both the mouth and nose with your mouth, and place your free hand very lightly on the child's chest. Use small puffs of air rather than big breaths. Feel the chest inflate as you blow, and listen for exhaled air. Repeat once every three seconds (twenty breaths per minute).

Broken Bones

If you suspect that a person has broken a leg, do not move him or her unless there is immediate danger.

1. Check for signs of breathing. If there is none or breathing is very weak, administer mouth-to-mouth resuscitation.

2. If the person is bleeding, apply direct pressure on the site of the wound.

3. Try to keep the victim warm and calm.

4. Do not try to push a broken bone back into place if it is sticking out of the skin. You can apply a moist dressing to prevent it from drying out.

5. Do not try to straighten out a fracture.

6. Do not allow the victim to walk.

7. Splint unstable fractures to prevent painful motion.

Burns

1. If fire caused the burn, cool the affected area with water to stop the burning process.

2. Remove the victim's garments and jewelry and cover him or her with clean sheets or towels.

3. Call for help immediately.

4. If chemicals caused the burn, wash the affected area with cool water for at least 20 minutes. Chemical burns of the eye require immediate medical attention after flushing with water for 20 minutes.

Choking

A person with anything stuck in the throat and blocking the airway can stop breathing, lose consciousness, and die within four to six minutes. A universal signal of distress because of choking is clasping the throat with one or both hands. Other signs are an inability to talk and noisy, difficult breathing. You need to take immediate action, but NEVER slap the victim's back. This could make the obstruction worse.

If the victim can speak, cough, or breathe, do not interfere. Coughing alone may dislodge the foreign object. If the choking continues without lessening, call for medical help.

If the victim cannot speak, cough, or breathe but is conscious, use the Heimlich maneuver, as follows

1. Stand behind the victim (who may be seated or standing) and wrap your arms around his or her waist.
2. Make a fist with one hand and place the thumb side of your fist against the victim's abdomen, just above the navel. Grasp your fist with your other hand and press into his or her abdomen with a quick, upward thrust. Do not exert any pressure against the rib cage with your forearms.
3. Repeat this procedure until the victim is no longer choking or loses consciousness.
4. If the person is lying face down, roll the victim over. Facing the person, kneel with your legs astride his or her hips. Put the heel of one hand below the rib cage and place your other hand on top. Press into the abdomen with a quick, upward thrust. Repeat thrusts as needed.
5. If you start choking when you're by yourself, place your fist below your rib cage and above your navel. Grasp this fist with your other hand and press into your abdomen with a quick, upward thrust. You also can lean over a fixed, horizontal object, such as a table edge or chair back, and press your upper abdomen against it with a quick, upward thrust. Repeat as needed until you dislodge the object.

If the Victim Is Unconscious

1. Place him or her on the ground and give mouth-to-mouth resuscitation as described earlier.
2. If the victim does not start breathing and air does not seem to be going into his or her lungs, roll the victim onto his or her back and give one or more manual thrusts: Place one of your hands on top of the other with the heel of the bottom hand in the middle of the abdomen, slightly above the navel and below the rib cage. Press into the abdomen with a quick, upward thrust. Do not push to either side. Repeat six to ten times as needed.
3. Clear the airway. Hold the victim's mouth open with one hand and use your thumb to depress the tongue. Make a hook with the index finger of your other hand and, using a gentle, sweeping motion, reach into the victim's throat and feel for a swallowed foreign object in the airway.
4. Repeat the following steps in this sequence:
   • Six to ten abdominal thrusts

• Probe in mouth
• Try to inflate lungs
• Repeat

5. If the victim suddenly seems okay, but no foreign material has been removed, take him or her directly to the hospital. A foreign object, such as a fish or chicken bone or other jagged object, could do internal damage as it passes through the victim's system.

If the Victim Is a Child

1. If the child is coughing, do nothing. The coughing alone may dislodge the object.
2. If the airway is blocked and the child is panicky and fighting for breath, do *NOT* probe the airway with your fingers to clear an unseen foreign object. You might push the material back into the airway, worsening the obstruction.
3. For an infant younger than a year, hang the child over your arm so that the head is lower than the trunk. Using the heel of your hand, administer four firm blows high on the back between the shoulder blades. For a bigger child, follow the same procedure, but invert the child over your knee rather than your arm.
4. After four back blows, perform four chest thrusts (the Heimlich maneuver as described above).

Drowning

A person can die of drowning four to six minutes after breathing stops. Although prevention is the wisest course, follow these steps in case of a drowning emergency:

1. Get the victim out of the water fast. Be extremely cautious, because a drowning person may panic and grasp at a rescuer, endangering that individual as well. If possible, push a branch or pole within the victim's reach.
2. If the victim is unconscious, use a flotation device if at all possible. Carefully place the person on the device. Once out of the water, place the victim on his or her back.
3. If the victim is not breathing, start mouth-to-mouth resuscitation. Continue until the person can breathe unassisted or help arrives. (Note that it may take an hour or two for a drowning victim to resume independent breathing.) Do not leave the victim alone for any reason.
4. Once the person is breathing without assistance, even if he or she is still coughing, you need only stay nearby until professional help arrives.

Electrical Shock

1. If you suspect that an electrical shock has knocked a person unconscious, approach very carefully. Do not touch the victim unless the electricity has been turned off.
2. Shut off the power at the plug, circuit breaker, or fuse box. Simply shutting off an appliance does not remove the shock hazard. Use a dry stick to move a wire or downed power line from the victim. Keep in mind that you also are in danger until the power is off.
3. If the person's breathing is weak or has stopped, follow the steps for mouth-to-mouth resuscitation.
4. Even if the victim returns to consciousness, call for medical help. While waiting, cover the victim with a blanket or coat to keep him or her warm. Place a blanket underneath the body if the surface is cold. Be sure the person lies flat if conscious, with legs raised. If the victim is unconscious, place him or her on one side, with a pillow supporting the head. Do not give the victim anything to eat or drink.
5. Electrical burns can extend deep into the tissue, even when they appear minor. Do not put butter, household remedies, or sprays on burns without a doctor's instruction. Do not use ice or cold water on an electrical burn that is more than 2 inches across.

Heart Attack

Chest pain can be caused by indigestion, strained muscles, or lung infections. The warning signs of a heart attack are:

- Intense pain that lasts for more than two minutes, produces a tight or crushing feeling, is centered in the chest, or spreads to the neck, jaw, shoulder, or arm

- Shortness of breath that is worse when the person lies flat and improves when the person sits

- Heavy sweating

- Nausea or vomiting

- Irregular pulse

- Pale or bluish skin or lips

- Weakness

- Severe anxiety, feeling of doom

If an individual develops these symptoms:

1. Call for emergency medical help immediately.

2. Have the person sit up or lie in a semi-reclining position. Loosen tight clothing. Keep him or her comfortably warm.
3. If the person loses consciousness, turn on his or her back and check for breathing and pulse. If vomiting occurs, turn the victim's head to one side and clean the mouth.
4. If the person has medicine for angina pectoris (chest pain) and is conscious, help him or her take it.
5. If the person is unconscious, and you are trained to perform cardiopulmonary resuscitation (CPR), check for a pulse at the wrist or neck. If there is none, begin CPR in conjunction with mouth-to-mouth resuscitation. Do not attempt CPR unless you are trained. It is not a technique you can learn from a book.

Poisoning

Many common household substances, including glue, aspirin, bleaches, and paint, can be poisonous. Make sure you know the emergency numbers for the Poison Control Center and Fire Department Rescue Squad. Keep them near your telephone. Be prepared to provide the following information:

- The kind of substance swallowed and how much was swallowed

- If a child or adult swallowed the substance

- Symptoms

- Whether or not vomiting has occurred

- Whether you gave the person anything to drink

- How much time it will take to get to an emergency room

The Poison Control Center or rescue team will tell you whether or not to induce vomiting or neutralize a swallowed poison. Here are some additional guidelines:

1. Always assume the worst if a small child has swallowed or might have swallowed something poisonous. Call the local Poison Control Center or emergency number (911 in many areas). Keep the suspected item or container with you to answer questions.
2. Do not give any medications unless a physician or the Poison Control Center instructs you to do so.
3. Do not follow the directions for neutralizing poisons on the container unless a doctor or the Poison Control Center confirms that they are appropriate measures to take.
4. If the child is conscious, give moderate doses of water to dilute the poison.

5. If a poisoning victim is unconscious, make sure he or she is breathing. If not, give mouth-to-mouth resuscitation. Do not give anything by mouth or attempt to stimulate the person. Call for emergency help immediately.

6. If the person is vomiting, make sure he or she is in a position in which he or she cannot choke on what is brought up.

7. While vomiting is the fastest way to expel swallowed poisons from the body, never try to induce vomiting if the person has swallowed any acid or alkaline substance, which can cause burns of the face, mouth, and throat (examples include ammonia, bleach, dishwasher detergent, drain and toilet cleaners, lye, oven cleaners, or rust removers), or petroleum-like products, which produce dangerous fumes that can be inhaled during vomiting (examples include floor polish, furniture wax, gasoline, kerosene, lighter fluid, turpentine, and paint thinner).

A Consumer's Guide to Medical Tests

✔ **What They Tell the Doctor**
✔ **How Often You Need Them**
✔ **What to Do About Abnormal Results**

Do you wonder what the doctor sees when he looks into your eyes with that little light or what it means when your blood or urine test is normal? In this section we cover some of the most common tests your doctor does, what they tell, and how often they should be done.

General Information

• Always ask your doctor what tests are being done, why they are being ordered, what they involve, and what the results mean.

• No test is foolproof. If a result is unexpected, whether normal or abnormal, your doctor should repeat the test before making any decisions.

• Modern X-ray machines expose you to a minuscule amount of radiation. Nevertheless, be sure to tell the physician or X-ray technician if there is even a chance you may be pregnant.

• Often a doctor orders a test because that is the only way to prove you do not have a disease.

Allergy Skin Testing

• Skin testing is still the most reliable method.

• The physician either pricks your skin 20 to 40 or more times to introduce a tiny bit of potentially allergic material or injects a small amount.

• Children who are frightened by multiple needle sticks and are unlikely to sit still for as long as necessary may have blood (RAST) tests instead.

What results mean

If you develop redness or a hivelike bump around an area, you are probably allergic to the injected substance. Sometimes you can avoid the offending material, but

things like pollen and dust are everywhere. Your allergist may recommend desensitizing shots to reduce your reaction. The results of skin tests won't be reliable if you take antihistamines within 48 hours of the test.

How often to be tested

Skin tests are necessary only if you cannot get allergy relief from other measures such as over-the-counter medications, reducing mold and dust in the house, and staying away from animals.

Blood Pressure Reading

• High blood pressure, a major cause of stroke and heart attacks, usually causes no symptoms.

• The upper number in a reading—the systolic—refers to peak amount of pressure generated when your heart pumps blood, the lower number—the diastolic—measures the least amount of pressure.

What results mean

Most doctors today think the lower the pressure the better, which means a reading of 120/80 or less. Because the mere anxiety of having your blood pressure taken can cause a mild elevation, your doctor will want to repeat an abnormal test, ideally on a different day, before diagnosing high blood pressure.

How often to be tested

Everyone—no matter how healthy—should have a blood-pressure reading taken at least once a year, more often if you have high blood pressure.

Blood Tests

• Blood may be taken from either a finger prick or, more commonly, a vein in your arm.

• See below for information on cholesterol testing, which is also done from a blood sample.

Complete Blood Count (CBC)

This is the most commonly performed of all blood tests.

What results mean

A low red-cell count, called anemia, can be caused by something as simple as too little iron in your diet, as complex as an abnormality in your digestion, or as serious as a bone marrow problem or silent bleeding. Iron deficiency is the most frequent cause, with women who menstruate and limit their intake of red meat at the greatest risk. If your doctor diagnoses this problem, ask about making dietary changes as well as taking iron supplements.

A high white-cell count, a measure of the body's defenses against infection, usually indicates some kind of infection. Depending on the type of cell that predominates, your doctor may be able to identify whether you have a bacterial or viral infection.

Platelets, the first participants in blood clotting, may be decreased because of a viral infection, abnormal bleeding, or for no identifiable reason.

Chemistry Panels (Chem 12 or 18, SMA 12 or 24)

Kidney, bone, liver, pancreas, prostate, and some glandular functions are screened by these tests.

What results mean

An abnormality may signal a problem that needs treatment. Because accuracy decreases when many tests are run together, any specific abnormal test should be repeated, especially if unexpected.

CAT (Computerized Axial Tomography) Scan

- A CAT scan is 100 times more sensitive than an X ray.

- You lie as motionless as possible in a large tube while an X-ray beam travels 360 degrees around you. The test takes about an hour.

What results mean

The test can help diagnose such conditions as tumors, blood clots, cysts, and bleeding in the brain as well as in various other organs.

Cholesterol Test/Lipoprotein Profile

- Anyone can have a high cholesterol level, but you are more apt to be at risk if there is a family history of early heart attacks, strokes, or high blood cholesterol.

- Your doctor will look at total blood cholesterol, high-density lipoprotein (HDL, the "good" cholesterol that prevents cholesterol from sticking to your blood vessels), low-density lipoprotein (LDL, the "bad" cholesterol that does the reverse), and triglycerides.

What results mean

Experts today think optimum total cholesterol levels are below 200 mg/dL of blood. Persistently high cholesterol values will prompt your doctor to advise dietary and lifestyle changes—less fat intake, more exercise—and perhaps medication. Optimal LDL levels are less than 100 mg/dL, and optimal HDL levels are 60 mg/dL or higher.

How often to be tested

If your cholesterol level is under 200 and your LDL level is under 130, repeat the test every five years. If your test is borderline, repeat it annually. (Note that the test should be taken when you have not eaten for at least twelve hours.)

If you have a family history of cholesterol problems, have your children tested annually from age 2; if you don't, have them tested around age 10 and every few years thereafter. Children under 2 should not be given a low-cholesterol diet; they need extra fat to make brain tissue and hormones for growth.

Fundoscopy

- The doctor looks into your eye with a little light.

What results mean

The beginnings of cataracts may be visible, as well as irregularities in the blood vessels that indicate damage from high cholesterol (fatty deposits in the blood vessels), high blood pressure (narrowing and notching), diabetes, or other diseases. If the optic nerve is swollen, there may be excess pressure inside your skull.

What your doctor *cannot* see are the early signs of glaucoma, which can lead to blindness if not treated. Over age 20, have a pressure check for glaucoma from an ophthalmologist or optometrist every three years—or every year if you have a family history of glaucoma.

Heart Tests

- The following tests are listed from the simplest through the most complicated.
- Also see listings for blood pressure readings, cholesterol tests, and pulse.

Electrocardiogram (ECG, EKG)

A machine amplifies the electrical signals from your heart and records them on paper.

What results mean

An EKG can detect such things as an enlarged heart, abnormal levels of potassium or calcium, disease of the small vessels of the heart, or the source of an abnormal heart rhythm. It is a nonspecific test, however, and more advanced studies should be done if serious disease is suspected.

Echocardiogram

In this painless test sound waves are used to produce a picture of the heart in action on a TV-type screen.

What results mean

The test investigates the size of the heart chambers, the thickness of the walls, how the four heart valves are working, and the condition of the membrane surrounding the heart. Mitral valve prolapse, a common minor abnormality, often shows up on this test, as well as more serious problems.

Stress Test

Your heart rate, blood pressure, and EKG are constantly monitored as you exercise on a treadmill that goes faster and faster with a steeper and steeper incline. This test—also called an exercise tolerance test or treadmill test—should be performed in the presence of a cardiologist and in or near a hospital in case the strain causes heart problems that need emergency treatment. The test should be stopped immediately if you experience any light-headedness, chest pain, nausea, or palpitations.

What results mean

The increasing strain on the heart causes changes that can tell your doctor if you are at risk of a heart attack. This is because a blockage in the coronary arteries—the blood vessels that feed your heart muscle—may show up only during exercise.

Angiography

A dye is injected into various arteries, and X rays are taken.

What results mean

The doctor can detect blockages in the blood vessels that can lead to heart attack or stroke, as well as aneurysms (weakened spots in the blood-vessel walls). The test carries some risk of causing stroke.

Kidney Tests

The two tests listed here involve taking X rays. Ultrasound (similar to an echocardiogram) can also be used to outline the kidneys.

Intravenous Pyelogram (IVP)

After an iodine-containing substance is injected into a vein, X rays are taken at five-minute intervals to show the outlines of the kidney, ureter, and bladder.

What results mean

Tumors, kidney stones, and swelling of the kidney tissue can be seen, as well as blockage to urine flow or a mass that may be pressing on the kidney. A kidney that is not functioning will not appear on the X ray, and one in an abnormal position can be found.

Voiding Cystourethrogram (VCUG)

A technician will fill your bladder with a dye injected through a catheter and take X rays while you urinate.

What results mean

If you have recurrent urinary-tract infections, the test will show if there is a significant backup of urine from the bladder into the ureter, in which case daily antibiotics may be needed to prevent infection. Investigating recurrent urinary tract infections is particularly important for children.

Magnetic Resonance Imaging (MRI)

MRI uses no radiation but produces pictures of the brain that are much more detailed than those of a CAT scan.

What results mean

In addition to locating bleeding or tumors, as a CAT scan does, the test picks up subtle signs such as those of Parkinson's disease and multiple sclerosis in the brain or a herniated disc in the spinal column.

Mammography

- Only a small amount of radiation is used to take the mammogram. You usually stand up and put your breast on a photographic plate where it is compressed with a plastic shield or balloonlike device. It shouldn't hurt. If your breasts are tender at certain times in your menstrual cycle, schedule your mammogram when they are least sensitive.

- Mammograms can detect breast abnormalities at easily treated stages before you can feel them, but they are not foolproof. Examine your breasts monthly.

What results mean

Mammograms can detect cysts, abscesses, and tumors. Whether a mass is benign or malignant is hard to tell in the early stages, so abnormalities usually need to be biopsied or removed totally to determine treatment.

How often to be tested

Although there is controversy over the benefits of mammography for women under 50, many experts still recommend having a first mammogram between ages 35 and 40, followed by one every two years between 40 and 50, and yearly thereafter. If your mother or sister has had breast cancer, consult your doctor for an appropriate schedule. And if you have a lump, pain, or nipple discharge, have a mammogram right away, no matter what your age.

You also should have a breast examination by a doctor at least every three years between ages 20 and 40, and every year after 40.

Pap Smear

- A routine part of every gynecological examination.

- Your doctor takes a painless swab from the cervix and vaginal walls and sends it to a lab for analysis.

What results mean

Pap smears can detect not only cervical cancer but also inflammation and many infections, minor and more serious; they also provide important information about the state of your female hormones. A normal test is termed class I, and abnormal results are graded by degree into four classifications, with only the most severe—a class V test—signifying outright cancer. Treatment depends on the diagnosis and may range from doing nothing for a minor inflammation to, in rare cases, a hysterectomy for cancer. Because the error rate of Pap smears is high, the doctor should always repeat an abnormal test.

How often to be tested

Women who are on birth control pills and are sexually active should have a Pap smear every six months; other women should be checked every year.

Physical Examination

The routine physical exam generally includes a pulse and blood-pressure reading, measure of height and weight, blood tests (including a lipoprotein profile), fundoscopy, and sometimes other tests as well, such as a fecal occult blood test.

What results mean

A physical exam serves as a general measure of health and sometimes picks up early signs of disease.

How often to have a physical exam

Most doctors no longer recommend yearly physicals for everybody. A good schedule to follow instead is to have a complete checkup every four or five years under age 40, every three years between 40 and 50, every two years between 50 and 60, and every year after that. At any age, you should have more frequent examinations if you have chronic medical problems such as diabetes or high blood pressure, are obese, or smoke cigarettes.

Pulse

To take your own pulse, press two fingertips over the artery in your wrist, just below the base of the thumb. Count the beats in 20 seconds, then multiply by 3.

What results mean

The normal pulse rate—the speed at which your heart pumps blood—is 60–80 beats a minute; it should be regular, without skipped or extra beats. Abnormal rates can be due to thyroid problems (too high causes a fast rate, too low a slow one), heart problems, anxiety (even the stress of a physical exam), or weakness from an illness such as the flu or other problems.

The character of your pulse is also important. A discrepancy between the strength of the pulse on one side of the neck and the other may mean you are in danger of a stroke. A pulse that is abnormally strong and bounding can signal a problem with a heart valve. If the pulse is weak, you may have blockages in your blood vessels from diabetes, atherosclerosis (hardening of the arteries), or a variety of other disorders.

Stomach and Intestinal Tests

Though most of these tests are uncomfortable, they generally are not painful.

Barium Enema

Barium, a radioactive material, is instilled in your large intestine through a tube inserted into your anus. Because barium is constipating, drink fluids afterward. Don't be alarmed if you have white stools for a day or two.

What results mean

The doctor will be able to see tumors or polyps, any obstructions, and other abnormalities.

Colonoscopy and Sigmoidoscopy

In colonoscopy, for which you will be sedated, the doctor looks into the colon with a flexible tube inserted into your anus. The procedure is essentially the same for sigmoidoscopy, except that the doctor looks only into the lower third of the intestine.

What results mean

Your doctor can see where bleeding comes from, remove a polyp, or biopsy a mass.

Upper GI Series

You will be asked to down a drink of barium so that X rays can be taken of the esophagus, stomach, duodenum, and sometimes the small intestine.

What results mean

Your doctor can diagnose swallowing disorders, hiatus hernias, ulcers, tumors, and some inflammations of the stomach and small bowel.

Fecal Occult Blood Test (FOBT)

A small sample of stool that remains on the doctor's glove after a rectal exam or that is collected by you at home is tested for blood that is invisible to the eye.

What results mean

This test is done routinely as part of a regular checkup to detect the earliest sign of cancer of the colon. It is also part of an investigation of anemia or abdominal pain. If your test is positive, tell your doctor if you recently ate radishes, turnips, or red meat, took large doses of vitamin C or iron pills, or had a nosebleed. All of these things can produce misleading results.

Urinalysis

Urine can tell about the health not only of the kidneys but also of other organ systems.

What results mean

Specific gravity is the degree to which your urine is concentrated or diluted. If it is persistently too dilute, your doctor may ask for a first morning sample to see how well your kidneys concentrate your urine overnight. Urine that is too concentrated may indicate poor fluid intake, decreased kidney function, or dehydration from vomiting and diarrhea.

Acidity or alkalinity (pH) is useful information when there is a history or possibility of kidney stones, urinary tract infection, or kidney disease.

Glucose or sugar in the urine may mean you have diabetes. You will need a blood test to confirm the diagnosis, as some families filter sugar easily through their kidneys but do not have any disease. Inflammation of the pancreas and thyroid problems also may cause sugar in the urine.

Blood in the urine may mean infection, a stone, or an inflammation of the kidney. Excessive exertion such as running sometimes causes some blood to leak into the urine; this usually disappears after resting.

Protein molecules are large and under normal conditions should not filter into the urine. However, they may appear in small amounts in the urine after strenuous exercise or an illness, especially one with a fever. In large amounts, protein in the urine warrants a search for an underlying kidney problem.

Nitrites, substances produced when bacteria multiply, may be the earliest or only sign of an infection.

White blood cells may be present because of a urinary tract or vaginal infection.

X Ray

The simple X ray is a nonspecific test that is being replaced more and more by CAT scans, magnetic resonance imaging, and other tests.

What results mean

An X ray can detect such things as an enlarged heart, a broken bone, a sinus infection, or pneumonia.

Counting Your Calories and Fat Grams

Total calorie values for each item in this table were rounded to the nearest 5 calories (calories from fat and fat grams were not). The portion sizes are given in common household units and in grams. The portion size shown may not be the amount that you eat. If you choose larger or smaller portions than listed, increase or decrease the calorie and fat counts accordingly. Check nutrition labels on foods for additional information, including saturated fat, cholesterol, and sodium content.

Breads, Cereals, and Other Grain Products

Breads	Calories	Fat grams	Calories from fat
Bagel			
plain, 1, 3½" diam.	195	1	10
oat bran, 1, 3½"	180	1	8
poppy seed, 1, Sara Lee	190	1	9
Cracked-wheat bread, 1, 25 g slice	65	1	9
French bread, 1, 25 g slice	70	1	7
Pita bread			
white, 1, 6½" diam.	165		6
whole wheat, 1, 6½" diam.	170		15
Pumpernickel, 1, 32 g slice	80	1	9
Raisin, 1, 26 g slice	70	1	10
Rye, 1, 32 g slice	85	1	10
White			
regular, 1, 25 g slice	65	1	8
Wonder bread light, 2 slices, 45 g	80	1	9
Whole wheat			
regular, 1, 25 g slice	70	1	11
Wonder bread, 2 slices, 45 g	80	<1	14
Rolls			
Croissant, prepared w/butter, 1, 57 g	230	12	108
Dinner, 1, 28 g	85	2	19
Frankfurter or hamburger, 1, 43 g	125	2	20
French, 1, 38 g	105	2	15
Hard, 1 3½", 57 g	165	2	22
Quick breads, Biscuits, Muffins, Breakfast Pastries			
Biscuit			
plain, 2½" diam., 60 g	210	10	88
from dry mix, 3" diam., 57 g	190	7	62
from refrig. dough, 2½" diam., 27 g	95	4	36
Banana bread, 1 slice, 60 g	195	57	
Coffee cake			
cinnamon w/crumb topping, 63 g	265	15	132
butter streusel, Sara Lee, 41 g	160	7	63
Danish			
cheese, Sara Lee, individual, 36 g	130	8	72

	Calories	Fat grams	Calories from fat
cheese-filled, Entenmann's, fat-free 54 g	130	0	0
Doughnuts			
plain cake, 1, 47 g	200	11	97
glazed, 1, 45 g	190	10	93
English muffin, plain, 1, 57 g	135	1	9
Muffin			
blueberry, 1, 2½", 57 g	160	4	33
bran w/raisins, Dunkin' Donuts 1, 104 g	310	9	81
Pancake			
plain, from dry mix, 1, 56 g	200	1	9
plain, frozen Aunt Jemima, 3, 114 g	185	2	22
Waffle			
plain, 7" diam., 75 g	220	11	95
blueberry, frozen, Eggo, 2, 78 g	220	8	72
Breakfast Cereal			
All-Bran, ½ cup, 30 g	80	1	9
Bran flakes, ¾ cup, 28 g	100	1	9
Cheerios, 1¼ cup, 28 g	110	2	18
Corn flakes, 1 cup, 30 g	110	0	0
Cream of Wheat			
regular or instant, cooked, ⅔ cup, 168 g	100	0	0
instant, cooked, ⅔ cup, 161 g	100	<1	0
mix'n eat, 1 pkg., 28 g	100	0	0
Frosted Flakes, ¾ cup, 30 g	120	0	0
Frosted Mini-Wheats, 1 cup, 55 g	190	1	9
Grape-Nut Flakes, 1 cup, 28 g	100	1	9
Granola, date nut, Erewhon, ¼ cup, 28 g	130	6	50
Oatmeal			
reg., quick, or instant, cooked, 1 cup, 234 g	145	2	21
cinnamon & spice, instant , 1 pkg., 46 g	170	2	18
Raisin bran, 1 cup, 55 g	170	1	9
Rice Chex, 1 cup, 31 g	120	0	0
Rice Krispies, 1¼ cup, 30 g	110	0	0
Shredded wheat, Quaker	220	2	14
Special K, 1 cup, 30 g	110	0	0
Total, 1 cup, 28 g	100	1	9
Wheaties, 1 cup, 28 g	100	1	9
Pasta and Rice			
Macaroni			
cooked, plain, ½ cup, 65 g	95	<1	3
spinach, cooked, Ronzoni, ½ cup, 67 g	105	<1	4
Pasta			
fresh, cooked, plain, 1 cup, 170 g	225	2	16
homemade w/egg, cooked, 1 cup, 170 g	220	3	27
Ravioli, cheese, cooked, Contadina, ⅓ container, 190 g	270	11	99
Rice, cooked, ½ cup			
Brown, medium grain, 98 g	110	1	7
White, glutinous, 120 g	115	<1	2
White, long grain instant, 82 g	80	<1	1

Pasta and Rice	Calories	Fat grams	Calories from fat
White, medium grain, 93 g	120	<1	2
Wild rice, 82 g	85	<1	3
Spaghetti, cooked, plain, 1 cup, 140 g	155	<1	4

Crackers

	Calories	Fat grams	Calories from fat
Cheez-it, Sunshine, 24 crackers, 32 g	140	8	72
Finn-Crisp dark, 3 crackers, 15 g	60	0	0
Matzo, plain, 1, 28 g	110	<1	4
Ritz, Nabisco, 4 crackers, 14 g	70	4	36
Saltine, 10 crackers, 28 g	120	4	36
Soup or oyster, 4 crackers, 14 g	70	4	36
Triscuit, Nabisco, 6 crackers, 28 g	120	4	36

Fruits

Fruits

(calories in cooked and canned fruit include both fruit and liquid)

	Calories	Fat grams	Calories from fat
Apple, raw, sliced, ½ cup, 55 g	30	<1	2
Applesauce, ½ cup			
sweetened, 128 g	95	<1	2
unsweetened, 122 g	50	<1	1
Apricots			
canned, heavy syrup, 3 halves, 85 g	70	<1	1
canned, light syrup pack, 3 halves, 85 g	55	<1	0
dried, cooked without sugar, ½ cup, 125 g	105	<1	2
raw, 4 halves, 78 g	35	<1	3
Avocados			
California, 3", ½, 86 g	155	15	135
Florida, 3⅝", ½, 152 g	170	13	121
Banana, medium, 114 g	105	1	5
Blueberries, ½ cup			
frozen, unsweetened, 78 g	40	<1	4
frozen, sweetened, 115 g	95	1	5
raw, 72 g	40	<1	3
Cherries, ½ cup			
raw, sweet, 72 g	50	1	6
sweet, frozen, sweetened, 130 g	115	<1	2
sour red, frozen, unsweetened, 78 g	35	<1	3
Cranberry sauce, sweetened, ¼ cup, 70 g	110	0	0
Dates, dried, 10, 83 g	230	<1	3
Fruit cocktail, canned, ½ cup			
juice pack, 124 g	55	<1	0
heavy syrup, 128 g	95	<1	1
Grapefruit, raw, 3¾", ½, 118 g	40	<1	1
Melon, honeydew, cubed, ½ cup, 85 g	30	<1	1
Oranges, ½ cup			
mandarin, canned, light syrup, 122 g	80	0	0
raw, sections, 90 g	40	<1	1
Peaches			
canned, in juice, ½ cup, 77 g	55	0	0
canned, in light syrup, ½ cup, 77 g	70	<1	1
Pears			
canned, in light syrup, 1 half, 77 g	35	<1	1
dried, without added sugar, ½ cup, 128 g	165	<1	4

Pineapple	Calories	Fat grams	Calories from fat
canned, juice pack, ½ cup, 125 g	75	<1	1
raw, diced, ½ cup, 78 g	40	<1	3
Plums			
canned, juice pack, 3, 95 g	55	<1	0
raw, 2⅛" diam., 66 g	35	<1	4
Prunes			
dried, cooked, without sugar, ½ cup, 106 g	115	<1	2
dried, uncooked, 10, 84 g	200	<1	4
Raisins, seedless, ¼ cup, 41 g	125	<1	2
Raspberries, ½ cup			
frozen, unsweetened, 125 g	61	1	6
raw, 62 g	30	<1	3
Rhubarb, cooked, sweetened, ½ cup, 120 g	140	<1	1
Tangerines, sections, ½ cup, 98 g	45	<1	2
Watermelon, 10" x 1", 480 g	155	2	19

Juices

	Calories	Fat grams	Calories from fat
Apple juice or cider, 1 cup, 249 g	120	0	0
Apricot nectar, canned, ¾ cup, 188 g	105	<1	2
Cranberry juice cocktail, ¾ cup, 190 g	110	<1	2
Grape juice			
bottled, ¾ cup, 188 g	110	0	0
from frozen concentrate, ¾ cup, 188 g	96	<1	2
Lemonade, ¾ cup			
homemade, prepared w/sugar, 186 g	90	0	0
from frozen concentrate, 186 g	75	<1	0
Orange juice, ¾ cup			
fresh, 186 g	85	<1	3
from frozen concentrate, 187 g	85	<1	1
Pineapple juice, canned, ¾ cup, 188 g	105	<1	1
Prune juice, canned, ¾ cup, 192 g	135	<1	1
Snapple, 1 bottle			
Dixie Peach, 295 g	140	0	0
Lemonade, 240 g	110	0	0
Passion Supreme, 309 g	160	0	0
Pink Grapefruit Cocktail, 249 g	120	0	0
V-8 juice, canned, ¾ cup, 182 g	35	0	0

Vegetables

	Calories	Fat grams	Calories from fat
Alfalfa sprouts, raw, 1 cup, 33 g	10	<1	2
Artichoke, cooked, medium, 120 g	60	<1	2
Asparagus, ½ cup			
canned, drained, 120 g	25	1	7
cooked, drained, 90 g	20	<1	3
Bean sprouts, Mung, raw, ½ cup, 52 g	15	<1	1
Beet greens, cooked, drained, ½ cup, 72 g	20	<1	1
Beets, ½ cup			
canned, sliced, drained, 85 g	25	<1	1
cooked, sliced, drained, 85 g	35	<1	1
Broccoli, ½ cup			
frozen florets, cooked, 71 g	20	0	0
raw, chopped, 44 g	10	<1	1
Brussels sprouts, cooked, drained, ½ cup, 78 g	30	<1	4
Cabbage, ½ cup			
Chinese bok choy, shredded, raw, 35 g	5	<1	1
shredded, raw, 35 g	10	<1	1
shredded, cooked, drained, 75 g	15	<1	3

Vegetables	Calories	Fat grams	Calories from fat
Carrots			
frozen, sliced, cooked, drained, ½ cup, 73 g	25	<1	1
raw, 7½" x 1⅛", 72 g	30	<1	1
Cauliflower, ½ cup			
frozen, cooked, drained, 90 g	15	<1	2
raw, 1" pieces, 50 g	10	<1	1
Celery, raw			
cooked, drained, ½ cup, 75 g	15	<1	1
raw, 7½ in x 1¼", 40 g	5	<1	1
Corn, cooked			
canned, yellow, cream style, ½ cup, 128 g	90	1	5
canned, solids & liquid, ½ cup, 128 g	80	1	5
frozen, white, cooked, drained, ½ cup, 82 g	65	<1	1
on the cob, drained, 1 ear, 140 g	85	1	9
Cucumber, raw, sliced, ½ cup, 52 g	10	<1	1
Eggplant			
cooked, drained, 1" pieces, ½ cup, 48 g	15	<1	1
in tomato sauce, 1 cup, 231 g	75	<1	3
Green beans, ½ cup			
canned, drained, 68 g	25	0	0
cooked, drained, 62 g	20	<1	2
frozen, French style 85 g	25	0	0
raw, snap, 55 g	15	<1	1
Kale, cooked, drained, ½ cup, 65 g	20	<1	2
Lettuce			
iceberg, ¼ of a 6" head, 135 g	20	<1	2
looseleaf, shredded, ½ cup, 28 g	5	<1	1
romaine, shredded, ½ cup, 28 g	5	<1	4
Lima beans, cooked, drained, ½ cup, 85 g	105	<1	2
Mushrooms			
canned, pieces, drained, ½ cup, 78 g	20	<1	2
raw, whole, 1, 18 g	5	<1	1
shiitake, cooked, ½ cup, 73 g	40	<1	1
Onions			
canned, solids & liquid, 1", 63 g	10	<1	1
raw, chopped, ½ cup, 80 g	30	<1	1
Peas, green, ½ cup			
frozen, cooked, drained, 80 g	60	<1	2
raw, 72 g	50	<1	3
Peppers, sweet, red or green, ½ cup			
cooked, drained, 68 g	20	<1	1
raw, 50 g	15	<1	1
Potatoes			
baked, w/skin, 4¾" x 2⅓", 156 g	220	<1	2
boiled, no skin, 2½ inch diameter, 135 g	115	<1	1
hash browns, Ore-Ida frozen, 1 patty, 85 g	70	<1	0
mashed, w/whole milk, ½ cup, 105 g	80	1	6
scalloped, frozen, Stouffer's, ½ pkg., 165 g	135	6	52
Tater Tots, frozen, Ore-Ida, 1¼ cup, 85 g	160	7	63
Spinach, ½ cup			
frozen, cooked, drained, 95 g	25	<1	2
raw, chopped, 28 g	5	<1	1
Squash, ½ cup			
summer, cooked, drained, 90 g	20	<1	3
winter, baked cubes, 102 g	40	1	6
Sweet potatoes			
baked in skin, 5" x 2", 114 g	115	<1	1
canned, mashed, 128 g	130	<1	2

	Calories	Fat grams	Calories from fat
Tomato sauce, canned, ½ cup, 112 g	35	<1	2
Tomatoes, ½ cup			
canned, stewed, 103 g	35	0	0
raw, chopped, 90 g	20	<1	3
Turnip greens, cooked, drained, ½ cup, 72 g	15	<1	2
Turnips, cooked, mashed, ½ cup, 115 g	20	<1	1

Meat, Poultry, Fish, and Alternates

(Serving sizes are cooked, edible parts.)

Beef

	Calories	Fat grams	Calories from fat
Beef liver, 3 oz., 85 g			
braised	135	4	37
pan-fried	185	7	61
Corned beef, canned, 1 oz., 28 g	70	4	38
Ground beef, broiled, medium, 3 oz., 85 g			
extra lean	220	14	125
ground chuck	230	16	141
regular	245	18	158
Roast beef, 3 oz., 85 g			
bottom round, lean & fat	160	6	56
eye of round, lean & fat	195	11	98
pot roast, lean & fat	280	20	182
rib, lean & fat	300	24	216
tip round, lean & fat	160	7	60
Sirloin, broiled, lean & fat, 3 oz., 85 g	165	6	55
Veal, loin, lean only, roasted, 3 oz., 85 g	150	6	53

Lamb

	Calories	Fat grams	Calories from fat
Ground lamb, broiled, 3 oz., 85 g	240	17	150
Leg of lamb, lean & fat roasted, 3 oz., 85 g	250	18	158
Shoulder chop, lean & fat, braised, 3 oz., 85 g	295	20	185

Pork

	Calories	Fat grams	Calories from fat
Bacon, thick, broiled, 1 slice, 10 g	55	4	40
Bacon, Canadian, grilled, 1 slice, 23 g	45	2	18
Ham			
center slice, 3 oz., 85 g	170	11	99
canned, lean, 3 oz., 85 g	100	4	35
canned, regular, 3 oz., 85 g	190	13	116
Pork chop, loin, broiled, 3 oz., 85 g	205	11	100
Pork loin ribs, braised, 3 oz., 85 g	250	18	165
Pork roast, center loin, 3 oz., 85 g	200	11	103
Pork roast, sirloin, 3 oz., 85 g	175	8	72
Pork shoulder, roasted, 3 oz., 85 g	245	20	180

Sausage and Luncheon Meats

	Calories	Fat grams	Calories from fat
Bologna, 1 slice, 28 g			
beef & pork	90	8	72
turkey	55	4	40
Braunschweiger, 1 slice, 18 g	65	6	52
Chicken breast			
Oscar Mayer, roasted, 1 slice, 28 g	25	<1	3
Healthy Choice, roasted, 3 slices, 28 g	30	<1	4
Ham, boiled, 1 slice, 21 g	20	1	9
Salami			
beef, 1 slice, 23 g	60	5	43
turkey, 10% fat, 1 oz., 28 g	45	3	24

A32

Sausage and Luncheon Meats	Calories	Fat grams	Calories from fat
Sausage, summer, beef, 1 slice, 23 g	70	6	54
Turkey			
Oscar Mayer, roasted, 1 slice, 28 g	25	1	7
Oscar Mayer, fat-free, smoked, 4 slices, 52 g	40	<1	3
Poultry			
Chicken breast, ½ breast			
boneless, w/out skin, roasted, 86 g	140	3	28
boneless, w/skin, flour fried, 98 g	220	9	78
Chicken drumstick, 1			
w/out skin, roasted, 72 g	75	2	22
w/skin, roasted, 81 g	110	6	52
Chicken liver, simmered, ½ cup, 70 g	110	4	34
Chicken, thigh, 1			
w/out skin, roasted, 71 g	110	6	51
w/skin, roasted, 81 g	155	10	86
Turkey, ground, cooked, 1 patty, 82 g	195	11	97
Turkey, roasted			
dark meat w/out skin, diced, ½ cup, 64 g	120	5	42
dark meat w/skin, 3 oz., 85 g	190	10	88
light meat w/out skin diced, ½ cup, 64g	100	2	19
light meat w/skin, 3 oz., 85 g	170	7	64
Turkey liver, simmered, ½ cup, 70 g	120	4	38
Fish and Shellfish			
Anchovies, canned in oil, drained, 5, 20 g	45	2	17
Clams, canned, drained, ½ cup, 80 g	120	2	14
Fish fillets			
breaded, frozen, 2, 99 g	280	19	171
breaded, Healthy Choice, 1, 99 g	160	5	45
Flounder, cooked, dry heat, 3 oz., 85 g	100	1	12
Halibut, cooked, dry heat, 3 oz., 85 g	120	2	22
Salmon 3 oz., 85 g			
Chinook, cooked, dry heat	195	11	102
Chum, cooked, dry heat	130	4	37
Coho, cooked, moist heat	155	6	57
Sardines, Atlantic, canned in oil, drained solids, 2, 24 g	50	3	25
Sea Bass, cooked, dry heat, 3 oz., 85 g	105	2	20
Shrimp, cooked			
breaded & fried, 4, 30 g	75	4	33
moist heat, large, 4 22 g	20	<1	2
Tuna, light, canned in water, ½ cup, 74 g	85	1	5
Eggs			
Fried, whole, 1, 46 g	90	7	62
Hard-cooked, whole, 1, 50 g	80	5	48
Poached, 1 whole, , 50 g	75	5	45
Scrambled, w/marg. & whole milk, 1, 64 g	105	8	7
Soft-boiled, whole, 1, 50 g	80	6	50
Whites, raw, 1, 33 g	15	0	0
Beans and Peas			
Baked beans, canned			
pork & beans, tomato sauce, ½ cup, 114 g	100	1	13
w/pork, molasses & sugar, ½ cup, 126 g	190	6	58
Black-eyed peas, ½ cup			
canned, solids & liquid, 120 g	90	1	6
cooked, drained, ½ cup, 82 g	80	<1	3
Chickpeas (garbanzos), canned, ½ cup, 120 g	145	1	12
Black beans, cooked, ½ cup, 86 g	115	<1	4
Kidney beans, cooked, ½ cup, 88 g	110	<1	4
Lima beans, cooked, drained, ½ cup, 85 g	105	<1	2
Navy beans, cooked, ½ cup, 91 g	130	1	5
Refried beans, canned, ½ cup, 126 g	135	1	12
Nuts and Seeds			
Almonds, unblanched			
dried, 3 Tbs., 28 g	165	15	133
dry roasted, 3 Tbs., 26 g	150	13	119
Cashews, dry roasted, 3 Tbs., 28 g	165	13	118
Coconut, dried, sweetened, flaked, 2 Tbs., 9 g	45	3	27
Peanut butter, 2 Tbs., 32 g	190	14	126
Peanuts, roasted			
dry roasted, 3 Tbs., 28 g	165	14	125
honey roasted, 3 Tbs., 28 g	170	14	126
Pecans, dried, ½ cup, 28 g	190	19	173
Pine nuts, dried, 1 Tbs., 10 g	50	5	46
Pistachios, dry roasted, 3 Tbs., 28 g	170	15	135
Sesame seeds			
Tahini, raw kernels, 1 Tbs., 15 g	85	7	65
dried, kernels, 1 Tbs., 8 g	45	4	39
Sunflower seeds, dry roasted, 3 Tbs., 28 g	165	14	127
Walnuts, dried, ¼ cup, 28 g	180	18	158
Meat Substitutes			
Burger, vegetarian			
Vege burger, Natural Touch, 1, 64 g	140	6	54
Veggie Sizzler, nonfat, Soy Boy, 1, 85 g	90	0	0
Hot dog, Not Dogs, 1, 43 g	105	5	45
Tofu			
fried, 2¾ x 1 x ½", 29 g	80	6	53
regular, ½ cup, 124 g	95	6	53

Dairy Products

Cheese	Calories	Fat grams	Calories from fat
American, light, 1 slice, 28g	70	4	36
Blue, crumbled (not packed), ¼ cup, 34 g	120	10	87
Brie, 1 oz., 28 g	95	8	70
Cheddar			
1" cube, 17 g	70	6	51
light, 1 slice, 28 g	70	4	36
Colby, 10 oz., 28 g	110	9	79
Cottage cheese, ½ cup			
creamed, large curd, 113 g	115	5	46
dry curd, 73 g	60	<1	3
low-fat, 1% fat, 113 g	80	1	10
Cream cheese, 2 Tbs.			
light, Philadelphia brand, 28 g	60	5	45
regular, 30 g	105	10	94
whipped, Philadelphia brand, 28 g	100	10	90
Feta, 1 oz., 28 g	75	6	54
Mozzarella, 1 oz., 28 g			
regular	80	6	54
part skim	70	4	40

Cheese	Calories	Fat grams	Calories from fat
Parmesan, grated, 1 Tbs., 5 g	25	2	14
Swiss			
1" cube, 15 g	55	4	37
light, 1 slice, 28 g	70	3	27
Cream			
Half & half, 1 Tbs., 15 g	20	2	16
Heavy, whipping, 1 Tbs., 15 g	50	6	48
Sour cream			
cultured, 2 Tbs., 24 g	50	5	45
light, 50% less fat, 2 Tbs., 30 g	40	2	22
Whipped cream, pressurized, 1 Tbs., 3 g	10	1	6
Imitation Cream Products			
Coffee creamers			
nondairy, liquid, Coffee Rich, 1 Tbs., 14 g	25	1	13
nondairy, liquid, Int'l Delight, 1 Tbs., 15 g	45	2	14
Sour cream			
imitation, cultured, nondairy, 2 Tbs., 28 g	60	5	49
imitation, nonbutterfat, 2 Tbs., 24 g	45	4	36
powdered, Coffee-Mate, 1 tsp., 2 g	10	1	6
Whipped topping			
nondairy, pressurized, 2 Tbs., 9 g	25	2	19
nondairy, frozen, Cool Whip, 1 Tbs., 4 g	10	1	7
Milk			
Buttermilk, 1% fat, 1 cup, 245 g	100	2	19
Chocolate milk, 1 cup, 250 g			
low-fat, 1% fat	160	2	22
whole	210	8	76
Condensed, sweetened, 2 Tbs., 38 g	125	3	30
Evaporated, canned, 2 Tbs., 32 g			
low-fat	30	1	5
skim	25	<1	1
whole	40	2	21
Low-fat, 1% fat, 1 cup, 244 g	100	3	23
Skim, 1 cup, 245 g	85	<1	4
Whole, 3.3% fat, 1 cup, 244 g	150	8	73
Yogurt			
Fruit flavors, custard, Yoplait, 1 cont., 170 g	190	4	36
Fruit-on-the-bottom, low-fat, 1 cont., 226 g	230	3	27
Plain, 1 cont., 226 g			
low-fat	145	4	32
nonfat	125	<1	4

Soups

Canned Soups

(Canned, condensed soups are prepared with water, unless otherwise noted.)

	Calories	Fat grams	Calories from fat
Bean & ham, Healthy Choice, ½ can, 228 g	220	4	36
Beef broth, ready-to-serve, 1 cup, 240 g	15	1	5
Black bean, Healthy Valley, 1 cup, 240 g	110	0	0
Chicken broth, ready-to-serve, ½ can, 249 g	30	3	27
Chicken noodle, Campbell's, 1 cup, 226 g	60	2	18
Chicken rice, 1 cup, 241 g	60	2	17

Clam chowder, New England	Calories	Fat grams	Calories from fat
frozen, Stouffer's 1 cup, 227 g	180	9	81
prepared w/skim milk, 1 cup, 233 g	100	2	18
prepared w/water, Campbell's, 1 cup, 224 g	80	2	20
Cream of Chicken, 1 cup, 244 g	110	7	62
Cream of mushroom, 1 cup			
prepared w/water, 244 g	130	9	81
prepared w/whole milk, 248 g	205	14	122
Minestrone			
prepared w/water, 1 cup, 241 g	80	3	23
ready-to-serve, Hain, ½ can, 270 g	160	3	27
Tomato, 1 cup			
prepared w/water, 244 g	85	2	17
prepared w/whole milk, 248 g	160	6	54
Vegetable			
prepared w/water, 1 cup, 241 g	90	1	9
ready-to-serve, Pritikin, ½ can, 209 g	70	0	0
Dried or Dehydrated Soups			
Black bean, Nile Spice, 1 container, 309 g	180	1	5
Chicken vegetable, 1 cup, 251 g	50	1	7
Cream of chicken, 1 cup, 261 g	105	5	48
Mushroom, 1 cup, 253 g	95	1	44
Onion, 1 pkg., 7 g	20	<1	4
Split pea, 1 cup, 271 g	135	2	14
Tomato, 1 cup, 265 g	105	2	22

Desserts, Snack Foods, and Candy

Cakes

	Calories	Fat grams	Calories from fat
Angel food, 1⁄12 of 10" tube, 50 g	130	<1	1
Boston Cream Pie, 1⁄6 of 20 oz., 92 g	230	8	70
Carrot cake, Sara Lee, snack size, 1, 52 g	180	7	63
Cheesecake, plain, 1⁄6 of 17 oz., 80 g	255	18	160
Cupcake, 1			
chocolate, Hostess, 46 g	170	5	45
yellow, w/icing, 36 g	130	4	34
Devil's food, w/icing, 1⁄6 of 9", 69 g	235	8	72
Fruitcake, 1 slice, 34 g	140	4	35
Pound cake, Sara Lee, 1⁄10 of cake, 30 g	130	7	63
Yellow cake, w/icing, 1⁄8 of 8 oz., 64 g	240	9	84

Cookies and Bars

Brownies, chocolate	Calories	Fat grams	Calories from fat
frozen, Weight-Watchers, 1, 36 g	100	3	27
from mix, 2" square, 33 g	140	7	59
Chocolate chip			
Chips Ahoy!, 3, 32 g	160	8	72
refrigerated, Pillsbury, 2, 31 g	140	7	59
Creme sandwich, Nabisco, 2, 28 g	140	6	54
Fig bar, 2, 31 g	110	2	21
Gingersnaps, Sunshine, 6, 28 g	120	4	36
Graham crackers, 4, 1½" squares, 28 g	120	2	18
Oatmeal raisin, Barbara's, 2, 38 g	160	7	63
Oreo, Nabisco, 2, 28 g	100	4	36

Cookies and Bars	Calories	Fat grams	Calories from fat
Shortbread, 1⅝" square, 4, 32 g	160	8	69
Vanilla wafers, Nabisco, 7, 28 g	120	4	36
Pies			
Apple, ⅛ of 9" pie, 155 g	410	19	175
Blueberry, ⅛ of 9" pie, 147 g	360	17	157
Cherry, ⅛ of 9" pie, 180 g	485	22	198
Chocolate cream, ⅛ of 9" pie, 142 g	400	23	206
Custard, ⅛ of 9" pie, 127 g	260	11	102
Lemon meringue, ⅛ of 9" pie, 127 g	360	16	147
Pumpkin, ⅛ of 9" pie, 155 g	315	14	130
Other Desserts			
Custard, baked, ½ cup, 141 g	150	7	60
Frozen yogurt, vanilla, ½ cup			
Häagen-Dazs, 98 g	160	2	22
Yoplait, soft, 72 g	90	3	27
Gelatin, Jell-O, ½ cup, 140 g	80	0	0
Ice cream, vanilla, ½ cup			
regular, 10% fat, 66 g	135	7	65
Häagen-Dazs, 106 g	260	17	153
Ice cream, chocolate, ½ cup			
regular, 10% fat, 66 g	145	7	65
Häagen-Dazs, 106 g	270	17	153
Ice milk sandwich, Weight Watchers, 78 g	160	4	36
Juice bars			
Strawberry, Fruit'n Juice, Dole, 74 g	70	0	0
Strawberry, Welch's, 85 g	80	0	0
Puddings, from mix, prepared w/2% milk			
butterscotch, ½ cup, 148 g	150	2	20
chocolate, ½ cup, 147 g	150	2	20
tapioca, ½ cup, 141 g	145	2	22
vanilla, ½ cup, 144 g	140	2	20
Sherbet, ½ cup, 87 g	135	2	17
Snack Foods			
Corn chips, ¾ cup, 28 g	155	9	85
Crackers (see Crackers)			
Nuts (see Nuts and Seeds)			
Popcorn			
air-popped, 1 cup, 8 g	30	<1	3
microwave, natural flavor, 1 cup, 8 g	35	2	18
Potato chips, 1 cup, 28 g	150	10	90
Pretzels			
Dutch, twisted, 2¾", 2, 32 g	120	1	10
Sticks, 2½ x ⅛", 60, 30 g	115	1	9
Twists, thin, Rold Gold, 10, 28 g	110	1	9
Candy			
Caramel, plain, ¾ inch, 8 g	30	1	6
Fudge, chocolate, 1 cu inch, 17 g	65	1	13
Gum drops, 8, 28 g	110	0	0
Hard candy, 5, 28 g	105	0	0
Jellybeans, 10 large or 26 small, 28 g	105	<1	1
Hershey's Kisses, 6, 28 g	150	9	81
Lollipops, 1, 28 g	110	0	0

Beverages

(Milk and juices are in Dairy Products and Fruits sections.)

Carbonated Sodas	Calories	Fat grams	Calories from fat
Cola, 1½ cup, 370 g	150	<1	0
Diet cola, w/aspartame, 1½ cup, 355 g	4	0	0
Gingerale, 1½ cup, 366 g	125	0	0
Grape soda, 1½ cup, 372 g	160	0	0
Lemon-lime, 1½ cup, 368 g	145	0	0
Orange soda, 1½ cup, 372 g	180	0	0
Root beer, 1½ cup, 370 g	150	0	0
Coffee and Tea			
Coffee			
brewed, 1 cup, 235 g	5	<1	0
brewed, decaffeinated, 1 cup, 240 g	3	0	0
instant, 1 cup, 240 g	5	0	0
Tea, brewed, 1 cup 237 g	2	<1	0
Tea, brewed herb, unflavored, 1 cup, 236 g	2	<1	0
Tea, iced, instant, lemon flavored			
sweetened w/aspartame, 1 cup, 259 g	2	0	0
sweetened w/sugar, made w/4 tsp., 23 g	85	<1	0
Alcoholic Beverages			
Beer, 1½ cup, 355 g			
light	100	0	0
regular	145	0	0
nonalcoholic	50	0	0
Gin, Rum, Whiskey, or Vodka,			
80 proof, 1 jigger, 42 g	95	0	0
Wine, 1 glass			
red, 147 g	105	0	0
white, 147 g	100	0	0
Wine cooler, 1 glass, 360 g	175	<1	0
Wine, dessert, 1 glass			
dry, 59 g	75	0	0
sweet, 59 g	90	0	0

Fats, Oils, and Condiments

Fats and Oils	Calories	Fat grams	Calories from fat
Butter			
regular or unsalted, 1 tsp., 5 g	35	4	37
whipped, 1 Tbs., 11 g	80	9	80
Margarine			
spread, tub, 1 Tbs., 14 g	75	9	75
stick, 1 Tbs., 14 g	100	11	100
Oil			
corn, 1 Tbs., 14 g	120	14	122
olive, 1 Tbs., 14 g	120	14	122
vegetable spray, 1¼ seconds, 1 g	5	1	5
Salad dressing			
blue cheese, 1 Tbs., 15 g	75	8	72
French 1 Tbs., 16 g	65	6	57
French, low-calorie, 1 Tbs., 16 g	20	1	9
Italian, 1 Tbs., 15 g	70	7	64
Italian, low calorie, 1 Tbs., 16 g	15	1	12
mayonnaise-like, 1 Tbs., 15 g	55	5	43
thousand island, 1 Tbs., 16 g	60	6	50

Condiments	Calories	Fat grams	Calories from fat
Barbecue sauce, 1 Tbs., 15g	15	<1	3
Catsup, 1 Tbs., 15 g	15	<1	0
Gravy, canned			
au jus, ¼ cup, 60 g	10	<1	1
beef, ¼ cup, 58 g	30	1	12
chicken, ¼ cup, 60 g	45	3	30
turkey, ¼ cup, 60 g	30	1	11
Horseradish, prepared, 1 tsp., 5 g	2	<1	0
Mustard, prepared, 1 tsp., 5 g	4	<1	2
Olives			
black, canned, small, 3, 10 g	10	1	9
green, medium, 4, 13 g	15	2	14
green, stuffed, 10, 34 g	35	4	34
Pickles			
dill, kosher spears, 1, 28 g	5	0	0
sweet, gherkins, small, 2½", 2, 30 g	40	<1	0
Relish, sweet pickle, 2 Tbs., 30 g	40	<1	1
Soy sauce, tamari, 1 Tbs., 18 g	10	<1	0
Tartar sauce, 1 Tbs., 14 g	75	8	68

Sugar, Jams, and Jellies

	Calories	Fat grams	Calories from fat
Chocolate syrup			
fudge-type, 2 Tbs., 42 g	145	6	51
thin-type, 2 Tbs., 38 g	82	<1	3
Honey, 1 Tbs., 21 g	65	0	0
Jams and preserves, 1 Tbs., 20 g	50	<1	0
Jellies, 1 Tbs., 19 g	50	<1	0
Maple syrup, 2 Tbs., 40 g	105	<1	1
Sugar			
brown, unpacked, 1 cup, 145 g	545	0	0
white, granulated, 1 tsp., 4 g	15	0	0

Fast Foods

Burgers and Sandwiches

Burger King	Calories	Fat grams	Calories from fat
Big Fish	700	41	370
Broiler Chicken	550	29	260
Double Cheeseburger with Bacon	640	39	350
Hamburger	330	15	140
Whopper	640	39	350
McDonald's			
Big Mac	530	28	250
Filet-O-Fish	360	16	150
Hamburger	270	10	90
McChicken	570	30	270
McGrilled Chicken	510	30	270
Wendy's			
Big Bacon Classic	610	33	290
Chicken Club	500	23	200
Grilled Chicken Sandwich	310	8	70
Hamburger, with everything	420	20	180

Salads, Fries, and Miscellaneous

(Salad values are given for salads without dressing.)

Burger King	Calories	Fat grams	Calories from fat
Broiled Chicken Salad	200	10	90
French fries, medium	370	20	180
Garden Salad	100	5	45
Salad dressing, 30 g, thousand island	140	12	110
Salad dressing, 30 g, ranch	180	19	170
Salad dressing, 30 g, reduced-calorie Italian	15	<1	5
McDonald's			
Chef Salad	210	11	100
Fajita Chicken Salad	160	6	60
French fries, large	450	22	200
French fries, small	210	10	90
Salad dressing, 1 pkg., blue cheese	190	17	150
Salad dressing, 1 pkg., lite vinaigrette	50	2	20
Salad dressing, 1 pkg., ranch	180	19	170
Pizza Hut			
Breadsticks, 5	770	25	223
Buffalo wings, 12	565	35	310
Cheese pizza, ⅛ of med., thin crust	205	8	75
Cheese pizza, ⅛ of med., pan pizza	260	11	98
Pepperoni pizza, ⅛ of med., thin crust	215	10	69
Veggie Lover's, ⅛ of med., thin crust	185	7	61
Wendy's			
Baked potato, plain	310	0	0
Baked potato w/chili and cheese	620	24	220
Baked potato w/sour cream and chives	380	6	60
Deluxe Garden Salad	110	6	50
Salad dressing, 2 Tbs., blue cheese	170	19	170
Salad dressing, 2 Tbs., fat-free French	30	0	0
Salad dressing, 2 Tbs., ranch	90	10	90

Desserts

Burger King	Calories	Fat grams	Calories from fat
Dutch apple pie	300	15	140
McDonald's			
Baked apple pie	260	13	120
Cookies	260	9	80
Pizza Hut			
Dessert pizza, ⅛ of med.	245	5	46
Wendy's			
Chocolate chip cookies, 1, 57 g	270	11	100

Glossary

abscess A localized accumulation of pus and disintegrating tissue.

absorption The passage of substances into or across membranes or tissues.

abstinence Voluntary refrainment from sexual intercourse.

acid rain Rain with a high concentration of acids produced by air pollutants emitted during the combustion of fossil fuels and the smelting of ores; damages plant and animal life and buildings.

acquired immunodeficiency syndrome (AIDS) The final stages of HIV infection, characterized by a variety of severe illnesses and decreased levels of certain immune cells.

active stretching A technique that involves stretching a muscle by contracting the opposing muscle.

acupuncture A Chinese medical practice of puncturing the body with needles inserted at specific points to relieve pain or cure disease.

acute injuries Physical injuries, such as sprains, bruises, and pulled muscles, which result from sudden traumas, such as falls or collisions.

adaptive response The body's attempt to reestablish homeostasis or stability.

addiction A behavioral pattern characterized by compulsion, loss of control, and continued repetition of a behavior or activity in spite of adverse consequences.

additive Characterized by a combined effect that is equal to the sum of the individual effects.

additives Substances added to foods to enhance certain qualities, such as appearance, taste, or freshness.

adoption The legal process for becoming the parent to a child of other biological parents.

advance directives Documents that specify individual's preferences regarding treatment in a medical crisis.

aerobic circuit training Combining aerobic and strength exercises to build both cardiorespiratory fitness and muscular strength and endurance.

aerobic exercise Physical activity in which sufficient or excess oxygen is continually supplied to the body.

alcohol abuse Continued use of alcohol despite awareness of social, occupational, psychological, or physical problems related to its use, or use of alcohol in dangerous ways or situations, such as before driving.

alcohol dependence Development of a strong craving for alcohol due to the pleasurable feelings or relief of stress or anxiety produced by drinking.

alcoholism A chronic, progressive, potentially fatal disease characterized by impaired control of drinking, a preoccupation with alcohol, continued use of alcohol despite adverse consequences, and distorted thinking, most notably denial.

allergy A hypersensitivity to a particular substance in one's environment or diet.

allopathic medicine Conventional or orthodox Western medicine.

allostasis The body's ability to adapt to constantly changing environments.

altruism Acts of helping or giving to others without thought of self-benefit.

Alzheimer's disease A progressive deterioration of intellectual powers due to physiological changes within the brain; symptoms include diminishing ability to concentrate and reason, disorientation, depression, apathy, and paranoia.

amenorrhea The absence or suppression of menstruation.

amino acids Organic compounds containing nitrogen, carbon, hydrogen, and oxygen; the essential building blocks of proteins.

amnion The innermost membrane of the sac enclosing the embryo or fetus.

amphetamine Any of a class of stimulants that trigger the release of epinephrine, which stimulates the central nervous system; users experience a state of hyper-alertness and energy, followed by a crash as the drug wears off.

anabolic steroids Drugs derived from testosterone and approved for medical use, but often used by athletes to increase their musculature and weight.

anaerobic exercise Physical activity in which the body develops an oxygen deficit.

androgyny The expression of both masculine and feminine traits.

anemia A condition characterized by a marked reduction in the number of circulating red blood cells or in hemoglobin, the oxygen-carrying component of red blood cells.

angina pectoris A severe, suffocating chest pain caused by a brief lack of oxygen to the heart.

angioplasty Surgical repair of an obstructed artery by passing a balloon catheter through the blood vessel to the area of disease and then inflating the catheter to compress the plaque against the vessel wall.

anorexia nervosa A psychological disorder in which refusal to eat and/or an extreme loss of appetite leads to malnutrition, severe weight loss, and possibly death.

antagonistic Opposing or counteracting.

antibiotics Substances produced by microorganisms, or synthetic agents, that are toxic to other types of microorganisms; in dilute solutions, used to treat infectious diseases.

antidepressant A drug used primarily to treat symptoms of depression.

antioxidants Substances that prevent the damaging effects of oxidation in cells.

antiviral drug A substance that decreases the severity and duration of a viral infection if taken prior to or soon after onset of the infection.

anxiety A feeling of apprehension and dread, with or without a known cause; may range from mild to severe and may be accompanied by physical symptoms.

anxiety disorders A group of psychological disorders involving episodes of apprehension, tension, or uneasiness, stemming from the anticipation of danger and sometimes accompanied by physical symptoms, which cause significant distress and impairment to an individual.

aorta The main artery of the body, arising from the left ventricle of the heart.

appetite A desire for food, stimulated by anticipated hunger, physiological changes within the brain and body, the availability of food, and other environmental and psychological factors.

arrhythmia Any irregularity in the rhythm of the heartbeat.

arteriosclerosis Any of a number of chronic diseases characterized by degeneration of the arteries and hardening and thickening of arterial walls.

arthritis Inflammation of the joints.

artificial insemination The introduction of viable sperm into the vagina by artificial means for the purpose of inducing conception.

assertive Behaving in a confident manner to make your needs and desires clear to others in a nonhostile way.

asthma A disease or allergic response characterized by bronchial spasms and difficult breathing.

atherosclerosis A form of arteriosclerosis in which fatty substances (plaque) are deposited on the inner walls of arteries.

atrial fibrillation A condition characterized by an irregular, abnormally rapid heartbeat.

atrium (plural **atria**) Either of the two upper chambers of the heart, which receive blood from the veins.

attention deficit/hyperactivity disorder (ADHD) A spectrum of difficulties in controlling motion and sustaining attention, including hyperactivity, impulsivity, and distractibility.

autoimmune Resulting from the attack on body tissue by an immune system that fails to recognize the tissue as self.

autonomy The ability to draw on internal resources; independence from familial and societal influences.

autoscopy The sensation of one's self being outside its body, often experienced by individuals in near-death medical crises.

aversion therapy A treatment that attempts to help a person overcome a dependence or bad habit by making the person feel disgusted or repulsed by that habit.

axon The long fiber that conducts impulses from the neuron's nucleus to its dendrites.

axon terminal The ending of an axon, from which impulses are transmitted to a dendrite of another neuron.

ayurveda A traditional Indian medical treatment involving meditation, exercise, herbal medications, and nutrition.

bacteria (singular, **bacterium**) One-celled microscopic organisms; the most plentiful pathogens.

bacterial vaginosis A vaginal infection caused by overgrowth and depletion of various microorganisms living in the vagina, resulting in a malodorous white or gray vaginal discharge.

ballistic stretching Rapid bouncing movements.

barbiturates Antianxiety drugs that depress the central nervous system, reduce activity and induce relaxation, drowsiness, or sleep; often prescribed to relieve tension and treat epileptic seizures or as a general anesthetic.

barrier contraceptives Birth-control devices that block the meeting of egg and sperm, either by physical barriers, such as condoms, diaphragms, or cervical caps, or by chemical barriers, such as spermicide, or both.

basal body temperature The body temperature upon waking, before any activity.

basal metabolic rate (BMR) The number of calories required to sustain the body at rest.

behavior therapy Psychotherapy that emphasizes application of the principles of learning to substitute desirable responses and behavior patterns for undesirable ones.

benign prostatic hypertrophy Enlargement of the prostate gland, resulting in a pinching of the urethra.

benzodiazepines Antianxiety drugs that depress the central nervous system, reduce activity and induce relaxation, drowsiness, or sleep; often prescribed to relieve tension, muscular strain, sleep problems, anxiety, and panic attacks; also used as an anesthetic and in the treatment of alcohol withdrawal.

bidis Skinny, sweet-flavored cigarettes.

binge drinking For a man, having five or more alcoholic drinks at a single sitting; for a woman, having four drinks or more at a single sitting.

binge eating The rapid consumption of an abnormally large amount of food in a relatively short time.

biofeedback A technique of becoming aware, with the aid of external monitoring devices, of internal physiological activities in order to develop the capability of altering them.

bipolar disorder Severe depression alternating with periods of manic activity and elation.

bisexual Sexually oriented toward both sexes.

blended family A family formed when one or both of the partners bring children from a previous union to the new marriage.

blood-alcohol concentration (BAC) The amount of alcohol in the blood, expressed as a percentage.

body composition The relative amounts of fat and lean tissue (bone, muscle, organs, water) in the body.

body mass index (BMI) A mathematical formula that correlates with body fat; the ratio of weight to height squared.

bone-marrow transplantation A cancer treatment involving high doses of radiation or chemotherapy during which the marrow is destroyed and then replaced with healthy bone marrow.

botulism Possibly fatal food poisoning, caused by a type of bacterium that grows and produces its toxin in the absence of air and is found in improperly canned food.

bradycardia An abnormally slow heart rate, under 60 beats per minute.

breech birth A birth in which the infant's buttocks or feet pass through the birth canal first.

bulimia nervosa Episodic binge eating, often followed by forced vomiting or laxative abuse, and accompanied by a persistent preoccupation with body shape and weight.

bupropion A drug, also known as Zyban, for treating nicotine addiction that is an alternative to the nicotine patch.

burnout A state of physical, emotional, and mental exhaustion resulting from constant or repeated emotional pressure.

caesarean delivery The surgical procedure in which an infant is delivered through an incision made in the abdominal wall and uterus.

calorie The amount of energy required to raise the temperature of 1 gram of water by 1 degree Celsius. In everyday usage related to the energy content of foods and the energy expended in activities, a calorie is actually the equivalent of a thousand such calories, or a kilocalorie.

candidiasis An infection of the yeast *Candida albicans,* commonly occurring in the vagina, vulva, penis, and mouth and causing burning, itching, and a whitish discharge.

capillary A minute blood vessel that connects an artery to a vein.

carbohydrates Organic compounds, such as starches, sugars, and glycogen, that are composed of carbon, hydrogen, and oxygen, and are sources of bodily energy.

carbon monoxide A colorless, odorless gas produced by the burning of gasoline or tobacco; displaces oxygen in the hemoglobin molecules of red blood cells.

carcinogen A substance that produces cancerous cells or enhances their development and growth.

cardiopulmonary resuscitation (CPR) A method of artificial stimulation of the heart and lungs; a combination of mouth-to-mouth breathing and chest compression.

cardiorespiratory fitness The ability of the heart and blood vessels to circulate blood through the body efficiently.

celibacy Abstention from sexual activity; can be partial or complete, permanent or temporary.

cell-mediated The portion of the immune response that protects against parasites, fungi, cancer cells, and foreign tissue, primarily by means of T cells, or lymphocytes.

certified social worker A person who has completed a two-year graduate program in counseling people with mental problems.

cervical cap A thimble-sized rubber or plastic cap that is inserted into the vagina to fit over the cervix and prevent the passage of sperm into the uterus during sexual intercourse; used with a spermicidal foam or jelly, it serves as both a chemical and a physical barrier to sperm.

cervix The narrow, lower end of the uterus that opens into the vagina.

chanchroid A soft, painful sore or localized infection usually acquired through sexual contact.

chemoprevention The use of natural or synthetic substances to reduce the risk of developing cancer.

chiropractic A method of treating disease, primarily through manipulating the bones and joints to restore normal nerve function.

chlamydial infections A sexually transmitted disease caused by the bacterium *Chlamydia trachomatis,* often asymptomatic in women, but sometimes characterized by urinary pain; if undetected and untreated, may result in pelvic inflammatory disease (PID).

chlorinated hydrocarbons Highly toxic pesticides, such as DDT and chlordane, that are extremely resistant to breakdown; may cause cancer, birth defects, neurological disorders, and damage to wildlife and the environment.

cholesterol An organic substance found in animal fats; linked to cardiovascular disease, particularly atherosclerosis.

chronic fatigue syndrome (CFS) A cluster of symptoms whose cause is not yet known; a primary symptom is debilitating fatigue.

chronic obstructive lung disease (COLD) Any one of several lung diseases characterized by obstruction of breathing, including emphysema and chronic bronchitis.

circumcision The surgical removal of the foreskin of the penis.

cirrhosis A chronic disease, especially of the liver, characterized by a degeneration of cells and excessive scarring.

clitoris A small erectile structure on the female, corresponding to the penis on the male.

club drugs Illegally manufactured psychoactive drugs that have dangerous physical and psychological effects.

cocaine A white crystalline powder extracted from the leaves of the coca plant which stimulates the central nervous system and produces a brief period of euphoria followed by a depression.

codependence An emotional and psychological behavioral pattern in which the spouses, partners, parents, children, and friends of individuals with addictive behaviors allow or enable their loved ones to continue their self-destructive habits.

cognitive therapy A technique used to identify an individual's beliefs and attitudes, recognize negative thought patterns, and educate in alternative ways of thinking.

cohabitation Two people living together as a couple, without official ties such as marriage.

coitus interruptus The removal of the penis from the vagina before ejaculation.

colpotomy Surgical sterilization by cutting or blocking the fallopian tubes through an incision made in the wall of the vagina.

coma A state of total unconsciousness.

companion-oriented marriage A marital relationship in which the partners share interests, activities, and domestic responsibilities.

complementary and alternative medicine (CAM) A term used to apply to all health-care approaches, practices, and treatments not widely taught in medical schools, not generally used in hospitals, and not usually reimbursed by medical insurance companies.

complementary proteins Incomplete proteins that, when combined, provide all the amino acids essential for protein synthesis.

complete proteins Proteins that contain all the amino acids needed by the body for growth and maintenance.

complex carbohydrates Starches, including cereals, fruits, and vegetables.

computer vision syndrome A condition caused by computer use marked by tired and sore eyes, blurred vision, headaches, and neck, shoulder, and back pain.

conception The merging of a sperm and an ovum.

conditioning The gradual building up of the body to enhance one or more of the three main components of physical fitness: flexibility, cardiorespiratory or aerobic fitness, and muscular strength and endurance.

condom A latex sheath worn over the penis during sexual acts to prevent conception and/or the transmission of disease; some condoms contain a spermicidal lubricant.

congestive heart failure Inability of the heart to pump at normal capacity, resulting in decreased blood flow throughout the body, collection of blood fluids in the lungs, and pulmonary congestion.

constant-dose combination pill An oral contraceptive that releases synthetic estrogen and progestin at constant levels throughout the menstrual cycle.

contraception The prevention of conception; birth control.

coronary angiography A diagnostic test in which a thin tube is threaded through the blood vessels of the heart, a dye is injected, and X rays are taken to detect blockage of the arteries.

coronary bypass Surgical correction of a blockage in a coronary artery by grafting an artery from the patient's leg or chest wall onto the damaged artery to detour blood around the blockage.

corpus luteum A yellowish mass of tissue that is formed, immediately after ovulation, from the remaining cells of the follicle; it secretes estrogen and progesterone for the remainder of the menstrual cycle.

Cowper's glands Two small glands that discharge into the male urethra; also called bulbourethral glands.

crib death *See* sudden infant death syndrome (SIDS).

cross-training Alternating two or more different types of fitness activities.

crucifers Plants, including broccoli, cabbage, and cauliflower, that contain large amounts of fiber, proteins, and indoles.

culture The set of shared attitudes, values, goals, and practices of a group that are internalized by an individual within the group.

cunnilingus Sexual stimulation of a woman's genitals by means of oral manipulation.

cystitis Inflammation of the urinary bladder.

daily values (DV) Reference values developed by the FDA specifically for use on food labels.

decibel (dB) A unit for measuring the intensity of sounds.

deleriants Chemicals, such as solvents, aerosols, glue, cleaning fluids, petroleum products, and some anesthetics, that produce vapors with psychoactive effects when inhaled.

delirium tremens (DTs) The delusions, hallucinations, and agitated behavior following withdrawal from long-term chronic alcohol abuse.

dementia Deterioration of mental capability.

dendrites Branching fibers of a neuron that receive impulses from axon terminals of other neurons and conduct these impulses toward the nucleus.

depression In general, feelings of unhappiness and despair; as a mental illness, also characterized by an inability to function normally

depressive disorders A group of psychological disorders involving pervasive and sustained depression.

dermatitis Any inflammation of the skin.

detoxification The supervised removal of a poisonous or harmful substance (such as a drug) from the body; a therapy for alcoholics in which they are denied alcohol in a controlled environment.

diabetes mellitus A disease in which the inadequate production of insulin leads to failure of the body tissues to break down carbohydrates at a normal rate.

diagnostic-related group (DRG) A category of conditions requiring hospitalization for which the cost of care has been determined prior to a client's hospitalization.

diaphragm A bowl-like rubber cup with a flexible rim that is inserted into the vagina to cover the cervix and prevent the passage of sperm into the uterus during sexual intercourse; used with a spermicidal foam or jelly, it serves as both a chemical and a physical barrier to sperm.

diastole The period between contractions in the cardiac cycle, during which the heart relaxes and dilates as it fills with blood.

dietary reference intakes (DRI) A set of values for the dietary nutrient intakes of healthy people in the United States and Canada. These values are used for planning and assessing diets and include Estimated Average Requirements, Recommended Dietary Allowances, Adequate Intakes, and Tolerable Upper Intake levels.

dilation and evacuation (D and E) A medical procedure in which the contents of the uterus are removed through the use of instruments.

distress A negative stress that may result in illness.

do-not-resuscitate (DNR) An advance directive expressing an individual's preference that resuscitation efforts not be made during a medical crisis.

drug Any substance, other than food, that affects bodily functions and structures when taken into the body.

drug abuse The excessive use of a drug in a manner inconsistent with accepted medical practice.

drug misuse The use of a drug for a purpose (or person) other than that for which it was medically intended.

dyathanasia The act of permitting death by the removal or ending of any extraordinary efforts to sustain life; passive euthanasia.

dynamic flexibility The ability to move a joint quickly and fluidly through its entire range of motion with little resistance.

dysfunctional Characterized by negative and destructive patterns of behavior between partners or between parents and children.

dysmenorrhea Painful menstruation.

dyspareunia A sexual difficulty in which a woman experiences pain during sexual intercourse.

dysthymia Frequent, prolonged mild depression.

eating disorders Bizarre, often dangerous patterns of food consumption, including anorexia nervosa and bulimia nervosa.

ecosystem A community of organisms sharing a physical and chemical environment and interacting with each other.

ecstasy (MDMA) A synthetic compound, also known as methylenedioxymethamphetamine, that is similar in structure to methamphetamine and has both stimulant and hallucinogenic effects.

ectopic pregnancy A pregnancy in which the fertilized egg has implanted itself outside the uterine cavity, usually in the fallopian tube.

ejaculation The expulsion of semen from the penis.

ejaculatory duct The canal connecting the seminal vesicles and vas deferens.

electrocardiogram (ECG, EKG) A graphic record of the electric current associated with heartbeats.

electromagnetic fields (EMFs) The invisible electric and magnetic fields generated by an electrically charged conductor.

embryo An organism in its early stage of development; in humans, the embryonic period lasts from the second to the eighth week of pregnancy.

emergency contraception Types of oral contraceptive pills usually taken within 72 hours after intercourse that can prevent pregnancy.

emotional health The ability to express and acknowledge one's feelings and moods.

emotional intelligence A term used by some psychologists to evaluate the capacity of people to understand themselves and relate well with others.

enabling To unwittingly contribute to a person's addictive or abusive behavior. Components of enabling include shielding or covering up for an abuser/addict; controlling them; taking over responsibilities; rationalizing addictive behavior; or cooperating with them.

endocrine disruptors Synthetic chemicals that interfere with the ways that hormones work in humans and wildlife.

endocrine system The group of ductless glands that produce hormones and secrete them directly into the blood for transport to target organs.

endometrium The mucous membrane lining the uterus.

endorphins Mood-elevating, pain-killing chemicals produced by the brain.

endurance The ability to withstand the stress of continued physical exertion.

environmental tobacco smoke Secondhand cigarette smoke; the third leading preventable cause of death.

epididymis That portion of the male duct system in which sperm mature.

epidural block An injection of anesthesia into the membrane surrounding the spinal cord to numb the lower body during labor and childbirth.

epilepsy A variety of neurological disorders characterized by sudden attacks (seizures) of violent muscle contractions and unconsciousness.

ergogenic aids Dietary supplements that purport to boost strength and enhance athletic performance, such as androstenedione and creatine.

erogenous Sexually sensitive.

essential nutrients Nutrients that the body cannot manufacture for itself and must obtain from food.

estrogen The female sex hormone that stimulates female secondary sex characteristics.

ethyl alcohol The intoxicating agent in alcoholic beverages; also called ethanol.

eustress Positive stress, which stimulates a person to function properly.

euthanasia Any method of painlessly causing death for a terminally ill person.

failure rate The number of pregnancies that occur per year for every 100 women using a particular method of birth control.

fallopian tubes The pair of channels that transport ova from the ovaries to the uterus; the usual site of fertilization.

false negative A diagnostic test result that falsely indicates the absence of a particular condition.

false positive A diagnostic test result that falsely indicates the presence of a particular condition.

family A group of people united by marriage, blood, or adoption, residing in the same household, maintaining a common culture, and interacting with one another on the basis of their roles within the group.

fellatio Sexual stimulation of a man's genitals by means of oral manipulation.

fertilization The fusion of the sperm and egg nuclei.

fetal alcohol effects (FAE) Milder forms of FAS, including low birthweight, irri-tability as newborns, and permanent mental impairment as a result of the mother's alcohol consumption during pregnancy.

fetal alcohol syndrome (FAS) A cluster of physical and mental defects in the newborn, including low birthweight, smaller-than-normal head circumference, intrauterine growth retardation, and permanent mental impairment caused by the mother's alcohol consumption during pregnancy.

fetus The human organism developing in the uterus from the ninth week until birth.

fiber Indigestible materials in food that lower blood cholesterol or facilitate digestion and elimination.

flexibility The range of motion allowed by one's joints; determined by the length of muscles, tendons, and ligaments attached to the joints.

folate Various chemical forms of a water-soluble B vitamin that can be obtained from a diet high in vegetables and citrus fruit.

folic acid A form of folate used in vitamin supplements and fortified foods.

food allergies Hypersensitivities to particular foods.

food toxicologists Specialists who detect toxins in food and treat the conditions toxins produce.

frostbite The freezing or partial freezing of skin and tissue just below the skin, or even muscle and bone; more severe than frostnip.

frostnip Sudden blanching or lightening of the skin on hands, feet, and face, resulting from exposure to high wind speeds and low temperatures.

fungi (singular, **fungus**) Organisms that reproduce by means of spores.

gallstones Clumps of solid material, usually cholesterol, that form in bile stored in the gallbladder.

gamma globulin The antibody-containing portion of the blood fluid (plasma).

GBL gamma butyrolactone The main ingredient in gamma hydroxybutyrate (GHB), also known as the "date rape drug"; once ingested, GBL converts to GHB and can cause the ingestor to lose consciousness.

gender Maleness or femaleness, as determined by a combination of anatomical and physiological factors, psychological factors, and learned behaviors.

gene therapy A cancer treatment involving the insertion of genes into a patient.

general adaptation syndrome (GAS) The sequenced physiological response to a stressful situation; consists of three stages: alarm, resistance, and exhaustion.

generalized anxiety disorder (GAD) An anxiety disorder characterized as chronic distress.

generic Refers to products without trade names that are equivalent to other products protected by trademark registration.

GHB gamma hydroxybutyrate A brain messenger chemical that stimulates the release of human growth hormone; commonly abused for its high and its alleged ability to trim fat and build muscles. Also known as "blue nitro" or the "date rape drug."

gingivitis Inflammation of the gums.

glia Support cells for neurons in the brain and spinal cord that separate the brain from the bloodstream, assist in the growth of neurons, speed transmission of nerve impulses, and eliminate damaged neurons.

gonadotropins Gonad-stimulating hormones produced by the pituitary gland.

gonorrhea A sexually transmitted disease caused by the bacterium *Neisseria gonorrhoeae;* symptoms include discharge from the penis; women are generally asymptomatic.

guided imagery An approach to stress control, self-healing, or motivating life changes by means of visualizing oneself in the state of calmness, wellness, or change.

gum disease Inflammation of the gum and bones that hold teeth in place.

hallucinogen A drug that causes hallucinations.

hashish A concentrated form of a drug, derived from the cannabis plant, containing the psychoactive ingredient TCH, which causes a sense of euphoria when inhaled or eaten.

health A state of complete well-being, including physical, psychological, spiritual, social, intellectual, and environmental components.

health maintenance organization (HMO) An organization that provides health services on a fixed-contract basis.

health promotion An educational and informational process in which people are helped to change attitudes and behaviors in an effort to improve their health.

heat cramps Painful muscle spasms caused by vigorous exercise accompanied by heavy sweating in the heat.

heat exhaustion Faintness, rapid heart beat, low blood pressure, an ashen appearance, cold and clammy skin, and nausea, resulting from prolonged sweating with inadequate fluid replacement.

heat stress Physical response to prolonged exposure to high temperature; occurs simultaneously with or after heat cramps.

heat stroke A medical emergency consisting of a fever of at least 105°F, hot dry skin, rapid heartbeat, rapid and shallow breathing, and elevated or lowered blood pressure, caused by the breakdown of the body's cooling mechanism.

helminth A parasitic roundworm or flatworm.

hemoglobin The oxygen-transporting component of red blood cells; composed of heme and globin.

hepatitis An inflammation and/or infection of the liver caused by a virus, often accompanied by jaundice.

herbal medicine An ancient form of medical treatment using substances derived from trees, flowers, ferns, seaweeds, and lichens to treat disease.

hernia The abnormal protrusion of an organ or body part through the tissues of the walls containing it.

herpes simplex A condition caused by one of the herpes viruses and characterized by lesions of the skin or mucous membranes; herpes virus type 2 is sexually transmitted and causes genital blisters or sores.

heterosexual Primary sexual orientation toward members of the other sex.

holistic An approach to medicine that takes into account body, mind, emotions, and spirit.

holographic will A will wholly in the handwriting of its author.

home health care Provision of medical services and equipment to patients in the home to restore or maintain comfort, function, and health.

homeopathy A system of medical practice that treats a disease by administering dosages of substances that would in healthy persons produce symptoms similar to those of the disease.

homeostasis The body's natural state of balance or stability.

homocysteine A naturally occurring amino acid that has recently been identified as a risk factor for heart disease.

homosexual Primary sexual orientation toward members of the same sex.

hormone Substance released in the blood that regulates specific bodily functions.

hormone replacement therapy (HRT) The use of supplemental hormones during and after menopause.

hospice A homelike health-care facility or program committed to supportive care for terminally ill people.

host A person or population that contracts one or more pathogenic agents in an environment.

hostile or offensive environment A workplace made hostile, abusive, or unbearable by persistent inappropriate behaviors of coworkers or supervisors.

human immunodeficiency virus (HIV) A type of virus that causes a spectrum of health problems, ranging from a symptomless infection to changes in the immune system, to the development of life-threatening diseases because of impaired immunity.

human papilloma virus (HPV) A pathogen that causes genital warts and increases the risk of cervical cancer.

humoral A portion of the immune response that provides lifelong protection against bacterial or viral infections, such as mumps, by means of antibodies whose production is triggered by the release of antigens upon first exposure to the infectious agent.

hunger The physiological drive to consume food.

hypertension High blood pressure occurring when the blood exerts excessive pressure against the arterial walls.

hypothermia An abnormally low body temperature; if not treated appropriately, coma or death could result.

hysterectomy The surgical removal of the uterus.

hysterotomy A procedure in which the uterus is surgically opened and the fetus inside it removed.

immune deficiency Partial or complete inability of the immune system to respond to pathogens.

immunity Protection from infectious diseases.

immunotherapy A series of injections of small but increasing doses of an allergen, used to treating allergies.

implantation The embedding of the fertilized ovum in the uterine lining.

impotence A sexual difficulty in which a man is unable to achieve or maintain an erection.

incomplete proteins Proteins that lack one or more of the amino acids essential for protein synthesis.

incubation period The time between a pathogen's entrance into the body and the first symptom.

indemnity A form of insurance that pays a major portion of medical expenses after a deductible amount is paid by the insured person.

indoles Naturally occurring chemicals found in foods such as winter squash, carrots, and crucifers; may help lower cancer risk.

infertility The inability to conceive a child.

infiltration A gradual penetration or invasion.

inflammation A localized response by the body to tissue injury, characterized by swelling and the dilation of the blood vessels.

inflammatory bowel disease (IBD) A digestive disease that causes frequent and intense diarrhea, abdominal pain, gas, fever, and rectal bleeding. Crohn's disease is an inflammation anywhere in the digestive tract, and ulcerative colitis causes severe ulcers in the inner lining of the colon and rectum.

informed consent Permission (to undergo or receive a medical procedure or treatment) given voluntarily, with full knowledge and understanding of the procedure or treatment and its possible consequences.

inhalants Substances that produce vapors having psychoactive effects when sniffed.

insoluble fiber Fiber that increases bulk in feces, prevents constipation and diverticulosis, and may lower the risks of heart disease and stroke. May be found in wheat and corn bran, leafy greens, and the skins of fruits and root vegetables.

integrative medicine An approach that combines traditional medicine with alternative/complementary therapies.

intercourse Sexual stimulation by means of entry of the penis into the vagina; coitus.

interpersonal therapy (IPT) A technique used to develop communication skills and relationships.

intimacy A state of closeness between two people, characterized by the desire and ability to share one's innermost thoughts and feelings with each other either verbally or nonverbally.

intoxication Maladaptive behavioral, psychological, and physiologic changes that occur as a result of substance abuse.

intramuscular Into or within a muscle.

intrauterine device (IUD) A device inserted into the uterus through the cervix to prevent pregnancy by interfering with implantation.

intravenous Into a vein.

ionizing radiation A form of energy emitted from atoms as they undergo internal change.

irradiation Exposure to or treatment by some form of radiation.

irritable bowel syndrome A digestive disease caused by intestinal spasms, resulting in frequent need to defecate, nausea, cramping, pain, gas, and a continual sensation of rectal fullness.

isokinetic Having the same force; exercise with specialized equipment that provides resistance equal to the force applied by the user throughout the entire range of motion.

isometric Of the same length; exercise in which muscles increase their tension without shortening in length, such as when pushing an immovable object.

isotonic Having the same tension or tone; exercise requiring the repetition of an action that creates tension, such as weight lifting or calisthenics.

kidney stones Formations of calcium salts or minerals that form in the kidneys; may be passed out of the body in urine, surgically removed, or decomposed by high-frequency sound waves.

labia majora The fleshy outer folds that border the female genital area.

labia minora The fleshy inner folds that border the female genital area.

labor The process leading up to birth: effacement and dilation of the cervix; the movement of the baby into and through the birth canal, accompanied by strong contractions; and contraction of the uterus and expulsion of the placenta after the birth.

lacto-vegetarians People who eat dairy products as well as fruits and vegetables (but not meat, poultry, or fish).

Lamaze method A method of childbirth preparation taught to expectant parents to help the woman cope with the discomfort of labor; combines breathing and psychological techniques.

laparoscopy A surgical sterilization procedure in which the fallopian tubes are observed with a laparoscope inserted through a small incision, and then cut or blocked.

laparotomy A surgical sterilization procedure in which the fallopian tubes are cut or blocked through an incision made in the abdomen.

licensed clinical social worker (LCSW). See certified social worker.

lipoprotein A compound in blood that is made up of proteins and fat; a high-density lipoprotein (HDL) picks up excess cholesterol in the blood; a low-density lipoprotein (LDL) carries more cholesterol and deposits it on the walls of arteries.

listeria A bacterium commonly found in deli meats, hot dogs, and soft cheeses that can cause an infection called listeriosis.

living will A written statement providing instructions for the use of life-sustaining procedures in the event of terminal illness or injury.

lochia The vaginal discharge of blood, mucus, and uterine tissue that occurs after birth.

locus of control An individual's belief about the source of power and influence over his or her life.

lumpectomy The surgical removal of a breast tumor and its surrounding tissue.

Lyme disease A disease caused by a bacterium carried by a tick; it may cause heart arrhythmias, neurological problems, and arthritis symptoms.

lymph nodes Small tissue masses in which some immune cells are stored.

mainstream smoke The smoke inhaled directly by smoking a cigarette.

major depression Sadness that does not end.

male pattern baldness The loss of hair at the vertex, or top, of the head.

malpractice The failure of a doctor or other health-care professional to provide appropriate and skillful medical or surgical treatment.

mammography A diagnostic X-ray exam used to detect breast cancer.

managed care Health-care services and reimbursement predetermined by third-party insurers.

marijuana The drug derived from the cannabis plant, containing the psychoactive ingredient THC, which causes a mild sense of euphoria when inhaled or eaten.

marriage and family therapist A psychiatrist, psychologist, or social worker who specializes in marriage and family counseling.

massage therapy A therapeutic method of using the hands to rub, stroke, or knead the body to produce positive effects on an individual's health and well-being.

mastectomy The surgical removal of an entire breast.

masturbation Manual (or nonmanual) self-stimulation of the genitals, often resulting in orgasm.

medical abortion Method of ending a pregnancy within 9 weeks of conception using hormonal medications that cause expulsion of the fertilized egg.

medical history The health-related information collected during the interview of a client by a health-care professional.

meditation A group of approaches that use quiet sitting, breathing techniques, and/or chanting to relax, improve concentration, and become attuned to one's inner self.

menarche The onset of menstruation at puberty.

meningitis An extremely serious, potentially fatal illness that attacks the membranes around the brain and spinal cord; caused by the bacterium *Neisseria meningitis.*

menopause The complete cessation of ovulation and menstruation for twelve consecutive months.

menstruation Discharge of blood from the vagina as a result of the shedding of the uterine lining at the end of the menstrual cycle.

mental disorder Behavioral or psychological syndrome associated with distress or disability or with a significantly increased risk of suffering death, pain, disability, or loss of freedom.

mental health The ability to perceive reality as it is, to respond to its challenges, and to develop rational strategies for living.

meta-analysis Summarization and review of research in a particular area to evaluate the results of several large clinical trials in a uniform manner.

metastasize To spread to other parts of the body via the bloodstream or lymphatic system.

microwaves Extremely high frequency electromagnetic waves that increase the rate at which molecules vibrate, thereby generating heat.

migraine headache Severe headache resulting from the constriction, then dilation of blood vessels within the brain; sometimes accompanied by vomiting and nausea.

mindfulness A method of stress reduction that involves experiencing the physical and mental sensations of the present moment.

minerals Naturally occurring inorganic substances, small amounts of some being essential in metabolism and nutrition.

minilaparotomy A surgical sterilization procedure in which the fallopian tubes are cut or sealed by electrical coagulation through a small incision just above the pubic hairline.

minipill An oral contraceptive containing a small amount of progestin and no estrogen, which prevents contraception by making the mucus in the cervix so thick that sperm cannot enter the uterus.

miscarriage A pregnancy that terminates before the twentieth week of gestation; also called spontaneous abortion.

mitral valve prolapse A condition in which a valve in the heart is abnormally long and floppy, which can cause heart murmurs.

mononucleosis An infectious viral disease characterized by an excess of white blood cells in the blood, fever, bodily discomfort, a sore throat, and kidney and liver complications.

monophasic pill *See* constant-dose combination pill.

mons pubis The rounded, fleshy area over the junction of the female pubic bones.

mood A sustained emotional state that colors one's view of the world for hours or days.

multiphasic pill An oral contraceptive that releases different levels of estrogen and progestin to mimic the hormonal fluctuations of the natural menstrual cycle.

multiple chemical sensitivity (MCS) A sensitivity to low-level chemical exposures from ordinary substances, such as perfumes and tobacco smoke, that results in physiological responses such as chest pain, depression, dizziness, fatigue, and nausea. Also known as environmentally triggered illness.

muscular fitness The amount of strength and level of endurance in the body's muscles.

mutagen An agent that causes alterations in the genetic material of living cells.

mutation A change in the genetic material of a cell or cells that is brought about by radiation, chemicals, or natural causes.

myocardial infarction (MI) A condition characterized by the dying of tissue areas in the myocardium, caused by interruption of the blood supply to those areas; the medical name for a heart attack.

naturopathy An alternative system of treatment of disease that emphasizes the use of natural remedies such as sun, water, heat, and air. Therapies may include dietary changes, steam baths, and exercise.

near-death experiences *See* autoscopy *and* transcendence.

negligence The failure to act in a way that a reasonable person would act.

neoplasm Any tumor, whether benign or malignant.

nephrosis A cluster of symptoms indicating chronic damage to the kidneys.

neuron The basic working unit of the brain, which transmits information from the senses to the brain and from the brain to specific body parts; each nerve cell consists of an axon, an axon terminal, and dendrites.

neuropsychiatry The study of the brain and mind.

neurotransmitters Chemicals released by neurons that stimulate or inhibit the action of other neurons.

nicotine The addictive substance in tobacco; one of the most toxic of all poisons.

nocturnal emissions Ejaculations while dreaming; wet dreams.

non-exercise activity thermogenesis (NEAT) The process of burning calories through nonvolitional activities such as walking and gardening,

nongonococcal urethritis (NGU) Inflammation of the urethra caused by organisms other than the gonococcus bacterium.

nonopioids Chemically synthesized drugs that have sleep-inducing and pain-relieving properties similar to those of opium and its derivatives.

norms The unwritten rules regarding behavior and conduct expected or accepted by a group.

nucleus The central part of a cell, contained in the cell body of a neuron.

nutrients Elements in food that the body cannot produce on its own, which are essential for growth, repair, and energy.

nutrition The science devoted to the study of dietary needs for food and the effects of food on organisms.

obesity The excessive accumulation of fat in the body; a condition of having a BMI of 30 or above.

obsessive-compulsive disorder (OCD) An anxiety disorder characterized by obsessions and/or compulsions that impair one's ability to function and form relationships.

oncogene A gene that, when activated by radiation or a virus, may cause a normal cell to become cancerous.

opioids Drugs that have sleep-inducing and pain-relieving properties, including opium and its derivatives and nonopioid, synthetic drugs.

optimism The tendency to seek out, remember, and expect pleasurable experiences.

oral contraceptives Preparations of synthetic hormones that inhibit ovulation; also referred to as birth control pills or simply the pill.

organic Term designating food produced with, or production based on the use of, fertilizer originating from plants or animals, without the use of pesticides or chemically formulated fertilizers.

organic phosphates Toxic pesticides that may cause cancer, birth defects, neurological disorders, and damage to wildlife and the environment.

orgasm A series of contractions of the pelvic muscles occurring at the peak of sexual arousal.

osteopathy The manipulation of the spine and other structural parts of the body to treat disorders.

osteoporosis A condition common in older people in which the bones become increasingly soft and porous, making them susceptible to injury.

outcomes The ultimate impacts of particular treatments or absence of treatment.

ovary The female sex organ that produces egg cells, estrogen, and progesterone.

over-the-counter (OTC) drugs Medications that can be obtained legally without a prescription from a medical professional.

overloading Method of physical training involving increasing the number of repetitions or the amount of resistance gradually to work the muscle to temporary fatigue.

overtrain Working muscles too intensely or too frequently, resulting in persistent muscle soreness, injuries, unintended weight loss, nervousness, and an inability to relax.

overuse injuries Physical injuries to joints or muscles, such as strains, fractures, and tendinitis, which result from overdoing a repetitive activity.

overweight A condition of having a BMI between 25.0 and 29.9.

ovo-lacto-vegetarians People who eat eggs, dairy products, and fruits and vegetables (but not meat, poultry, or fish).

ovulation The release of a mature ovum from an ovary approximately 14 days prior to the onset of menstruation.

ovulation method A method of birth control based on the observation of changes in the consistency of the mucus in the vagina to predict ovulation.

ovum (plural, **ova**) The female gamete (egg cell).

oxytocin A hormone that has been linked to one's ability to bond with others; also plays a key role in inducing labor during childbirth.

panic attack A short episode characterized by physical sensations of lightheadedness, dizziness, hyperventilation, and numbness of extremities, accompanied by an inexplicable terror, usually of a physical disaster such as death.

panic disorder An anxiety disorder in which the apprehension or experience of recurring panic attacks is so intense that normal functioning is impaired.

Pap smear A test in which cells removed from the cervix are examined under a microscope for signs of cancer; also called a Pap test.

passive stretching A stretching technique in which an external force or resistance (your body, a partner, gravity, or a weight) helps the joints move through their range of motion.

pathogen A microorganism that produces disease.

PCP (phencyclidine) A synthetic psychoactive substance that produces effects similar to other psychoactive drugs when swallowed, smoked, sniffed, or injected, but may also trigger unpredictable behavioral changes.

pelvic inflammatory disease (PID) An inflammation of the internal female genital tract, characterized by abdominal pain, fever, and tenderness of the cervix.

penis The male organ of sex and urination.

percutaneous transluminal coronary angioplasty (PTCA) A procedure for unclogging arteries; also called balloon angioplasty.

perimenopause The period from a woman's first irregular cycles to her last menstruation.

perinatology The medical specialty concerned with the diagnosis and treatment of pregnant women with high-risk conditions and their fetuses.

perineum The area between the anus and vagina in the female and between the anus and scrotum in the male.

periodontitis Severe gum disease in which the tooth root becomes infected.

persistent vegetative state A state of being awake and capable of reacting to physical stimuli, such as light, while being unaware of pain or other environmental stimuli.

phobia An anxiety disorder marked by an inordinate fear of an object, a class of objects, or a situation, resulting in extreme avoidance behaviors.

physical dependence The physiological attachment to, and need for, a drug.

physical fitness The ability to respond to routine physical demands, with enough reserve energy to cope with a sudden challenge.

phytochemicals Chemicals such as indoles, coumarins, and capsaicin, which exist naturally in plants and have disease-fighting properties.

placenta An organ that develops after implantation and to which the embryo attaches, via the umbilical cord, for nourishment and waste removal.

plaque The sludgelike substance that builds up on the inner walls of arteries; the sticky film of bacteria that forms on teeth.

pneumonia An inflammation of the lungs caused by infection or irritants.

pollutant A substance or agent in the environment, usually the by-product of human industry or activity, that is injurious to human, animal, or plant life.

pollution The presence of pollutants in the environment.

polyabuse The misuse or abuse of more than one drug.

postpartum depression The emotional downswing that occurs after having a baby due to hormonal changes, physical exhaustion, and psychological pressures.

posttraumatic stress disorder (PTSD) The repeated reliving of a trauma through nightmares or recollection.

potentiating Making more effective or powerful.

preconception care Health care to prepare for pregnancy.

precycling The use of products that are packaged in recycled or recyclable material.

preferred provider organization (PPO) A group of physicians contracted to provide health care to members at a discounted price.

premature ejaculation A sexual difficulty in which a man ejaculates so rapidly that his partner's satisfaction is impaired.

premature labor Labor that occurs after the twentieth week but before the thirty-seventh week of pregnancy.

premenstrual dysphoric disorder (PMDD) A disorder that causes symptoms of psychological depression during the last week of the menstrual cycle.

premenstrual syndrome (PMS) A disorder that causes physical discomfort and psychological distress prior to a woman's menstrual period.

prevention Information and support offered to help healthy people identify their health risks, reduce stressors, prevent potential medical problems, and enhance their well-being.

primary care Ambulatory or outpatient care provided by a physician in an office, emergency room, or clinic.

progesterone The female sex hormone that stimulates the uterus, preparing it for the arrival of a fertilized egg.

progestin-only pill *See* minipill.

progressive relaxation A method of reducing muscle tension by contracting, then relaxing certain areas of the body.

proof The alcoholic strength of a distilled spirit, expressed as twice the percentage of alcohol present.

prostate gland A structure surrounding the male urethra that produces a secretion that helps liquefy the semen from the testes.

prostatitis Inflammation of the prostate gland.

protection Measures that an individual can take when participating in risky behavior to prevent injury or unwanted risks.

protein A substance that is basically a compound of amino acids; one of the essential nutrients.

protozoa Microscopic animals made up of one cell or a group of similar cells.

psoriasis A chronic skin disorder caused by stress, skin damage, or illness and resulting in scaly, deep-pink, raised patches on the skin.

psychiatric drugs Medications that regulate a person's mental, emotional, and physical functions to facilitate normal functioning.

psychiatric nurse A nurse with special training and experience in mental health care.

psychiatrist Licensed medical doctor with additional training in psychotherapy, psychopharmacology, and treatment of mental disorders.

psychoactive Mood-altering.

psychodynamic Interpreting behaviors in terms of early experiences and unconscious influences.

psychological dependence The emotional or mental attachment to the use of a drug.

psychologists Mental health-care professionals who have completed doctoral or graduate programs in psychology and are trained in a variety of psychotherapeutic techniques, but who are not medically trained and do not prescribe medications.

psychoneuroimmunology A scientific field that explores the relationships between and among the mind, the central nervous system, and the immune system.

psychoprophylaxis *See* Lamaze method.

psychotherapy Treatment designed to produce a response by psychological rather than physical means, such as suggestion, persuasion, reassurance, and support.

psychotropic Mind-affecting.

pyelonephritis Inflammation of the kidney.

quackery Medical fakery; unproven practices claiming to cure diseases or solve health problems.

quid pro quo A form of harassment in which a person in power or authority makes unwanted sexual advances as a condition for receiving a job, promotion, or favor.

rape Sexual penetration of a female or a male by means of intimidation, force, or fraud.

rapid-eye-movement (REM) sleep Regularly occurring periods of sleep during which the most active dreaming takes place.

receptors Molecules on the surface of neurons on which neurotransmitters bind after their release from other neurons.

Recommended Dietary Allowances (RDA) The average daily amount of a nutrient considered adequate to meet the known nutrient needs of practically all healthy people; a goal for dietary intake by individuals.

recycling The processing or reuse of manufactured materials to reduce consumption of raw materials.

reflexology A treatment based on the theory that massaging certain points on the foot or hand relieves stress or pain in corresponding parts of the body.

refractory period The period of time following orgasm during which the male cannot experience another orgasm.

rehabilitation medicine The use of surgical procedures, medication, and physical therapy to improve the condition of patients with disabling conditions such as blindness, deafness, and arthritis.

reinforcement Reward or punishment for a behavior that will increase or decrease one's likelihood of repeating the behavior.

relapse prevention An alcohol recovery treatment method that focuses on social skills training to develop ways of preventing or minimizing a relapse.

relative risk The risk of developing cancer in persons with a certain exposure or trait compared to the risk in persons who do not have the same exposure or trait.

rep (or repetition) In weight training, a single performance of a movement or exercise.

repetitive motion injury (RMI) Inflammation of or damage to a part of the body due to repetition of the same movements.

rescue marriage A marital relationship in which one partner has had a traumatic childhood and views marriage as a way of healing the past.

resting heart rate The number of heartbeats per minute during inactivity.

reuptake Reabsorption by the originating cell of neurotransmitters that have not connected with receptors and have been left in synapses.

rhythm method A birth-control method in which sexual intercourse is avoided during those days of the menstrual cycle in which fertilization is most likely to occur.

romantic marriage A marital relationship in which sexual passion never fades.

rubella An infectious disease that may cause birth defects if contracted by a pregnant woman; also called German measles.

satiety A feeling of fullness after eating.

saturated fat A chemical term indicating that a fat molecule contains as many hydrogen atoms as its carbon skeleton can hold. These fats are normally solid at room temperature.

schizophrenia A general term for a group of mental disorders with characteristic psychotic symptoms, such as delusions, hallucinations, and disordered thought patterns during the active phase of the illness, and a duration of at least six months.

scrotum The external sac or pouch that holds the testes.

secondary sex characteristics Physical changes associated with maleness or femaleness, induced by the sex hormones.

self-actualization A state of wellness and fulfillment that can be achieved once certain human needs are satisfied; living to one's full potential.

self-efficacy Belief in one's ability to accomplish a goal or change a behavior.

self-esteem Confidence and satisfaction in oneself.

self-talk Repetition of positive messages about one's self-worth to learn more optimistic patterns of thought, feeling, and behavior.

semen The viscous whitish fluid that is the complete male ejaculate; a combination of sperm and secretions from the prostate gland, seminal vesicles, and other glands.

seminal vesicles Glands in the male reproductive system that produce the major portion of the fluid of semen.

set A person's expectations or preconceptions about a situation or experience; mind-set.

set-point theory The proposition that every person has an unconscious control system for keeping body fat (and therefore weight) at a predetermined level, or set point.

sets In weight training, the number of repetitions of the same movement or exercise.

sex Maleness or femaleness, resulting from genetic, structural, and functional factors.

sexual addiction A preoccupation with sex so intense and chronic that an individual cannot have a normal sexual relationship with a spouse or lover; sexual compulsion.

sexual coercion Sexual activity forced upon a person by the exertion of psychological pressure by another person.

sexual compulsion *See* sexual addiction.

sexual dysfunction The inability to react emotionally and/or physically to sexual stimulation in a way expected of the average healthy person or according to one's own standards.

sexual health The integration of the physical, emotional, intellectual, and social aspects of sexual being in ways that are positively enriching and that enhance personality, communication, and love.

sexuality The behaviors, instincts, and attitudes associated with being sexual.

sexually transmitted diseases (STDs) Any of a number of diseases that are acquired through sexual contact.

sidestream smoke The smoke emitted by a burning cigarette and breathed by everyone in a closed room, including the smoker; contains more tar and nicotine than mainstream smoke.

simple carbohydrates Sugars; like all carbohydrates, they provide the body with glucose.

smog A grayish or brownish fog caused by the presence of smoke and/or chemical pollutants in the air.

social isolation A feeling of unconnectedness with others caused by and reinforced by infrequency of social contacts.

social phobia A severe form of social anxiety marked by extreme fears and avoidance of social situations.

soluble fiber Fiber that lowers blood cholesterol and may help control blood sugar levels. May be found in oats, beans, barley, and the pulp of many fruits and vegetables.

sperm The male gamete produced by the testes and transported outside the body through ejaculation.

spermatogenesis The process by which sperm cells are produced.

spinal block An injection of anesthesia directly into the spinal cord to numb the lower body during labor and childbirth.

spiritual health The ability to identify one's basic purpose in life and to achieve one's full potential; the sense of connectedness to a greater power.

spiritual intelligence The capacity to sense, understand, and tap into ourselves, others, and the world around us.

static flexibility The ability to assume and maintain an extended position at one end point in a joint's range of motion.

static stretching A gradual stretch held for a short time of 10 to 30 seconds.

sterilization A surgical procedure to end a person's reproductive capability.

stimulant An agent, such as a drug, that temporarily relieves drowsiness, helps in the performance of repetitive tasks, and improves capacity for work.

strength Physical power; the maximum weight one can lift, push, or press in one effort.

stress The nonspecific response of the body to any demands made upon it; may be characterized by muscle tension and acute anxiety, or may be a positive force for action.

stressor Specific or nonspecific agents or situations that cause the stress response in a body.

stroke A cerebrovascular event in which the blood supply to a portion of the brain is blocked.

subcutaneous Under the skin.

suction curettage A procedure in which the contents of the uterus are removed by means of suction and scraping.

sudden infant death syndrome (SIDS) The unexplained death of an apparently healthy baby under one year of age during sleep.

synapse A specialized site at which electrical impulses are transmitted from the axon terminal of one neuron to a dendrite of another.

synergistic Characterized by a combined effect that is greater than the sum of the individual effects.

syphilis A sexually transmitted disease caused by the bacterium *Treponema pallidum,* and characterized by early sores, a latent period, and a final period of life-threatening symptoms including brain damage and heart failure.

systemic disease A pathologic condition that spreads throughout the body.

systole The contraction phase of the cardiac cycle.

tachycardia An abnormally rapid heart rate, over 100 beats per minute.

tamoxifen An estrogen-based medication that can help reduce the likelihood of developing cancer.

tar A thick, sticky dark fluid produced by the burning of tobacco, made up of several hundred different chemicals, many of them poisonous, some of them carcinogenic.

target heart rate Sixty to eighty-five percent of the maximum heart rate; the heart rate at which one derives maximum cardiovascular benefit from aerobic exercise.

teratogen Any agent that causes spontaneous abortion or defects or malformations in a fetus.

terminal illness An illness in which death is inevitable.

testes (singular, **testis**) The male sex organs that produce sperm and testosterone.

testosterone The male sex hormone that stimulates male secondary sex characteristics.

thallium scintigraphy A diagnostic test in which radioactive isotopes are injected into the bloodstream, and images of the rays emitted by the isotopes are captured and then translated into images of the heart as it pumps.

thanatology The discipline of humanitarian caregiving for critically ill patients and their grieving family members and friends.

toxic shock syndrome (TSS) A disease characterized by fever, vomiting, diarrhea, and often shock, caused by a bacterium that releases toxic waste products into the bloodstream.

toxicity Poisonousness; the dosage level at which a drug becomes poisonous to the body, causing either temporary or permanent damage.

traditional marriage A marital relationship in which the roles of the partners are distinct; defined by gender-based cultural norms and expectations.

trans fats Fats formed when liquid vegetable oils are processed to make table spreads or cooking fats, and also found in dairy and beef products; considered to be especially dangerous dietary fats.

transcendence The sense of passing into a foreign region or dimension, often experienced by a person near death.

transgendered Having a gender identity opposite one's biological sex; transsexual.

transient ischemic attack (TIA) A cerebrovascular event in which the blood supply to a portion of the brain is blocked temporarily; repeated attacks are predictors of more severe strokes.

trichomoniasis An infection of the protozoan *Trichomonas vaginalis;* females experience vaginal burning, itching, and discharge, but male carriers may be asymptomatic.

triglyceride A blood fat that flows through the blood after meals and is linked to increased risk of coronary artery disease.

tubal ligation The suturing or tying shut of the fallopian tubes to prevent pregnancy.

tubal occlusion The blocking of the fallopian tubes to prevent pregnancy.

tuberculosis A highly infectious bacterial disease that primarily affects the lungs and is often fatal.

tumor suppressor gene Gene that normally controls cell growth. Many cancers are linked to defects in a tumor suppressor gene.

twelve-step programs Self-help group programs based on the principles of Alcoholics Anonymous.

ulcer A lesion in, or an erosion of, the mucous membrane of an organ.

unsaturated fat A chemical term indicating that a fat molecule contains fewer hydrogen atoms than its carbon skeleton can hold. These fats are normally liquid at room temperature.

urethra The canal through which urine from the bladder leaves the body; in the male, also serves as the channel for seminal fluid.

urethral opening The outer opening of the thin tube that carries urine from the bladder.

urethritis Infection of the urethra.

uterus The female organ that houses the developing fetus until birth.

vagina The canal leading from the exterior opening in the female genital area to the uterus.

vaginal contraceptive film (VCF) A small dissolvable sheet saturated with spermicide that can be inserted into the vagina and placed over the cervix.

vaginal spermicide A substance that kills or neutralizes sperm, inserted into the vagina in the form of a foam, cream, jelly, or suppository.

vaginismus A sexual difficulty in which a woman experiences painful spasms of the vagina during sexual intercourse.

values The criteria by which one makes choices about one's thoughts and actions and goals and ideals.

vas deferens Two tubes that carry sperm from the epididymis into the urethra.

vasectomy A surgical sterilization procedure in which each vas deferens is cut and tied shut to stop the passage of sperm to the urethra for ejaculation.

vector A biological or physical vehicle that carries the agent of infection to the host.

vegans People who eat only plant foods.

ventricle Either of the two lower chambers of the heart, which pump blood out of the heart and into the arteries.

video display terminal (VDT) A screen or monitor that emits electromagnetic fields from all sides; these fields may lead to increased reproductive problems, miscarriages, low birthweights, and cataracts.

virus A submicroscopic infectious agent; the most primitive form of life.

visualization An approach to stress control, self-healing, or motivating life changes by means of guided, or directed, imagery.

vital signs Measurements of physiological functioning; specifically, temperature, blood pressure, pulse rate, and respiration rate.

vitamins Organic substances that are needed in very small amounts by the body and carry out a variety of functions in metabolism and nutrition.

waist-hip ratio The proportion of one's waist circumference to one's hip circumference.

wellness A state of optimal health.

withdrawal Development of symptoms that cause significant psychological and physical distress when an individual reduces or stops drug use.

zygote A fertilized egg.

Photography Credits

Index